ORAL PATHOLOGY:
A COMPREHENSIVE ATLAS AND TEXT

ORAL PATHOLOGY:

A COMPREHENSIVE ATLAS AND TEXT

SECOND EDITION

Sook-Bin Woo, DMD, MMSc
Associate Professor
Department of Oral Medicine, Infection, and Immunity
Harvard School of Dental Medicine
Boston, Massachusetts

Consultant Pathologist
Department of Pathology
Brigham and Women's Hospital
Boston, Massachusetts

Co-Director
Center for Oral Pathology
StrataDx
Lexington, Massachusetts

ELSEVIER

ELSEVIER

1600 John F. Kennedy Blvd.
Ste 1800
Philadelphia, PA 19103-2899

ORAL PATHOLOGY: A COMPREHENSIVE ATLAS AND TEXT
SECOND EDITION

ISBN: 978-0-323-39054-5

Previous edition copyrighted 2012.

Library of Congress Cataloging-in-Publication Data

Names: Woo, Sook-bin, author.
Title: Oral pathology : a comprehensive atlas and text / Sook-Bin Woo.
Description: Second edition. | Philadelphia, PA : Elsevier, [2017] | Includes bibliographical references and index.
Identifiers: LCCN 2016023952 | ISBN 9780323390545 (hardcover)
Subjects: | MESH: Mouth Diseases—pathology | Atlases
Classification: LCC RC815 | NLM WU 17 | DDC 616.3/1—dc23 LC record available at https://lccn.loc.gov/2016023952

Executive Content Strategist: William Schmitt
Senior Content Development Specialist: Anne Snyder
Publishing Services Manager: Patricia Tannian
Senior Project Manager: Cindy Thoms
Book Designer: Ryan Cook

Printed in the United States of America

Last digit is the print number: 9 8 7 6 5 4

This book is dedicated to my parents, who believe that education will lift us all,
and to John, Sook-Yee, Chi-kan, I-Hwei, and Sarah.

CONTRIBUTORS

Elizabeth A. Morgan, MD
Associate Pathologist
Department of Pathology
Brigham and Women's Hospital
Assistant Professor
Harvard Medical School
Boston, Massachusetts
Hematolymphoid Tumors of the Oral Cavity

Olga K. Weinberg, MD
Assistant Professor in Pathology
Harvard Medical School
Director of Hematopathology and Flow Cytometry
Boston Children's Hospital
Boston, Massachusetts
Hematolymphoid Tumors of the Oral Cavity

PREFACE

This atlas was written to serve pathologists in training, dermatopathologists, general pathologists, as well as dental and medical specialists interested in diseases of the oral mucosa, minor salivary gland, and jawbones. Specific and detailed diagnostic criteria are provided for the diagnosis of pathology in the oral cavity. For the clinician, medications used in the treatment of inflammatory oral disease and viral and fungal infections are provided in Appendices A and B, which have been expanded in this edition. The chapter on infectious diseases has also been expanded to include most fungal diseases in the mouth and parasitic diseases that have become more common as a result of population migration. A new chapter on oral lymphomas, the second most common malignancy in the oral cavity, has been added.

Advances in molecular pathology in soft tissue and bone tumors, as well as salivary gland tumors, have occurred in leaps and bounds and brought new understanding to diagnosis, tumor biology, etiopathogenesis, and treatment. The chapter on salivary gland tumors has been expanded and now includes molecular findings in salivary gland tumors as are known at this time. Similar molecular findings are now included for soft tissue tumors often encountered in the oral cavity, primary bone tumors, and some odontogenic tumors.

However, it is inflammatory diseases of the mucosa, salivary glands, and jawbones that constitute the bulk of oral and maxillofacial pathology. Diagnosis of these conditions requires a deep understanding of the "lives of lesions," as they evolve, resolve, and recur. Knowing the clinical presentation of oral mucosal disease is often essential for accurate diagnosis, especially for leukoplakia, the most common precancerous condition in the mouth. In this era of the ubiquitous smartphone, obtaining a photograph of a clinical lesion is simple and takes only seconds, and all clinicians should be encouraged to send in photographs of such lesions to the pathologist with whom they collaborate. Similarly, clinicians should be encouraged to send oral radiographs, including computerized tomograms for accurate diagnosis of intra-bony lesions.

Practicing and teaching pathology teaches me humility on a regular basis. I continue to enjoy being challenged by my trainees and residents, revisiting old concepts and hopefully, debunking myths, or at least trying to view lesions in light of new concepts of etiopathogenesis and new diagnostic technologies. Pathology is a specialty that has much to offer the life-long learner and the curious mind. I hope that you will find this atlas to be informative and useful in your daily clinical or pathology practice.

Acknowledgments

I am indebted to my colleagues and friends who contributed slides and images for this atlas and to clinician colleagues who contribute cases to our biopsy service and have steadfastly supported the oral and maxillofacial pathology training program at Harvard School of Dental Medicine. Some cases were retrieved from the files of the American Board of Oral and Maxillofacial Pathology and the now defunct Armed Forces Institute of Pathology. Grateful thanks are due to my colleagues at the Ohio State University, Columbus, Ohio; Oral Pathology Laboratories, Queens, New York; University of Florida, Gainesville, Florida; and in Guatemala for their study sets. This endeavor would be less than what it is without the patients who have shared their stories and insights about their diseases with me, and whose images appear within these pages; it is an honor to care for them.

Sook-Bin Woo, DMD, MMSc

CONTENTS

1 INTRODUCTION

CHAPTER CONTENTS

Pathology of the oral cavity affects the following structures: (1) the mucosa, (2) the salivary glands, and (3) the jaw bones. Lesions may extend into the oropharynx, sinuses, and the skin. As such, the scope of practice of oral and maxillofacial pathology overlaps with otorhinolaryngologic pathology, dermatopathology, and bone pathology. The oral cavity is also the primary site for the development of lymphomas and many soft tissue tumors, and is also sometimes the location of metastatic tumors. This atlas focuses on pathology that is frequently seen in the oral cavity.

Unlike the skin, mucosal lesions in the oral cavity may manifest only in a limited number of ways—erythematous/erosive (from epithelial atrophy, vascular ectasia, and inflammation), white (from keratosis or underlying fibrosis), yellow/ulcerative (from fibrinous exudate), vesiculobullous (often erosive), pigmented, papillary, diffuse or nodular swelling, and mass. It is important for the pathologist to be familiar with clinical presentations of mucosal disease for accurate diagnosis. Clinical images (even those taken with a smartphone) or radiographic images are often indispensable for the diagnosis of mucosal lesions and osseous pathology, respectively.

ANATOMY

The oral mucosa varies clinically and histologically from site to site, and is divided into keratinized and nonkeratinized mucosa (Fig. 1.1). Specific oral conditions correlate with oral anatomy: for example, recurrent aphthous ulcers occur primarily on the nonkeratinized mucosa, whereas recrudescent herpes simplex virus infections occur almost exclusively on the keratinized mucosa (such as the hard palatal mucosa and keratinized gingiva) in immune-competent patients. The tongue dorsum (with the thickest epithelium in the oral cavity) but not ventrum (with thin epithelium) is specialized for gustatory, masticatory, and deglutition functions. Filiform papillae cover the entire surface of the dorsum. Taste buds are present within fungiform (on dorsum), circumvallate (8 to 14 on the posterior dorsum), and foliate (posterior lateral tongue) papillae but not within filiform papillae (Fig. 1.2). The lingual tonsil extends across the base of the tongue and may extend into the foliate papillae. The oral mucosa contains no submucosa per se because there is no muscularis mucosa or any other consistently recognizable histologic landmark that separates mucosa from submucosa. As such, the terms *papillary* (between rete ridges), *superficial*, and *deep lamina propria* are preferable to *submucosa*. In general, the epithelium of the oral cavity is much thicker than that of the skin (Table 1.1; Figs. 1.3–1.9). The keratinocytes are generally well glycogenated and may exhibit perinuclear halos; these should not be misdiagnosed as koilocytes. Muscle is present fairly superficially on the tongue and slightly deeper on the buccal and lip mucosa. Minor salivary glands are predominantly mucous, although serous acini and demilunes are frequently seen (Fig. 1.10); they are present everywhere in the mouth except on the keratinized gingiva (also known as "attached" gingiva because of its "attachment" to the periosteum and bone). Serous salivary glands with a smaller mucous component are frequently encountered on the anterior ventral tongue (glands of Blandin-Nuhn) and posterior lateral and dorsal tongue (glands of von Ebner), sometimes invested in muscle.

The subgemmal (gemma = Greek for bud) neurogenous plaque (also known as "subepithelial nerve plexus") is a normal nerve plexus located in the superficial lamina propria beneath the epithelium rich in taste buds and represent afferent fibers, and should not be mistaken for neurofibroma; ganglion cells are sometimes present (Fig. 1.11A–B). This neural plaque is positive for S100 protein, neurofilament protein, and PGP9.5 (Fig. 1.11C–D. It is often noted in biopsies from the posterior lateral tongue in the area of the foliate papillae but is not exclusive to that site. Infrequently, ganglion cells and neuroepithelial islands similar to the organ of Chievitz may be seen within this neurogenous plaque.

The juxtacortical organ of Chievitz is likely a remnant from embryogenesis and consists of small islands of benign epithelium with peripheral basal cells closely apposed to, or within nerve fibers (likely the buccal nerve) (Fig. 1.12). This organ may be located in the area of the pterygomandibular raphe, medial to the mandible,

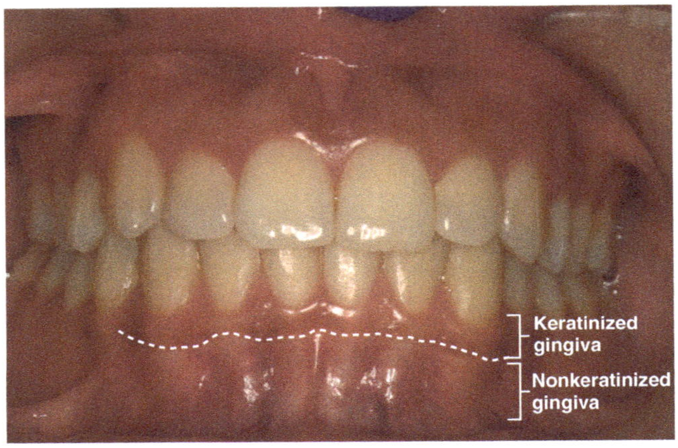

FIG 1.1 Gingival mucosa showing marginal and attached (keratinized) gingiva and nonattached (nonkeratinized) gingiva.

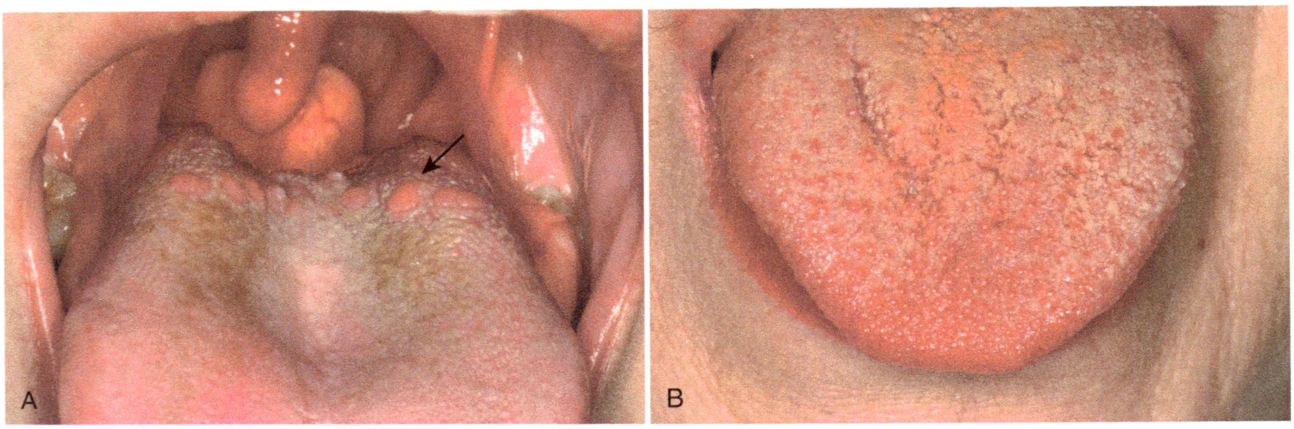

FIG 1.2 (A) Tongue showing filiform papillae (generalized "fur") and circumvallate papillae *(arrow)*, as well as epiglottis behind the uvula. (B) Tongue with inflamed fungiform papillae (small red papules).

TABLE 1.1 Histology of Oral Mucosa at Different Sites

Site	Appearance
Nonkeratinized mucosa (thick) Buccal mucosa Labial mucosa	Buccal and labial mucosa are contiguous and similar (see Fig. 1.3) Epithelium 15–25 cells thick Broad, tapered rete ridges Loose fibrovascular tissue in the lamina propria or corium; muscle at the base
Nonkeratinized mucosa (intermediate) Nonattached gingiva/alveolar mucosa	Nonattached gingiva/alveolar mucosa Intermediate in thickness between buccal mucosa and floor of mouth
Nonkeratinized mucosa (thin) Floor of mouth Ventral tongue Soft palate/fauces	Floor of mouth and ventral tongue are contiguous and similar to soft palate (see Fig. 1.4) Epithelium 10–15 cells thick Short or poorly formed rete ridges Ventral tongue in the anterior and posterior often contains serous salivary glands (glands of Blandin-Nuhn and von Ebner, respectively) (see Fig. 1.5)
Keratinized mucosa Hard palatal mucosa Attached gingiva	Hard palatal mucosa and attached gingiva are similar (see Fig. 1.6) Thin layer of orthokeratin with thin granular layer Epithelium 15–25 cells thick Gingiva has more tapered, slender rete ridges; may see odontogenic rests of Serres (see Fig. 1.7) Dense fibrous tissue and periosteum at the base Hard palatal mucosa often has fatty tissue investing neurovascular bundles and minor salivary glands
Keratinized and specialized mucosa Tongue dorsum	Moderate-to-thick layer of parakeratin Filiform papillae are keratin spires surrounded by bacterial colonies (see Fig. 1.8) Epithelium 20–30 cells thick Fungiform, circumvallate, and foliate papillae are fibrovascular polypoid structures containing taste buds (see Fig. 1.9); subgemmal neurogenous plaque are usually present in the lamina propria Posterior dorsum and lateral tongue contain lingual tonsils Skeletal muscle is superficial

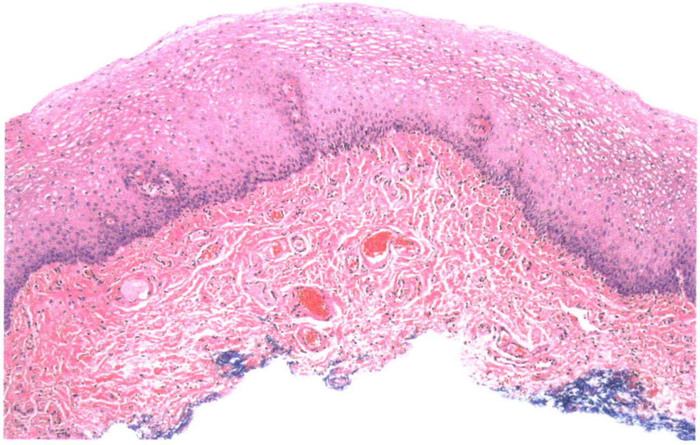

FIG 1.3 Normal buccal mucosa: nonkeratinized stratified squamous epithelium 15 to 25 cells thick; perinuclear halos are present because of glycogen.

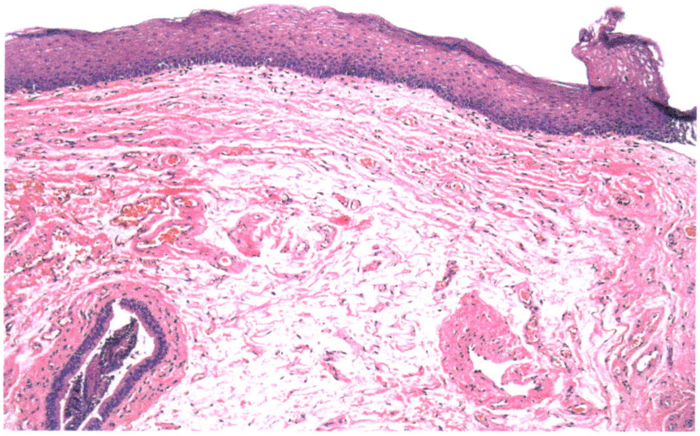

FIG 1.4 Normal floor of mouth: thin, nonkeratinized stratified squamous epithelium with poorly formed rete ridges.

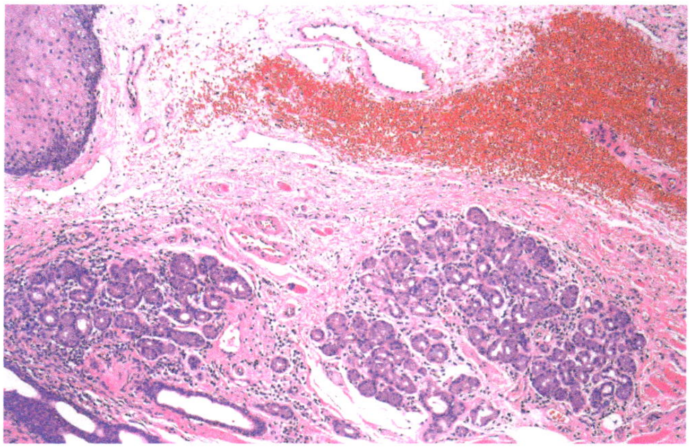

FIG 1.5 Mostly serous glands of von Ebner in the posterior tongue.

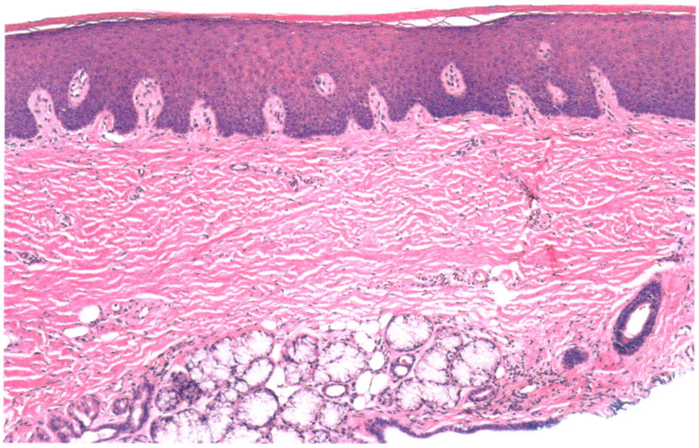

FIG 1.6 Normal hard palatal mucosa: thin layer of orthokeratin, epithelium 15 to 20 cells thick, dense lamina propria, and salivary glands.

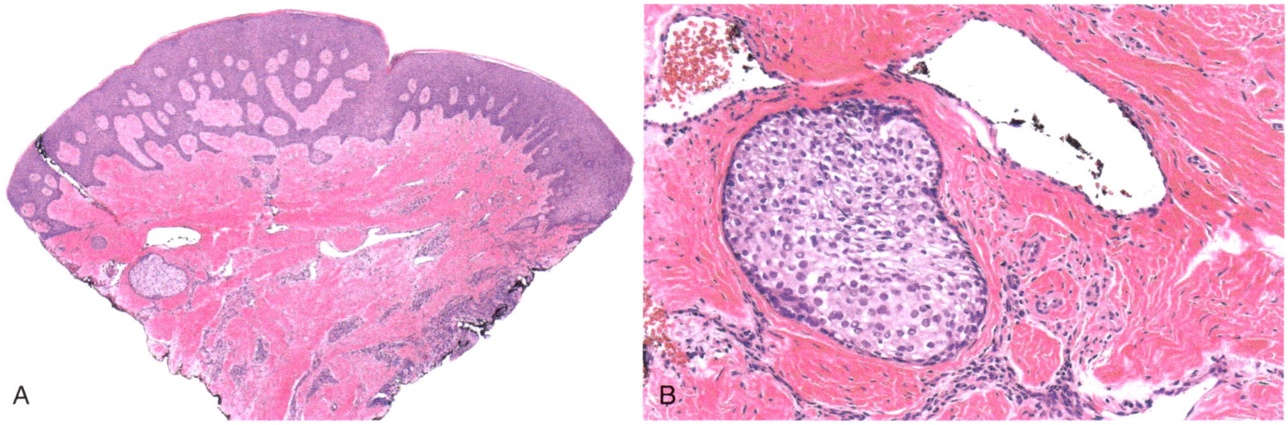

FIG 1.7 (A) Gingiva is thinly orthokeratinized and 15 to 25 cells thick with tapered rete ridges. (B) Odontogenic rest of Serres contains many clear cells.

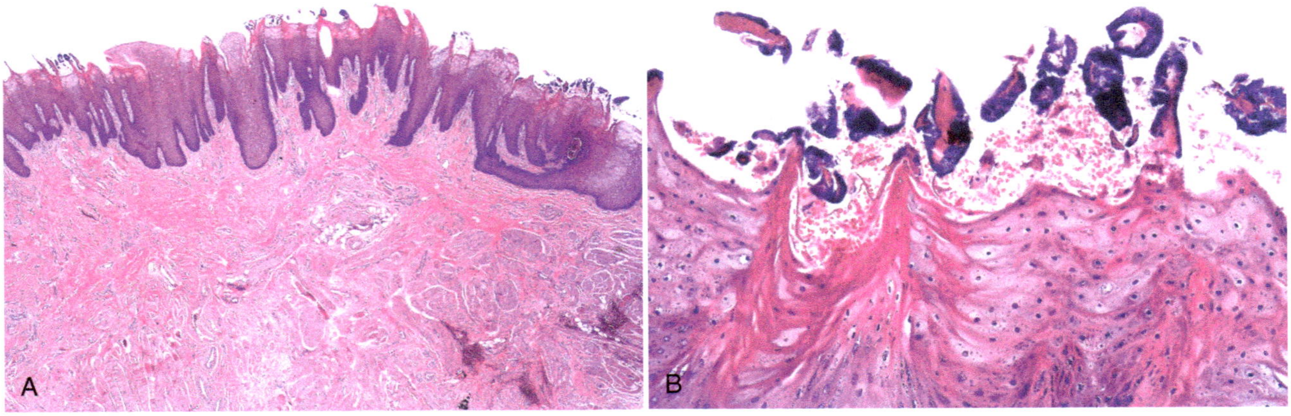

FIG 1.8 (A) Tongue dorsum: thick epithelium with abundant muscle. (B) Tongue dorsum: filiform papillae composed of parakeratin spires with bacterial colonies.

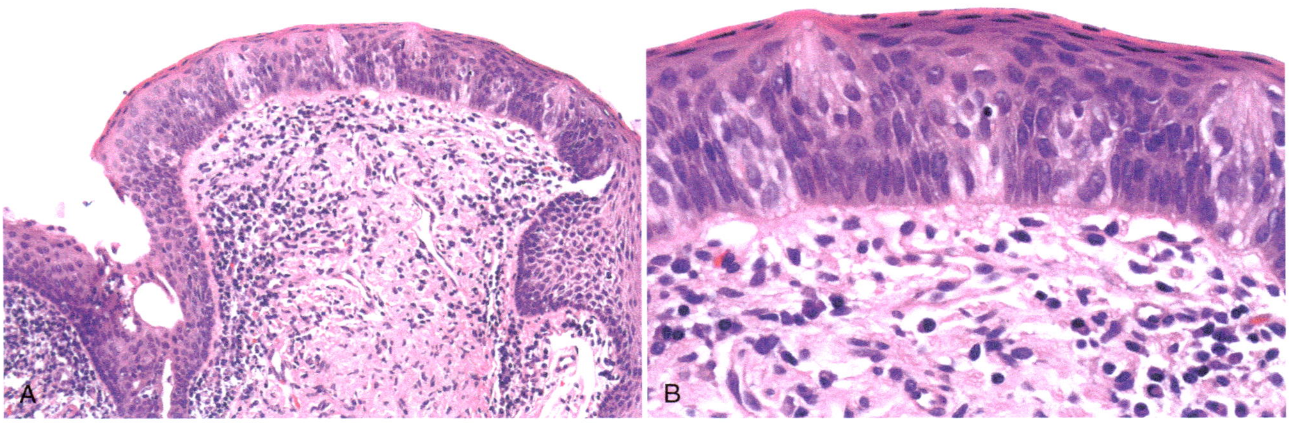

FIG 1.9 (A) Fungiform papilla with taste buds in the epithelium and many nerve fibers in the lamina propria. (B) Taste buds: flask-shaped clusters of sustentacular and gustatory sensory cells.

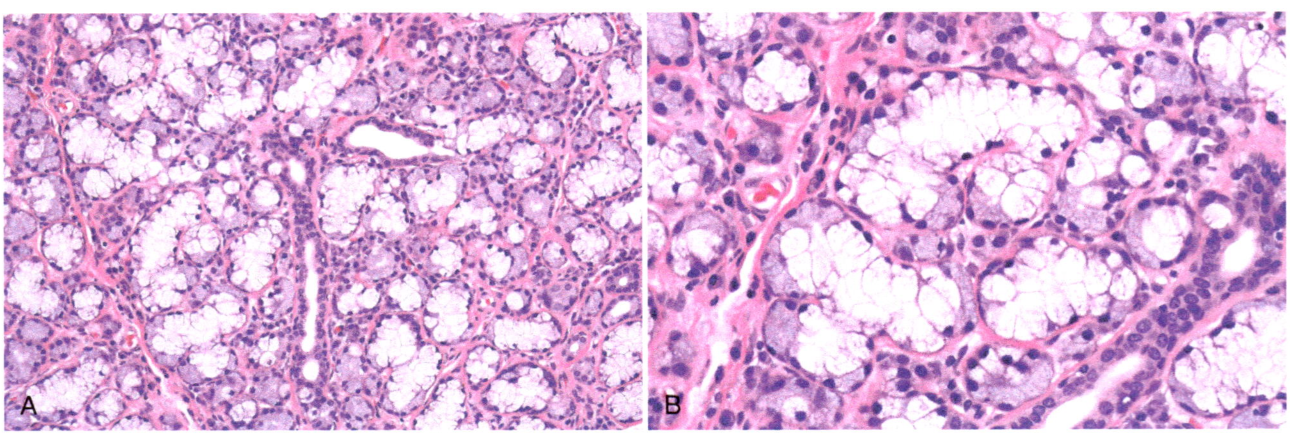

FIG 1.10 (A) Mucous glands of the lower lip with some serous acini. (B) Serous acinar cells in caplike demilune arrangement over mucous acini.

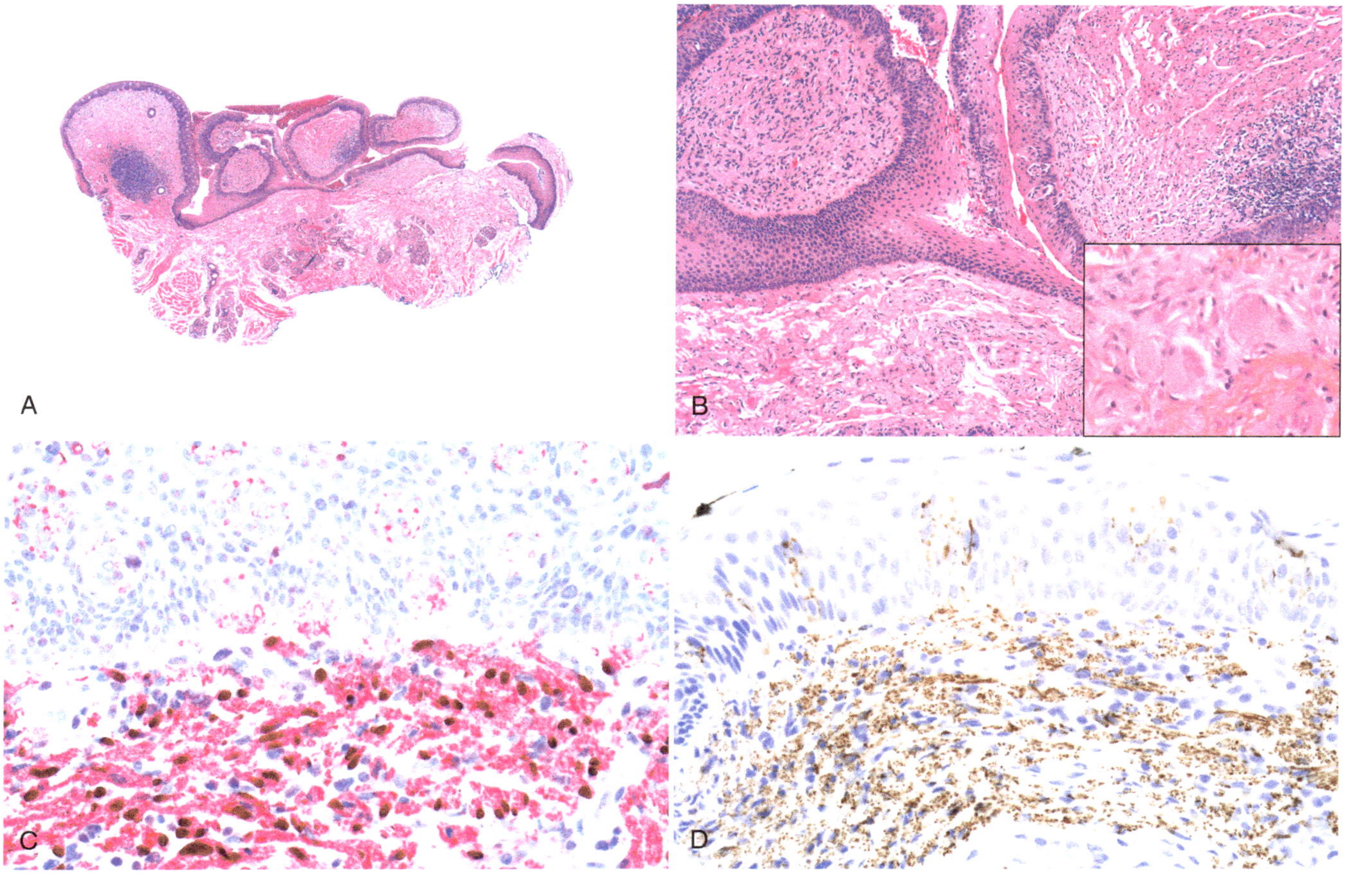

FIG 1.11 Subgemmal neurogenous plaque. (A) Foliate papillae of tongue with serous glands. (B) Numerous taste buds in the epithelium and subepithelial neural plexus with ganglion cells *(inset)*. (C) Spindle cells anc taste buds are positive for S-100 protein. (D) Spindle cells and taste buds are positive for neurofilament protein.

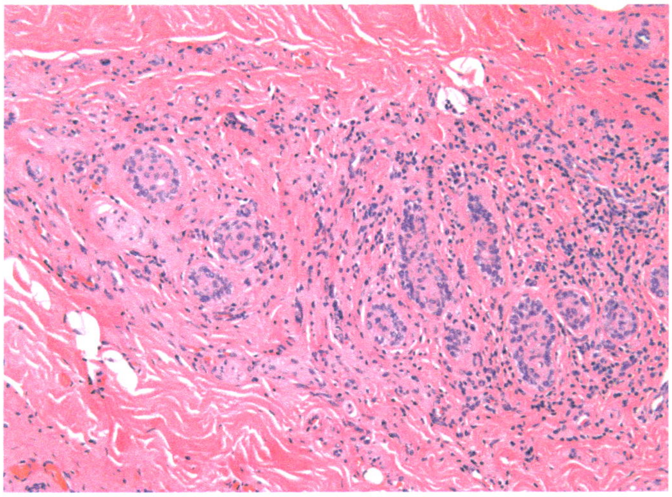

FIG 1.12 Juxtacortical organ of Chievitz composed of nests of benign epithelium with closely associated nerve fibers.

and may extend toward the opening of the parotid duct. These structures must not be misinterpreted as perineural invasion by carcinomas in the vicinity.

TEETH

Teeth are made up mostly of tubular dentin that is capped by a thin shell of very hard enamel overlying the crown of the tooth. The root of the tooth is surrounded by a thin layer of cementum (Fig. 1.13). The periodontal membrane attaches to the cementum on one side and the alveolar bone on the other, allowing for slight movement of teeth within the bone. This membrane contains Sharpey fibers rich in type III (argyrophilic reticulin fibers) and type VI collagen. Although Sharpey fibers has been used to refer almost exclusively to these fibers of the periodontal membrane, they are also present in muscle-bone and periosteum-bone anchorage elsewhere in the body.

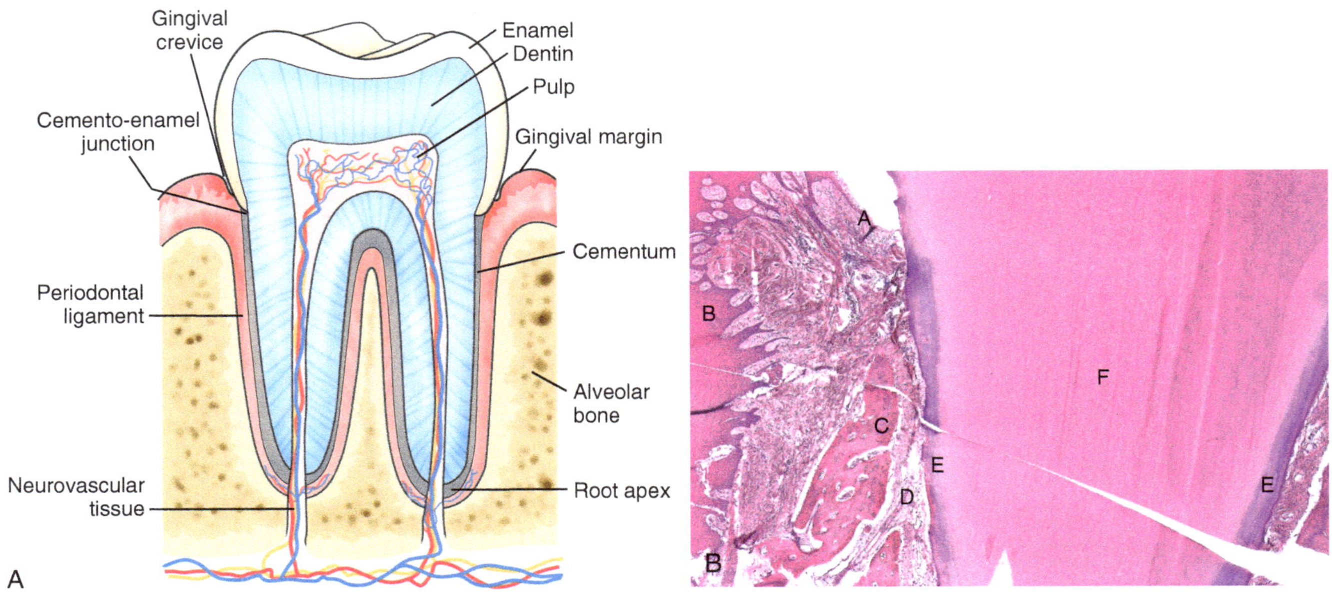

FIG 1.13 (A) Diagram of a tooth in bone. (B) Tooth showing crevicular epithelium *(A)*, surface epithelium *(B)*, alveolar bone *(C)*, collagenous periodontal ligament *(D)*, cementum *(E)*, and dentin *(F)*.

Enamel (ectodermal in nature) is 96% mineral (carbonate apatite crystals) and 4% organic material and water. The organic material consists of noncollagenous proteins called amelogenins (90%), enamelin, and ameloblastin. Mature tubular dentin is composed of 70% inorganic material (hydroxyapatite), 20% organic material, and 10% water. The organic base is composed of 90% collagen (mainly type I), noncollagenous proteins such as dentin phosphoprotein, dentin sialoprotein, and dentin matrix protein-1, as well as bone matrix proteins such as osteocalcin, osteopontin, and bone sialoprotein. Dentin is deposited by the odontoblast (of ectomesenchymal derivation) and wraps around an odontoblastic process that traverses the entire thickness of the dentin from the pulp where the odontoblast resides, to the enamel or cementum. Cementum is closest to bone in composition, with 45% to 50% hydroxyapatite and 50% collagen and noncollagenous matrix proteins. Type I collagen constitutes 90% of the nonmineral portion of cementum; noncollagenous proteins include bone sialoprotein, osteocalcin, dentin sialoprotein, and dentin matrix protein-1.

Tooth Numbering System and Nomenclature

There are three commonly used nomenclatures for tooth identification. In the American Dental Association (ADA) system each tooth is identified by one number (#1 to #32 starting from the right maxillary third molar moving clockwise when facing the patient) (Fig. 1.14). Palmer notation (used mainly by the British) and the system adopted by the Fédération Dentaire Internationale (FDI) use a single number for each of the eight teeth in a quadrant, starting from the central incisor (#1) moving posteriorly to the third molar (#8). In the FDI system, a qualifier is added for the specific quadrant in which the tooth is located also in a clockwise fashion; quadrant 1 is right maxilla, 2 is left maxilla, 3 is left mandible, and 4 is right mandible. For example, tooth #12 by the ADA system is the left maxillary first premolar or bicuspid. By Palmer notation, this is designated left upper 4 or |4, and by the FDI system it is tooth 24 (quadrant 2, tooth #4).

The terms *facial*, *buccal*, and *labial* refer to the aspect of the gingiva or teeth that are in contact with the labial/lip or buccal mucosa and oriented outwards. Conversely, the terms *palatal* and *lingual* are used for aspects that are oriented inwards toward the palate or the tongue.

DIAGNOSIS AND MANAGEMENT

For macules or larger lesions, biopsies using a 3- to 5-mm skin punch provide tissue that is easy to orient for processing; primary closure with one to two sutures is readily achieved (Fig. 1.15A–B). Small papules or nodules should be excised with a shave biopsy or an elliptical wedge excision (Fig. 1.15C). The hard palatal mucosa/gingiva abuts the periosteum and as such, is not amenable to primary closure after biopsy; the use of silver nitrate or aluminum chloride to control hemostasis is preferable (Fig. 1.15D). Laser removal of lesions for evaluation of dysplasia is not recommended because of the difficulty of evaluating margins with laser cautery artifact. For the purposes of the clinician, Appendices A and B at the end of the book provide the most commonly used medications for definitive treatment of mucosal diseases and common infections and agents for topical pain control.

SOME BASIC GUIDELINES

The histopathologic features of inflammatory mucosal disorders depend on the stage at which the lesion is biopsied (evolving or resolving) and whether it has been treated. The "typical" or "classic" histology for many inflammatory conditions is seen in untreated, fully evolved lesions, an infrequent occurrence. As such, a range of

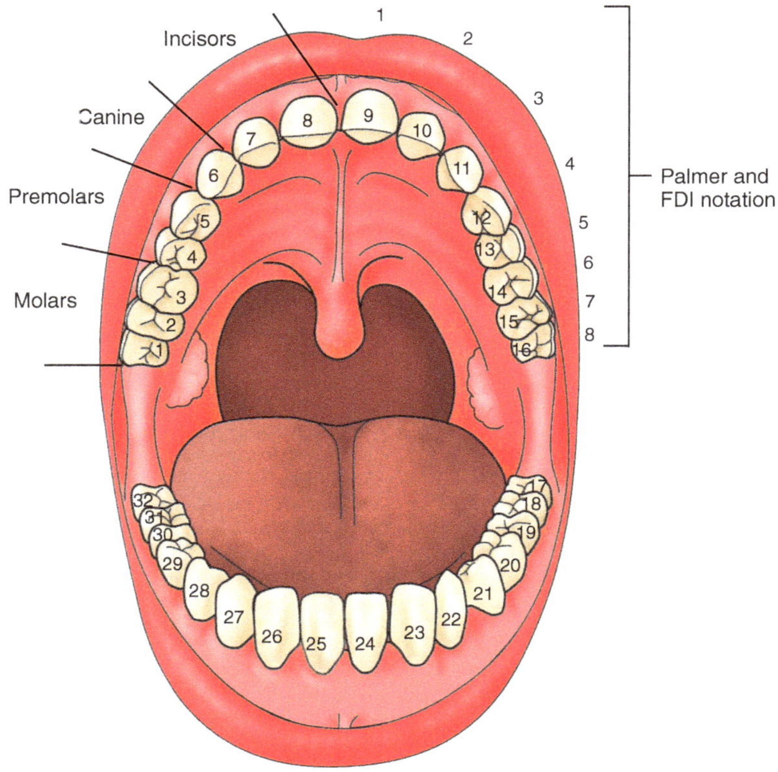

FIG 1.14 Tooth numbering system: #1 to #32 (American Dental Association); #1 to #8 (British Palmer notation and European Fédération Dentaire Internationale [FDI] system).

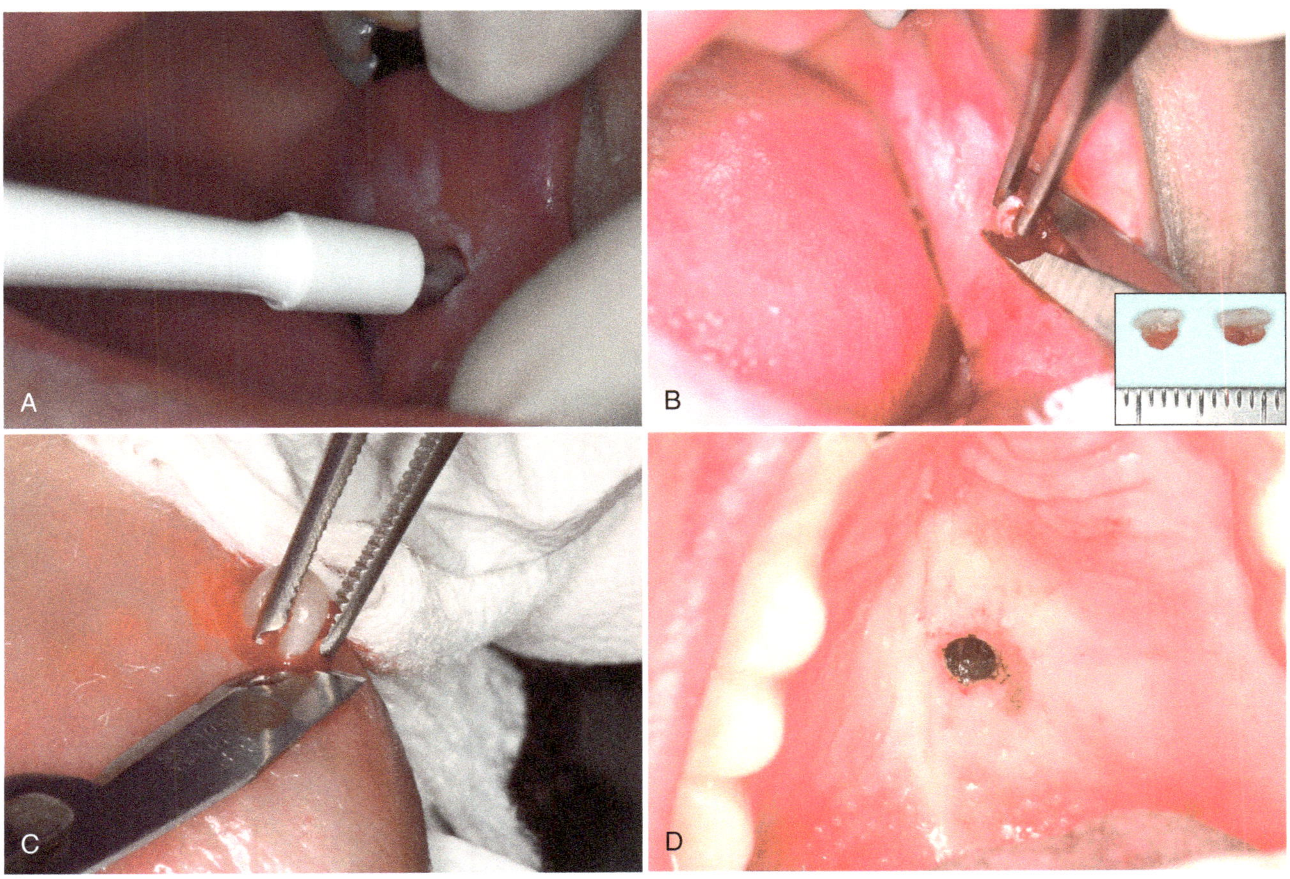

FIG 1.15 (A) Punch biopsy: inserting the skin punch. (B) Punch biopsy: cutting the tissue at the base; bisected punch biopsy specimen *(inset)*. (C) Shave biopsy of a fibroma with scalpel blade parallel to the mucosal surface. (D) Silver nitrate to seal punch biopsy site on the palatal mucosa.

histopathologic features is presented for inflammatory lesions in this atlas.

Dysplastic conditions are probably the most challenging for the pathologist, because the clinical appearance of the lesion plays an important role in the accurate diagnosis of dysplasia. To this end, clinicians are encouraged to send a photograph (even a smartphone image) of the lesion with the biopsy. Many dysplastic oral lesions show architectural rather than cytologic evidence of dysplasia. These concepts are covered in depth in Chapter 11.

The teeth and salivary glands are adnexa of the oral cavity in the same way that hair and sweat glands are skin adnexa. As such, there are histopathologic similarities among odontogenic, salivary gland, skin adnexal, and breast neoplasms. Teeth and salivary glands are derived from the same primordium and it is therefore not surprising that primary salivary gland tumors may occur as primary tumors within the jawbones. The diagnosis of odontogenic cysts and tumors and primary intraosseous lesions can be accurately rendered only if radiographic images are provided.

Finally, a few words on terminology. The oral mucosa has no submucosa per se as mentioned previously, because it lacks a muscularis mucosae. There is only lamina propria, superficial and deep, and even then, the demarcation between the two is somewhat arbitrary. The term *hard palatal mucosa* is preferable to hard palate, because the hard palate is the bony plate to which mucosa is attached. Similarly, *mandibular* and *maxillary mucosa* are preferable to mandible and maxilla (implying bone) if one is referring to the mucosa overlying the bone. The term *parakeratosis* is used without the modifying "hyper" because all parakeratin is abnormal in the oral cavity, except on the tongue dorsum, which contains parakeratotic filiform papillae, so that hyperparakeratosis would be appropriate only for tongue dorsum lesions. The term *hyperkeratosis* is preferred over *hyperorthokeratosis* in keeping with usage by general pathologists and dermatopathologists.

REFERENCES

Aaron JE. Periosteal Sharpey's fibers: a novel bone matrix regulatory system? *Front Endocrinol (Lausanne)*. 2012;3:1-10.

Gueiros LA, Leon JE, Leao JC, et al. Subgemmal neurogenous plaque: clinical and microscopic evaluation of 7 cases. *Oral Surg Oral Med Oral Pathol Oral Radiol Endod.* 2009;108:920-924.

McDaniel RK. Subepithelial nerve plexus (with ganglion cells) associated with taste buds. *Oral Surg Oral Med Oral Pathol Oral Radiol Endod.* 1999;87:605-609.

Nanci A. *Ten Cate's Oral Histology: Development, Structure and Function.* 7th ed. St. Louis: Mosby; 2008.

Palazzolo MJ, Fowler CB, Magliocca KR, Gnepp DR. Neuroepithelial structures associated with the subepithelial nerve plexus of taste buds: a fortuitous finding resembling the juxtaoral organ of Chievitz. *Oral Surg Oral Med Oral Pathol Oral Radiol.* 2014;117:497-501.

Pantanowitz L, Balogh K. Significance of the juxtaoral organ (of Chievitz). *Head Neck.* 2003;25:400-405, discussion.

Triantafyllou A, Coulter P. Structural organization of subgemmal neurogenous plaques in foliate papillae of tongue. *Hum Pathol.* 2004;35:991-999.

2 DEVELOPMENTAL AND CONGENITAL CONDITIONS

CHAPTER CONTENTS

Definitions

Choristoma: An overgrowth of tissues that is mature and found in an area where such tissue is not usually present, such as an osseous or cartilaginous choristoma of the tongue.

Hamartoma: An overgrowth of tissue that is mature and normally found in that area, such as a leiomyomatous hamartoma.

Nevus: An overgrowth of tissue that is normally found in the skin or oral mucosa, such as melanocytic, epidermal, or vascular nevus.

Epithelial Lesions

Developmental macular epithelial conditions fall into three categories: diffuse white lesions, diffuse red lesions, and nevi that may be mucosa-colored or pigmented. Diffuse white lesions are often dyskeratotic and represent oral manifestations of genodermatoses, of which the most well-known is the Cannon white sponge nevus that involves mucosal sites only. Dyskeratosis congenita results in keratotic skin lesions and oral dysplastic leukoplakias. Oral lesions of pachyonychia congenita are rarely biopsied, because the diagnosis is established via skin biopsies. Oral lesions of hereditary mucoepithelial dysplasia, a condition of defective expression of cytoskeleton junctional elements, presents as erythematous plaques.

Macular Epithelial Lesions

WHITE SPONGE NEVUS (CANNON WHITE SPONGE NEVUS)

Clinical Findings

- Lesions are noted in the first two decades of life and persist throughout life. The skin is not involved, although there may be esophageal, upper airway, and genital involvement.
- The buccal mucosa (the most commonly affected site) appears white to gray, folded, painless, edematous, and spongy. The tongue, lip mucosa, and floor of the mouth may also be involved (Fig. 2.1).

Etiopathogenesis and Histopathologic Features

White sponge nevus is a rare, autosomal dominant condition resulting from a mutation of the helical domain on keratins K4 (chromosome 12q) and K13 (chromosome 17q), leading to keratin instability and abnormal tonofilament aggregation. There may be abnormal degradation of K13 protein and abnormal ubiquitination.

- Variable parakeratosis and acanthosis with a "spongy appearance" are noted. The last is caused by cytoplasmic vacuolation (partly due to glycogen) and not spongiosis. There is minimal to no inflammation (Fig. 2.2A–C).
- Perinuclear eosinophilic condensations of keratin and dyskeratotic cells are the sine qua non for diagnosis (Fig. 2.2D). Rare cases exhibit epidermolytic hyperkeratosis.

Differential Diagnosis

- Chronic frictional keratosis of the buccal mucosa, a very common condition, exhibits parakeratosis, acanthosis, and keratinocytic edema but not perinuclear keratin condensations (see Chapter 10).
- Hereditary benign intraepithelial dyskeratosis (see later) exhibits dyskeratosis and "cell-within-a-cell" structures but not perinuclear condensations.

Management and Prognosis

- There is no effective treatment. Patients who purportedly respond to antibiotic or chlorhexidine therapy are likely to have some other entity, such as frictional keratoses, which typically wax and wane.

REFERENCES

Aloi FG, Molinero A. White sponge nevus with epidermolytic changes. *Dermatologica*. 1988;177:323-326.

Atkinson JC, Harvey KE, Domingo DL, et al. Oral and dental phenotype of dyskeratosis congenita. *Oral Dis*. 2008;14:419-427.

Cai W, Jiang B, Feng T, et al. Expression profiling of white sponge nevus by RNA sequencing revealed pathological pathways [published correction appears in *Orphanet J Rare Dis*. 2015;10:119.]. *Orphanet J Rare Dis*. 2015;10:72.

Lourenco SV, Boggio PA, Fezzi FA, et al. Dyskeratosis congenita—report of a case with emphasis on gingival aspects. *Pediatr Dermatol*. 2009;26:176-179.

Morris R, Gansler TS, Rudisil MT, Neville B. White sponge nevus: diagnosis by light microscopic and ultrastructural cytology. *Acta Cytol*. 1988;32:357-361.

Pradeep AR, Nagaraja C. Pachyonychia congenita with unusual dental findings: a case report. *Oral Surg Oral Med Oral Pathol Oral Radiol Endod*. 2007;104:89-93.

Rugg EL, McLean WH, Allison WE, et al. A mutation in the mucosal keratin K4 is associated with oral white sponge nevus. *Nat Genet*. 1995;11:450-452.

Terrinoni A, Candi E, Oddi S, et al. A glutamine insertion in the 1A alpha helical domain of the keratin 4 gene in a familial case of white sponge nevus. *J Invest Dermatol*. 2000;114:388-391.

Treister N, Lehmann LE, Cherrick I, et al. Dyskeratosis congenita vs. chronic graft versus host disease: report of a case and a review of the literature. *Oral Surg Oral Med Oral Pathol Oral Radiol Endod*. 2004;98:566-571.

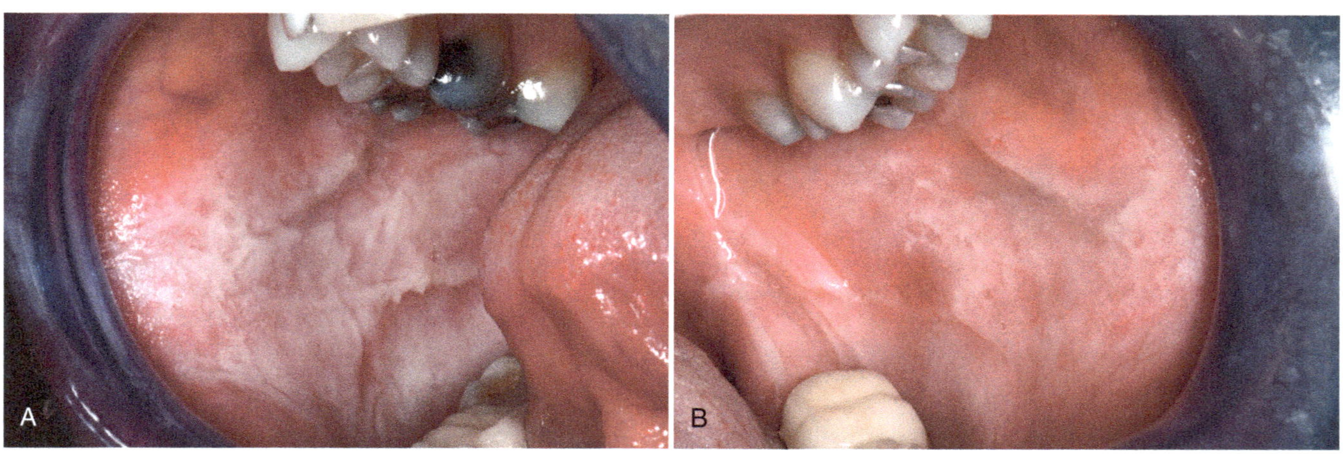

FIG 2.1 (A) and (B) White sponge nevus: diffuse, boggy white plaques of the buccal mucosa present bilaterally. *(Courtesy Dr. Carl Allen, The Ohio State University, Columbus, Ohio.)*

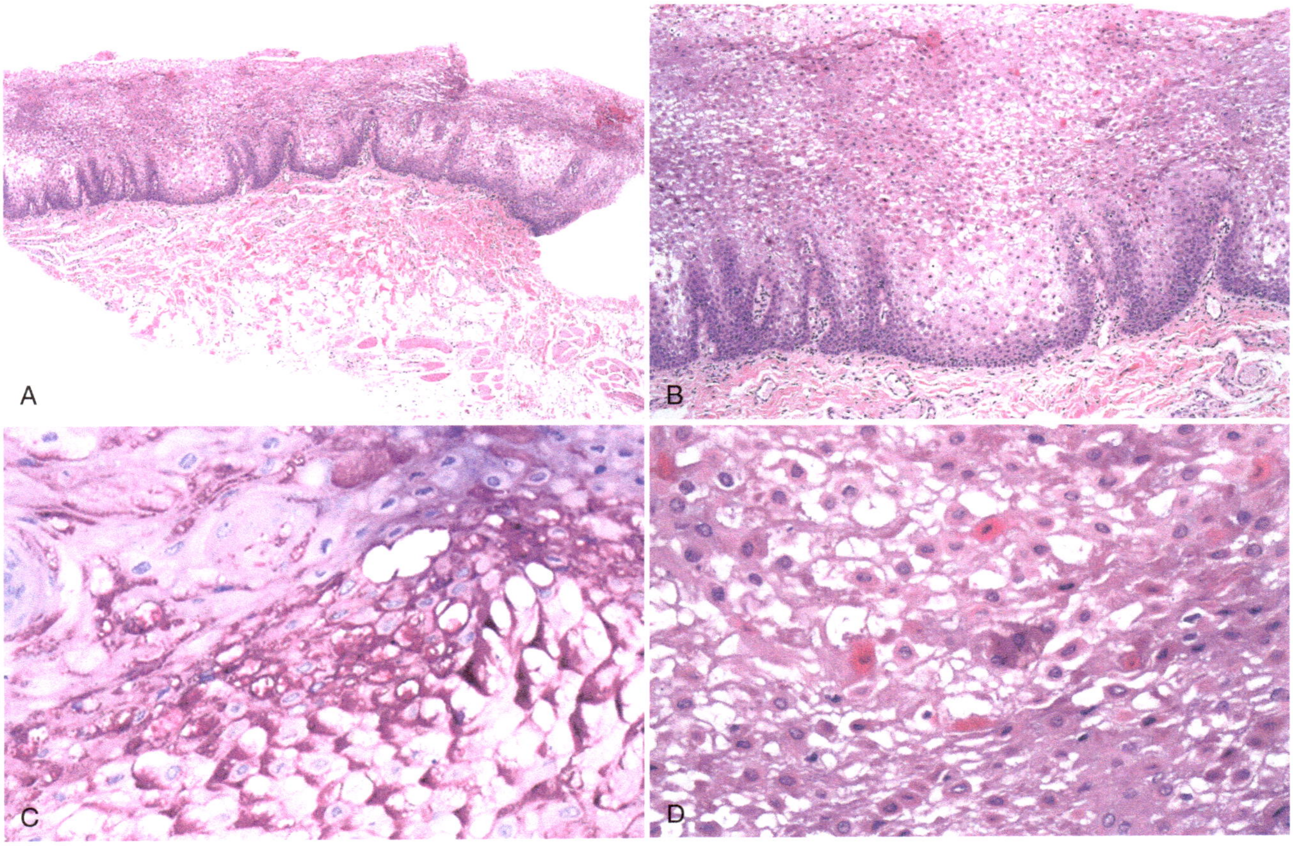

FIG 2.2 White sponge nevus. (A) The epithelium exhibits acanthosis with a pale "spongy" appearance. (B) The pale epithelium is caused by intracellular vacuolation and dyskeratosis that spares the basal cells. (C) There is positive periodic acid–Schiff staining of intracytoplasmic granules typical for glycogen. (D) Perinuclear eosinophilic condensations and intracytoplasmic vacuolation (not spongiosis).

HEREDITARY BENIGN INTRAEPITHELIAL DYSKERATOSIS

Clinical Findings

- This is diagnosed in the first two decades of life and affects Haliwa-Saponi Native Americans in North Carolina and their descendants (usually on the east coast of the United States), although sporadic cases exist. The skin is not affected.
- The oral mucosa exhibits diffuse, thickened, painless, spongy white plaques similar to white sponge nevus.
- Eye lesions are present as gelatinous plaques on bulbar conjunctiva in a perilimbic location.

Etiopathogenesis and Histopathologic Features

Hereditary benign intraepithelial dyskeratosis is an autosomal dominant condition resulting from a duplication on chromosome 4q35.

- Parakeratosis, acanthosis, and many dyskeratotic "tobacco" cells (so called because of their brown color seen in Papanicolaou stains) are located in the upper epithelium. Sometimes these dyskeratotic cells are surrounded by epithelial cells, resulting in a cell-within-a-cell appearance (Fig. 2.3).

Differential Diagnosis

- White sponge nevus shows perinuclear keratin condensations.
- Darier disease or warty dyskeratoma is acantholytic with dyskeratosis but without the cell-within-a-cell appearance.

Management and Prognosis

- There is no effective treatment.

REFERENCES

Allingham RR, Seo B, Rampersaud E, et al. Duplication in chromosome 4q35 is associated with hereditary benign intraepithelial dyskeratosis. *Am J Hum Genet.* 2001;68:491-494.

Cummings TJ, Dodd LG, Eedes CR, Klintworth GK. Hereditary benign intraepithelial dyskeratosis: an evaluation of diagnostic cytology. *Arch Pathol Lab Med.* 2008;132:1325-1328.

Haisley-Royster CA, Allingham RR, Klintworth GK, Prose NS. Hereditary benign intraepithelial dyskeratosis: report of two cases with prominent oral lesions. *J Am Acad Dermatol.* 2001;45:634-636.

Jham BC, Mesquita RA, Aguiar MC, Carmo MA. Hereditary benign intraepithelial dyskeratosis: a new case? *J Oral Pathol Med.* 2007;36:55-57.

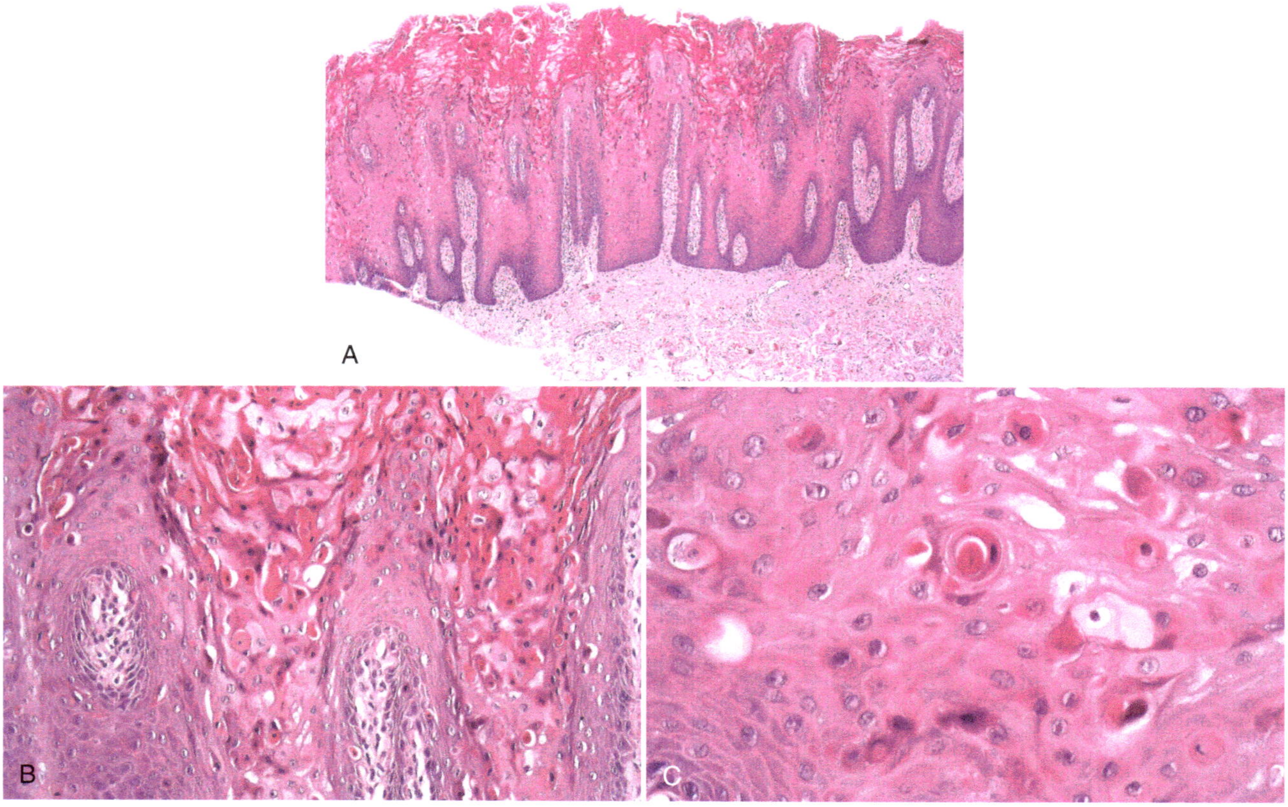

FIG 2.3 Hereditary benign intraepithelial dyskeratosis. (A) Parakeratosis and acanthosis with dyskeratosis. (B) Prominent dyskeratosis within the superficial keratinocytes. (C) Dyskeratotic cells with "cell-within-a-cell" morphology.

KERATOSIS FOLLICULARIS (DARIER DISEASE, DARIER-WHITE DISEASE)

Darier disease in the mouth does not occur in the absence of skin lesions. A localized papule or nodule with similar histopathology is known as *warty dyskeratoma* or *focal acantholytic dyskeratosis* and is discussed in Chapter 10.

Clinical Findings

- Onset occurs in first and second decades of life with lesions on the palatal mucosa, gingiva, or tongue, all keratinized sites. White, painless, keratotic papules (seen in mild disease) or plaques, and cobblestoning of the oral mucosa (seen in more severe disease) are noted in 10% to 50% of patients with skin disease (Fig. 2.4). Up to one-third of cases exhibit parotid or submandibular swelling that is likely due to strictures and obstruction.

Etiopathogenesis and Histopathologic Features

Darier disease is an autosomal dominant disorder associated with a mutation of the *ATP2A2* gene, which encodes sarcoendoplasmic Ca^{2+}-ATPase isoform 2. This protein is involved in the transport of calcium from the cytoplasm into the endoplasmic reticulum as well as posttranslational protein processing required for proper functioning of desmosomes and keratin. The mutation results in dyscohesion.

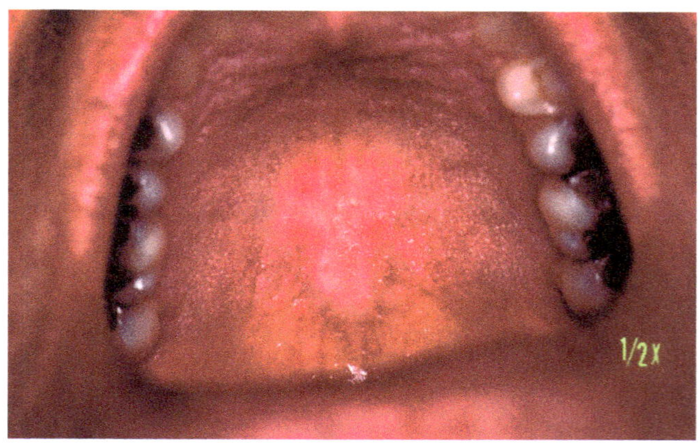

FIG 2.4 Darier disease: diffuse, pebbly white papules on the hard palate. *(From Frezzini C, Cedro M, Leao JC, Porter S. Darier disease affecting the gingival and oral mucosal surfaces. Oral Surg Oral Med Oral Pathol Oral Radiol Endod. 2006;102:e29–e33.)*

- Skin biopsies show marked parakeratosis, acanthosis, dyskeratosis presenting as rounded eosinophilic bodies (corps ronds) as well as spindled eosinophilic structures (grains).

Management and Prognosis

- Darier disease is managed with topical steroids, retinoids, calcineurin inhibitors, diclofenac sodium, laser therapy, and photodynamic therapy.

REFERENCES

Adams AM, Macleod RI, Munro CS. Symptomatic and asymptomatic salivary duct abnormalities in Darier's disease: a sialographic study. *Dentomaxillofac Radiol.* 1994;23:25-28.

Burge SM, Wilkinson JD. Darier-White disease: a review of the clinical features in 163 patients. *J Am Acad Dermatol.* 1992;27:40-50.

Frezzini C, Cedro M, Leao JC, Porter S. Darier disease affecting the gingival and oral mucosal surfaces. *Oral Surg Oral Med Oral Pathol Oral Radiol Endod.* 2006;102:e29-e33.

Macleod RI, Munro CS. The incidence and distribution of oral lesions in patients with Darier's disease. *Br Dent J.* 1991;171:133-136.

Raszewska-Famielec M, Dudra-Jastrzębska M, Borzęcki A, Chodorowskaf G. Darier-White disease treated with fractional CO_2 laser in two cases. *Dermatol Ther.* 2015;28:254-257.

Savignac M, Simon M, Edir A, et al. SERCA2 dysfunction in Darier disease causes endoplasmic reticulum stress and impaired cell-to-cell adhesion strength: rescue by Miglustat. *J Invest Dermatol.* 2014;134: 1961-1970.

HEREDITARY MUCOEPITHELIAL DYSPLASIA

Clinical Findings

- Usually diagnosed in childhood, this disorder is characterized by perineal and oral erythema, nonscarring alopecia, and eye abnormalities. Patients may also have keratosis follicularis, airway disease, and recurrent infections.
- Bright red demarcated plaques of the gingiva and hard palatal mucosa, angular cheilitis, and fissured tongue are seen. The dentition is normal (Fig. 2.5A).

Etiopathogenesis and Histopathologic Features

Hereditary mucoepithelial dysplasia is an autosomal condition (although there are also sporadic cases) resulting from abnormalities in gap junctions and desmosome formation, leading to epithelial dyscohesion. The responsible gene has yet to be identified.

- There is variable papillomatosis, dyscohesion, dyskeratosis, vacuolations within keratinocytes, and lack of intercellular bridges. Dyskeratotic cells are sometimes seen within keratinocytes, giving a cell-within-a-cell appearance (Fig. 2.5B).
- Ultrastuctural examination reveals a reduced number of desmosomes and internalized gap junctions.

Management and Prognosis

- There is no effective treatment.

REFERENCES

Boralevi F, Haftek M, Vabres P, et al. Hereditary mucoepithelial dysplasia: clinical, ultrastructural and genetic study of eight patients and literature review. *Br J Dermatol.* 2005;153:310-318.

Hernández-Martín A, Colmenero I, Torrelo A. Hereditary mucoepithelial dysplasia: report of two sporadic cases. *Pediatr Dermatol.* 2012;29:311-315.

Witkop CJ Jr, White JG, King RA, et al. Hereditary mucoepithelial dysplasia: a disease apparently of desmosome and gap junction formation. *Am J Hum Genet.* 1979;31:414-427.

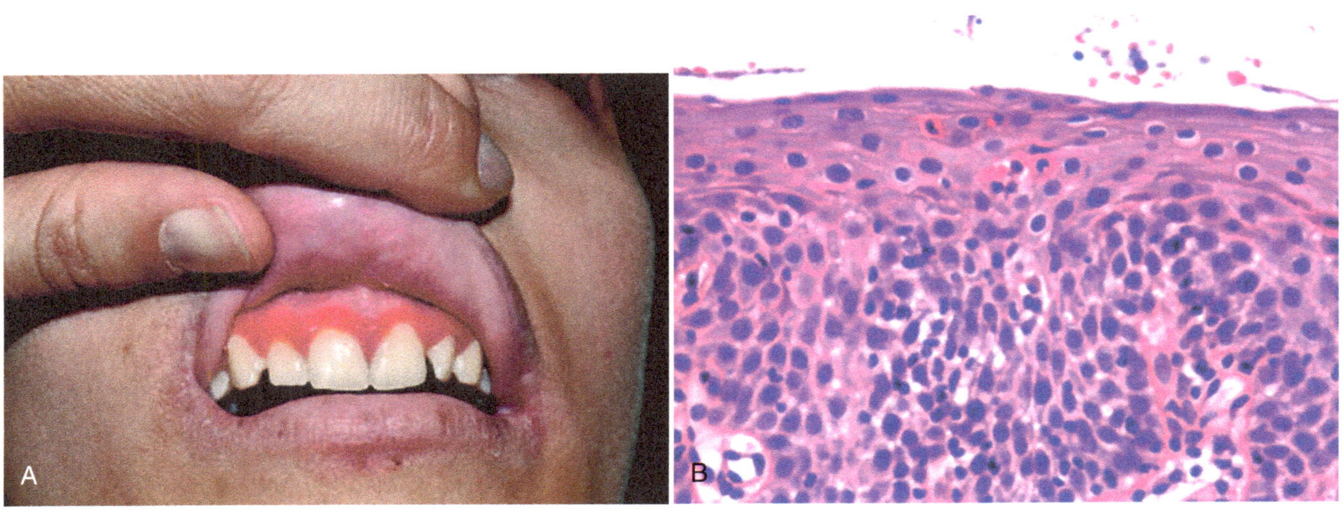

FIG 2.5 Hereditary mucoepithelial dysplasia. (A) Demarcated erythema of the gingiva. (B) Gingival tissue biopsy sample showing scattered dyskeratotic keratinocytes and spongiosis. *(From Hernández-Martín A, Colmenero I, Torrelo A. Hereditary mucoepithelial dysplasia: report of two sporadic cases. Pediatr Dermatol. 2012;29:311–315.)*

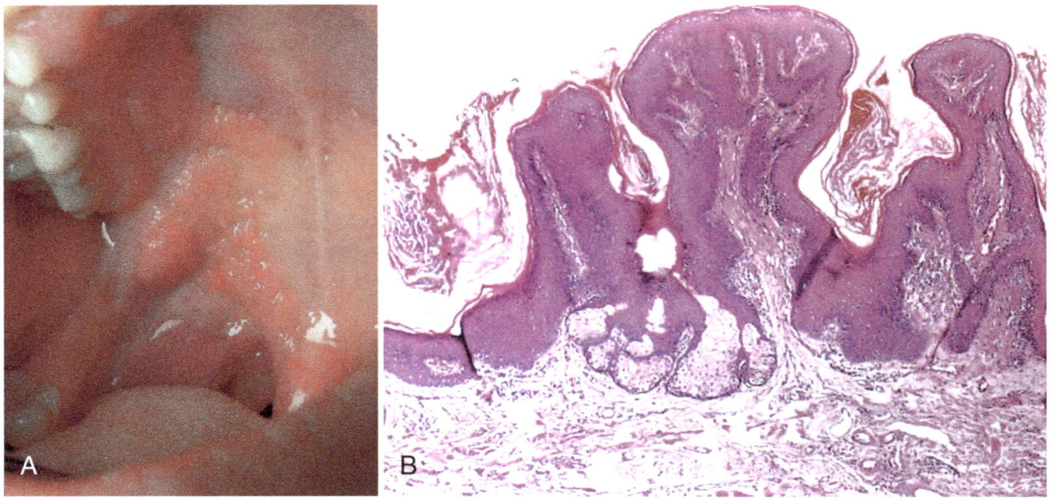

FIG 2.6 Oral linear epidermal nevus. (A) Palatal mucosa with linear verrucous mucosal plaque ipsilateral to cutaneous lesion. (B) Oral mucosa exhibiting hyperkeratosis, papillary acanthosis, and sebaceous glands. *(From Ozçelik D, Parlak AH, Oztürk A, et al. Unilateral linear verrucous epidermal nevus of the face and the oral mucosa. Plast Reconstr Surg. 2005;115:17e–19e.)*

ORAL LINEAR EPIDERMAL NEVUS (ORAL LINEAR VERRUCOUS NEVUS, NEVUS UNIUS LATERIS)

Clinical Findings

- Generally noted in infancy or childhood, linear pigmented and verrucous papules and plaques occur unilaterally on the skin.
- The corresponding oral papillary plaques may be extensive and multifocal. These are mucosa colored in a unilateral distribution or sometimes at the midline. The lips, tongue, and palatal mucosa are the most common sites. Infrequently, there may be missing teeth or enamel hypoplasia. Oral lesions rarely occur without skin lesions (Fig. 2.6).

Etiopathogenesis and Histopathologic Features

Linear epidermal nevi are hamartomatous malformations of the epidermis that tend to follow skin tension lines (of Blaschko), possibly resulting from abnormal migration patterns of embryonic cells. Oral involvement is uncommon.

- Hyperkeratosis and papillary acanthosis are present, sometimes with sebaceous glands.

Differential Diagnosis

- Squamous papillomas and condylomas are solitary lesions and unassociated with linear skin lesions.
- Verruca vulgaris exhibits large keratohyalin granules and is also a solitary lesion.
- Sporadic epidermal nevus (extremely rare) in the mouth exhibits a demarcated area of epithelial proliferation with pilosebaceous units and sometimes other adnexal structures.

Management and Prognosis

- Excision or laser ablation is performed for oral lesions. Skin cases may recur.

REFERENCES

Haberland-Carrodeguas C, Allen CM, Lovas JG, et al. Review of linear epidermal nevus with oral mucosal involvement – series of five new cases. *Oral Dis.* 2008;14:131-137.

Hickman RE, Eveson JW, Cawson RA. Nevus unius lateris and intraoral verrucous nevi. *Oral Surg Oral Med Oral Pathol.* 1988;66:226-229.

Ozçelik D, Parlak AH, Oztürk A, et al. Unilateral linear verrucous epidermal nevus of the face and the oral mucosa. *Plast Reconstr Surg.* 2005;115:17e-19e.

Tesi D, Ficarra G. Oral linear epidermal nevus: a review of the literature and report of two new cases. *Head Neck Pathol.* 2010;4:139-143.

EPIDERMAL NEVUS (EPIDERMAL CHORISTOMA)

Clinical Findings

- This usually occurs within the first 3 months of life, presenting as brown plaques or macules, usually on the tongue, although some cases occur in adults. It differs from linear epidermal nevus in that it is unassociated with an overlying epidermal nevus.

Etiopathogenesis and Histopathologic Features

Oral epidermal nevus represents a developmental overgrowth of tissues, such as mature pilosebaceous units and other skin adnexa, that one would not normally see in the oral cavity. If only sebaceous units are present, the term *epidermal nevus* is more appropriate because sebaceous glands are frequently seen as Fordyce granules in the oral cavity.

- Hyperkeratosis, hypergranulosis, melanosis of basal cells without melanocytic hyperplasia, and pilosebaceous and other adnexal structures are noted within the lamina propria.

Differential Diagnosis

- Sebaceous hyperplasia (hyperplastic Fordyce granules) is often seen in adults.

Management and Prognosis

- Excision is curative.

REFERENCES

Azorin D, Enriquez de Salamanca J, de Prada I, et al. Congenital melanotic macules and sebaceous choristoma arising on the tongue of a newborn: epidermal choristoma? *J Cutan Pathol.* 2005;32:251-253.

Chi AC, Mapes IL, Javed T, Neville BW. Epidermal choristoma of the oral cavity: report of 2 cases of an extremely rare entity. *J Oral Maxillofac Surg.* 2010;68:451-455.

Curto-Barredo L, Vicente A, Rovira C, et al. Epidermal choristoma of the tongue mimicking a congenital melanotic macule. *Pediatr Dermatol.* 2015;32:536-538.

Yoshioka I, Marutsuka K, Igawa K, et al. Epidermal choristoma arising on the midline gingiva as a congenital epulis: a case report. *J Craniomaxillofac Surg.* 2012;40:812-814.

Nodular or Tumor-Like Lesions

FORDYCE GRANULES, SEBACEOUS HYPERPLASIA, ADENOMA, AND CHORISTOMA

Clinical Findings

- Fordyce granules: these are usually noted in adults, present in up to 60% of the population, and appear as 1- to 3-mm yellowish papules, frequently located on the posterior buccal mucosa and vermilion of the lips, but they may be seen at any site. They are usually bilateral and symmetric (Fig. 2.7).
- Sebaceous hyperplasia and adenoma: these are larger, yellowish papules and nodules seen at the same sites as Fordyce granules.
- Sebaceous choristoma: these are papules or nodules usually located in the midline of the tongue in the area of the foramen cecum.

Etiopathogenesis and Histopathologic Features

Fordyce granules are considered normal structures in the mouth. They can become hyperplastic and adenomatous. Patients with Muir-Torre syndrome who present with skin sebaceous tumors and internal malignancy have a high prevalence of sebaceous hyperplasia.

- Fordyce granules: these consist of mature sebaceous glands with a single germinative layer and may or may not open onto the mucosa via a duct lined by squamous epithelium. Sebocytes have central nuclei and vacuolated cytoplasm. Hair and *Demodex folliculorum* have been reported (Fig. 2.8).
- Sebaceous hyperplasia: this consists of at least 15 sebaceous lobules (this number is somewhat arbitrary) opening into a central duct lined by squamous epithelium (Fig. 2.9). The duct may become cystically dilated (Fig. 2.10).
- Sebaceous adenoma: this consists of many sebaceous lobules with proliferation of germinative basaloid cells at the periphery of the lobules.

Differential Diagnosis

- Some salivary gland neoplasms show foci of sebaceous differentiation, with the majority of the tumor representing a recognizable salivary gland neoplasm.

Management and Prognosis

- Excision of sebaceous hyperplasia and adenoma is curative. Very rarely, sebaceous carcinomas arise in the oral cavity.

REFERENCES

Azevedo RS, Almeida OP, Netto JN, et al. Comparative clinicopathological study of intraoral sebaceous hyperplasia and sebaceous adenoma. *Oral Surg Oral Med Oral Pathol Oral Radiol Endod.* 2009;107:100-104.

Daley TD. Intraoral sebaceous hyperplasia: diagnostic criteria. *Oral Surg Oral Med Oral Pathol Oral Radiol Endod.* 1993;75:343-347.

Franklin CD, Underwood JC. Demodex infestation of oral mucosal sebaceous glands. *Oral Surg Oral Med Oral Pathol.* 1986;61:80-82.

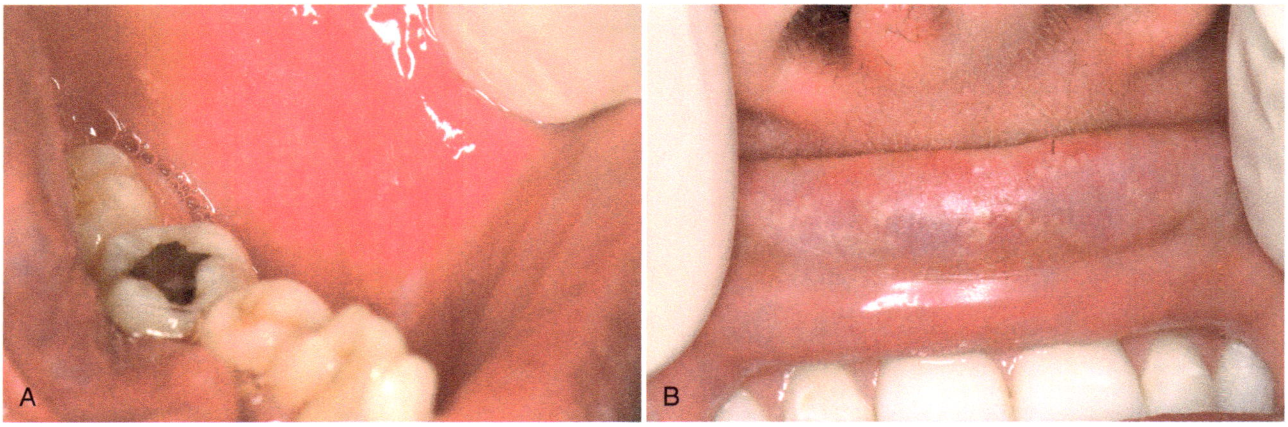

FIG 2.7 Fordyce granules. (A) Yellow papules on the left buccal mucosa. (B) Yellow papules on the upper vermilion.

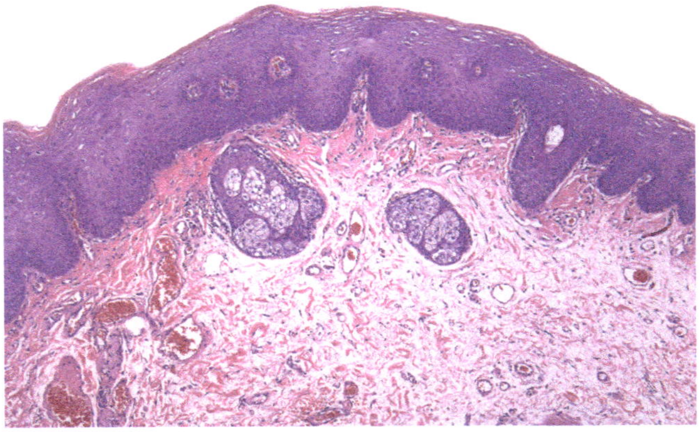

FIG 2.8 Fordyce granules: two sebaceous glands in the lamina propria.

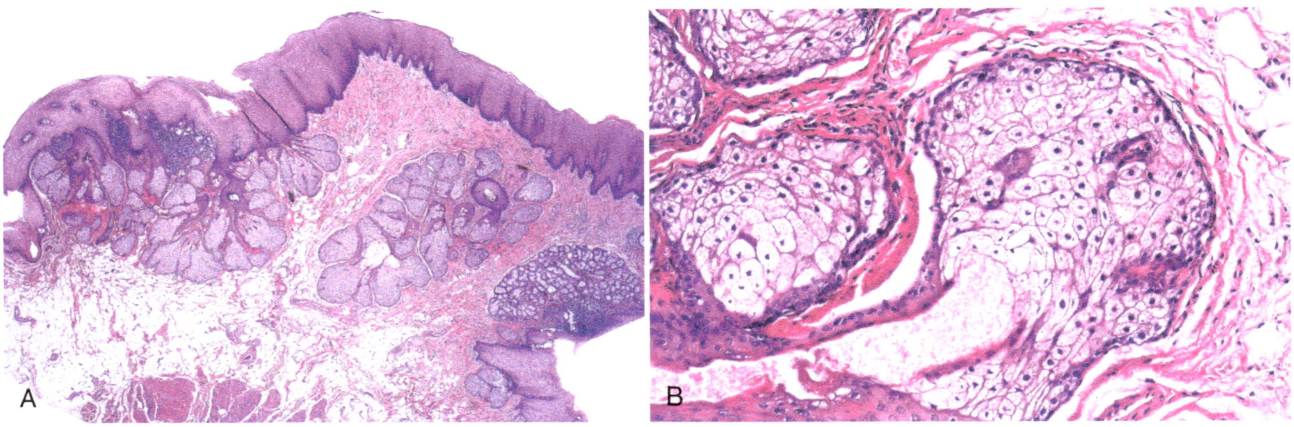

FIG 2.9 Sebaceous hyperplasia. (A) Many lobules of sebaceous glands in the lamina propria without hyperplasia of the germinative layer. (B) Mature sebocytes, secretions within the duct and no proliferation of germinative cells.

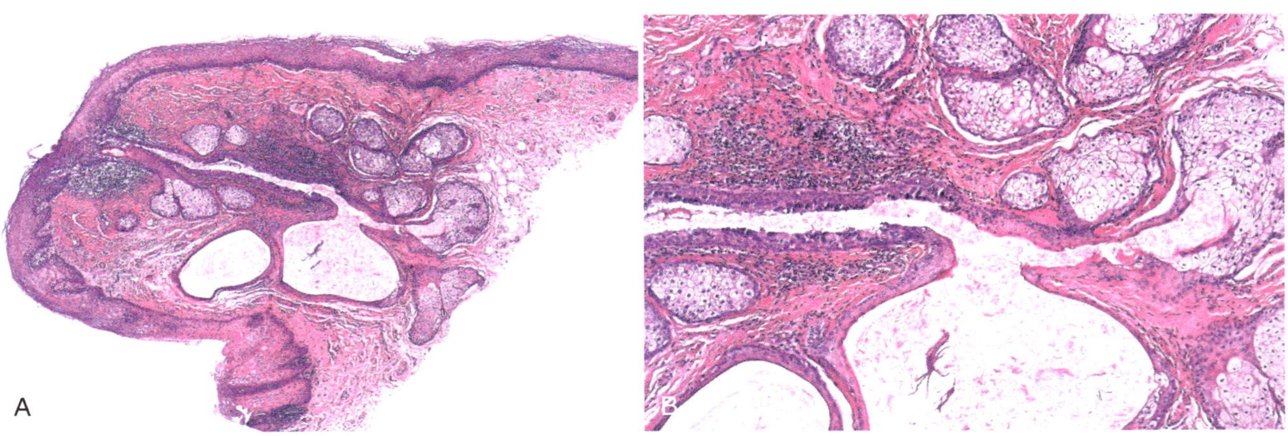

FIG 2.10 Sebaceous hyperplasia. (A) Lobular proliferation of sebaceous glands with ducts opening into the oral cavity. (B) Cystically dilated ducts and mature sebocytes.

Kaminagakura E, Andrade CR, Rangel AL, et al. Sebaceous adenoma of oral cavity: report of case and comparative proliferation study with sebaceous gland hyperplasia and Fordyce's granules. *Oral Dis.* 2003;9:323-327.
Ponti G, Meschieri A, Pollio A, et al. Fordyce granules and hyperplastic mucosal sebaceous glands as distinctive stigmata in Muir-Torre syndrome patients: characterization with reflectance confocal microscopy. *J Oral Pathol Med.* 2015;44:552-557.
Rowe ME, Khorsandi AS, Urken GR, Wenig BM. Intraoral sebaceous carcinoma metastatic to the lung and subcutis: case report and discussion of the literature. *Head Neck.* 2016;38:E20-E24.

CONGENITAL GRANULAR CELL TUMOR (CONGENITAL GRANULAR CELL EPULIS)

Clinical Findings

- This tumor occurs in the newborn and has a strong 8–10:1 female predilection. It appears as a pink, pedunculated mass on the alveolar ridge mucosa and occurs three times more frequently on the maxillary ridge mucosa (Fig. 2.11). Synchronous lesions may be present, and some may regress. They rarely manifest at extragingival sites.

Etiopathogenesis and Histopathologic Features

Congenital granular cell tumor is a mesenchymal tumor of uncertain etiopathogenesis. Ultrastructurally, there are numerous lysosomes, subplasmalemmal dense bodies, pinocytotic vesicles containing precollagenous material, and intracytoplasmic laminin and fibronectin suggestive of pericytic or myofibroblastic differentiation.

- There are sheets of cells with well-defined cell borders; pale, granular cytoplasm; and nuclei with dispersed chromatin and small nucleoli. There are prominent arborizing vessels, and the epithelium is atrophic with no pseudoepitheliomatous hyperplasia (Fig. 2.12).

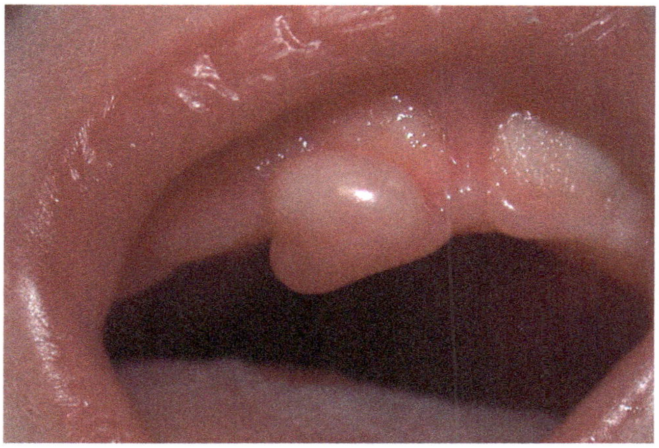

FIG 2.11 Congenital granular cell tumor presenting as a maxillary gingival mass. *(Courtesy Dr. Bonnie Padwa, Harvard School of Dental Medicine, Boston, Mass.)*

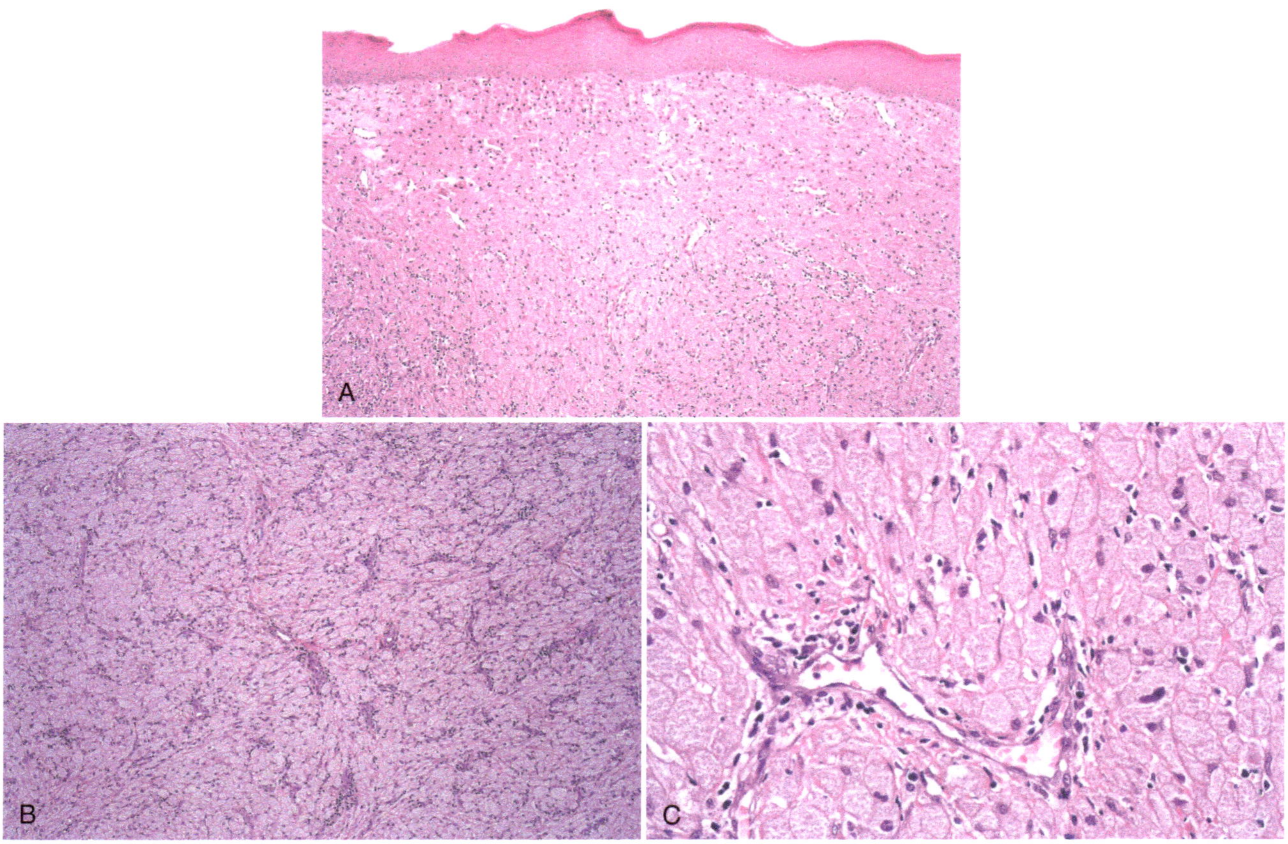

FIG 2.12 Congenital granular cell tumor. (A) Sheets of granular cells without epithelial hyperplasia. (B) Sheets of granular cells with many arborizing vessels. (C) Cells with granular cytoplasm, defined cell borders, and small nuclei with inconspicuous nucleoli.

- Cells are S100-negative but CD68-, NK1/C3-, and PGP-9.5-positive; 40% are neuron-specific enolase–positive.

Differential Diagnosis

- Conventional granular cell tumor is positive for S100 protein without prominent arborizing vessels.
- Primitive polypoid granular cell tumor shares the same immunohistochemical profile, has an epithelial collarette, and exhibits cytologic atypia.

Management and Prognosis

- Excision is curative. Some cases show spontaneous regression.

REFERENCES

Bhatia SK, Goyal A, Ritwik P, Rai S. Spontaneous regression of a congenital epulis in a newborn. *J Clin Pediatr Dent.* 2013;37:297-299.

Childers EL, Fanburg-Smith JC. Congenital epulis of the newborn: 10 new cases of a rare oral tumor. *Ann Diagn Pathol.* 2011;15:157-161.

Damm DD. Investigation into the histogenesis of congenital epulis of the newborn. *Oral Surg Oral Med Oral Pathol.* 1993;76:205-212.

Kaiserling E, Ruck P, Xiao JC. Congenital epulis and granular cell tumor: a histologic and immunohistochemical study. *Oral Surg Oral Med Oral Pathol Oral Radiol Endod.* 1995;80:687-697.

Kupers AM, Andriessen P, van Kempen MJ, et al. Congenital epulis of the jaw: a series of five cases and review of literature. *Pediatr Surg Int.* 2009;25:207-210.

Lack EE, Worsham GF, Callihan MD, et al. Gingival granular cell tumors of the newborn (i.e., congenital "epulis"): a clinical and pathologic study of 21 patients. *Am J Surg Pathol.* 1981;5:37-46.

Vered M, Dobriyan A, Buchner A. Congenital granular cell epulis presents an immunohistochemical profile that distinguishes it from the granular cell tumor of the adult. *Virchows Arch.* 2009;454:303-310.

OSSEOUS, CARTILAGINOUS, AND OSTEOCHONDROMATOUS CHORISTOMA

Clinical Findings

- Osseous choristoma: this is seen in young adults, and it has a 3:1 female predilection. More than 90% present as a mass or nodule, usually on the dorsum (most common site) or lateral tongue, near the foramen cecum. The buccal mucosa is the second most common site.
- Cartilaginous choristoma: this is seen in young adults with equal gender predilection. More than 80% present as a mass or nodule in the dorsal or lateral tongue (most common site).

Etiopathogenesis and Histopathologic Features

These choristomas may represent a developmental malformation arising from multipotent stem cells in the soft tissues or from ossification of branchial arch remnants. However, they may also represent metaplastic bone or cartilage formation due to trauma such as within a traumatic fibroma or within a lipoma (osteolipoma).

- Osseous choristoma: this consists of a discrete proliferation of mature lamellar bone (sometimes with mature adipose or hematopoietic tissue). Mature cartilage may be present (Fig. 2.13).

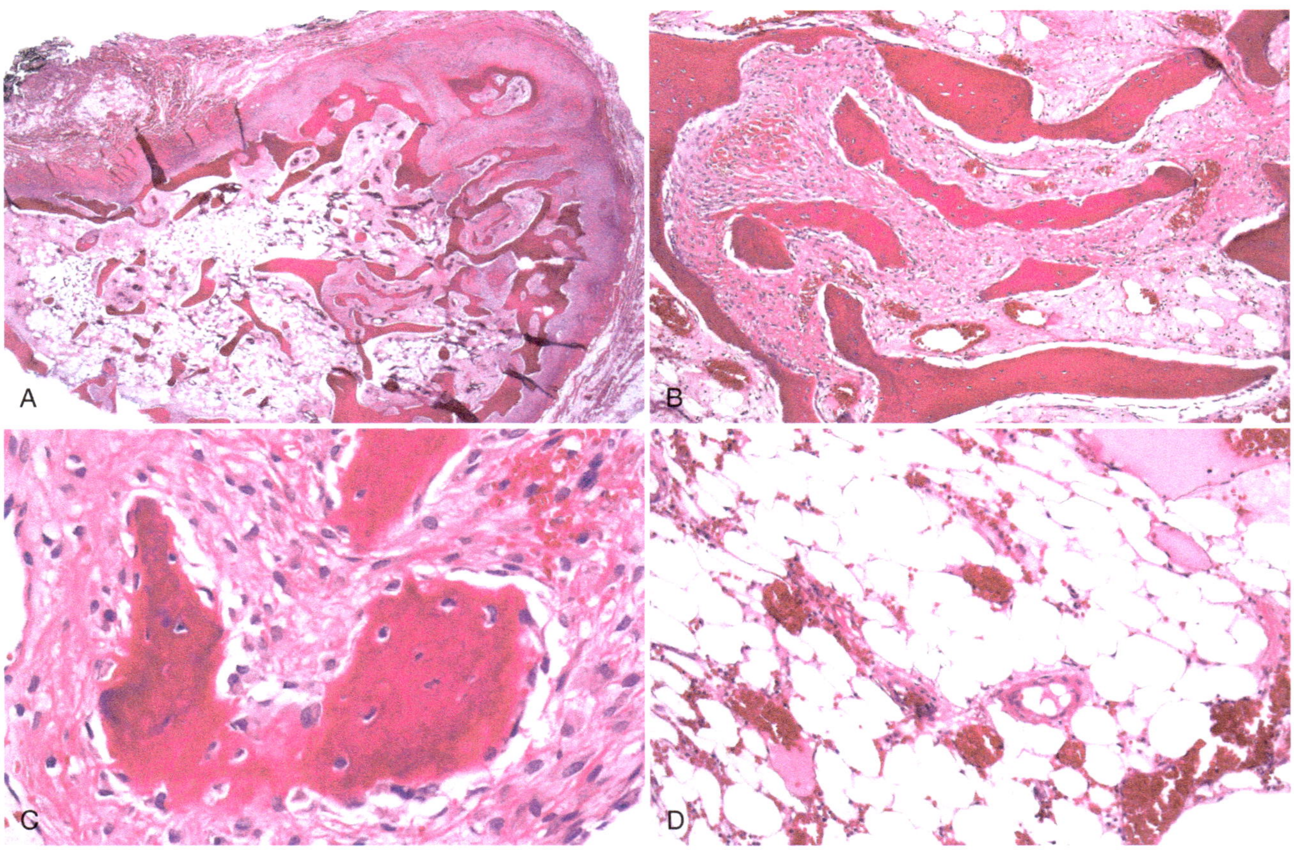

FIG 2.13 Osteolipomatous choristoma. (A) Encapsulated mass of cellular fibrous tissue, viable lamellar bone, and mature fat. (B) Cellular fibrous tissue containing many plump fibroblasts and woven bone. (C) Woven bone with osteocytes and surrounding plump fibroblasts. (D) Mature lipocytes are present.

- Cartilaginous choristoma: consists of mature hyaline cartilage, sometimes with spindle cell proliferation or primitive mesenchyme. Mature bone may be present.

Differential Diagnosis

- Myoepithelioma or pleomorphic adenoma with bone and cartilage production also consists of ductal structures and myoepithelial cells that are p63- or p40-positive (see Chapter 13).
- Metaplastic cartilage is often seen in denture-related fibrous hyperplasias in the maxillary vestibule and in the nasopalatine duct area.
- Myositis ossificans exhibits a distinct "zoning" phenomenon with a central cellular area of spindle cells gradually forming osteoid and more mature lamellar bone at the periphery.
- Ectomesenchymal chondromyxoid tumor (which may represent a soft tissue myoepithelioma) has a specific histopathologic and immunohistochemical profile (see Chapter 5).

Management and Prognosis

- Excision is curative.

REFERENCES

Andressakis DD, Pavlakis AG, Chrysomali E, Rapidis AD. Infected lingual osseous choristoma: report of a case and review of the literature. *Med Oral Patol Oral Cir Bucal.* 2008;13:E627-E632.

Chou LS, Hansen LS, Daniels TE. Choristomas of the oral cavity: a review. *Oral Surg Oral Med Oral Pathol.* 1991;72:584-593.

Kamburoglu K, Ozen T, Sencimen M, et al. Osseous choristoma of the submandibular region: case report. *Dentomaxillofac Radiol.* 2009; 38:489-492.

Lin CC, Chen CH, Chen YK, et al. Osseous choristoma of oral cavity – report of two cases and review of the literature. *Kaohsiung J Med Sci.* 1998;14:727-733.

Norris O, Mehra P. Chondroma (cartilaginous choristoma) of the tongue: report of a case. *J Oral Maxillofac Surg.* 2012;70:643-646.

GINGIVAL FIBROMATOSIS

Clinical Findings

- This is often first noted in the first decade of life during eruption of permanent teeth. There is diffuse overgrowth of dense, firm, pink, gingival tissue of the mandible and/or maxilla (Fig. 2.14).
- Localized versions occur, especially in the area of the maxillary tuberosity, bilaterally.
- Gingival fibromatosis is associated with some syndromes (such as Zimmerman-Laband, Rutherford, Ramon, and Cross syndromes). Syndromic patients may also be taking medications used to control seizures (eg, phenytoin), and these can aggravate the gingival hyperplasia. Syndromic patients often also present with periodontal disease, hyperhydrosis, and cognitive disabilities.

Etiopathogenesis and Histopathologic Features

The gene for the nonsyndromic, autosomal dominant form is associated with a *SOS1* mutation. However, the disease is heterogeneous, with some cases showing autosomal recessive transmission. There is increased production and reduced metabolism of collagen and ground substance, possibly because of reduced matrix metalloproteinase activity mediated by transforming growth factor β1.

- There is a proliferation of densely collagenous, fibrous tissue with benign, plump, spindled and stellate fibroblasts (Fig. 2.15). Rete ridges are long and slender and interconnect. There is minimal inflammation.

Differential Diagnosis

- Hyaline fibromatosis syndrome is an autosomal recessive condition that consists of a mild form formerly known as *juvenile hyaline fibromatosis*, a moderate form

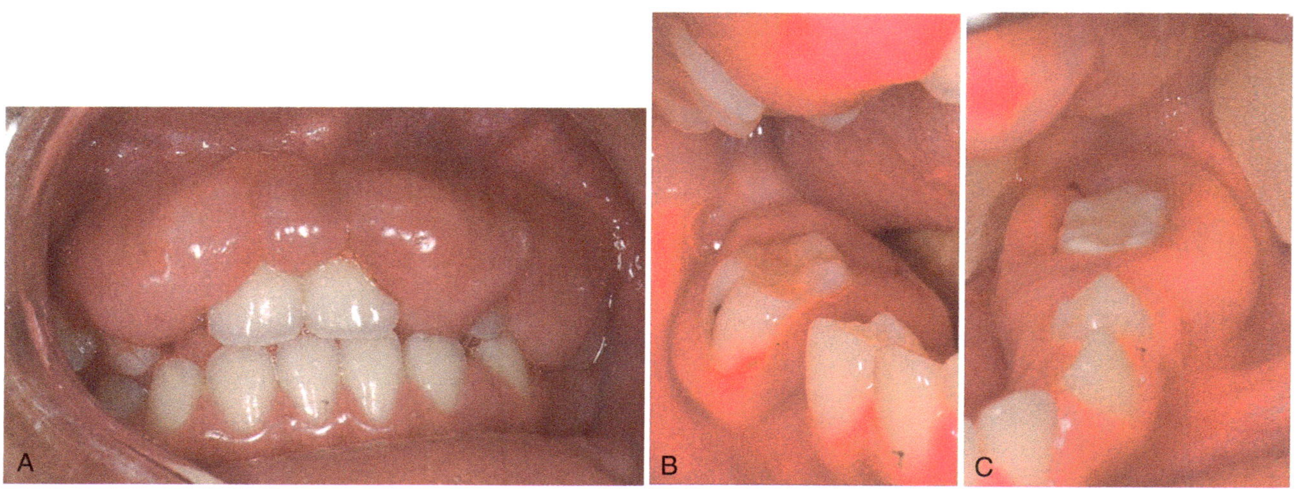

FIG 2.14 Gingival fibromatosis in one patient. (A) Bulky symmetric overgrowth of the maxillary gingiva. (B) Overgrowth of the right mandibular gingiva. (C) Overgrowth of the left mandibular gingiva. *(Courtesy Nalton Ferraro, DMD, MD, Boston Children's Hospital, Boston, Mass.)*

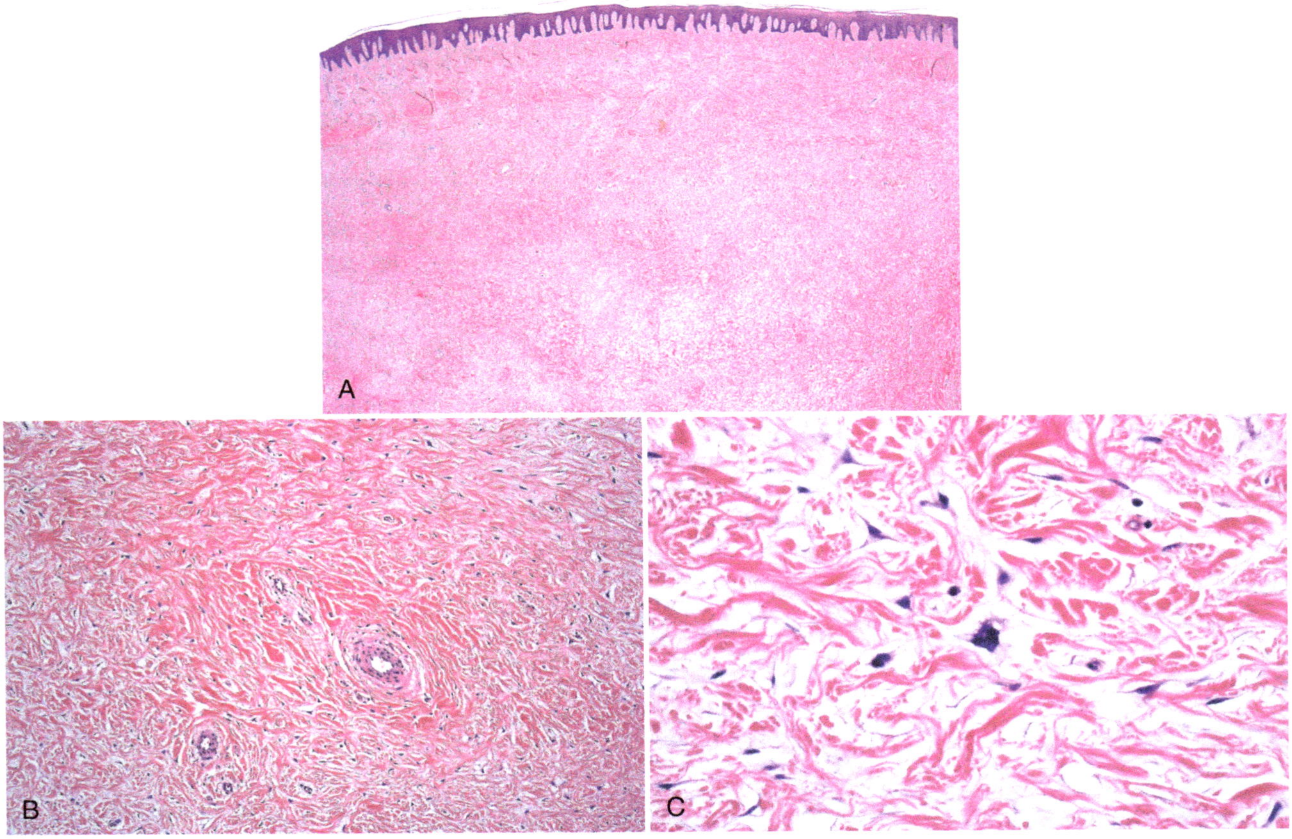

FIG 2.15 Gingival fibromatosis. (A) Marked proliferation of dense, fibrocollagenous tissue with slight epithelial hyperplasia. (B) Dense collagen with small vessels. (C) Stellate, spindled, and multinucleated fibroblasts.

that includes bone lesions and joint contractures, and a severe form formerly known as *infantile systemic hyalinosis* with visceral involvement, recurrent infections, and poor survival. All cases exhibit gingival overgrowth composed of densely hyalinized, paucicellular stromal deposits that resemble chondroid material or amyloid. There is a mutation in the *ANTXR2* gene (formerly called the *capillary morphogenesis factor 2 gene*) (Fig. 2.16).

- Myofibroma is cellular with a fasciculated pattern often with zoning, and cells are positive for smooth muscle actin.

Management and Prognosis

- Excision and recontouring help esthetics, and maintenance of good oral hygiene (with use of antimicrobial oral rinses) reduces the severity of recurrences.

REFERENCES

Breen GH, Addante R, Black CC. Early onset of hereditary gingival fibromatosis in a 28-month-old. *Pediatr Dent.* 2009;31:286-288.

Casavecchia P, Uzel MI, Kantarci A, et al. Hereditary gingival fibromatosis associated with generalized aggressive periodontitis: a case report. *J Periodontol.* 2004;75:770-778.

Denadai R, Raposo-Amaral CE, Bertola D, et al. Identification of 2 novel *ANTXR2* mutations in patients with hyaline fibromatosis syndrome and proposal of a modified grading system. *Am J Med Genet A.* 2012; 158A:732-742.

Hakkinen L, Csiszar A. Hereditary gingival fibromatosis: characteristics and novel putative pathogenic mechanisms. *J Dent Res.* 2007;86: 25-34.

Lim AA, Kozakewich HP, Feingold M, Padwa BL. Juvenile hyaline fibromatosis: report of a case and comparison with infantile systemic hyalinosis. *J Oral Maxillofac Surg.* 2005;63:271-274.

Nibali L, Medlar A, Stanescu H, et al. Linkage analysis confirms heterogeneity of hereditary gingival fibromatosis. *Oral Dis.* 2013;19: 100-105.

Nofal A, Sanad M, Assaf M, et al. Juvenile hyaline fibromatosis and infantile systemic hyalinosis: a unifying term and a proposed grading system. *J Am Acad Dermatol.* 2009;61:695-700.

Shieh JT, Swidler P, Martignetti JA, et al. Systemic hyalinosis: a distinctive early childhood-onset disorder characterized by mutations in the anthrax toxin receptor 2 gene (*ANTRX2*). *Pediatrics.* 2006;118: e1485-e1492.

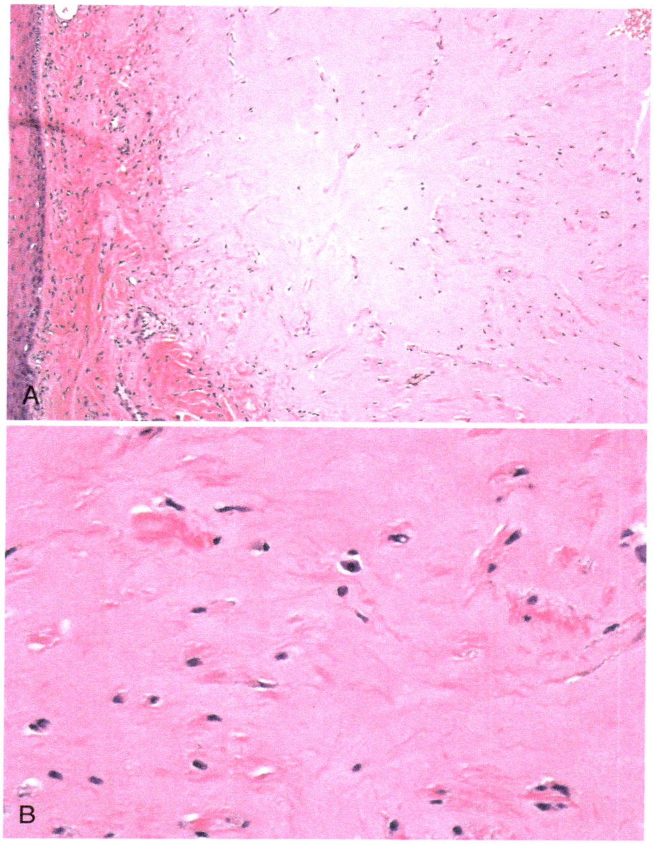

FIG 2.16 Hyaline fibromatosis syndrome. (A) Amorphous, eosinophilic deposits in the gingiva. (B) Plump polygonal cells within chondroid-like material.

GASTROINTESTINAL AND BRAIN HETEROTOPIA

Clinical Findings

- Infants or children present with a mass that may be cystic and located in the midline of the tongue or floor of the mouth or near the foramen cecum associated with sinus tracts. Many gastrointestinal heterotopias are cystic ("foregut cyst").

Etiopathogenesis and Histopathologic Features

Gastrointestinal and brain heterotopias are likely caused by entrapped or displaced undifferentiated endodermal or neuroectodermal tissues, respectively, that subsequently differentiate in a multidirectional pattern.

- Gastrointestinal heterotopia: this is usually cystic and lined by epithelium typical of the cardiac, fundic, or pyloric regions of the stomach with parietal and Paneth cells. They may also be lined by squamous epithelium (believed to duplicate the esophageal lining) as well as colonic and/or ciliated epithelium, and pancreatic tissue may be identified. Some cases are solid (Fig. 2.17).
- Brain heterotopia: glia, astrocytes, oligodendrocytes, ependymal tissue, choroid plexus–like tissue, and, rarely, neuronal tissue are identified. This is often associated with cleft palate (Fig. 2.18).

Differential Diagnosis

- Salivary duct cyst is lined by cuboidal, columnar, and/or squamous epithelium, often with mucous cells, and salivary glands are usually present in the adjacent tissues.

Management and Prognosis

- Excision is curative.

REFERENCES

Chou LS, Hansen LS, Daniels TE. Choristomas of the oral cavity: a review. *Oral Surg Oral Med Oral Pathol.* 1991;72:584-593.

Khunamornpong S, Yousukh A, Tananuvat R. Heterotopic gastrointestinal and pancreatic tissue of the tongue: a case report. *Oral Surg Oral Med Oral Pathol Oral Radiol Endod.* 1996;81:576-579.

Martins F, Hiraki KR, Mimura MA, et al. Heterotopic gastrointestinal mucosa in the oral cavity of adults. *Oral Surg Oral Med Oral Pathol Oral Radiol.* 2013;115:e51-e54.

Sun LS, Sun ZP, Ma XC, Li TJ. Glial choristoma in the oral and maxillofacial region: a clinicopathologic study of 6 cases. *Arch Pathol Lab Med.* 2008;132:984-988.

Zhang Q, Luo CY, Huang Y, Wang YJ. Heterotopic central nervous system tissue arising in the palatopharyngeal region associated with cleft palate: case report. *Br J Oral Maxillofac Surg.* 2014;52:e4-e6.

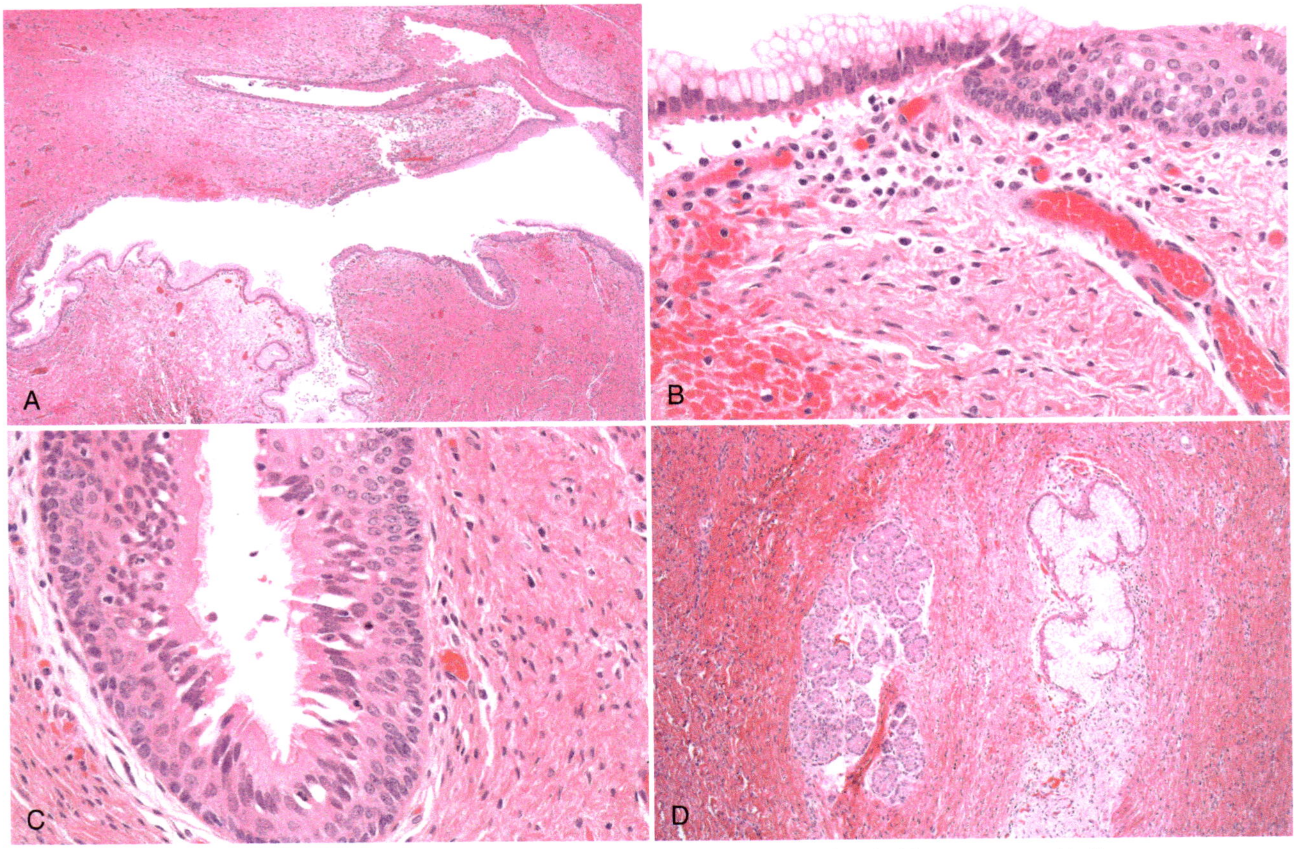

FIG 2.17 Heterotopic gastrointestinal cyst. (A) The cyst is lined by uniformly thin squamous epithelium and mucous cells. (B) Transition between stratified squamous and mucous cells (resembling gastric lining). (C) Ciliated epithelium is frequently encountered. (D) Islands of pancreatic tissue are present within the cyst wall. *(A, Courtesy Dr. Lee Slater, Scripps Institute, San Diego, Calif.)*

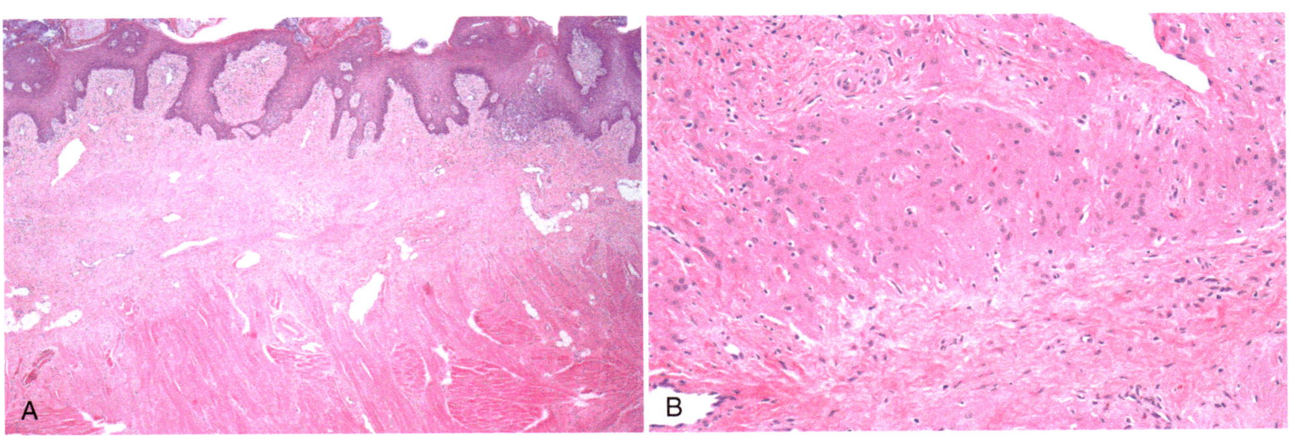

FIG 2.18 Heterotopic brain tissue. (A) Pale epithelioid cells lying within the tongue lamina propria above skeletal muscle. (B) Glial tissue.

LYMPHANGIOMA OF THE ALVEOLAR RIDGE IN THE NEONATE

Clinical Findings

- Four percent of infants, almost exclusively Black, exhibit this congenital disorder. Multiple dome-shaped, 3- to 4-mm, bluish, fluid-filled vesicles are noted in the posterior maxillary and mandibular alveolar ridge.

Etiopathogenesis and Histopathologic Features

The etiopathogenesis is unknown, and this condition is more likely to represent lymphatic ectasia.

- Typical endothelium-lined spaces filled with amorphous, eosinophilic material are noted, and odontogenic rests may be present.

Differential Diagnosis

- This is indistinguishable from lymphatic ectasia or lymphangioma circumscriptum found in older patients, except for the clinical presentation.

Management and Prognosis

- No treatment is required, because these malformations regress by 6 months of age.

REFERENCES

FitzGerald K, Barry S, Fleming P. Alveolar lymphangioma in infants: report of two cases. *J Ir Dent Assoc.* 2009;55:144-145.

Friend GW, Harris EF, Mincer HH, et al. Oral anomalies in the neonate, by race and gender, in an urban setting. *Pediatr Dent.* 1990;12:157-161.

Wilson S, Gould AR, Wolff C. Multiple lymphangiomas of the alveolar ridge in a neonate: case study. *Pediatr Dent.* 1986;8:231-234.

LINGUAL THYROID

Clinical Findings

- There is a bimodal distribution in the first to second decades and fifth to sixth decades of life, with a 3–4:1 female predilection. Patients often report a globus sensation and sometimes dysphagia and airway obstruction. The majority of patients are hypothyroid, and a minority euthyroid. Hyperthyroidism is rare.
- The majority of cases present as a soft mass in the area of the foramen cecum or between the foramen cecum and the epiglottis in the midline posterior to the circumvallate papillae. Scintigraphy using technetium-99m or radioactive iodine reveals positive uptake.

Etiopathogenesis and Histopathologic Features

Lingual thyroid represents remnants of thyroid tissue or an entire undescended thyroid due to dysembryogenesis. It is located anywhere along the path of descent of the thyroid from the midline base of the tongue to the pretracheal position and is the only thyroid tissue in many cases. Lingual thyroid tissue is present in 10% of autopsy specimens. Increased demand for thyroid hormone in puberty and adulthood leads to increased thyroid-stimulating hormone levels and growth of ectopic thyroid tissue.

- There is mature or embryonic thyroid tissue with microfollicular, macrofollicular, or adenomatous changes (Fig. 2.19). There may be an associated thyroglossal duct.
- Follicular, papillary, and medullary carcinomas have been reported with a less pronounced gender predilection.

Management and Prognosis

- Most cases are treated with either partial or total excision when symptomatic. If this represents undescended thyroid, removal leads to hypothyroidism and requires repletion. Biopsy may lead to excessive bleeding.

REFERENCES

Adelchi C, Mara P, Melissa L, et al. Ectopic thyroid tissue in the head and neck: a case series. *BMC Res Notes.* 2014;7:790.

Chou LS, Hansen LS, Daniels TE. Choristomas of the oral cavity: a review. *Oral Surg Oral Med Oral Pathol.* 1991;72:584-593.

Kamat MR, Kulkarni JN, Desai PB, Jussawalla DJ. Lingual thyroid: a review of 12 cases. *Br J Surg.* 1979;66:537-539.

Noussios G, Anagnostis P, Goulis DG, et al. Ectopic thyroid tissue: anatomical, clinical, and surgical implications of a rare entity. *Eur J Endocrinol.* 2011;165:375-382.

Rahbar R, Yoon MJ, Connolly LP, et al. Lingual thyroid in children: a rare clinical entity. *Laryngoscope.* 2008;118:1174-1179.

Sturniolo G, Violi MA, Galletti B, et al. Differentiated thyroid carcinoma in lingual thyroid. *Endocrine.* 2016;51:189-198.

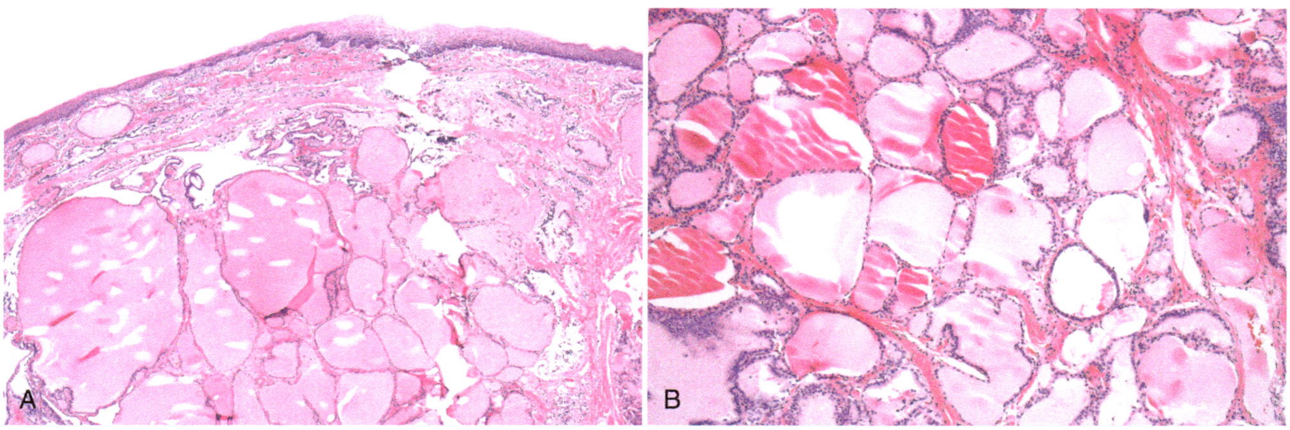

FIG 2.19 Lingual thyroid. (A) Mass of thyroid tissue with overlying oral epithelium. (B) Normal thyroid follicles filled with colloid. *(A, Courtesy Dr. Harry Kozakewich, Harvard Medical School, Boston, Mass.)*

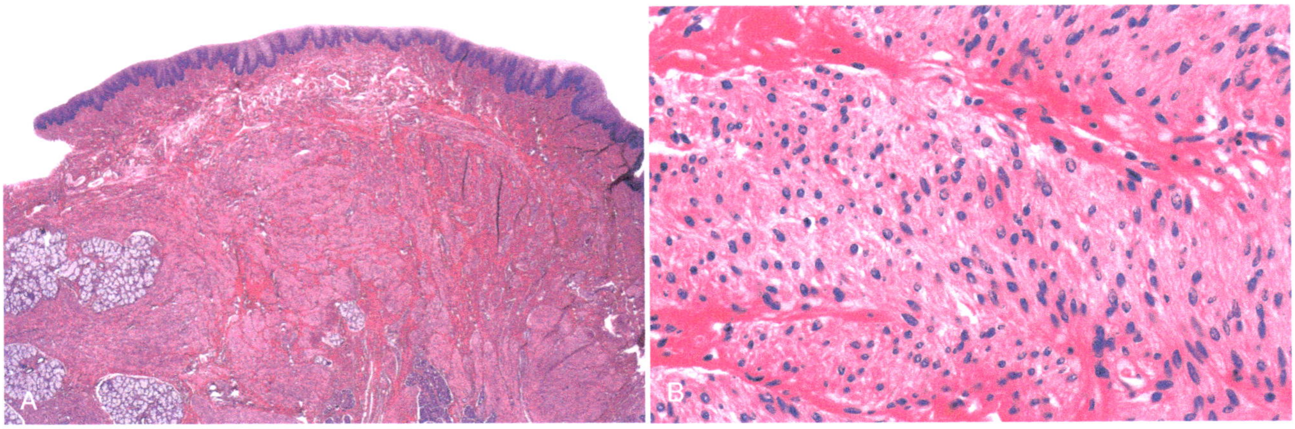

FIG 2.20 Leiomyomatous hamartoma of the tongue. (A) Unencapsulated mass of spindle cells within the tongue surrounding salivary glands. (B) Spindled smooth muscle cells with abundant, pale eosinophilic cytoplasm.

LEIOMYOMATOUS HAMARTOMA

Clinical Features

- This is usually noted within the first year of life and presents as a soft, painless polypoid mass, usually on the tongue and anterior maxillary/palatal mucosa in the area of the nasopalatine foramen.

Etiopathogenesis and Histopathologic Features

Leiomyomatous hamartoma is a developmental malformation of smooth muscle.

- There is a nonencapsulated proliferation of fusiform and spindled smooth muscle cells that express HHF-35, smooth muscle actin, and desmin, but not S100 protein (Fig. 2.20).

Differential Diagnosis

- Myofibroma is a more extensive and cellular lesion with sweeping fascicles of tumor cells exhibiting a zoning phenomenon.

Management and Prognosis

- Excision is curative.

REFERENCES

Iida S, Kishino M, Senoo H, et al. Multiple leiomyomatous hamartoma in the oral cavity. *J Oral Pathol Med.* 2007;36:241-244.

Semba I, Kitano M, Mimura T. Gingival leiomyomatous hamartoma: immunohistochemical and ultrastructural observations. *J Oral Pathol Med.* 1993;22:468-470.

Takeda Y, Satoh M, Nakamura S, Matsumoto D. Congenital leiomyomatous epulis: a case report with immunohistochemical study. *Pathol Int.* 2000;50:999-1002.

Wang HL, Chiang FY, Tai CF, et al. Lingual leiomyomatous hamartoma with bifid tip and ankyloglossia in a patient without oral-facial-digital syndrome: a case report and literature review. *World J Surg Oncol.* 2013;11:230.

Cystic Lesions

ORAL LYMPHOEPITHELIAL CYST (BENIGN LYMPHOEPITHELIAL CYST)

Clinical Findings

- The majority of cases occur in the fourth to sixth decades of life, and there is a 2:1 female predilection. They appear as yellowish, painless, soft nodules with 80% to 90% of cases occurring on the posterior ventral-lateral tongue, the floor of the mouth, the hard palatal mucosa, and the soft palate. Cysts are filled with cheesy, keratinaceous material (Fig. 2.21A).

Etiopathogenesis and Histopathologic Features

Lymphoepithelial cysts may arise from entrapped embryonic epithelial remnants of surface epithelium, metaplastic salivary ducts or from blocked crypts of lingual or ectopic tonsils. They are histologically indistinguishable from parotid lymphoepithelial cysts often seen in patients with HIV infection (see Fig. 2.21B).

- The cyst lining is composed of parakeratotic, stratified squamous epithelium that is generally uniformly 5–10 cells thick, often with prominent lymphocyte exocytosis reminiscent of the reticulated epithelium of the tonsils. Infrequently, mucous cells are noted or the epithelium is respiratory in nature. The cyst is surrounded partially or completely by a mantle of lymphocytes that may exhibit germinal centers. The lumen is filled with keratinaceous material (Figs. 2.22 and 2.23).

Differential Diagnosis

- Hyperplastic lingual tonsils are not as obviously cystic, although blockage of the crypt opening often leads to retention of secretions, and the two may become indistinguishable (Figs. 2.24 and 2.25).

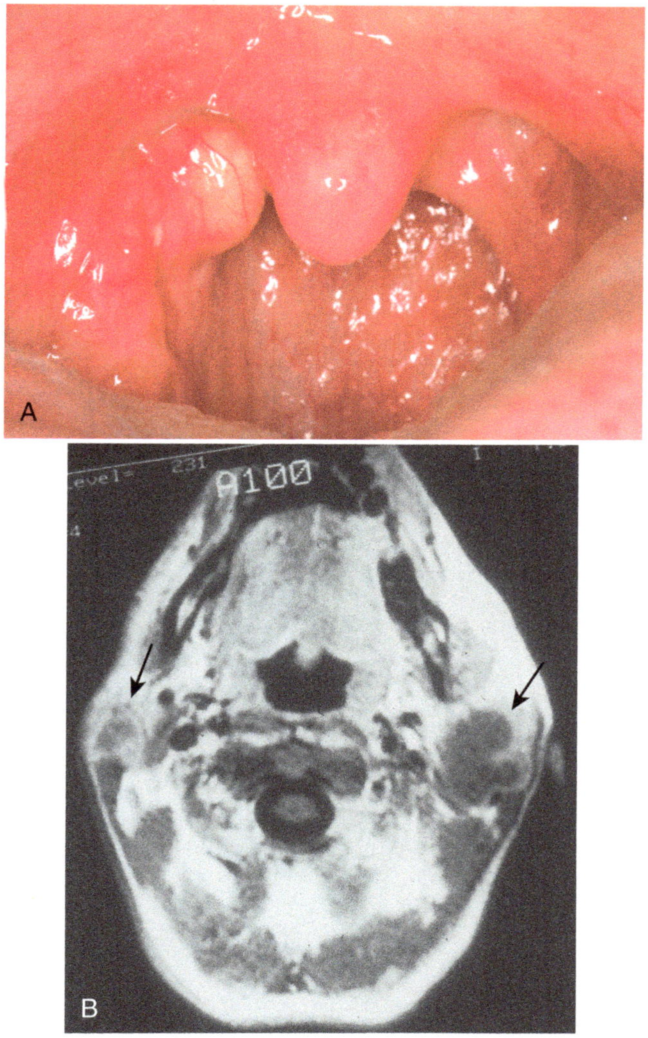

FIG 2.21 (A) Lymphoepithelial cyst of the right tonsillar pillar presenting as a yellow nodule. (B) Bilateral lymphoepithelial cysts of the parotid (*arrows*) in a patient with HIV/AIDS.

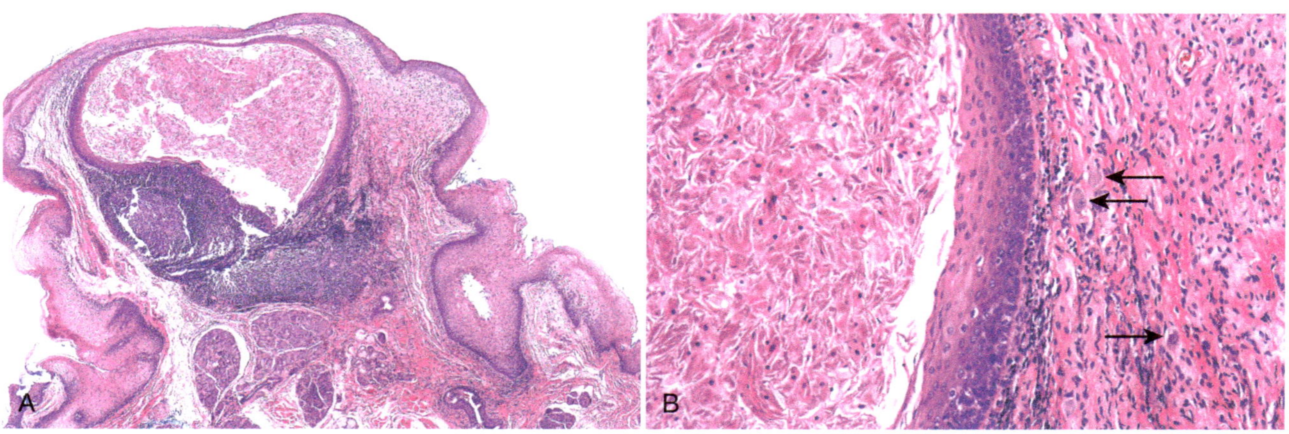

FIG 2.22 Oral lymphoepithelial cyst. (A) The cyst is filled with keratin and partially surrounded by lymphoid tissue. (B) The cyst is lined by parakeratotic, stratified squamous epithelium. Note the ganglion-like cells surrounded by neural tissue typical of a subgemmal neurogenous plaque (*arrows*).

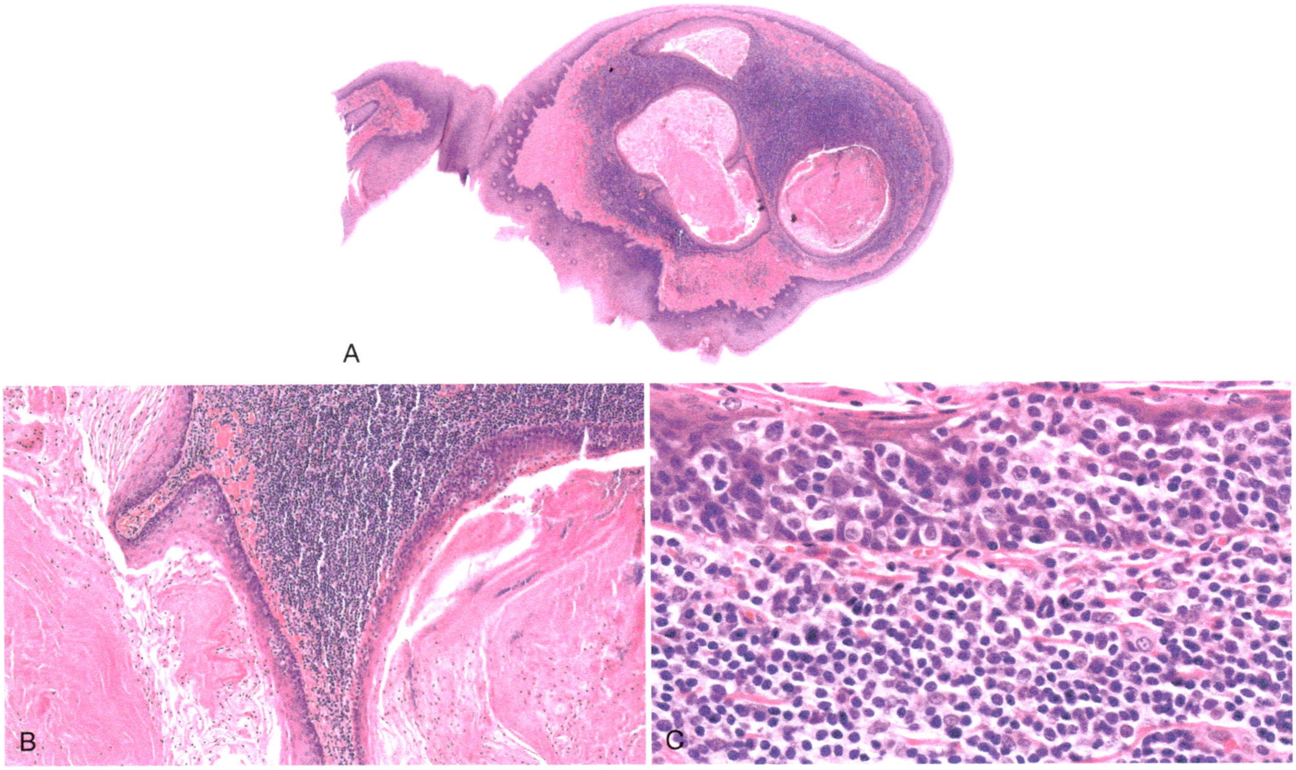

FIG 2.23 Oral lymphoepithelial cyst. (A) This convoluted cyst appears multicystic and is almost entirely surrounded by lymphocytes. (B) The cyst is lined by uniformly thin parakeratotic stratified squamous epithelium. (C) Parts of the cyst lining exhibit marked lymphocyte exocytosis, resulting in a reticulated appearance of the epithelium.

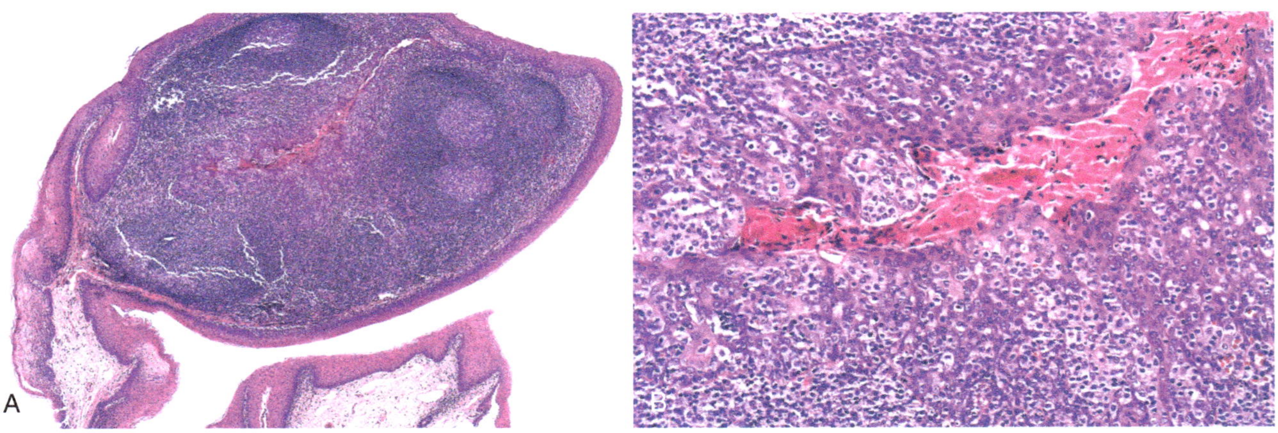

FIG 2.24 Hyperplastic lingual tonsil. (A) The tonsillar crypt is surrounded by lymphoid tissue exhibiting follicular hyperplasia. (B) There is retained parakeratin in the crypt and marked lymphocyte exocytosis within reticulated epithelium.

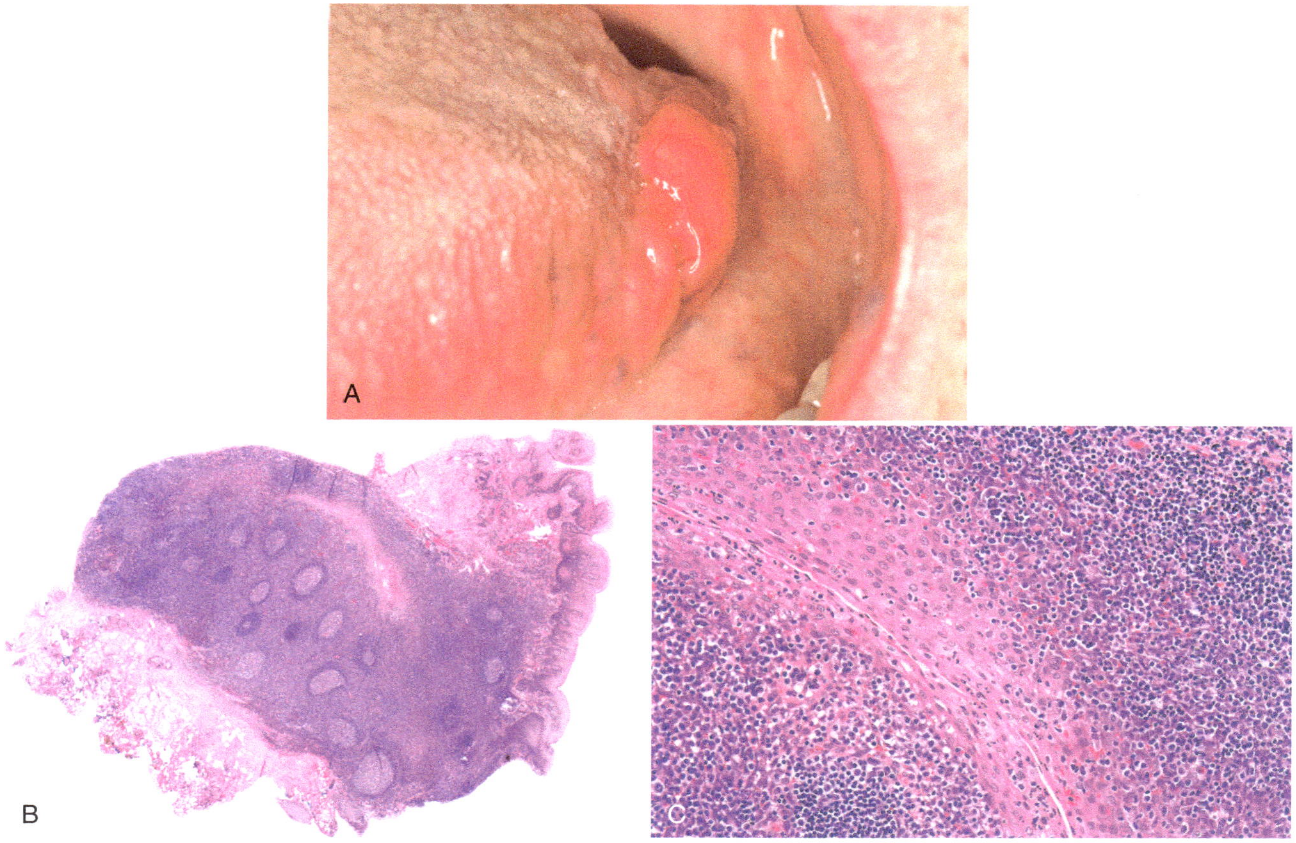

FIG 2.25 Hyperplastic lingual tonsil. (A) Sessile protuberance in the left posterolateral tongue. (B) and (C) Histological images of the lesion shown in (A). (B) Benign follicular hyperplasia of lymphoid tissue surrounds a crypt. (C) The crypt epithelium exhibits prominent leukocyte exocytosis with reticulated epithelium similar to the lining of a lymphoepithelial cyst.

- Salivary duct cysts often exhibit oncocytic metaplasia without a lymphocytic mantle.
- An epithelial inclusion cyst is orthokeratotic and does not exhibit a lymphocytic mantle.

Management and Prognosis

- Excision is curative.

REFERENCES

Buchner A, Hansen LS. Lymphoepithelial cysts of the oral cavity: a clinicopathologic study of thirty-eight cases. *Oral Surg Oral Med Oral Pathol.* 1980;50:441-449.

Chaudhry AP, Yamane GM, Scharlock SE, et al. A clinico-pathological study of intraoral lymphoepithelial cysts. *J Oral Med.* 1984;39: 79-84.

Wu L, Cheng J, Maruyama S, et al. Lymphoepithelial cyst of the parotid gland: its possible histopathogenesis based on clinicopathologic analysis of 64 cases. *Hum Pathol.* 2009;40:683-692.

Yang X, Ow A, Zhang CP, et al. Clinical analysis of 120 cases of intraoral lymphoepithelial cyst. *Oral Surg Oral Med Oral Pathol Oral Radiol.* 2012;113:448-452.

EPIDERMOID (EPITHELIAL INCLUSION), DERMOID, AND TERATOID CYST

Clinical Findings

- These occur mainly in children and young adults and may be congenital. There is a 3:1 male predilection. They appear as dome-shaped, doughy, painless yellow nodules and masses, usually in the midline of the floor of the mouth and often located above the geniohyoid or between the geniohyoid and mylohyoid. Rare cases occur on the buccal mucosa (Fig. 2.26).

Etiopathogenesis and Histopathologic Features

The epithelium arises from displaced epithelium or entrapped epithelial rests during embryonic fusion of the first and second pharyngeal arches. There has been a suggestion to combine the terms *epidermoid*, *dermoid*, and *teratoid cysts* into a single term, *congenital germline fusion cyst.*

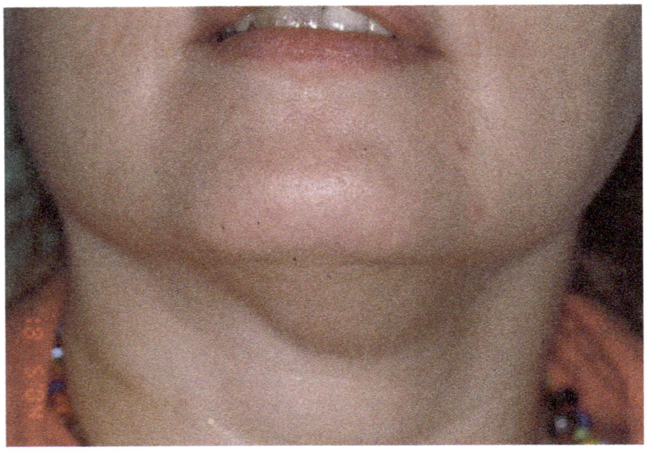

FIG 2.26 Dermoid cyst: soft tissue swelling located beneath the mylohyoid.

- Epidermoid cyst (most common): this is lined by orthokeratinized, stratified squamous epithelium 5–10 cells thick with abundant keratin in the lumen (Fig. 2.27). Rupture results in a foreign body granulomatous reaction. Adnexal structures are not present.
- Dermoid cyst: this is similar to an epidermoid cyst but contains hair follicles, sebaceous glands, or eccrine structures (Fig. 2.28).

Differential Diagnosis

- Some gastrointestinal heterotopias are cystic and lined by epithelium typical of the cardiac, fundic, or pyloric regions of the stomach with parietal and Paneth cells, or of colonic epithelium.
- Salivary duct cyst is a retention cyst of the excretory salivary duct and exhibits squamous, mucous, and ciliated cell metaplasia.

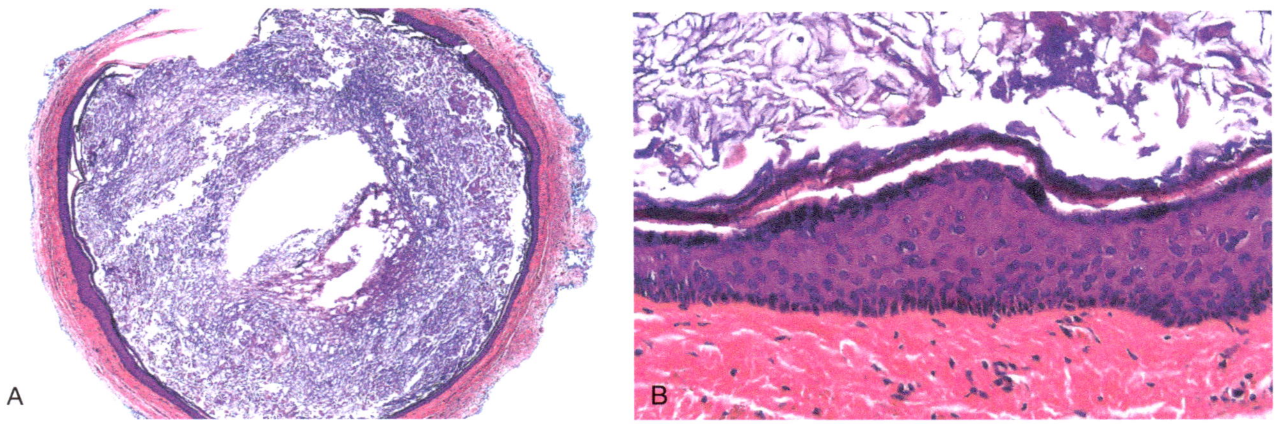

FIG 2.27 Epidermoid cyst. (A) The cyst is lined by uniformly thin stratified squamous epithelium and is filled with keratin. (B) The lining is orthokeratinized stratified squamous epithelium that is uniformly thin with a prominent granular cell layer.

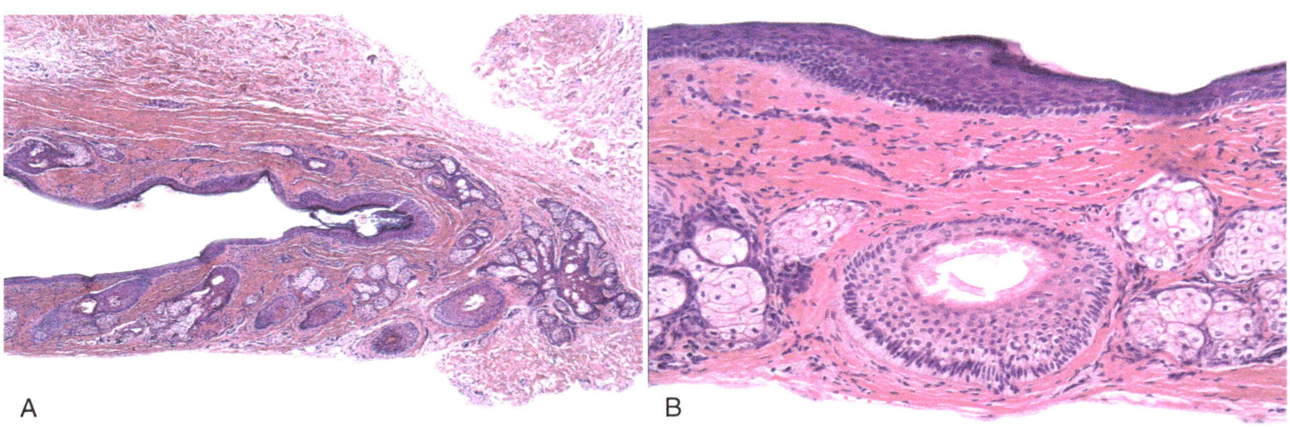

FIG 2.28 Dermoid cyst. (A) The cyst has pilosebaceous units in the wall. (B) The lining is orthokeratinized stratified squamous epithelium that is uniformly thin with a granular layer and pilosebaceous units in the wall.

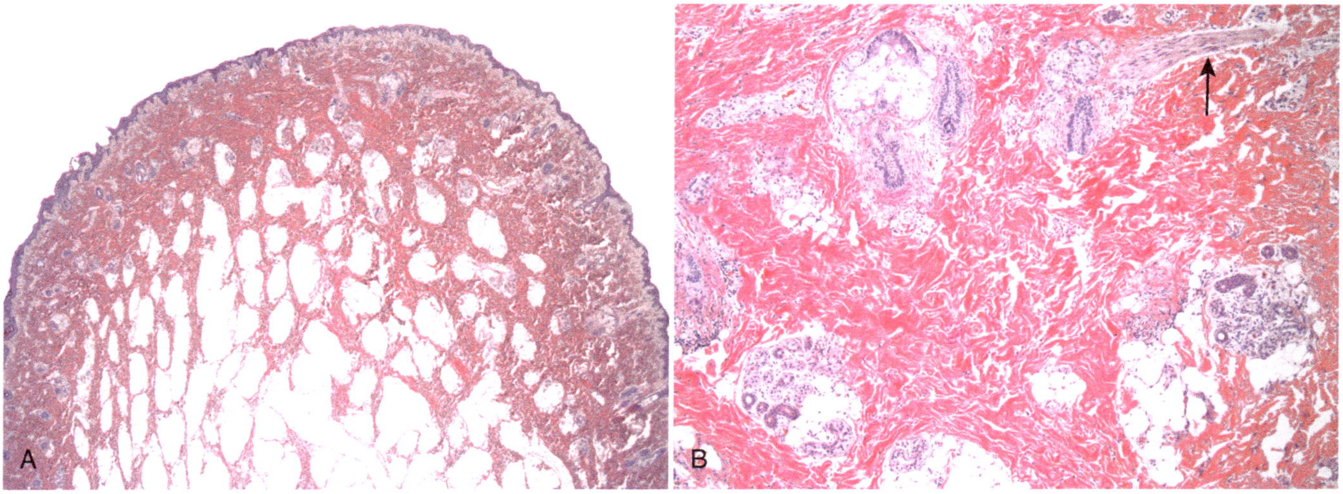

FIG 2.29 Dermoid tumor (hairy polyp). (A) The nodule is covered by epidermis with pilosebaceous units and abundant mature adipose tissue. (B) Pilosebaceous units, eccrine glands, and smooth muscle are present (*arrow*) *(Courtesy Dr. Harry Kozakewich, Harvard Medical School, Boston, Mass.)*

- Keratocystic odontogenic tumors (odontogenic keratocyst) have been reported to occur infrequently within the soft tissues, especially those of the buccal mucosa. These are invariably parakeratinized.
- Dermoid tumor (dermoid or hairy polyp) is a polypoid bigerminal tumor usually located on the soft palate and covered by skin with adnexal structures and a mesodermal component such as fat, cartilage, or muscle (Fig. 2.29). Teratoid tumor (a cystic version exists), teratoma, and epignathus are trigerminal and must also demonstrate ecto-, meso-, and endodermal components in increasing degrees of maturity and duplication of organs, with the most extreme form being *fetus in fetu*.

Management and Prognosis

- Excision is curative.

REFERENCES

Dutta M, Roy S, Ghatak S. Naso-oropharyngeal choristoma (hairy polyps): an overview and current update on presentation, management, origin and related controversies. *Eur Arch Otorhinolaryngol.* 2015;272:1047-1059.

Gordon PE, Faquin WC, Lahey E, Kaban LB. Floor-of-mouth dermoid cysts: report of 3 variants and a suggested change in terminology. *J Oral Maxillofac Surg.* 2013;71:1034-1041.

Kaminagakura E, Almeida JD, Carvalho YR, et al. Keratocyst of the buccal mucosa: case report and immunohistochemical comparative study with sporadic intraosseous keratocystic odontogenic tumor. *Oral Surg Oral Med Oral Pathol Oral Radiol.* 2013;116:e387-e392.

Longo F, Maremonti P, Mangone GM, et al. Midline (dermoid) cysts of the floor of the mouth: report of 16 cases and review of surgical techniques. *Plast Reconstr Surg.* 2003;112:1560-1565.

Maeda Y, Suenaga H, Sugiyama M, et al. Clinical presentation of epignathus teratoma with cleft palate; and duplication of cranial base, tongue, mandible, and pituitary gland. *J Craniofac Surg.* 2013;24:1486-1491.

Pentenero M, Marino R, Familiari U, Gandolfo S. Choristoma involving the floor of the mouth and the anterior tongue: a case of teratoid cyst with gastric and respiratory epithelia. *J Oral Maxillofac Surg.* 2013;71:1706-1711.

PALATAL AND GINGIVAL CYST OF THE NEONATE

Clinical Findings

- These are present in the newborn. They present as yellowish, milia-like, soft papules on the midline of the palatal mucosa, the junction of hard and soft palate, or the gingiva (usually maxillary), with a frequency of 10% to 86%. Palatal cysts are by far the most common (Fig. 2.30).

Etiopathogenesis and Histopathologic Features

Cysts in the midline of the palate (Epstein pearls) and gingiva (original Bohn nodules) are likely epithelial inclusion cysts formed from entrapped embryonic epithelium during fusion of palatal shelves, and from dental lamina rests, respectively. The ones at the junction of the hard and soft palate are likely caused by blocked excretory salivary ducts. It may be more appropriate to refer to these as *palatal* or *gingival cysts* of the neonate.

- These are simple cysts lined by three to five layers of stratified squamous epithelium, often filled with keratin.

Management and Prognosis

- Biopsy is not indicated, because these cysts exteriorize on their own.

REFERENCES

Cizmeci MN, Kanburoglu MK, Kara S, Tatli MM. Bohn's nodules: peculiar neonatal intraoral lesions mistaken for natal teeth. *Eur J Pediatr.* 2014;173:403.

George D, Bhat SS, Hegde SK. Oral findings in newborn children in and around Mangalore, Karnataka State, India. *Med Princ Pract.* 2008;17:385-389.

Paula JD, Dezan CC, Frossard WT, et al. Oral and facial inclusion cysts in newborns. *J Clin Pediatr Dent.* 2007;31:127-129.

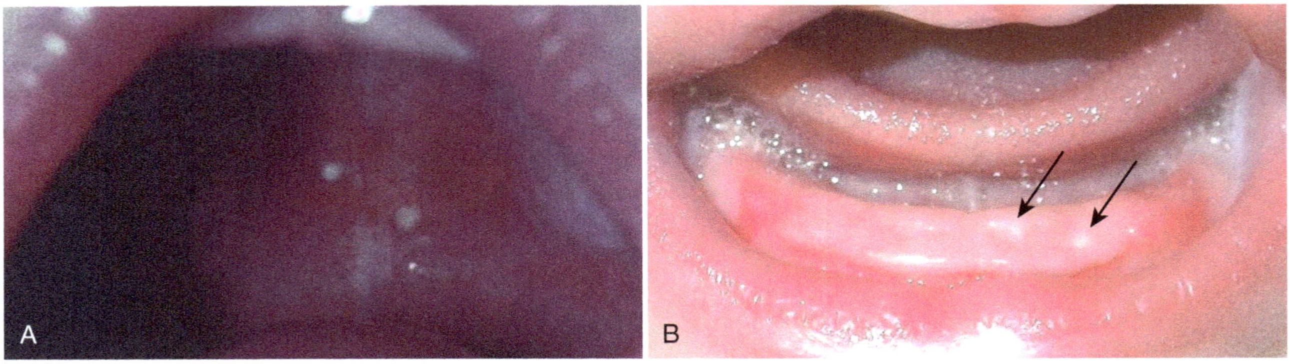

FIG 2.30 (A) Palatal cysts of the newborn: milia-like yellow papules of the palate. (B) Gingival dental lamina cyst of the newborn: cysts of the left mandibular ridge (*arrows*). *(A, Courtesy Dr. Bonnie Padwa, Harvard School of Dental Medicine, Boston, Mass; B, Courtesy Dr. Catherine Flaitz, The University of Texas Dental Branch at Houston, Tex.)*

CYST OF THE INCISIVE PAPILLA

Clinical Findings

- This cyst presents as a swelling, usually less than 1 cm, of the incisive papilla, without underlying bone involvement (Fig. 2.31).

Etiopathogenesis and Histopathologic Features

The epithelium likely derives from rests of the nasopalatine duct within soft tissues.

- This cyst is lined by ciliated, pseudostratified columnar epithelium with mucous cells, flattened low cuboidal epithelium, or two to five layers of nonkeratinized, stratified squamous epithelium. Neurovascular bundles may or may not be present, and there is variable inflammation (Fig. 2.32).

Differential Diagnosis

- Nasopalatine duct cyst has similar histology but is present within bone (see Chapter 16).

Management and Prognosis

- Excision is curative.

REFERENCE

Brown FH, Houston GD, Lubow RM, Sagan MA. Cyst of the incisive (palatine) papilla: report of a case. *J Periodontol.* 1987;58:274-275.

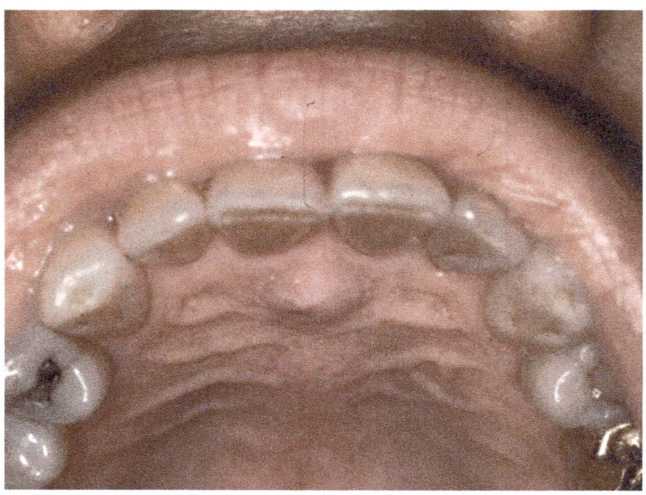

FIG 2.31 Cyst of the incisive papilla: sessile, soft papule on the incisive papilla.

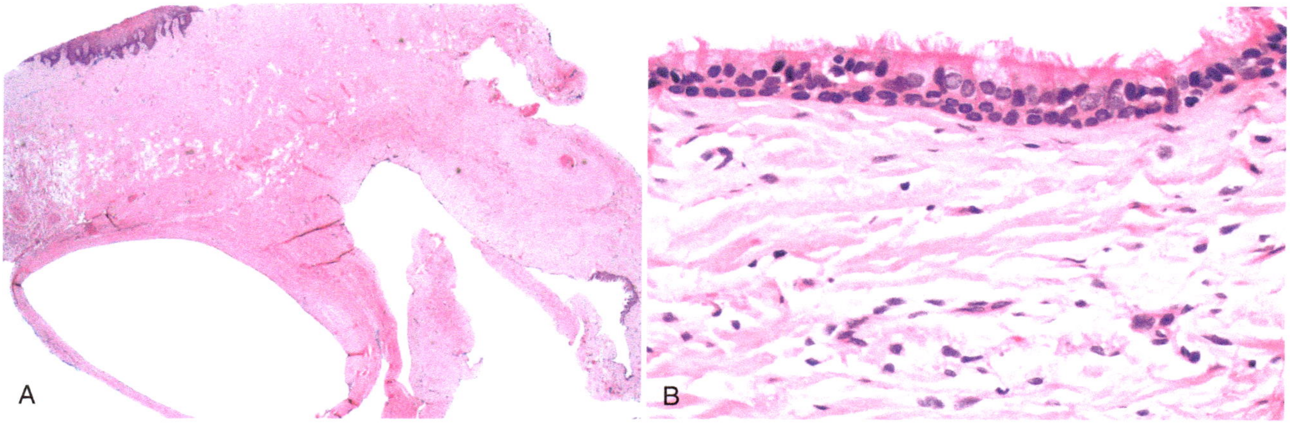

FIG 2.32 Cyst of the incisive papilla. (A) A cyst is present within the deep lamina propria. (B) The cyst is lined by pseudostratified columnar and ciliated epithelium with mucous cells.

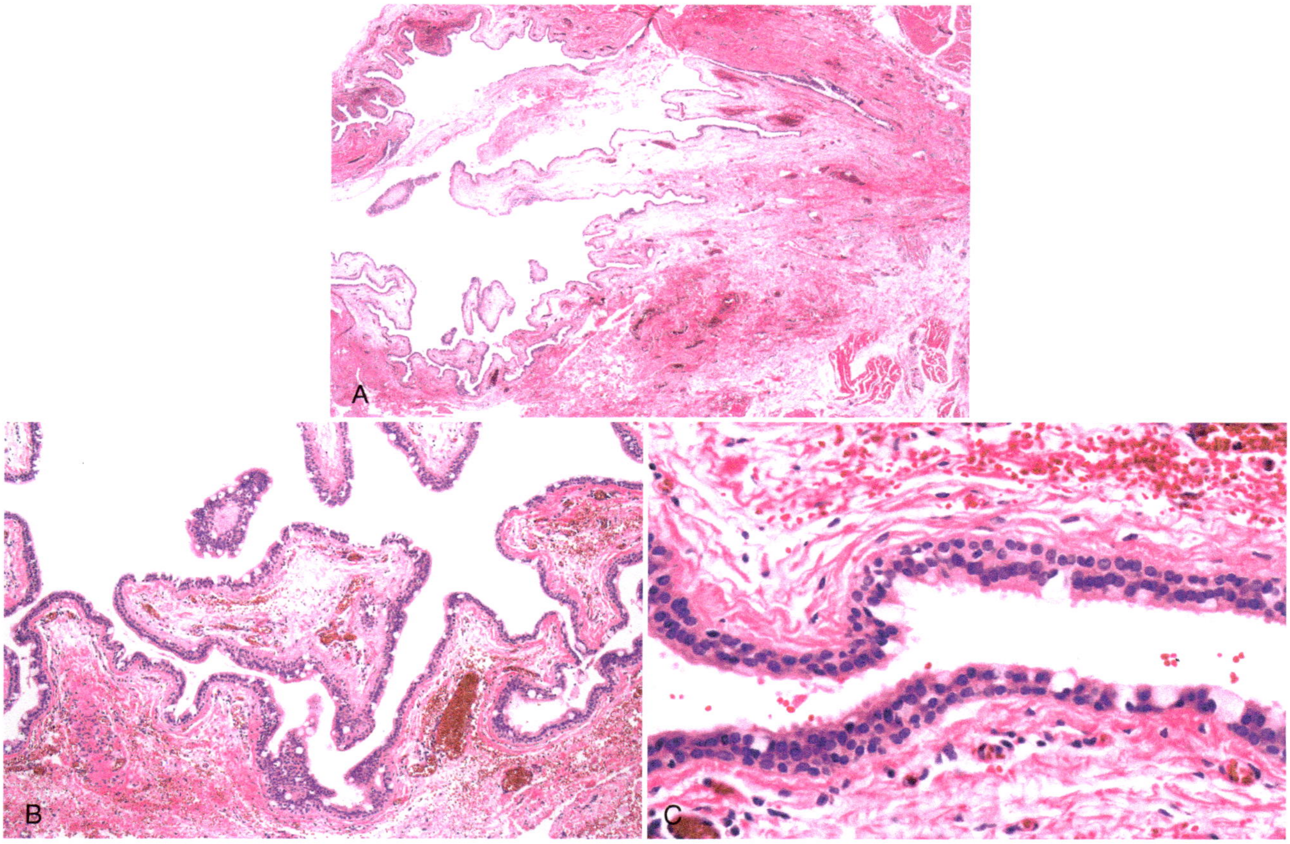

FIG 2.33 Nasolabial cyst. (A) The cyst is lined by uniformly thin epithelium with muscle within the wall. (B) The cyst is lined by uniformly thin epithelium containing mucous cells. (C) Ciliated columnar and cuboidal epithelium with mucous cells present.

NASOLABIAL CYST (NASOALVEOLAR CYST, KLESTADT CYST)

Clinical Findings

- This cyst is usually noted in the fifth decade of life and has a 3 : 1 female predilection. There is a soft, painless, fluctuant swelling of the upper lip (usually on the left side) in the area of the nasolabial fold, often causing effacement of the fold and elevation of the ala of the nose. Up to 10% of cases are bilateral, and the underlying bone is not involved.

Etiopathogenesis and Histopathologic Features

The epithelium of the nasolabial cyst is likely derived from remnants of the nasolacrimal duct.

- The cyst is lined by low, cuboidal, pseudostratified, columnar ciliated epithelium with mucous cells, nonkeratinized stratified squamous epithelium, or a mixture of all three (Fig. 2.33).

Differential Diagnosis

- Epidermoid (epithelial inclusion) cysts of the skin are orthokeratinized with a granular layer.

Management and Prognosis

- Excision is curative.

REFERENCES

Perez AJ, Castle JT. Nasolabial cyst. *Head Neck Pathol.* 2013;7: 155-158.

Sethukumar P, Taghi A, Kuchai R. A rare case of bilateral nasolabial cysts. *BMJ Case Rep.* 2015;2015:bcr2014203543.

Sheikh AB, Chin OY, Fang CH, et al. Nasolabial cysts: a systematic review of 311 cases. *Laryngoscope.* 2016;126:60-66.

Yuen HW, Julian CY, Samuel CL. Nasolabial cysts: clinical features, diagnosis, and treatment. *Br J Oral Maxillofac Surg.* 2007;45: 293-297.

3 NONINFECTIOUS PAPILLARY LESIONS

CHAPTER CONTENTS

INFLAMMATORY PAPILLARY HYPERPLASIA OF THE PALATAL MUCOSA

Clinical Findings

- This occurs in adults wearing maxillary dentures and is occasionally seen in patients with high-arched palates and mouth-breathing habit. Patients may report sensitivity, especially if associated with candidiasis, and the denture may act as a fomite (Fig. 3.1).
- Pebbly excrescences occur on the palatal vault in a diffuse, symmetric distribution.

Etiopathogenesis and Histopathologic Features

Papillary hyperplasia of the palatal mucosa results from chronic irritation due to dentures or from mouth-breathing that leads to reactive hyperplasia of tissues.

- Proliferation of fibrovascular tissue occurs in nodules with a variable lymphoplasmacytic infiltrate. The overlying epithelium may be hyperplastic and exhibit spongiosis and leukocyte exocytosis. Pseudoepitheliomatous hyperplasia may be seen (Figs. 3.2–3.4).
- The presence of spongiotic pustules should always raise suspicion for candidiasis and periodic acid–Schiff staining with diastase should be performed.

Differential Diagnosis

- Inflamed squamous papilloma is usually solitary and pedunculated.
- Human papillomavirus–associated papillary lesions or condylomas contain koilocytes (see Chapter 4).

Management and Prognosis

- Excision or laser ablation of lesions must be accompanied by a denture reline or fabrication of new dentures. Lesions may recur if the denture continues to fit poorly.
- If present, candidiasis can be effectively treated with topical antifungals (eg, antifungal and steroid cream applied to the denture base [see Appendix B]). The dentures should also be disinfected with chlorhexidine, nystatin, sodium benzoate, or other effective disinfectant.

REFERENCES

Canger EM, Celenk P, Kayipmaz S. Denture-related hyperplasia: a clinical study of a Turkish population group. *Braz Dent J.* 2009;20:243-248.

Kaplan I, Vered M, Moskona D, et al. An immunohistochemical study of p53 and PCNA in inflammatory papillary hyperplasia of the palate: a dilemma of interpretation. *Oral Dis.* 1998;4:194-199.

Poulopoulos A, Belazi M, Epivatianos A, et al. The role of *Candida* in inflammatory papillary hyperplasia of the palate. *J Oral Rehabil.* 2007;34:685-692.

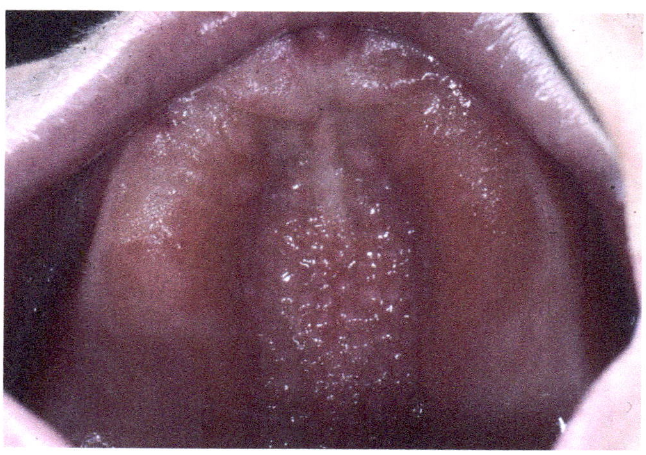

FIG 3.1 Inflammatory papillary hyperplasia of the palatal mucosa. *(Courtesy Dr. Sadru Kabani, Boston, Mass.)*

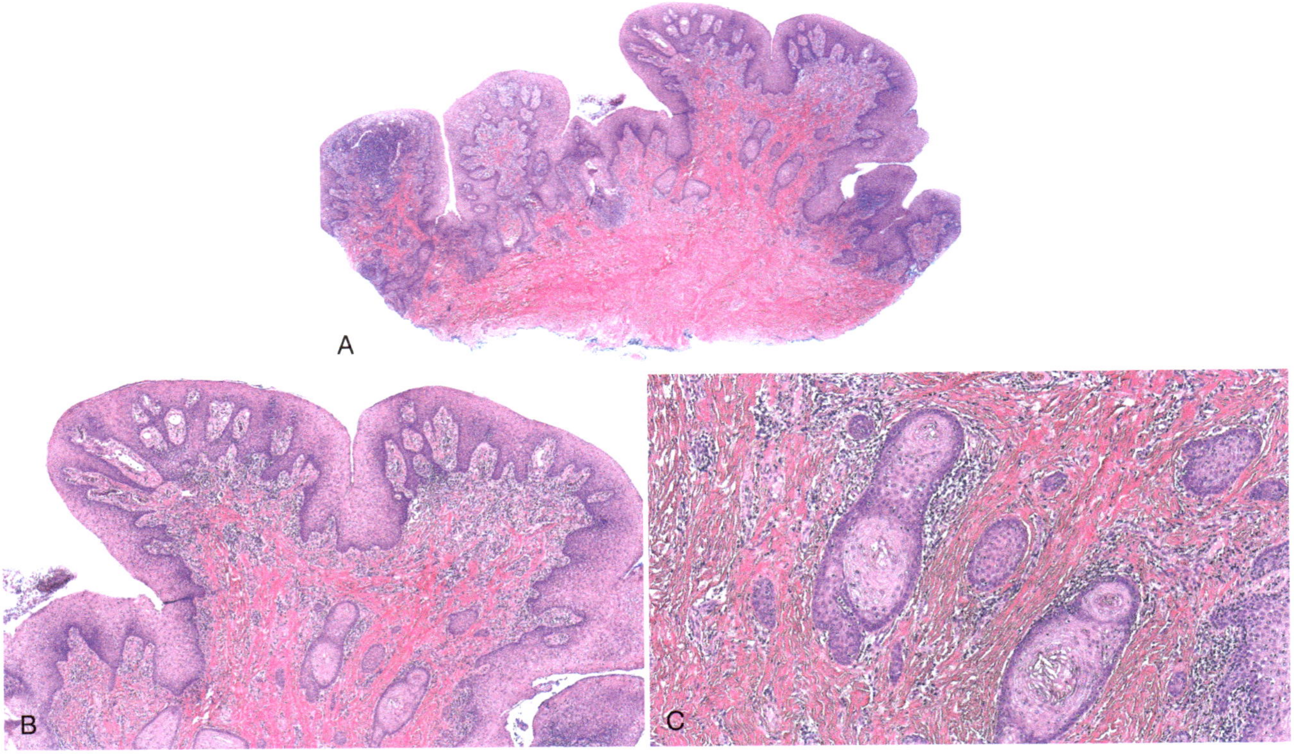

FIG 3.2 Inflammatory papillary hyperplasia of the palatal mucosa. (A) Papillary proliferation of fibrous tissue and epithelium. (B) Fibroepithelial and pseudoepitheliomatous hyperplasia with chronic inflammation. (C) Islands of benign epithelial cells.

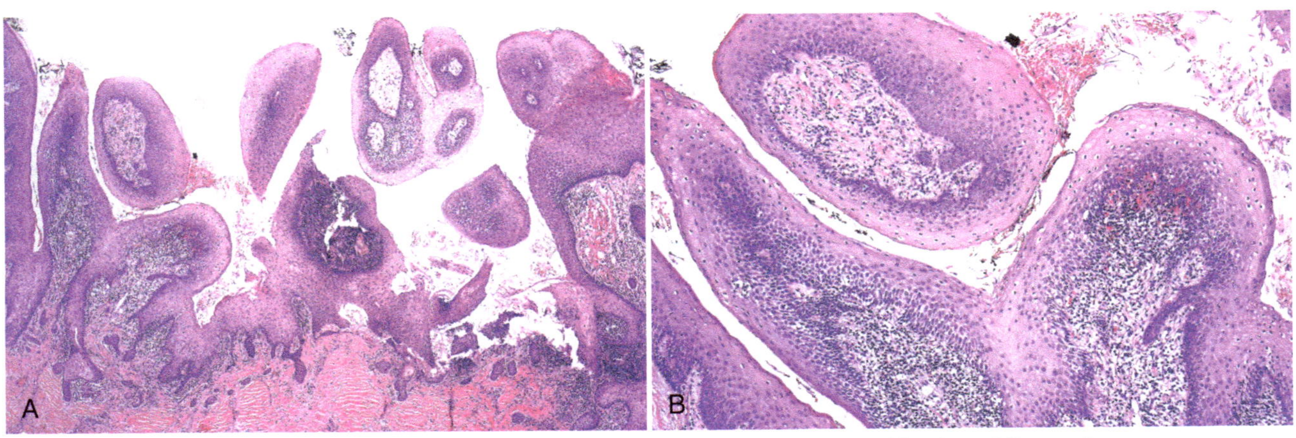

FIG 3.3 Inflammatory papillary hyperplasia of the palate. (A) Papillary proliferation of fibrous tissue and epithelium. (B) Papillary structures, spongiosis, and chronic inflammation.

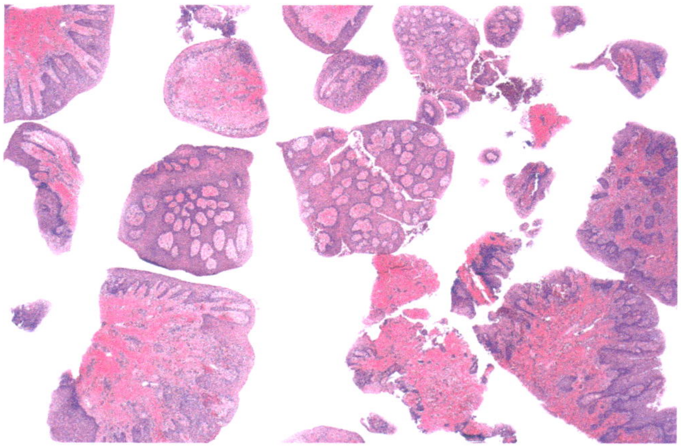

FIG 3.4 Inflammatory papillary hyperplasia composed of a benign papillary proliferation of fibrous tissue and epithelium with chronic inflammation (curetted specimen).

VERRUCIFORM XANTHOMA

Clinical Findings

- This occurs most frequently in the fifth and sixth decades of life with equal gender predilection. It occurs as a discrete, nontender, yellowish, or mucosa-colored plaque with a pebbly, warty appearance, although some are flat. Seventy-five percent are located on the keratinized tissues of the gingiva and hard palatal mucosa, with the tongue and buccal mucosa being the next most common sites (Fig. 3.5).
- This may be seen in areas of mucosa or skin exhibiting damage to the epithelium, such as from trauma, and inflammatory conditions such as lichen planus, pemphigus vulgaris, epidermolysis bullosa, and chronic graft-versus-host disease. It is less commonly associated with carcinoma in situ, invasive carcinoma, chronic lymphedema, and congenital epidermal nevi.

Etiopathogenesis and Histopathologic Features

Verruciform xanthoma is a reactive lesion believed to be a histiocytic response to products of epithelial breakdown, although some believe that it is accumulation of lipid-laden macrophages that induces the epithelial proliferation. Resident and reparative macrophages are involved. A subset of cutaneous cases shows mutation of the 3β-hydroxysteroid dehydrogenase gene, which is important in cholesterol biosynthesis.

- There is a benign papillary proliferation of stratified squamous epithelium with elongated rete ridges, generally of the same length and confluent at the tips (Figs. 3.6A and 3.7A). Infrequently, lesions have a flat surface (Fig. 3.8A).
- There is parakeratosis with a brightly eosinophilic hue, parakeratin plugs, and keratin squames on the surface and within crypts. Neutrophilic exocytosis and spongiosis are often present. Foamy macrophages (positive for CD68, CD163, and NKIC3; negative for S100) fill the lamina propria (Fig. 3.9; see Figs. 3.6–3.8). When inflamed, there may be minimal parakeratosis (Fig. 3.10).

Differential Diagnosis

- Verrucous hyperplasia (a dysplastic lesion) exhibits hyperkeratosis or parakeratosis and variable cytologic atypia without foamy macrophages.
- Granulomatous lichen planus exhibits a band of lymphocytes and histiocytes at the interface with squamatized basal cells without papillomatosis (see Chapter 8).

Management and Prognosis

- Excision is the treatment of choice. Lesion tends not to recur even if incompletely excised.

REFERENCES

Blankenship DW, Zech L, Mirzabeigi M, Venna S. Verruciform xanthoma of the upper-extremity in the absence of chronic skin disease or syndrome: a case report and review of the literature. *J Cutan Pathol.* 2013;40:745-752.

de Andrade BA, Agostini M, Pires FR, et al. Oral verruciform xanthoma: a clinicopathologic and immunohistochemical study of 20 cases. *J Cutan Pathol.* 2015;42:489-495.

Ide F, Obara K, Yamada H, et al. Cellular basis of verruciform xanthoma: immunohistochemical and ultrastructural characterization. *Oral Dis.* 2008;14:150-157.

Mehra S, Li L, Fan CY, et al. A novel somatic mutation of the 3β-hydroxysteroid dehydrogenase gene in sporadic cutaneous verruciform xanthoma. *Arch Dermatol.* 2005;141:1263-1267.

Mohsin SK, Lee MW, Amin MB, et al. Cutaneous verruciform xanthoma: a report of five cases investigating the etiology and nature of xanthomatous cells. *Am J Surg Pathol.* 1998;22:479-487.

Philipsen HP, Reichart PA, Takata T, Ogawa I. Verruciform xanthoma—biological profile of 282 oral lesions based on a literature survey with nine new cases from Japan. *Oral Oncol.* 2003;39:325-336.

Rawal SY, Kalmar JR, Tatakis DN. Verruciform xanthoma: immunohistochemical characterization of xanthoma cell phenotypes. *J Periodontol.* 2007;78:504-509.

Shahrabi Farahani S, Treister NS, Khan Z, Woo SB. Oral verruciform xanthoma associated with chronic graft-versus-host disease: a report of five cases and a review of the literature. *Head Neck Pathol.* 2011;5:193-198.

Zegarelli DJ, Aegarelli-Schmidt EC, Zegarelli EV. Verruciform xanthoma: a clinical, light microscopic, and electron microscopic study of two cases. *Oral Surg Oral Med Oral Pathol.* 1974;38:725-734.

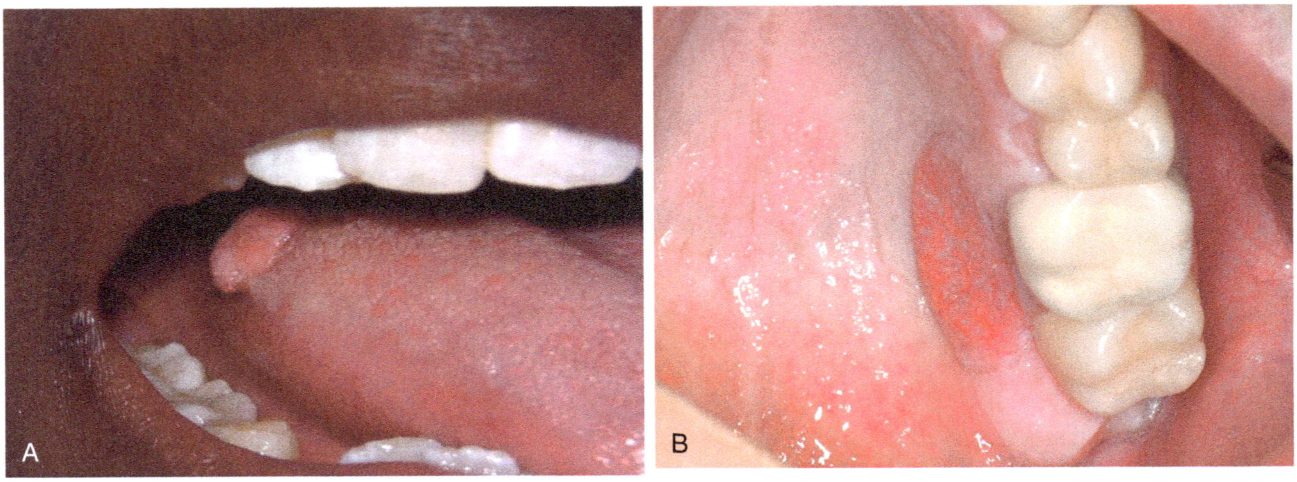

FIG 3.5 Verruciform xanthoma. (A) Papillary nodule of the right lateral tongue. *(Reprinted from Shahrabi Farahani S, Treister NS, Khan Z, Woo SB. Oral verruciform xanthoma associated with chronic graft-versus-host disease: a report of five cases and a review of the literature. Head Neck Pathol. 2011;5:193–198.)* (B) Papillary plaque of the left hard palatal mucosa. *(Courtesy Dr. John Wright, Baylor College of Dentistry, Dallas, Tex.)*

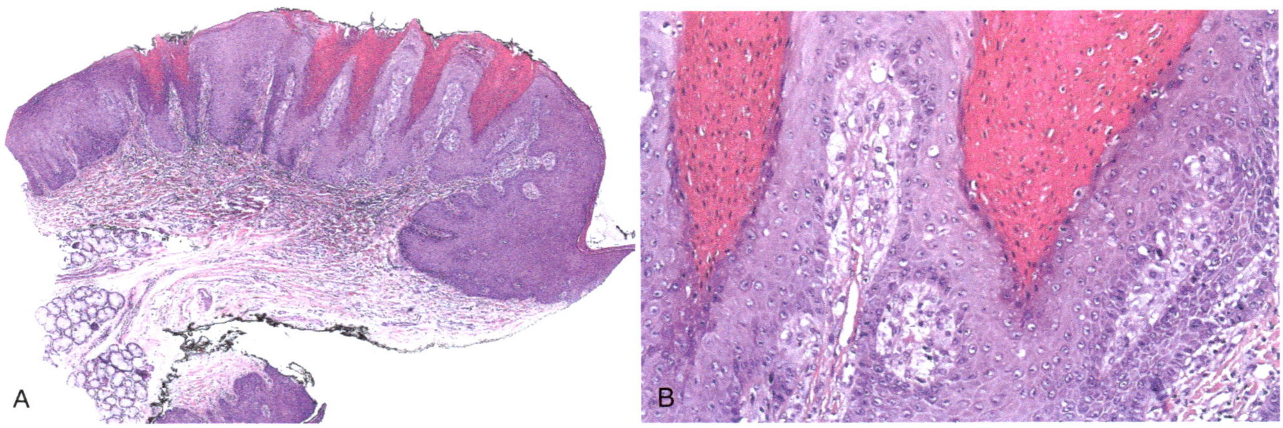

FIG 3.6 Verruciform xanthoma. (A) Brightly eosinophilic keratin, parakeratin plugs, and papillary acanthosis. (B) Compact parakeratosis and foamy macrophages in the lamina propria.

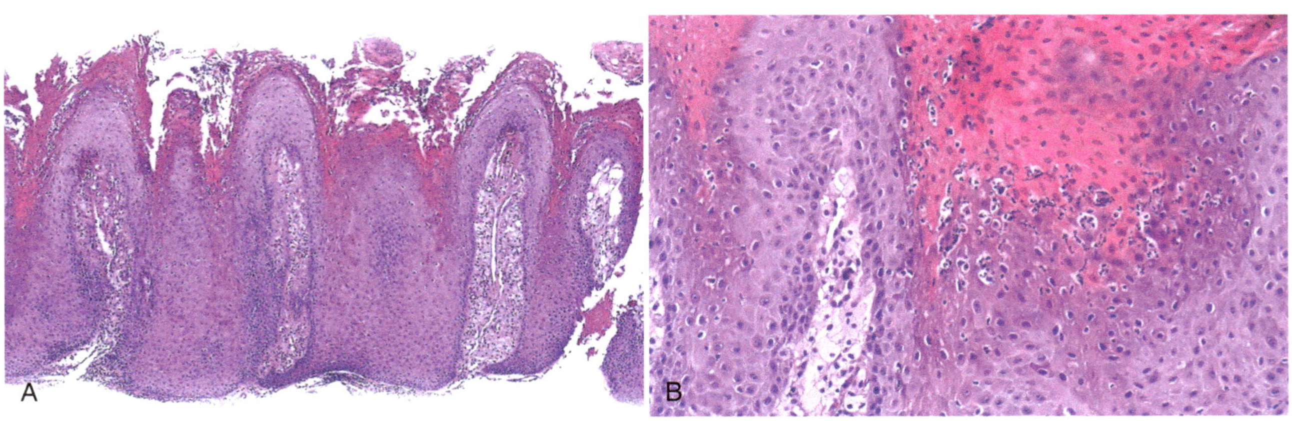

FIG 3.7 Verruciform xanthoma. (A) Parakeratosis, papillary epithelial hyperplasia, keratin squames, and rete ridges of equal length. (B) Parakeratosis, spongiotic pustules, and foamy macrophages within the lamina propria.

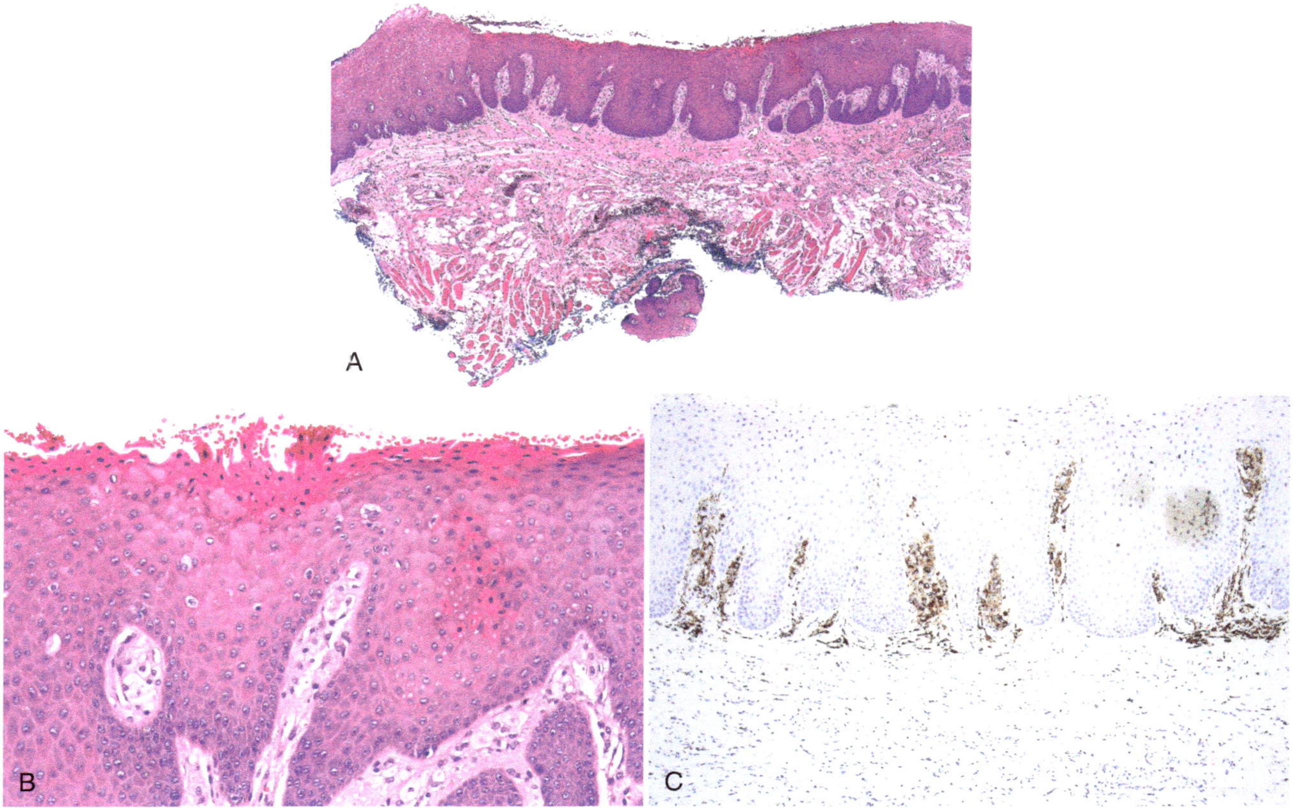

FIG 3.8 Verruciform xanthoma. (A) Parakeratosis and acanthosis without papillomatosis. (B) Parakeratosis and foamy macrophages. (C) CD68+ macrophages in the papillary lamina propria.

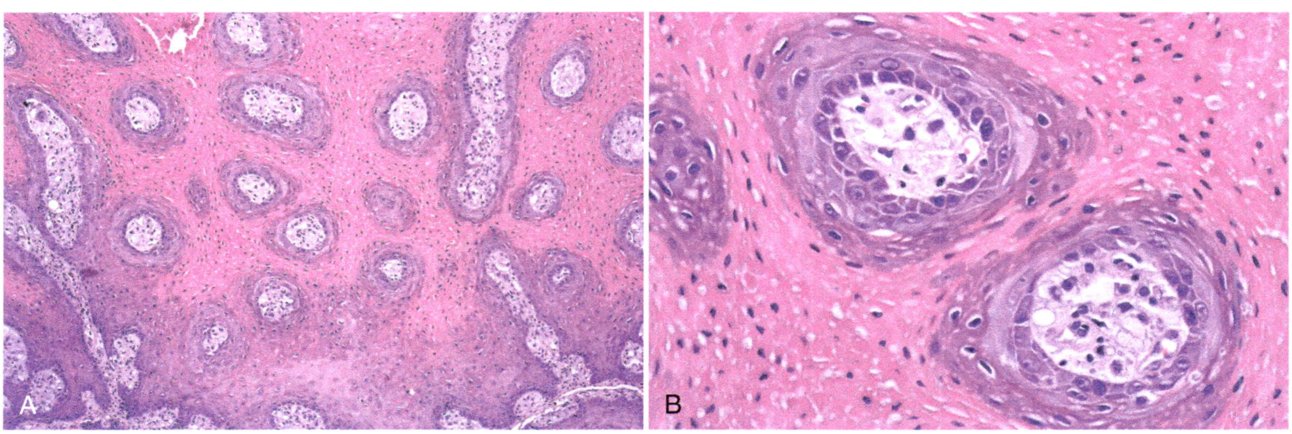

FIG 3.9 Verruciform xanthoma. (A) Sectioned tangentially (ie, *en face*) with brightly eosinophilic parakeratin. (B) Xanthoma cells in the lamina propria.

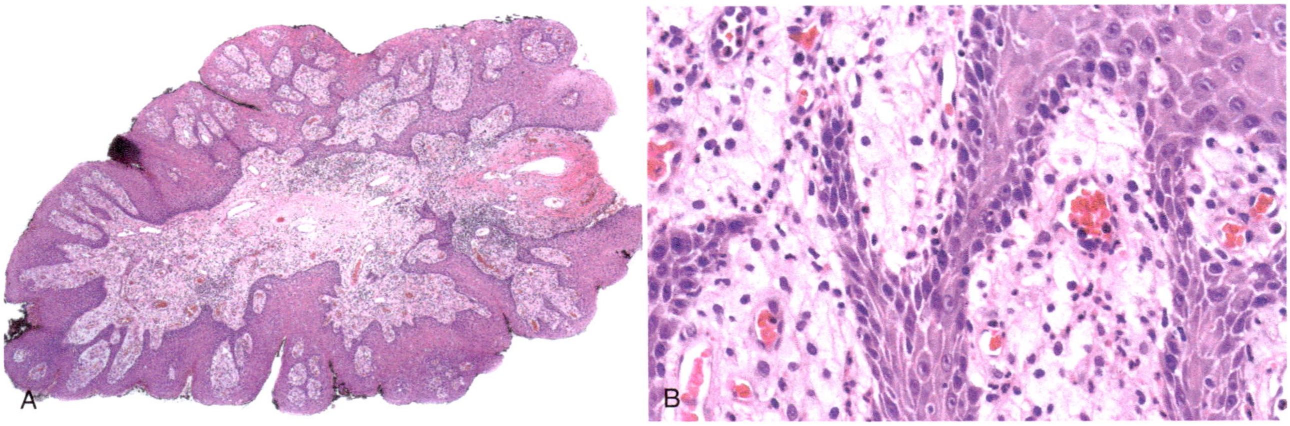

FIG 3.10 Verruciform xanthoma. (A) Papillary epithelial hyperplasia with minimal parakeratosis and chronic inflammation. (B) Foamy macrophages and inflammatory cells.

LOCALIZED JUVENILE SPONGIOTIC GINGIVAL HYPERPLASIA

Clinical Findings

- More than 90% occur between 5 and 15 years of age, and there is a 2:1 male predominance. They occur mostly on the maxillary anterior facial gingiva (84%), and 15% of patients have orthodontic hardware on the teeth.
- There is an erythematous, often pebbly, nontender plaque measuring less than 1 cm on the marginal gingiva, and the condition may be multifocal (Fig. 3.11).

Etiopathogenesis and Histopathologic Features

Localized juvenile spongiotic gingival hyperplasia is a reactive lesion likely related to trauma and local irritation. It is unclear if the epithelial proliferation originates from the crevicular or junctional epithelium.

- There is a pedunculated or sessile benign papillary (may be subtle) proliferation of nonkeratinized stratified squamous epithelium exhibiting prominent spongiosis and leukocyte exocytosis, with many dilated, congested vessels and many plasma cells (Fig. 3.12).
- The epithelium is positive for CK19, and p16INK4A positivity may be noted. Human papillomavirus has not been consistently identified.

Differential Diagnosis

- Some lesions may represent an inflamed squamous papilloma. The gingiva is a common location for this, and the age group is also supportive (Fig. 3.13).

Management and Prognosis

- Excision is the treatment of choice, and the lesion recurs in approximately 10% of cases.

REFERENCES

Argyris PP, Nelson AC, Papanakou S, et al. Localized juvenile spongiotic gingival hyperplasia featuring unusual p16INK4A labeling and negative human papillomavirus status by polymerase chain reaction. *J Oral Pathol Med.* 2015;44:37-44.

Chang JY, Kessler HP, Wright JM. Localized juvenile spongiotic gingival hyperplasia. *Oral Surg Oral Med Oral Pathol Oral Radiol Endod.* 2008;106:411-418.

Darling MR, Daley TD, Wilson A, Wysocki GP. Juvenile spongiotic gingivitis. *J Periodontol.* 2007;78:1235-1240.

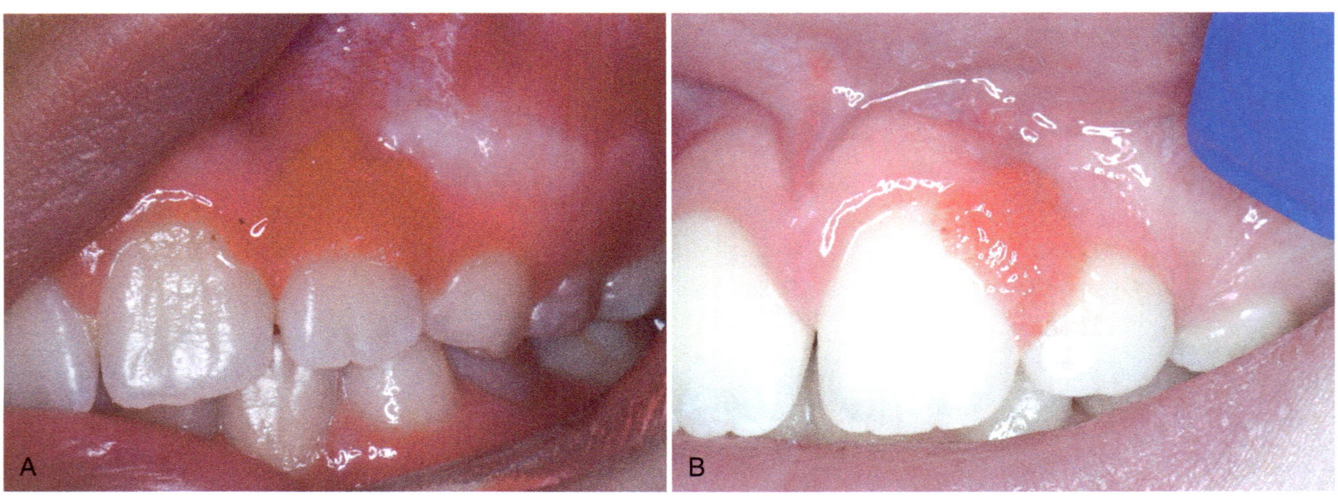

FIG 3.11 Juvenile localized spongiotic gingival hyperplasia (A). Pebbly erythematous plaque of the facial gingiva (B). *(A, Courtesy Dr. Jeffrey Stone, private practice, Lowell, Mass; B, Courtesy Dr. Andrew Abela, private practice, Winchester, Mass.)*

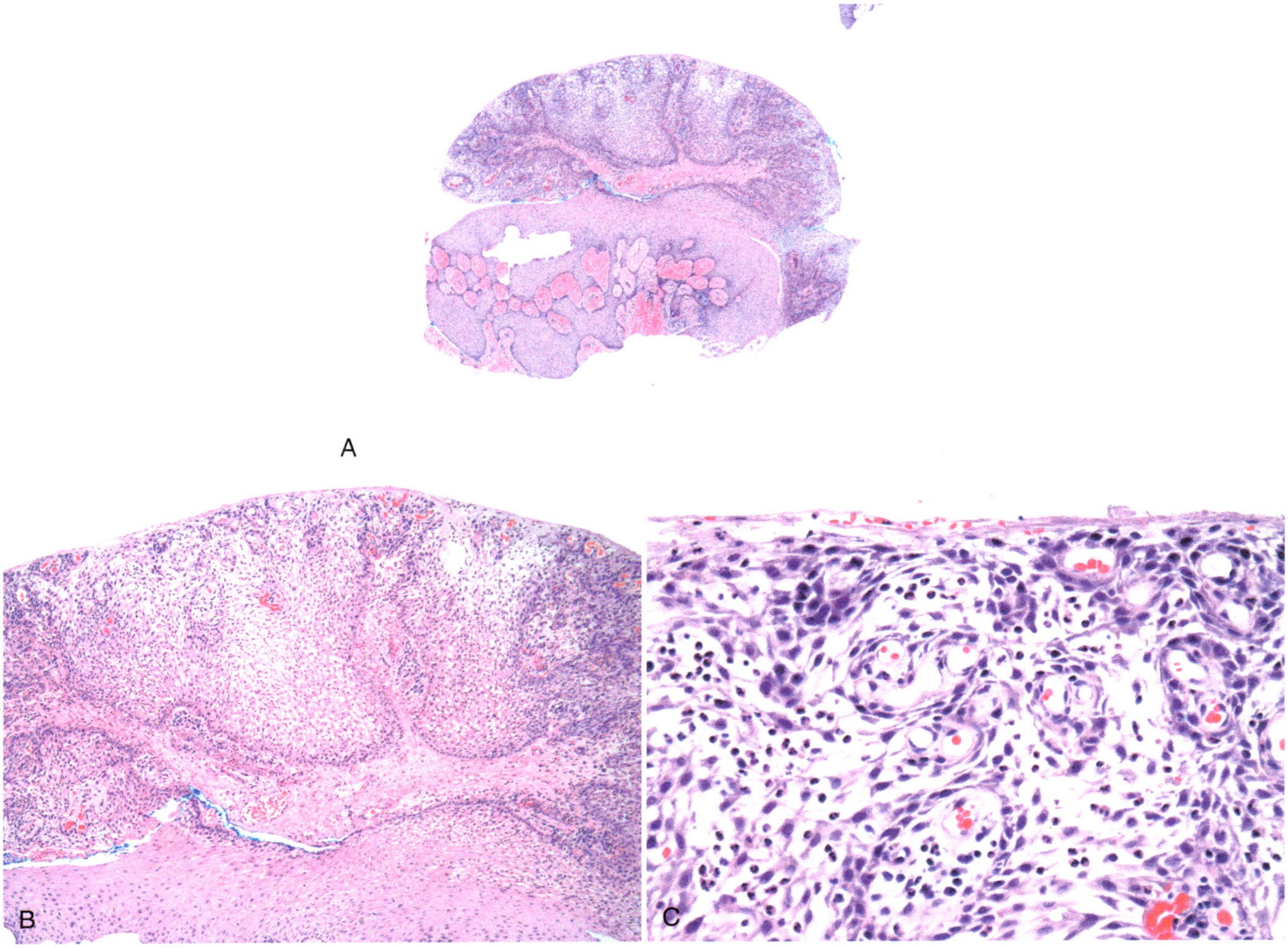

FIG 3.12 Juvenile localized spongiotic gingival hyperplasia. (A) Proliferation of nonkeratinized stratified squamous epithelium on a peduncle. (B) Marked spongiosis and leukocyte exocytosis. (C) Marked spongiosis, leukocyte exocytosis, and superficial congested capillaries.

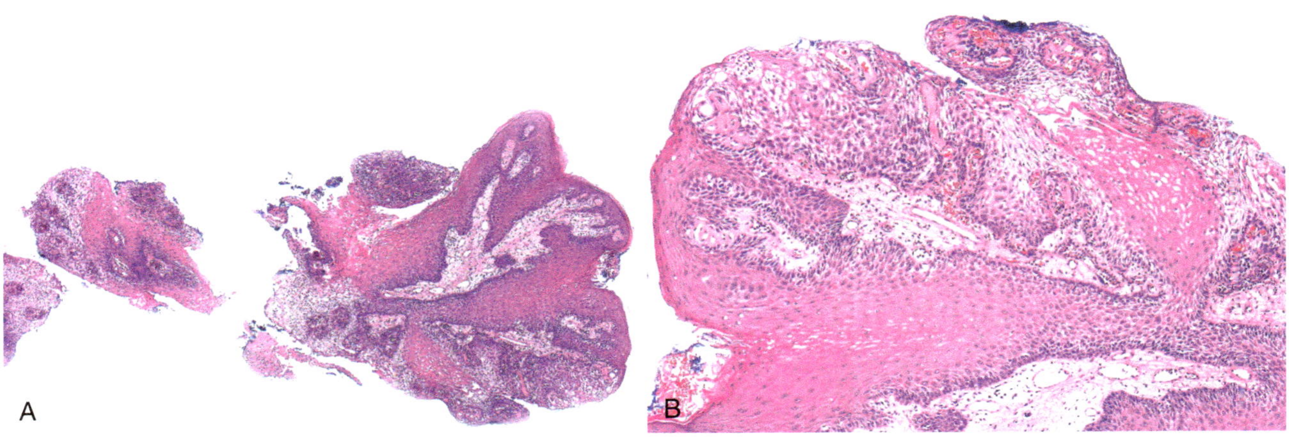

FIG 3.13 (A) Papilloma associated with juvenile localized spongiotic gingival hyperplasia. (B) Transition between intact noninflamed papilloma and spongiotic lesion.

4 BACTERIAL, VIRAL, FUNGAL, AND OTHER INFECTIOUS CONDITIONS

CHAPTER CONTENTS

Besides the common bacterial, fungal, and viral infections of the oral cavity, an infection that occurs in any part of the body may manifest in the mouth, including mycobacterial, treponemal, and protozoal infections, although they are uncommon and rarely occur *initially* in the mouth. In many parts of the world, syphilitic and protozoal infections are on the rise. Polymicrobial bacterial infections in the mouth are common and are generally not subject to biopsy, because most of these are related to dental caries and periodontal infections. Actinomycosis is one bacterial infection that is seen on biopsy with some frequency.

ACTINOMYCOSIS

In the medical literature, the five common sites for actinomycosis are cervicofacial, pulmonary, ileocecal, genitourinary, and central nervous system. The least well-recognized, and yet fairly common, infection involving the jawbones and oral soft tissues is discussed here.

Clinical Findings

- This occurs in adults in the fifth and sixth decades of life, and patients are infrequently immunocompromised.
- The most common manifestation is a periapical radiolucency, painless (80% of cases) or painful, in a root canal–treated or grossly carious tooth (Fig. 4.1A). It may also be associated with impacted teeth, periodontitis around natural teeth, or periimplantitis around dental implants. Approximately 20% of cases involve the soft tissues only, and mandibular tooth infection may lead to cutaneous fistulae and cervicofacial actinomycosis (see Fig. 4.1B).
- A sinus tract (gingival parulis) and suppuration are almost always present, and yellowish "sulfur granules" or "grains" representing masses of bacteria may be noted during the curettage (Fig. 4.2).
- The presence of actinomycetes colonies within tonsillar crypts may predispose patients to obstructive tonsillar hypertrophy; this is not considered a form of actinomycosis.

Etiopathogenesis and Histopathologic Features

Actinomyces are gram-positive microaerophilic, obligate, or facultative filamentous bacteria. There are several species, such as *Actinomyces israelii* (most common in infections), *A. odontolyticus, A. naeslundii, A. gerencseriae,* and *A. viscosus.* They cause suppurative lesions and enter the bone through a carious tooth or through periodontal pockets.

- Abundant granulation tissue is present with abscesses and acute and chronic inflammation.
- "Sulfur granules" are composed of round-to-ovoid masses of filamentous bacteria with a peripheral eosinophilic rim, often with eosinophilic radiating "clubs" (Splendore-Hoeppli phenomenon) surrounded by neutrophils (Fig. 4.3A–B). Bacteria are gram-positive, gram-variable (variable gram-positive staining along the filament), and argyrophilic (see Fig. 4.3C–D).
- Concomitant radicular cyst, periapical granuloma, dentigerous cyst, or other pathosis is usually present.
- Clumps of actinomycetes alone without the eosinophilic fringe (representing the host response) are not sufficient for the diagnosis.

Differential Diagnosis

- Actinomycotic colonies (without the eosinophilic border) are a common component of dental plaque

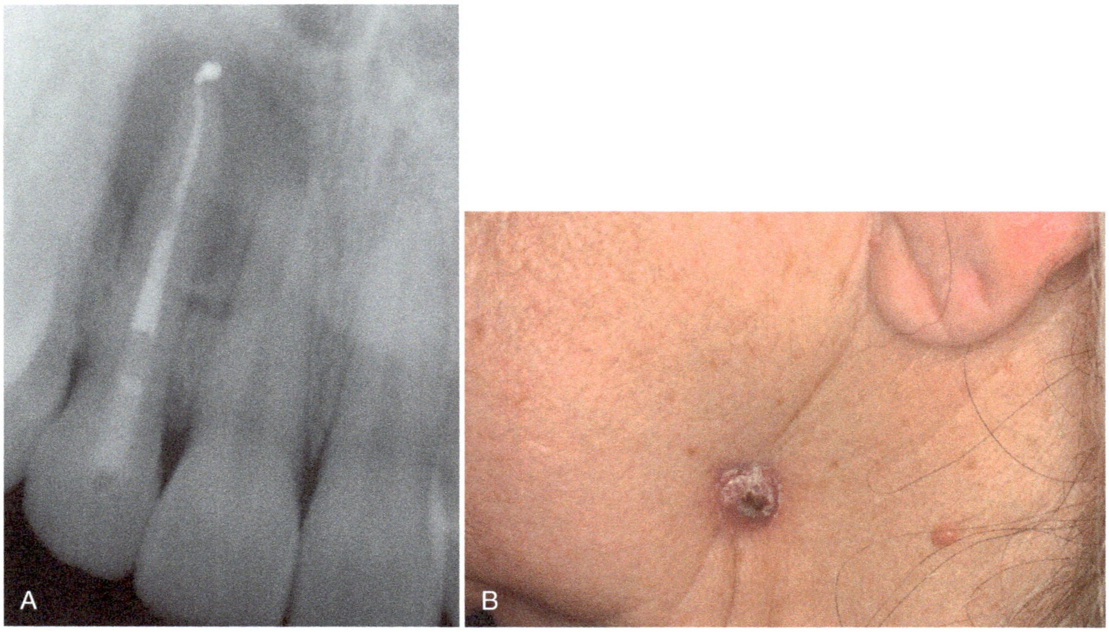

FIG 4.1 (A) Periapical actinomycosis manifesting within an apical radicular cyst after root canal therapy. (B) Actinomycosis from a carious mandibular molar resulting in cutaneous sinus tract. *(A, Courtesy Dr. Michael Joseph, private practice, Worcester, Mass.)*

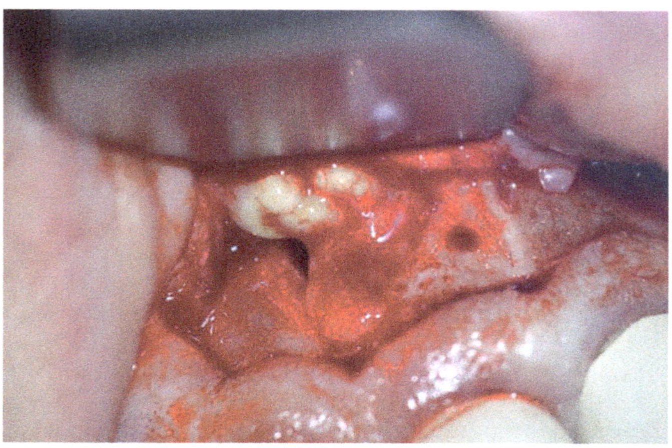

FIG 4.2 Periapical actinomycosis with yellow sulfur granules. *(Courtesy Dr. Christopher Allen, private practice, Traverse City, Mich.)*

that often contaminates oral biopsy specimens and do not represent actinomycosis in the absence of suppuration and clinical signs.

- Masses of actinomycotic organisms are often found on the surface of exposed bony sequestra, such as in osteoradionecrosis or medication-related osteonecrosis of the jaws. This phenomenon represents surface colonization only (biofilm) (see Chapter 17).

Management and Prognosis

- Curettage, 2 to 3 weeks of antibiotics (eg, amoxicillin, doxycycline, or clindamycin), and removal of the original source of infection (eg, carious or impacted tooth) is curative. Prolonged antibiotic therapy is not indicated for conventional periapical actinomycosis.

REFERENCES

Brook I. Actinomycosis: diagnosis and management. *South Med J.* 2008;101:1019-1023.

Kaplan I, Anavi K, Anavi Y, et al. The clinical spectrum of *Actinomyces*-associated lesions of the oral mucosa and jawbones: correlations with histomorphometric analysis. *Oral Surg Oral Med Oral Pathol Oral Radiol Endod.* 2009;108:738-746.

Kutluhan A, Salvız M, Yalçıner G, et al. The role of the *Actinomyces* in obstructive tonsillar hypertrophy and recurrent tonsillitis in pediatric population. *Int J Pediatr Otorhinolaryngol.* 2011;75:391-394.

Kuyama K, Fukui K, Ochiai E, et al. Identification of the actinomycete 16S ribosomal RNA gene by polymerase chain reaction in oral inflammatory lesions. *Oral Surg Oral Med Oral Pathol Oral Radiol.* 2013;116:485-491.

LeCorn DW, Vertucci FJ, Rojas MF, et al. In vitro activity of amoxicillin, clindamycin, doxycycline, metronidazole, and moxifloxacin against oral *Actinomyces. J Endod.* 2007;33:557-560.

Lo Muzio L, Favia G, Lacaita M, et al. The contribution of histopathological examination to the diagnosis of cervico-facial actinomycosis: a retrospective analysis of 68 cases. *Eur J Clin Microbiol Infect Dis.* 2014;33:1915-1918.

Tang G, Samaranayake LP, Yip HK, et al. Direct detection of *Actinomyces* spp. from infected root canals in a Chinese population: a study using PCR-based, oligonucleotide-DNA hybridization technique. *J Dent.* 2003;31:559-568.

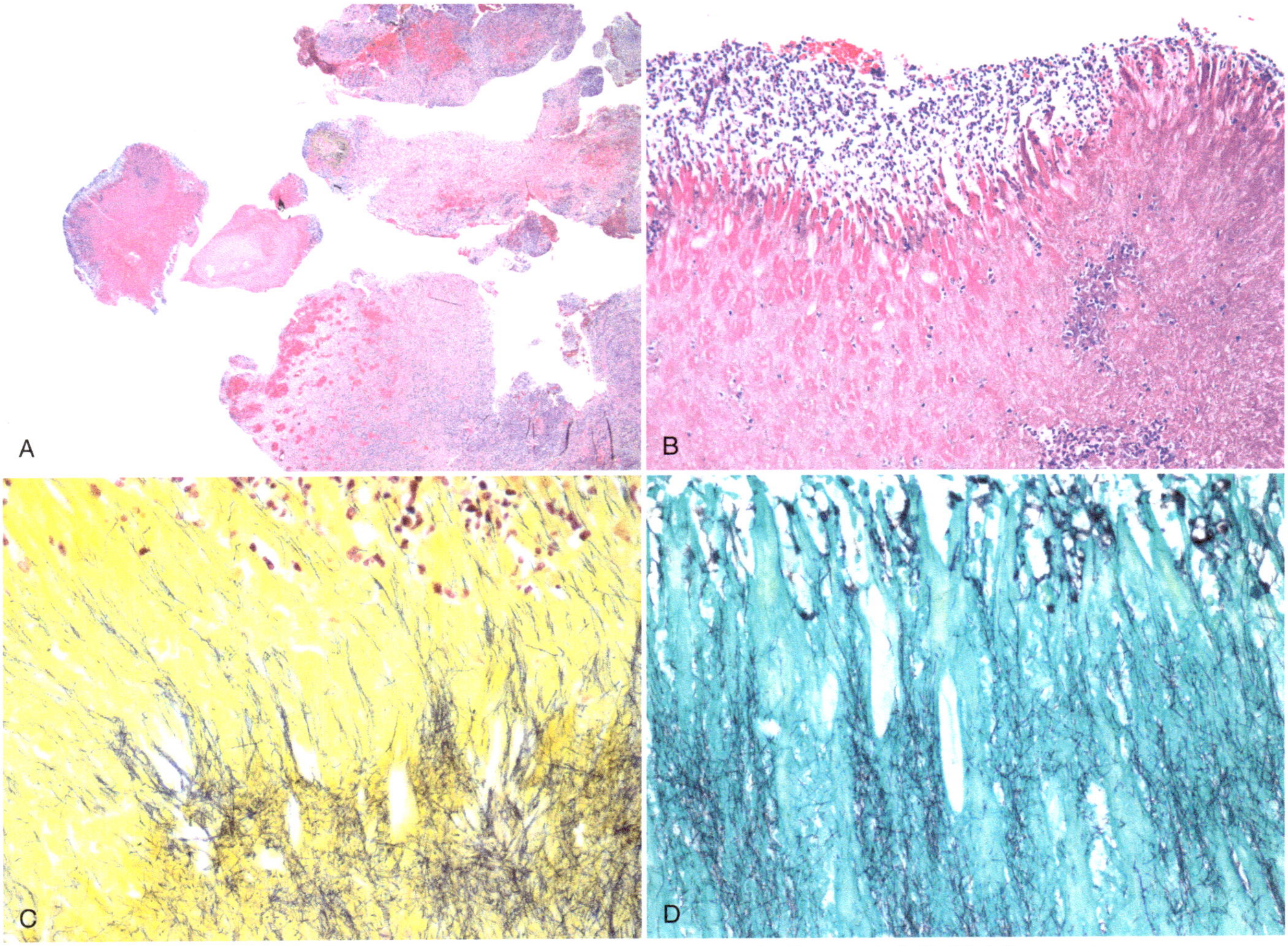

FIG 4.3 Periapical actinomycosis. (A) Periapical granuloma and sulfur granule (*left*). (B) Sulfur granule with typical radiating morphology (Splendore-Hoeppli phenomenon) and suppuration. (C) Sulfur granule showing inconsistent Gram staining along the filament (Gram variability) (Brown and Brenn stain). (D) Sulfur granule containing slender argyrophilic filaments (methenamine silver stain).

HERPESVIRUS INFECTIONS

Table 4.1 shows the eight herpesviruses that are pathogenic in humans. Primary infection is generally subclinical or results in only mild constitutional symptoms. All herpesviruses establish latency for the lifetime of the host after a primary infection, with periodic reactivation. Most adults in the United States are seropositive for many of the herpesviruses. Kaposi sarcoma is discussed in Chapter 6.

HERPES SIMPLEX VIRUS AND VARICELLA ZOSTER INFECTION

These two herpesvirus infections result in painful ulcers and blisters of the oral mucosa and skin.

Clinical Findings

- Primary herpetic gingivostomatitis is the most common herpesvirus infection in the first three decades of life. There is a viral prodrome followed by an acute onset of multiple, painful, clustered, and subsequently coalescent ulcers on any mucosal surface, but frequently on the lip mucosa, tongue, and gingiva. Most cases are associated with herpes simplex virus (HSV)-1 and some with HSV-2 (Fig. 4.4A–B)
- Recrudescent infection in healthy hosts: herpes labialis (fever blisters or cold sores) on the lip is the most common presentation; less common sites are the keratinized mucosa of the hard palatal mucosa and attached gingiva. There are painful, 2- to 3-mm clustered and coalescent ulcers with scalloped borders often induced by injury (eg, sunburn) or trauma (eg, dental procedures) (see Fig. 4.4C–E).
- Recrudescent infection in immunocompromised hosts: ulcers occur anywhere on the oral mucosa and may appear aphthous-like if on the nonkeratinized mucosa (see Fig. 4.4F).
- At least 70% of cases of erythema multiforme are induced by HSV reactivation (see Chapter 8).
- Primary varicella-zoster virus (VZV) infection exhibits vesicles on the skin and also in the mouth that rupture to form ulcers. Reactivation of VZV tends to occur in older adults, in immunocompromised hosts, and

TABLE 4.1 Herpesvirus Infections

Herpesvirus Type	Disease Manifestation
HHV-1 Herpes simplex virus-1 Alpha virus	Oral cavity: Primary herpetic gingivostomatitis and recrudescent herpes stomatitis or herpes labialis Genital herpes, eczema herpeticum, herpes whitlow, herpes gladiatorum, ocular herpes, herpes encephalitis, disseminated infection
HHV-2 Herpes simplex virus-2 Alpha virus	Although usually found on skin and mucosa below the waist (genital herpes), may also be found in the mouth with lesions identical to those of HSV-1, neonatal infection, herpetic whitlow (also see HHV-1 above)
HHV-3 Varicella-zoster virus Alpha virus	Oral cavity: Primary infection exhibits oral ulcers; recrudescent infection is facial or oral shingles along the distribution of the trigeminal nerve and is usually unilateral Primary infection is chickenpox; skin shingles are common on the trunk
HHV-4 Epstein-Barr virus Gamma virus	Oral cavity: Hairy leukoplakia occurs in patients with HIV/AIDS, organ transplant recipients, or other immunocompromised hosts, as well as those on immunosuppressive agents; rarely occurs in the healthy host Epstein-Barr virus mucocutaneous ulcer in immunosuppressed or immunosenescent host Infectious mononucleosis, Burkitt lymphoma, nasopharyngeal carcinoma, central nervous system lymphoma, post-transplant lymphoproliferative disorder, Hodgkin lymphoma, plasmablastic lymphoma
HHV-5 Cytomegalovirus Beta virus	Oral cavity: Penetrating oral ulcers; organism may be a bystander noted in other ulcerative lesions Infectious mononucleosis–like syndrome, retinitis, gastroenteritis, hepatitis, pneumonitis
HHV-6 Beta virus	No documented oral findings Roseola infantum, exanthema subitum
HHV-7 Beta virus	No documented oral findings Roseola infantum, exanthema subitum
HHV-8 Kaposi sarcoma herpesvirus Gamma virus	Oral cavity: Kaposi sarcoma Skin and visceral Kaposi sarcoma, primary effusion lymphoma, multicentric Castleman disease

HHV, Human herpes virus.

in those on new biologic therapies such as tumor necrosis factor inhibitors.

- Herpes zoster is present as linear blisters and ulcers in a dermatomal distribution on the skin along the course of a sensory nerve, as well as in the oral cavity and facial skin corresponding to the distribution of the trigeminal nerve (Fig. 4.5). Postherpetic neuropathy occurs frequently and can be chronic and debilitating.

Etiopathogenesis and Histopathologic Features

HSV and VZV are DNA viruses that are cytotoxic to epithelial cells. After primary infection, latency is established in sensory ganglia and peripherally at mucosal sites. Reactivation of HSV leads to asymptomatic shedding, which is the primary means of transmission. Some reactivations present with painful lesions as noted above (also referred to as *recrudescence*).

- Multinucleated giant epithelial cells at the edge of the ulcer exhibit "nuclear molding," and there is acute and chronic inflammation. Nuclei contain "ground-glass" amphophilic Cowdry inclusions; similar cells are noted if the edge of the ulcer is scraped (Tzanck test), and the presence of HSV or VZV may be confirmed by immunohistochemical studies (Fig. 4.6).
- A biopsy of only the center of the ulcer without epithelium may not show viral inclusions and cannot be presumed to be negative for HSV or VZV infection.
- Positive cultures for HSV should be correlated with clinical findings because asymptomatic shedding (induced by trauma, illness, or stress) is a frequent occurrence.

Differential Diagnosis

- Inflammatory reactions and the epithelium adjacent to an ulcer may contain multinucleated giant epithelial cells, but these cells have abundant cytoplasm, no nuclear molding, dispersed chromatin and no Cowdry inclusions, although nucleoli may be prominent (see Chapter 11).

Management and Prognosis

- Primary HSV infections, or recrudescent HSV infections in immunocompromised patients, as well as herpes zoster infections, are managed with supportive care, hydration, pain control, and systemic therapy with acyclovir, valacyclovir, or famciclovir (see Appendix B).
- Herpes labialis may be successfully managed with a 1- or 2-day course of valacyclovir or famciclovir, topical acyclovir, penciclovir, or docosanol (Appendix B). The use of sunscreen often prevents recrudescent herpes labialis induced by sun damage.

REFERENCES

Arain N, Paravastu SC, Arain MA. Effectiveness of topical corticosteroids in addition to antiviral therapy in the management of recurrent herpes labialis: a systematic review and meta-analysis. *BMC Infect Dis.* 2015;15:82.

Eisen D. The clinical characteristics of intraoral herpes simplex virus infection in 52 immunocompetent patients. *Oral Surg Oral Med Oral Pathol Oral Radiol Endod.* 1998;86:432-437.

Elad S, Zadik Y, Hewson I, et al. A systematic review of viral infections associated with oral involvement in cancer patients: a spotlight on *Herpesviridae*. *Support Care Cancer.* 2010;18:993-1006.

Weathers DR, Griffin JW. Intraoral ulcerations of recurrent herpes simplex and recurrent aphthae: two distinct clinical entities. *J Am Dent Assoc.* 1970;81:81-87.

Woo SB, Challacombe SJ. Management of recurrent oral herpes simplex infections. *Oral Surg Oral Med Oral Pathol Oral Radiol Endod.* 2007;103(suppl S12):e1-e18.

Woo SB, Lee SF. Oral recrudescent herpes simplex virus infection. *Oral Surg Oral Med Oral Pathol Oral Radiol Endod.* 1997;83:239-243.

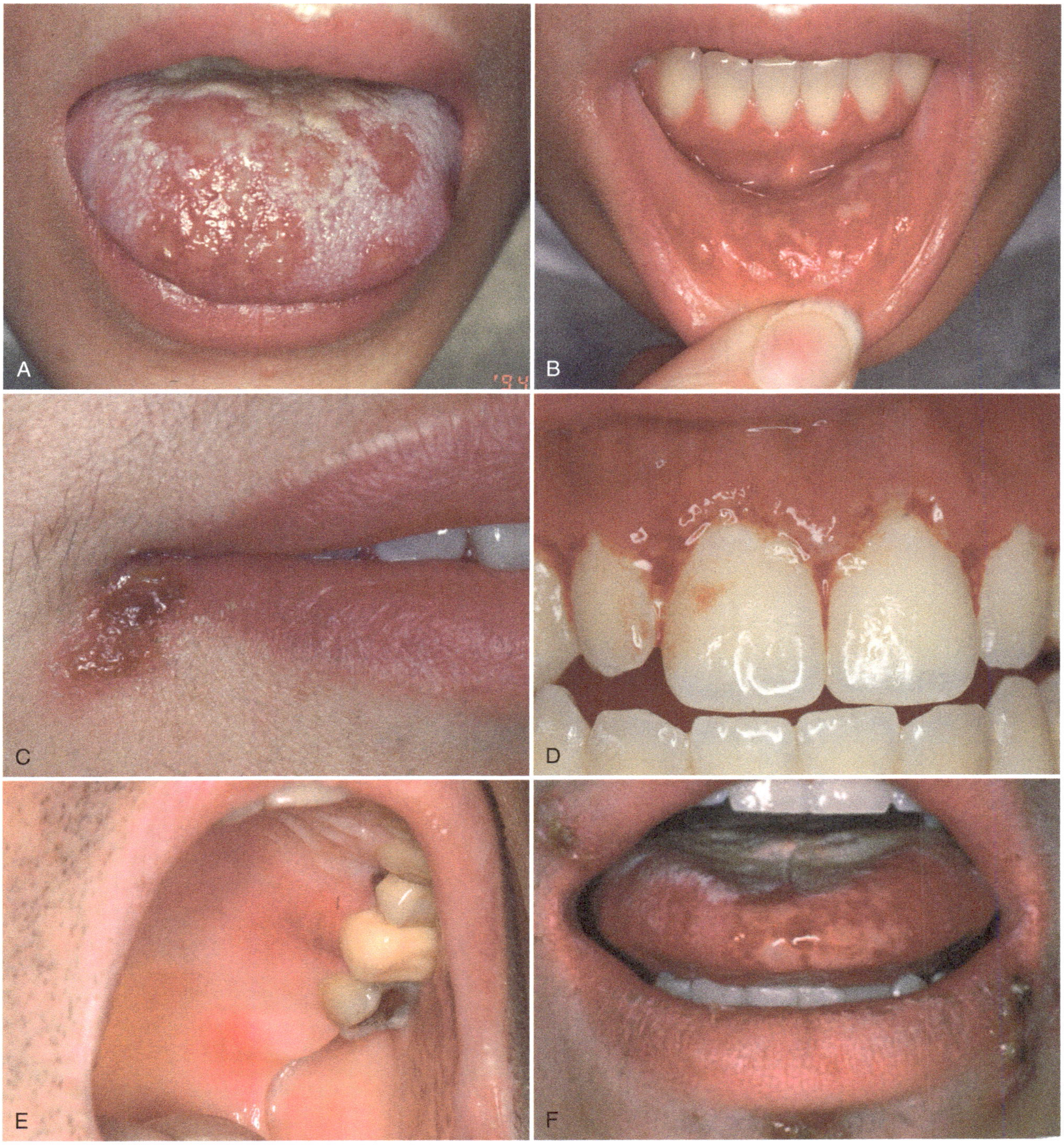

FIG 4.4 Herpes simplex virus infection. (A) Primary infection with coalescent ulcers on the tongue dorsum. (B) Ulcers on the nonkeratinized lip mucosa and marginal gingiva of same patient as in A. (C) Recrudescent herpes labialis in immunocompetent host. (D) Recrudescent herpes simplex on the marginal gingiva in an immunocompetent host. (E) Recrudescent herpes simplex on the hard palatal mucosa. (F) Recrudescent herpes simplex virus ulcer of the ventral tongue and skin in a patient with cancer.

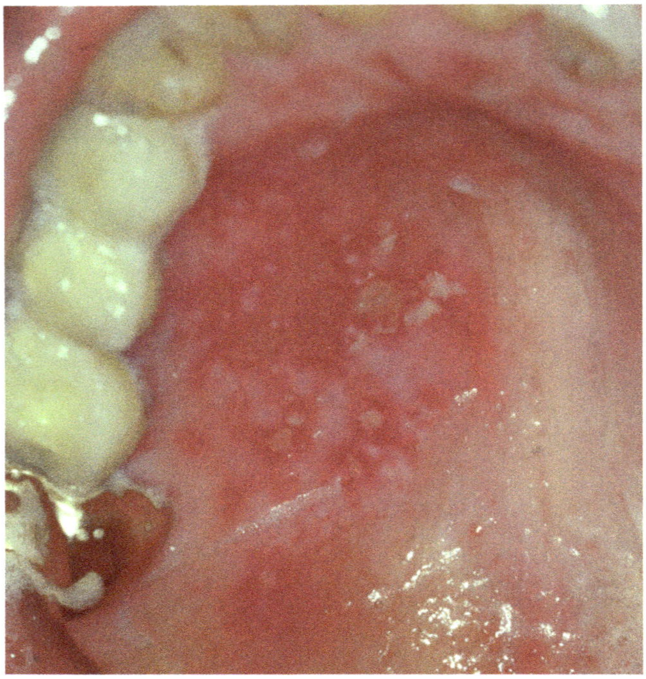

FIG 4.5 Recrudescent varicella zoster infection: oral shingles exhibiting coalescent ulcers of the right hard palatal mucosa.

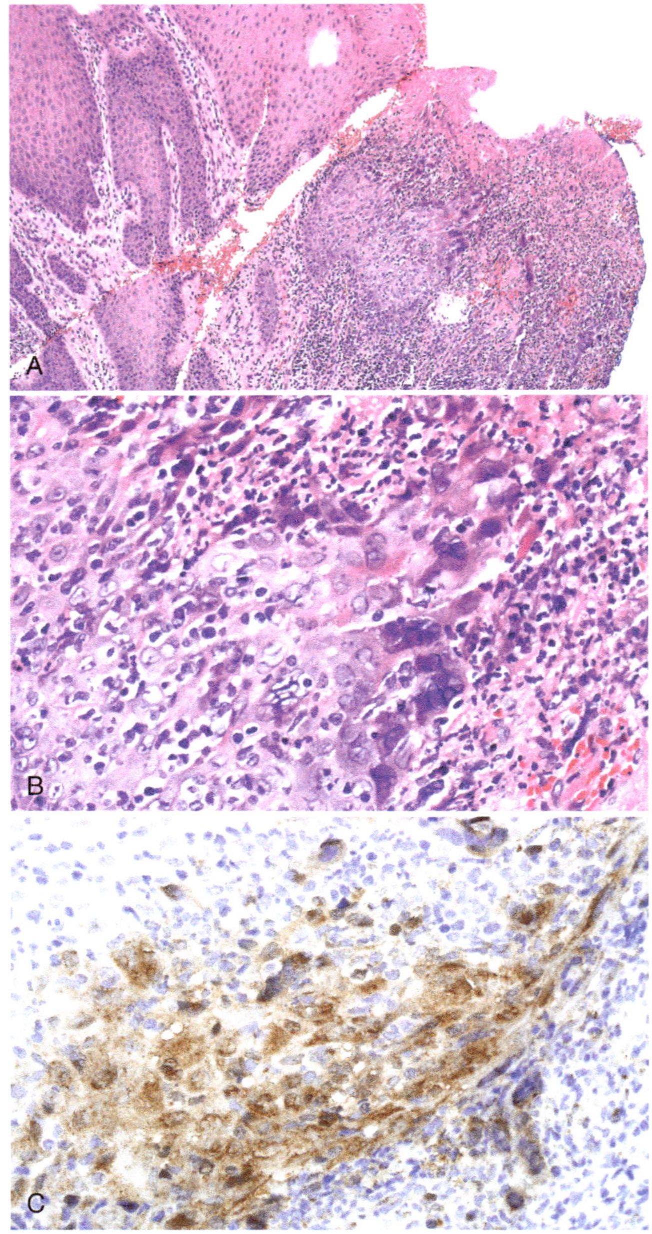

FIG 4.6 Herpes simplex virus (HSV) infection. (A) Oral mucosa with ulceration and hematoxyphilic cells at the ulcer edge. (B) Multinucleated epithelial cells with nuclear molding and Cowdry inclusions. (C) Immunohistochemical study confirms the presence of HSV-1.

HAIRY LEUKOPLAKIA

Hairy leukoplakia is caused by the Epstein-Barr virus (EBV), and the term *leukoplakia* as used in this context does not connote any tendency for dysplasia or malignancy.

Clinical Findings

- Hairy leukoplakia occurs most commonly in immunocompromised individuals, especially those with HIV/AIDS with low CD4 counts, in organ transplant recipients, and in patients on steroid inhalers. Cases have been reported in healthy patients, usually older adults, possibly due to immunosenescence.
- Hairy leukoplakia presents as a white, painless, linear lesion or plaque, usually on the lateral border of tongue, and cases are usually bilateral. Classically, white linear lesions run perpendicular to the long axis of the tongue (Fig. 4.7).

Etiopathogenesis and Histopathologic Features

EBV establishes latency in peripheral blood pre-Langerhans cells that migrate into the epithelium as Langerhans cells, where the virus is reactivated and leads to productive replication.

- There is variable parakeratosis with or without bacterial colonization, similar to factitial keratosis; candidal hyphae and/or spores are present, often in the absence of spongiotic pustules (Figs. 4.8 and 4.9A).
- Sharp demarcation of parakeratin from the subjacent pale, edematous superficial keratinocytes is characteristic. Virally infected cells show central Cowdry inclusions ("ground-glass," homogeneous, amphophilic nuclear mass consisting of virions) with margination ("beading") of chromatin against the nuclear membrane (see Figs. 4.8B and 4.9B). Such findings are readily identified on exfoliative cytology.
- In situ hybridization studies show nuclear positivity for Epstein-Barr–encoded RNA (EBER); Epstein-Barr nucleic acid, and latent membrane protein (LMP) may be also positive (see Fig. 4.9C).
- Ultrastructurally, there are herpesvirus-sized particles in the center of the nucleus (Cowdry inclusion) with chromatin margination at the periphery (Fig. 4.9D).

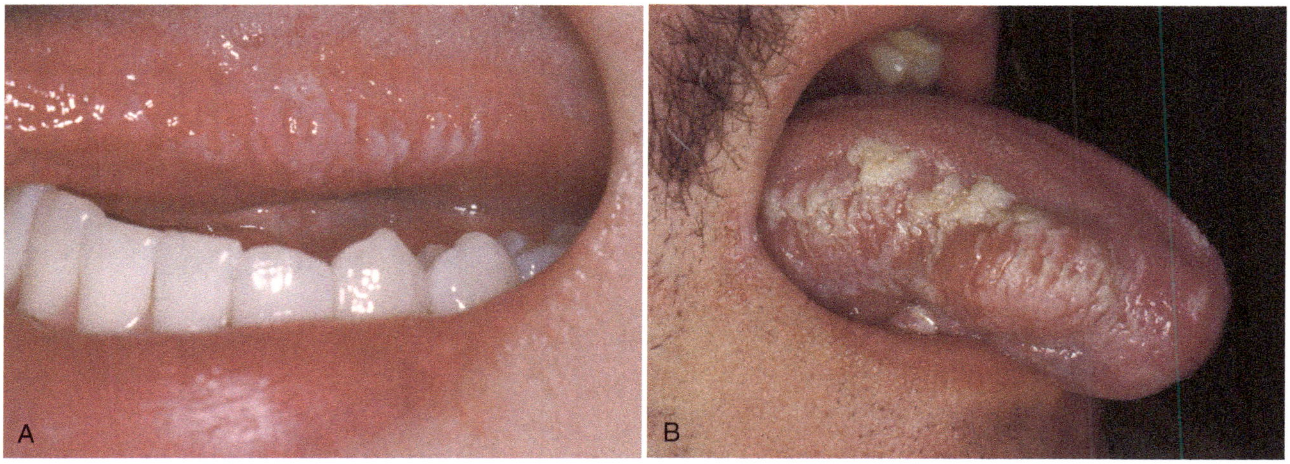

FIG 4.7 Hairy leukoplakia. (A) Typical vertical fissures on lateral border of tongue. (B) White plaque and fissures, likely with secondary candidiasis.

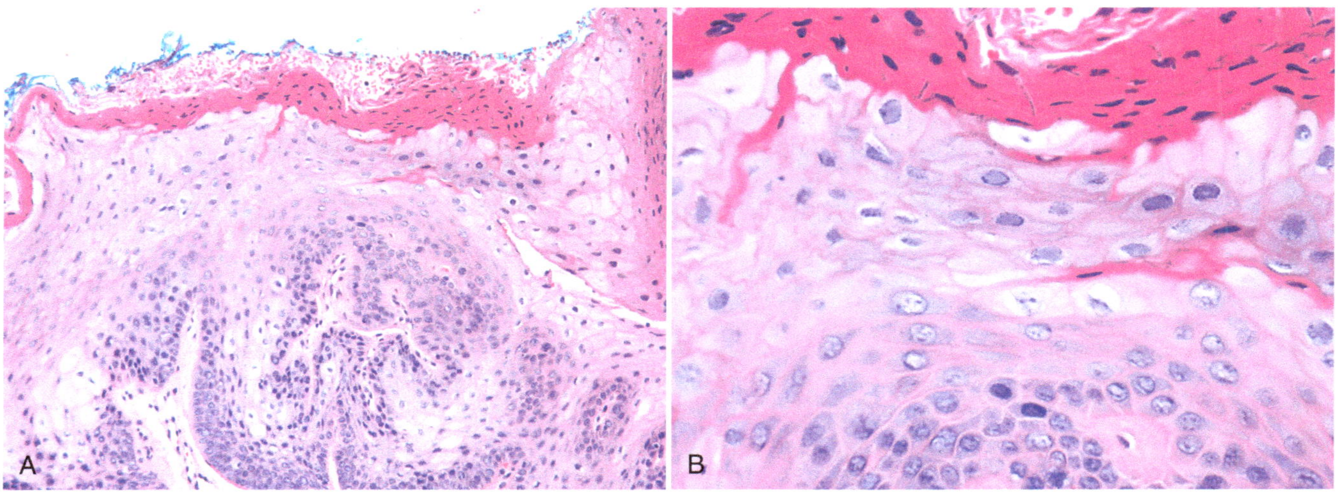

FIG 4.8 Hairy leukoplakia. (A) Oral mucosa with parakeratosis and acanthosis. (B) There is candidal colonization without spongiotic pustules and keratinocytes exhibit peripheral condensation of chromatin surrounding smudgy central Cowdry inclusions.

Differential Diagnosis

- Factitial/frictional keratosis due to bite trauma does not show Cowdry inclusions or chromatin margination and is negative for EBV by in situ hybridization (Fig. 4.10).

Management and Prognosis

- Adjustment of antiretroviral therapy or reduction of immunosuppressive therapy in post–organ transplant patients may resolve lesions, and candidiasis should be treated (Appendix B).
- Cases may resolve with a combination of topical antiherpetic medications (such as 1% penciclovir or 5% acyclovir cream/ointment), valacyclovir, and 25% podophyllin resin.
- Hairy leukoplakia may be the first indication of HIV-positive status.

REFERENCES

Bhayat A, Yengopal V, Rudolph M. Predictive value of group I oral lesions for HIV infection. *Oral Surg Oral Med Oral Pathol Oral Radiol Endod*. 2010;109:720-723.

Casiglia J, Woo SB. Oral hairy leukoplakia as an early indicator of Epstein-Barr virus-associated post-transplant lymphoproliferative disorder. *J Oral Maxillofac Surg*. 2002;60:948-950.

Chambers AE, Conn B, Pemberton M, et al. Twenty-first-century oral hairy leukoplakia—a non–HIV-associated entity. *Oral Surg Oral Med Oral Pathol Oral Radiol*. 2015;119:326-332.

Fraga-Fernández J, Vicandi-Plaza B. Diagnosis of hairy leukoplakia by exfoliative cytologic methods. *Am J Clin Pathol*. 1992;97:262-266.

Moura MD, Haddad JP, Senna MI, et al. A new topical treatment protocol for oral hairy leukoplakia. *Oral Surg Oral Med Oral Pathol Oral Radiol Endod*. 2010;110:611-617.

Walling DM, Ray AJ, Nichols JE, et al. Epstein-Barr virus infection of Langerhans cell precursors as a mechanism of oral epithelial entry, persistence, and reactivation. *J Virol*. 2007;81:7249-7268.

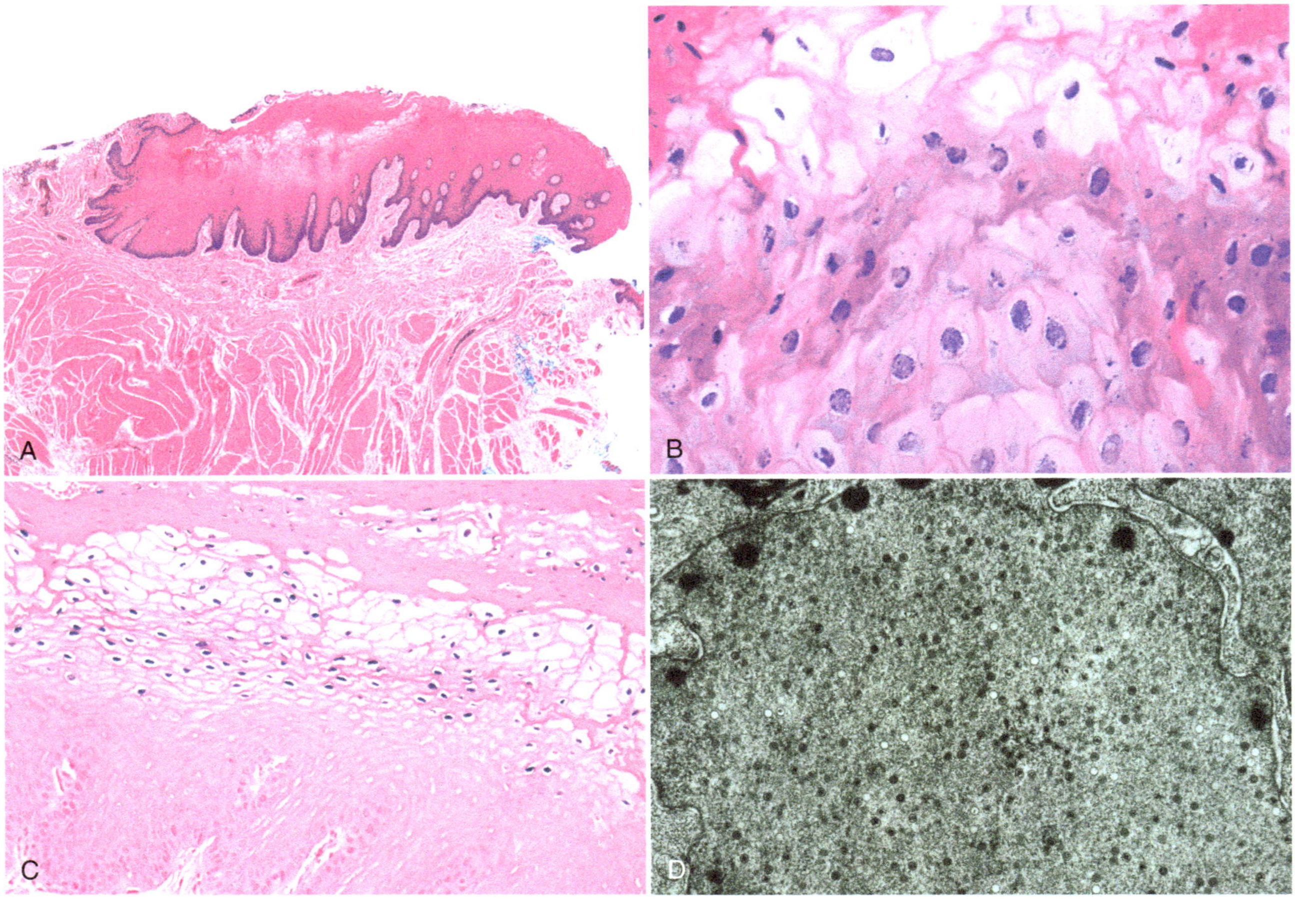

FIG 4.9 Hairy leukoplakia. (A) Oral mucosa with parakeratosis and underlying band of pale, ballooned cells. (B) Keratinocytes exhibit peripheral condensation of chromatin, coarsely clumped chromatin, and smudgy Cowdry inclusions. (C) In situ hybridization study shows nuclear positivity for Epstein-Barr virus–encoded mRNA. (D) Electron photomicrograph showing peripheral condensation of chromatin ("beading") and nucleus filled with virions that constitute the Cowdry inclusion.

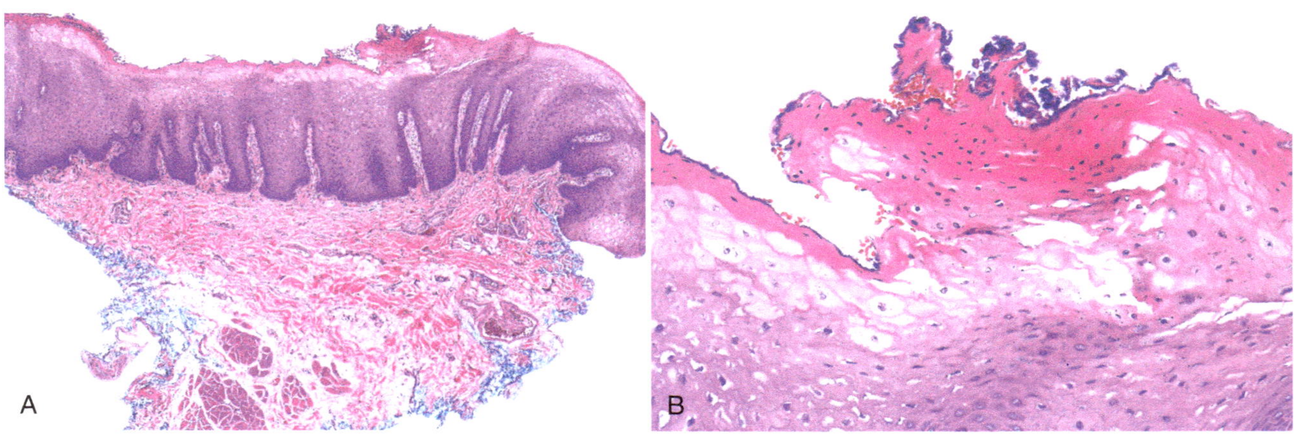

FIG 4.10 Frictional/factitial parakeratosis. (A) Oral mucosa with parakeratosis and underlying band of pale cells and acanthosis. (B) There is no evidence of Cowdry inclusions or chromatin margination can be seen.

EPSTEIN-BARR VIRUS MUCOCUTANEOUS ULCER

Clinical Findings

- This occurs in patients on immunosuppressive medications for autoimmune diseases (such as methotrexate for rheumatoid arthritis), in post–organ transplant patients, and in patients in the eighth decade of life and older (age-related immunosenescence).
- It presents as a nonhealing ulcer of the oral mucosa (tongue and tonsils are most common sites), skin, or gastrointestinal tract.

Etiopathogenesis and Histopathologic Features

This is believed to arise from reactivation of latent EBV infection due to immunocompromise or immunosenescence.

- There is deep ulcer with a polymorphous infiltrate of lymphocytes, plasma cells, eosinophils, atypical immunoblast-like lymphocytes, and Hodgkin-like cells or Reed-Sternberg–like cells (Fig. 4.11A–B)
- There are sheets of CD20+ cells also positive for CD30, MUM-1, and PAX-5. Atypical cells are CD20-, EBER-, and LMP1+ and occasionally CD15-, CD45-, Bcl-2 and Bcl-6 (Fig. 4.11C–D). The infiltrate is CD10- and BCL6–, and scattered CD3 cells are present, often in a band at the base of the ulcer.
- Some cases show light chain restriction or T-cell receptor gene rearrangements or other restricted T-cell responses.

Differential Diagnosis

- Traumatic ulcerative granuloma with stromal eosinophilia does not generally show atypical Reed-Sternberg cells but may have many eosinophils, lymphocytes, and histiocytes. Older reports of CD30+ traumatic ulcerative granulomas may have been cases of EBV mucocutaneous ulcers.

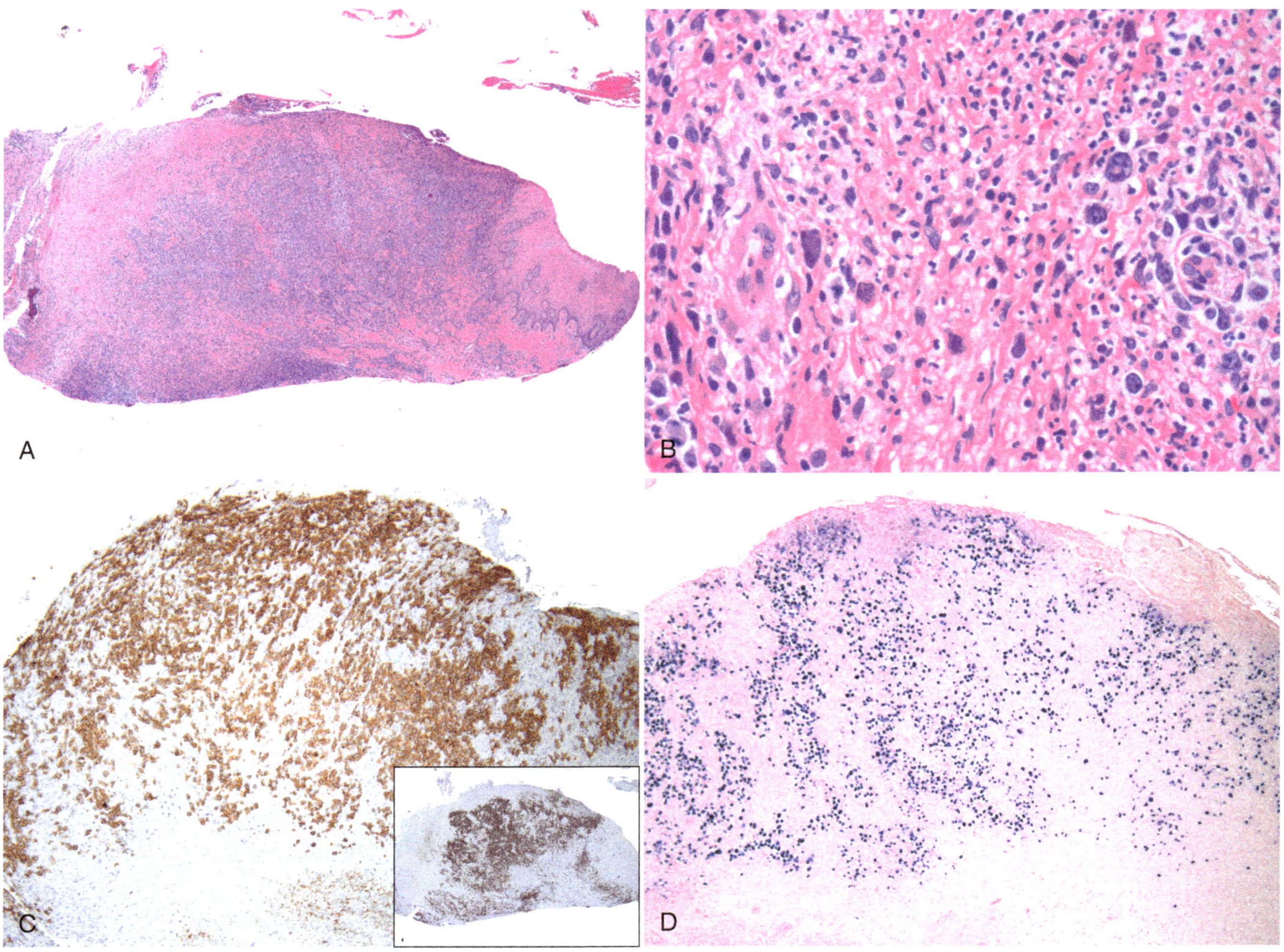

FIG 4.11 Epstein-Barr virus mucocutaneous ulcer. (A) Ulcerated mucosa with an intense, deep lymphocytic infiltrate. (B) The infiltrate is polymorphous and contains atypical Hodgkin-like cells with convoluted nuclear outlines. (C) Lymphocytes are positive for CD30 and CD20 (*inset*, CD20). (D) Lymphocytes are positive for Epstein-Barr–encoded RNA. *(Courtesy Dr. Indraneel Bhattacharyya, University of Florida, Gainesville, Fla.)*

Management and Prognosis

- Reduction in immunosuppressive therapy regresses lesions, and cases associated with immunosenescence often show spontaneous regression. Some cases require treatment with chemotherapy, radiation, mycophenolate mofetil, or rituximab, and none have resulted in disease-related death.

REFERENCES

Dojcinov SD, Venkataraman G, Raffeld M, et al. EBV positive mucocutaneous ulcer—a study of 26 cases associated with various sources of immunosuppression. *Am J Surg Pathol.* 2010;34:405-417.

Hart M, Thakral B, Yohe S, et al. EBV-positive mucocutaneous ulcer in organ transplant recipients: a localized indolent posttransplant lymphoproliferative disorder. *Am J Surg Pathol.* 2014;38:1522-1529.

CYTOMEGALOVIRUS INFECTION

Clinical Findings

- Neonates and immunocompromised individuals are generally affected, especially those with HIV/AIDS or organ transplant (especially kidney and hematopoietic stem cell transplant) recipients. Serious morbidities include retinitis, gastrointestinal ulcers, encephalitis, hepatitis, and pneumonitis.
- This occurs as a large, usually solitary, painful ulcer on the oral mucosa (Fig. 4.12). Cytomegalovirus (CMV) antigenemia may be present.

Etiopathogenesis and Histopathologic Features

Smooth muscle cells, endothelial cells, myeloid precursor cells, and immature Langerhans cells of the mucosa are sites of latency and replication. CMV-infected cells may also represent an incidental finding ("passenger") in an ulcer caused by another agent, such as HSV, and may be seen in clinically normal skin.

- Mucosal ulceration is present, and large, ballooned cells are noted within the endothelium or stromal cells. These cells contain "owl-eye" nuclei because of prominent eosinophilic nucleoli as well as dark pink granules in the cytoplasm (Fig. 4.13A–C). Biopsies must be of sufficient depth for diagnosis.
- In situ hybridization studies for CMV show nuclear positivity (see Fig. 4.13D).
- Quantitative polymerase chain reaction (PCR) on blood samples, as well as CMV antigenemia (pp65 antigen in leukocytes), is helpful in diagnosis.

Differential Diagnosis

- EBV-associated mucocutaneous ulcers exhibit atypical, large, immunoblast-like B cells and Reed-Sternberg–like cells that are EBER- and CD30+.

Management and Prognosis

- Ganciclovir and valganciclovir are the conventional treatments; newer medications include letermovir and maribavir.

REFERENCES

Daudén E, Fernández-Buezo G, Fraga J, et al. Mucocutaneous presence of cytomegalovirus associated with human immunodeficiency virus infection: discussion regarding its pathogenetic role. *Arch Dermatol.* 2001;137:443-448.

Griffiths P, Lumley S. Cytomegalovirus. *Curr Opin Infect Dis.* 2014;27:554-559.

Meer S, Altini M. Cytomegalovirus co-infection in AIDS-associated oral Kaposi's sarcoma. *Adv Dent Res.* 2006;19:96-98.

Tarkan JL, Woo SB, Pavlakis M, et al. Spotting the owl: surreptitious cytomegalovirus disease in a renal transplant recipient. *Clin Transplant.* 2008;22:391-395.

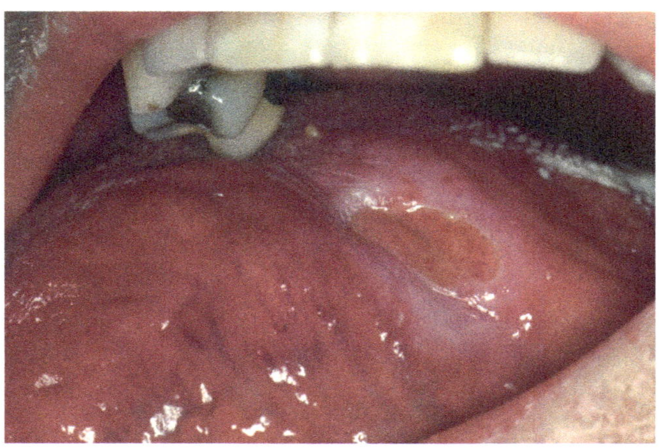

FIG 4.12 Cytomegalovirus-infected ulcer of the left ventral tongue.

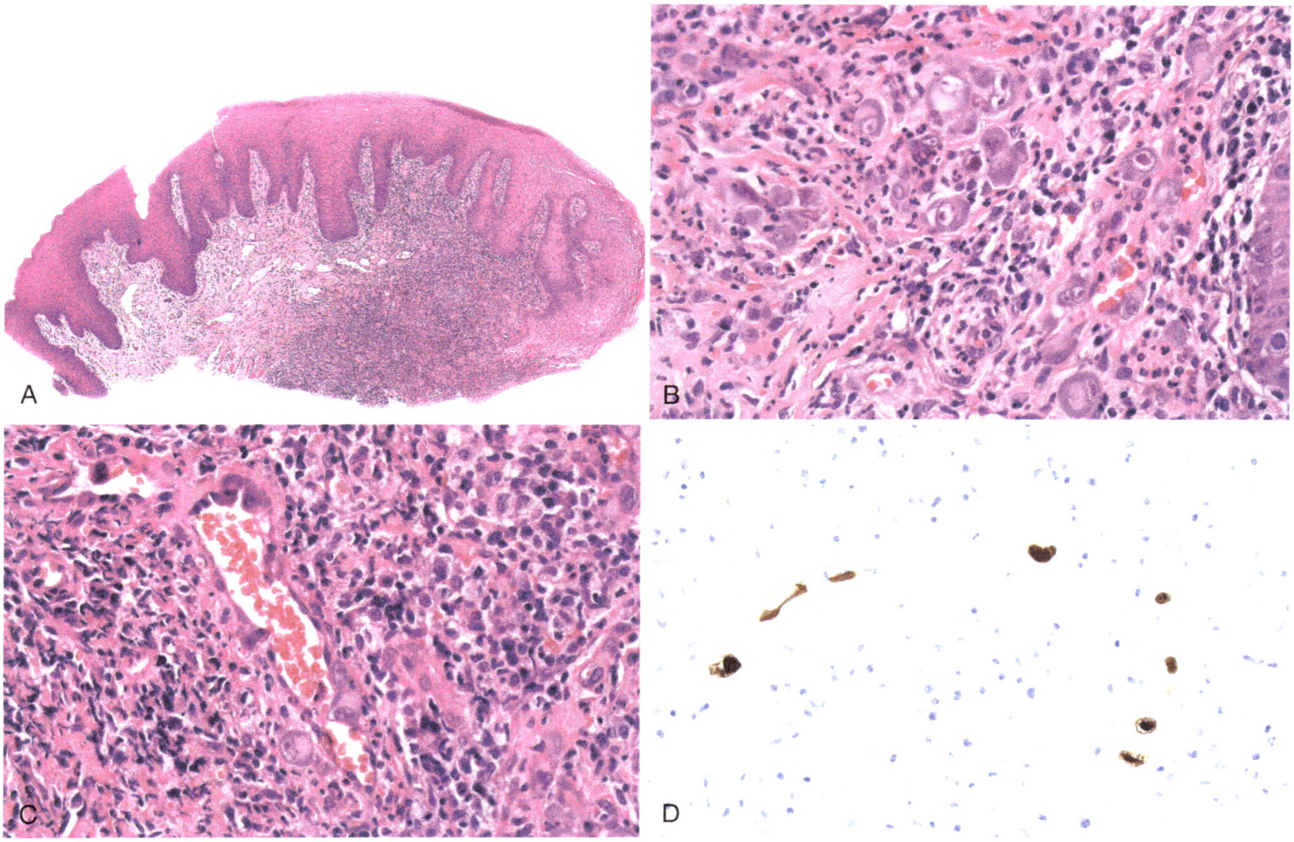

FIG 4.13 Cytomegalovirus (CMV) infection. (A) The oral mucosa is ulcerated (ulcer at *bottom*). (B) Ballooned cells with large nuclei and prominent red nucleoli ("owl eye"), as well as slightly granular amphophilic cytoplasm, can be seen. (C) There is involvement of endothelial cells by CMV. (D) In situ hybridization study positive for CMV.

HUMAN PAPILLOMAVIRUS–RELATED BENIGN LESIONS

Squamous papilloma, verruca vulgaris, condyloma acuminatum, and Heck disease (focal epithelial hyperplasia) are discussed together because of their similarities in clinical presentation and histopathology.

Clinical Findings

- These tend to occur in young patients, and all present as painless, exophytic, papillary/verrucous or papular, white or pink, sessile or pedunculated growths on the mucosa.
- Squamous papilloma: this is often seen on the soft palate or tongue and may be white or pink (Fig. 4.14A).
- Verruca vulgaris: this is often on the gingiva, lips, and palatal mucosa and is almost always white (Fig. 4.14B).
- Condyloma acuminatum: this is usually seen in immunocompromised patients (and sometimes in immunocompetent patients) as single or multiple papular or papillary lesions (Fig. 4.14C–E).
- Heck disease: there are multiple papules/nodules or papillary lesions (less common) on the mucosa of the lips and tongue, often seen in young persons (first and second decades of life) living in crowded conditions in South and Central America, with a prevalence of up to 13%. It is also common in Africa, the Middle East, in patients with HIV/AIDS, and sporadically in North America (see Fig. 4.14F). The condition tends to regress with age.

Etiopathogenesis and Histopathologic Features

These lesions are related to human papillomavirus infection. In situ hybridization and PCR studies have allowed these to be characterized more accurately. Condylomas may result from sexual transmission, vertical transmission (maternal-fetal), or through salivary transmission.

- See Table 4.2 and Figs. 4.15–4.25 for histopathologic features.

Differential Diagnosis

- See Table 4.2.
- Acanthosis nigricans exhibits papillomatosis and acanthosis without involvement by human papillomavirus and the malignant form may be an indicator of visceral malignancy (Fig. 4.26). The benign form is associated with obesity, insulin-resistant diabetes mellitus, or may be medication-induced.

Text continued on p. 58

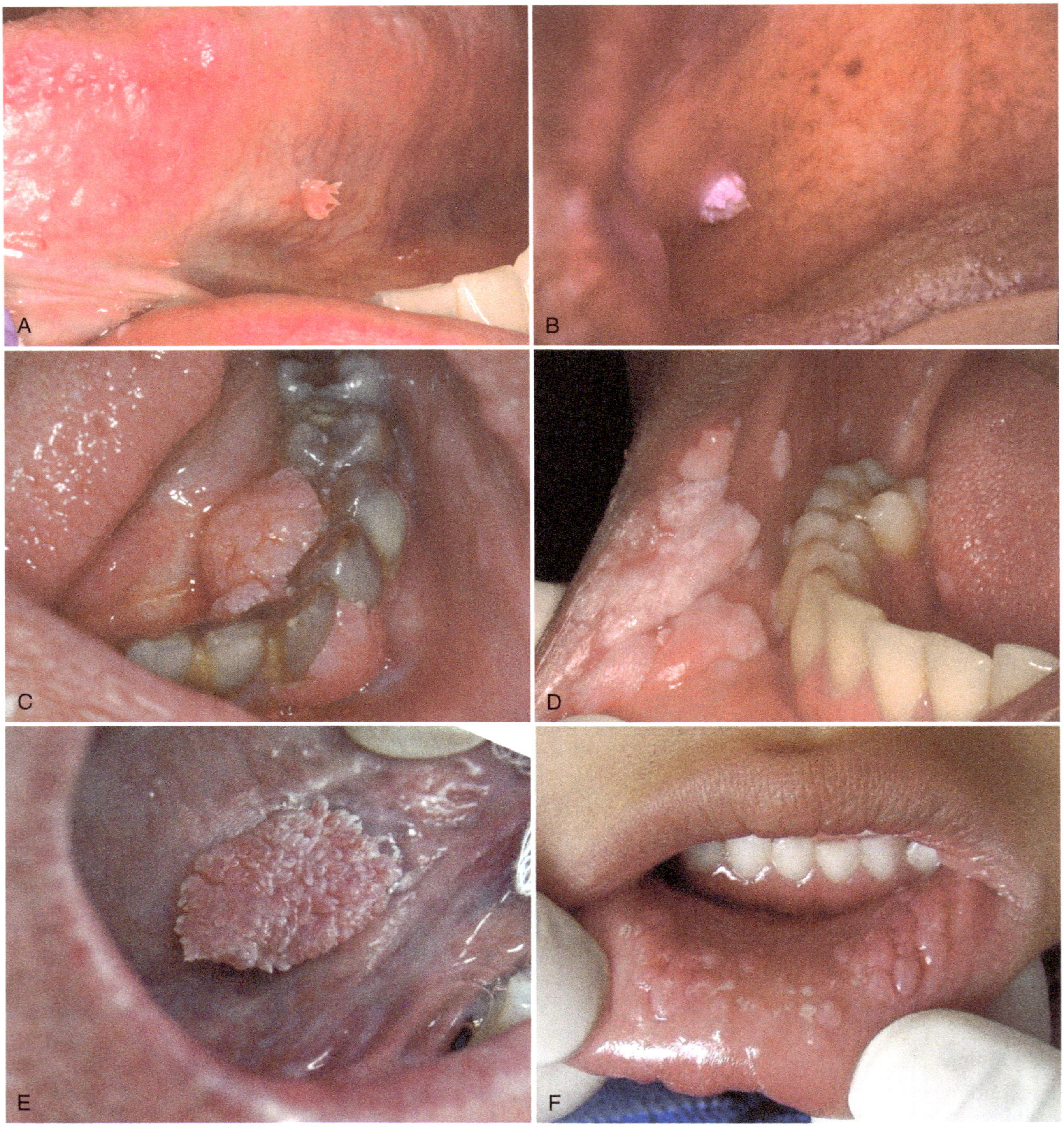

FIG 4.14 (A) Squamous papilloma of the left ventral tongue. (B) Verruca vulgaris of the right hard palatal mucosa. (C) Condyloma acuminatum (one of many) in a patient after lung transplant. (D) Condyloma acuminata in a patient with HIV/AIDS. (E) Pedunculated condyloma acuminatum in a healthy patient. (F) Heck disease in a child from Guatemala. *(A, Courtesy Dr. Mark Lerman, Lecturer, Harvard School of Dental Medicine, Boston, Mass; B, Courtesy Dr. John Lovas, Dalhousie University, Halifax, Nova Scotia, Canada; D, Courtesy Dr. Mark Lerman, Harvard School of Dental Medicine, Boston, Mass; E, Courtesy Dr. Sherwin Kershman, private practice, Houston, Tex; F, Courtesy Dr. Roman Carlos, Guatemala City, Guatemala.)*

TABLE 4.2 Histopathologic Features and Differential Diagnosis for Squamous Papilloma, Verruca Vulgaris, and Condyloma Acuminatum

Condition	HPV Subtype[a]	Histopathologic Features	Differential Diagnosis
Squamous papilloma (see Figs. 4.15–4.18)	6, 11	• Papillary epithelial hyperplasia in thin ribbons with variable parakeratosis or hyperkeratosis • Soft palate and ventral tongue lesions exhibit prominent keratinocyte edema with minimal keratin; koilocytes are infrequently seen • Fibrovascular cores are edematous or hyalinized • Inflammation often leads to spongiosis, loss of keratin, and basal cell hyperplasia	• Giant cell fibroma has stellate-shaped, giant, and multinucleated fibroblasts • Papillary epithelial dysplasia exhibits significant cytologic atypia that is not reactive in nature
Verruca vulgaris (see Figs. 4.19–4.22)	1, 2, 4, 57	• Papillary epithelial hyperplasia with hyperkeratosis, large keratohyaline granules, and axial inclination of peripheral rete ridges • Koilocytes[b] are usually present • Inflammation may lead to significant reactive atypia, parakeratosis, and dyskeratosis (especially lip and cutaneous lesions)	• Irritated seborrheic keratosis exhibits a basaloid cell proliferation with pseudohorn cysts • Inverted follicular keratosis resembles irritated seborrheic keratosis and tends to follow the orientation of the hair follicle
Condyloma acuminatum (see Figs. 4.23 and 4.24)	6, 11	• Pronounced papillary epithelial hyperplasia with little keratin and large bulbous rete ridges • Koilocytes[b] are always seen and basal cell hyperplasia is often present	• Verrucous hyperplasia is broad-based with hyperkeratosis or parakeratosis and bulbous rete ridges with variable cytologic atypia/dysplasia • Verrucous carcinoma has an endophytic as well as exophytic growth pattern and is parakeratotic
Heck disease (see Fig. 4.25)	13, 32, 55 1, 6, 11, 16, 19	• Epithelial hyperplasia often without papillary features forming elongated, sometimes bulbous rete ridges • Koilocytes[b] and mitosoid bodies (karyorrhectic cells with coarse, fragmented chromatin) are characteristic and represent HPV cytopathic effect.	

[a]Not seen in every case.
[b]Koilocytes exhibit irregular, twisted nuclear outlines and nuclear hyperchromatism; perinuclear halos alone are not sufficient for the diagnosis.
HPV, Human papillomavirus.

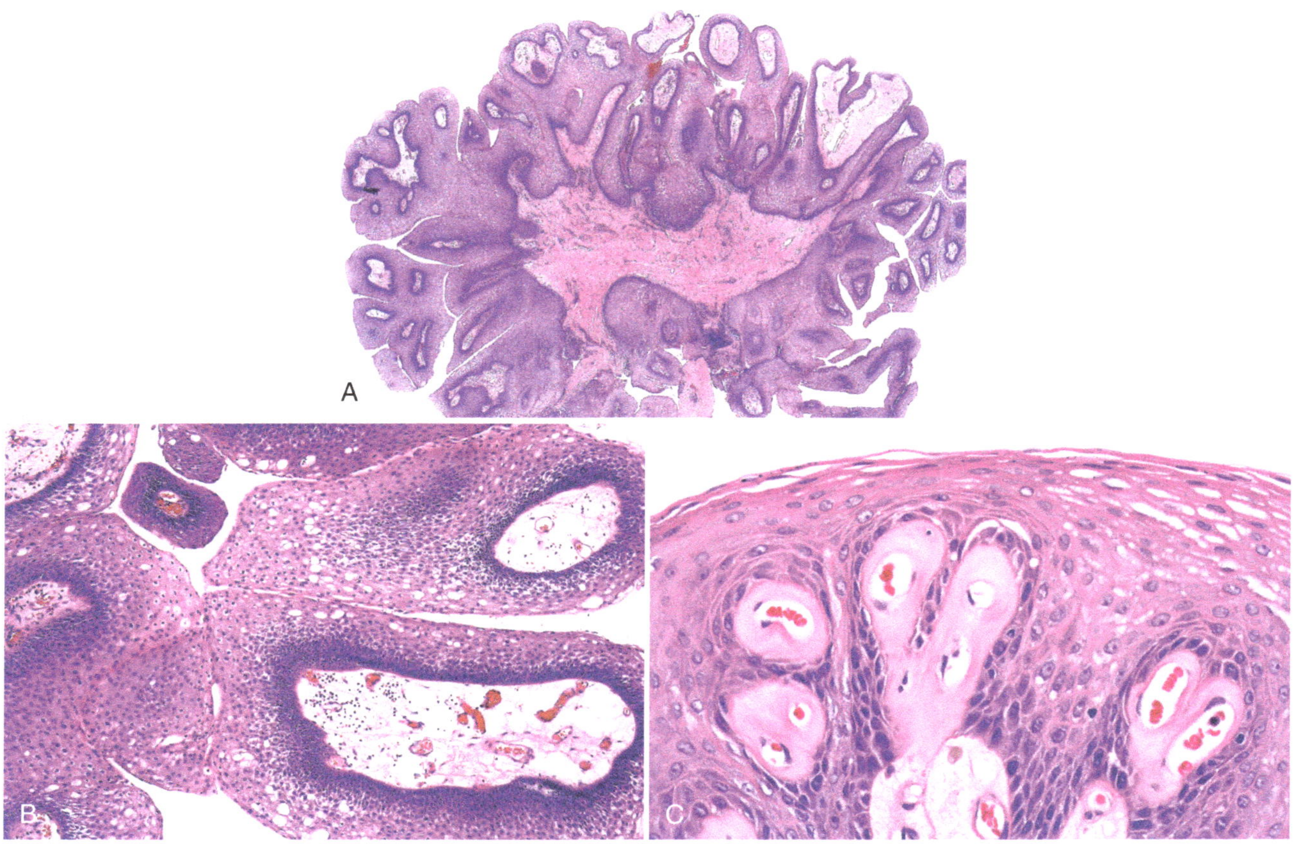

FIG 4.15 Irritated squamous papillomas of soft palate. (A) Soft palate papillomas typically have little keratin. (B) Spongiosis, basal cell hyperplasia, and edematous fibrovascular cores can be seen. (C) Fibrovascular cores may exhibit hyalinization.

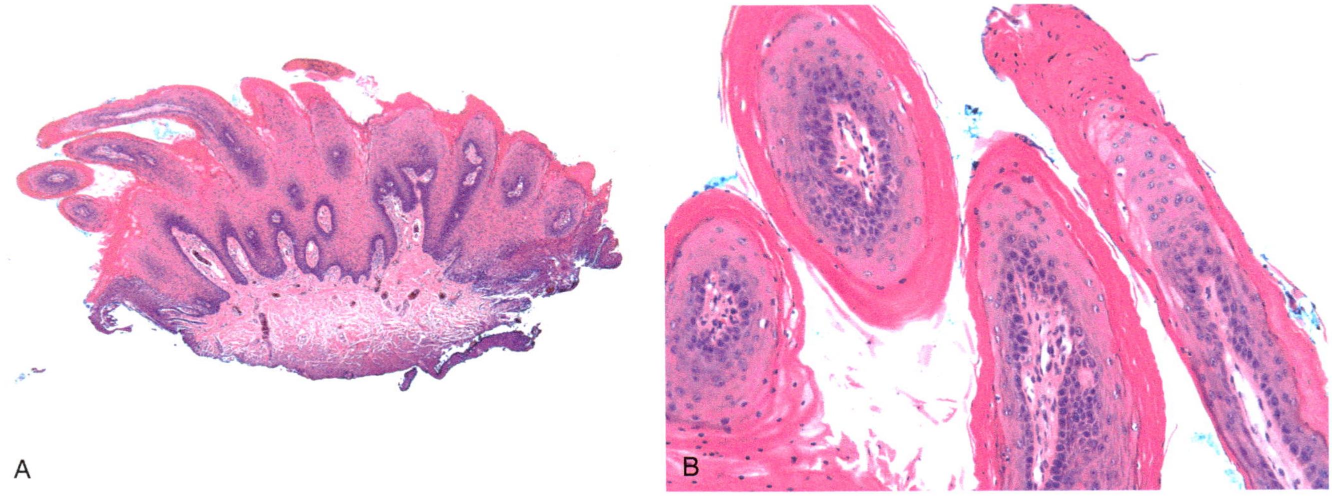

FIG 4.16 Squamous papilloma of the tongue. (A) Papillary epithelial hyperplasia with parakeratosis. (B) Fibrovascular cores contain dilated capillaries.

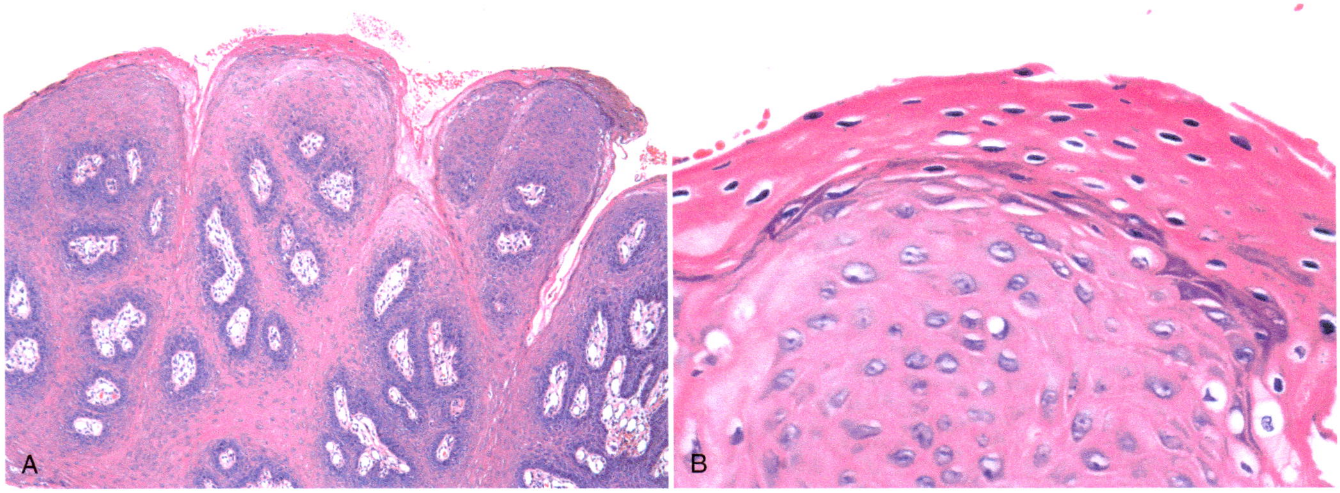

FIG 4.17 Squamous papilloma. (A) Parakeratosis and benign epithelial hyperplasia. (B) Koilocytes are present with perinuclear halos and crenated, hyperchromatic nuclei.

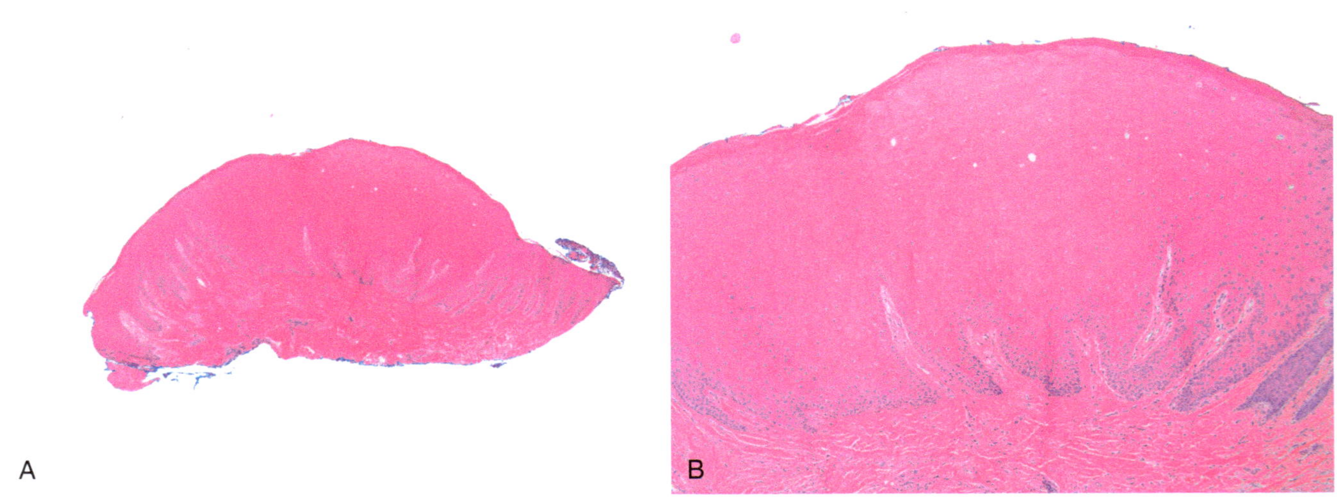

FIG 4.18 Early squamous papillomas. (A) Acanthosis with axial inclination of rete ridges at the periphery can be seen. (B) Early fibrovascular cores are present.

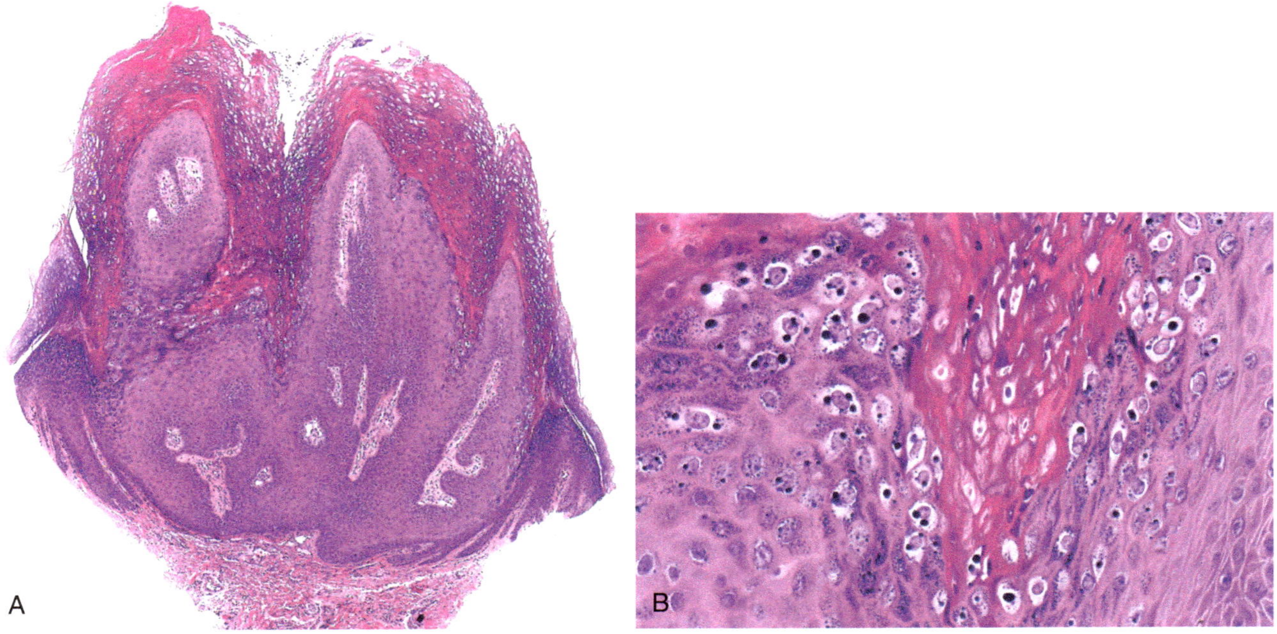

FIG 4.19 Verruca vulgaris. (A) Hyperkeratosis and papillary epithelial hyperplasia with axial inclination of rete ridges. (B) Coarse keratohyaline granules.

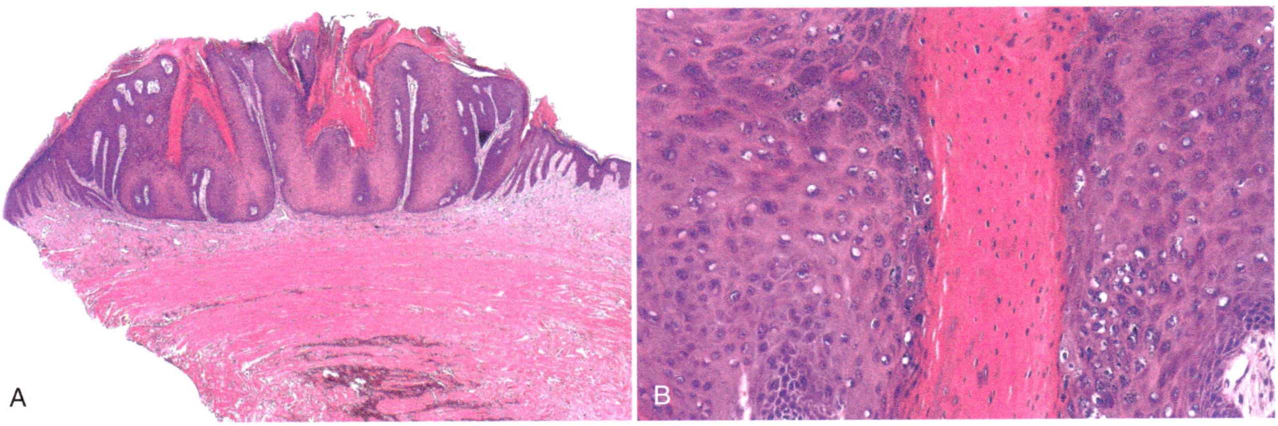

FIG 4.20 Traumatized verruca vulgaris. (A) Hyperkeratosis, parakeratosis, and papillary epithelial proliferation forming bulbous rete ridges with peripheral axial inclination. (B) Parakeratosis and small keratohyaline granules.

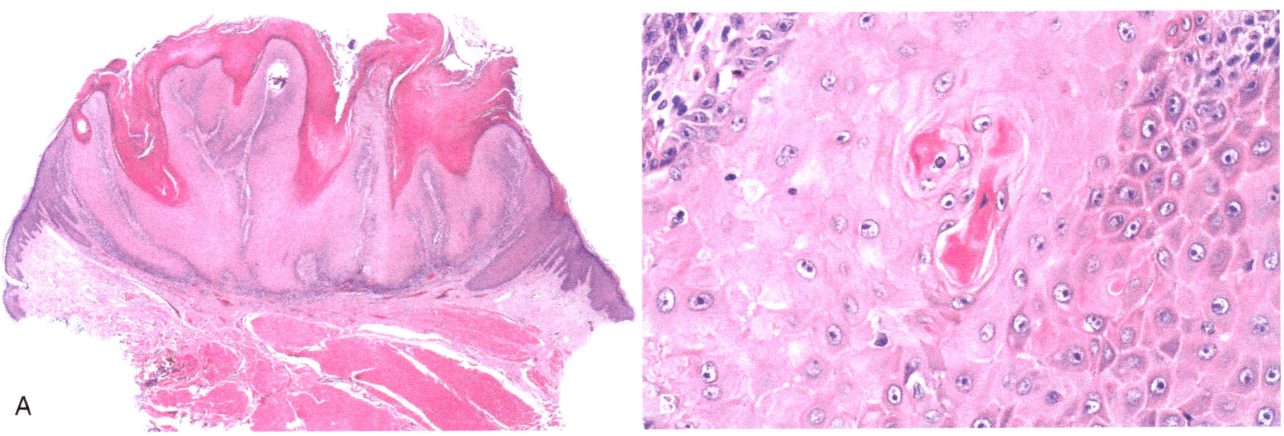

FIG 4.21 Traumatized and inflamed verruca vulgaris. (A) Parakeratosis, papillary epithelial hyperplasia with bulbous rete ridges with peripheral axial inclination. (B) Reactive epithelial atypia and dyskeratosis.

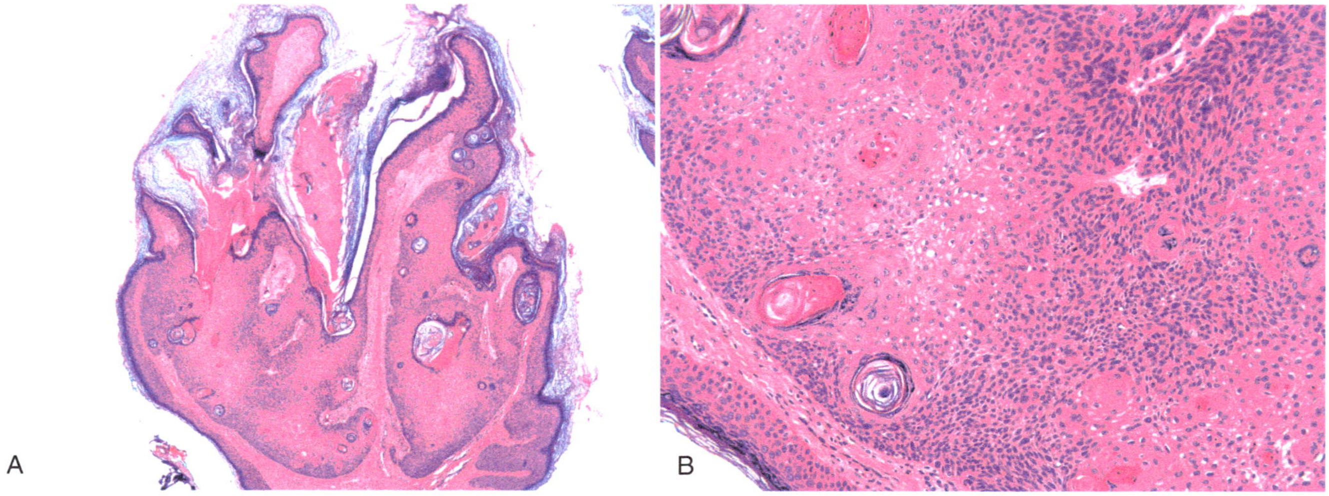

FIG 4.22 Irritated seborrheic keratosis. (A) Hyperkeratosis and papillary and endophytic epithelial hyperplasia forming bulbous rete ridges. (B) Many basaloid cells, dyskeratotic cells, squamous eddies, and pseudohorn cysts are present.

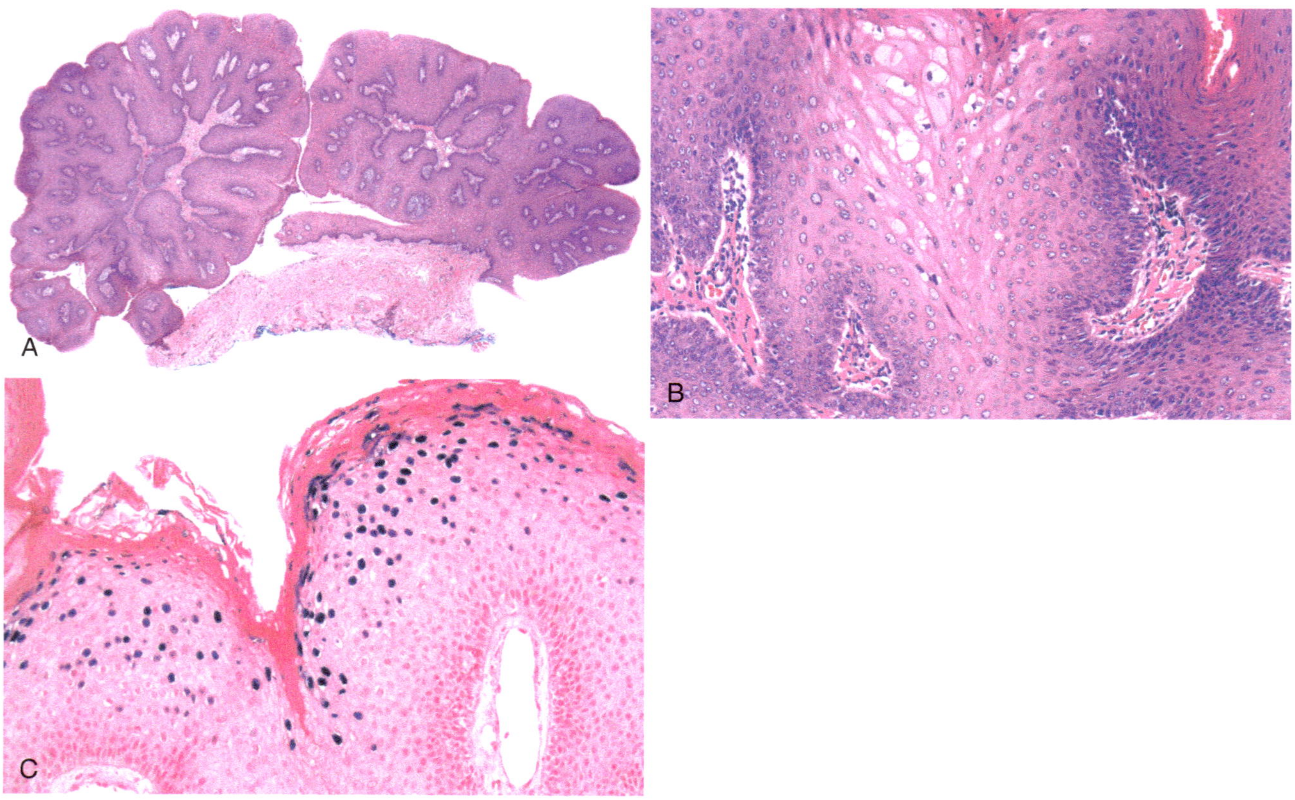

FIG 4.23 Condyloma acuminatum. (A) Parakeratosis and papillary epithelial hyperplasia with bulbous rete ridges. (B) Mild basal cell hyperplasia and subtle koilocytes. (C) In situ hybridization is positive for low-risk human papillomavirus subtypes.

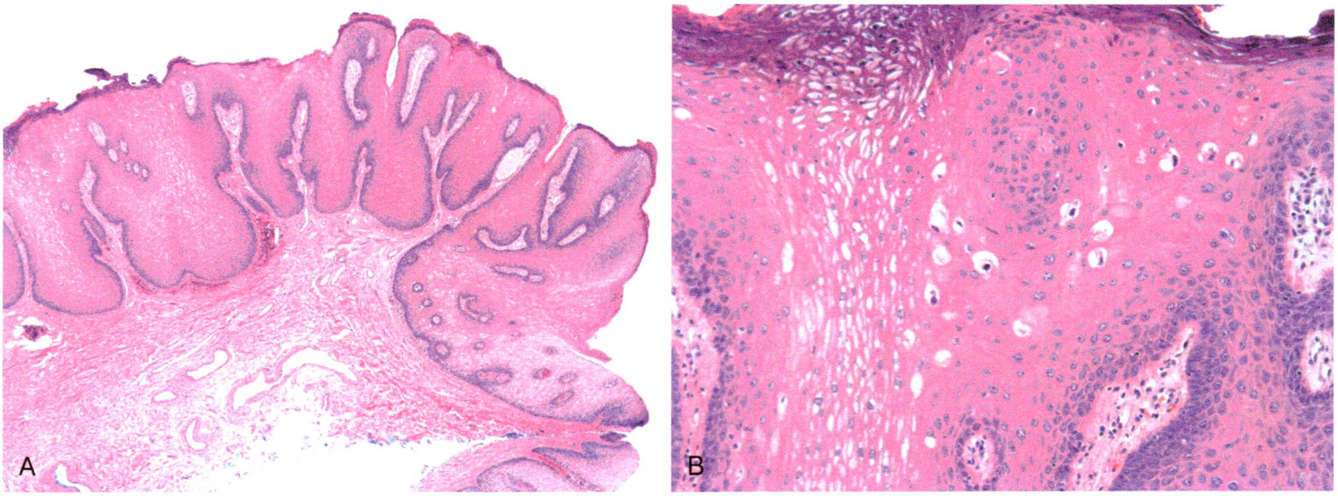

FIG 4.24 Condyloma acuminatum. (A) Parakeratosis and papillary and endophytic epithelial hyperplasia forming bulbous rete ridges. (B) Koilocytes are readily identified.

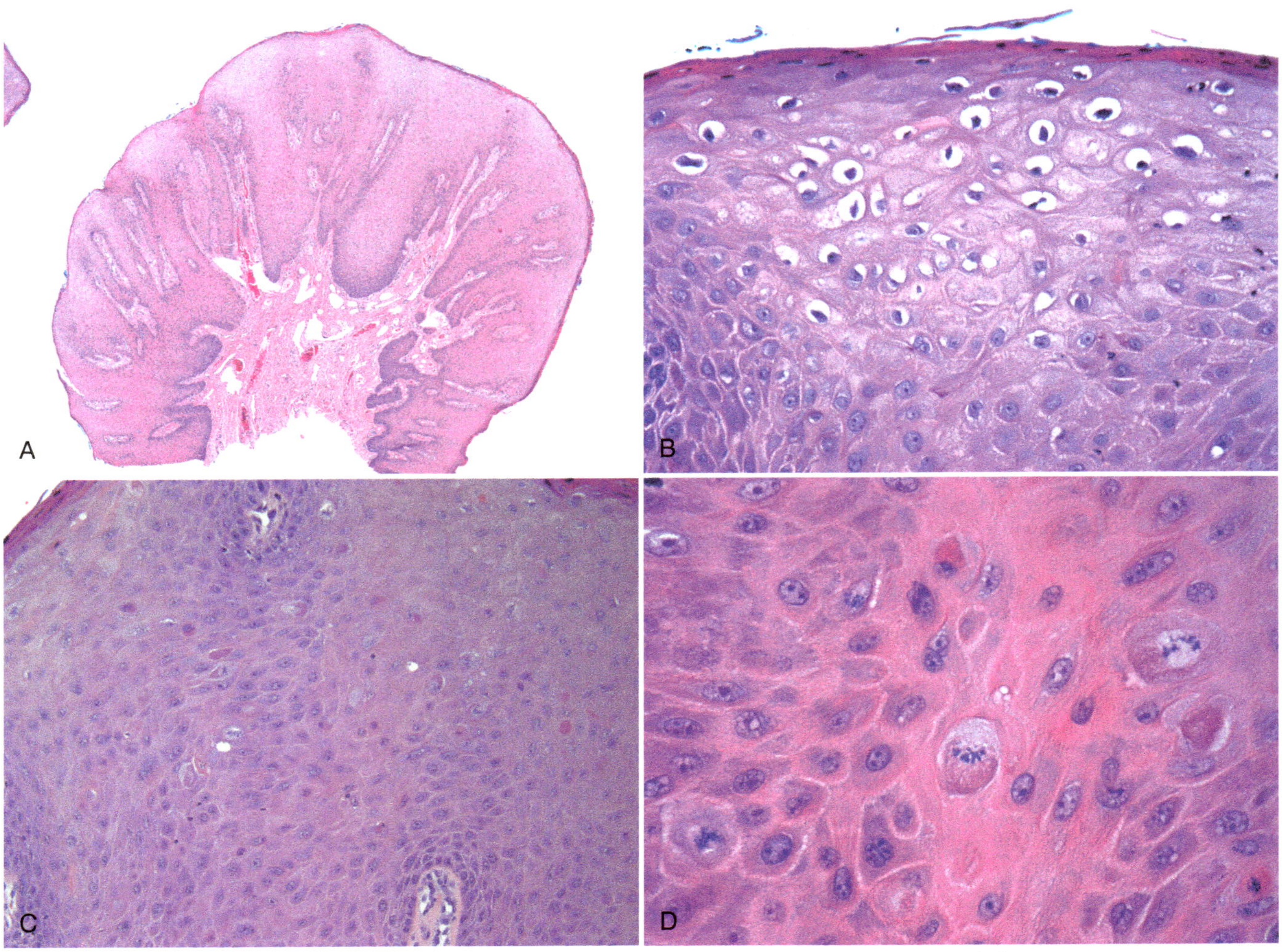

FIG 4.25 Heck disease. (A) Parakeratosis and benign epithelial hyperplasia. (B) Many koilocytes are present. (C) Karyorrhectic and apoptotic cells are noted throughout the epithelium. (D) Many karyorrhectic cells and brightly eosinophilic apoptotic cells are present.

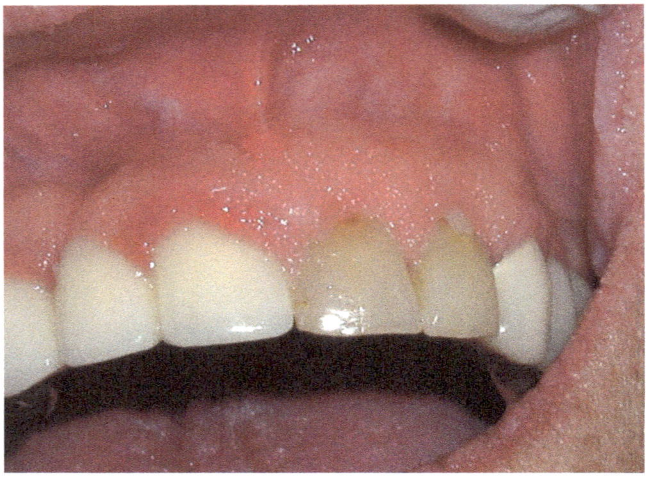

FIG 4.26 Acanthosis nigricans: diffuse papillomatosis of the anterior maxillary facial gingiva. *(From Damm DD, Roddy SC, White DK. Diffuse oral papillomatosis with corrugated lesions of the skin. Oral Surg Oral Med Oral Pathol Oral Radiol Endod. 2008;106:630–636.)*

Management and Prognosis

- Excision is the treatment of choice if lesions are solitary. Viral particles have been identified in laser plumes.
- Imiquimod may be useful for vermilion lesions, but it is difficult to keep the medication localized for intraoral applications.

REFERENCES

Abbey LM, Page DG, Sawyer DR. The clinical and histopathologic features of a series of 464 oral squamous papillomas. *Oral Surg Oral Med Oral Pathol.* 1980;49:419-428.

Anderson KM, Perez-Montiel D, Miles L, et al. The histologic differentiation of oral condyloma acuminatum from its mimics. *Oral Surg Oral Med Oral Pathol Oral Radiol Endod.* 2003;96:420-428.

Chrysomali E, Piperi E, Sklavounou-Andrikopoulou A. Oral acanthosis nigricans in chronic hepatitis B with a 21-year follow up. *J Dermatol.* 2011;38:1172-1176.

Cuberos V, Perez J, Lopez CJ, et al. Molecular and serological evidence of the epidemiological association of HPV 13 with focal epithelial hyperplasia: a case-control study. *J Clin Virol.* 2006;37:21-26.

Damm DD, Roddy SC, White DK. Diffuse oral papillomatosis with corrugated lesions of skin. *Oral Surg Oral Med Oral Pathol Oral Radiol Endod.* 2008;106:630-636.

González LV, Gaviria AM, Sanclemente G, et al. Clinical, histopathological and virological findings in patients with focal epithelial hyperplasia from Colombia. *Int J Dermatol.* 2005;44:274-279.

Said AK, Leao JC, Fedele S, Porter S. Focal epithelial hyperplasia—an update. *J Oral Pathol Med.* 2013;42:435-442.

Stojanov IJ, Woo SB. Human papillomavirus and Epstein-Barr virus associated conditions of the oral mucosa. *Semin Diagn Pathol.* 2015;32:3-11.

Syrjänen S. Current concepts on human papillomavirus infections in children. *APMIS.* 2010;118:494-509.

Zunt SL, Tomich CE. Oral condyloma acuminatum. *J Dermatol Surg Oncol.* 1989;15:591-594.

MOLLUSCUM CONTAGIOSUM

Molluscum contagiosum has a prevalence of 3% to 8%. Cases are transmitted by close physical contact through a breach in the skin (or mucosa) and fomites.

Clinical Findings

- These are most common in children under age 5 years and present as fleshy, dome-shaped papules with an umbilicated center containing yellowish, curdy material. Most patients have more than 15 lesions, which occur most frequently on the trunk and limbs; one-third occur in the skin of the head and neck, including perioral skin (Fig. 4.27). Intraoral lesions are uncommon.
- Patients with atopic dermatitis tend to have more lesions, and there is some association with swimming in public pools.
- Patients with immunocompromise or HIV/AIDS have severe outbreaks or giant lesions.

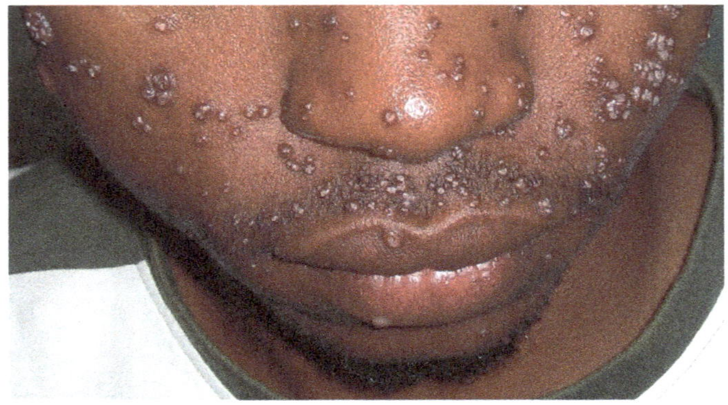

FIG 4.27 Molluscum contagiosum presenting as multiple umbilicated papules of the facial skin and lips in a patient with HIV/AIDS. *(Courtesy Dr. Adam Lipworth, Division of Dermatology, Brigham and Women's Hospital, Boston, Mass.)*

Etiopathogenesis and Histopathologic Features

Molluscum contagiosum is caused by the *molluscum contagiosum* virus, a large DNA virus of the *Poxviridae* family and *Molluscipox* genus. There are four subtypes, of which subtypes 1 and 2 are the most common, with subtype 2 being more common in those who are immunocompromised or have HIV/AIDS.

- There is endophytic acanthosis, often with the formation of a crateriform lesion where the keratinocytes of the middle and upper thirds of the epithelium contain intracytoplasmic molluscum bodies (or Henderson-Paterson bodies) that are basophilic or purplish-pink, and displace the nucleus (Fig. 4.28).

Management and Prognosis

- In healthy patients, cases generally resolve spontaneously within 12–18 months.
- Treatment modalities include curettage, cryotherapy, tretinoin, imiquimod, and pulsed dye laser therapy.

REFERENCES

Chen X, Anstey AV, Bugert JJ. *Molluscum contagiosum* virus infection. *Lancet Infect Dis.* 2013;13:877-888.

Cribier B, Scrivener Y, Grosshans E. Molluscum contagiosum: histologic patterns and associated lesions. A study of 578 cases. *Am J Dermatopathol.* 2001;23:99-103.

de Carvalho CH, de Andrade AL, de Oliveira DH, et al. Intraoral molluscum contagiosum in a young immunocompetent patient. *Oral Surg Oral Med Oral Pathol Oral Radiol.* 2012;114:e57-e60.

Ishikawa MK, Arps DP, Chow C, et al. Histopathological features of molluscum contagiosum other than molluscum bodies. *Histopathology.* 2015;67:836-842.

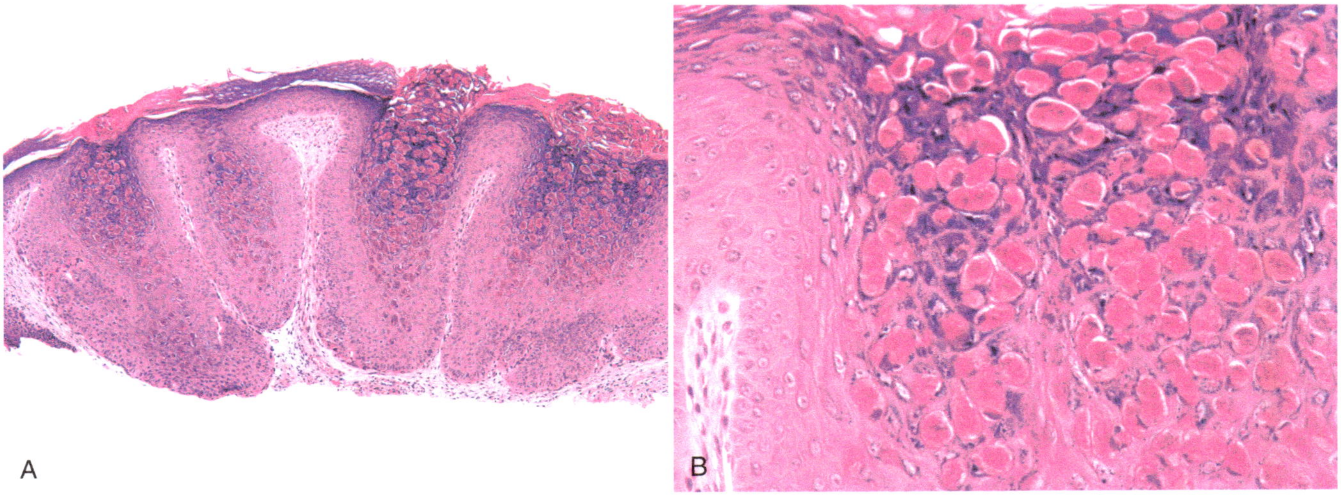

FIG 4.28 Molluscum contagiosum. (A) Endophytic epithelial hyperplasia with many viral inclusions. (B) Large, purple-pink molluscum bodies fill the cytoplasm and push the nucleus to the side.

CANDIDIASIS (CANDIDOSIS)

This is the most common fungal infection in the mouth.

Clinical Findings

Oral candidiasis has several clinical presentations.

- Thrush or pseudomembranous candidiasis: this presents as curdy, white papules and plaques with surrounding erythema that may or may not wipe off, associated with mouth soreness or sensitivity (Fig. 4.29A–B).
- Erythematous candidiasis: this presents as a sore erythematous area, without white papules, often outlined by the shape of a denture (referred to as *denture stomatitis*). It may also present as linear erythematous gingivitis in patients with HIV/AIDS (see Fig. 4.29C–D).
- Angular cheilitis: there is pain, cracking, fissuring, and maceration of the corners of the mouth, usually bilaterally. It is often seen in denture wearers where dentures do not adequately support the soft tissues, as well as in vitamin B12 and iron deficiencies (see Fig. 4.29E).
- Hyperplastic candidiasis: this occurs as white plaques and is often seen in mucocutaneous disease, endocrinopathies, and immunosuppression. It is common on the commissures bilaterally and often is associated with hairy leukoplakia.
- Median rhomboid glossitis (central papillary atrophy of tongue): this is an erythematous, ovoid, or rhomboid, sometimes nodular, plaque of the midline dorsum of the tongue, anterior to the circumvallate papillae (see Fig. 4.29F).
- Diffuse candidiasis on the tongue dorsum: this diffuse, red-and-white lesion on the tongue dorsum is often associated with similar "kissing" lesions on the palatal mucosa (see Fig. 4.29G–H).

Etiopathogenesis and Histopathologic Features

Oral candidiasis is an opportunistic infection that is caused by *Candida albicans* or other candidal species when there is (1) alteration of the local oral milieu (such as from hyposalivation), (2) local immunosuppression (such as use of topical antibiotics or corticosteroids), and (3) systemic use of antibiotics or immunosuppression. Because *Candida* is a commensal in 20% to 50% of the population, a positive culture in itself is not diagnostic for candidiasis. Scraping the lesion and use of either potassium hydroxide or standard cytology stains to identify hyphae is diagnostic, as is a biopsy (Fig. 4.29I).

- Parakeratosis, epithelial hyperplasia (often psoriasiform), neutrophilic exocytosis and spongiotic pustules, reactive epithelial atypia, vascular ectasia, and variable lymphocytic infiltrate are present (Fig. 4.30A–C). Candidal hyphae and/or spores are seen with periodic acid–Schiff stain with diastase digestion or methenamine silver stain (see Fig. 4.30D). Some cases exhibit epithelial atrophy (Fig. 4.31).
- Median rhomboid glossitis: there is loss of filiform papillae with spongiotic pustules and candidal hyphae. The median raphe is a hyalinized band seen only in the midline of the tongue dorsum (Fig. 4.32).

Differential Diagnosis

- Epithelial dysplasia with secondary candidiasis may be difficult to differentiate from candidiasis with reactive atypia (see Fig. 4.31B); however, effective treatment returns the mucosa to normal in cases of candidiasis with reactive atypia.
- Spongiotic pustules are also seen in (see relevant sections):
  - Benign migratory glossitis/stomatitis (see Chapter 8)
  - Edge of an ulcer or erosion (see Chapter 7)
  - Irritant contact stomatitis (see Chapter 7)
  - Oral psoriasis (extremely rare)
- *Geotrichum candidum* (causing geotrichosis) forms short septate hyphae.

Management and Prognosis

- Topical antifungal agents (without or without a topical steroid) and systemic antifungal medications are listed in Appendix B. Topical medications may be associated

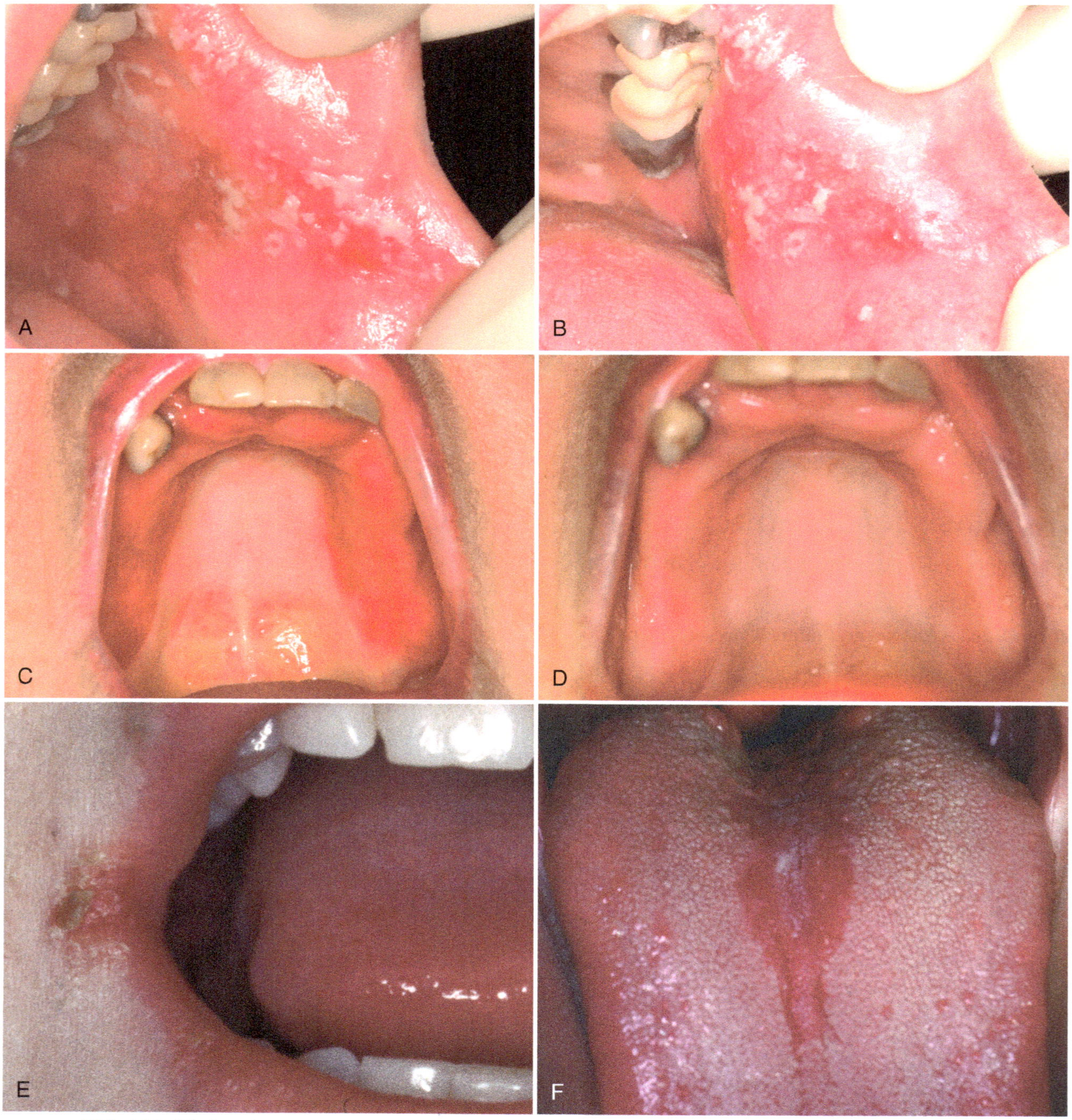

FIG 4.29 (A) Pseudomembranous candidiasis: white plaques and erythema. (B) Pseudomembranous candidiasis: lesion shown in A scrapes off. (C) Erythematous candidiasis: erythema in the outline of denture. (D) Erythematous candidiasis: same patient as in C after treatment with nystatin and triamcinolone paste applied to denture. (E) Angular cheilitis. (F) Median rhomboid glossitis.

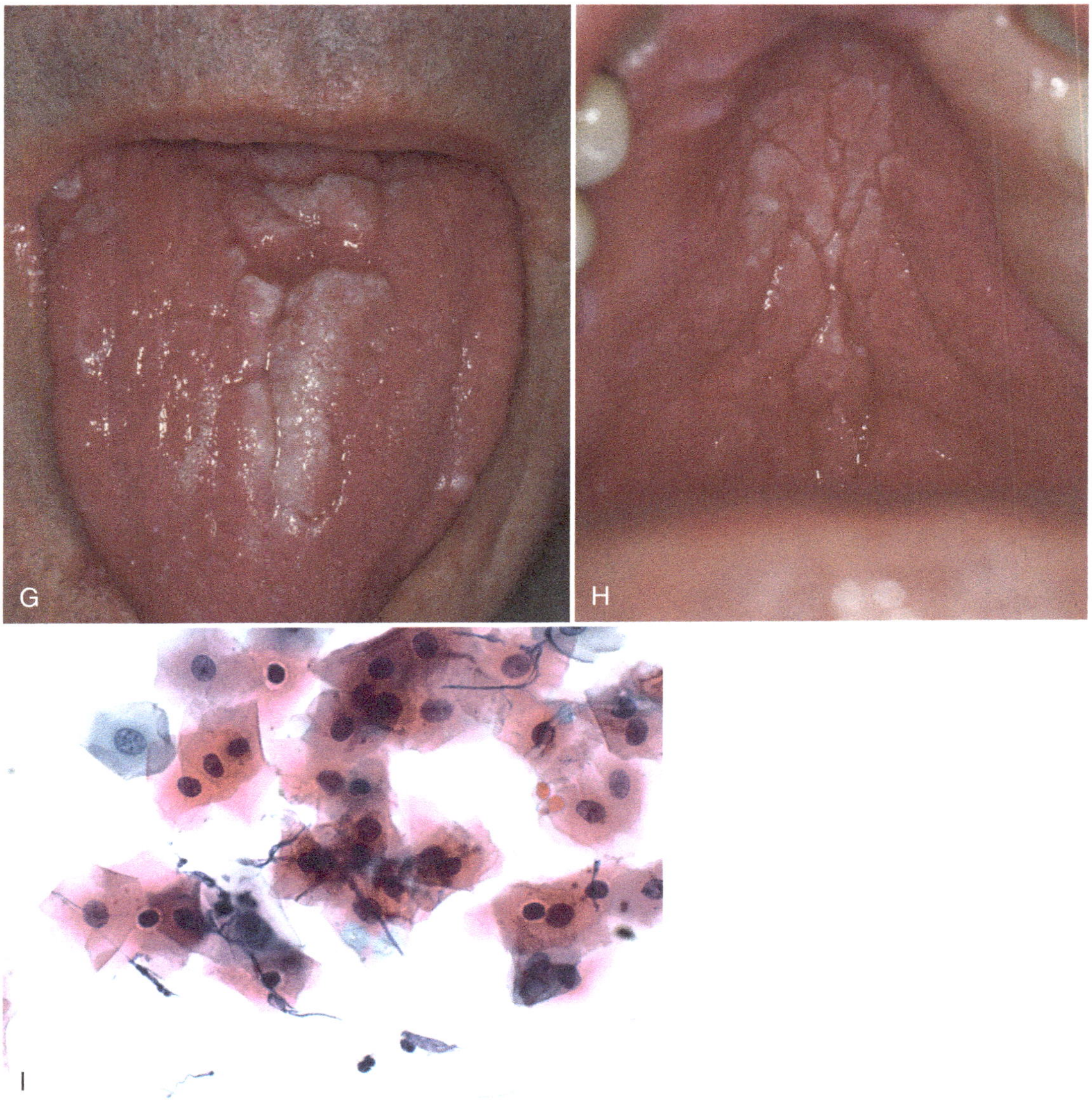

FIG 4.29, cont'd (G) Diffuse candidiasis of the tongue dorsum with "kissing lesion" on the palatal mucosa. (H) Same patient as in G, with palatal candidiasis. (I) Scraping of lesion for cytology reveals many candidal hyphae.

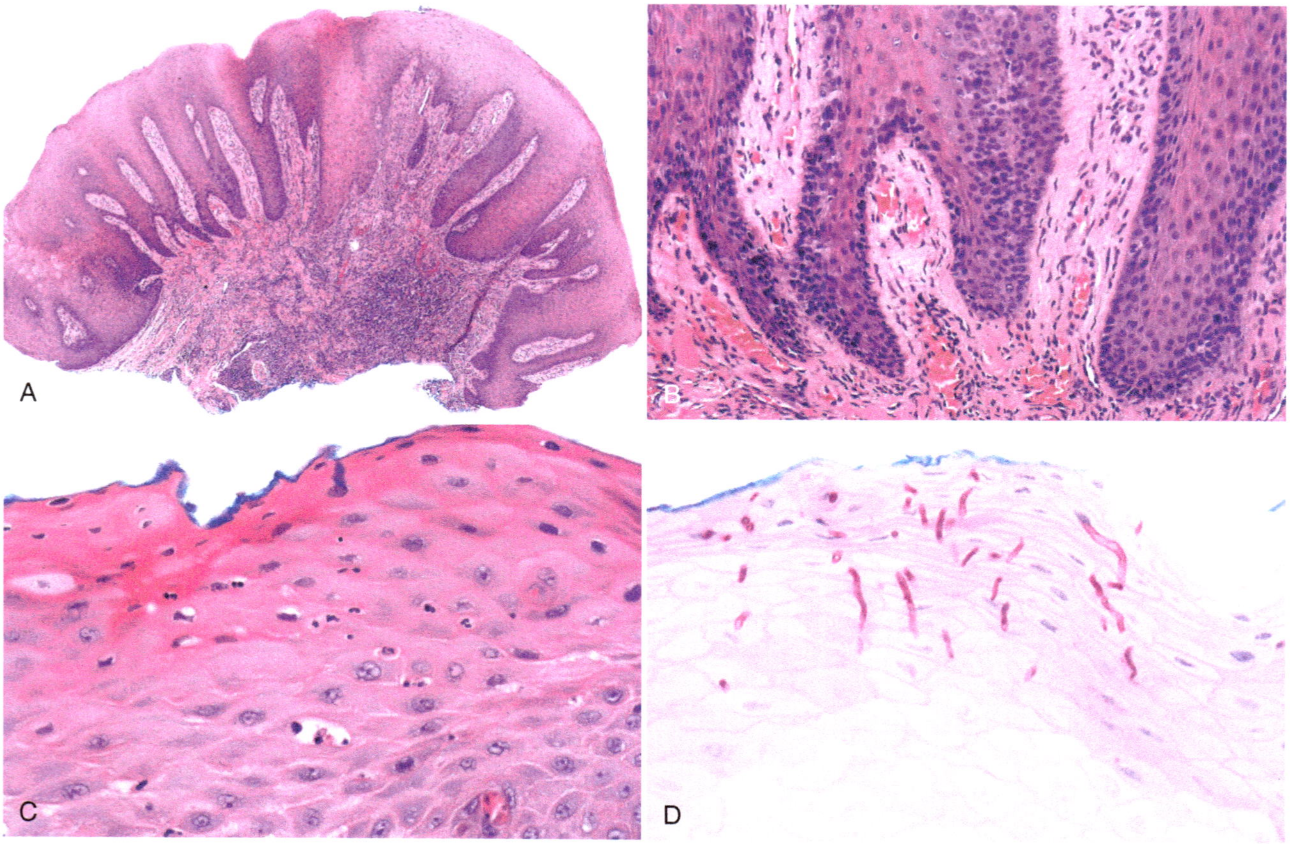

FIG 4.30 Candidiasis. (A) Psoriasiform epithelial hyperplasia with chronic inflammation. (B) Mild reactive epithelial atypia. (C) Neutrophilic exocytosis and early spongiotic pustules. (D) Periodic acid–Schiff stain with diastase digestion reveals candidal hyphae.

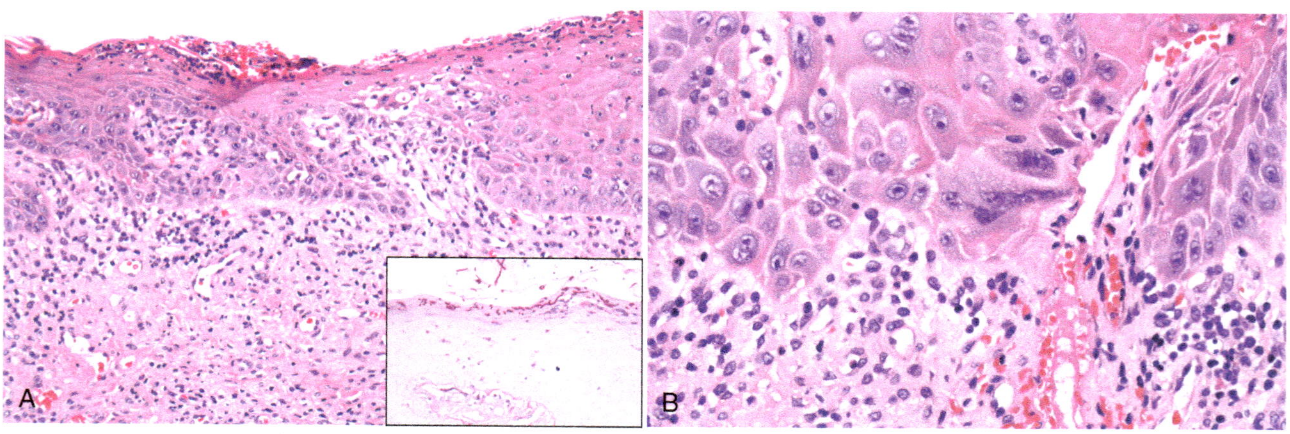

FIG 4.31 Candidiasis. (A) Parakeratosis, epithelial atrophy, spongiotic pustules, and chronic inflammation. Periodic acid–Schiff stain with diastase digestion reveals candidal hyphae (*inset*). (B) Reactive epithelial atypia with multinucleated epithelial cells with abundant cytoplasm.

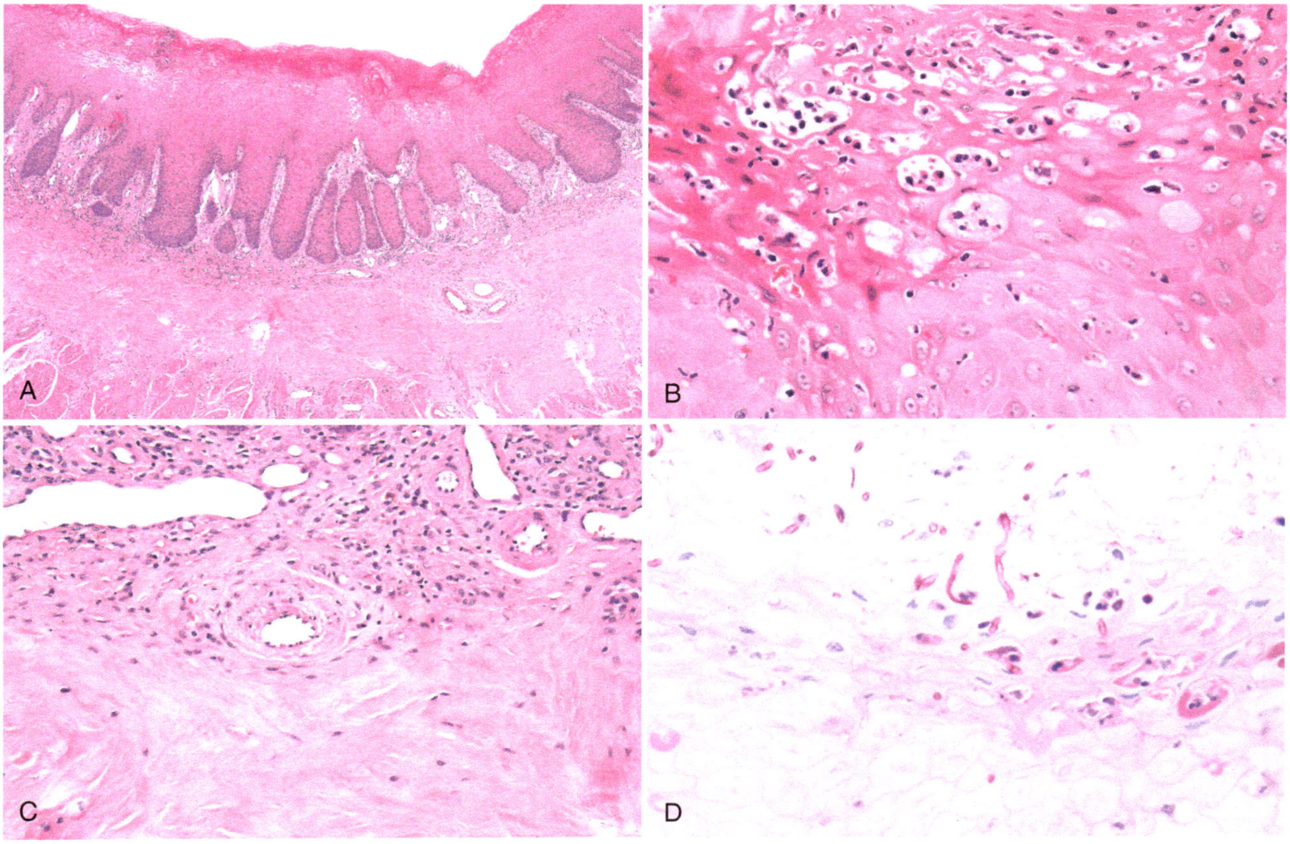

FIG 4.32 Median rhomboid glossitis. (A) Parakeratosis, atrophy of filiform papillae, psoriasiform epithelial hyperplasia, and hyaline median raphe. (B) Many spongiotic pustules are present. (C) Densely hyalinized median raphe identifies this site as midline dorsum of tongue. (D) Periodic acid–Schiff stain with diastase digestion reveals many candidal hyphae.

with poor compliance because of the need for frequent dosing.

- *Staphylococcus aureus* is present in up to 30% of patients with angular cheilitis, and topical erythromycin is helpful if lesions are recalcitrant.

REFERENCES

Akpan A, Morgan R. Oral candidiasis. *Postgrad Med J*. 2002;78:455-459.

Bonifaz A, Vázquez-González D, Macías B, et al. Oral geotrichosis: report of 12 cases. *J Oral Sci*. 2010;52:477-483.

Dias AP, Samaranayake LP. Clinical, microbiological and ultrastructural features of angular cheilitis lesions in Southern Chinese. *Oral Dis*. 1995;1:43-48.

Pienaar ED, Young T, Holmes H. Interventions for the prevention and management of oropharyngeal candidiasis associated with HIV infection in adults and children. *Cochrane Database Syst Rev*. 2010;(11):CD003940.

Sitheeque MA, Samaranayake LP. Chronic hyperplastic candidosis/candidiasis (candidal leukoplakia). *Crit Rev Oral Biol Med*. 2003;14:253-267.

Wright BA. Median rhomboid glossitis: not a misnomer. *Oral Surg Oral Med Oral Pathol*. 1978;46:806-814.

DEEP FUNGAL INFECTIONS

A deep fungal infection infrequently may have its first presentation in the oral cavity; if so, a work-up must be undertaken to identify concomitant systemic or skin involvement. Only the more common ones are discussed here.

Clinical Findings

- Deep fungal infections present as ulcers, or indurated, granular, vegetating plaques and nodules of the oral mucosa, and concomitant lung, lymph node, and skin disease may be present. Lesions may be penetrating and necrotic, resulting in "midline destructive disease" of the palatal mucosa, leading to oronasal or oroantral perforation.
- Immunocompromised patients with cancer, neutropenia, and/or HIV/AIDS, as well as those who are post–organ transplantation, are particularly susceptible to disseminated disease, as are those on new biologic agents such as tumor necrosis factor-alpha.
- There are three endemic mycoses in the United States:
  - Histoplasmosis caused by *Histoplasma capsulatum* is endemic in the Ohio-Mississippi Valley, and the organism is found in the soil and in bird and bat droppings.
  - North American blastomycosis caused by *Blastomyces dermatitidis* is endemic in the Mid-Atlantic States and southwestern states bordering the Mississippi Valley. The organism is found in soil, and, as such, this infection often affects agricultural and construction workers. Sixty to eighty percent have oral and skin manifestations that resemble pyoderma gangrenosum.

- Coccidioidomycosis ("valley fever") caused by *Coccidioides immitis* is endemic in the San Joaquin Valley in California. The organism is found in soil, and, as such, this infection also primarily affects agricultural workers. *Coccidioides posadasii* is endemic in the southwestern United States and South and Central America.
- Paracoccidioidomycosis is caused by *Paracoccidioides brasiliensis,* a soil saprophyte. It is common in South America, where 80% to 90% of cases are chronic (Fig. 4.33).
- Cryptococcosis is caused by *Cryptococcus neoformans.* It is often found in bird droppings and often causes meningitis in patients with HIV/AIDS and in organ transplant recipients.
- Mucormycoses are often caused by *Rhizopus, Mucor,* and *Lichtheimia* (the most common genera causing disease), and these are found in soil and decaying vegetation. They are seen most frequently in patients with diabetes mellitus (especially if ketoacidotic) as orbitorhinocerebral disease, as well as in patients with hematologic malignancies who undergo chemotherapy or allogeneic hematopoietic stem cell transplantation. The mortality rate is 60% to 90%. A black eschar is a typical presentation.
- Aspergillosis is caused by *Aspergillus fumigatus* or *A. flavus* and is usually found in decaying vegetation. It often affects patients with hematologic malignancies and post–organ transplantation, with an up to 50% mortality rate. It is also seen in immunocompetent patients. Lesions present as black, necrotic plaques resembling malignancy. Inhaled *Aspergillus* may lead to noninvasive allergic fungal sinusitis in patients who are atopic and have a history of allergic sinusitis.
- Identification of the organism is done by biopsy, histochemical staining, immunohistochemistry, culture, enzyme immunoassay, PCR, and serology, such as for galactomannan and β-D-glucan, as well as by identification of antigens in serum and urine.

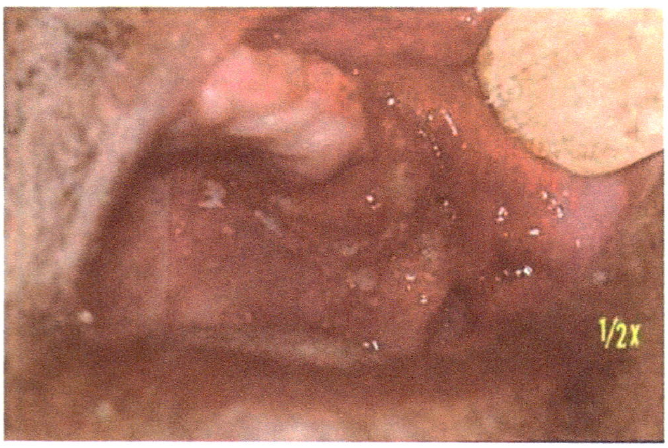

FIG 4.33 Oral paracoccidioidomycosis: ulcerated and erythematous lesion of palatal mucosa. *(Courtesy Dr. Roman Carlos, Guatemala City, Guatemala.)*

Etiopathogenesis and Histopathologic Features

Most of these organisms cause granulomatous (often necrotizing) inflammation, although granulomas are not seen as frequently in mucormycosis. All are positive with methenamine silver stain. Pulmonary disease is one of the primary manifestations. Hematologic dissemination or direct inhalation and inoculation onto the oral mucosa lead to oral lesions.

- Histoplasmosis: there is granulomatous inflammation, sometimes with necrosis. Organisms are small, narrow-based budding yeast forms that are abundant within macrophages (Fig. 4.34).
- North American blastomycosis: there is pseudoepitheliomatous hyperplasia with suppuration and thick-walled fungi with multiple asymmetric, broad-based budding yeast cells (Fig. 4.35).
- Coccidioidomycosis: there is pseudoepitheliomatous hyperplasia with granulomatous inflammation and often suppuration, and thick-walled spherules with endospores are characteristic (Fig. 4.36).

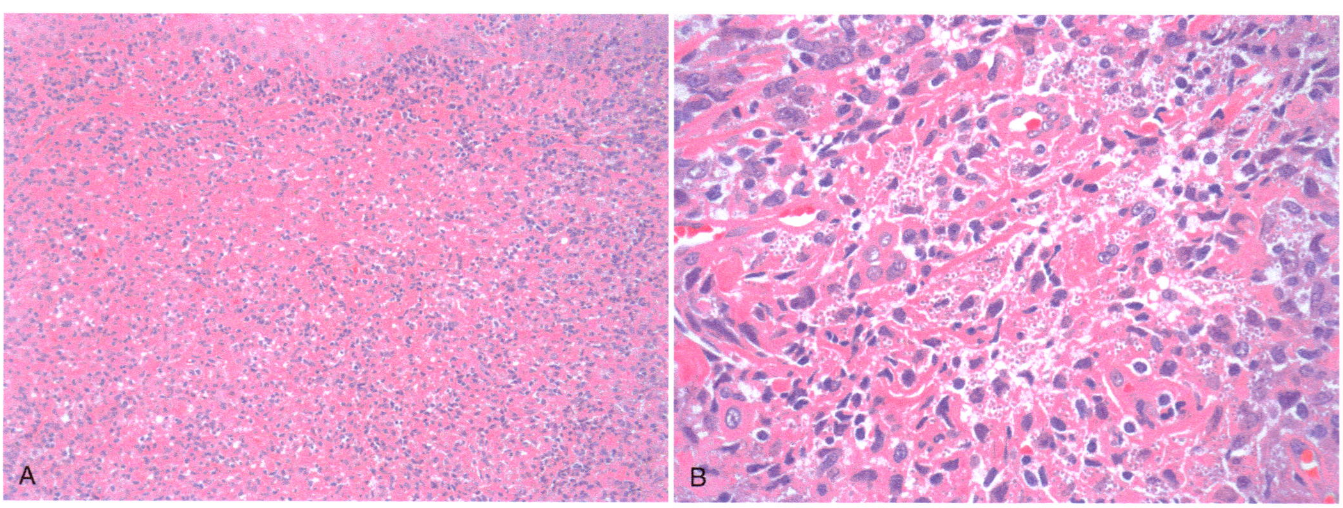

FIG 4.34 Histoplasmosis. (A) There are sheets of macrophages present in the lamina propria. (B) There are numerous organisms, dot-like, within macrophages. *(A and B, Courtesy Dr. Lee Slater, Scripps University, San Diego, Calif.)*

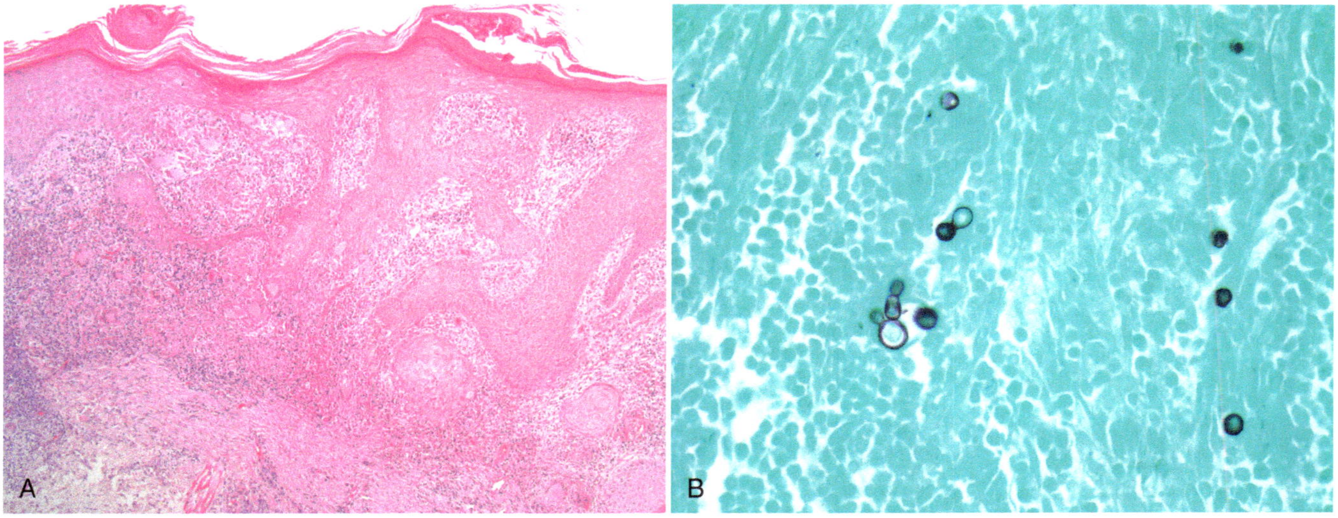

FIG 4.35 North American blastomycosis. (A) Pseudoepitheliomatous hyperplasia with many granulomas and multinucleated giant cells. (B) Organisms are broad-based budding yeasts (methenamine silver stain). *(Courtesy Dr. Dan Milner, Harvard Medical School, Boston, Mass.)*

- Paracoccidioidomycosis: there is pseudoepitheliomatous hyperplasia with suppuration and budding yeast cells with a "ship's wheel" or "Mickey Mouse ears" appearance (Fig. 4.37).
- Cryptococcosis: there is granulomatous inflammation with narrow-based budding yeast cells that have thick mucopolysaccharide capsules that stain strongly with mucicarmine (Fig. 4.38).
- Mucormycosis: this does not usually lead to granuloma formation, and the organism is ribbon-like with right-angle branching. Angioinvasion leads to necrosis (Fig. 4.39).
- Aspergillosis: there is granulomatous inflammation with suppuration, and angioinvasion leads to necrosis. Organisms are slender and show acute-angle branching (Fig. 4.40). Invasive *Aspergillus* within the tissues must be differentiated from two other conditions in the sinus: (1) Allergic fungal sinusitis leads to abundant "allergic" eosinophilic mucin containing a few fungal forms (usually of the dematiaceous family, such as *Bipolaris* or *Curvularia*), many eosinophils, and often Charcot-Leyden crystals; and (2) chronic, noninvasive fungal sinusitis leads to colonization of the sinus by masses of fungi, resulting in a mycetoma or "fungus ball" (usually *Aspergillus*) with little mucin (Fig. 4.41).

Differential Diagnosis

- Pseudoepitheliomatous hyperplasia must be differentiated from squamous cell carcinoma, which exhibits epithelial proliferation but with significant cytologic atypia and evidence of invasion.
- Sarcoidosis produces nonnecrotizing granulomas, as does Crohn disease, but organisms would not be identified (see Fig. 8.13 in Chapter 8).

Management

- Treatment is with surgical excision of the infected tissue and antimicrobial therapy with amphotericin B, itraconazole, voriconazole, posaconazole, isavuconazole, and echinocandins.

REFERENCES

Almeida OP, Jacks J Jr, Scully C. Paracoccidioidomycosis of the mouth: an emerging deep mycosis. *Crit Rev Oral Biol Med.* 2003;14:377-383.

Bernardeschi C, Foulet F, Ingen-Housz-Oro S, et al. Cutaneous invasive aspergillosis: retrospective multicenter study of the French Invasive-Aspergillosis Registry and literature review. *Medicine (Baltimore).* 2015;94:e1018.

Bonifaz A, Macias B, Paredes-Farrera F, et al. Palatal zygomycosis: experience of 21 cases. *Oral Dis.* 2008;14:569-574.

Fernandez-Flores A, Saeb-Lima M, Arenas-Guzman R. Morphological findings of deep cutaneous fungal infections. *Am J Dermatopathol.* 2014;36:531-553, quiz 554-556.

Granville L, Chirala M, Cernoch P, et al. Fungal sinusitis: histologic spectrum and correlation with culture. *Hum Pathol.* 2004;35:474-481.

Guarner J, Brandt ME. Histopathologic diagnosis of fungal infections in the 21st century. *Clin Microbiol Rev.* 2011;24:247-280.

Henao-Martínez AF, Beckham JD. Cryptococcosis in solid organ transplant recipients. *Curr Opin Infect Dis.* 2015;28:300-307.

Hernández SL, López De Blanc SA, Sambuelli RH, et al. Oral histoplasmosis associated with HIV infection: a comparative study. *J Oral Pathol Med.* 2004;33:445-450.

Marques SA. Fungal infections of the mucous membrane. *Dermatol Ther.* 2010;23:243-250.

Mignogna MD, Fortuna G, Leuci S, et al. Mucormycosis in immunocompetent patients: a case-series of patients with maxillary sinus involvement and a critical review of the literature. *Int J Infect Dis.* 2011;15:e533-e540.

Parish JM, Blair JE. Coccidioidomycosis. *Mayo Clin Proc.* 2008;83:343-348, quiz 348-349.

Petrikkos G, Skiada A, Lortholary O, et al. Epidemiology and clinical manifestations of mucormycosis. *Clin Infect Dis.* 2012;54(suppl 1):S23-S34.

Reder PA, Neel HB 3rd. Blastomycosis in otolaryngology: review of a large series. *Laryngoscope.* 1993;103:53-58.

Roden MM, Zaoutis TE, Buchanan WL, et al. Epidemiology and outcome of zygomycosis: a review of 929 reported cases. *Clin Infect Dis.* 2005;41:634-653.

Smith JA, Kauffman CA. Endemic fungal infections in patients receiving tumour necrosis factor-alpha inhibitor therapy. *Drugs.* 2009;69:1403-1415.

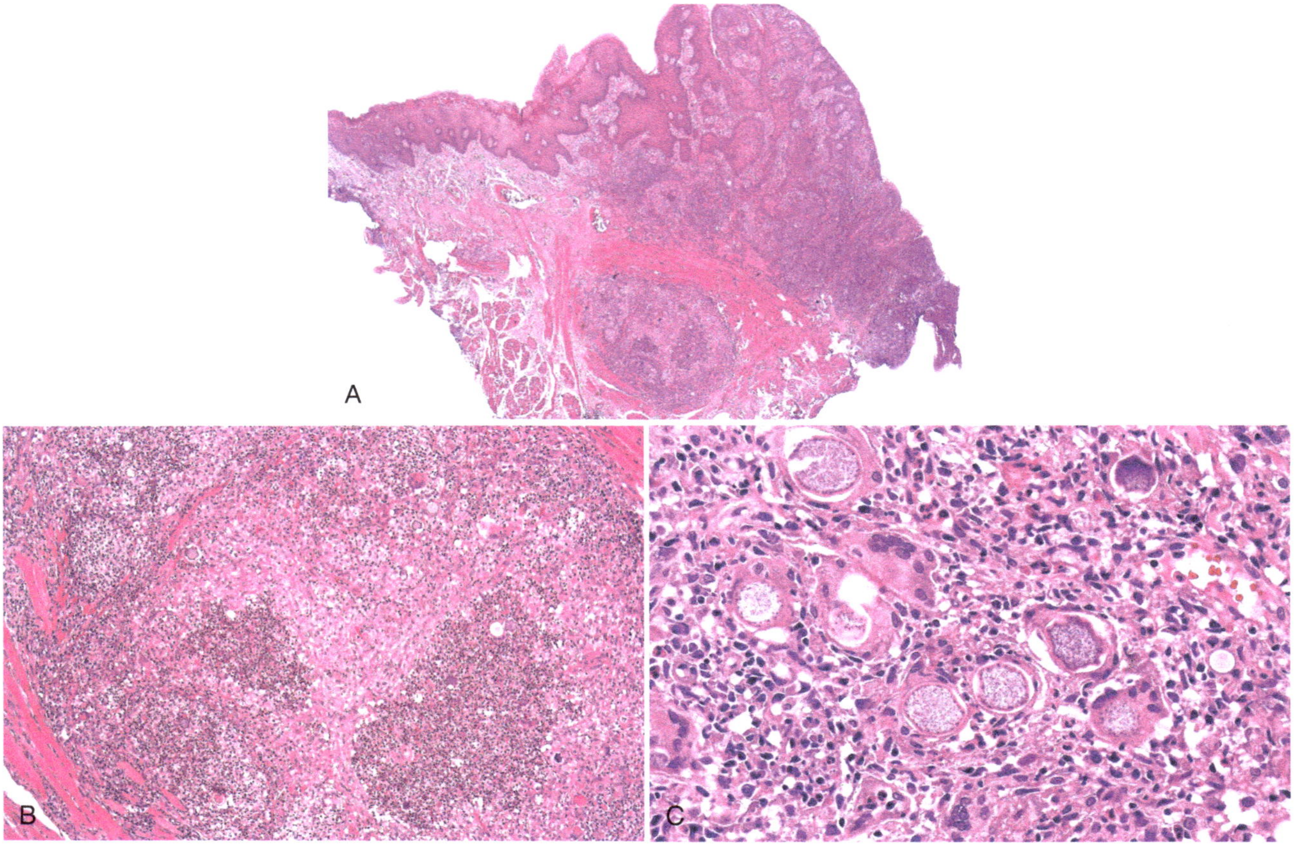

FIG 4.36 Coccidioidomycosis. (A) Pseudoepitheliomatous hyperplasia and granulomatous inflammation involving muscle. (B) Necrotizing and suppurative granulomatous inflammation. (C) Granulomas with large spherules containing many endospores. *(Courtesy Dr. Roman Carlos, Guatemala City, Guatemala.)*

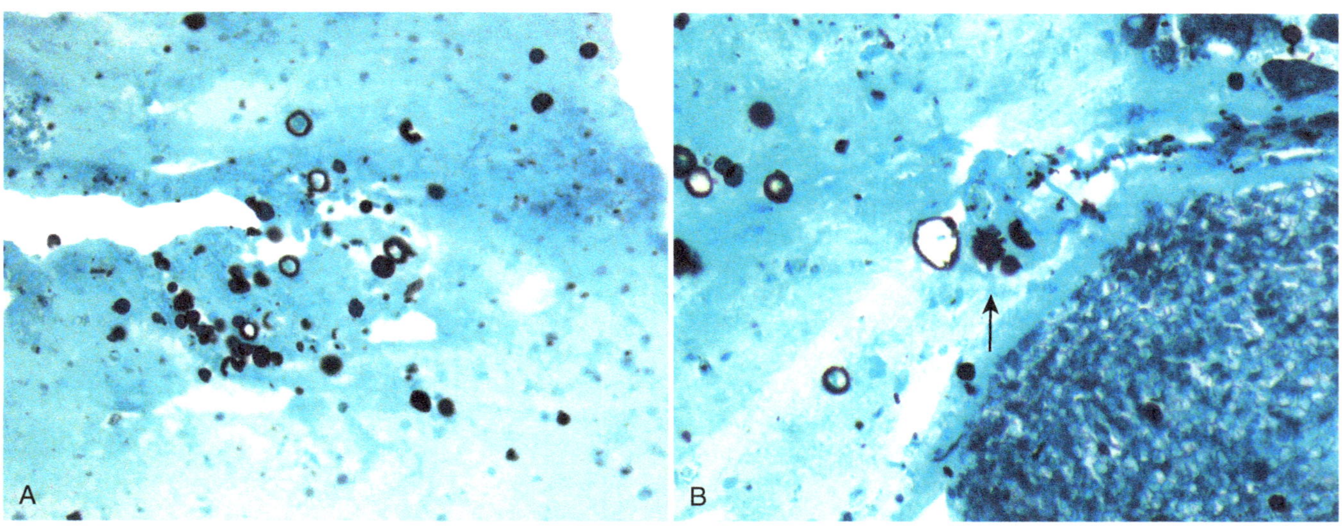

FIG 4.37 Paracoccidioidomycosis. (A) Budding yeast forms that are methenamine silver–positive. (B) Typical circumferential budding of yeasts giving rise to a "ship's wheel" appearance (*arrow*) (methenamine silver stain). *(Courtesy Dr. Dan Milner, Harvard Medical School, Boston, Mass.)*

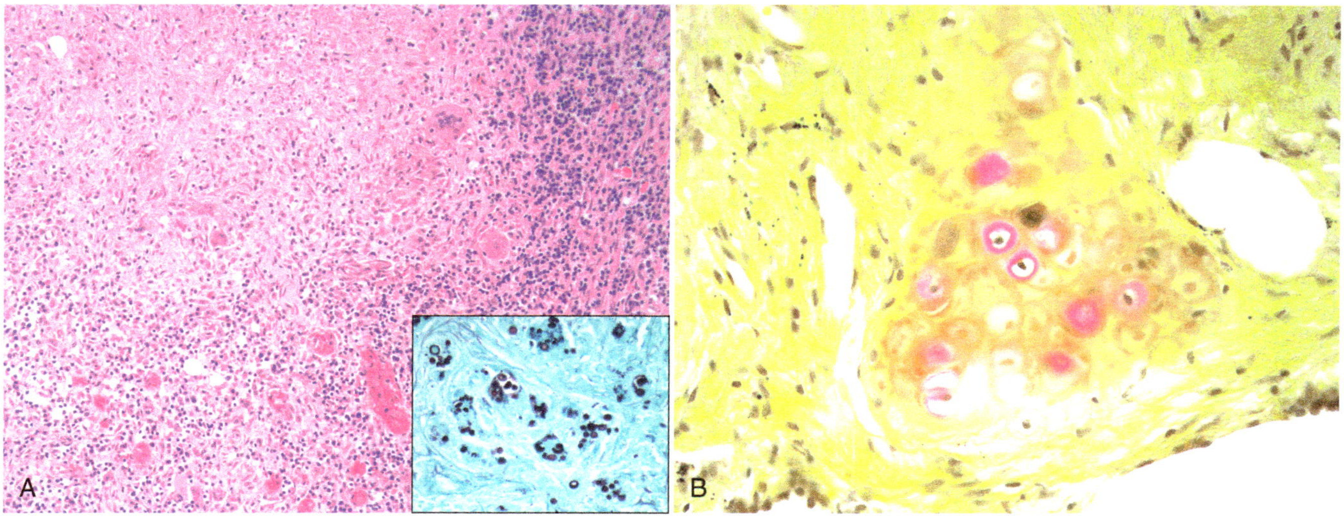

FIG 4.38 Cryptococcosis. (A) Granulomatous inflammation with budding yeast forms with thick capsules (*inset*, methenamine silver stain). (B) Organisms showing thick, mucicarmine-positive walls (mucicarmine stain) *(Courtesy Dr. Dan Milner, Harvard Medical School, Boston, Mass.)*

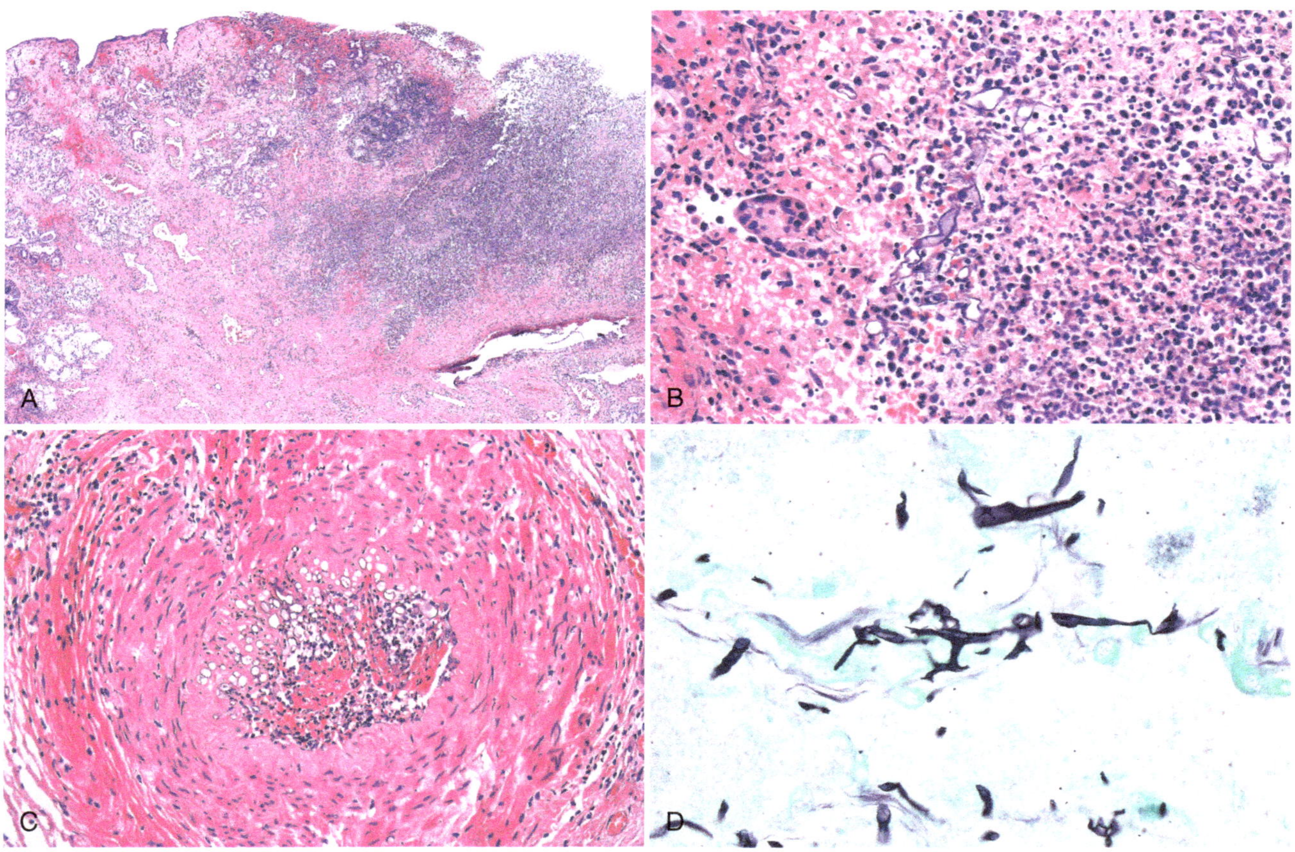

FIG 4.39 Mucormycosis. (A) Sinus mucosa exhibiting areas of necrosis and ulceration. (B) Ribbon-like fungi within area of necrosis. (C) Artery with fungi within the wall. (D) Ribbon-like organism with right-angled branching (methenamine silver stain). *(A, Courtesy Dr. Dan Milner, Harvard Medical School, Boston, Mass.)*

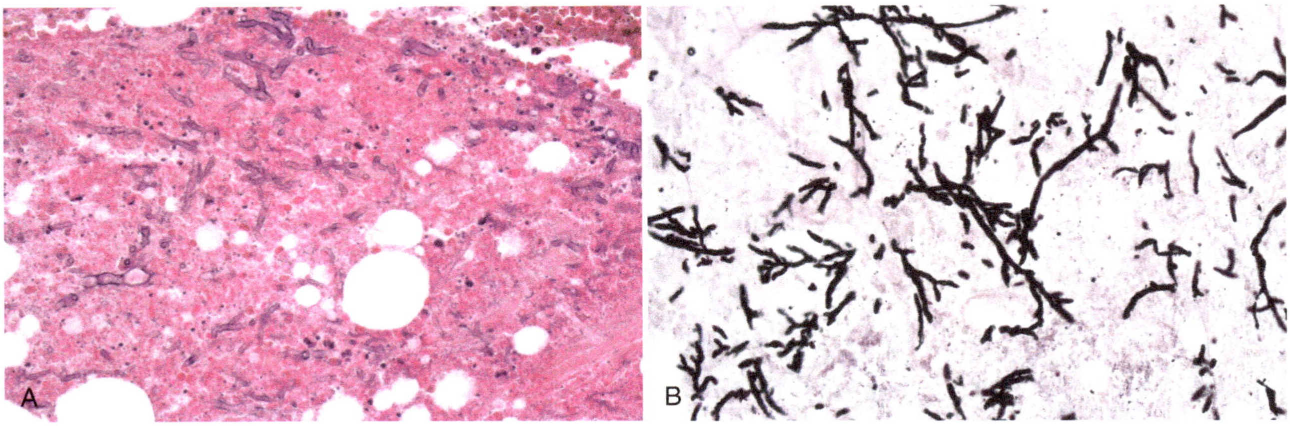

FIG 4.40 Aspergillosis. (A) Fungi within area of necrosis. (B) Fungal hyphae with acute-angled branching (methenamine silver stain). *(A, Courtesy Dr. Dan Milner, Harvard Medical School, Boston, Mass.)*

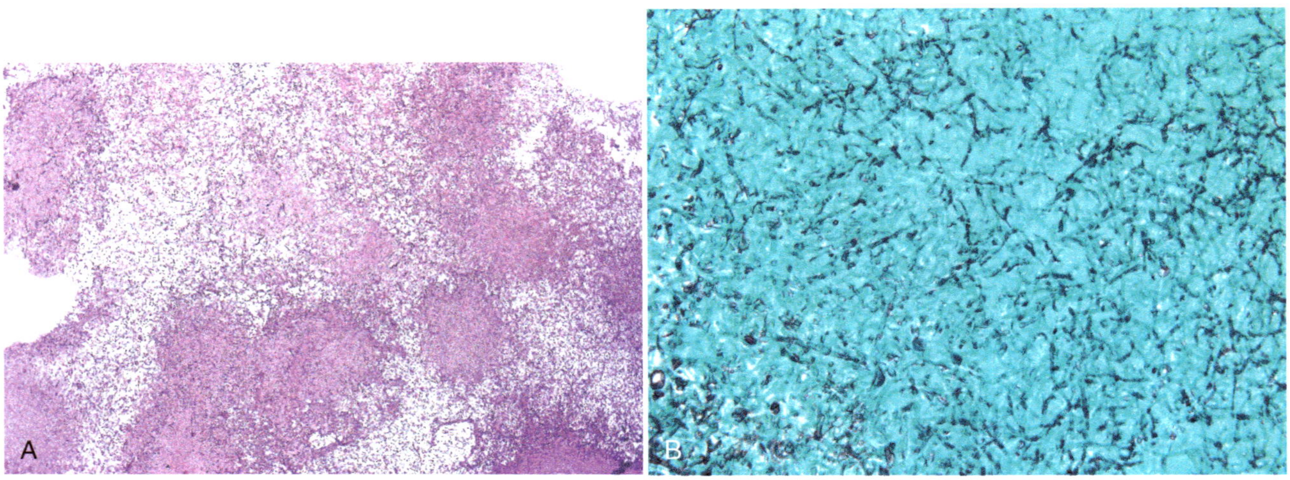

FIG 4.41 Mycetoma of chronic noninvasive fungal sinusitis. (A) Mass of fungi within the sinus, not invading the soft tissues. (B) Tangled masses of silver-positive fungal hyphae (methenamine silver stain).

TUBERCULOSIS

Tuberculosis is the second most common cause of death from a single infectious agent worldwide, after HIV/AIDS. Up to 10 million new cases are diagnosed each year, and approximately 0.5 million patients have multidrug-resistant tuberculosis. Those who are sick with HIV/AIDS are more likely to contract this illness. While oral lesions are noted in less than 5% of patients with pulmonary tuberculosis, the prevalence of primary oral tuberculosis may be as high as 30%.

Clinical Findings

- Tuberculosis usually occurs in the second to fourth decades of life and presents as an ulcer of the oral mucosa or osteolytic lesions within the jawbones, with some patients exhibiting tuberculous lymphadenitis (scrofula) and salivary gland involvement (Fig. 4.42). Tuberculosis is seen in those living in crowded conditions.
- Systemic symptoms include productive cough, fever, night sweats, and weight loss.
- Reactivation of latent tuberculosis infection is a significant adverse effect of the use of tumor necrosis factor-alpha inhibitors, and patients to be placed on such medications should be screened for tuberculosis. Organ transplant recipients are also at risk for reactivation of latent infection.
- Some helpful tests include performing the tuberculin skin (Mantoux) test, chest radiography to identify pulmonary lesions, and the QuantiFERON-TB Gold In-Tube test (QIAGEN, Valencia, Calif), an interferon-γ release assay, this test being positive for both active and latent infections. Cultures take several weeks to confirm positivity or negativity.

Etiopathogenesis and Histopathologic Features

Primary infection is in the lungs due to inhaled infected particles, and oral mucosal involvement is likely due to direct inoculation of sputum onto an oral ulcer. The

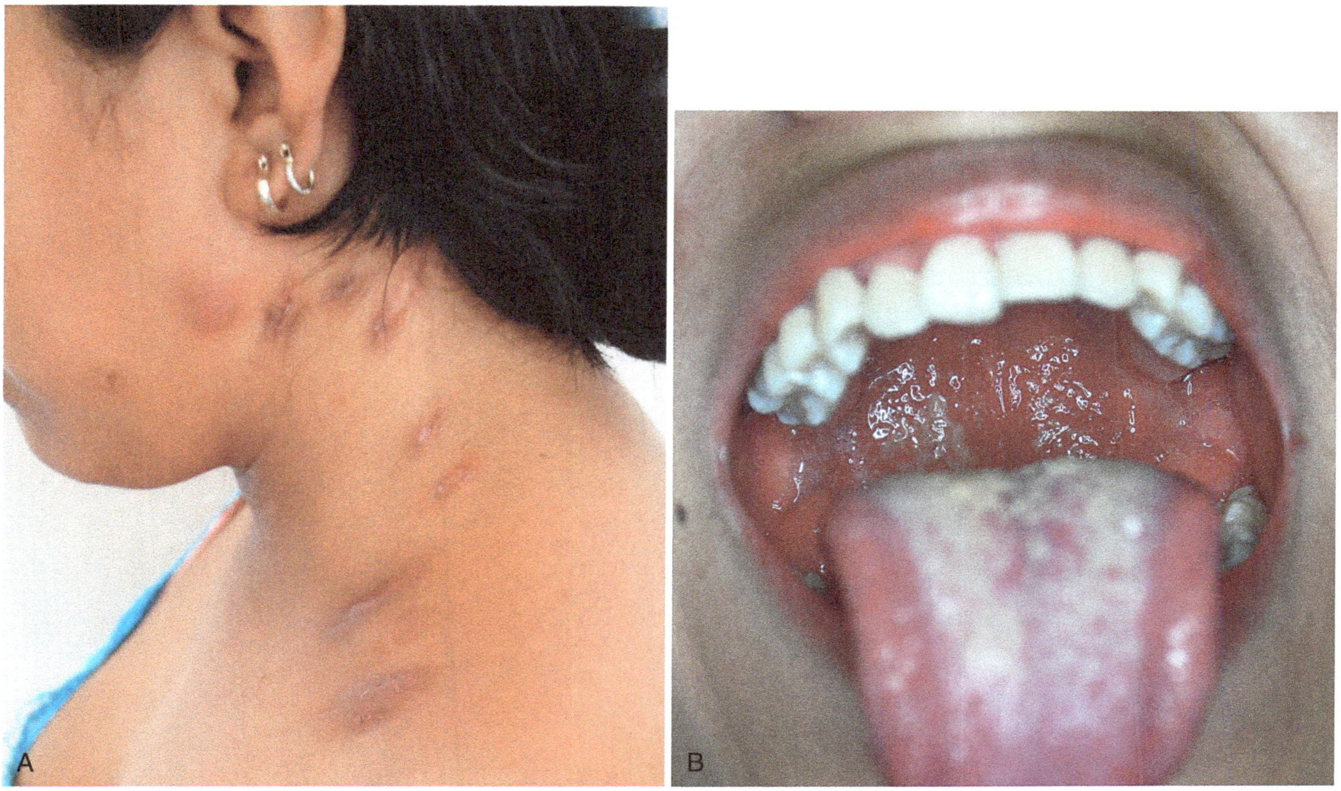

FIG 4.42 (A) Tuberculosis of the cervical nodes (scrofula) and skin. (B) Tuberculosis of the soft palate presenting as ulceration and erythema. *(Courtesy Dr. Roman Carlos, Guatemala City, Guatemala.)*

mycobacterium incites a type IV hypersensitivity reaction mediated through Th1 responses. The most common pathogen is *Mycobacterium tuberculosis*, a facultative intracellular bacterium that can persist in macrophages as well as extracellularly, possibly within areas of necrosis, the reservoirs for latent infection.

- Necrotizing granulomas containing tiny, rod-shaped, acid-fast bacilli are identified with Ziehl-Neelsen or Kinyoun stain (Fig. 4.43). Langhans-type giant cells with nuclei aligned in a horseshoe pattern are often seen, but these are also seen in other granulomatous conditions.
- PCR is a more sensitive diagnostic test if bacilli are not seen on microscopy.

Differential Diagnosis

- Other infectious granulomatous conditions, such as deep fungal infections, are identified with methenamine silver stain.
- *M. leprae* results in similar granulomatous inflammation. The organism is identified with the Fite stain. Orofacial lesions of leprosy are usually seen in lepromatous leprosy and consist of mucocutaneous macules and nodules, facial deformity, atrophy of nasal spine, and facial nerve involvement (Fig. 4.44).

Management

- Therapy is with pyrazinamide, isoniazid, rifampin, ethambutol, and rifapentine, usually for many months, although there are now many multidrug-resistant strains. Latent infections are treated with the same medications with a different dosing regimen.

REFERENCES

Andrade NN, Mhatre TS. Orofacial tuberculosis—a 16-year experience with 46 cases. *J Oral Maxillofac Surg*. 2012;70:e12-e22.

de Abreu MA, Michalany NS, Weckx LL, et al. The oral mucosa in leprosy: a clinical and histopathological study. *Braz J Otorhinolaryngol*. 2006;72:312-316.

Haroon N, Inman RD. Infectious complications of biological therapy. *Curr Opin Rheumatol*. 2009;21:397-403.

Kakisi OK, Kechagia AS, Kakisis IK, et al. Tuberculosis of the oral cavity: a systematic review. *Eur J Oral Sci*. 2010;118:103-109.

Mignogna MD, Muzio LL, Favia G, et al. Oral tuberculosis: a clinical evaluation of 42 cases. *Oral Dis*. 2000;6:25-30.

Orme IM. A new unifying theory of the pathogenesis of tuberculosis. *Tuberculosis*. 2014;94:8-14.

Sidhu A, Verma G, Humar A, Kumar D. Outcome of latent tuberculosis infection in solid organ transplant recipients over a 10-year period. *Transplantation*. 2014;98:671-675.

Taheri JB, Mortazavi H, Moshfeghi M, et al. Oro-facial manifestations of 100 leprosy patients. *Med Oral Patol Oral Cir Bucal*. 2012;17:e728-e732.

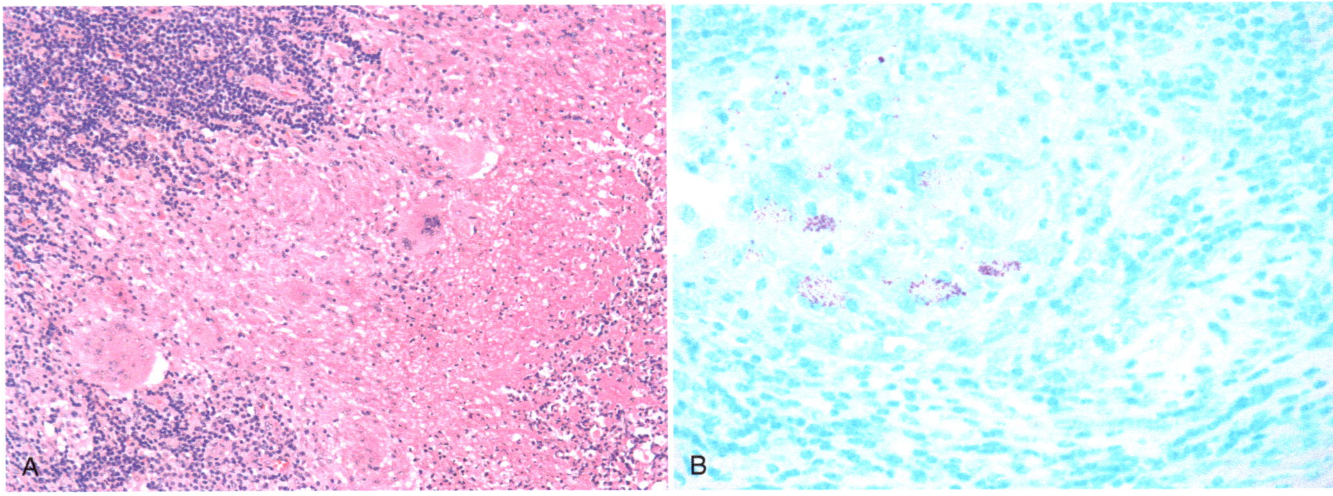

FIG 4.43 Oral tuberculosis. (A) Necrotizing granulomatous inflammation of the mandibular vestibule in a patient with chronic lymphocytic leukemia. (B) Presence of tiny acid-fast bacilli (Ziehl-Neelsen stain).

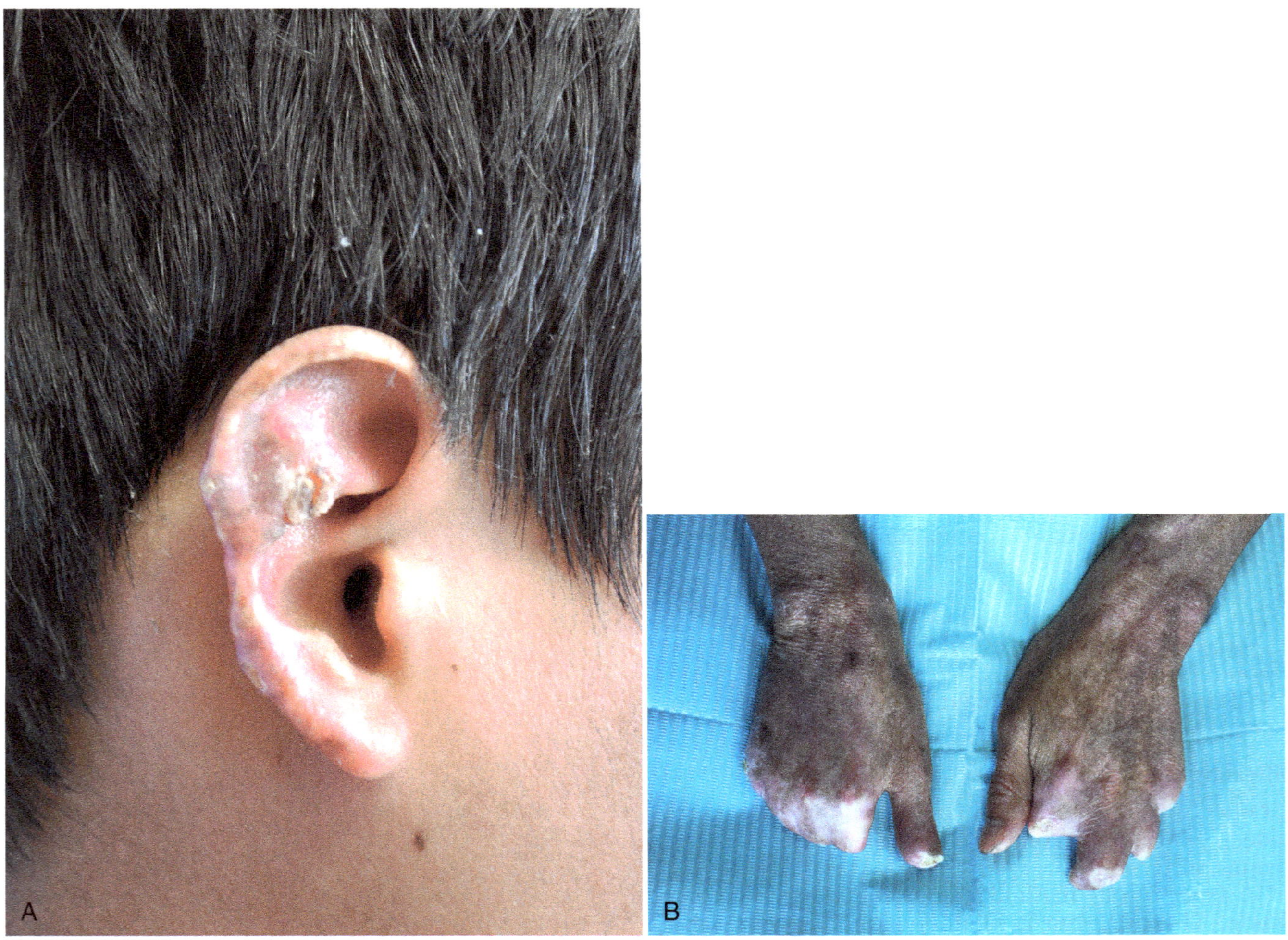

FIG 4.44 Leprosy. (A) Lesions of the skin of the pinna. (B) Autoamputation of digits. *(Courtesy Dr. Roman Carlos, Guatemala City, Guatemala.)*

SYPHILIS

The number of cases of both primary and secondary syphilis doubled between 2000 and 2013. Ninety-one percent of all cases occur in men, mostly in men who have sex with men. The behavior associated with the increase of acquired syphilis also increases the likelihood of acquiring and transmitting HIV.

Clinical Findings

- Primary syphilis (chancre): this occurs within 2 to 8 weeks at the site of inoculation. The most common extragenital site is the mouth, where it appears as a painless ulcer (Fig. 4.45A).
- Secondary syphilis: this occurs within 2 to 12 weeks as a result of hematogenous spread and manifests as whitish-grayish plaques, usually of the soft palate and tongue ("mucous patch"), or as serpiginous "snail track" ulcers, and an erythematous skin rash that mimics other skin conditions (see Fig. 4.45B). Condyloma latum occurs on the skin and genitalia.
- Tertiary syphilis: one-third of patients who are untreated develop gummas, which are ulcerated nodules or penetrating ulcers, especially of the palatal mucosa, appearing as midline destructive disease. Syphilitic endarteritis of organs results in organ-specific disease, and the eyes, aorta, and central nervous system are usually affected.
- Congenital syphilis: this is typified by deafness, notched incisors, "mulberry molars," rhagades (fissuring of the corners of the mouth), saddle nose deformity, and interstitial keratitis.
- Screening tests used to evaluate for the presence of antibodies include the nontreponemal tests, such as Venereal Disease Research Laboratory and rapid plasma reagin tests. Confirmation is achieved with a fluorescence treponemal antibody absorption test, *Treponema pallidum* particle agglutination assay, microhemagglutination, enzyme immunoassays, rapid point-of-care tests (such as dark-field microscopy to identify live organisms), and PCR.

Etiopathogenesis and Histopathologic Features

The spirochete responsible for this sexually transmitted disease is *Treponema pallidum*. The best-characterized stage histopathologically is secondary syphilis, because that is the most frequent presentation before a diagnosis is established.

- Primary lesions: these are ulcers with many lymphocytes and plasma cells, swollen endothelial cells, and perivascular plasma cell infiltrates. In the skin, most of the spirochetes are located in the dermis, at the dermal-epidermal junction, and around blood vessels.
- Secondary lesions: the epithelium exhibits parakeratosis, spongiosis, and leukocyte exocytosis and may be hyperplastic or atrophic, with necrotic keratinocytes. A lymphoplasmacytic infiltrate is present in a lichenoid band in the lamina propria and around blood vessels that may show endarteritis with swollen endothelial cells. Seventy percent of cases show a perineural plasma cell infiltrate (Fig. 4.46A–D). Granulomas may be present even at this stage; in the skin, organisms are found at sites similar to primary lesions but also within the epidermis.
- Tertiary syphilis: granulomas are noted, and organisms are generally present in small numbers.
- Thin, threadlike, "cork-screw" organisms are identified in both the epithelium and lamina propria with Warthin-Starry, modified Steiner, or Dieterle stain, or by immunohistochemistry, which has much better sensitivity (see Fig. 4.46E–F).

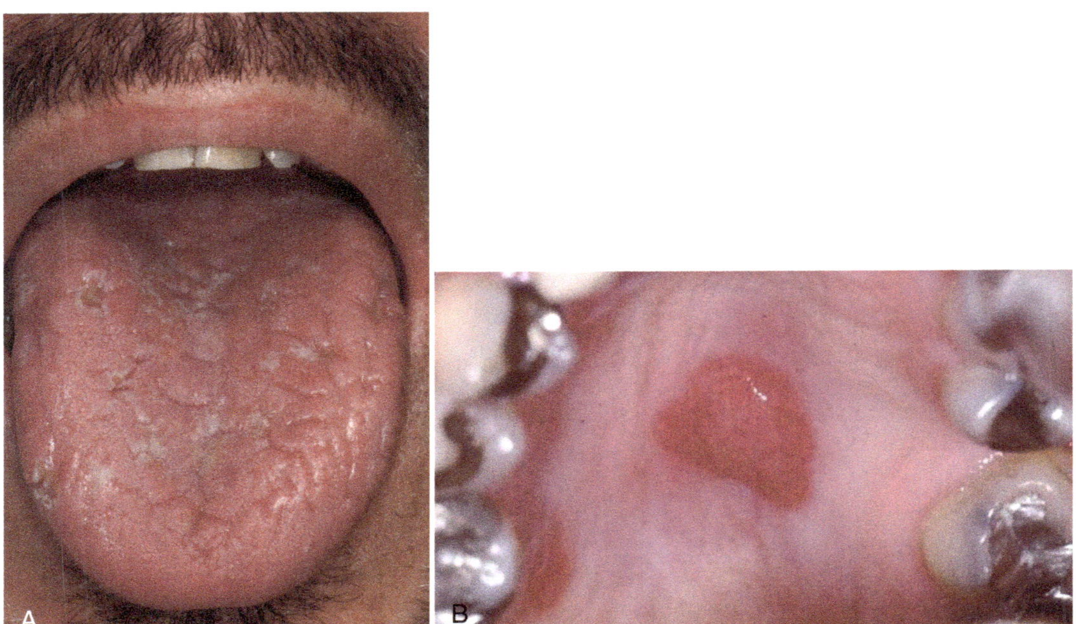

FIG 4.45 (A) Primary syphilitic chancres of the right posterior tongue dorsum in an HIV-positive patient. (B) Secondary syphilis lesion of the palatal mucosa. *(A, Courtesy Dr. Brian Shumway, University of Louisville School of Dentistry, Louisville, Ky; B, Courtesy Dr. Roman Carlos, Guatemala City, Guatemala.)*

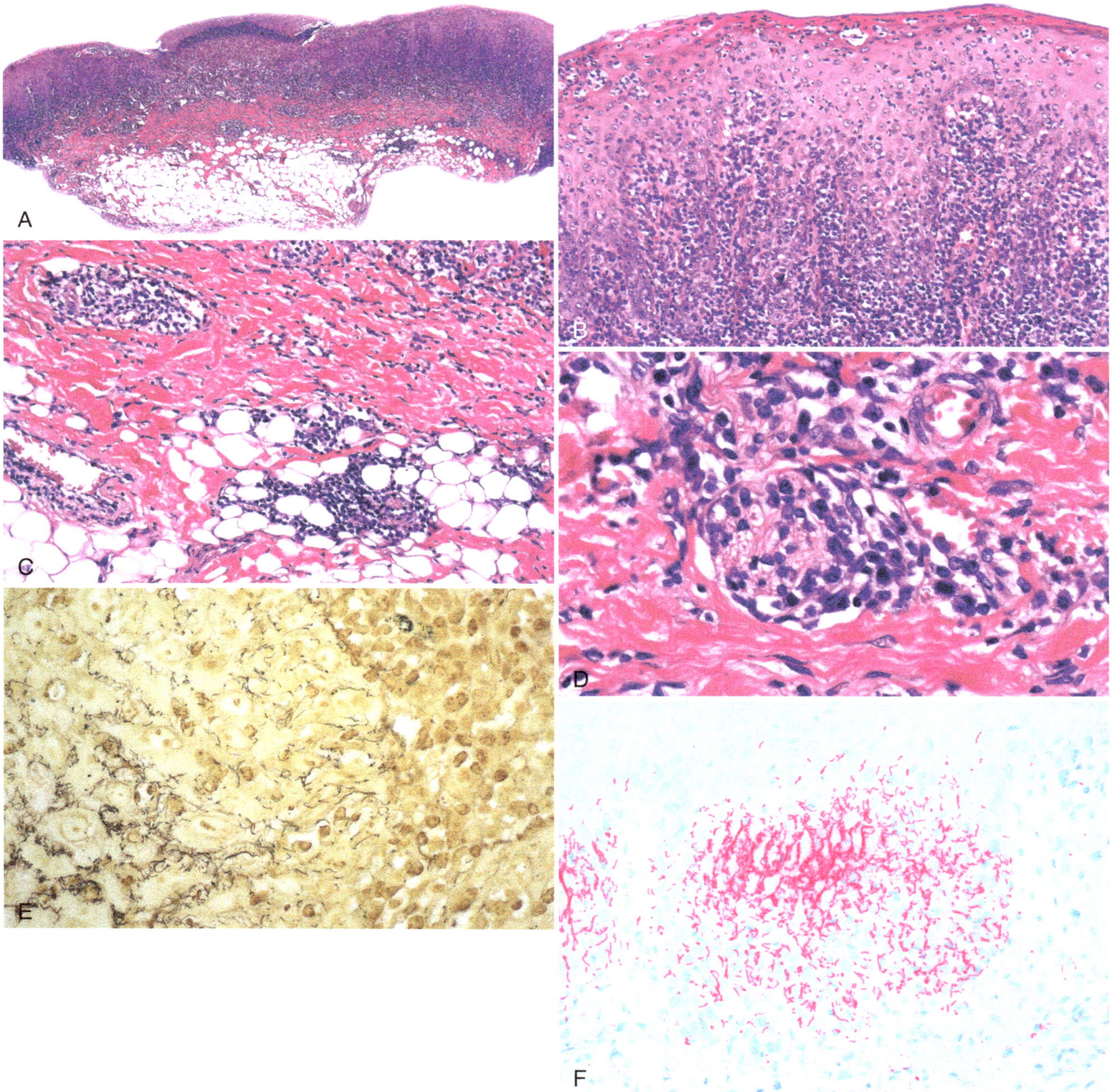

FIG 4.46 Secondary syphilis. (A) Ulceration and dense chronic inflammatory infiltrate at the interface (lichenoid pattern) and around blood vessels. (B) Parakeratosis and acute and chronic inflammation within the epithelium and plasma cells in lamina propria with occasional necrotic keratinocytes. (C) Plasma cells are present within fat and around vessels. (D) Perivascular and perineural lymphoplasmacytic infiltrate. (E) Corkscrew, threadlike spirochetes mostly within the lamina propria (modified Steiner stain). (F) Thready organisms within the epithelium and lamina propria typical for secondary syphilis (immunohistochemical study).

Differential Diagnosis

- Identification of the organism is the key to diagnosis, because the mucosal inflammatory lesion appears nonspecific.

Management

- Intramuscular penicillin G is the treatment of choice. Tetracycline, doxycycline, and azithromycin are also effective.

REFERENCES

Barrett AW, Villarroel Dorrego M, Hodgson TA, et al. The histopathology of syphilis of the oral mucosa. *J Oral Pathol Med.* 2004;33:286-291.

Ficarra G, Carlos R. Syphilis: the renaissance of an old disease with oral implications. *Head Neck Pathol.* 2009;3:195-206.

Flamm A, Parikh K, Xie Q, et al. Histologic features of secondary syphilis: a multicenter retrospective review. *J Am Acad Dermatol.* 2015;73:1025-1030.

Hoang MP, High WA, Molberg KH. Secondary syphilis: a histologic and immunohistochemical evaluation. *J Cutan Pathol.* 2004;31:595-599.

Leuci S, Martina S, Adamo D, et al. Oral syphilis: a retrospective analysis of 12 cases and a review of the literature. *Oral Dis.* 2013;19: 738-746.

Martín-Ezquerra G, Fernandez-Casado A, Barco D, et al. *Treponema pallidum* distribution patterns in mucocutaneous lesions of primary and secondary syphilis: an immunohistochemical and ultrastructural study. *Hum Pathol.* 2009;40:624-630.

Patton ME, Su JR, Nelson R, et al. Primary and secondary syphilis—United States, 2005-2013. *MMWR Morb Mortal Wkly Rep.* 2014;63:402-406.

Seña AC, White BL, Sparling PF. Novel *Treponema pallidum* serologic tests: a paradigm shift in syphilis screening for the 21st century. *Clin Infect Dis.* 2010;51:700-708.

Siqueira CS, Saturno JL, de Sousa SC, da Silveira FR. Diagnostic approaches in unsuspected oral lesions of syphilis. *Int J Oral Maxillofac Surg.* 2014;43:1436-1440.

LEISHMANIASIS

Leishmaniasis is endemic in over 70 countries, and 90% of cases occur in Afghanistan, Algeria, Brazil, Pakistan, Peru, Saudi Arabia, and Syria. It is also prevalent in India, Bangladesh, Nepal, and Sudan. Approximately 2 million new cases are diagnosed each year. It may present as a cutaneous, mucosal, or generalized visceral infection (kala-azar) and is potentially fatal. Mucocutaneous leishmaniasis is characterized by chronic, latent, and metastatic behavior, especially to the head and neck and oral and nasopharyngeal tissues. Persistent infection is one of the hallmarks of this disease.

Clinical Findings

- Leishmaniasis affects those in the fifth to sixth decades of life and has a 3–5 : 1 male predilection. The lesions present as painful ulcers, ulcerated nodules, areas of erythema and swelling in the mouth, and sometimes as midline destructive disease of the palatal mucosa. Patients with HIV/AIDS are susceptible to this infection.
- Involvement of the nasal mucosa and nasopharynx is common, and patients experience dysphagia, dysphonia, and dyspnea with destructive lesions at those sites.
- Skin lesions present as ulcers and ulcerated nodules, and visceral involvement is associated with systemic symptoms of fever, weakness, night sweats, and weight loss.

Etiopathogenesis and Histopathologic Features

Leishmania are protozoal parasites that spend part of their life cycle in the gut of the sand fly vector as promastigotes. After they are deposited in the skin of vertebrate hosts, they differentiate into amastigotes that multiply within macrophages. Many species exist; common ones include *Leishmania major*, *L. tropica*, and *L. aethiopica* (Old World infections); *L. infantum* and *L. chagasi* (infections seen around the Mediterranean); and *L. mexicana* and *L. braziliensis* (New World infections).

- There is marked pseudoepitheliomatous hyperplasia and many foamy macrophages, lymphocytes, and plasma cells, with granulomas are present in up to 60% of cases. Macrophages contain the amastigotes, which have a round nucleus and rod-shaped kinetoplast, well seen on Giemsa stains (Fig 4.47).
- PCR readily identifies organisms.

Differential Diagnosis

- Deep fungal infections are differentiated by the morphology of the organisms on special stains and by PCR and culture. Histoplasmosis also shows many small, dotlike, intracytoplasmic organisms that stain for silver and not Giemsa.
- Lymphoproliferative disease may have similar large, macrophage-like cells and many inflammatory cells, and a careful search must be made for amastigotes, especially if the patient is from or has travelled to an area where leishmaniasis is endemic.
- Wegener granulomatosis often shows a mixed inflammatory infiltrate with granulomas, but would not show the organisms.
- Nuclear debris from breakdown of inflammatory cells produces small, round bodies that vary in size. These are referred to as *pyronin bodies* (Fig. 4.48).

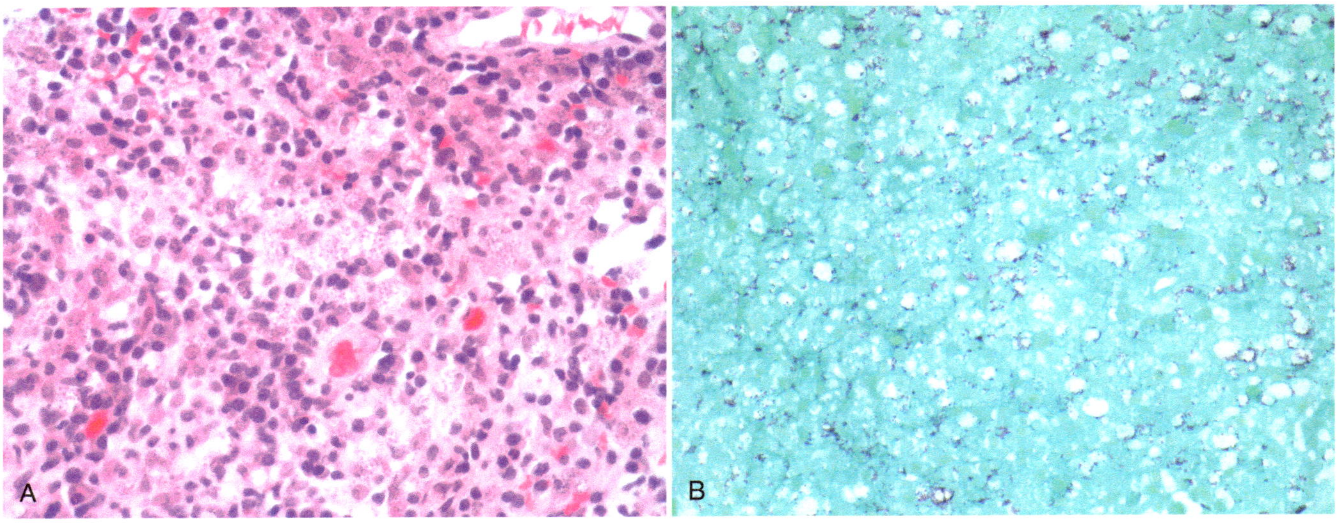

FIG 4.47 Leishmaniasis. (A) Macrophages in the lamina propria contain many tiny, intracytoplasmic, dotlike amastigotes. (B) Giemsa staining shows amastigotes.

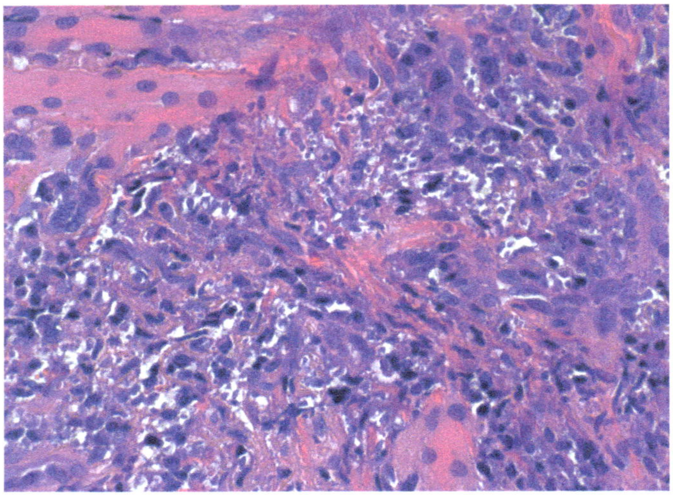

FIG 4.48 Nuclear debris (pyronin bodies) should not be mistaken for infective organisms.

Management and Prognosis

- Treatment is with parenteral or intralesional pentavalent antimonial drugs, paromomycin cream, pentamidine, miltefosine, fluconazole, and amphotericin B.

REFERENCES

Aoun J, Habib R, Charaffeddine K, et al. Caseating granulomas in cutaneous leishmaniasis. *PLoS Negl Trop Dis.* 2014;8:e3255.

Crovetto-Martínez R, Aguirre-Urizar JM, Orte-Aldea C, et al. Mucocutaneous leishmaniasis must be included in the differential diagnosis of midline destructive disease: two case reports. *Oral Surg Oral Med Oral Pathol Oral Radiol.* 2015;119:e20-e26.

Mignogna MD, Celentano A, Leuci S, et al. Mucosal leishmaniasis with primary oral involvement: a case series and a review of the literature. *Oral Dis.* 2015;21:e70-e78.

Reithinger R, Dujardin JC, Louzir H, et al. Cutaneous leishmaniasis. *Lancet Infect Dis.* 2007;7:581-596.

Saab J, Fedda F, Khattab R, et al. Cutaneous leishmaniasis mimicking inflammatory and neoplastic processes: a clinical, histopathological and molecular study of 57 cases. *J Cutan Pathol.* 2012;39:251-262.

5 FIBROUS, GINGIVAL, LIPOCYTIC, AND MISCELLANEOUS TUMORS

CHAPTER CONTENTS

Fibrous Lesions

FIBROMA ("BITE" OR "IRRITATION" FIBROMA, FIBROEPITHELIAL OR FIBROVASCULAR POLYP), AND GIANT CELL FIBROMA

Clinical Findings

- Fibroma: This consists of a dome-shaped nodule or papule that may be white/keratotic, mucosa-colored, or ulcerated; it is located in areas readily traumatized by biting (i.e., buccal mucosa, lateral tongue, and lower lip mucosa) or on the gingiva where plaque accumulates (Fig. 5.1A–D).
- Giant cell fibroma: This often has a papillary surface and 90% are located on the gingiva (50% of cases), tongue, and palatal mucosa; a similar histopathologic condition is referred to as the retrocuspid papilla, which occurs on the lingual attached gingiva of the mandibular cuspids, usually bilaterally (Fig. 5.1E).
- Multiple fibromas of the gingiva, buccal mucosa, and tongue are often seen in tuberous sclerosis complex (associated with a mutation in *TSC1* or *TSC2*), while sclerotic fibromas are seen in Cowden syndrome (part of PTEN hamartoma tumor syndrome).

Etiopathogenesis and Histopathologic Features

Conventional fibroma is a reactive fibrosis/scar (similar to a hypertrophic scar on the skin) from bite trauma and is not a true neoplasm.

- Fibroma: the nodule consists of a proliferation of fibrocollagenous tissue associated with variable vascularity, neurovascular hyperplasia, parakeratosis or hyperkeratosis, ulceration, inflammation, and epithelial hyperplasia or atrophy (Figs. 5.2 to 5.4); myxoid/mucinous change may be present (Fig. 5.5).
- Giant cell fibroma: nodules often have a papillary or bosselated surface with acanthosis forming spiky, sawtooth shaped rete ridges; there are many giant, stellate, bi- and multinucleate fibroblasts that sometimes show cytoplasmic positivity for smooth muscle actin, suggesting differentiation toward myofibroblasts; some of these cells have been shown to be factor XIIIa+; dense collagen and mast cells are often present similar to fibrous papule of the nose (Figs. 5.6 and 5.7).
- Solitary sclerotic fibroma (storiform collagenoma): the nodule contains hyalinized bands of dense collagen with a storiform pattern, usually demarcated from the surrounding soft tissue; there are stellate and fusiform fibroblasts, and clusters of stellate mononuclear cells appearing as multinucleate cells; clefts between

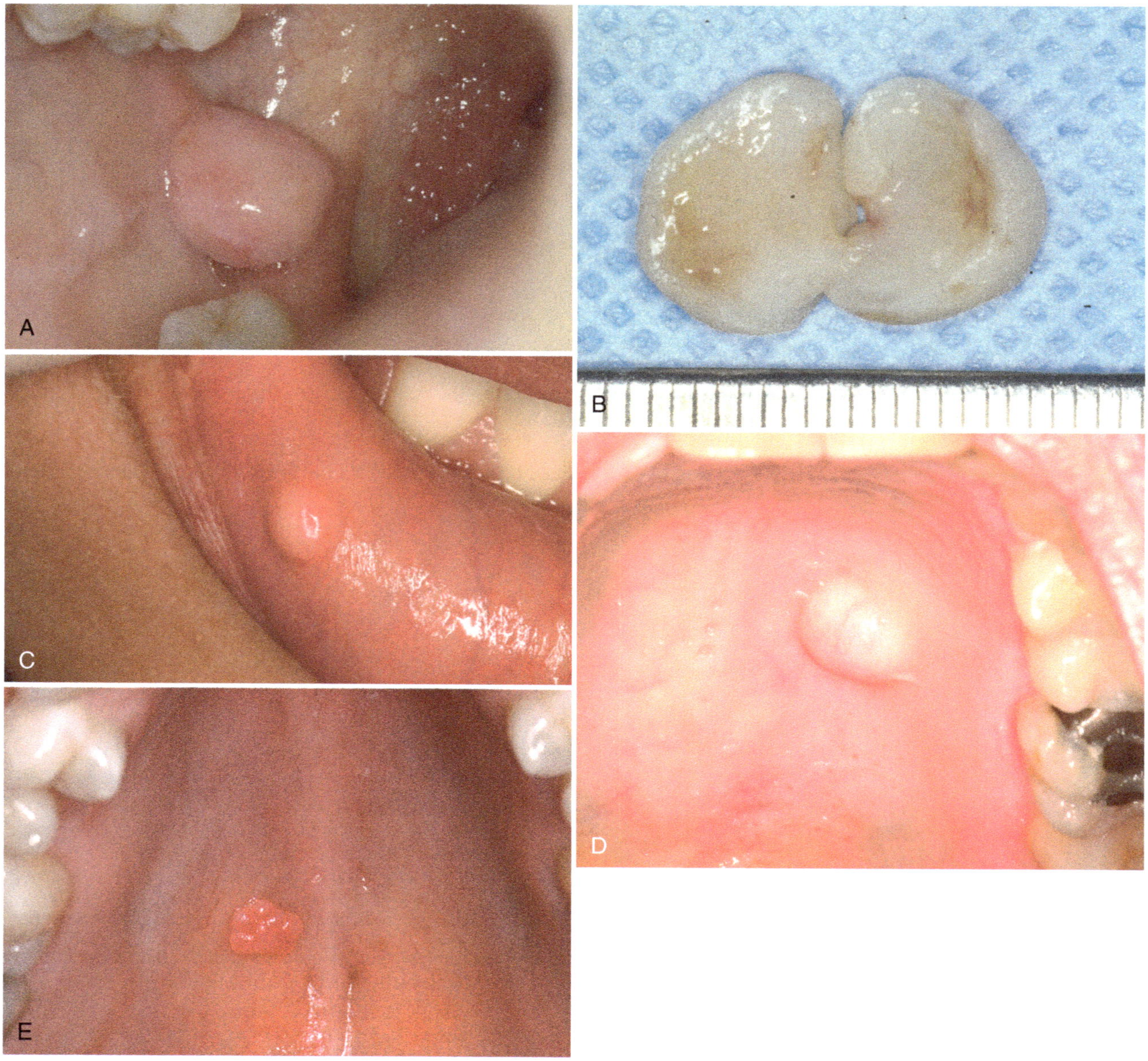

FIG 5.1 (A) Fibroma of right buccal mucosa. (B) Cut surfaces of fibroma, dense and white. (C) Fibroma of the lower lip mucosa. (D) Sclerotic fibroma of the palate. (E) Giant cell fibroma on the palatal mucosa. *(Courtesy Dr. Carl Allen, The Ohio State University, Columbus, Ohio.)*

collagen fibers are a distinctive feature; a giant cell version is recognized that contains bizarre, true multinucleate giant cells (Fig. 5.8); lesions are positive for CD34, CD99, and occasionally factor XIIIa; multiple sclerotic fibromas are associated with Cowden syndrome.
- Fibromas of the anterior hard palatal mucosa often contain cartilage and branches of the nasopalatine neurovascular bundle (Fig. 5.9).

Differential Diagnosis

- Desmoplastic fibroblastoma (collagenous fibroma) contains spindled and stellate fibroblasts but in an edematous to fibromyxoid stroma, and are likely true neoplasms because gene rearrangements have been identified.

Management and Prognosis

- Excision is curative although continued irritation and trauma may lead to recurrence.

REFERENCES

Alawi F, Freedman PD. Sporadic sclerotic fibroma of the oral soft tissues. *Am J Dermatopathol.* 2004;26:182-187.

de Sousa SF, Caldeira PC, Grossmann Sde M, de Aguiar MC, Mesquita RA. Desmoplastic fibroblastoma (collagenous fibroma): a case identified in the buccal mucosa. *Head Neck Pathol.* 2011;5:175-179.

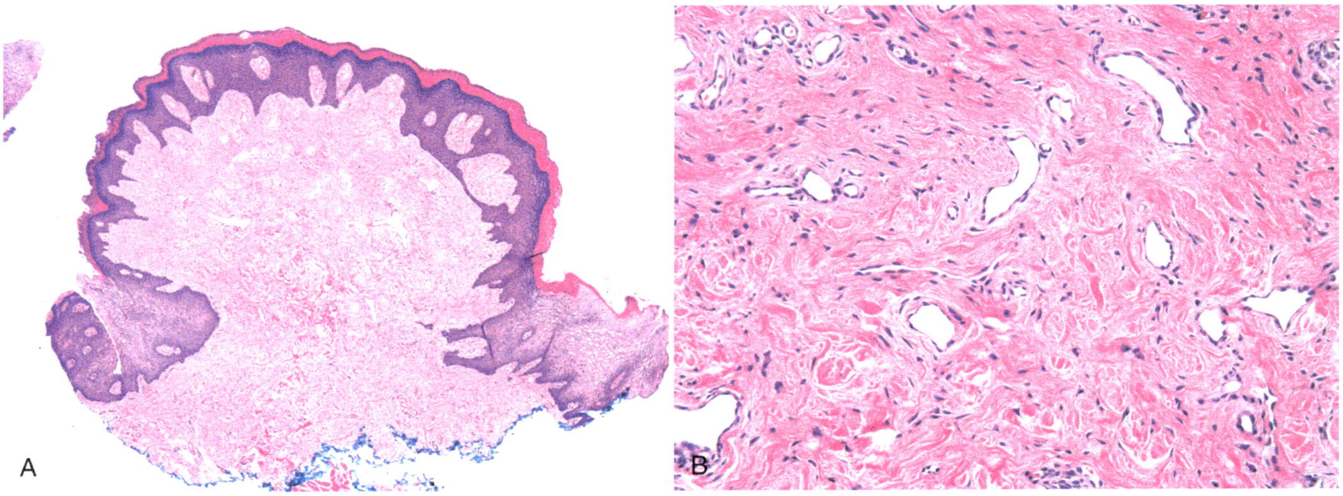

FIG 5.2 (A) Fibroma with frictional keratosis. (B) Dense collagenous tissue with dilated capillaries.

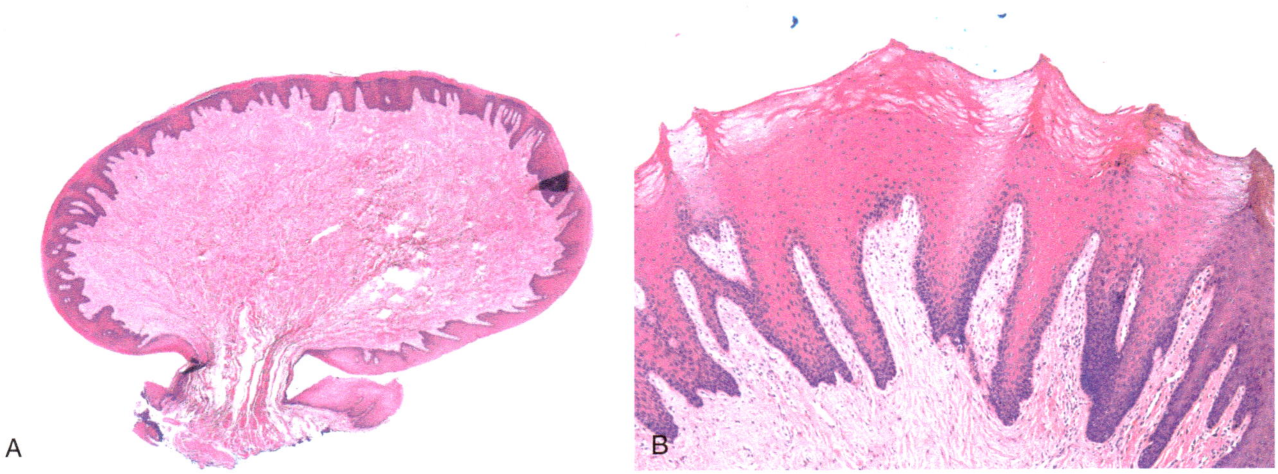

FIG 5.3 (A) Fibroma with frictional parakeratosis. (B) Fibroma with frictional parakeratotic chevrons.

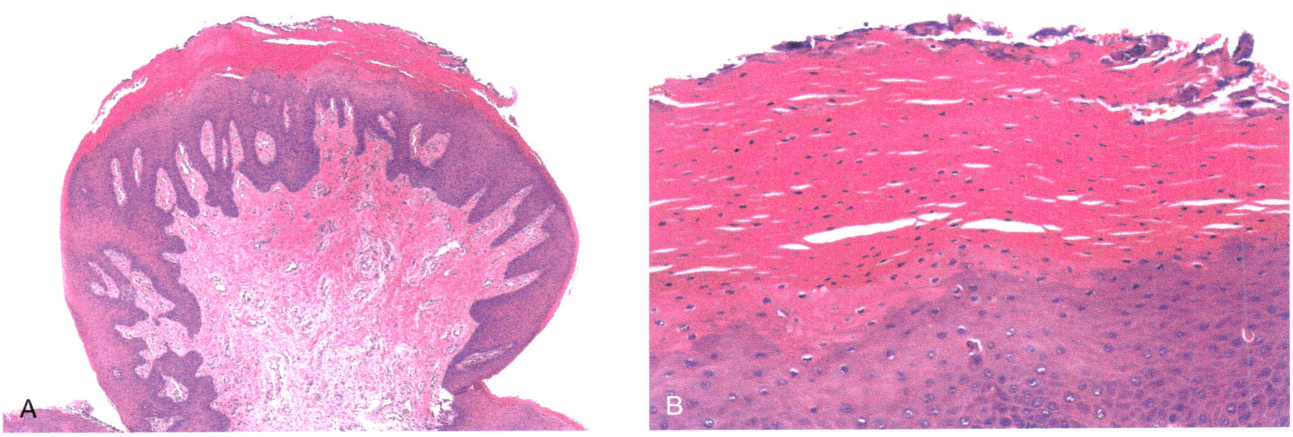

FIG 5.4 (A) Fibroma with frictional hyperkeratosis. (B) Parakeratosis and bacterial colonies typical for frictional/factitial keratosis.

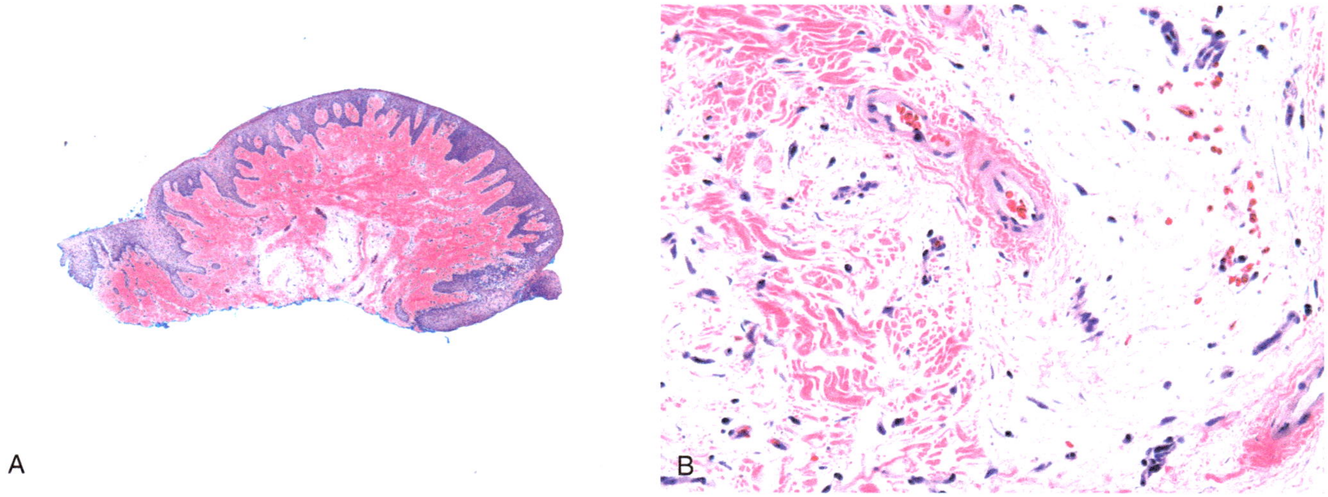

FIG 5.5 (A) Fibroma with focal myxoid/mucinous change. (B) Areas of dense collagen interspersed with myxoid/mucinous areas with mild chronic inflammation.

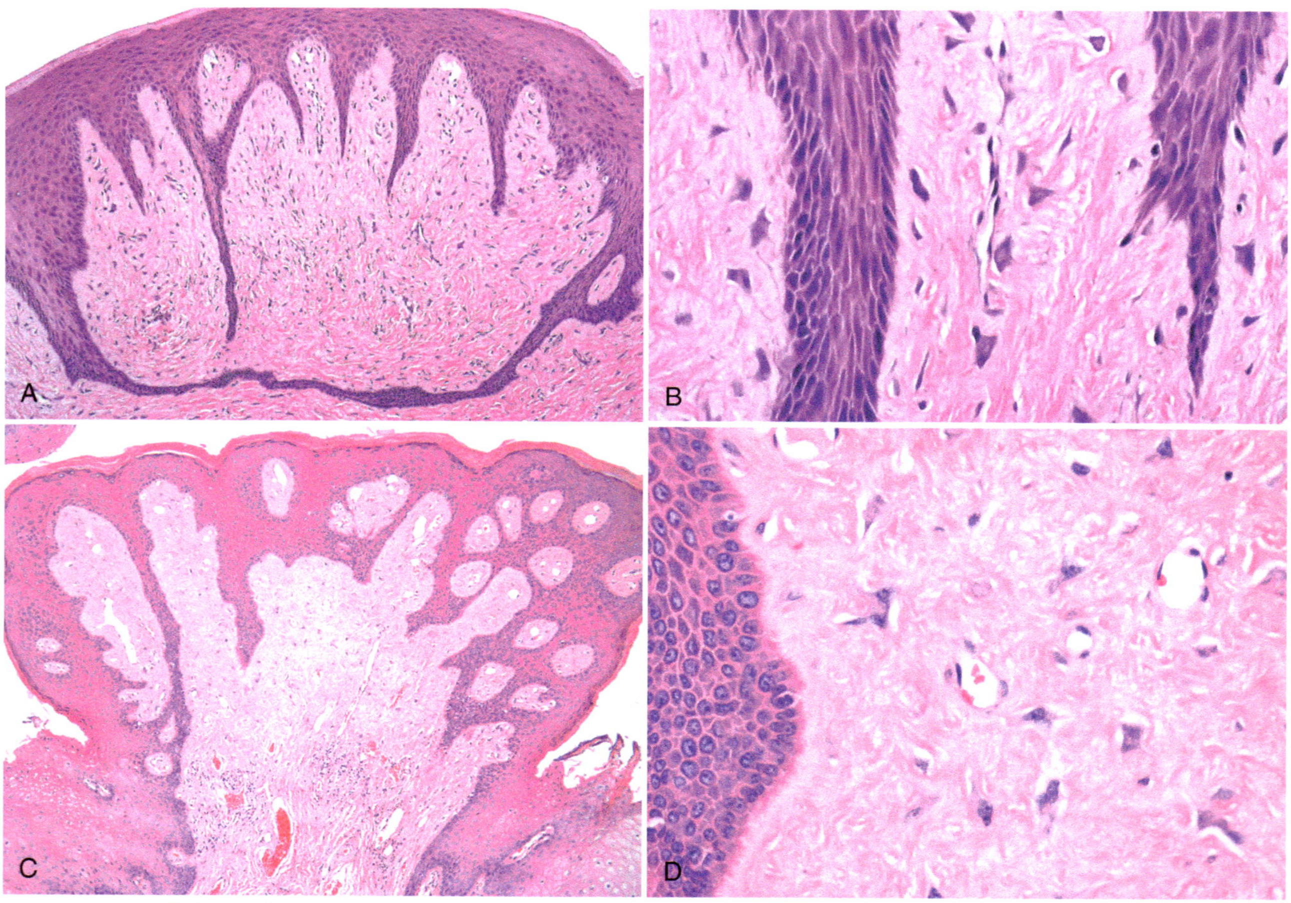

FIG 5.6 Giant cell fibroma. (A) Fibrous nodule with spiky rete ridges and dense collagen. (B) Stellate and multinucleate fibroblasts. (C) Nodule with bosselated surface and tapered interlacing rete ridges. (D) Stellate and multinucleate fibroblasts.

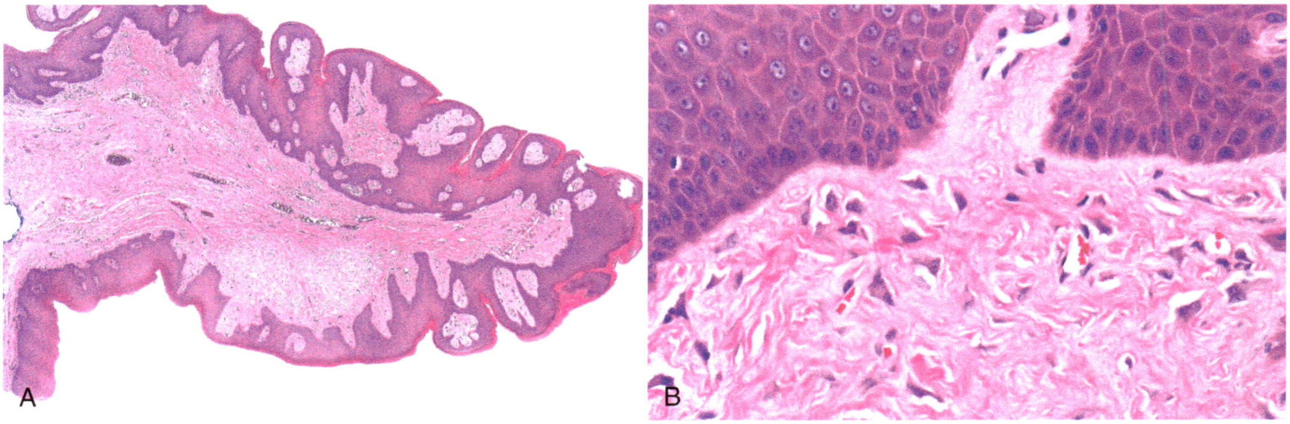

FIG 5.7 Giant cell fibroma. (A) Fibrous nodule with papillary surface. (B) Giant and binucleate fibroblast-like cells and dense collagen.

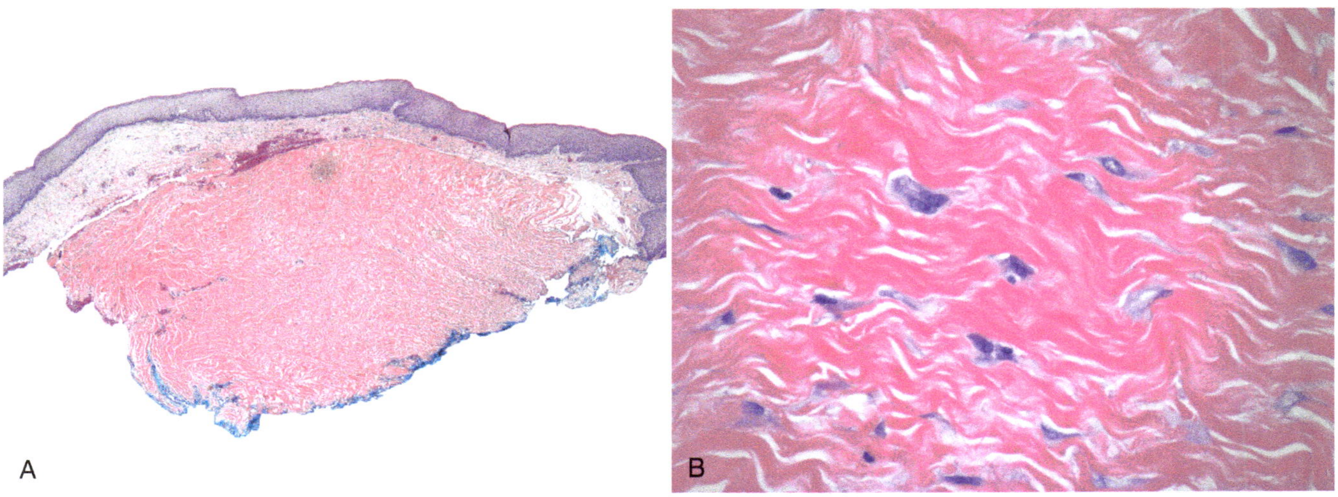

FIG 5.8 Sclerotic fibroma. (A) Well-demarcated nodule of dense, hyalinized collagen. (B) Stellate and fusiform fibroblasts with tissue clefts.

Fernandez-Flores A. Solitary oral fibromas of the tongue show similar morphologic features to fibrous papule of the face: a study of 31 cases. *Am J Dermatopathol.* 2010;32:442-447.

Hedin CA, Gerner L, Larsson A. The retrocuspid papilla and factor XIIIa: an epidemiologic and histomorphologic study. *Scand J Dent Res.* 1994;102:290-294.

Houston GD. The giant cell fibroma: a review of 464 cases. *Oral Surg Oral Med Oral Pathol.* 1982;53:582-587.

Magnusson BC, Rasmusson LG. The giant cell fibroma. A review of 103 cases with immunohistochemical findings. *Acta Odontol Scand.* 1995;53:293-296.

Metcalf JS, Maize JC, LeBoit PE. Circumscribed storiform collagenoma (sclerosing fibroma). *Am J Dermatopathol.* 1991;13:122-129.

Ramos D, Monteagudo C, Carda C, et al. Ultrastructural and immunohistochemical characterization of the so-called giant multinucleate cells in cutaneous collagenomas. *Histopathology.* 2002;41:134-143.

Rapini RP, Golitz LE. Sclerotic fibromas of the skin. *J Am Acad Dermatol.* 1989;20:266-271.

Santos PP, Nonaka CF, Pinto LP, de Souza LB. Immunohistochemical expression of mast cell tryptase in giant cell fibroma and inflammatory fibrous hyperplasia of the oral mucosa. *Arch Oral Biol.* 2011;56:231-237.

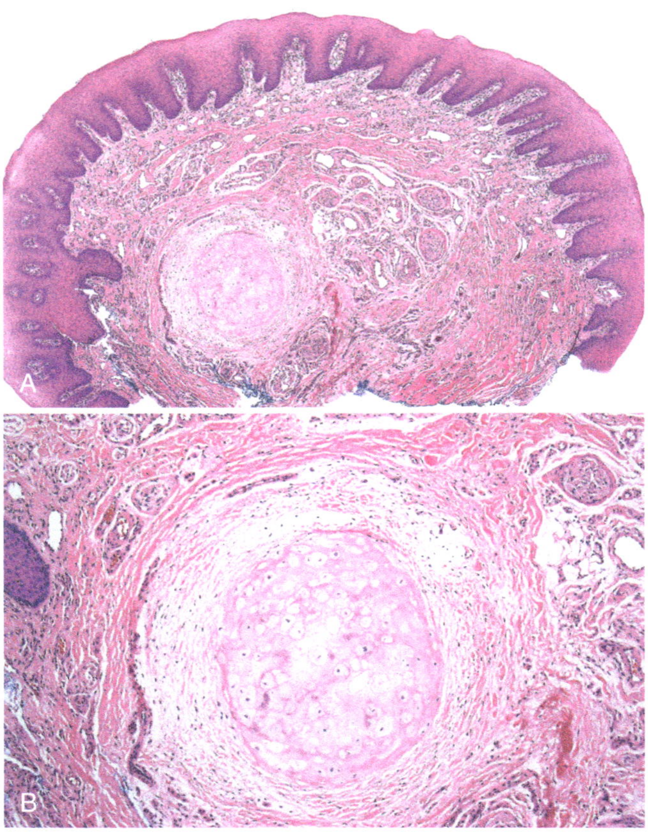

FIG 5.9 Fibroma of anterior palatal mucosa. (A) Nodule containing hyaline cartilage and neurovascular bundles. (B) Mature hyaline cartilage.

Gingival Masses

Gingival nodules may represent one of the following:

- Reactive/inflammatory gingival nodules, solitary or diffuse; these are by far the most common
- Peripheral (extraosseous) odontogenic cysts and tumors (see Chapters 14 and 15)
- Soft tissue tumors (such as nerve sheath or smooth muscle tumors discussed in Chapter 6)
- Extension of intrabony lesions into the gingiva
- Metastatic tumors to the gingiva

REACTIVE/INFLAMMATORY GINGIVAL NODULES

Clinical Findings

- Peripheral ossifying fibromas and pyogenic granulomas tend to occur in young patients in the second to fourth decades, but all occur as nodular masses on the marginal gingiva adjacent to teeth or dental implants, often in the maxillary anterior region; fibromas are pink, while pyogenic granulomas and peripheral giant cell granulomas are dusky purple; they may be painful if ulcerated, and if vascular will bleed; the underlying bone may show "saucerization" (especially with peripheral giant cell granuloma) (Fig. 5.10).
- Peripheral giant cell granuloma is the least common and tends to occur in older adults > 50 years.
- Parulis ("gum boil" or sinus tract) occurs on the attached gingiva and has a punctum and an underlying tract that leads to the infected tooth.
- Up to 5% of pregnant women develop gingival pyogenic granulomas (granuloma gravidarum or oral pregnancy tumor).
- Multiple gingival fibromas may be seen in tuberous sclerosis complex and Cowden syndrome (usually sclerotic fibromas).

Etiopathogenesis and Histopathologic Features

Multipotent cells in the gingival tissues when traumatized or irritated (usually by accumulation of dental calculus or bacterial plaque, rough edges of restorations, or the presence of implants) differentiate toward endothelial cells, fibroblasts, osteoblasts, or osteoclast-like cells, giving rise to four distinct histologic entities or combinations thereof. Estrogen and progesterone causes overexpression of vascular endothelial growth factor in granuloma gravidarum. See Table 5.1 and Figs. 5.11–5.19 for histopathologic features.

- A parulis (sinus tract) consists of a mass of edematous granulation tissue with many acute and chronic inflammatory cells and tracts lined by neutrophils (Figs. 5.20 and 5.21).

Differential Diagnosis

- A parulis may be mistaken for a mucocele (which does not occur on the attached gingiva) if the edematous tissue is mistaken for extravasated mucin.
- Infantile hemangioma may look similar to pyogenic granuloma but it is a developmental malformation and is almost always positive for glucose transporter-1 (GLUT-1) (Fig. 5.22).
- Peripheral odontogenic fibroma produces dentinoid rather than cementum, and epithelial islands are always present distinguishing this from peripheral ossifying fibroma (see later).
- Aggressive central (intraosseous) giant cell granuloma may erode through bone and radiographs differentiates it from a peripheral (extraosseous) lesions (see Chapter 17).

Management and Prognosis

- Excision is the treatment of choice, although if underlying irritating factors such as dental plaque are not removed the recurrence rate is 15% to 20%; anecdotal data suggests that pyogenic granulomas in teenagers may exhibit multiple recurrences.
- Granuloma gravidarum may resolve postpartum but may also sclerose and become a gingival fibroma.

REFERENCES

Andrikopoulou M, Chatzistamou I, Gkilas H, et al. Assessment of angiogenic markers and female sex hormone receptors in pregnancy tumor of the gingiva. *J Oral Maxillofac Surg.* 2013;71:1376-1381.

Buchner A, Hansen LS. The histomorphologic spectrum of peripheral ossifying fibroma. *Oral Surg Oral Med Oral Pathol.* 1987;63:452-461.

Text continued on p. 87

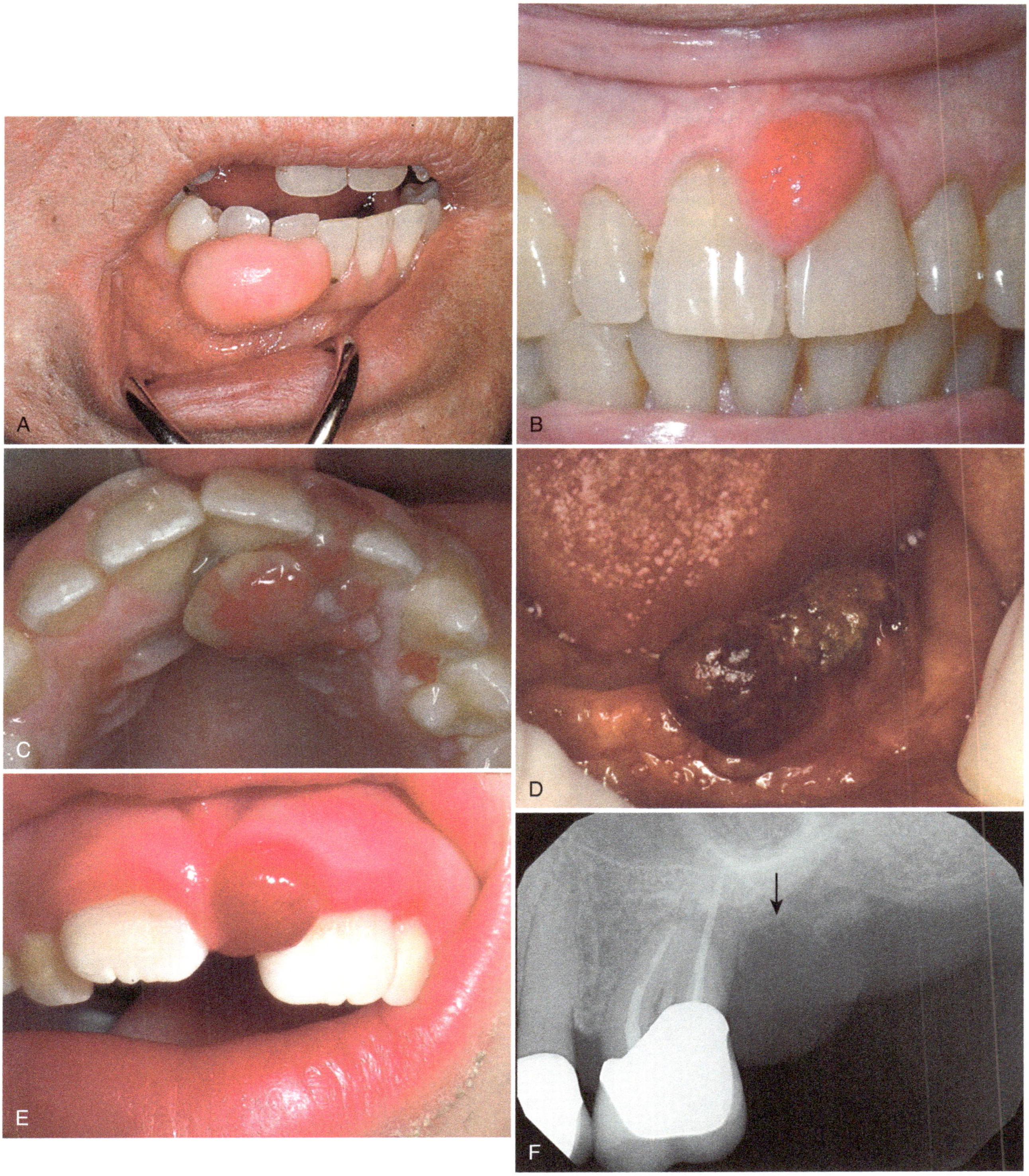

FIG 5.10 (A) Gingival fibroma. (B) Peripheral ossifying fibroma. (C) Pyogenic granuloma with ulceration. (D) Pyogenic granuloma of the mandibular ridge at an extraction site. (E) Peripheral giant cell granuloma. (F) Peripheral giant cell granuloma causing saucerization of bone (*arrow*). *(A, Courtesy Dr. Greg Sarka, private practice, Waterville, Me; B, Courtesy Dr. David Feinerman, private practice, Boynton Beach, Fla; C, Courtesy Dr. Jeffrey Freedman, private practice, Lexington, Mass; E, Courtesy Dr. Shelly Abramawitz, Children's Hospital Boston, Boston, Mass.)*

TABLE 5.1 Reactive Gingival Nodules

Diagnosis	Histopathology
Fibroma (fibrovascular hyperplasia/ polyp)	• Nodule of fibrous tissue with scattered vessels and variable edema and inflammation; crevicular epithelium with underlying plasma cells are often seen (see Fig. 5.11)
Giant cell fibroma	• Densely collagenous fibrous tissue and overlying epithelium forms spiky rete ridges; stellate and multinucleate fibroblast–like cells are present (see Fibroma section)
Pyogenic granuloma (see also Chapter 6)	• Lobular or nonlobular proliferation of endothelial cells and small, dilated capillaries; often ulcerated and inflamed (see Figs. 5.12A, 5.13) • Endothelial cells show reactive atypia sometimes with focal "hobnail" pattern, enlarged nuclei with prominent nucleoli and some mitotic activity (see Fig. 5.12B–C) • May see fibrosis depending on stage of organization
Peripheral ossifying fibroma (fibroma with osseous metaplasia)	• Cellular proliferation of spindled fibroblast-like cells with deposition of osteoid, woven bone with variable osteoblastic rimming, cementum droplets or cementicles (psammoma body–like) (see Figs. 5.14A–C and 5.15); sometimes lamellar bone is present • Spindle cells have ovoid nuclei, dispersed chromatin and inconspicuous nucleoli (see Fig. 5.14D); sometimes only subtle or minimal osteoid deposition is present (Fig. 5.16) • There may be clusters of multinucleate giant cells similar to peripheral giant cell granuloma (see Fig. 5.17) • Bone morphogenetic protein has been identified in the spindled fibroblast-like cells
Peripheral giant cell granuloma	• Proliferation of mononuclear and multinucleate giant cells (osteoclast-like or foreign body type) usually in sheets; giant cells contain 10–20 evenly-distributed nuclei; mitoses may be seen in mononuclear cells; fresh hemorrhage and hemosiderin deposits are usually present especially beneath the grenz zone (see Figs. 5.18 and 5.19) • May see concomitant osseous metaplasia similar to peripheral ossifying fibroma • Giant cells are positive for TRAP, RANK and osteoprotegrin

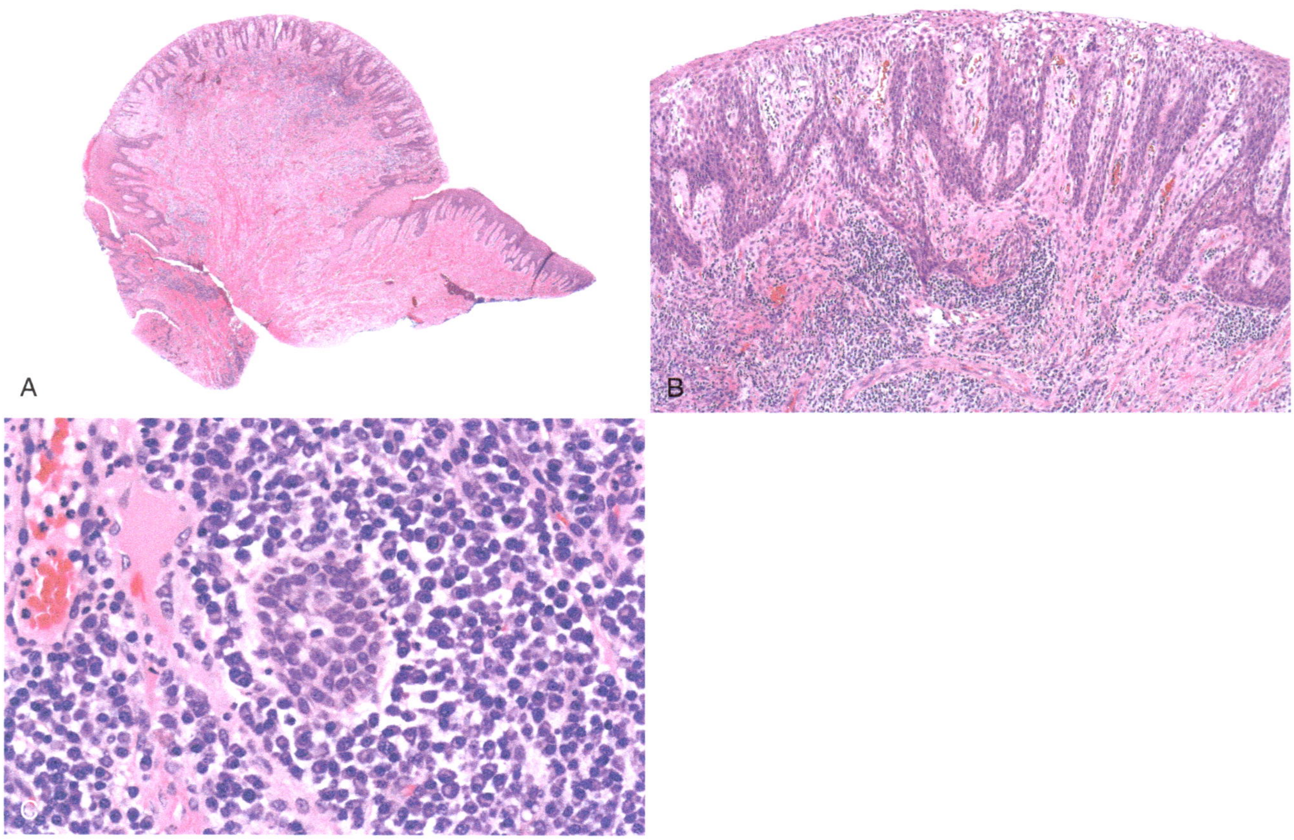

FIG 5.11 Gingival fibroma/inflammatory fibrous hyperplasia. (A) Fibrous nodule with chronic inflammation. (B) Acanthosis, spongiosis, and chronic inflammation. (C) Dense plasma cell infiltrate is a common feature.

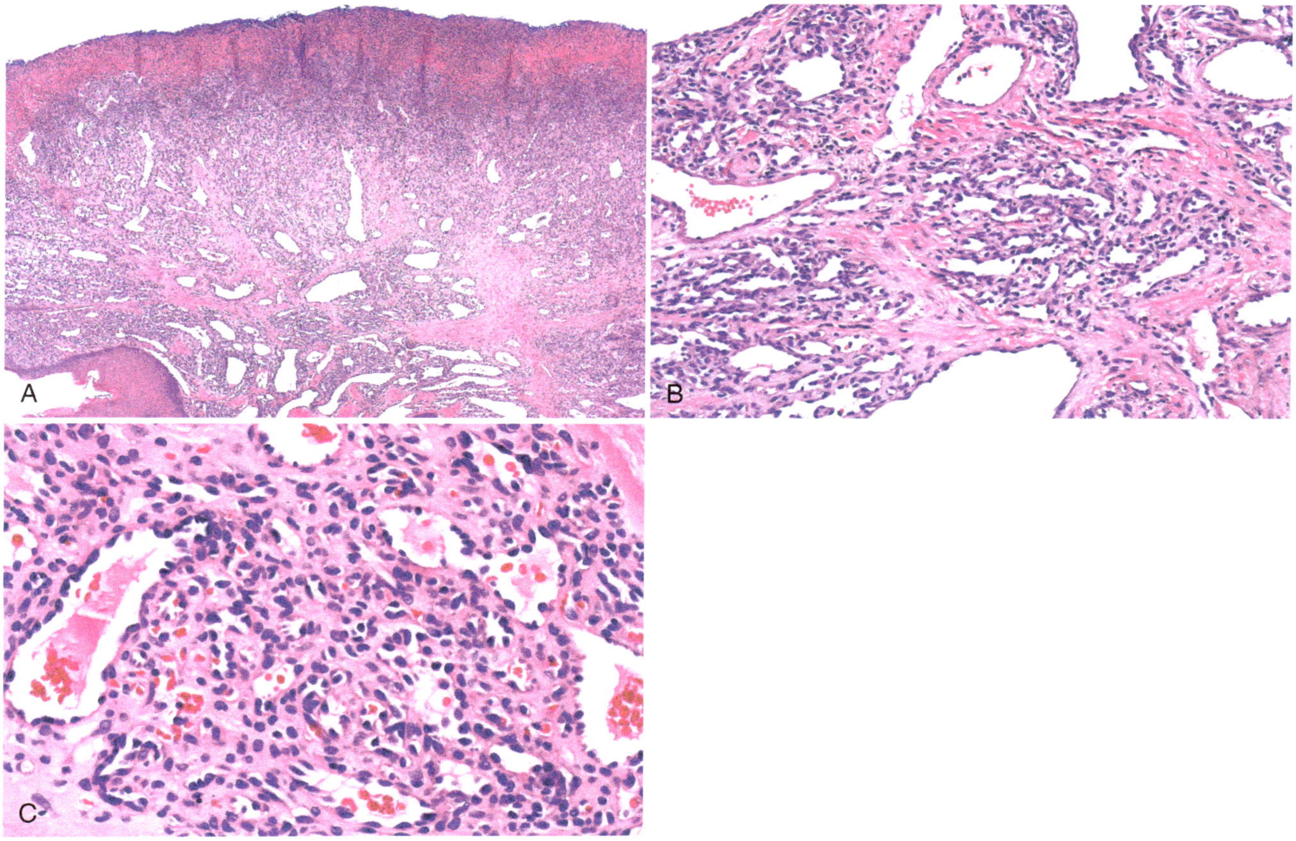

FIG 5.12 Granuloma gravidarum. (A) Vaguely lobular proliferation of capillaries, ulcerated. (B) Proliferation of endothelial cells and dilated capillaries with slight hobnailing of nuclei. (C) More cellular areas focally.

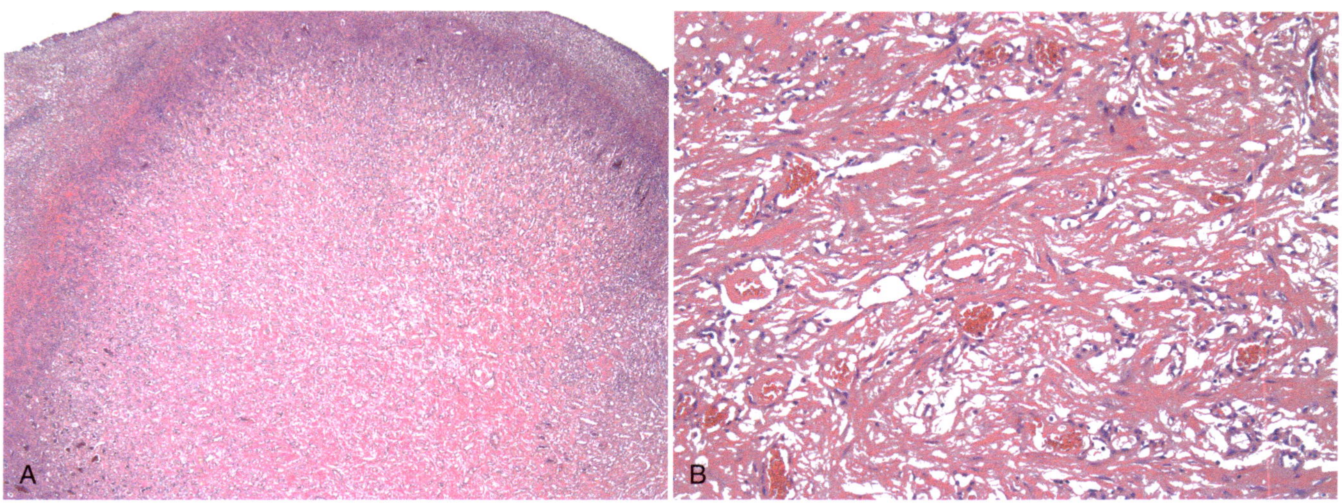

FIG 5.13 Pyogenic granuloma with early sclerosis. (A) Nonlobular proliferation of endothelial cells and capillaries with intervening fibrous tissue. (B) Fibrous tissue insinuates between and replaces endothelial cells and vessels.

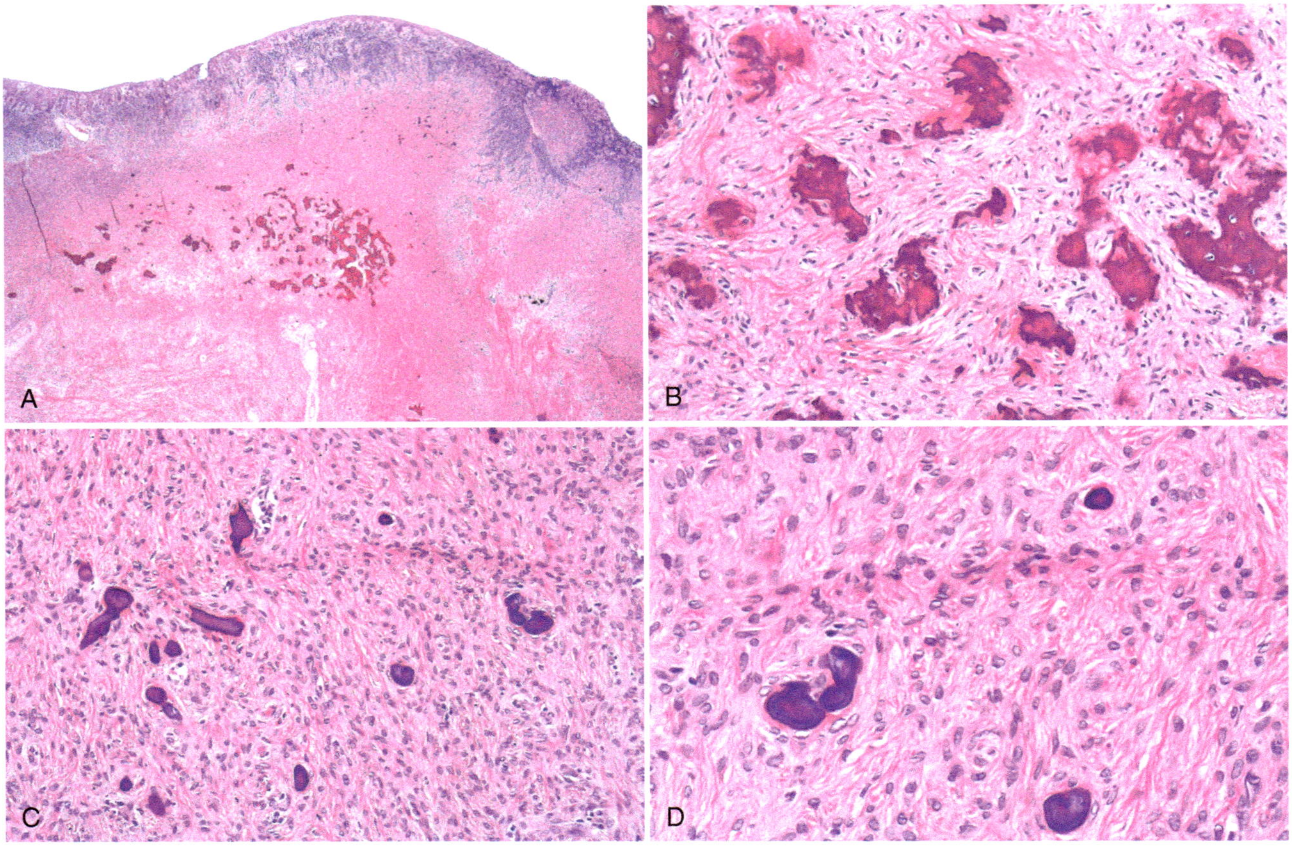

FIG 5.14 Peripheral ossifying fibroma. (A) Mass of cellular fibrous tissue with superficial cementum droplet (cementicle) deposition and woven bone deeper in the tissue. (B) Cellular proliferation of fibroblast-like spindle cells with deposition of woven bone with osteoid rim. (C) Deposition of cementum droplets (cementicles). (D) Cementum droplets with lamellar (psammomatoid) appearance.

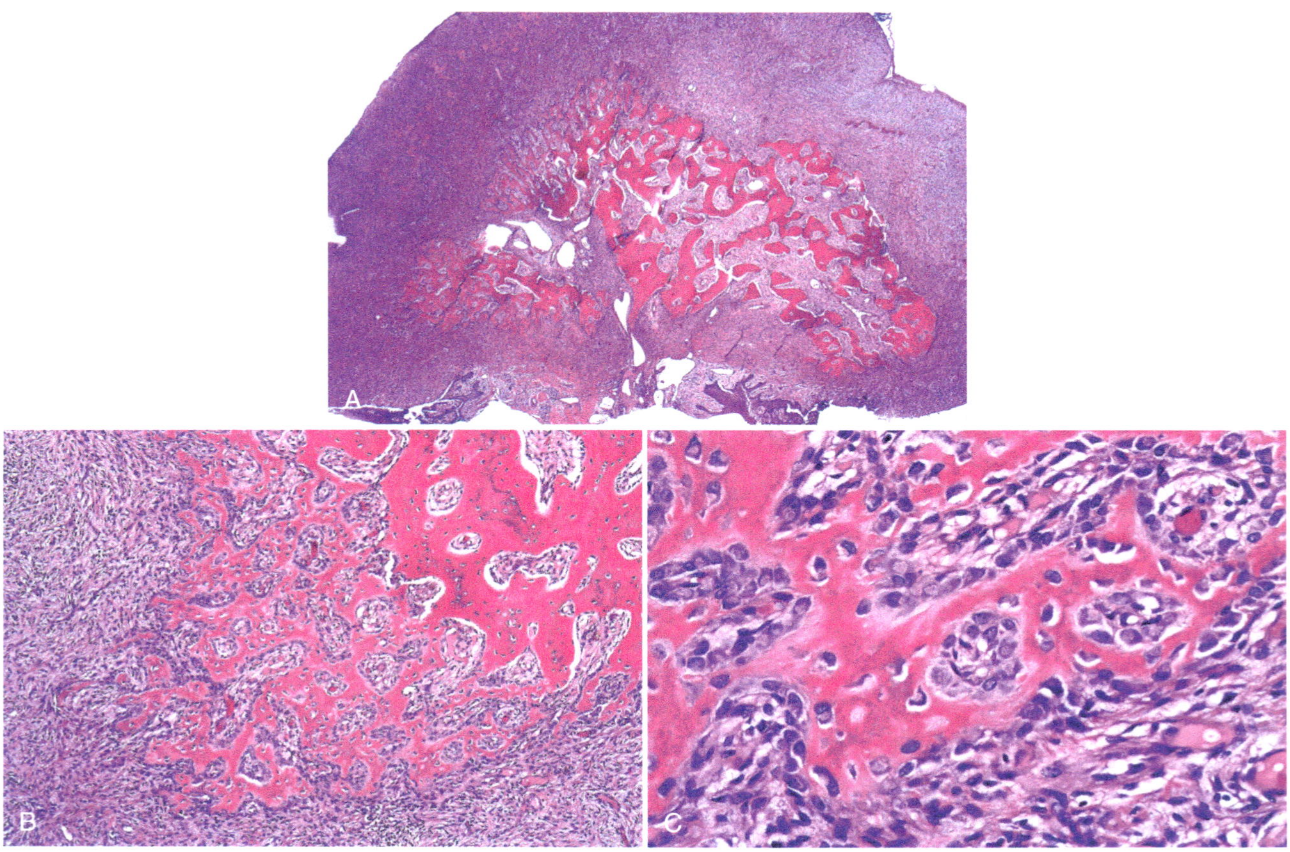

FIG 5.15 Peripheral ossifying fibroma. (A) Nodule of cellular fibrous tissue with abundant woven bone. (B) Cellular proliferation of spindle cells forming osteoid and woven bone. (C) Osteoid rimmed by layers of osteoblasts with plump osteocytes.

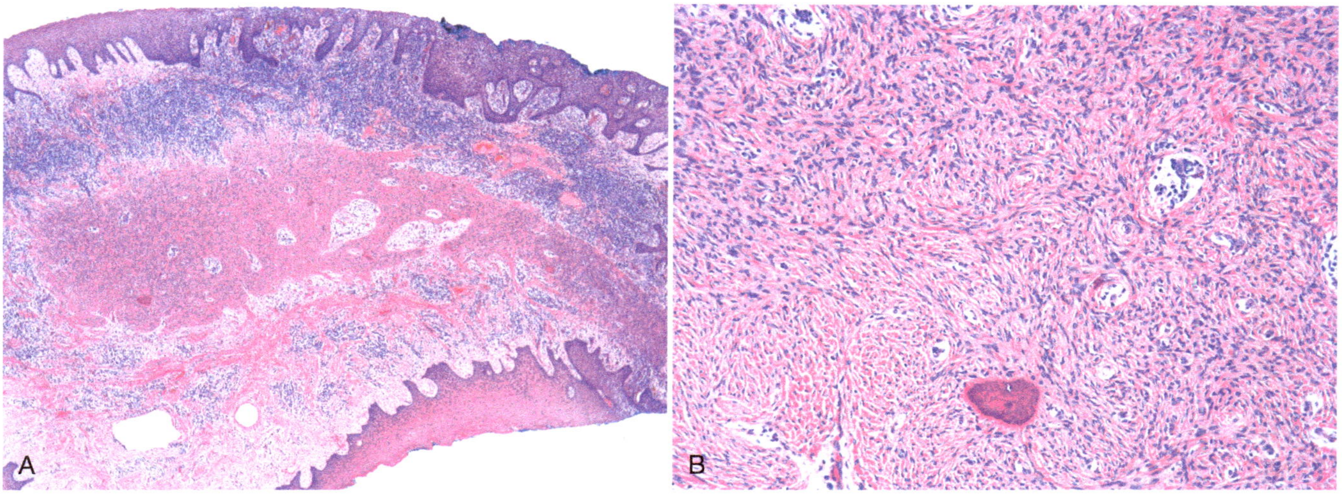

FIG 5.16 Peripheral ossifying fibroma. (A) Cellular proliferation of plump spindle cells with one focus of calcification. (B) Spindle cells have a storiform pattern with one focus of calcification.

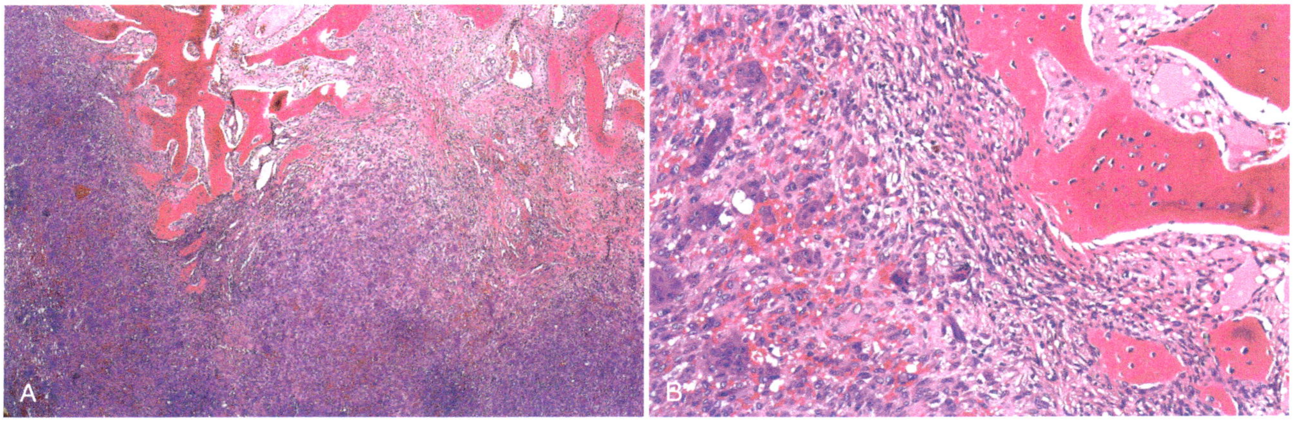

FIG 5.17 Peripheral ossifying fibroma and peripheral giant cell granuloma. (A) Sheets of giant cells and woven bone. (B) Woven bone formation and clusters of osteoclast-like giant cells and mononuclear cells in a hemorrhagic stroma.

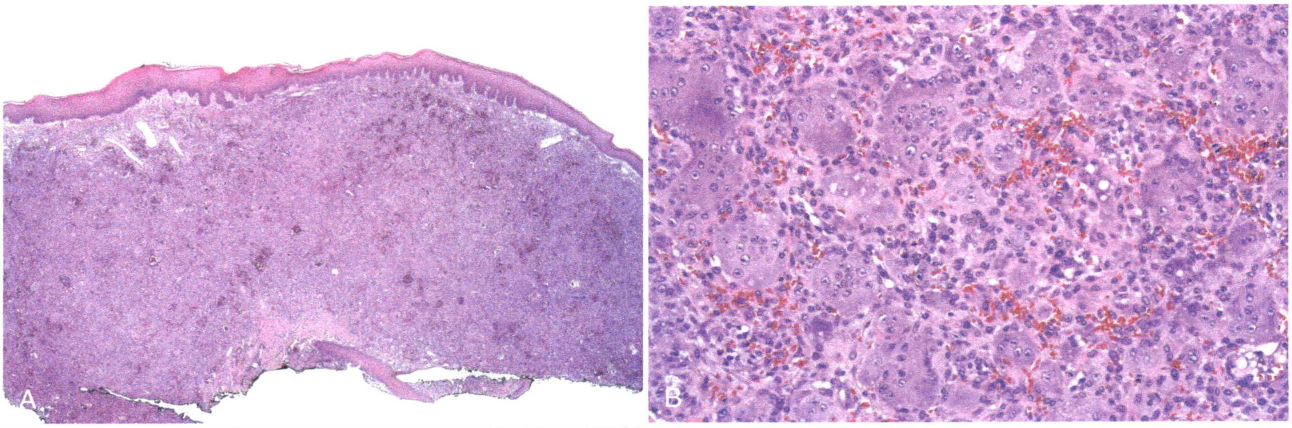

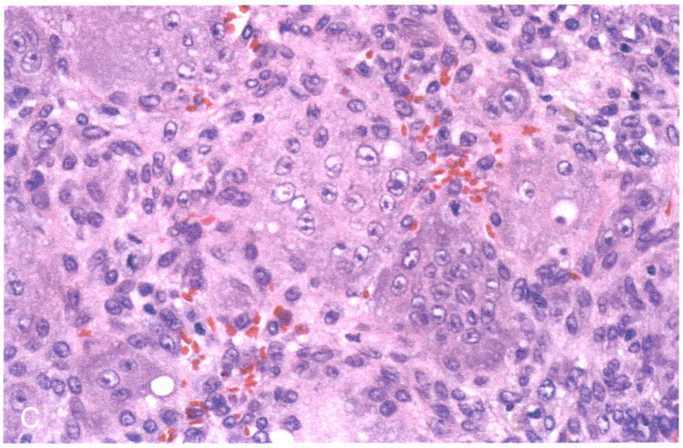

FIG 5.18 Peripheral giant cell granuloma. (A) Cellular tumor abuts the epithelium focally. (B) Sheets of multinucleate giant cells and mononuclear cells in vascular stroma. (C) Multinucleate giant cells and occasional mitoses in stromal cells.

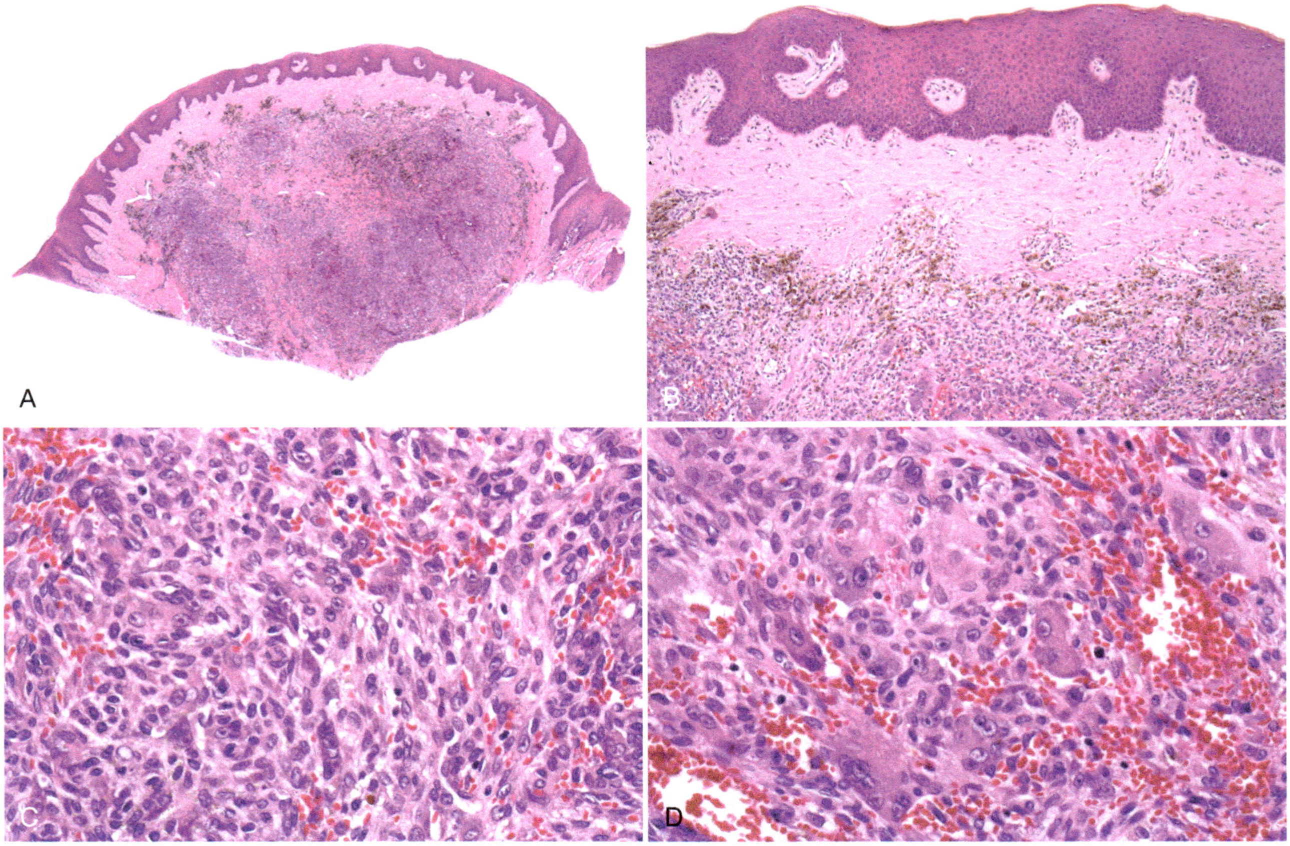

FIG 5.19 Peripheral giant cell granuloma. (A) Cellular tumor with grenz zone. (B) Hemosiderin and siderophages are prominent at the periphery of the lesion. (C) Many spindled mononuclear cells with hemorrhage. (D) Multinucleate giant cells and spindled mononuclear cells.

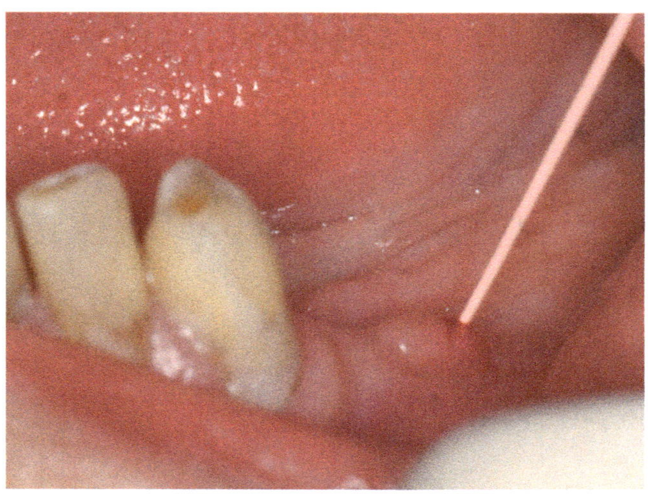

FIG 5.20 Parulis (sinus tract) of the gingiva with gutta-percha tracer.

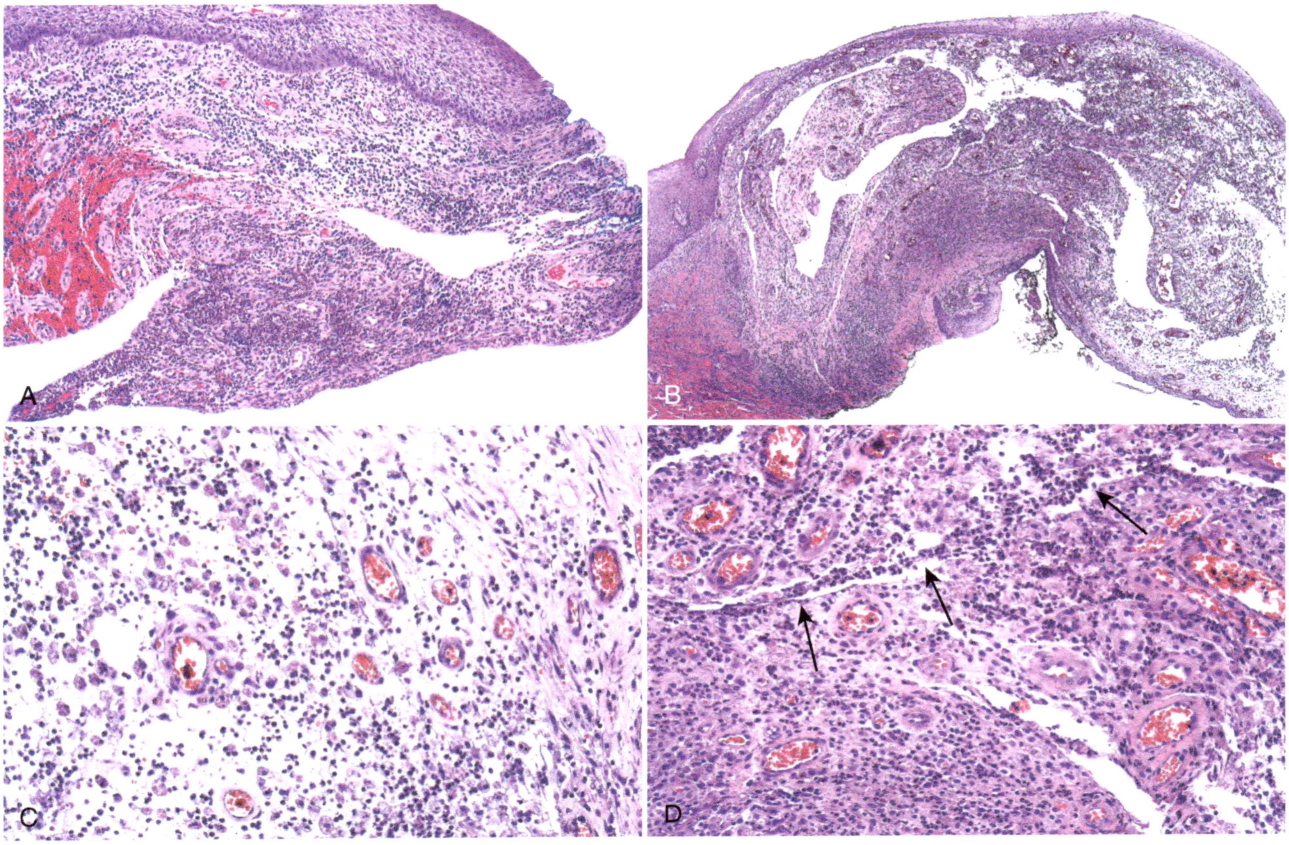

FIG 5.21 Parulis. (A) Edematous granulation tissue with linear tract communicating with the surface. (B) Edematous granulation tissue with linear spaces/tracts. (C) Edematous granulation tissue with foamy macrophages and acute and chronic inflammation, often misdiagnosed as a mucocele. (D) Tract filled with and lined by neutrophils (*arrows*).

Buchner A, Shnaiderman-Shapiro A, Vered M. Relative frequency of localized reactive hyperplastic lesions of the gingiva: a retrospective study of 1675 cases from Israel. *J Oral Pathol Med.* 2010;39:631-638.

de Oliveira DH, da Silveira EJ, de Medeiros AM, et al. Study of the etiopathogenesis and differential diagnosis of oral vascular lesions by immunoexpression of GLUT-1 and HIF-1alpha. *J Oral Pathol Med.* 2014;43:76-80.

Epivatianos A, Antoniades D, Zaraboukas T, et al. Pyogenic granuloma of the oral cavity: comparative study of its clinicopathological and immunohistochemical features. *Pathol Int.* 2005;55:391-397.

Fanourakis G, Lazaris AC, Krithinakis S, et al. Expression of receptor activator of NF-kappaB ligand and osteoprotegerin in peripheral giant cell granulomas of the jaws. *J Oral Pathol Med.* 2010;39:687-689.

Giunta JL. Gingival fibrous nodule. *Oral Surg Oral Med Oral Pathol Oral Radiol Endod.* 1999;88:451-454.

Gordon-Nunez MA, de Vasconcelos Carvalho M, Benevenuto TG, et al. Oral pyogenic granuloma: a retrospective analysis of 293 cases in a Brazilian population. *J Oral Maxillofac Surg.* 2010;68:2185-2188.

Johann AC, Salla JT, Gomez RS, et al. GLUT-1 in oral benign vascular lesions. *Oral Dis.* 2007;13:51-55.

Lester SR, Cordell KG, Rosebush MS, et al. Peripheral giant cell granulomas: a series of 279 cases. *Oral Surg Oral Med Oral Pathol Oral Radiol.* 2014;118:475-482.

Ono A, Tsukamoto G, Nagatsuka H, et al. An immunohistochemical evaluation of BMP-2, -4, osteopontin, osteocalcin and PCNA between ossifying fibromas of the jaws and peripheral cemento-ossifying fibromas on the gingiva. *Oral Oncol.* 2007;43:339-344.

Yuan K, Wing LY, Lin MT. Pathogenetic roles of angiogenic factors in pyogenic granulomas in pregnancy are modulated by female sex hormones. *J Periodontol.* 2002;73:701-708.

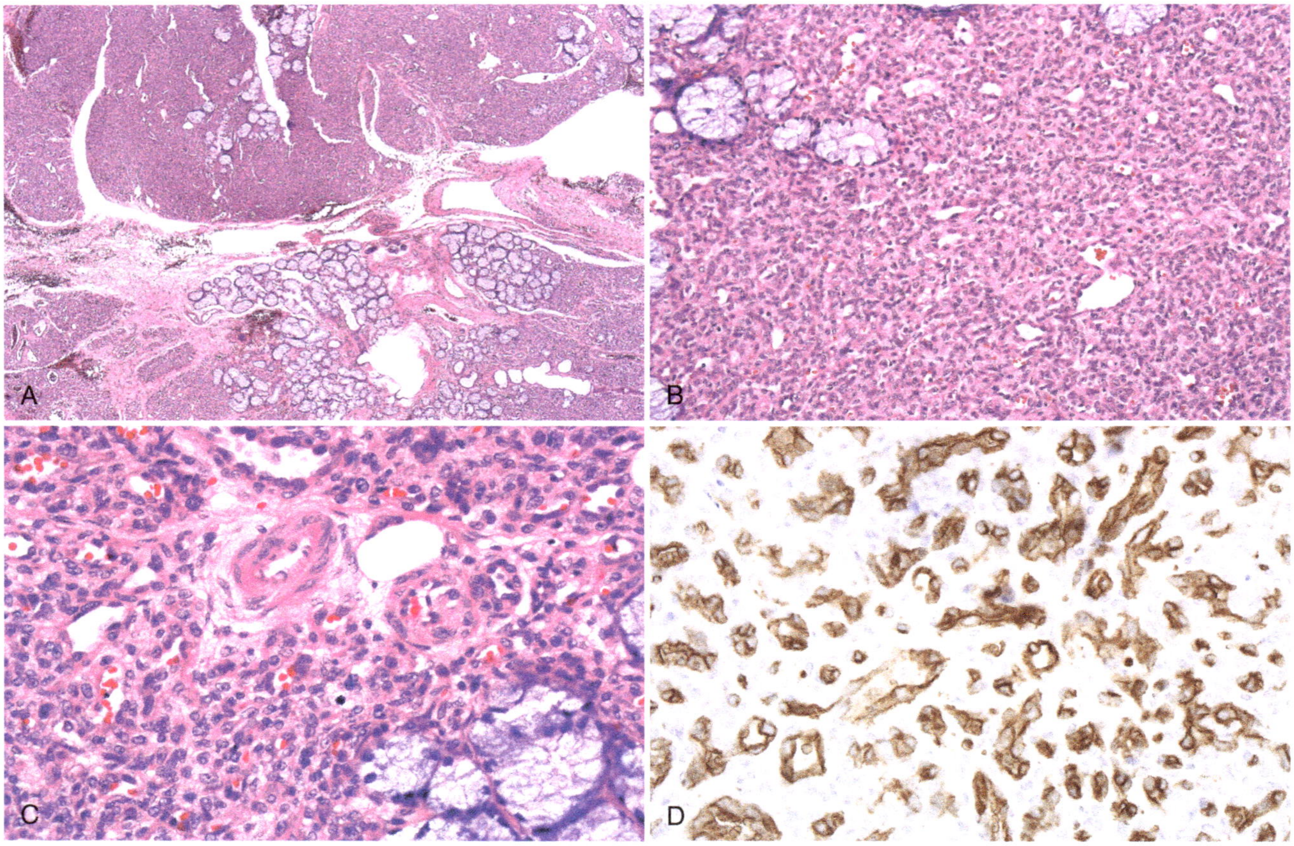

FIG 5.22 Infantile hemangioma of buccal mucosa. (A) Proliferation of endothelial cells that surround minor salivary glands. (B) Cellular proliferation of endothelial cells and capillaries. (C) Occasional mitoses noted. (D) Cytoplasmic positivity for glucose transporter-1 (GLUT-1). *(A, Courtesy Dr. Harry Kozakewich, Harvard Medical School, Boston, Mass.)*

DIFFUSE/MULTIFOCAL GINGIVAL HYPERPLASIA

Clinical Findings

- This is seen in patients with poor oral hygiene and/or undergoing hormonal changes (eg, puberty and pregnancy), and in patients on medications such as phenytoin, valproic acid, calcium channel blockers, cyclosporine, and rarely tacrolimus.
- There is a diffuse often slightly nodular enlargement of the gingiva of varying severity (Fig. 5.23A–B); leukemic infiltrates may have a similar clinical appearance (see Fig. 5.23C)

Etiopathogenesis and Histopathologic Features

Bacterial plaque induces the proliferation of fibroblasts, and hormones such as progesterone exacerbate this. Medications cause upregulation of TGF-β and a reduction in metalloproteinases, leading to accumulation of matrix. Recent research suggests that medication-induced gingival hyperplasia is caused by the medications inhibiting cellular folate uptake resulting in decreased collagenase activity and matrix degradation.

- There is fibrovascular hyperplasia with epithelial atrophy or acanthosis and variable chronic inflammation usually plasmacytic; cytoid bodies sometimes are present if there is prominent spongiosis (Fig. 5.24); phenytoin-associated lesions tend to be more fibrotic, whereas the other medication-induced gingival hyperplasias are more vascular; the gingival epithelium often loses its normal keratin layer from inflammation.
- "Test-tube" rete ridges have been reported in gingival lesions caused by phenytoin, but these are nonspecific and may also be seen in patients with conventional nonmedication-associated gingival hyperplasia.

Differential Diagnosis

- The presence of an atypical infiltrate should raise suspicion for acute myeloid or monocytic leukemia (see Chapter 17).
- The presence of abundant eosinophilic fibrinous material (positive with phosphotungstic acid-hematoxylin) that fills the lamina propria should raise suspicion for membranous (formerly ligneous) gingivitis/periodontitis, an autosomal recessive disorder of plasminogen activator deficiency that also affects other mucous membranes (Figs. 5.25 and 5.26).

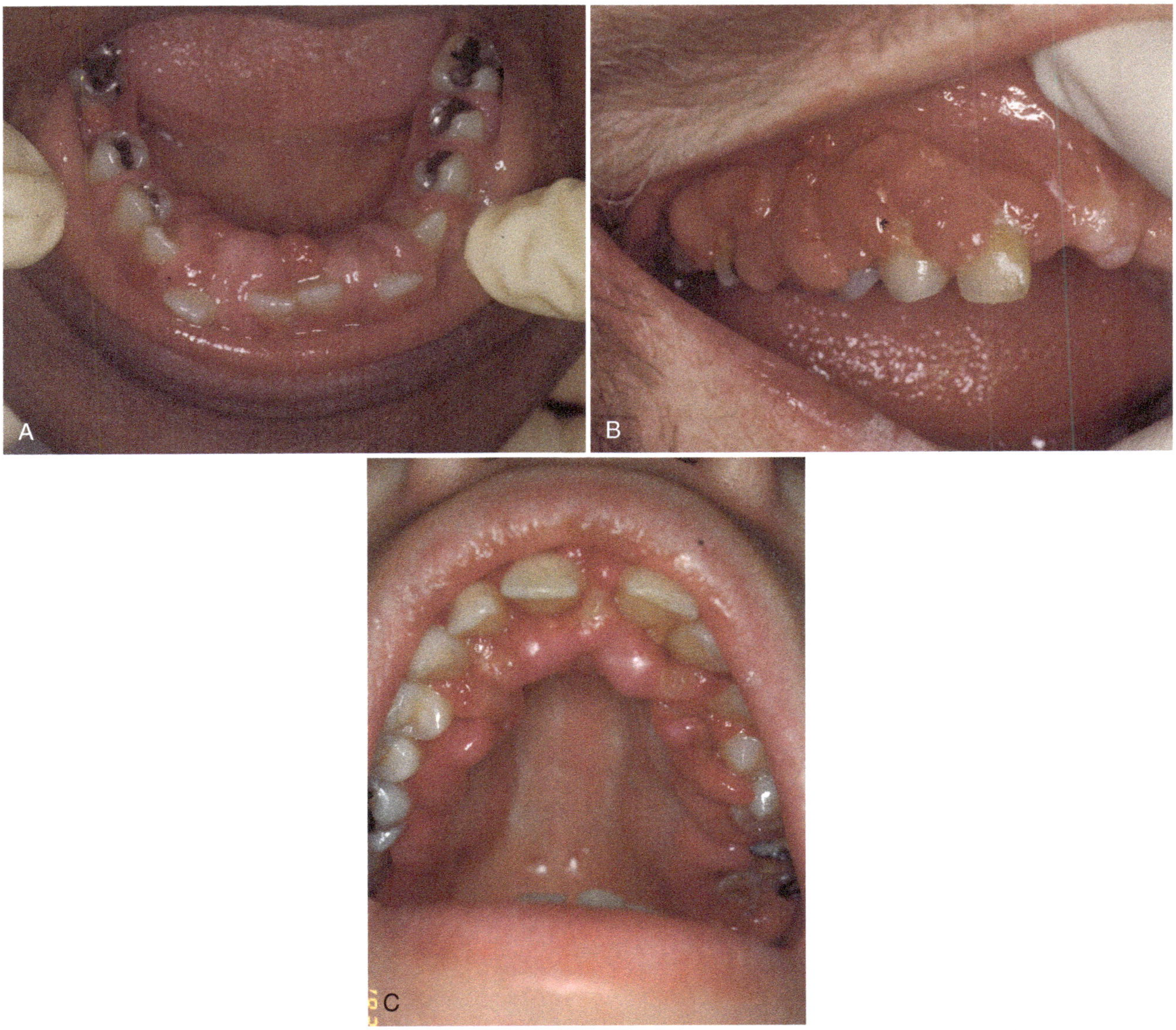

FIG 5.23 (A) Diffuse gingival hyperplasia secondary to phenytoin use. (B) Diffuse gingival hyperplasia secondary to nifedipine and cyclosporine use (postrenal transplantation). (C) Diffuse gingival enlargement from leukemic infiltrate.

Management and Prognosis

- Excision of hyperplastic tissue is the treatment of choice and subsequent maintenance of good oral hygiene; use of 0.12% chlorhexidine oral rinse, and low-dose doxycycline (20 mg) may reduce recurrence.

REFERENCES

Brown RS, Arany PR. Mechanism of drug-induced gingival overgrowth revisited: a unifying hypothesis. *Oral Dis.* 2015;21:e51-e61.

Fine G, Bauer K, Al-Mohaya M, Woo SB. Successful treatment of ligneous gingivitis with warfarin. *Oral Surg Oral Med Oral Pathol Oral Radiol Endod.* 2009;107:77-80.

Gunhan O, Gunhan M, Berker E, et al. Destructive membranous periodontal disease (ligneous periodontitis). *J Periodontol.* 1999;70:919-925.

Gunhan O, Avci A, Dereci O, et al. Extensive fibrin accumulation and accompanying epithelial changes in the pathogenesis of ligneous mucosal disease (ligneous periodontitis). *Am J Dermatopathol.* 2012;34:35-40.

Moffitt ML, Bencivenni D, Cohen RE. Drug-induced gingival enlargement: an overview. *Compend Contin Educ Dent.* 2013;34:330-336.

Trackman PC, Kantarci A. Molecular and clinical aspects of drug-induced gingival overgrowth. *J Dent Res.* 2015;94:540-546.

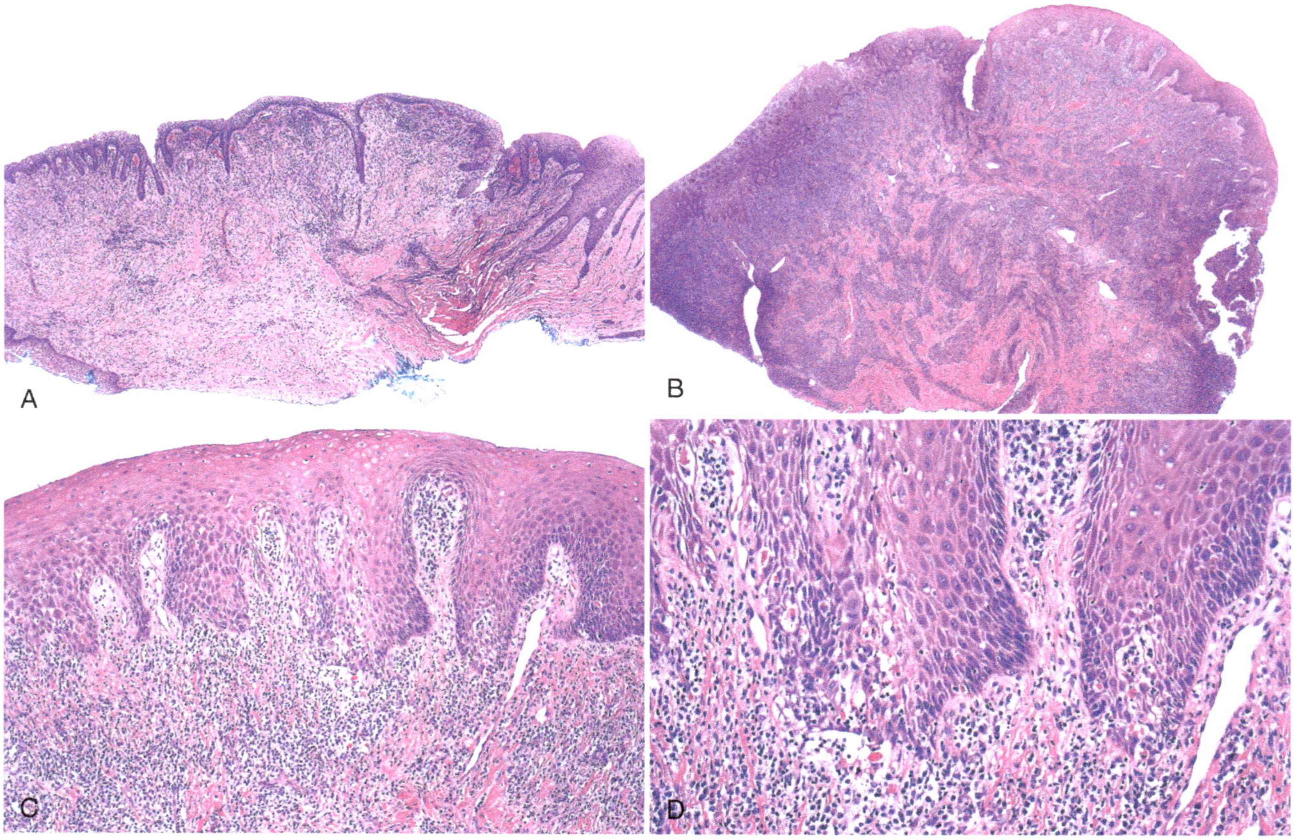

FIG 5.24 Gingival fibrous hyperplasia. (A) Fibrous tissue with epithelial atrophy and chronic inflammation. (B) Fibrous tissue with acanthosis and marked chronic inflammation. (C) Acanthosis with spongiosis. (D) Cytoid bodies present with many plasma cells.

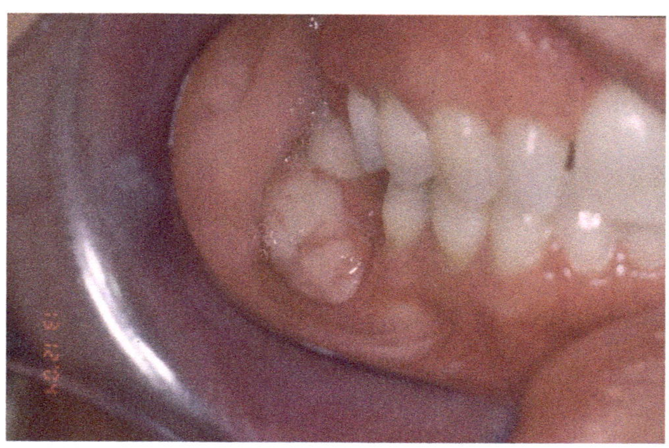

FIG 5.25 Membranous gingivitis/periodontitis manifesting as one of several yellowish (from fibrin) gingival nodules.

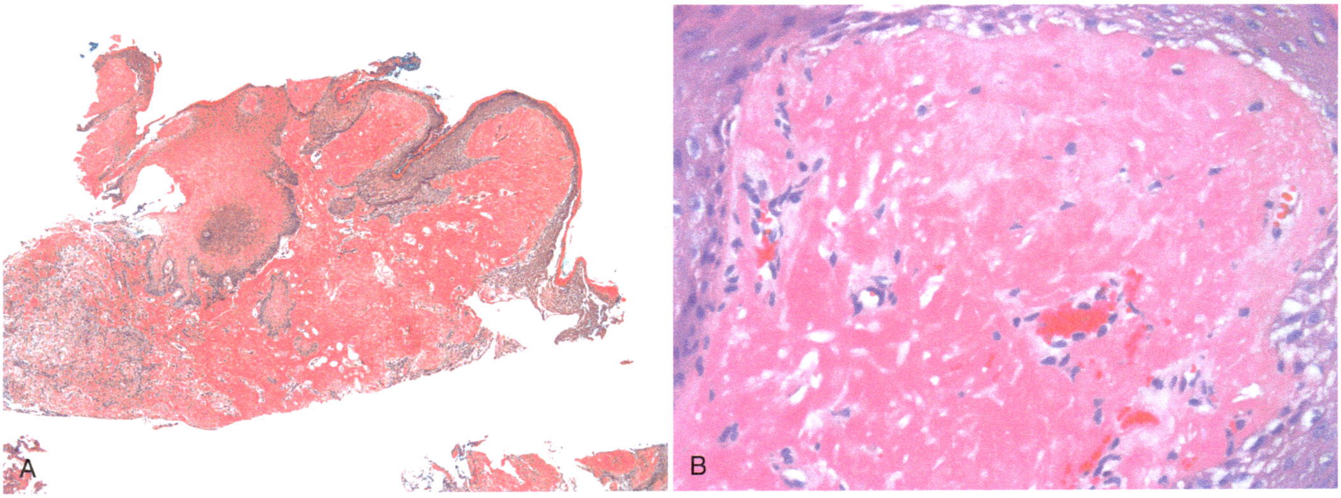

FIG 5.26 Membranous gingivitis/periodontitis. (A) The nodule consists of eosinophilic, amorphous material within the lamina propria. (B) Eosinophilic fibrinous material fills the lamina propria.

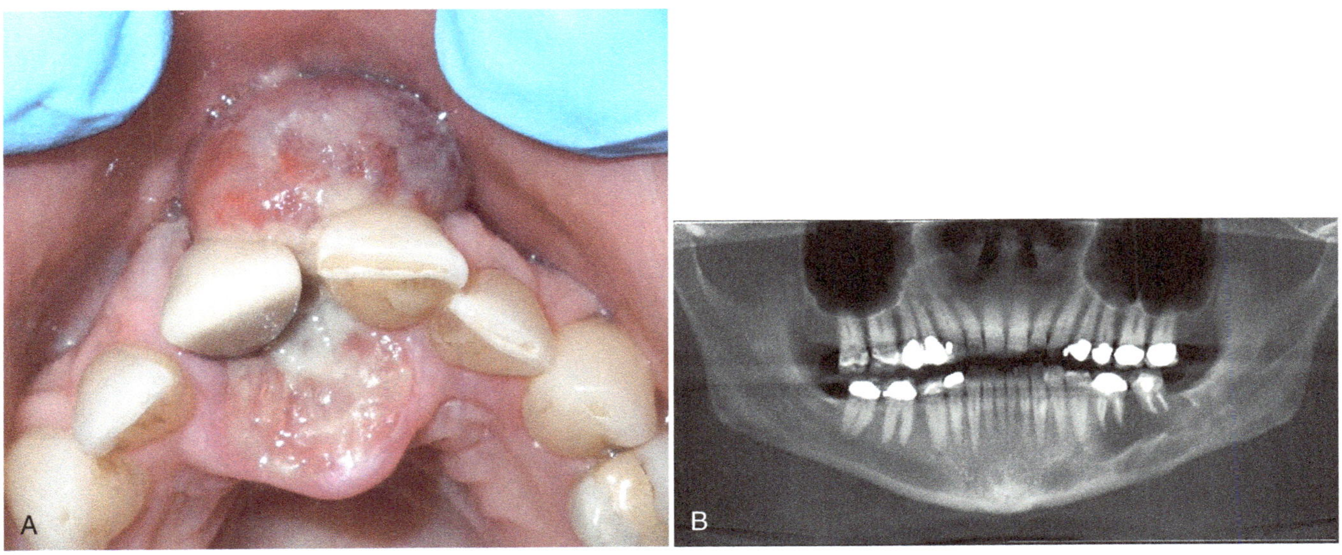

FIG 5.27 (A) Metastatic lung adenocarcinoma to the gingiva. (B) Metastatic renal cell carcinoma to the mandible. *(A, Courtesy Dr. Steven Young, private practice, Springfield, Mo; B, Courtesy Dr. Robert Schaedel, Boynton Beach, Fla.)*

GINGIVAL METASTASES

Two-thirds of metastases to the oral cavity occur to the jawbones (80% in the mandible) and one-third to the soft tissues, with the gingiva being the most common site, followed by the tongue.

Clinical Findings

- This occurs in older patients and gender predilection depends on the primary malignancy; it may present as a rapidly enlarging mass on the gingiva, may be associated with an underlying bone metastasis (radiolucency), or as a nonhealing extraction socket (Fig. 5.27); in 25% to 60% of cases, the gingival metastasis may be first indication that a malignancy is present.

Etiopathogenesis and Histopathologic Features

The most common primary sites for such metastases are lung, breast, prostate, kidney, and colon/rectum (Fig. 5.28).

Management and Prognosis

- As expected, the prognosis is extremely poor with few patients surviving more than 1 year, although this may change with new targeted therapies.

REFERENCES

D'Silva NJ, Summerlin DJ, Cordell KG, et al. Metastatic tumors in the jaws: a retrospective study of 114 cases. *J Am Dent Assoc.* 2006;137:1667-1672.

Hirshberg A, Shnaiderman-Shapiro A, Kaplan I, Berger R. Metastatic tumours to the oral cavity—pathogenesis and analysis of 673 cases. *Oral Oncol.* 2008;44:743-752.

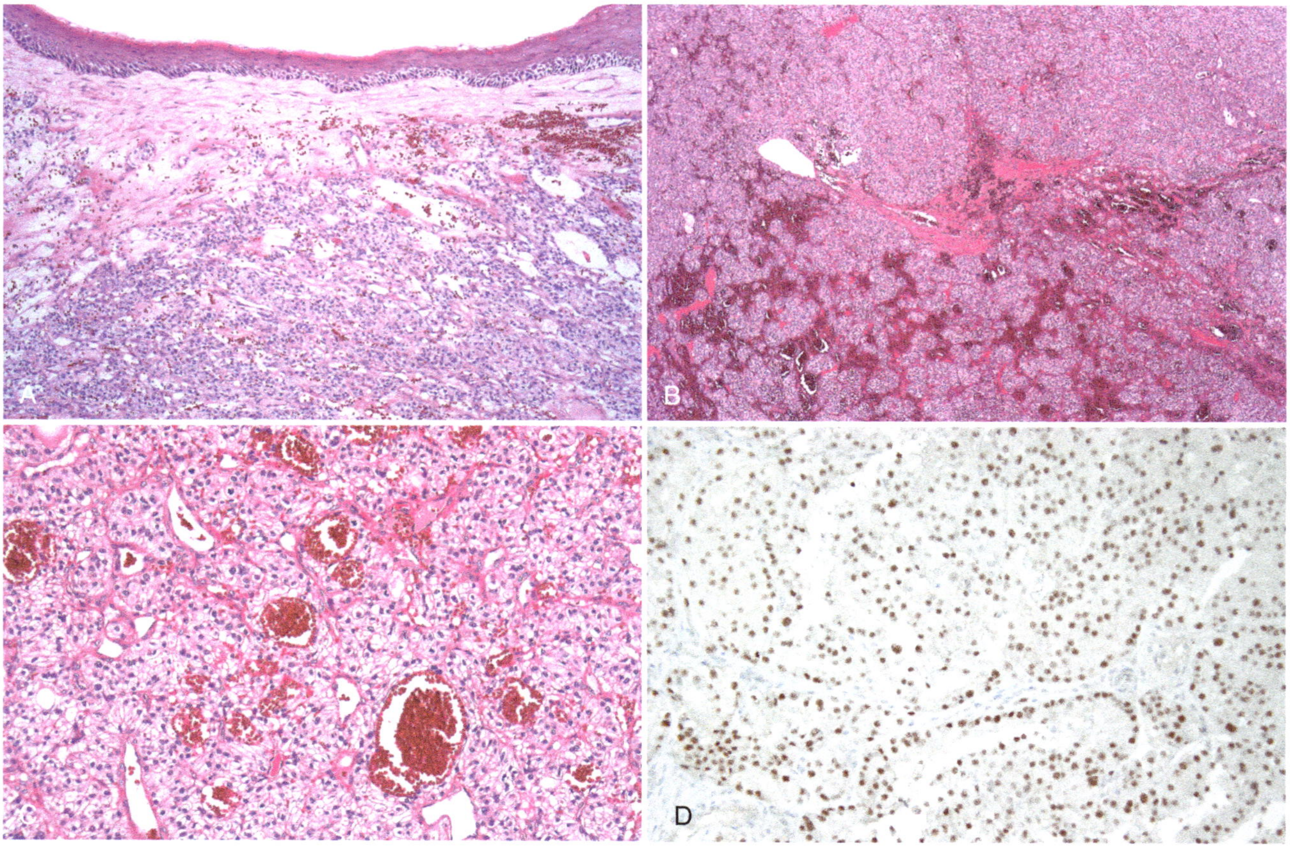

FIG 5.28 Metastatic renal cell carcinoma to the gingiva. (A) Tumor present within the gingival mucosa. (B) Tumor forms large lobules with nested tumor cells and abundant fresh hemorrhage. (C) Nests of clear cells surrounded by dilated vessels. (D) Diffuse nuclear positivity for PAX-8.

Denture-Associated Inflammatory Fibrous Hyperplasia (Epulis Fissuratum)

The term *epulis* refers to any mass on gingiva—inflammatory, neoplastic, or cystic—and is nonspecific.

Clinical Findings

- This occurs as a linear mass of tissue along the flange of a denture in the maxillary or mandibular buccal vestibule/sulcus or floor of the mouth, often with a fold in which the denture flange rests; the denture is loose and poorly fitting (Fig. 5.29) (see also Chapter 3).

Etiopathogenesis and Histopathologic Features

Fibrous tissue proliferates in reaction to trauma from movement of dentures on the mucosa.

- There is a fibroepithelial proliferation with a grossly fissured or papillary architecture with variable vascularity and a chronic inflammatory infiltrate (usually lymphocytic) that tends to be subepithelial; traumatic neuroma and myositis are often present (Fig. 5.30).
- Ulceration and pseudoepitheliomatous hyperplasia are not uncommon and the presence of spongiotic pustules necessitates a periodic acid–Schiff (PAS) stain with diastase digestion for identification of *Candida.*
- Cartilaginous and osseous metaplasias (sometimes with cytologic atypia) are sometimes seen (Cutright tumor) (Fig. 5.31); those found in maxillary fibrous hyperplasias are likely cartilaginous and are frequently encountered in the nasopalatine duct area.

Management and Prognosis

- Excision is curative if the denture is also relined or remade to reduce trauma to tissues.
- Treatment for candidiasis must include decontamination of the denture (see Appendix B).

REFERENCES

Canger EM, Celenk P, Kayipmaz S. Denture-related hyperplasia: a clinical study of a Turkish population group. *Braz Dent J.* 2009;20:243-248.

Cutright DE. Osseous and chondromatous metaplasia caused by dentures. *Oral Surg Oral Med Oral Pathol.* 1972;34:625-633.

Daley TD, Damm DD, Wysocki GP, Weir JC. Atypical cartilage in reactive osteocartilagenous metaplasia of the traumatized edentulous mandibular ridge. *Oral Surg Oral Med Oral Pathol Oral Radiol Endod.* 1997;83:26-29.

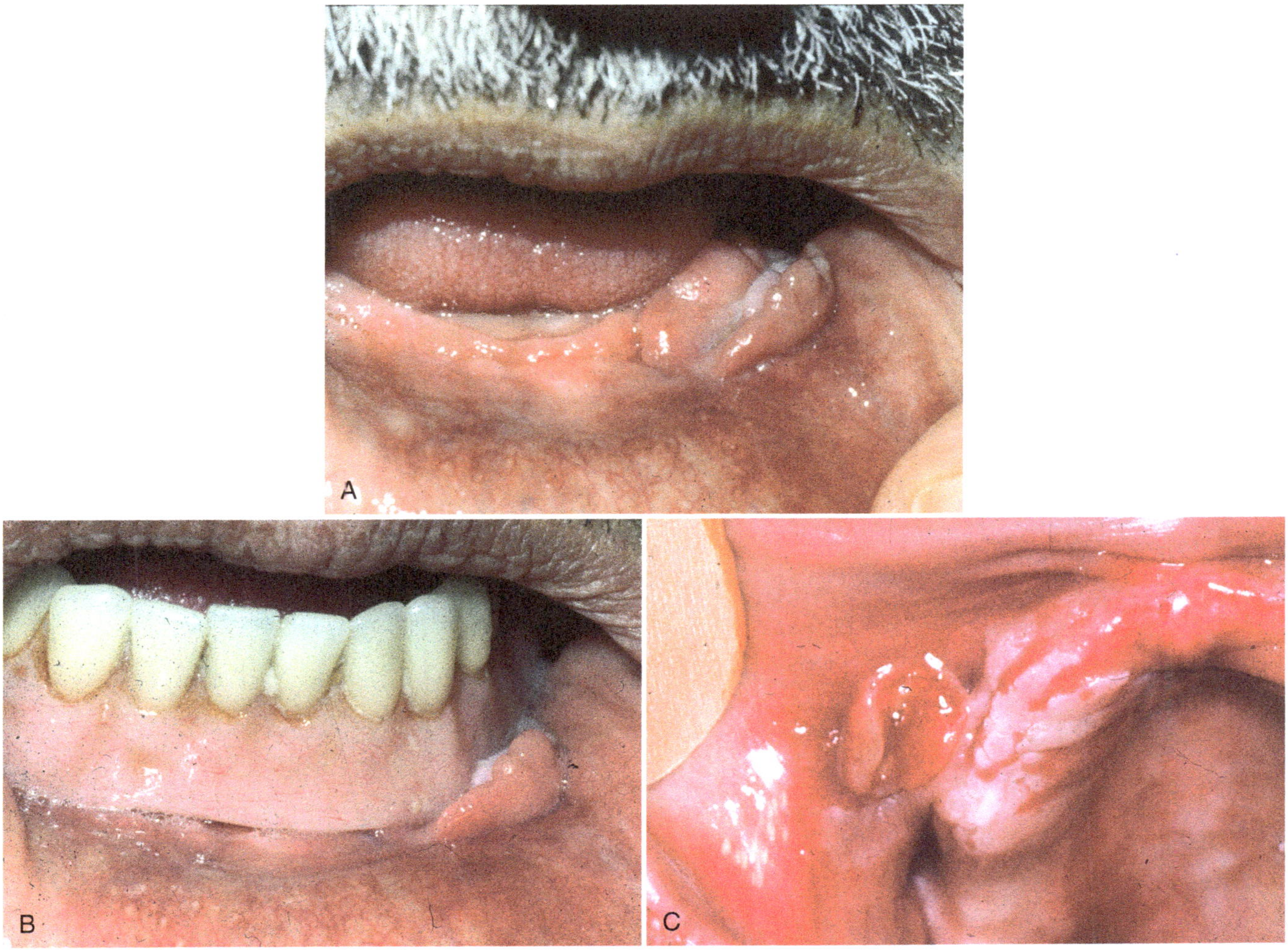

FIG 5.29 Denture-associated inflammatory fibrous hyperplasia. (A) Extraneous tissue has a fissure and papillary nodules. (B) Denture flange fits into the fissure. (C) Fissured fibrous hyperplasia and associated candidiasis.

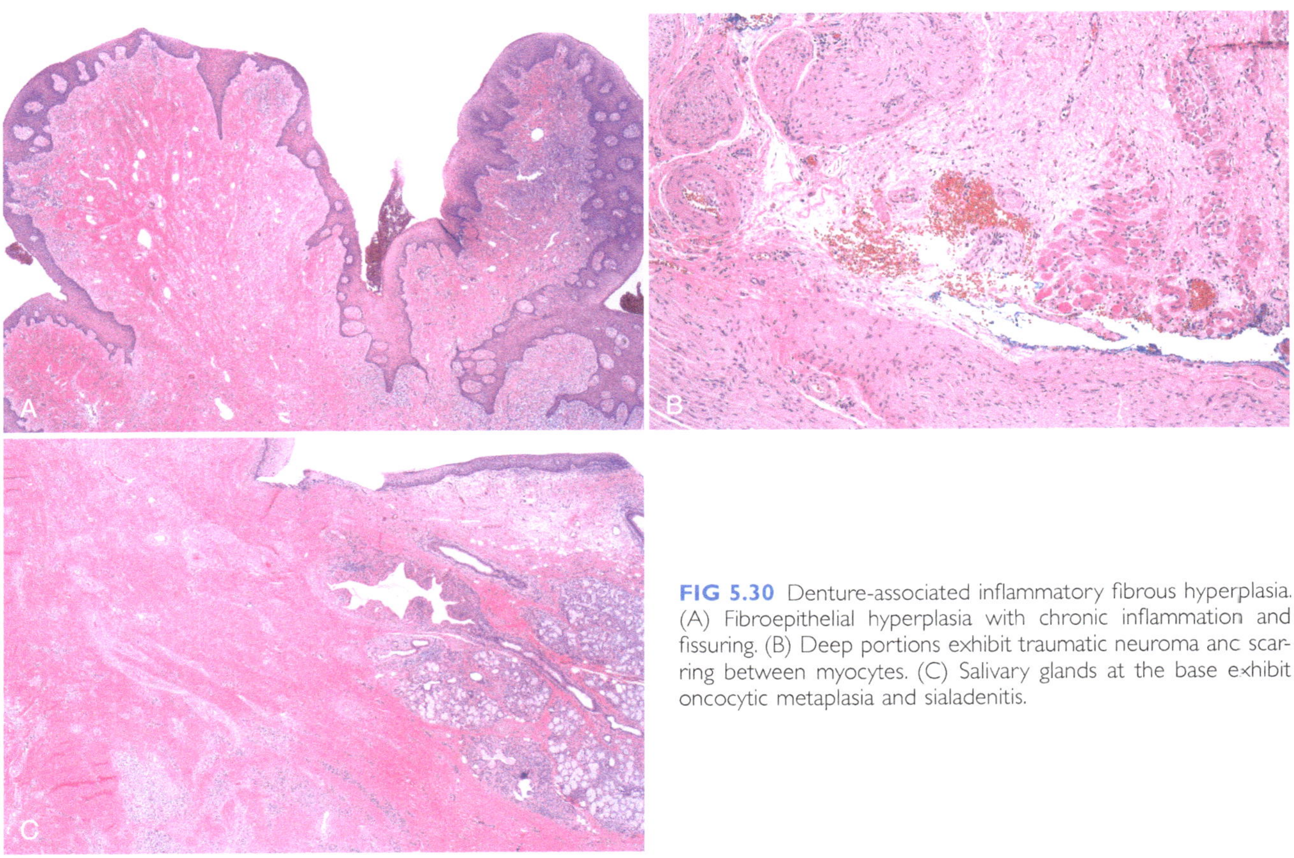

FIG 5.30 Denture-associated inflammatory fibrous hyperplasia. (A) Fibroepithelial hyperplasia with chronic inflammation and fissuring. (B) Deep portions exhibit traumatic neuroma anc scarring between myocytes. (C) Salivary glands at the base exhibit oncocytic metaplasia and sialadenitis.

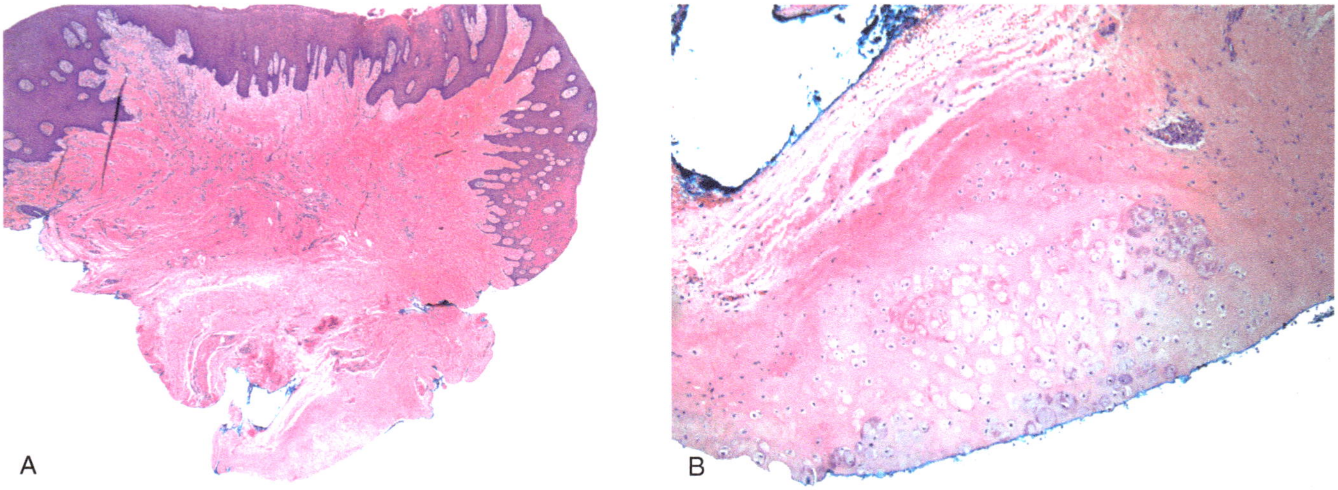

FIG 5.31 Denture-associated inflammatory fibrous hyperplasia. (A) Fibroepithelial hyperplasia with chronic inflammation and chondroid material at the base. (B) Mature hyaline cartilage is present within the fibrous tissue.

Lipocytic Lesions

LIPOMA

Clinical Findings

- This occurs in the fifth and sixth decades presenting as a yellowish, soft nodule often on the buccal mucosa, lips, and tongue (Fig. 5.32).

Etiopathogenesis and Histopathologic Features

True neoplasms arise from stem cells differentiating toward lipocytes, and in nonoral cases often show gene rearrangements on chromosome 12q. Pleomorphic lipoma, a variant of spindle cell lipoma, exhibits deletions in chromosome 13 or 16 and loss of retinoblastoma protein. Many so-called lipomas of the buccal mucosa represent herniation of the buccal fat pad.

- Thinly encapsulated lobules of mature lipocytes are sometimes separated by collagenous fibrous septa; lipocytes have evenly sized lipid vacuoles with no nuclear atypia; metaplastic bone (osteolipoma) or cartilage may be present (Figs. 5.33 and 5.34); the terms *lipofibroma* and *fibrolipoma* are sometimes used depending on whether fibrous or lipomatous tissue predominates, and lipomas may occur within muscle (intramuscular lipoma); unencapsulated tumors extensively and diffusely present in the buccinator muscle are more likely to represent herniation of the fat pad (Fig. 5.35).
- Spindle cell lipomas are true lipocytic neoplasms that are not uncommon in the oral cavity, and exhibit proliferation of bland spindle cells with mature lipocytes, ropy or wiry collagen, mucinous stroma, and mast cells (Fig. 5.36); cells are CD34+ (see Fig. 5.36C); pleomorphic lipoma is a variant of spindle cell lipoma with floret-type multinucleate cells.

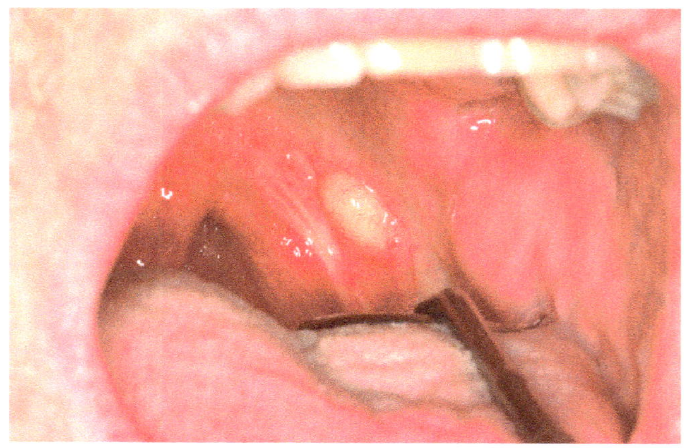

FIG 5.32 Lipoma of left soft palate.

Differential Diagnosis

- Lipocytic metaplasia may be seen in pleomorphic adenoma, but the spindled myoepithelial cells would be positive for keratin, smooth muscle actin, and p63.
- Traumatic and degenerative changes in fatty tissue may mimic lesions of atypical lipomatous tumors, and intramuscular lipomas may appear to be pseudoinvasive (Figs. 5.37 and 5.38); Lockhern cells (with nuclear pseudoinclusions) may be seen.

Management and Prognosis

- Excision is curative.

REFERENCES

Chen BJ, Marino-Enriquez A, Fletcher CD, Hornick JL. Loss of retinoblastoma protein expression in spindle cell/pleomorphic lipomas and cytogenetically related tumors: an immunohistochemical study with diagnostic implications. *Am J Surg Pathol.* 2012;36:1119-1128.

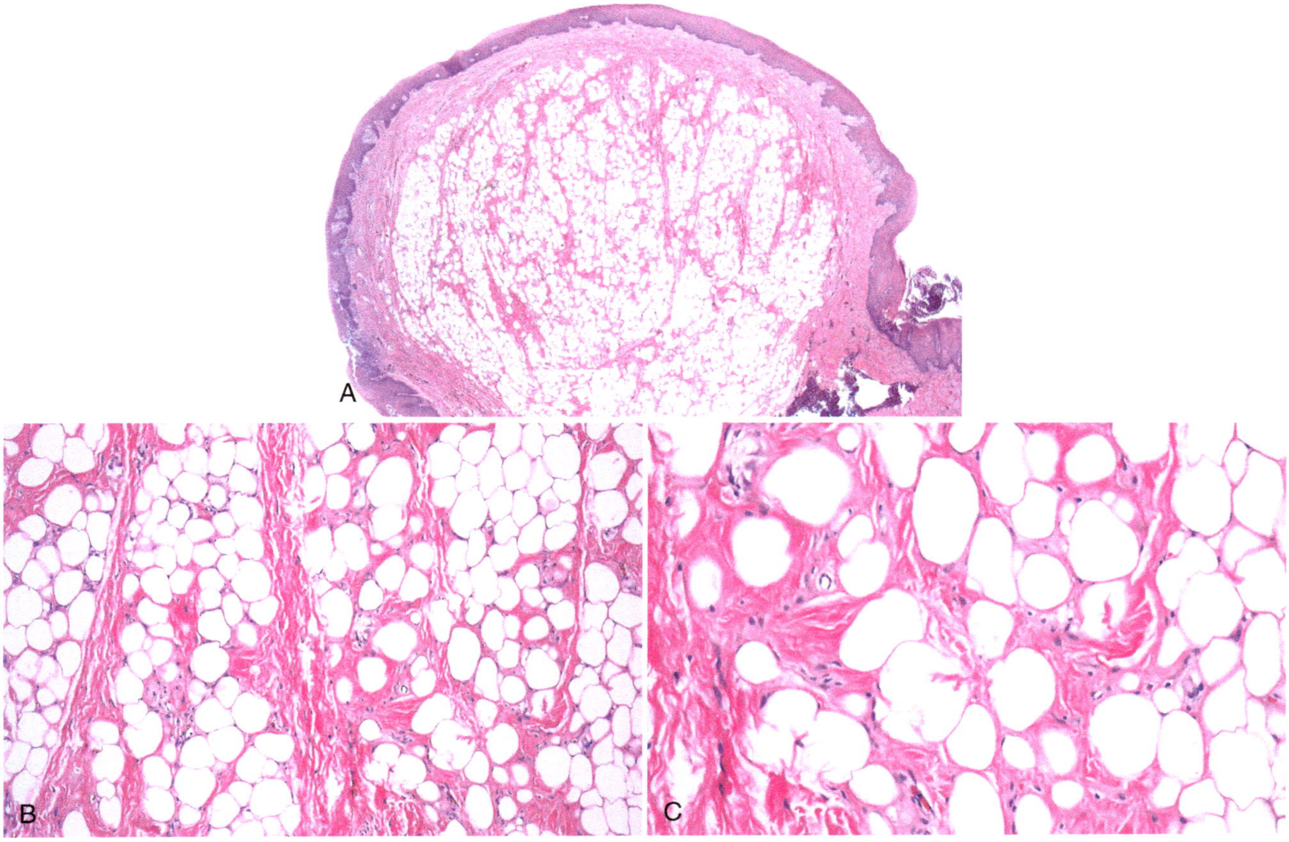

FIG 5.33 Lipoma. (A) Discrete nodule of lipocytes with bands of collagen. (B) Lipocytes with intervening bands of mature collagen. (C) Mature lipocytes with uniform lipid vacuoles and intervening fibrosis.

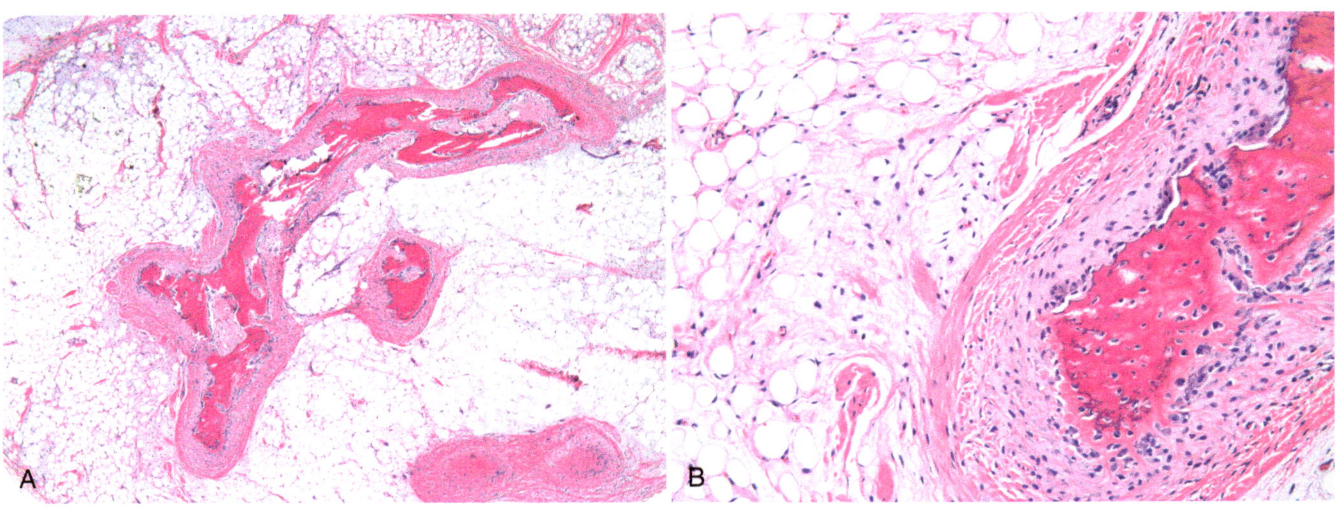

FIG 5.34 Osteolipoma. (A) Lipoma with osseous metaplasia. (B) Osteoid and woven bone with osteoclasts, surrounded by spindle cells.

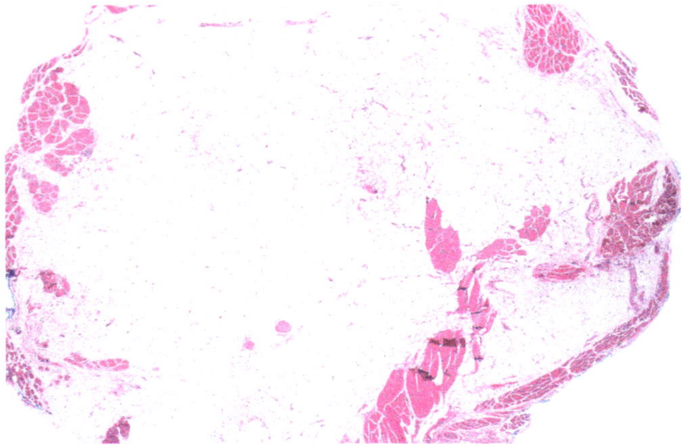

FIG 5.35 Herniation of buccal fat pad showing mature lipocytes diffusely within muscle fibers.

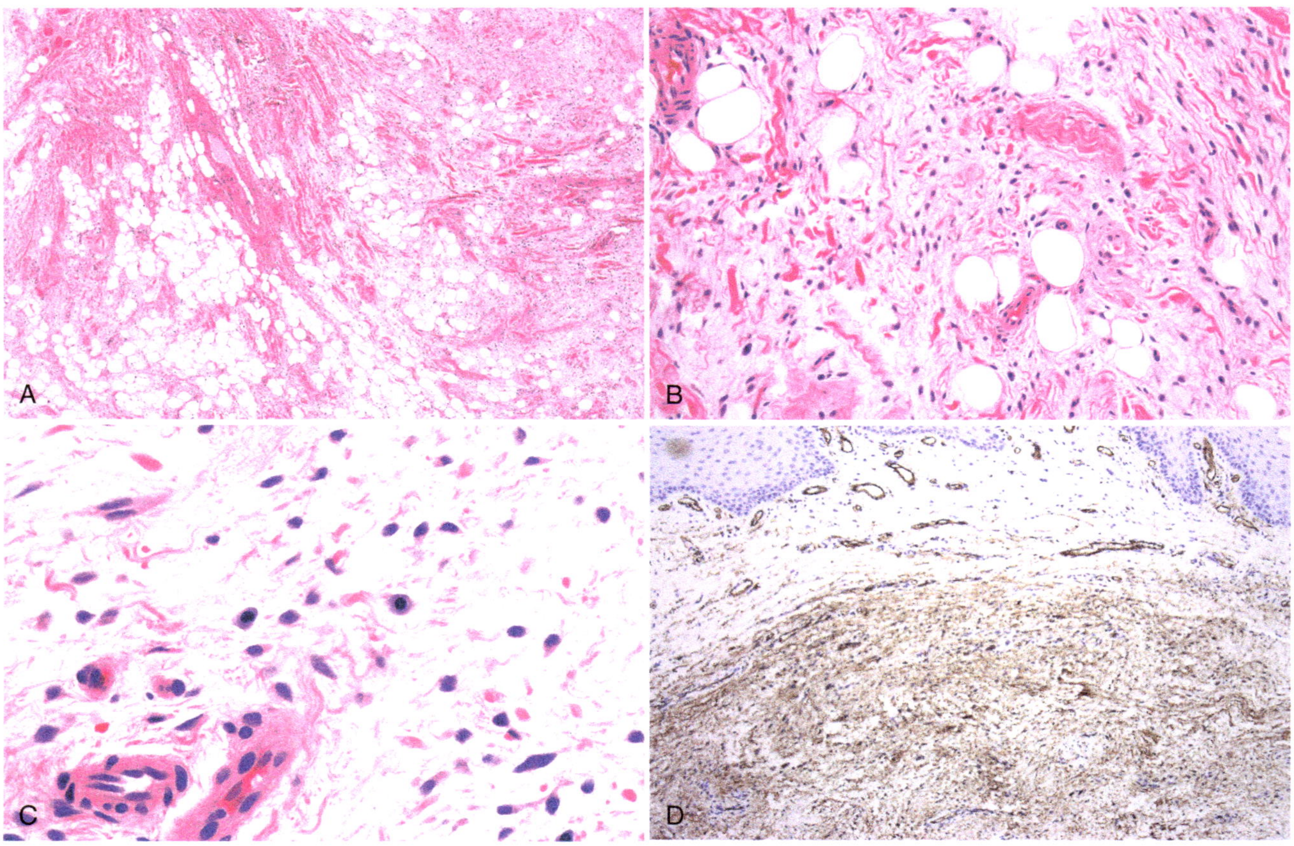

FIG 5.36 Spindle cell lipoma. (A) Mixture of mature lipocytes, spindle cells, and dense, ropy collagen. (B) Mature lipocytes, spindle cells, ropy collagen, and mast cells. (C) Spindle cells and mast cells. (D) Spindle cells are CD34+.

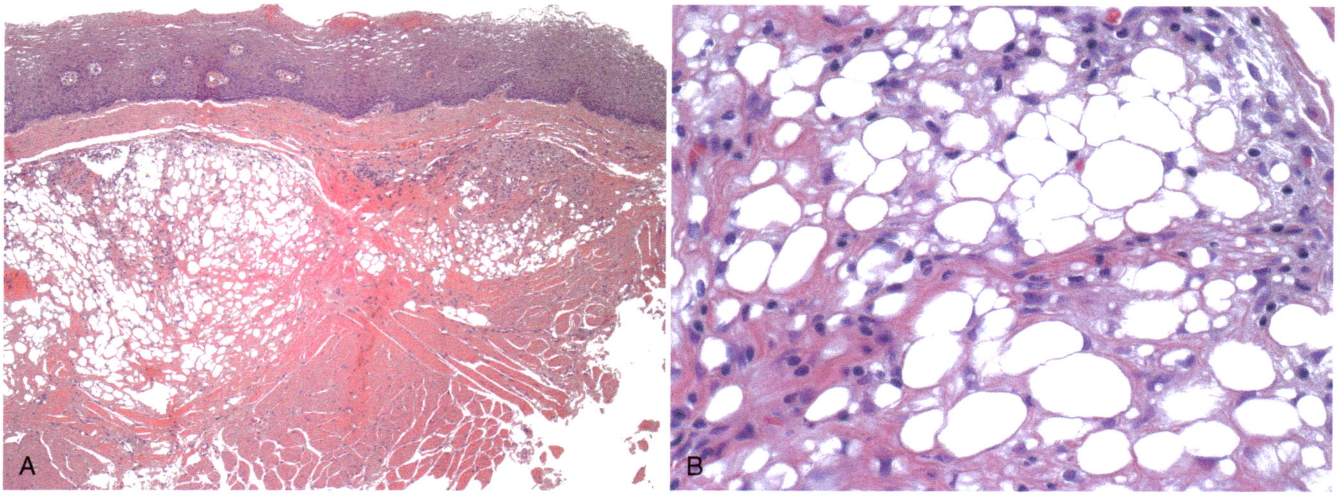

FIG 5.37 Traumatized lipoma. (A) Lipoma of tongue mucosa showing lipocytes of varying sizes with some fibrosis. (B) Lipoblast-like cells are noted with multiple vacuoles and indented nuclei (*middle and upper left*); Lockhern cells (with nuclear pseudoinclusions) are present.

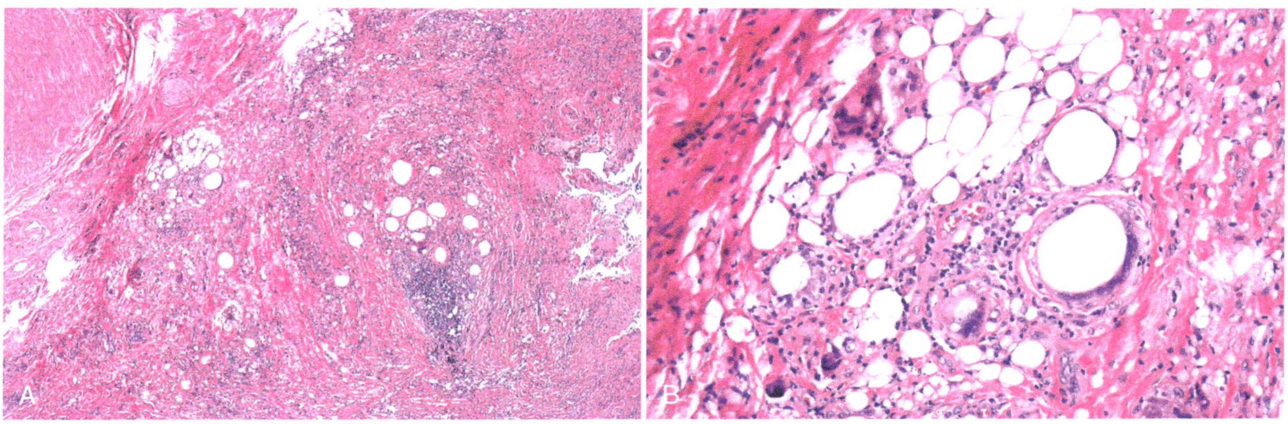

FIG 5.38 Lipid degeneration and inflammation. (A) Lipid vacuoles of varying sizes with fibrosis and chronic inflammation. (B) Small and large lipid vacuoles, some within multinucleate giant cells.

Doyle LA, Vivero M, Fletcher CD, et al. Nuclear expression of STAT6 distinguishes solitary fibrous tumor from histologic mimics. *Mod Pathol.* 2014;27:390-395.

Fregnani ER, Pires FR, Falzoni R, et al. Lipomas of the oral cavity: clinical findings, histological classification, and proliferative activity of 46 cases. *Int J Oral Maxillofac Surg.* 2003;32:49-53.

Furlong MA, Fanburg-Smith JC, Childers EL. Lipoma of the oral and maxillofacial region: site and subclassification of 125 cases. *Oral Surg Oral Med Oral Pathol Oral Radiol Endod.* 2004;98:441-450.

Lau SK, Bishop JA, Thompson LD. Spindle cell lipoma of the tongue: a clinicopathologic study of 8 cases and review of the literature. *Head Neck Pathol.* 2015;9:253-259.

Manor E, Sion-Vardy N, Joshua BZ, Bodner L. Oral lipoma: analysis of 58 new cases and review of the literature. *Ann Diagn Pathol.* 2011;15:257-261.

Rubin BP, Dal Cin P. The genetics of lipomatous tumors. *Semin Diagn Pathol.* 2001;18:286-293.

ATYPICAL LIPOMATOUS TUMOR

The most common malignant fat-producing tumor in the oral cavity is the atypical lipomatous tumor. Myxoid liposarcoma is a distant second in frequency of occurrence; dedifferentiated, spindle cell, and pleomorphic liposarcomas are rare.

Clinical Findings

This occurs in the fifth to seventh decades with slight male predominance, the majority occurring on the tongue and the buccal mucosa; it is a slow-growing, innocuous-appearing deep mucosal nodule.

Etiopathogenesis and Histopathologic Features

Atypical lipomatous tumor refers to a well-differentiated liposarcoma occurring on somatic soft tissue sites amenable to complete surgical excision such as the skin or mucosa. Tumors have distinctive ring chromosomes derived from 12q13(13–15); *MDM2* and *CDK4* are almost always amplified, with CDK4 being more specific.

- Most cases are lipoma-like and consist of a discrete but infiltrative proliferation of lipoblasts, lipocytes, and atypical spindle stromal cells; lipoblasts exhibit variation in the size of vacuoles and usually multivacuolation and have indented nuclei that are hyperchromatic and pleomorphic Lockhern cells with nuclear pseudoinclusions are often present but these may be seen in other tumors; there is insignificant mitotic activity and no necrosis or hemorrhage (Fig. 5.39).

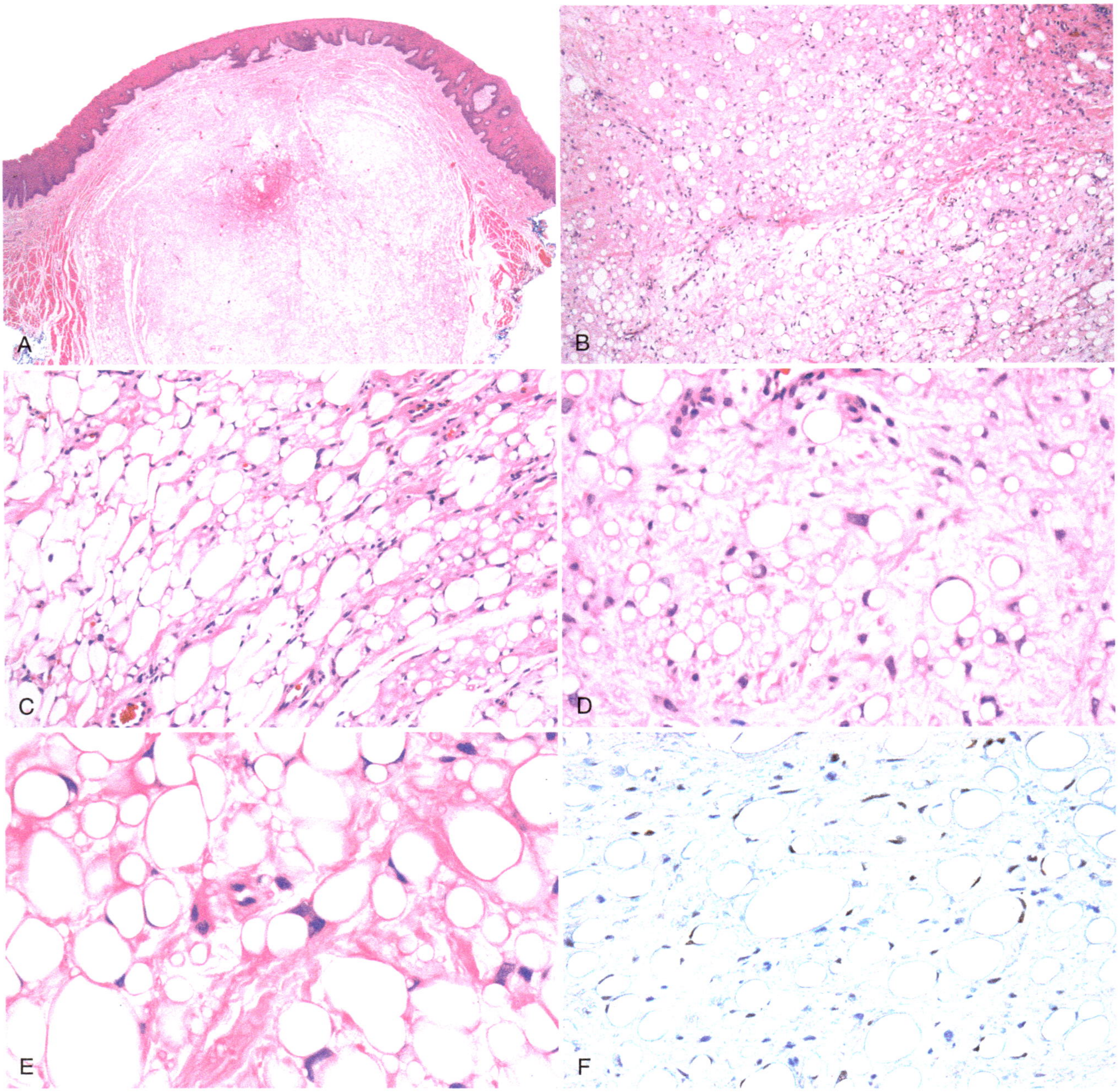

FIG 5.39 Atypical lipomatous tumor. (A) Lipocytic tumor with infiltrative borders. (B) Lipocytes with variably sized lipid vacuoles and spindle stromal cells with delicate collagen. (C) Lipid vacuoles of varying sizes. (D) Lipoblasts with nuclear pleomorphism and hyperchromasia. (E) Lipoblasts with indented, pleomorphic nuclei, some with nuclear pseudoinclusions (Lockhern cells). (F) Lipoblasts and stromal cells are positive for CDK4.

- Tumors may be sclerotic and rarely exhibit osseous, cartilaginous, or muscle metaplasia.
- *MDM2* and *CDK4* are consistently amplified and CD34 is negative; fluorescent in situ hybridization for MDM2 and CDK4 confirms the diagnosis.

Differential Diagnosis

Lipoblasts may be seen in spindle cell lipoma, pleomorphic lipoma, lipoblastoma, fat necrosis and degeneration, and silicone granulomas; however, they would be negative for *MDM2* and *CDK4* amplification.

Management and Prognosis

Wide excision is the treatment of choice and 10% to 15% recur, but they do not tend to metastasize.

REFERENCES

Dei Tos AP. Liposarcomas: diagnostic pitfalls and new insights. *Histopathology*. 2014;64:38-52.

Fanburg-Smith JC, Furlong MA, Childers EL. Liposarcoma of the oral and salivary gland region: a clinicopathologic study of 18 cases with emphasis on specific sites, morphologic subtypes, and clinical outcome. *Mod Pathol*. 2002;15:1020-1031.

Laco J, Mentzel T, Hornychova H, et al. Atypical lipomatous tumors of the tongue: report of six cases. *Virchows Arch.* 2009;455:383-388.
Nascimento AF, McMenamin ME, Fletcher CD. Liposarcomas/atypical lipomatous tumors of the oral cavity: a clinicopathologic study of 23 cases. *Ann Diagn Pathol.* 2002;6:83-93.

Miscellaneous Tumors

ORAL FOCAL MUCINOSIS

Clinical Findings

- This occurs most frequently in the fifth decade with a 2:1 female predilection and presents as a soft nodule of the gingiva (involved in 80% of cases) (Fig. 5.40).

Etiopathogenesis and Histopathologic Features

- Oral focal mucinosis may be a response to inflammation because reactive fibrous hyperplasia of the gingiva often shows myxoid change (see earlier).
- There is a nonencapsulated pool of mucinous or myxoid, alcianophilic ground substance with short bands of collagen; there are scattered S100 protein– spindle and stellate cells with trailing cytoplasmic processes and benign nuclei, and short bands of collagen; reticulin fibers are usually absent (Figs. 5.41 and 5.42).

Differential Diagnosis

- Soft tissue myxoma is a rare mesenchymal neoplasm that is encapsulated and may be difficult to distinguish from focal mucinosis but reticulin fibers are apparently more prominent; mucocutaneous myxomas are observed in Carney complex.
- Mucoceles have pools of mucin surrounded by granulation tissue containing muciphages.
- Spindle cells of myxoid neurofibroma are positive for neural markers such as S100 protein.
- Superficial angiomyxoma is a rare myxoid tumor that contains numerous blood vessels and CD34+ spindle cells, and may behave aggressively (Fig. 5.43).

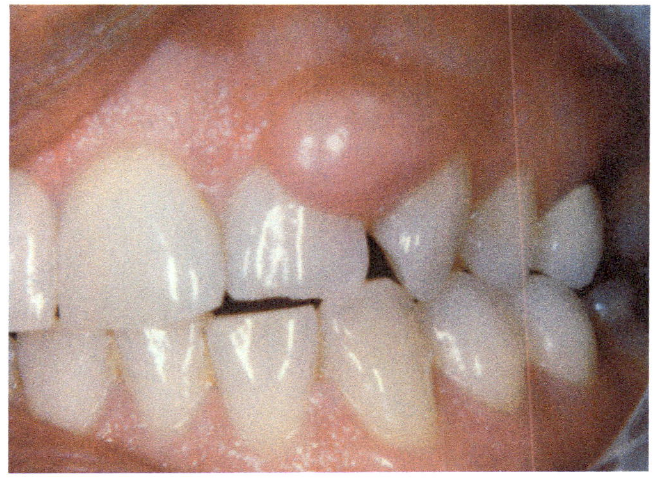

FIG 5.40 Oral focal mucinosis: soft, gelatinous nodule of the gingiva.

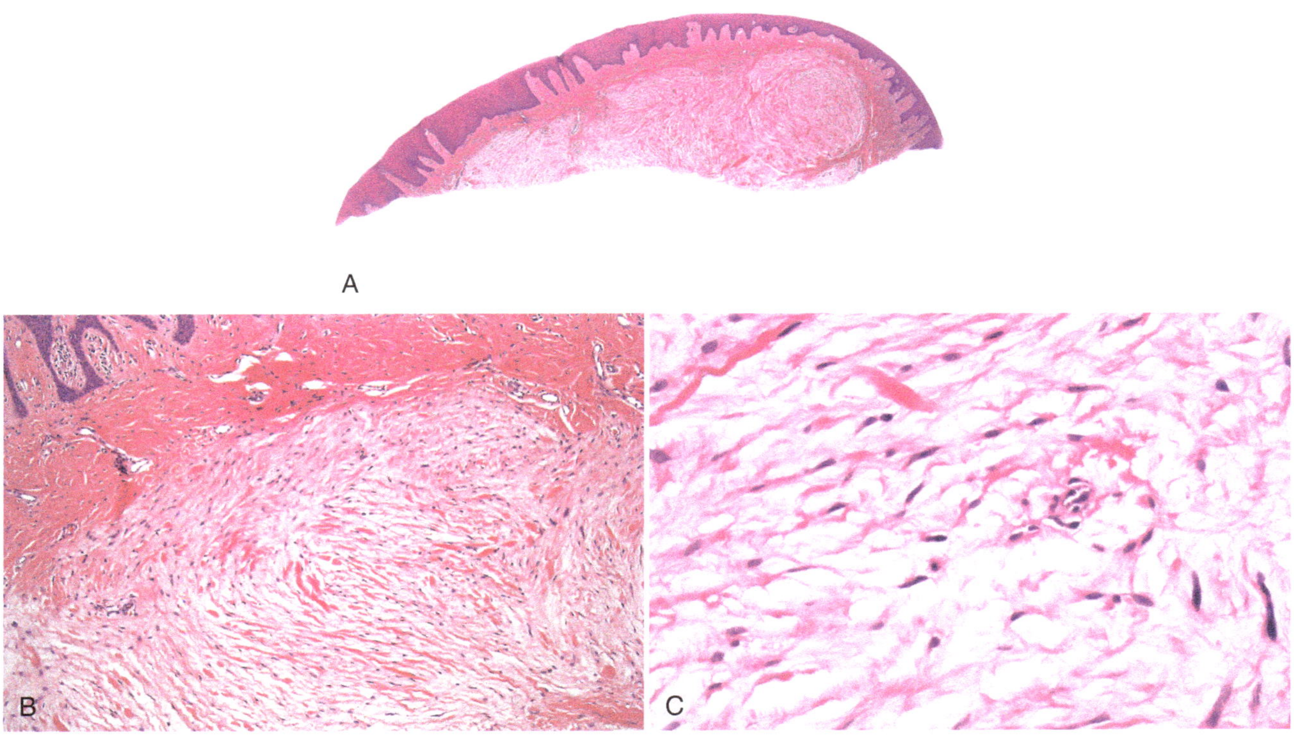

FIG 5.41 (A) Oral focal mucinosis of the gingiva. (B) Well-circumscribed pool of mucinous material with spindle cells and short bundles of collagen. (C) Spindle fibroblasts within myxoid/mucinous stroma.

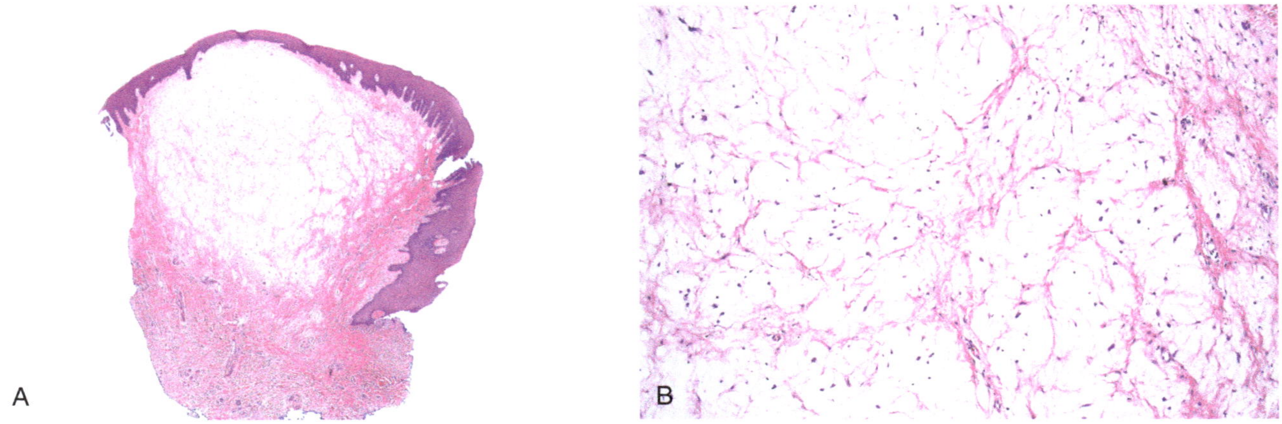

FIG 5.42 Oral focal mucinosis. (A) Nonencapsulated pools of mucinous material. (B) Mucinous material separated by thin collagen bands and stellate and spindle cells with a loculated pattern.

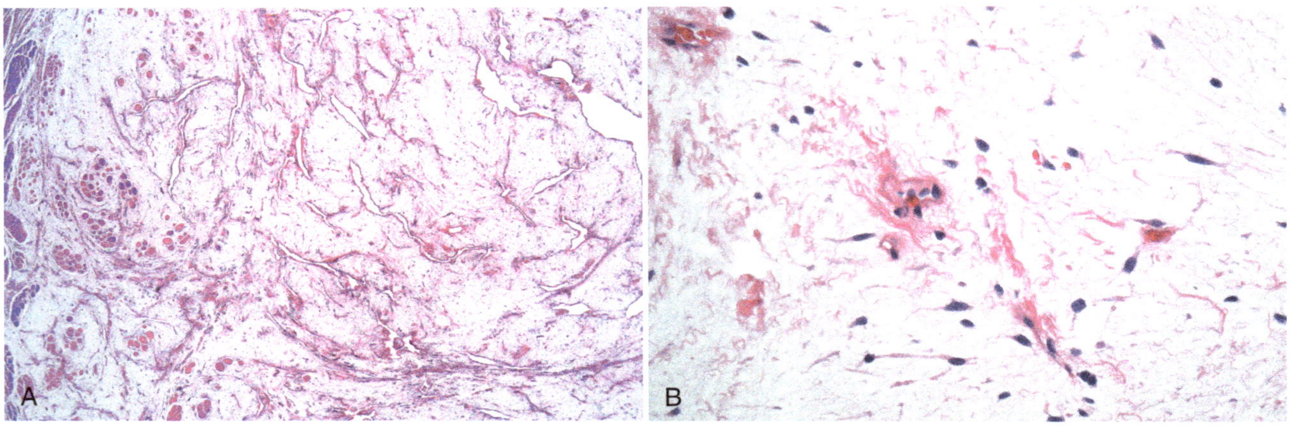

FIG 5.43 Soft tissue angiomyxoma of the oral mucosa. (A) Mucinous material, spindle cells, and dilated vessels infiltrating skeletal muscle fibers (*left*). (B) Spindled and stellate fibroblasts in mucinous stroma.

Management and Prognosis

- Excision is curative.

REFERENCES

Aldred MJ, Talacko AA, Ruljancich K, et al. Oral focal mucinosis: report of 15 cases and review of the literature. *Pathology*. 2003;35:393-396.

Buchner A, Merrell PW, Leider AS, Hansen LS. Oral focal mucinosis. *Int J Oral Maxillofac Surg*. 1990;19:337-340.

Calonje E, Guerin D, McCormick D, Fletcher CD. Superficial angiomyxoma: clinicopathologic analysis of a series of distinctive but poorly recognized cutaneous tumors with tendency for recurrence. *Am J Surg Pathol*. 1999;23:910-917.

Epivatianos A, Iordanidis S, Zaraboukas T. Myxoma of the oral soft tissues: report of a case and literature review. *J Oral Maxillofac Surg*. 2007;65:317-320.

Meer S, Beavon I. Intraoral superficial angiomyxoma. *Oral Surg Oral Med Oral Pathol Oral Radiol Endod*. 2008;106:e20-e23.

SOLITARY FIBROUS TUMOR

Clinical Findings

- This occurs mainly in the sixth decade and the most common sites are the buccal mucosa, maxillary or mandibular sulcus, lip, and tongue (Fig. 5.44).

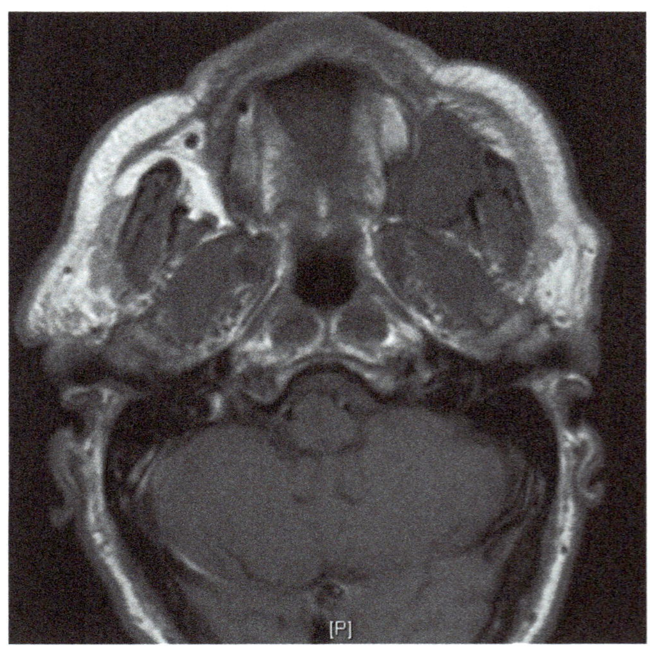

FIG 5.44 Solitary fibrous tumor: Magnetic resonance imaging showing mass of the left infratemporal fossa.

Etiopathogenesis and Histopathologic Features

Solitary fibrous tumor for the most part replaces the old term *hemangiopericytoma*. Gene fusion has been identified between NAB2-STAT6 on chromosome 12q13. Gene fusion variants are associated with different clinical subtypes.

- Tumors are circumscribed and may be encapsulated; cellular and fibrotic forms exist at two ends of the spectrum.
- The cellular variant, traditionally referred to as hemangiopericytoma, is monotonously cellular with spindle and ovoid cells that have indistinct cell borders, vesicular nuclei with small, inconspicuous nuclei, and sometimes pseudoinclusions; dilated stag-horn vessels are present that may show perivascular hyalinization (Fig. 5.45); less distinct hyper- and hypo-cellular areas are present.
- The fibrotic form exhibits areas of hypercellularity and hypocellularity referred to as "patternless" pattern and the stroma may be hyalinized or myxoid; spindle cells have the same morphology as the cellular variant (Fig. 5.46).
- Periductal hyalinization is seen if salivary glands are involved (Fig. 5.47A).
- Multinucleate tumor giant cells and mature lipocytes may be seen in the cellular variant, and amianthoid-like hyalinized bodies may be present (Fig. 5.47B–C).
- Spindle cells are CD34 and sometimes Bcl-2+ (see Fig. 5.46E); they are almost always STAT6+.
- Malignant solitary fibrous tumor exhibits increased cellularity, increased mitotic activity, and necrosis; dedifferentiation leads to anaplasia, loss of CD34 positivity, and expression of p53 and p16.

Differential Diagnosis

- Nerve sheath tumors consist of spindle cells with curvilinear nuclei that are S-100 protein+.
- Vascular neoplasms show a proliferation of spindle or epithelioid endothelial cells that form vessels with cytoplasmic positivity for CD31; intracellular lumina are not present in solitary fibrous tumors.
- Myopericytoma consists of a proliferation of spindle cells that often whorl concentrically around a central vessel with peripheral areas exhibiting perivascular spindle cell proliferation around smaller stag-horn vessels at the periphery; tumors are positive for smooth muscle actin (see Chapter 6).

Management and Prognosis

- Excision is curative and recurrence is uncommon.

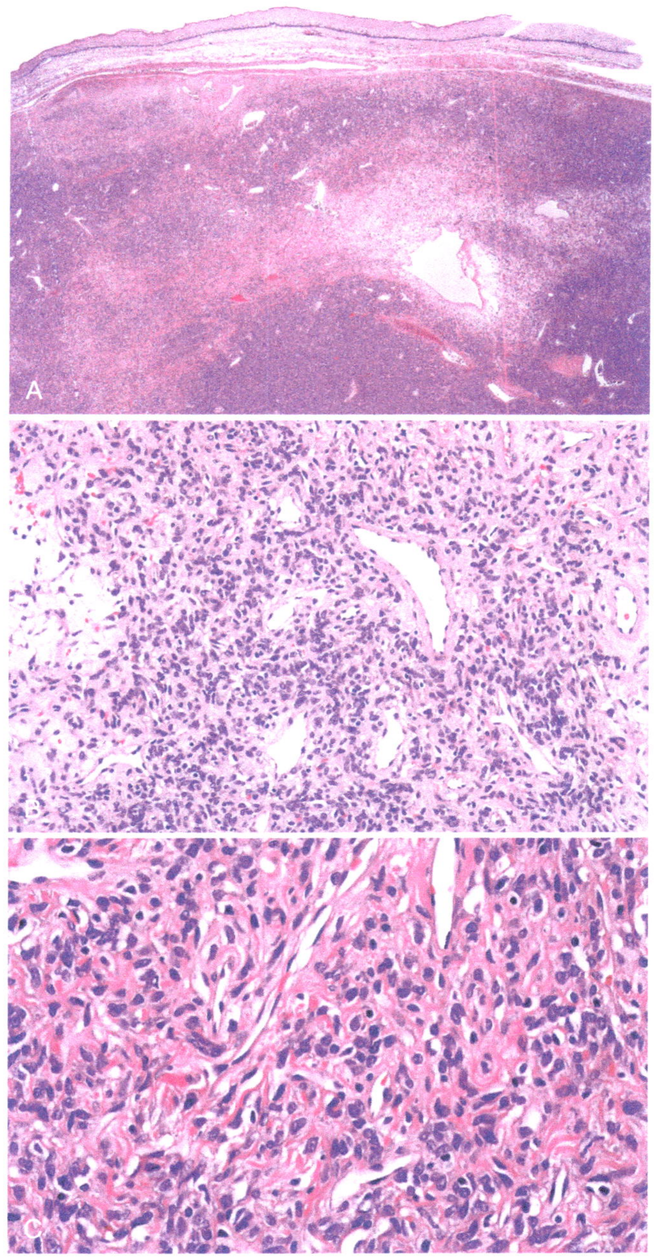

FIG 5.45 Solitary fibrous tumor, cellular type. (A) Cellular spindle cell proliferation with hypercellular and hypocellular areas and stag-horn vessels. (B) Dilated vessels surrounded by plump spindle cells. (C) Closely-packed spindle cells with plump round-to-ovoid benign nuclei.

REFERENCES

Alawi F, Stratton D, Freedman PD. Solitary fibrous tumor of the oral soft tissues: a clinicopathologic and immunohistochemical study of 16 cases. *Am J Surg Pathol.* 2001;25:900-910.

Chan JK. Solitary fibrous tumour—everywhere, and a diagnosis in vogue. *Histopathology.* 1997;31:568-576.

Dagrada GP, Spagnuolo RD, Mauro V, et al. Solitary fibrous tumors: loss of chimeric protein expression and genomic instability mark dedifferentiation. *Mod Pathol.* 2015;28:1074-1083.

Doyle LA, Vivero M, Fletcher CD, et al. Nuclear expression of STAT6 distinguishes solitary fibrous tumor from histologic mimics. *Mod Pathol.* 2014;27:390-395.

Ide F, Mishima K, Yamada H, et al. Perivascular myoid tumors of the oral region: a clinicopathologic re-evaluation of 35 cases. *J Oral Pathol Med.* 2008;37:43-49.

Lee JC, Fletcher CD. Malignant fat-forming solitary fibrous tumor (so-called "lipomatous hemangiopericytoma": clinicopathologic analysis of 14 cases. *Am J Surg Pathol.* 2011;35:1177-1185.

Mosquera JM, Fletcher CD. Expanding the spectrum of malignant progression in solitary fibrous tumors: a study of 8 cases with a discrete anaplastic component—is this dedifferentiated SFT? *Am J Surg Pathol.* 2009;33:1314-1321.

O'Regan EM, Vanguri V, Allen CM, et al. Solitary fibrous tumor of the oral cavity: clinicopathologic and immunohistochemical study of 21 cases. *Head Neck Pathol.* 2009;3:106-115.

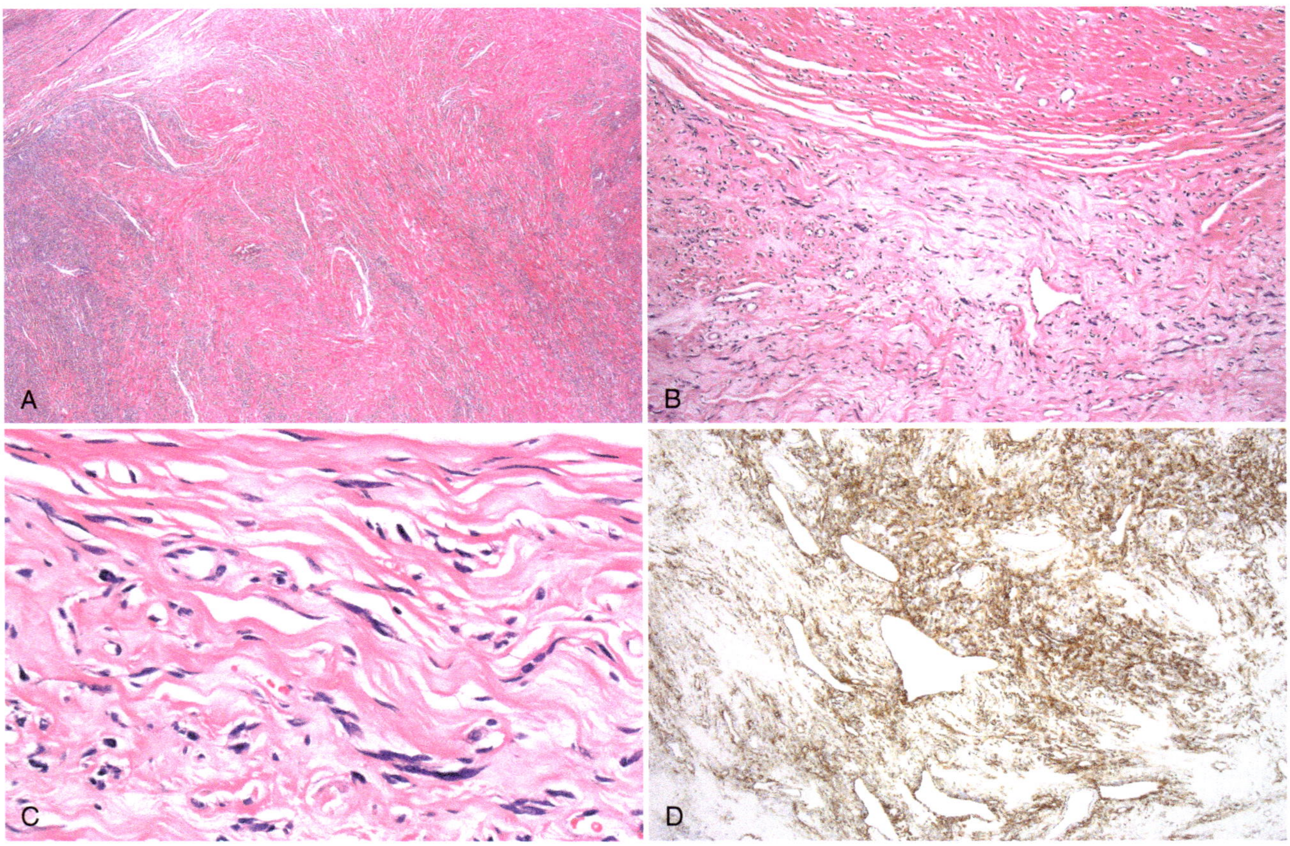

FIG 5.46 Solitary fibrous tumor, fibrotic type. (A) Mass of densely collagenous fibrous tissue. (B) Densely collagenous and hyalinized fibrous tissue (*top*) juxtaposed against delicately collagenous and vascular areas. (C) Some spindle cells have pleomorphic nuclei. (D) Cytoplasmic positivity for CD34 in hypercellular areas.

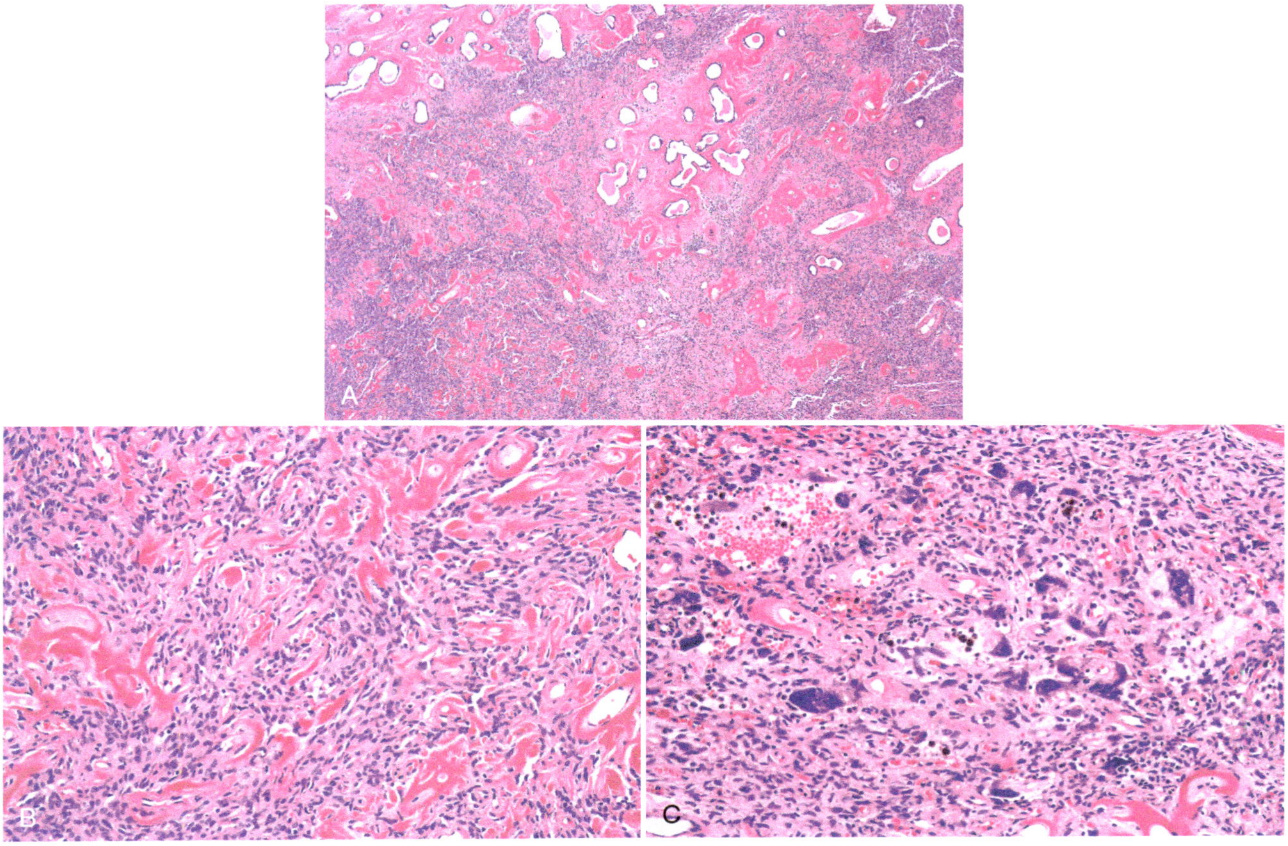

FIG 5.47 Solitary fibrous tumor, cellular type within a minor salivary gland. (A) Spindle cell proliferation with extensive hyalinization especially around salivary ducts. (B) Spindle cell proliferation with hyalinized amianthoid-like structures. (C) Multinucleate tumor cells are prominent in this tumor.

ECTOMESENCHYMAL CHONDROMYXOID TUMOR OF THE TONGUE

Clinical Findings

- This usually occurs in the fourth decade as a firm nodule on the dorsum tongue (usually anterior); other intraoral sites are rarely involved.

Etiopathogenesis and Histopathologic Features

It is uncertain what tissue this tumor attempts to recapitulate, although some believe that it may represent a soft tissue myoepithelioma. Approximately 25% and 45% of cases of this tumor and soft tissue myoepithelioma respectively, exhibit EWSR1 gene rearrangement.

- There is a circumscribed but not encapsulated lobular proliferation of polygonal, stellate, and spindle cells in a chondromyxoid stroma with tissue clefts and often muscle entrapment; pseudocystic, reticular, or solid patterns are recognized; cells have moderate eosinophilic cytoplasm and ovoid-to-round nuclei with dispersed chromatin and inconspicuous nucleoli, although nuclear pseudoinclusions, binucleation, and slight atypia may be seen; ductlike structures are usually absent (Figs. 5.48 and 5.49).
- There is consistent cytoplasmic positivity for glial fibrillary acidic protein (GFAP), S-100 protein, and vimentin; keratin (AE1/3), CD57, and smooth muscle actin are positive in 40% to 75% of cases; most cases are only weakly positive or negative for desmin, epithelial membrane antigen (EMA), smooth muscle myosin heavy chain, calponin, and p63.

Differential Diagnosis

- Myoepithelioma, soft tissue or otherwise, usually shows positivity for calponin and p63 and consistent positivity for keratin. Soft tissue myoepitheliomas also demonstrate *EWSR1* rearrangement.
- Pleomorphic adenoma contains ductal structures and is positive for myoepithelial markers.

Management and Prognosis

- Excision is usually curative; recurrence is possible if margins are involved.

REFERENCES

Allen CM. The ectomesenchymal chondromyxoid tumor: a review. *Oral Dis.* 2008;14:390-395.

Argyros PP, Bilodeau EA, Yancoskie AE, et al. A subset of ectomesenchymal chondromyxoid tumours of the tongue show EWSR1 rearrangements and are genetically linked to soft tissue myoepithelial neoplasms: a study of 11 cases. *Histopathol.* 2016;[epub ahead of print].

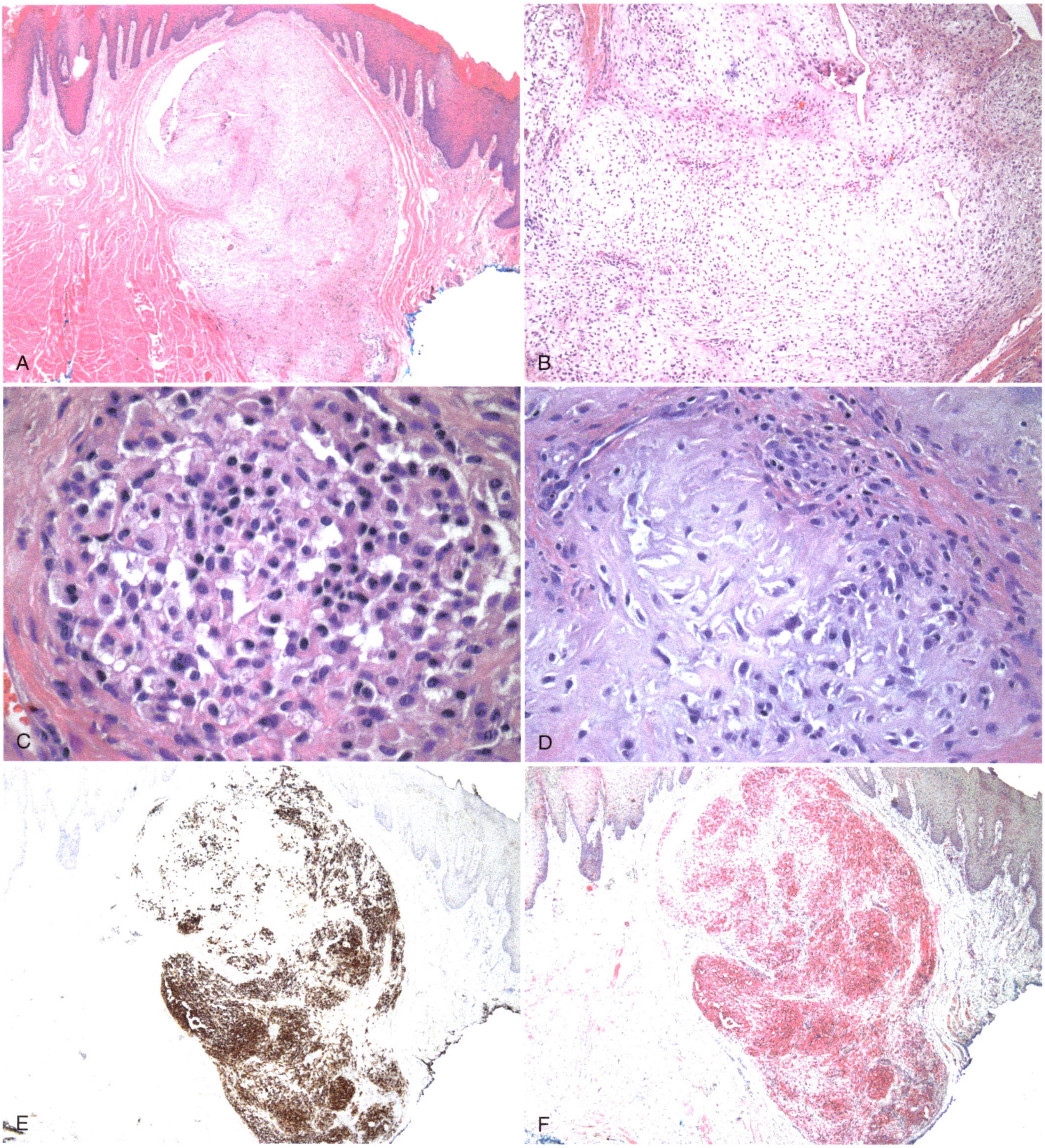

FIG 5.48 Ectomesenchymal chondromyxoid tumor of the tongue. (A) Discrete nonencapsulated myxoid nodule in the superficial and deep lamina propria. (B) There is a proliferation of spindle and epithelioid cells within myxochondroid stroma with tissue clefts. (C) Epithelioid cells have abundant eosinophilic cytoplasm and slightly pleomorphic nuclei. (D) Spindle cells are associated with myxochondroid stroma. (E) Glial fibrillary acidic protein (GFAP) is positive within many tumor cells (GFAP study). (F) S100 protein is present within many tumor cells (S100 protein study).

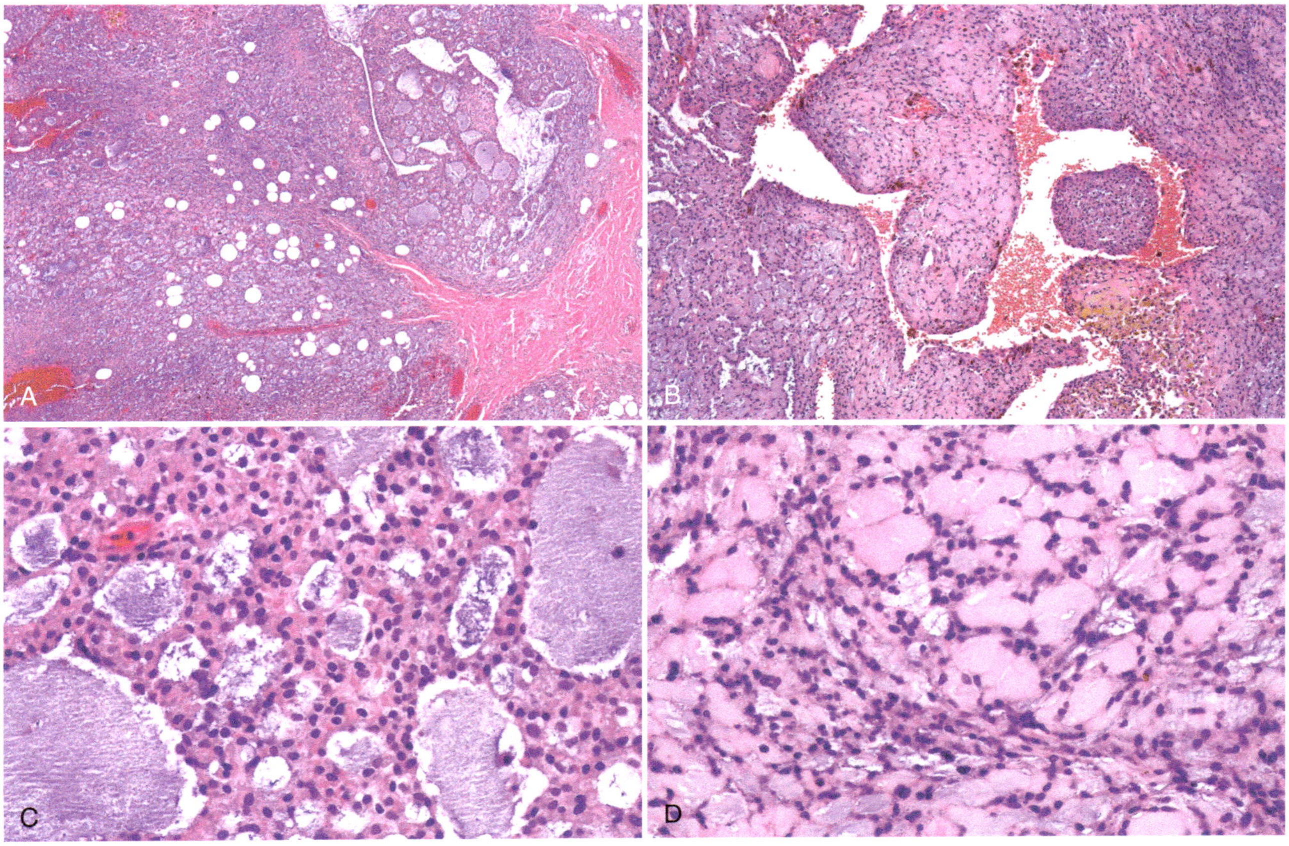

FIG 5.49 Ectomesenchymal chondromyxoid tumor of the tongue. (A) Lobules of tumor with a solid and pseudocystic pattern. (B) Chondromyxoid stroma with tissue clefting. (C) Microcystic pattern showing epithelioid cells with abundant eosinophilic cytoplasm and benign nuclei. (D) Epithelioid cells associated with eosinophilic chondroid material.

Jo VY, Fletcher CD. Myoepithelial neoplasms of soft tissue: an updated review of the clinicopathologic, immunophenotypic, and genetic features. *Head Neck Pathol.* 2015;9:32-38.

Seo SH, Shin DH, Kang HJ, et al. Reticulated myxoid tumor of the tongue: 2 cases supporting an expanded clinical and immunophenotypic spectrum of ectomesenchymal chondromyxoid tumor of the tongue. *Am J Dermatopathol.* 2010;32:660-664.

Smith BC, Ellis GL, Meis-Kindblom JM, Williams SB. Ectomesenchymal chondromyxoid tumor of the anterior tongue. Nineteen cases of a new clinicopathologic entity. *Am J Surg Pathol.* 1995;19:519-530.

Woo VL, Angiero F, Fantasia JE. Myoepithelioma of the tongue. *Oral Surg Oral Med Oral Pathol Oral Radiol Endod.* 2005;99:581-589.

AMYLOIDOMA

Amyloidosis is a spectrum of diseases where disordered folded proteins deposit within organs leading to organ-specific damage and impairment, and diagnosis depends on identification of the specific fibril precursor protein. Amyloidosis may be acquired or familial, localized or systemic. Systemic amyloidosis in monoclonal plasma cell dyscrasia is caused by AL (amyloid-light chain), in inflammatory conditions such as rheumatoid arthritis by AA (amyloid type A protein), and in dialysis-related amyloidosis by β2-microglobulin. Senile systemic amyloidosis with cardiac involvement is caused by transthyretin, and familial/hereditary amyloidosis is associated with a variety of proteins including apolipoproteins and transthyretin. Amyloid deposits are also noted in Alzheimer disease and late-stage diabetes mellitus.

Clinical Findings

- This occurs in older patients and the amyloid deposit or amyloidoma appears as a painless, yellowish, firm, waxy, deep mucosal nodule, often on the tongue, and most commonly associated with multiple myeloma, but sometimes without obvious etiology (Fig. 5.50); some patients exhibit diffuse macroglossia.
- Patients may present with hoarseness and dysphagia if the upper airway is affected, and there may be skin blistering and nail dystrophy.
- Minor salivary glands may show the presence of amyloid before it manifests elsewhere in the mouth.

Etiopathogenesis and Histopathologic Features

Amyloid consists of extracellular protein aggregates with a lamellar, cross-β-sheet structure, which is recognizable on x-ray diffraction and crystallographic studies. Glycosaminoglycan and the pentraxin protein serum amyloid P component are universal nonfibrillar proteins that play a role in fibrillogenesis and fibril persistence.

- There is deposition of pale, eosinophilic, amorphous material that is paucicellular, although lesions associated with plasma cell dyscrasia may show clusters of atypical plasma cells; a foreign body giant cell reaction may be present.

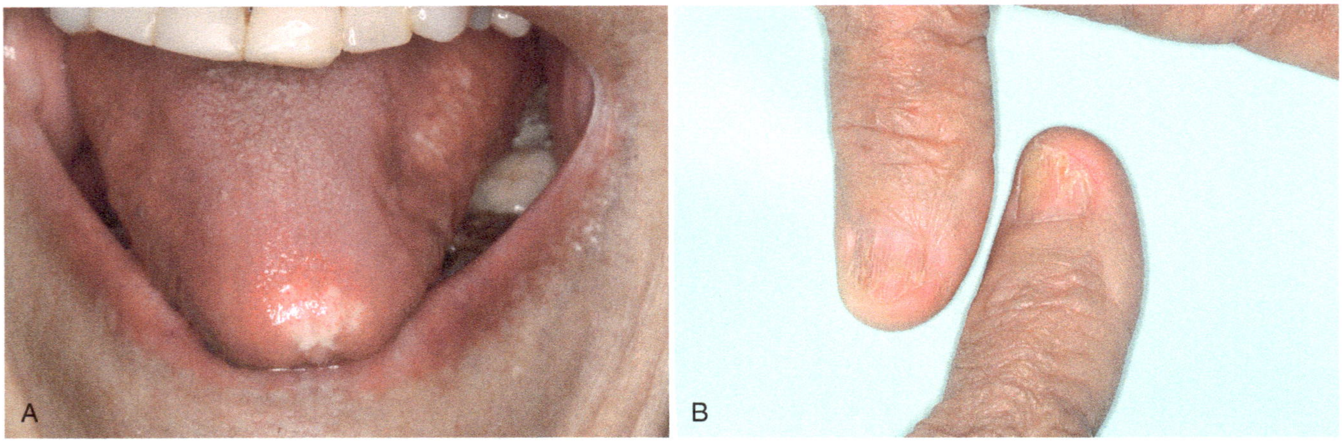

FIG 5.50 (A) Amyloid on the left lateral and tip of tongue presenting as yellow plaques in a patient with multiple myeloma. (B) Nail dystrophy is an uncommon but well-recognized manifestation of amyloidosis.

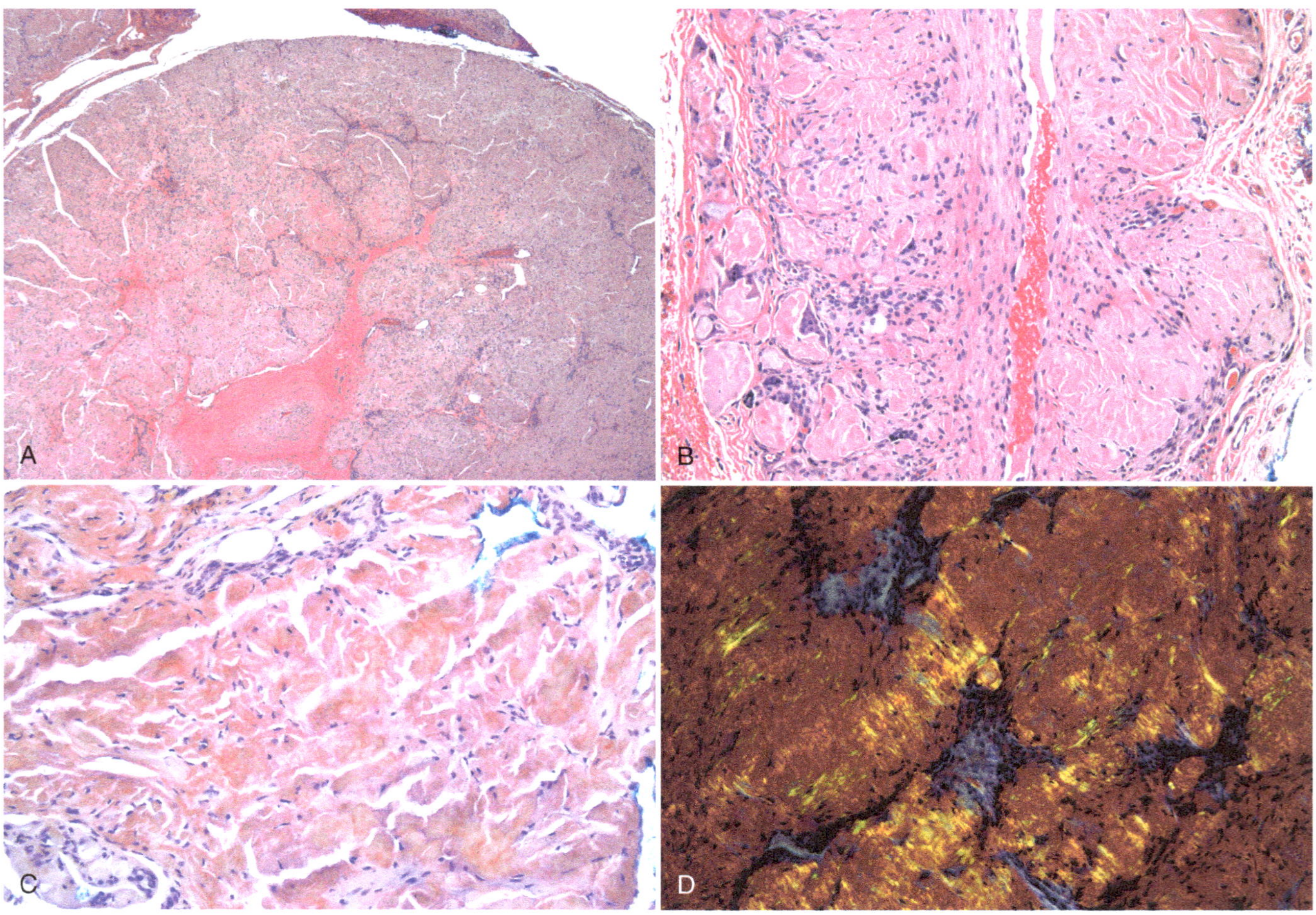

FIG 5.51 Amyloidoma. (A) Nodule composed of pale, eosinophilic amorphous material in the stroma. (B) Foreign body reaction is present around the amyloid. (C) Orange hue of amyloid with Congo red stain. (D) Apple-green birefringence noted with Congo red stain (Congo red in polarized light).

- The most commonly used stain for diagnosis is Congo red, which shows apple-green birefringence on polarized light (Fig. 5.51); other stains include crystal violet and thioflavin T.

Differential Diagnosis

- Smokeless tobacco lesions may be associated with amyloid-like hyalinized material within the lamina propria and salivary gland parenchyma, composed of altered collagen that is not congophilic.
- Fibrin deposits noted in membranous periodontitis stain with phosphotungstic acid-hematoxylin and not with Congo red.

Management and Prognosis

- All patients with oral amyloidomas should be referred for a work-up for systemic disease if this is not already known.
- Management depends on identification of the specific amyloid protein. Strategies include reducing production of the protein (eg, targeting neoplastic plasma cells or inflammation in rheumatoid arthritis), preventing aggregation of fibrils, and targeting specific components of the amyloid using monoclonal antibodies.

REFERENCES

Fujita Y, Tsuji-Abe Y, Sato-Matsumura KC, et al. Nail dystrophy and blisters as sole manifestations in myeloma-associated amyloidosis. *J Am Acad Dermatol.* 2006;54:712-714.

Gouvea AF, Ribeiro AC, Leon JE, et al. Head and neck amyloidosis: clinicopathological features and immunohistochemical analysis of 14 cases. *J Oral Pathol Med.* 2012;41:178-185.

Hirschfield GM. Amyloidosis: a clinico-pathophysiological synopsis. *Semin Cell Dev Biol.* 2004;15:39-44.

Penner CR, Muller S. Head and neck amyloidosis: a clinicopathologic study of 15 cases. *Oral Oncol.* 2006;42:421-429.

Pettersson T, Konttinen YT. Amyloidosis-recent developments. *Semin Arthritis Rheum.* 2010;39:356-368.

Stoopler ET, Sollecito TP, Chen SY. Amyloid deposition in the oral cavity: a retrospective study and review of the literature. *Oral Surg Oral Med Oral Pathol Oral Radiol Endod.* 2003;95:674-680.

Stoopler ET, Vogl DT, Alawi F, et al. The presence of amyloid in abdominal and oral mucosal tissues in patients initially diagnosed with multiple myeloma: a pilot study. *Oral Surg Oral Med Oral Pathol Oral Radiol Endod.* 2011;111:326-332.

6 VASCULAR, NEURAL, MUSCLE, AND MYOFIBROBLASTIC TUMORS

CHAPTER CONTENTS

Vascular Lesions

PYOGENIC GRANULOMA (LOBULAR CAPILLARY HEMANGIOMA)

Clinical Findings

- The majority of cases (80%) occur below 40 years of age with the highest prevalence in the second decade; it is often associated with local irritation or trauma and pregnant women may develop these on the gingiva (see Chapter 5).
- It appears as a purple-to-red nodule, sessile or pedunculated, usually on the gingiva (75%–80% of cases), lips (especially upper), and tongue, sometimes with a history of bleeding (Fig. 6.1A–C).
- Patients on cyclosporine after stem cell transplantation develop pyogenic granuloma-like lesions (fibrovascular polyps) on the buccal mucosa or tongue rather than the gingiva (Fig. 6.1D).

Etiopathogenesis and Histopathologic Features

Pyogenic granuloma is a reactive, nonneoplastic proliferation of endothelial cells and capillaries in response to local injury (such as plaque accumulation) where there is impaired wound healing and vascular growth driven by FLT4 (a tyrosine kinase receptor) and the nitric acid pathway. It is sometimes referred to as lobular capillary hemangioma, but unlike infantile capillary hemangioma, it does not react with glucose transporter-1 (GLUT-1).

- There is a proliferation of endothelial cells and capillaries (often dilated), often but not always in a lobular pattern, usually with overlying ulcer, and acute and chronic inflammation; mitotic figures are not

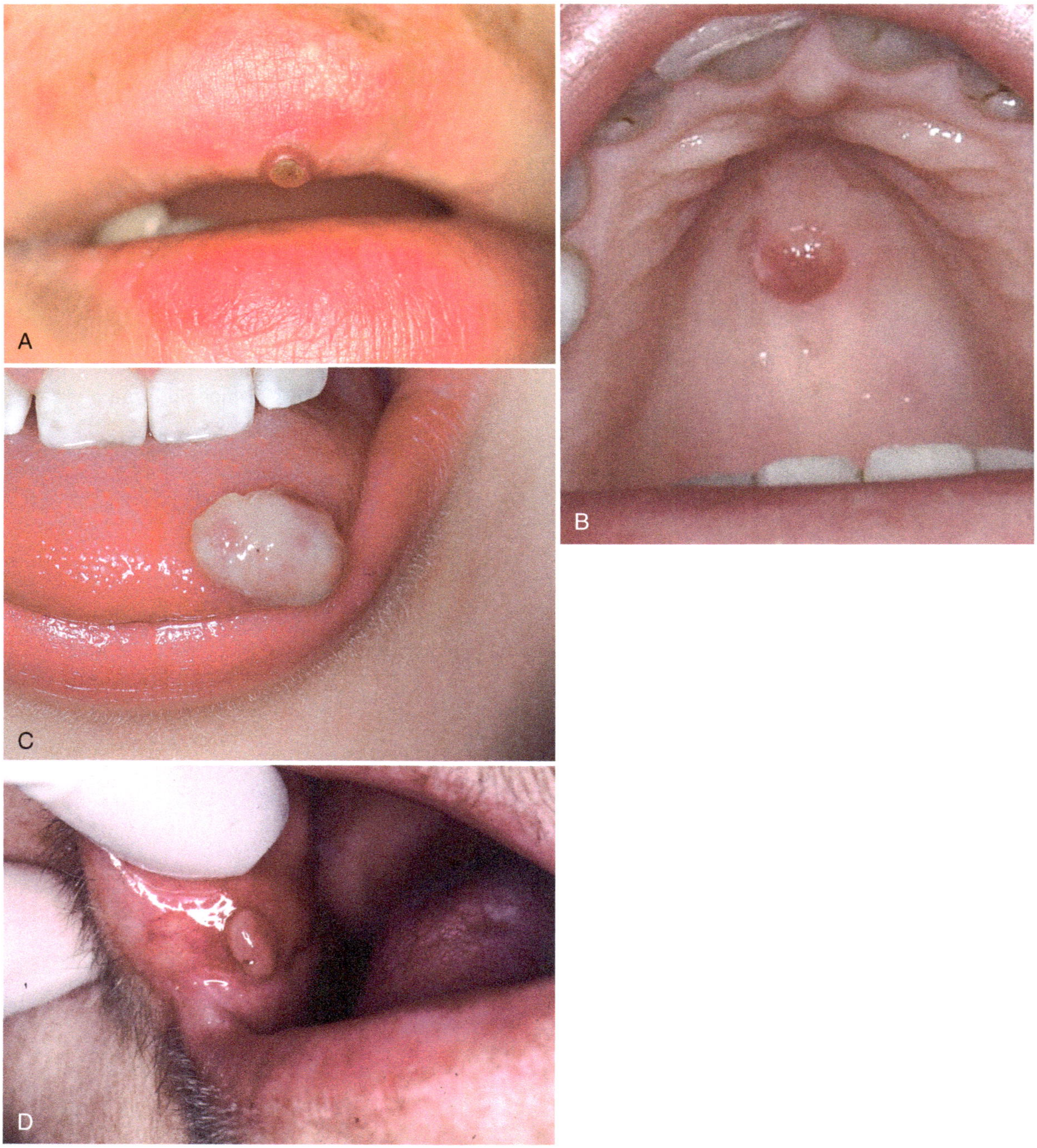

FIG 6.1 (A) Pyogenic granuloma of the upper vermilion. (B) Pyogenic granuloma of the hard palatal mucosa. (C) Pyogenic granuloma of the tongue, ulcerated. (D) Reactive fibrovascular polyp, cyclosporine-induced after stem cell transplantation.

uncommon (Figs. 6.2 and 6.3); capillaries are surrounded by smooth muscle actin (SMA)+ pericytes.

- Some lesions may show significant reactive atypia with hyperchromatic and pleomorphic nuclei (Fig. 6.4).
- Older lesions sclerose and become fibrous nodules or fibromas, especially those on the gingiva (Fig. 6.5).
- Lesions are CD31+ and CD34+ but GLUT-1−.

Differential Diagnosis

- Edematous polypoid masses of granulation tissue seen in stem cell transplant recipients on calcineurin inhibitors such as cyclosporine are better diagnosed as reactive fibrovascular hyperplasia or fibrovascular polyps.
- True infantile capillary hemangioma shows a cellular proliferation of endothelial cells and capillaries that are positive for GLUT-1+ and regress over time (see Fig. 5.22).

Management and Prognosis

- Excision is the treatment of choice with recurrence in 5% to 6% of cases.

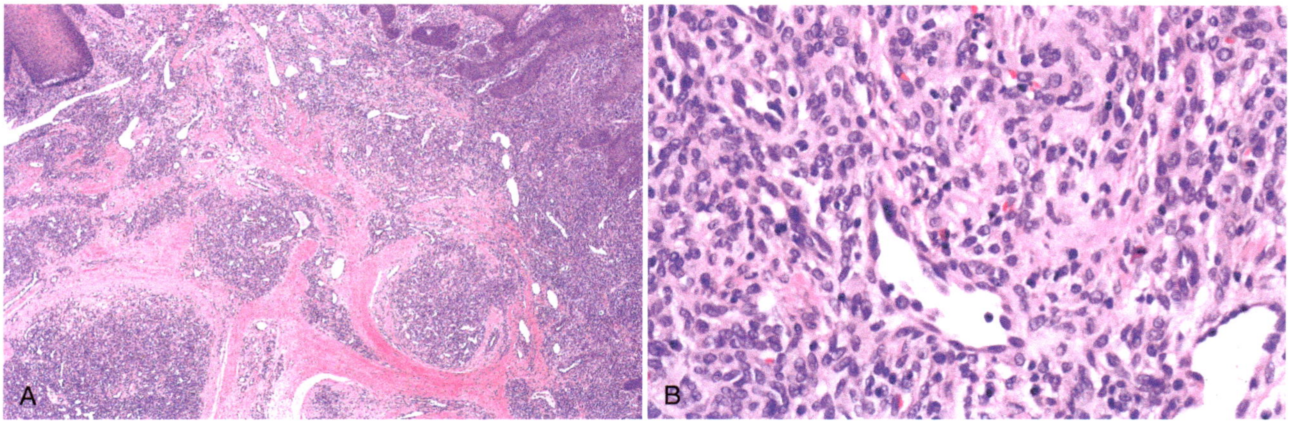

FIG 6.2 Pyogenic granuloma. (A) Typical lobular architecture with many dilated capillaries. (B) Cellular proliferation of endothelial cells and dilated capillaries.

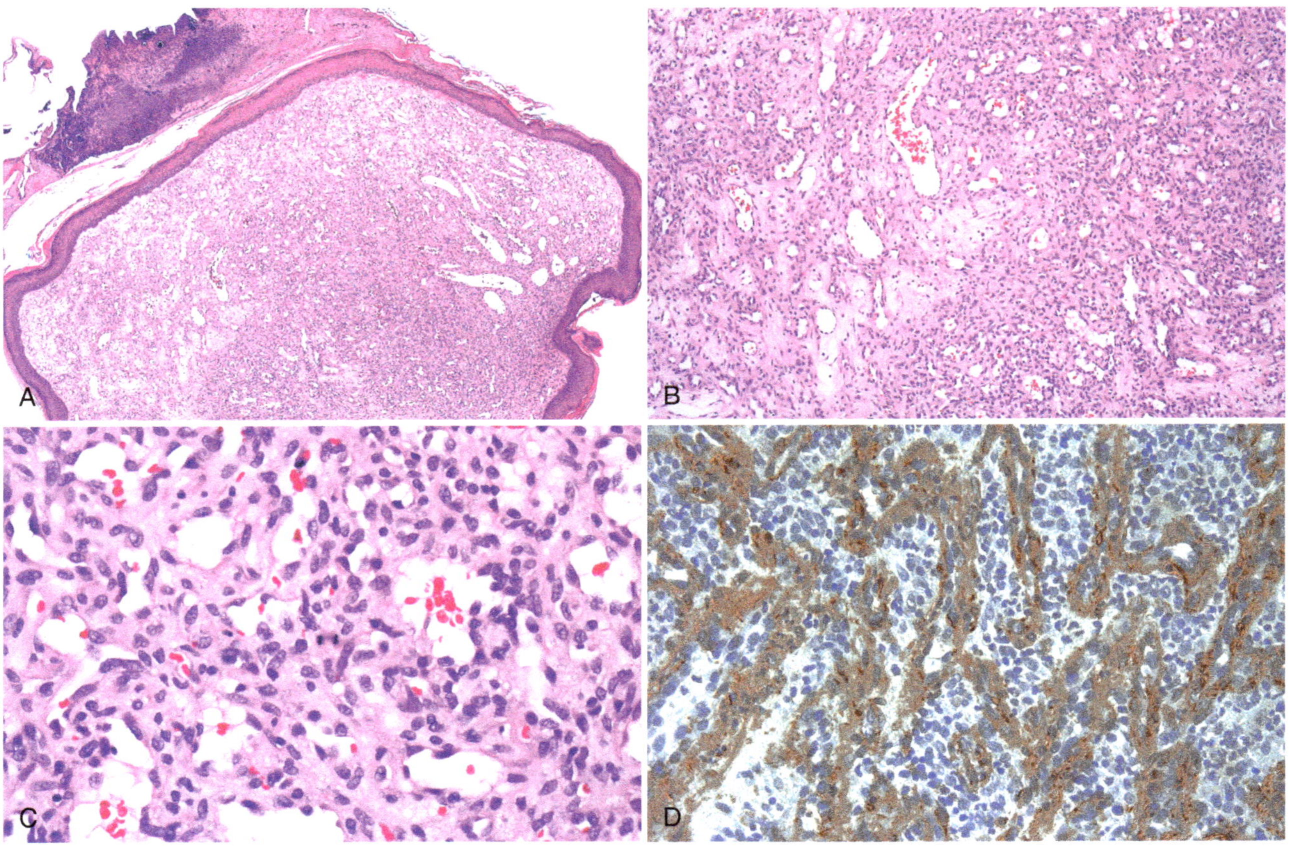

FIG 6.3 Pyogenic granuloma of lip. (A) Diffuse cellular proliferation of endothelial cells with dilated capillaries. (B) Variably dilated capillaries. (C) Benign endothelial cells and mitotic figure *(center)*. (D) Capillaries are surrounded by a layer of pericytes that are positive for smooth muscle actin.

REFERENCES

Al-Mohaya M, Treister N, Al-Khadra O, et al. Calcineurin inhibitor-associated oral inflammatory polyps after transplantation. *J Oral Pathol Med*. 2007;36:570-574.

Fishman SJ, Mulliken JB. Hemangiomas and vascular malformations of infancy and childhood. *Pediatr Clin North Am*. 1993;40:1177-2200.

Godfraind C, Calicchio ML, Kozakewich H. Pyogenic granuloma, an impaired wound healing process, linked to vascular growth driven by FLT4 and the nitric oxide pathway. *Mod Pathol*. 2013;26:247-255.

Gordon-Nunez MA, de Vasconcelos Carvalho M, Benevenuto TG, et al. Oral pyogenic granuloma: a retrospective analysis of 293 cases in a Brazilian population. *J Oral Maxillofac Surg*. 2010;68:2185-2188.

Johann AC, Salla JT, Gomez RS, et al. GLUT-1 in oral benign vascular lesions. *Oral Dis*. 2007;13:51-55.

Johncilla M, Jo V. Soft tissue tumors of the sinonasal tract. *Semin Diagn Pathol*. 2016;33:81-90.

North PE, Waner M, Mizeracki A, Mihm MC Jr. GLUT1: a newly discovered immunohistochemical marker for juvenile hemangiomas. *Hum Pathol*. 2000;31:11-22.

Renshaw AA, Rosai J. Benign atypical vascular lesions of the lip. A study of 12 cases. *Am J Surg Pathol*. 1993;17:557-565.

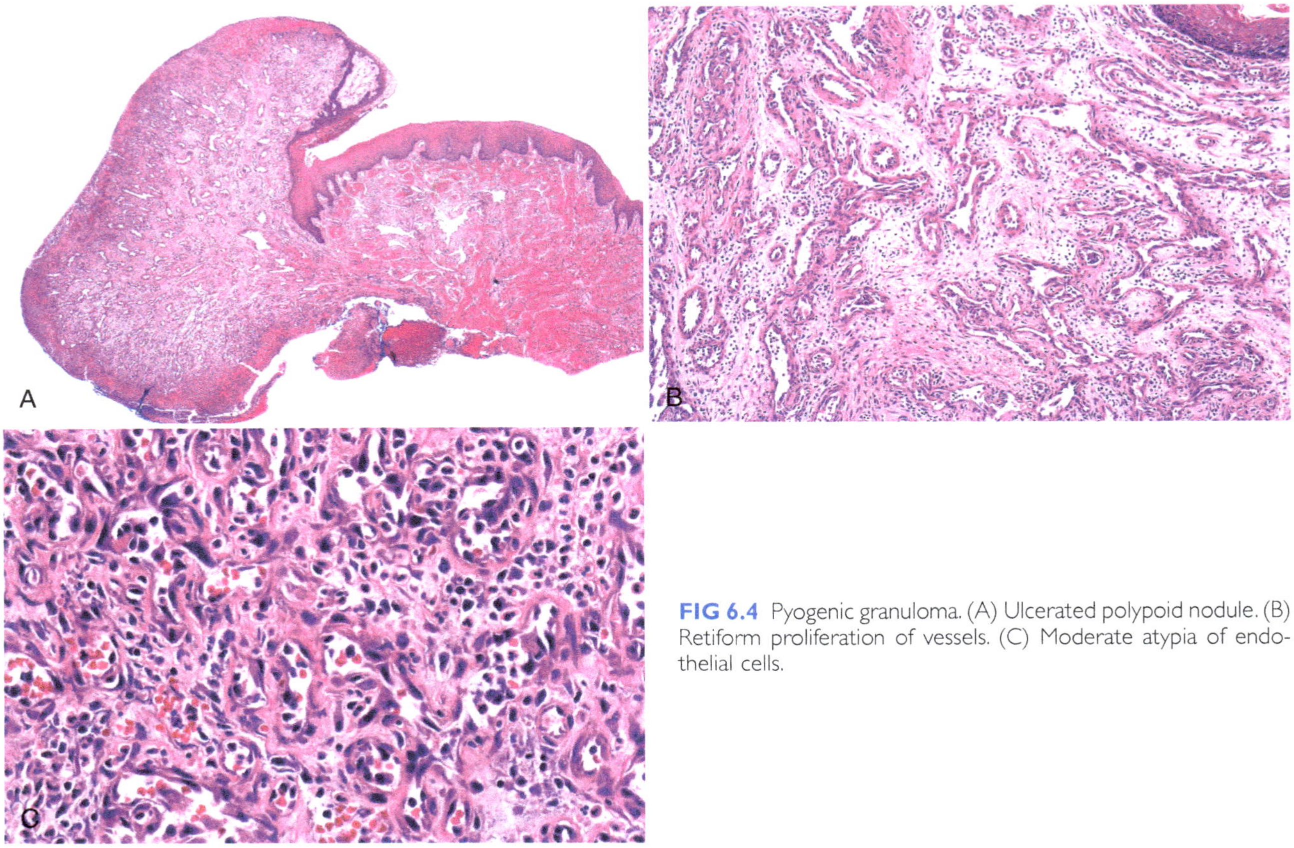

FIG 6.4 Pyogenic granuloma. (A) Ulcerated polypoid nodule. (B) Retiform proliferation of vessels. (C) Moderate atypia of endothelial cells.

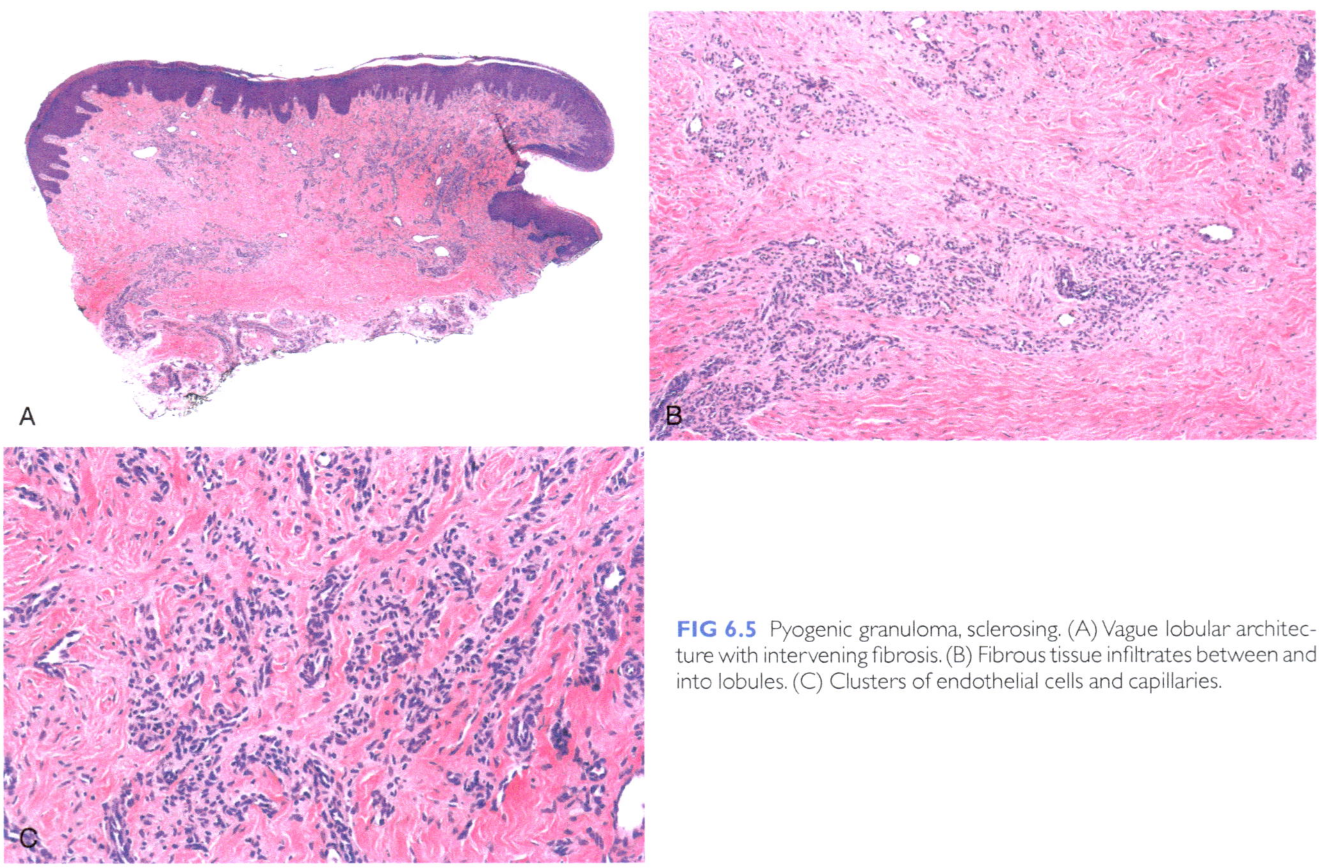

FIG 6.5 Pyogenic granuloma, sclerosing. (A) Vague lobular architecture with intervening fibrosis. (B) Fibrous tissue infiltrates between and into lobules. (C) Clusters of endothelial cells and capillaries.

VARIX (VENOUS LAKE), VASCULAR ANOMALY, AND VENOUS MALFORMATION

The term vascular anomaly as used by the International Society for the Study of Vascular Anomalies (ISSVA) encompasses vascular malformations (venous, capillary, lymphatic, and arteriovenous) in addition to vasoproliferative tumors such as infantile capillary hemangiomas. Intraoral vascular malformations are generally small; they occur with some frequency on the skin and subcutaneous tissues of the head and neck such as capillary malformation in Sturge-Weber syndrome affecting the skin, oral mucosa, eye, and central nervous system.

Clinical Findings

- Varix (venous lake): This occurs in middle-aged and older adults as a bluish bleb, from a few millimeters to 1 to 2 cm in size, located on the lips, tongue, or buccal mucosa; pressure causes blanching and this is demonstrated by pressing a glass slide onto the lesion so that the vessel empties (diascopy), although this can also be accomplished with a dental instrument; lesions may bleed (Fig. 6.6A–C).
- Bilateral lingual varicose veins of the ventral tongue are common in older adults (Fig. 6.6D).
- Simple venous malformation: These are larger bluish masses usually present at birth; in the oral cavity, they may occur in older patients and are usually several centimeters in size, often involving the underlying muscle; there may be significant deformity (Fig. 6.6E–F).

Etiopathogenesis and Histopathologic Features

A varix (venous lake) is a dilated venule that results from loss of elasticity of the muscle around venules (likely postcapillary venules) leading to dilatation of the lumen. Venous malformation is a low-flow lesion that is a developmental malformation of the veins that is caused by local defects of vascular morphogenesis and dysembryogenesis; such malformations are connected to the normal vasculature. They may occur as arteriovenous malformations and are best diagnosed by a thorough clinical examination and ultrasonographic and/or angiographic studies. What used to be known as cavernous hemangioma is now reclassified as a venous malformation by ISSVA.

- *Varix:* These are dilated, tortuous, thin-walled vessels with a variable but usually thin muscular coat; valve leaflets may be present (Figs. 6.7 and 6.8); thrombi in various stages of organization are often noted, sometimes with hyalinization, and Masson tumor (intravascular papillary endothelial hyperplasia) is sometimes seen; this is composed of small hyalinized globules containing small capillaries and is surrounded by endothelium (Figs. 6.9 and 6.10).
- *Venous malformation:* Many dilated venules of varying sizes are noted, sometimes intramuscular in location without a proliferation of endothelial cells (Figs. 6.11–6.13)

Differential Diagnosis

- Arteriovenous malformations exhibit the presence of arterioles, arteries, veins, and venules; these lesions have high flow and distinct ultrasonographic findings.
- Telangiectasia seen in limited systemic sclerosis (previously known as calcinosis-Raynaud phenomenon-esophageal dysmotility-sclerodactyly-telangiectasia [CREST] syndrome), an autoimmune condition characterized by anticentromere antibodies, and hereditary hemorrhagic telangiectasia, an autosomal dominant vascular dysplasia with *HHT-1, HHT-2,* or *SMAD4* mutations, consist of numerous dilated vessels in the lamina propria of the tongue or lips.

Management and Prognosis

- Excision is the treatment of choice for varices and small venous malformations; laser ablation and sclerotherapy are useful treatments for larger lesions.

REFERENCES

Buckmiller LM, Richter GT, Suen JY. Diagnosis and management of hemangiomas and vascular malformations of the head and neck. *Oral Dis.* 2010;16:405-418.

Eivazi B, Wiegand S, Teymoortash A, et al. Laser treatment of mucosal venous malformations of the upper aerodigestive tract in 50 patients. *Lasers Medical Sci.* 2010;25:571-576.

Govani FS, Shovlin CL. Hereditary haemorrhagic telangiectasia: a clinical and scientific review. *Eur J Hum Genet.* 2009;17:860-871.

Hedstrom L, Bergh H. Sublingual varices in relation to smoking and cardiovascular diseases. *Br J Oral Maxillofac Surg.* 2010;48:136-138.

Mulliken JB, Glowacki J. Hemangiomas and vascular malformations in infants and children: a classification based on endothelial characteristics. *Plast Reconstr Surg.* 1982;69:412-422.

Soares AB, Altemani A, Furuse C, et al. Intravascular papillary endothelial hyperplasia: report of 2 cases and immunohistochemical study. *Oral Surg Oral Med Oral Pathol Oral Radiol Endod.* 2008;106:708-711.

Stimpson P, Hewitt R, Barnacle A, et al. Sodium tetradecyl sulphate sclerotherapy for treating venous malformations of the oral and pharyngeal regions in children. *Int J Pediatr Otorhinolaryngol.* 2012;76:569-573.

Wassef M, Blei F, Adams D, et al. Vascular Anomalies Classification: Recommendations From the International Society for the Study of Vascular Anomalies. *Pediatrics.* 2015;136:e203-e214.

Text continued on p. 118

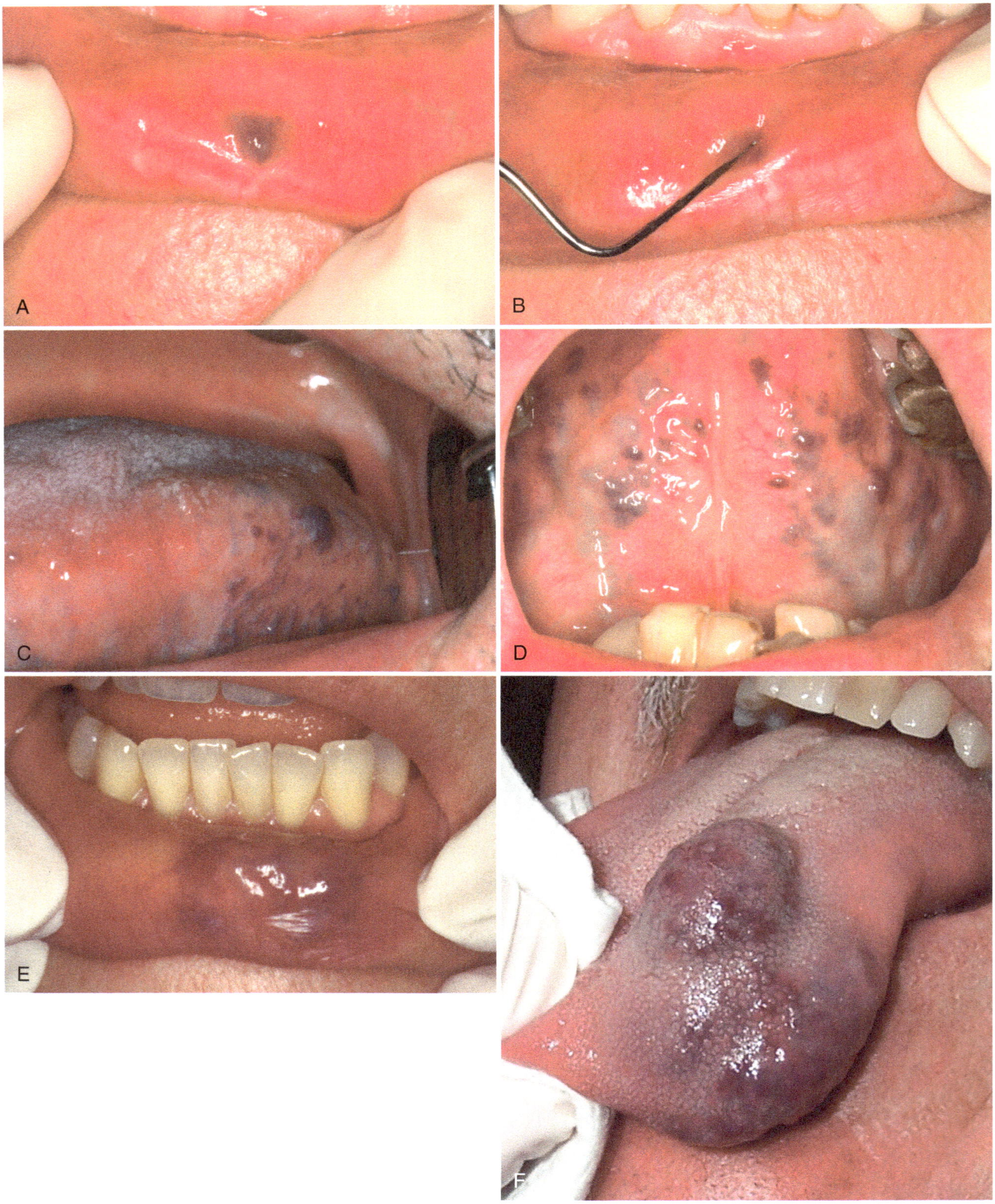

FIG 6.6 (A) Varix of the lower lip mucosa. (B) Same case as in A; varix blanches with pressure. (C) Varix of the left lateral tongue. (D) Bilateral lingual varices of the ventral tongue. (E) Venous malformation of lower lip mucosa. (F) Venous malformation of the left tongue. *(F, Courtesy Dr. David Feinerman, private practice, Boynton Beach, Fla.)*

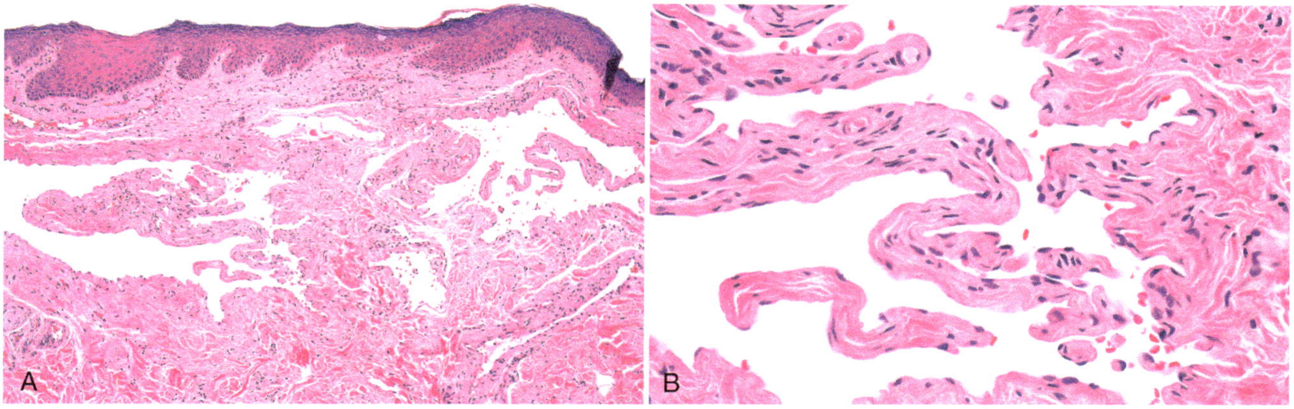

FIG 6.7 Varices. (A) Dilated vascular spaces. (B) Spaces are lined by a single layer of endothelium and valve leaflets are present.

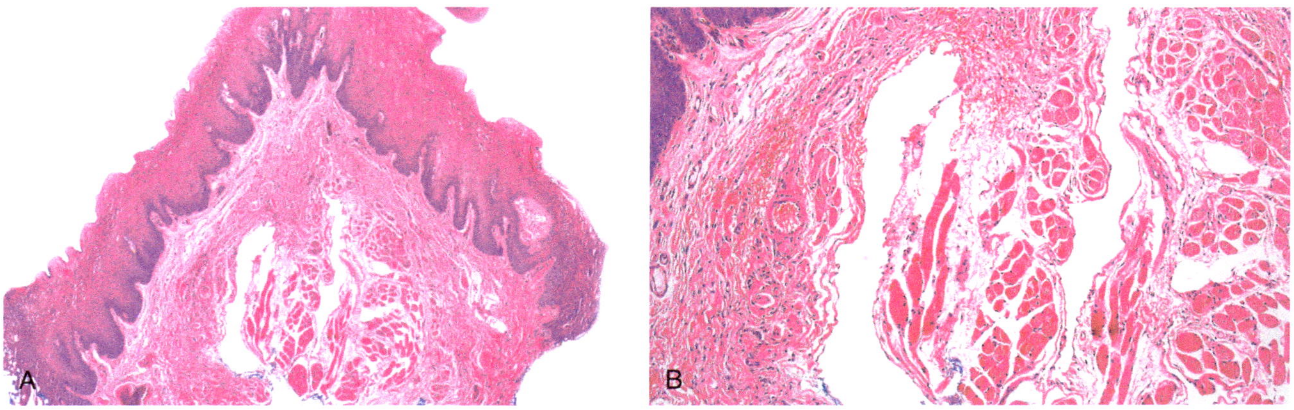

FIG 6.8 Varices. (A) Dilated venules within the muscle. (B) Dilated endothelium-lined space between skeletal muscle fibers.

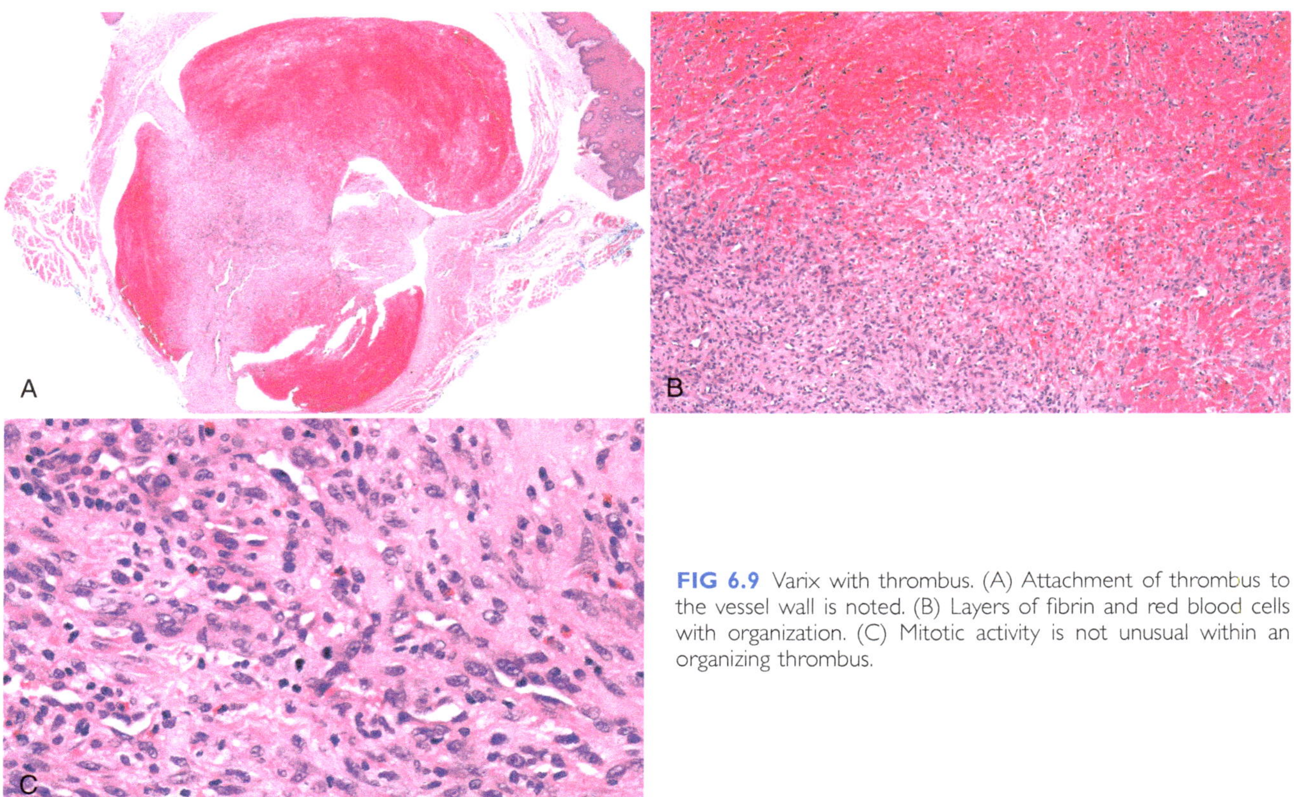

FIG 6.9 Varix with thrombus. (A) Attachment of thrombus to the vessel wall is noted. (B) Layers of fibrin and red blood cells with organization. (C) Mitotic activity is not unusual within an organizing thrombus.

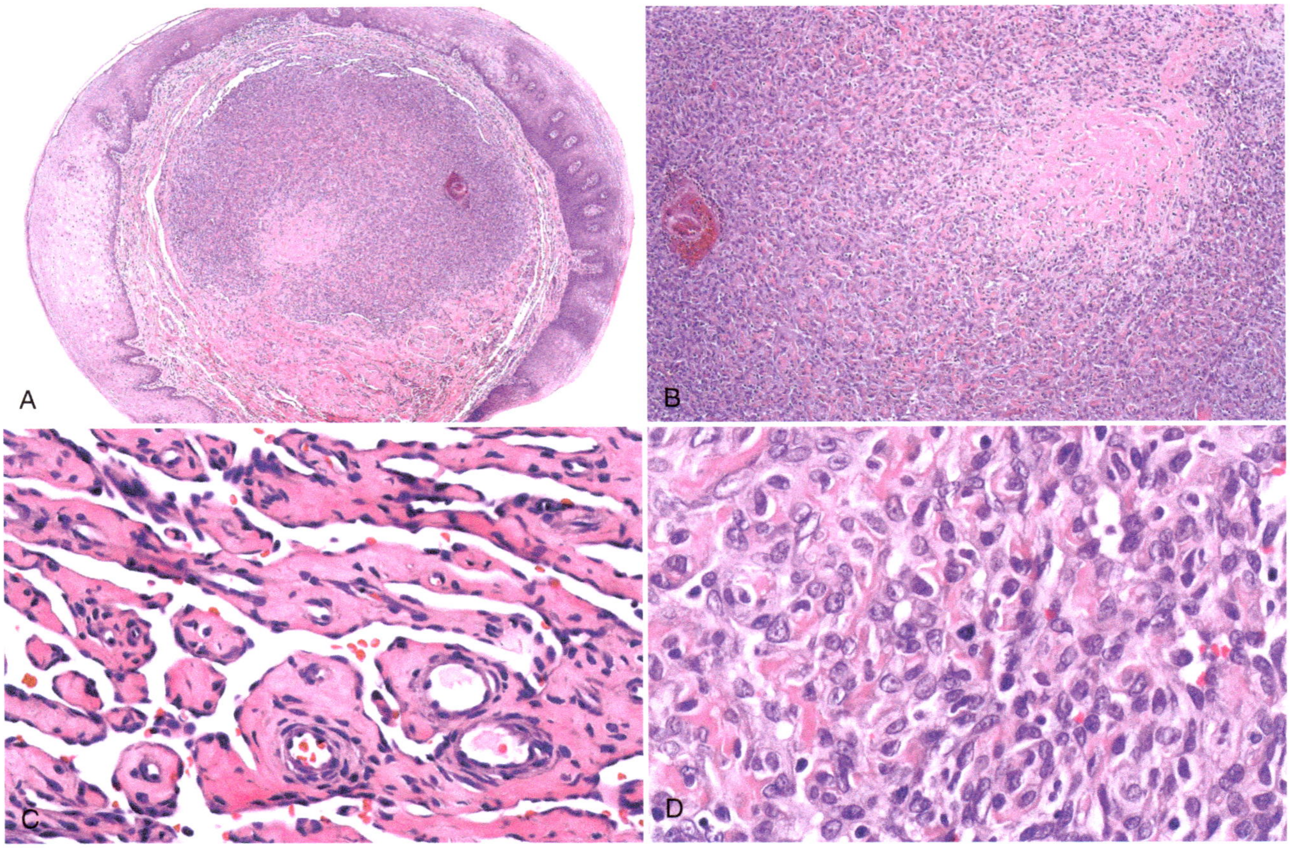

FIG 6.10 Organizing thrombus. (A) Markedly cellular nodule. (B) Nodule consists of mainly endothelial cells with remnants of the thrombus (*left*) and area of hyalinization (*right*). (C) Focus of Masson tumor. (D) Marked hypercellularity with mitotic figure.

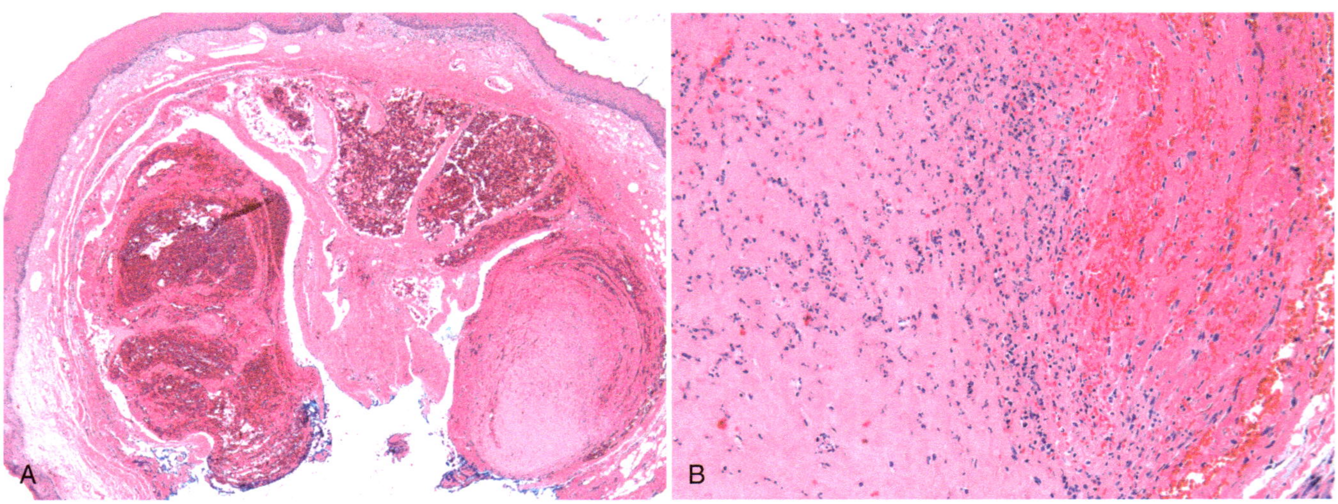

FIG 6.11 Venous malformation with thrombi. (A) Large dilated and congested venules with thrombus (*right*). (B) Thrombus with hyalinization.

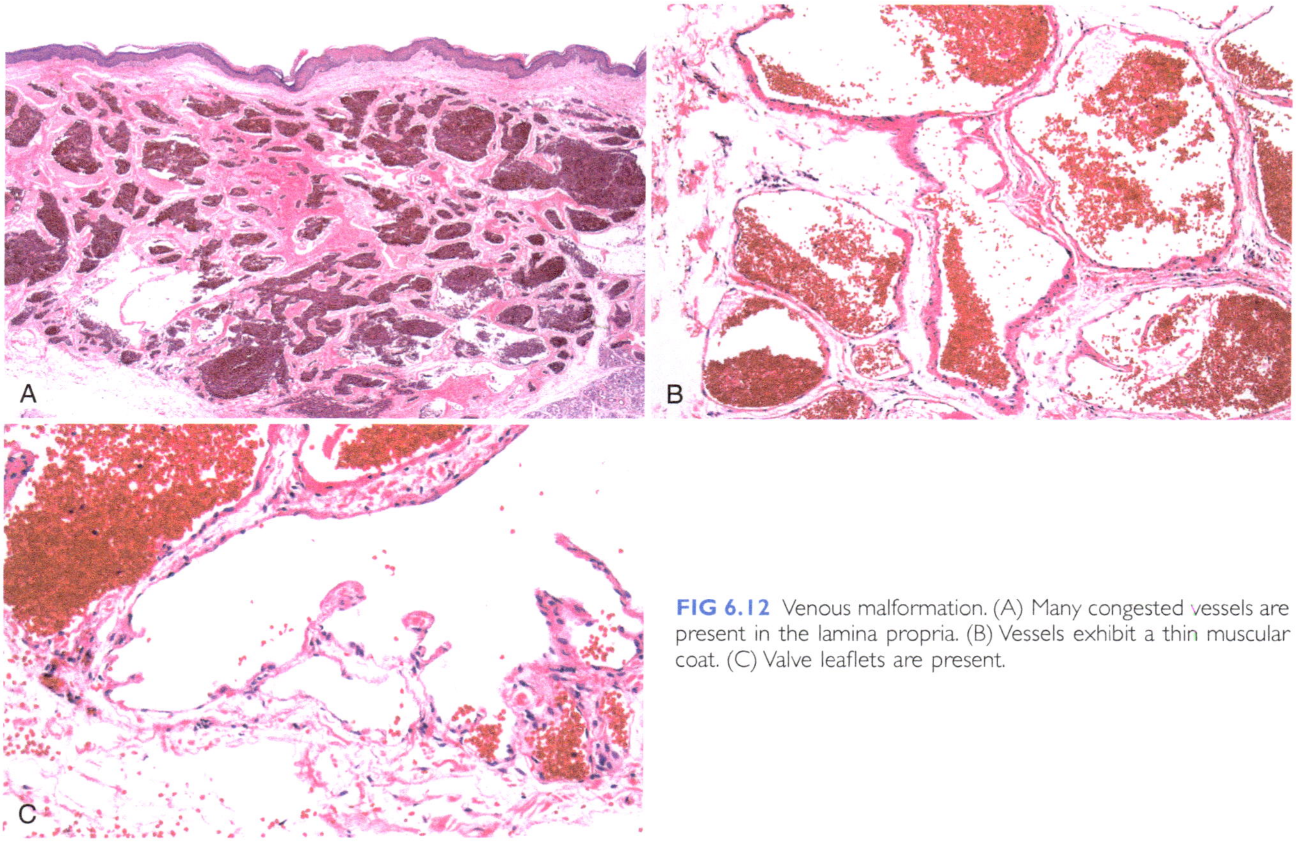

FIG 6.12 Venous malformation. (A) Many congested vessels are present in the lamina propria. (B) Vessels exhibit a thin muscular coat. (C) Valve leaflets are present.

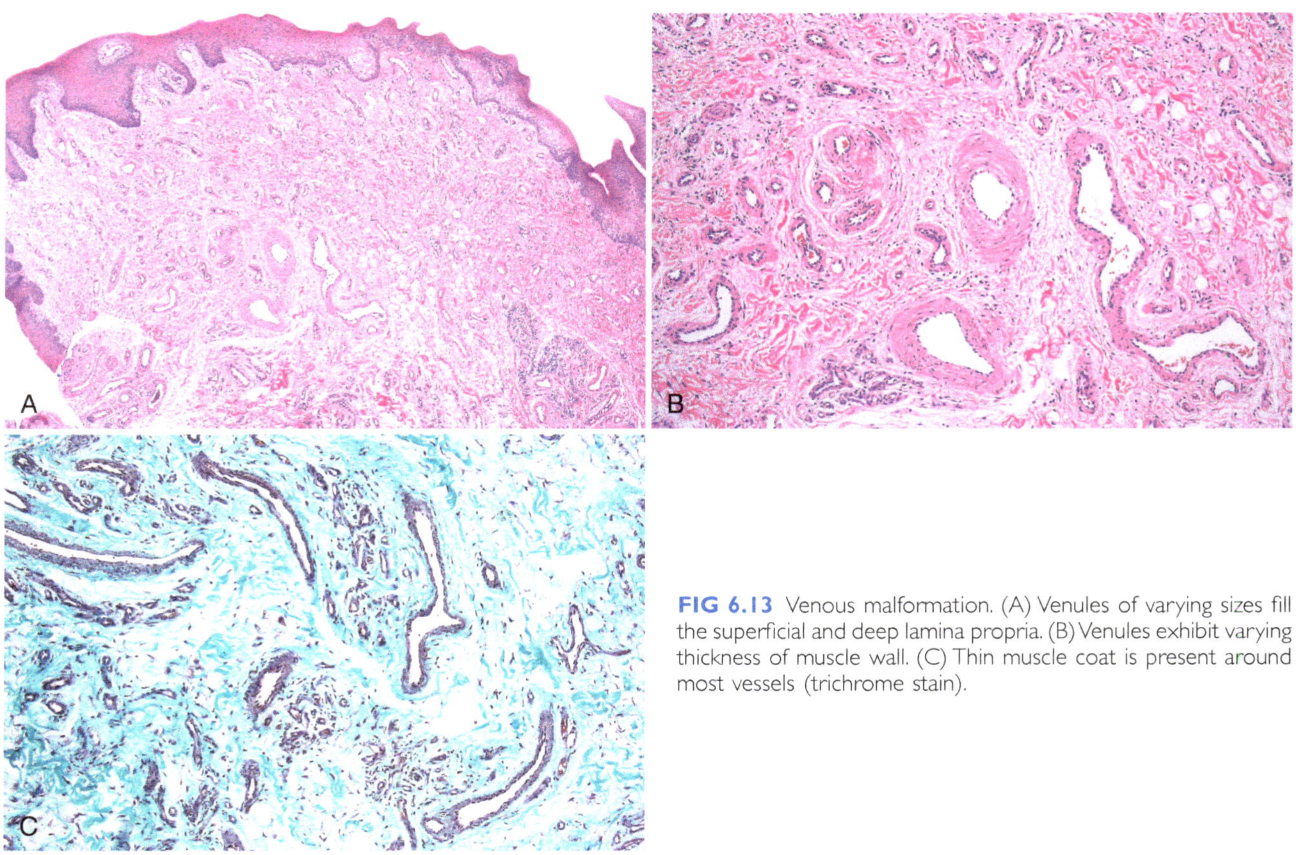

FIG 6.13 Venous malformation. (A) Venules of varying sizes fill the superficial and deep lamina propria. (B) Venules exhibit varying thickness of muscle wall. (C) Thin muscle coat is present around most vessels (trichrome stain).

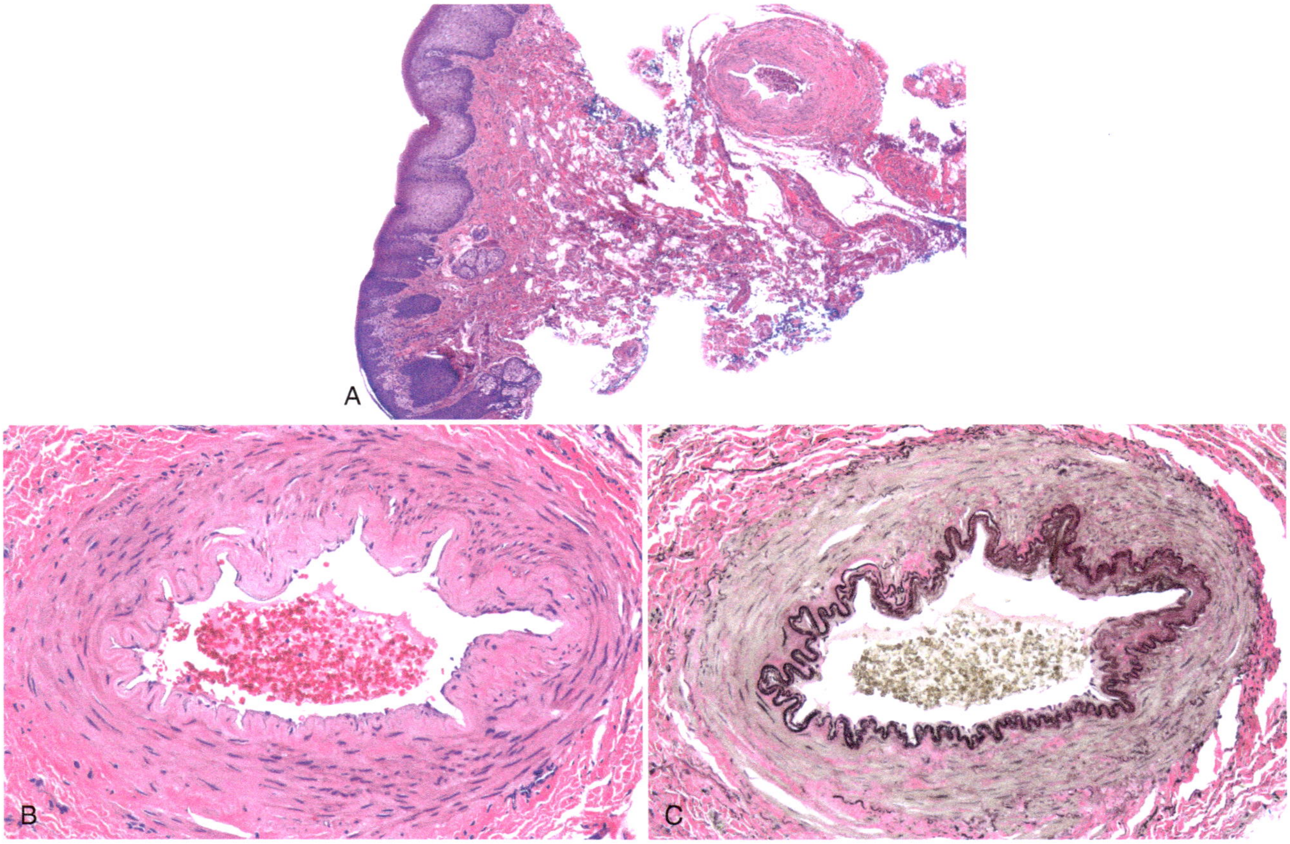

FIG 6.14 Caliber-persistent labial artery. (A) An artery is present in the deep lamina propria. (B) Artery with elastic lamina and thick muscle coat. (C) Elastin stain outlines the elastic lamina.

CALIBER-PERSISTENT LABIAL ARTERY

Clinical Findings

- The mean age of occurrence is in the sixth decade with equal gender distribution; there is a bluish, sometimes nodular, often vermiform, pulsatile lesion of the lip, with the lower lip involved twice as frequently; clinically it is often mistaken for mucocele.

Etiopathogenesis and Histopathologic Features

Caliber-persistent labial artery represents a branch of the labial artery that fails to reduce its caliber even in the superficial tissues.

- A normal artery with elastic lamina and thick muscular wall lies within the lamina propria, with an artery diameter-to-depth ratio of less than 1.6 (Fig. 6.14).

Management and Prognosis

- Trauma leads to pulsatile bleeding, and the biopsy is diagnostic; ultrasonographic imaging mitigates the need for a biopsy, but this is rarely performed because the clinical impression is usually that of mucocele, which is normally excised.

REFERENCES

Jaspers MT. Oral caliber-persistent artery. Unusual presentations of unusual lesions. *Oral Surg Oral Med Oral Pathol.* 1992;74:631-633.

Lovas JG, Rodu B, Hammond HL, et al. Caliber-persistent labial artery. A common vascular anomaly. *Oral Surg Oral Med Oral Pathol Oral Radiol Endod.* 1998;86:308-312.

Piccione MJ, Manganaro AM, Almony JS. Caliber-persistent labial artery: diagnosis and treatment—case report. *J Oral Maxillofac Surg.* 2010; 68:1987-1989.

Wortsman X, Calderon P, Arellano J, Orellana Y. High-resolution color Doppler ultrasound of a caliber-persistent artery of the lip, a simulator variant of dermatologic disease: case report and sonographic findings. *Int J Dermatol.* 2009;48:830-833.

LYMPHANGIOMA, LYMPHANGIECTASIA, AND LYMPHANGIOMA CIRCUMSCRIPTUM

Unlike cystic hygromas, lymphangiomas of the oral cavity are small and usually superficially located, and most represent lymphangiectasia. The term lymphangioma circumscriptum has been used for similar lesions of the skin.

Clinical Findings

- This occurs in children, teenagers, and young adults as clusters of translucent vesicular structures resembling "frog spawn," with at least 50% of cases occurring on the tongue (Fig. 6.15); congenital lesions occur on the alveolar ridge in neonates (see Chapter 2).

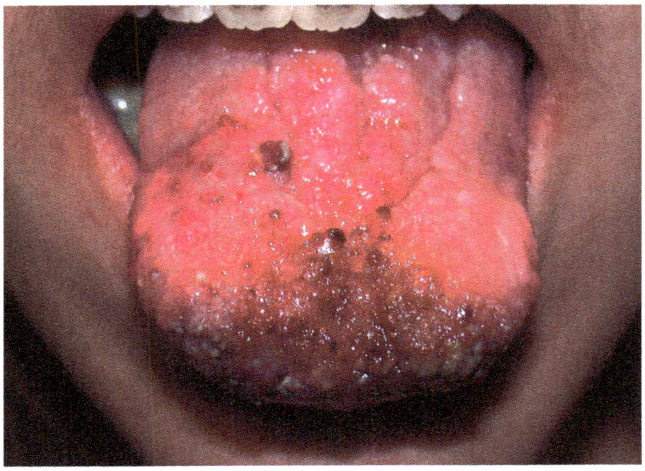

FIG 6.15 Lymphatic malformation of the tongue manifesting as clusters of hemorrhagic and ulcerated vesicles. *(Courtesy Dr. Bonnie Padwa, Harvard School of Dental Medicine, Boston, MA.)*

Etiopathogenesis and Histopathologic Features

Mutations in *PIK3CA* have been identified in extraoral lymphatic malformations and in sporadic syndromes associated with such malformative/overgrowth disorders (eg Klippel-Trenaunay syndrome), although it is unclear how such mutations that arise during embryogenesis produce these malformations.

- Dilated vascular spaces are lined by a single layer of endothelial cells (that are usually D2-40 [podoplanin]+) often with valve leaflets, and are filled with pale, wispy, or denser eosinophilic material; these typically abut the epithelium, which has a bosselated surface, and vascular channels may insinuate into the underlying muscle (Fig. 6.16); sometimes dilated venous channels are also present.

Differential Diagnosis

- Vessels of venous malformations have thin muscular coats and usually do not abut the epithelium.

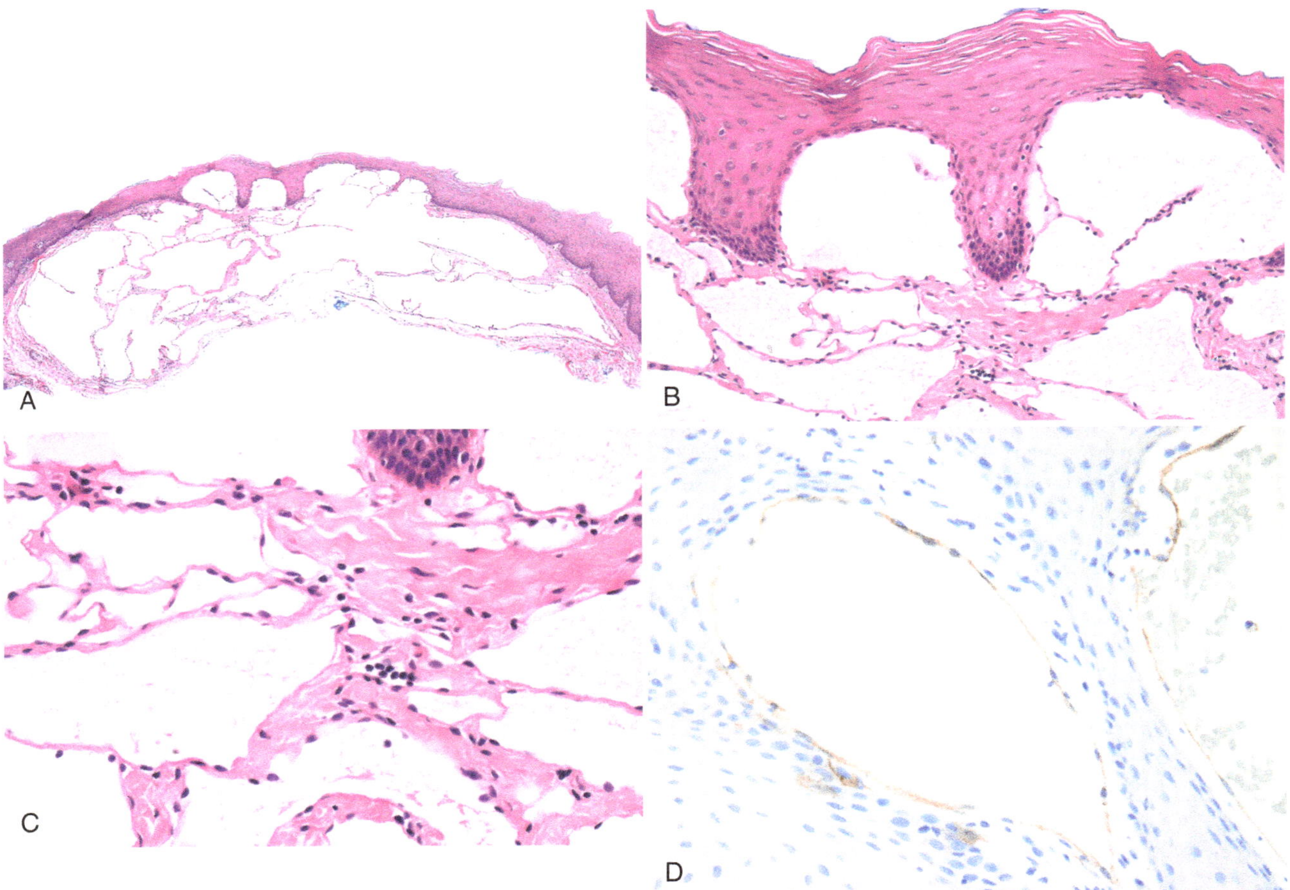

FIG 6.16 Lymphangioma circumscriptum. (A) Circumscribed collection of large vascular spaces within the superficial and deep lamina propria. (B) Vascular spaces abut the epithelium. (C) Vascular spaces are lined by a single layer of endothelial cells and filled with pale, wispy lymph. (D) Lymphatic endothelium showing cytoplasmic positivity for D2-40.

Management and Prognosis

- Excision or laser ablation is curative for small lesions, and embolization with debulking is the treatment for large lesions.

REFERENCES

Brennan TD, Miller AS, Chen SY. Lymphangiomas of the oral cavity: a clinicopathologic, immunohistochemical, and electron-microscopic study. *J Oral Maxillofac Surg.* 1997;55:932-935.

Itakura E, Yamamoto H, Oda Y, et al. VEGF-C and VEGFR-3 in a series of lymphangiomas: is superficial lymphangioma a true lymphangioma? *Virchows Arch.* 2009;454:317-325.

Kalpidis CD, Lysitsa SN, Kolokotronis AE, et al. Solitary superficial microcystic lymphatic malformation (lymphangioma circumscriptum) of the gingiva. *J Periodontol.* 2006;77:1797-1801.

Luks VL, Kamitaki N, Vivero MP, et al. Lymphatic and other vascular malformative/overgrowth disorders are caused by somatic mutations in PIK3CA. *J Pediatr.* 2015;166:1048-1054 e1–5.

EPITHELIOID HEMANGIOMA (HISTIOCYTOID HEMANGIOMA, ANGIOLYMPHOID HYPERPLASIA WITH EOSINOPHILIA)

Clinical Findings

This occurs in the third to fifth decade and is twice as common in males; it presents as a painless nodule with 90% occurring on the lips (the most common site), tongue or buccal mucosa, sometimes with a history of trauma.

Etiopathogenesis and Histopathologic Features

FOS gene rearrangement has been noted in only 5% of head and neck cases with the angiolymphoid hyperplasia pattern, and 43% and 59% in lesions in the extremities and bone, respectively. It may be that the head and neck cases with the angiolymphoid hyperplasia pattern may represent a reactive rather than neoplastic process associated with vascular injury as compared with classic and cellular types of epithelioid hemangioma.

Classic lesions exhibit a circumscribed, multilobular proliferation of capillaries and small vessels surrounding a larger damaged vessel; endothelial cells are plump, epithelioid, and contain abundant amphophilic cytoplasm, sometimes with an intracytoplasmic vacuole representing a rudimentary lumen; nuclei have dispersed chromatin and small nucleoli.

- There is a moderate to marked lymphocytic infiltrate and variable number of eosinophils (Fig. 6.17). There may be outward maturation with nests of epithelioid cells in the center, small-lumen vessels further out, and well-formed vessels at the periphery.
- Endothelial cells are positive for factor VIII–related antigen, CD31, CD34, and glucose transporter-1 (GLUT-1), and are negative for S100 protein.

Differential Diagnosis

- Kimura disease affects Asian men in the third and fourth decades and presents as nodules within the subcutaneous tissues of the head and neck, enlarged lymph nodes, or enlarged parotid gland; there is a patchy lymphocytic infiltrate with many germinal centers and eosinophils (Fig. 6.18).
- Epithelioid hemangioendothelioma consists of strands and cords of epithelioid and slightly atypical endothelial cells with abundant eosinophilic cytoplasm, prominent cytoplasmic vacuoles, and myxochondroid or hyaline stroma; well-formed vascular channels are usually absent.
- Epithelioid angiosarcoma consists of sheets of epithelioid cells with significant cytologic atypia and hyperchromasia.

Management and Prognosis

- Excision is curative.

REFERENCES

Fetsch JF, Sesterhenn IA, Miettinen M, Davis CJ Jr. Epithelioid hemangioma of the penis: a clinicopathologic and immunohistochemical analysis of 19 cases, with special reference to exuberant examples often confused with epithelioid hemangioendothelioma and epithelioid angiosarcoma. *Am J Surg Pathol.* 2004;28:523-533.

Gao Y, Chen Y, Yu GY. Clinicopathologic study of parotid involvement in 21 cases of eosinophilic hyperplastic lymphogranuloma (Kimura's disease). *Oral Surg Oral Med Oral Pathol Oral Radiol Endod.* 2006;102: 651-658.

Huang SC, Zhang L, Sung YS, et al. Frequent FOS gene rearrangements in epithelioid hemangioma: a molecular study of 58 cases with morphologic reappraisal. *Am J Surg Pathol.* 2015;39:1313-1321.

Sun ZJ, Zhang L, Zhang WF, et al. Epithelioid hemangioma in the oral mucosa: a clinicopathological study of seven cases and review of the literature. *Oral Oncol.* 2006;42:441-447.

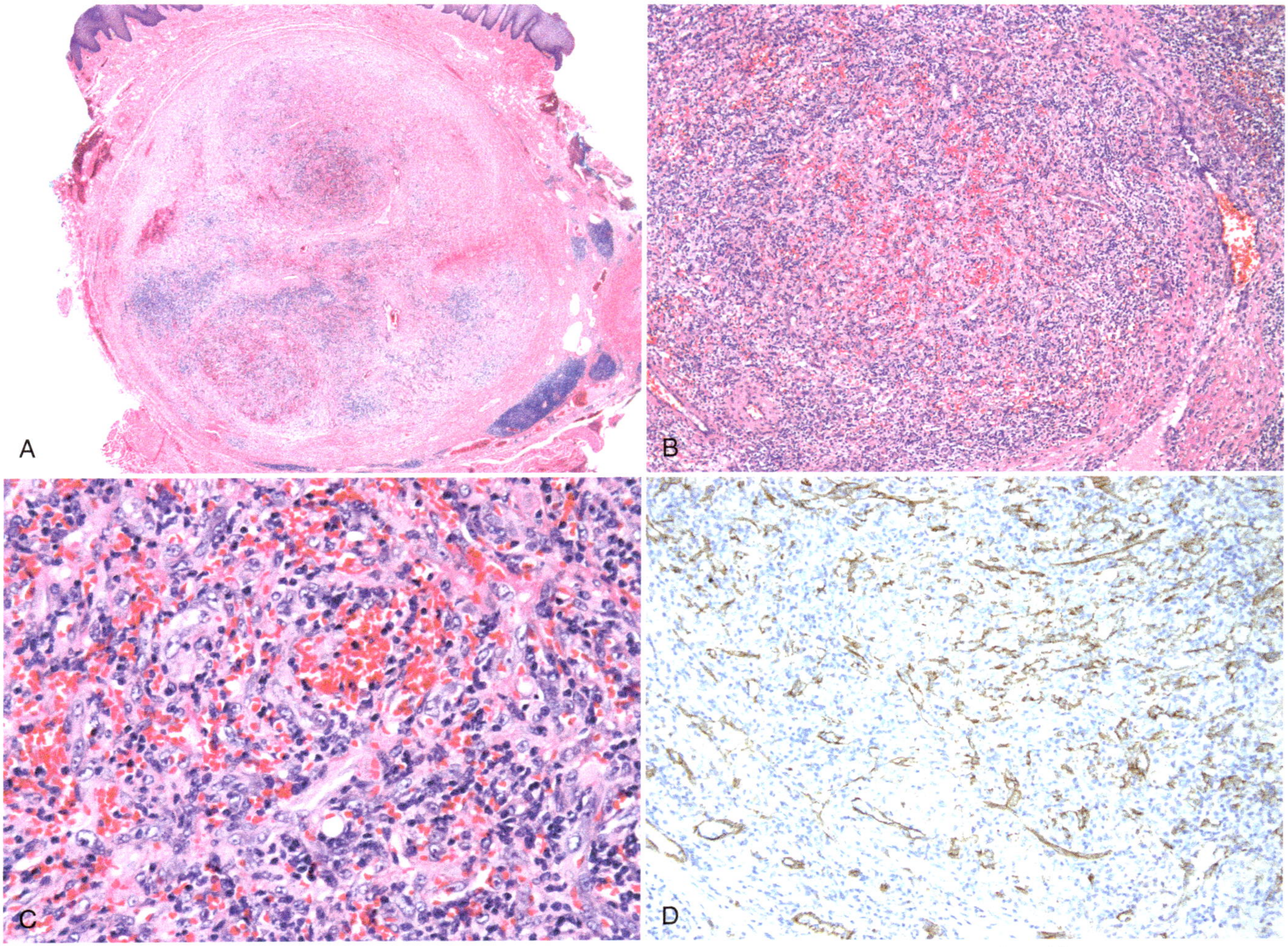

FIG 6.17 Epithelioid hemangioma. (A) Circumscribed multilobular cellular nodule with dilated large vessels in the center. (B) Many capillaries, epithelioid cells, and lymphocytes. (C) Epithelioid endothelial cells with large nuclei. (D) Cells show cytoplasmic positivity for CD31.

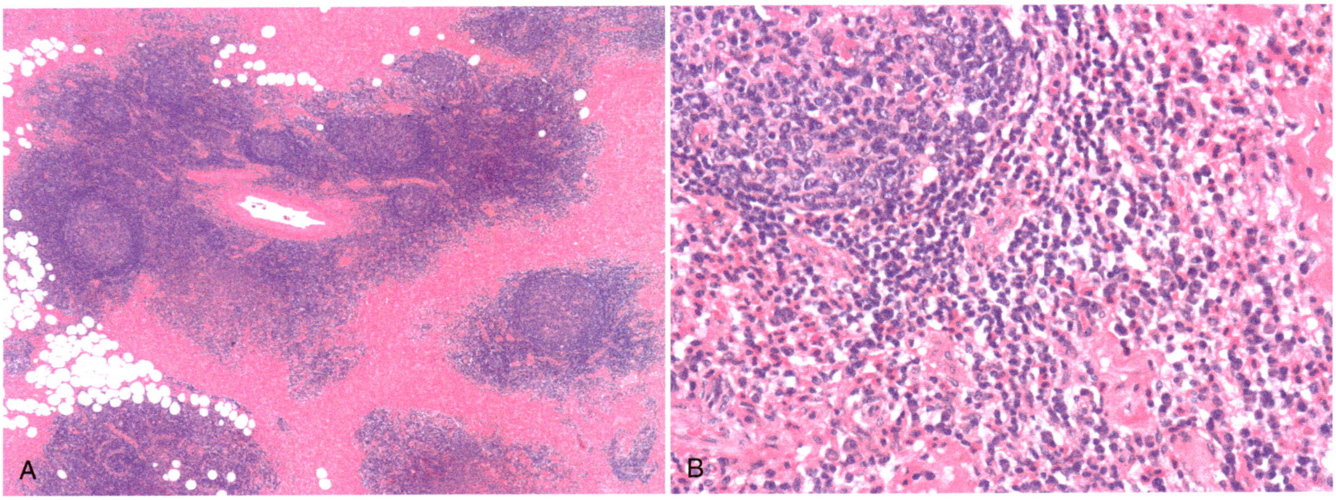

FIG 6.18 Kimura disease. (A) Fibrosis and a dense lymphocytic infiltrate with many germinal centers. (B) Germinal center, many lymphocytes, plasma cells, and eosinophils.

KAPOSI SARCOMA

Kaposi sarcoma is currently classified as a neoplasm of intermediate (nonmetastasizing) potential because of ambiguity regarding its biologic nature. It is associated with human herpesvirus-8 (HHV-8) infection.

Clinical Findings

There are four clinical presentations:

- Classic indolent type that involves the skin of the lower legs and sometimes the oral mucosa and viscera in older men of Mediterranean or Jewish descent.
- African endemic type that occurs in adults and children and involves the skin of the lower legs and lymph nodes, and tends to be progressive with the lymphadenopathic type being aggressive.
- Iatrogenic type that is associated with immunosuppression (especially after renal and lung transplantation) with localized or disseminated mucocutaneous lesions and sometimes visceral involvement; lesions may regress on reduction of immunosuppression.
- Epidemic type that is found in patients with HIV/AIDS with disseminated mucocutaneous lesions and sometimes visceral involvement; lesions may flare with antiretroviral therapy; this coexists with the endemic form in Africa; Kaposi sarcoma is an AIDS-defining illness.
- Lesions go through stages as follows: dusky red or purple macule (early patch stage), plaque (plaque stage), or nodular mass (tumor stage); the most common sites are maxillary gingiva, palatal mucosa, or tongue; infiltration of bone resulting in loosening of teeth (Fig. 6.19); oral involvement is seen in only 2% to 5% of nonepidemic cases and in 60% to 70% of patients with HIV/AIDS.
- Up to 60% of subjects who are seropositive for HHV-8 excrete this virus in saliva.
- Worsening of Kaposi sarcoma is one of the features of patients on antiretroviral therapy who develop immune reconstitution inflammatory syndrome (IRIS).

Etiopathogenesis and Histopathologic Features

Activity of Kaposi sarcoma-associated herpesvirus or HHV-8 infects and reprograms circulating mononuclear and endothelial "progenitor cells" to resemble lymphatic endothelium and to express D2-40 (podoplanin), and vascular endothelial growth factor receptor (VEGFR-3); there is also upregulation of HHV-8 gene products such as latency-associated nuclear antigen-1 (LANA-1); transmission may be through saliva rather than through blood or semen. However, not all patients who have been infected with HHV-8 develop Kaposi sarcoma.

- Most oral cavity cases are in the nodular stage and consist of a cellular proliferation of spindle cells in fascicles with slitlike vascular spaces, and abundant extravascular erythrocytes, hemosiderin and intra- and extracytoplasmic periodic acid–Schiff (PAS)-positive eosinophilic globules; nuclei are spindled with slight variation in size, dispersed chromatin, and small nucleoli; mitotic activity may be noted (Figs. 6.20 and 6.21A).
- Histologic variants have been identified such as anaplastic, lymphangioma-like, telangiectatic, glomeruloid, keloidal, and hyperkeratotic, although rarely in the mouth.
- Nuclear positivity for LANA-1 is diagnostic (Fig. 6.21B); spindle cells also exhibit cytoplasmic positivity for factor VIII–related antigen, CD31 (lower diagnostic sensitivity in tumor stage because it is removed by K5 protein produced by the virus), CD34, D2-40, PROX-1 and VEGFR-3, and also nuclear positivity for FLI-1 and BCL-2.

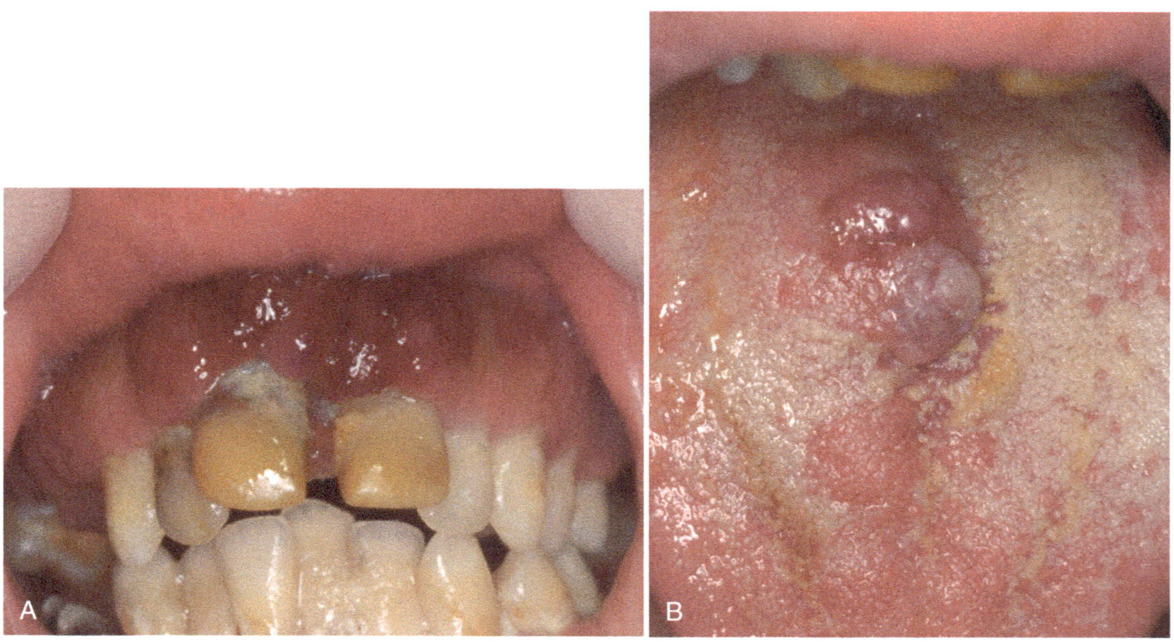

FIG 6.19 AIDS-associated Kaposi sarcoma. (A) Maxillary gingiva. (B) Tongue dorsum.

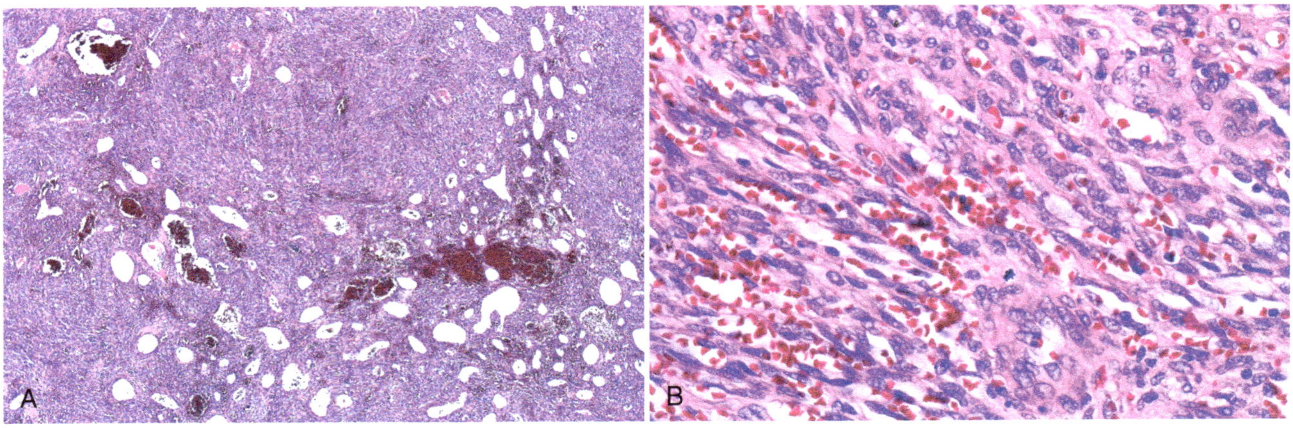

FIG 6.20 Kaposi sarcoma. (A) Cellular proliferation of spindle cells with dilated vascular spaces and abundant fresh hemorrhage. (B) Spindle cells surround slitlike spaces and show mild nuclear pleomorphism and mitotic activity; erythrocytes are present between spindle cells and within lumen.

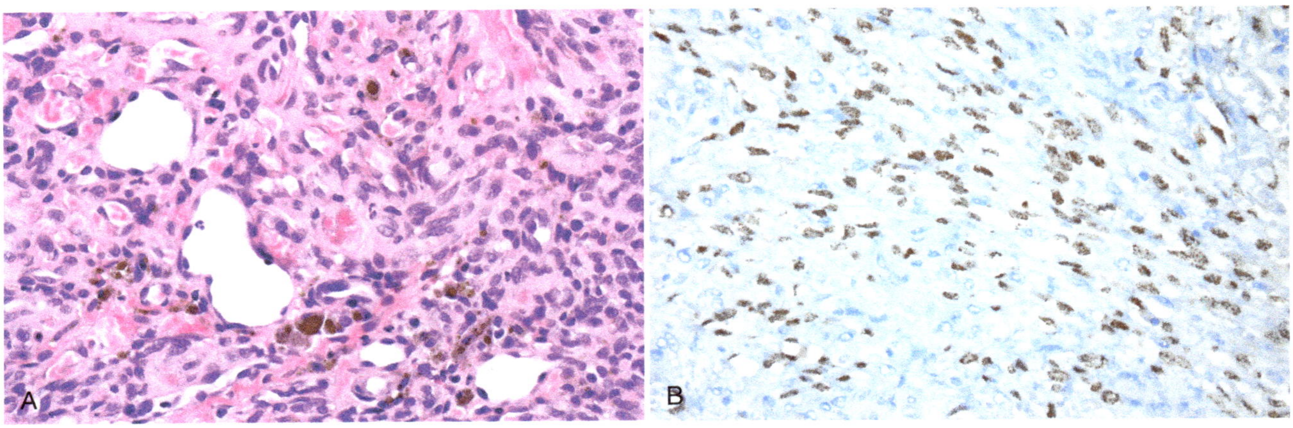

FIG 6.21 Kaposi sarcoma. (A) Plump spindle cells, eosinophilic globules, and abundant hemosiderin. (B) Positive immunostaining for nuclear HHV-8.

Differential Diagnosis

- The differential diagnosis of Kaposi sarcoma is vast and includes benign and malignant vasoformative and nonvasoformative spindle cell tumors. The presence of vascular markers and LANA-1 is diagnostic.

Management and Prognosis

- Oral lesions are successfully treated with excision, laser ablation, intralesional vinblastine therapy, and radiation; systemic therapy includes pegylated liposomal doxorubicin or daunorubicin; novel treatments include antiangiogenic agents such as bevacizumab, in addition to mammalian target of rapamycin (mTOR) inhibitors.
- Reduction in immunosuppression in posttransplantation patients with iatrogenic Kaposi sarcoma may lead to regression of tumors.

REFERENCES

Bagni R, Whitby D. Kaposi's sarcoma-associated herpesvirus transmission and primary infection. *Curr Opin HIV AIDS*. 2009;4:22-26.

Benevenuto de Andrade BA, Ramirez-Amador V, Anaya-Saavedra G, et al. Expression of PROX-1 in oral Kaposi's sarcoma spindle cells. *J Oral Pathol Med*. 2014;43:132-136.

Bunn BK, Carvalho Mde V, Louw M, et al. Microscopic diversity in oral Kaposi sarcoma. *Oral Surg Oral Surg Oral Med Oral Pathol Oral Radiol*. 2013;115:241-248.

Fletcher CD. The evolving classification of soft tissue tumours: an update based on the new WHO classification. *Histopathology*. 2006;48:3-12.

Folpe AL, Chand EM, Goldblum JR, Weiss SW. Expression of Fli-1, a nuclear transcription factor, distinguishes vascular neoplasms from potential mimics. *Am J Surg Pathol*. 2001;25:1061-1066.

Leidner RS, Aboulafia DM. Recrudescent Kaposi's sarcoma after initiation of HAART: a manifestation of immune reconstitution syndrome. *AIDS Patient Care STDS*. 2005;19:635-644.

Patrikidou A, Vahtsevanos K, Charalambidou M, et al. Non-AIDS Kaposi's sarcoma in the head and neck area. *Head Neck*. 2009;31:260-268.

Pauk J, Huang ML, Brodie SJ, et al. Mucosal shedding of human herpesvirus 8 in men. *N Engl J Med*. 2000;343:1369-1377.

Pugalagiri P, Muller S, Cox DP, et al. Lymphangioma-like Kaposi sarcoma of the oral mucosa. *Oral Surg Oral Med Oral Pathol Oral Radiol*. 2013;116:84-90.

Radu O, Pantanowitz L. Kaposi sarcoma. *Arch Pathol Lab Med*. 2013;137:289-294.

Ramirez-Amador V, Anaya-Saavedra G, Martinez-Mata G. Kaposi's sarcoma of the head and neck: a review. *Oral Oncol*. 2010;46:135-145.

Neural Tumors

Neural tumors are the most common benign spindle cell lesions in the oral cavity. Only the more common ones seen in the oral cavity will be discussed here. SOX-10, a transcription factor, is positive in most tumors with schwannian differentiation.

Clinical Findings

- Neural tumors present as a solitary nodule, most frequently on the tongue, lips (especially upper lip mucosa), and palatal mucosa (Fig. 6.22A).
- Traumatic neuromas are often painful and seen at sites of previous surgery or frequent trauma (eg, lower lip, tongue, and in the vicinity of the mental foramen in the edentulous mandible, the last from denture trauma).
- Multiple nodules on the lips and tongue strongly suggest mucosal neuromas of multiple endocrine neoplasia (MEN) type 2B.
- Neurofibroma, either solitary or multiple, may be associated with neurofibromatosis type 1, whereas schwannomas, especially vestibular schwannomas, are associated with neurofibromatosis type 2.

TRAUMATIC NEUROMA

Etiopathogenesis and Histopathologic Features

Traumatic partial or total severance of nerve fibers leads to first wallerian degeneration and subsequent axonal regeneration and remyelination with scar tissue.

- There are tangled nerve fibers of varying sizes, with some showing mucinous change or thickened perineurium with intervening fibrosis and scarring (Figs. 6.23 and 6.24A).
- Schwann cells are S-100 protein positive; neurofilament protein (NFP) highlights axons and the perineurium is positive for epithelial membrane antigen (EMA) and GLUT-1 (Fig. 6.24B).

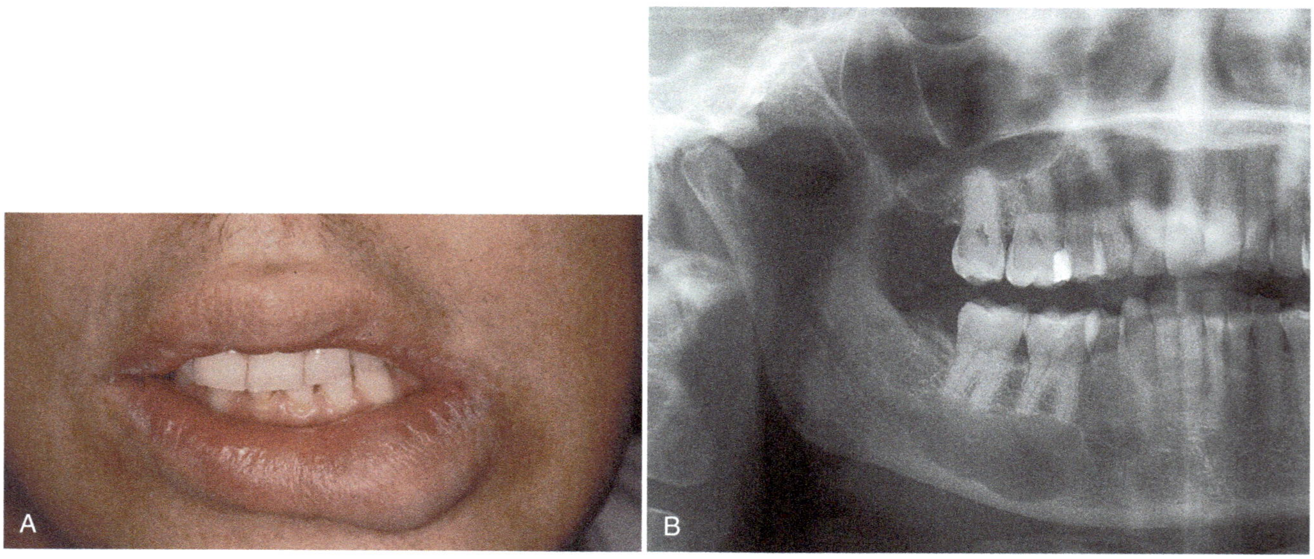

FIG 6.22 (A) Solitary neurofibroma of the lower lip. (B) Panoramic radiograph showing "blunderbuss" enlargement of the inferior alveolar canal secondary to a neural tumor.

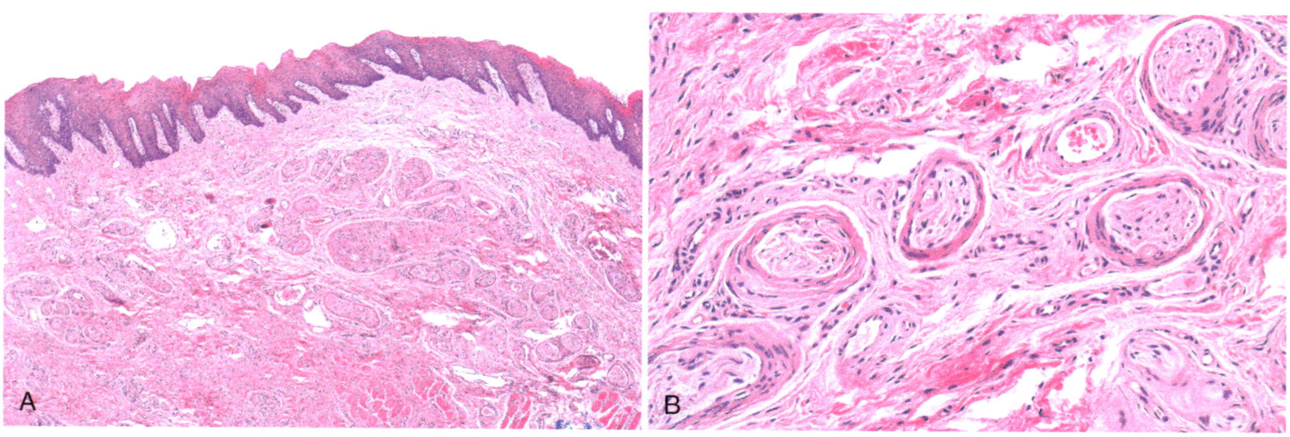

FIG 6.23 Traumatic neuroma. (A) Nerve fibers of varying sizes with fibrosis. (B) Nerve fibers with thickened endoneurium.

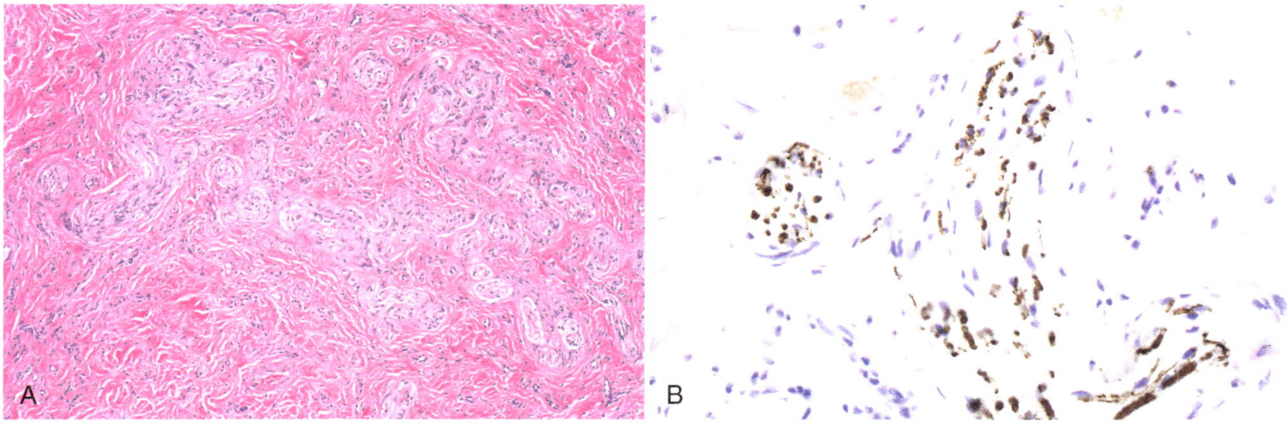

FIG 6.24 Traumatic neuroma. (A) Tangled nerve fibers with scarring. (B) Neurofilament protein positivity within neurites.

Differential Diagnosis

- Mucosal neuromas of MEN show hyperplasia of nerve fibers with thickened perineurium, but an absence of fibrosis and scarring.

Management and Prognosis

- Excision is curative.

REFERENCES

Chrysomali E, Papanicolaou SI, Dekker NP, Regezi JA. Benign neural tumors of the oral cavity: a comparative immunohistochemical study. *Oral Surg Oral Med Oral Pathol Oral Radiol Endod.* 1997;84:381-390.

Edwards M, Reid JS. Multiple endocrine neoplasia syndrome type IIb: a case report. *Int J Paediatr Dent.* 1998;8:55-60.

Foltan R, Klima K, Spackova J, Sedy J. Mechanism of traumatic neuroma development. *Med Hypotheses.* 2008;71:572-576.

Hirose T, Tani T, Shimada T, et al. Immunohistochemical demonstration of EMA/Glut1-positive perineurial cells and CD34-positive fibroblastic cells in peripheral nerve sheath tumors. *Mod Pathol.* 2003;16:293-298.

Jordan RC, Regezi JA. Oral spindle cell neoplasms: a review of 307 cases. *Oral Surg Oral Med Oral Pathol Oral Radiol Endod.* 2003;95:717-724.

Miettinen M, McCue PA, Sarlomo-Rikala M, et al. Sox10–a marker for not only schwannian and melanocytic neoplasms but also myoepithelial cell tumors of soft tissue: a systematic analysis of 5134 tumors. *Am J Surg Pathol.* 2015;39:826-835.

Salla JT, Johann AC, Garcia BG, et al. Retrospective analysis of oral peripheral nerve sheath tumors in Brazilians. *Braz Oral Res.* 2009;23:43-48.

Vora AR, Loescher AR, Craig GT, et al. A light microscopical study on the structure of traumatic neuromas of the human lingual nerve. *Oral Surg Oral Med Oral Pathol Oral Radiol Endod.* 2005;99:395-403.

NEUROFIBROMA

Etiopathogenesis and Histopathologic Features

- Neurofibroma arises within a nerve and represents a neoplastic proliferation of primarily Schwann cells with other components of a nerve such as fibroblasts, axons, and perineurial cells. Neurofibromas are usually solitary and sporadic; some (especially the plexiform type) are seen in patients with neurofibromatosis type 1 (NF1), an autosomal dominant disorder associated with an inactivating mutation in NF1 on chromosome 17. It is associated with other signs of neurofibromatosis such as café-au-lait macules, Lisch nodules, and multiple skin neurofibromas. Patients also show jaw abnormalities such as overgrowth of the alveolus and increased size of the coronoid notch.
- There is a nonencapsulated, discrete or diffuse proliferation of elongated and short spindle cells in a delicately collagenous stroma with variably (sometimes extensively) myxoid or mucinous background; cells have wavy cytoplasmic processes, indistinct cell borders, and curvilinear, comma-shaped or tadpole-shaped nuclei with inconspicuous nucleoli, and there may be slight nuclei atypia; mast cells are readily identified and neurites are often present (Figs. 6.25A–B and 6.26A–C).
- Diffuse neurofibroma infiltrates and entraps adjacent structures, although cells have the same morphology as conventional neurofibroma; Wagner-Meissner corpuscles are usually present (see Fig. 6.25C).
- Plexiform neurofibroma consists of tortuous nodules and cords of neural tissue that represent the unevenly enlarged and expanded nerve fascicle of neurofibromatosis.
- Spindle cells are positive for S100 protein and CD34 (Fig. 6.26D)
- Rarely, neurofibroma or other nerve sheath tumors may occur within the mandible involving the inferior alveolar nerve, leading to a "blunderbuss" appearance of the canal (see Fig. 6.22B).
- Dendritic cell neurofibroma is a variant that contains spindled type I cells with comma-shaped nuclei that surround large, polygonal, ganglion-like type II cells with dendritic processes, abundant pale cytoplasm, and vesicular nuclei with pseudoinclusions; pseudorosettes are present; both populations are S100+; the large cells are CD57+ and spindled cells show slight and variable positivity for glial fibrillary acidic protein (GFAP), microphthalmic transcription factor (MITF) and NFP (Fig. 6.27).

Differential Diagnosis

- Mucosal neuroma consists of nodules of tortuous and enlarged nerve fibers usually on the lips and tongue

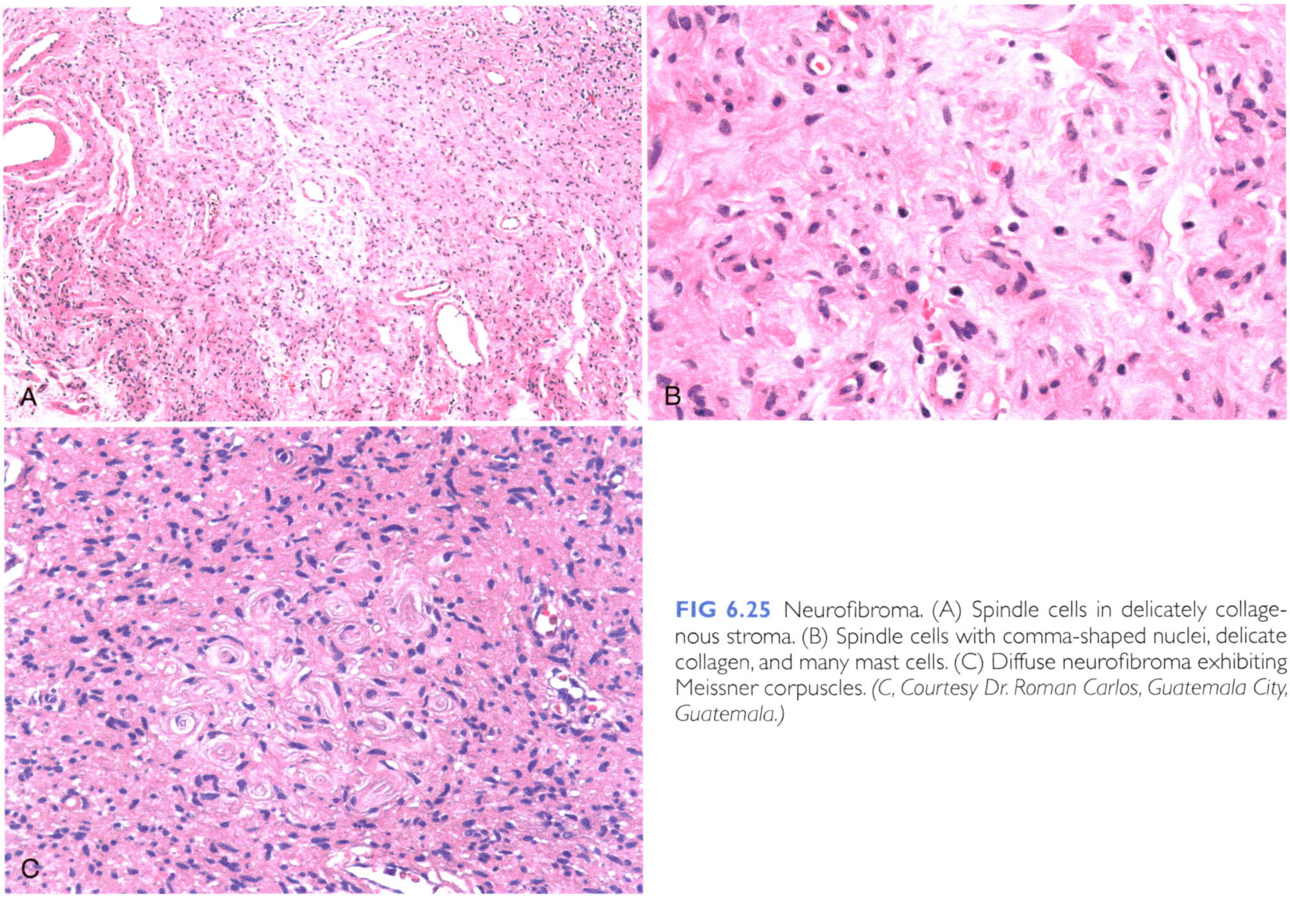

FIG 6.25 Neurofibroma. (A) Spindle cells in delicately collagenous stroma. (B) Spindle cells with comma-shaped nuclei, delicate collagen, and many mast cells. (C) Diffuse neurofibroma exhibiting Meissner corpuscles. *(C, Courtesy Dr. Roman Carlos, Guatemala City, Guatemala.)*

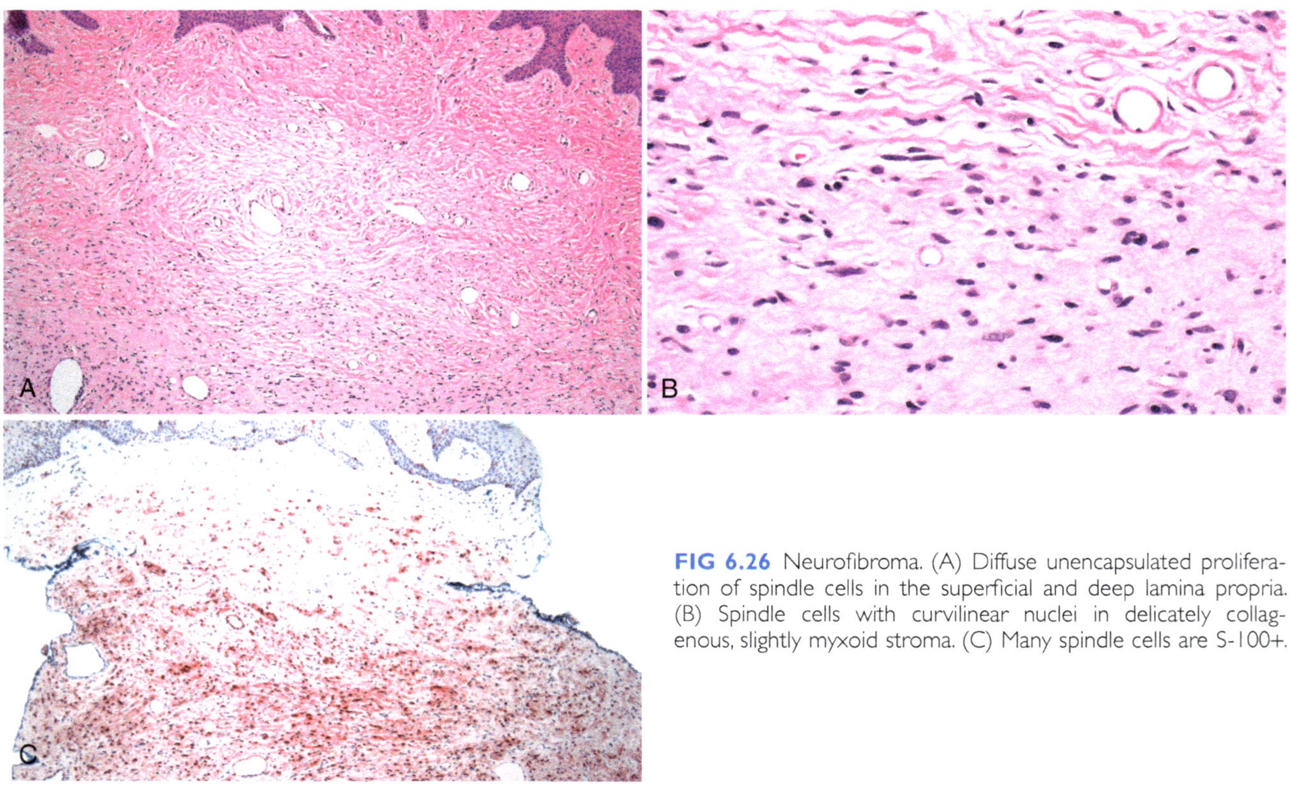

FIG 6.26 Neurofibroma. (A) Diffuse unencapsulated proliferation of spindle cells in the superficial and deep lamina propria. (B) Spindle cells with curvilinear nuclei in delicately collagenous, slightly myxoid stroma. (C) Many spindle cells are S-100+.

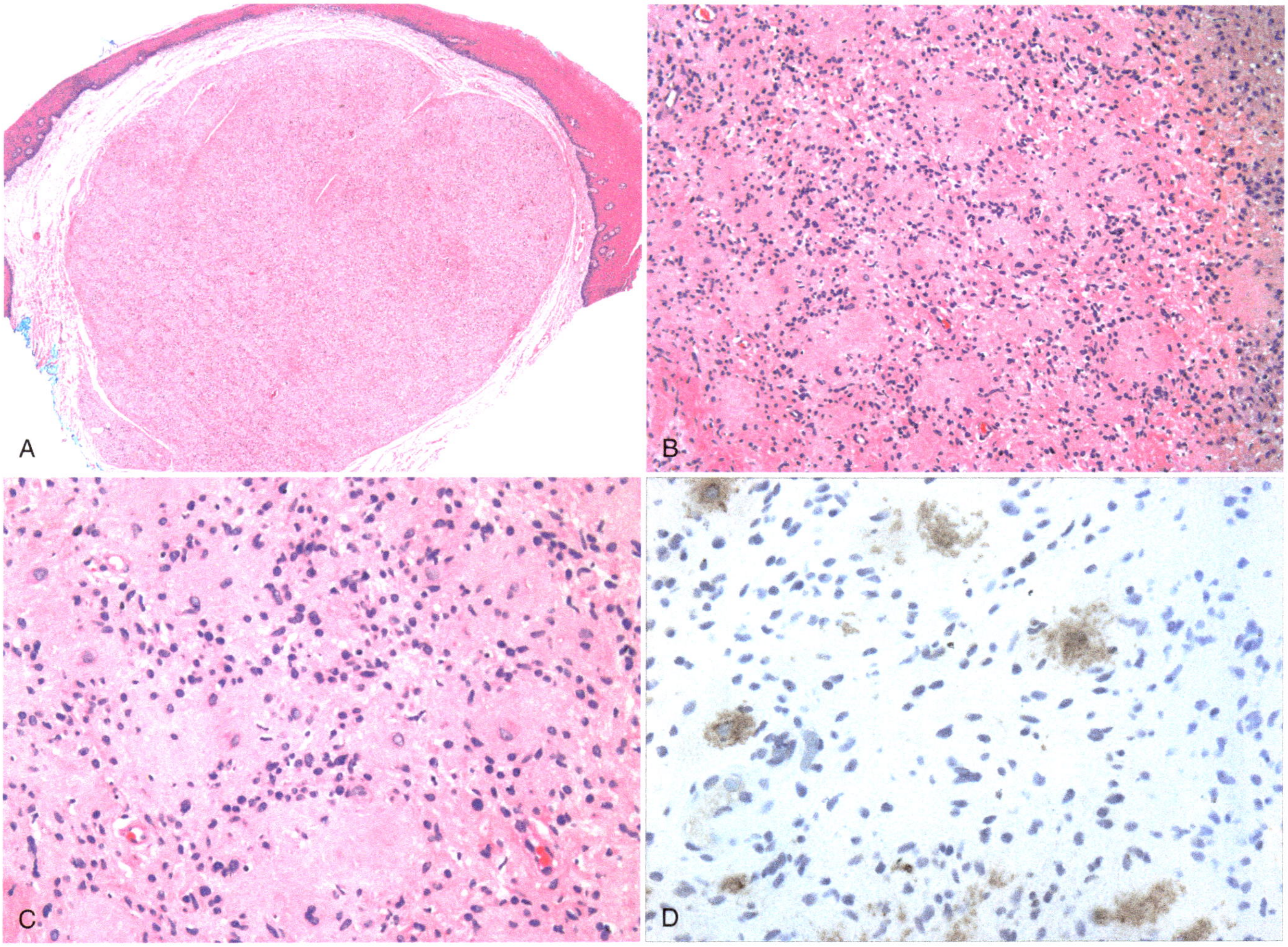

FIG 6.27 Dendritic cell neurofibroma. (A) Circumscribed nodule composed of spindle cells. (B) Pseudorosettes composed of spindle cells at the periphery and large, pale cells in the center. (C) Pseudorosette composed of spindle type I cells and larger, pale type II cells. (D) CD57 positivity within the larger pale cells.

(Fig. 6.28). It is associated with MEN type 2B, an autosomal dominant condition caused by a mutation in *RET* on chromosome 10; it is also associated with medullary thyroid carcinoma, pheochromocytomas (often bilateral), eyelid neuromas causing lid eversion, intestinal ganglioneuromatosis, and marfanoid phenotype.

- Nerve sheath myxomas are multilobular with intervening dense collagen bands; spindle and stellate cells may have a reticular pattern and are suspended in a myxoid matrix; cells are S100+ and GFAP+, and sometimes CD57+; this term is no longer used interchangeably with neurothekeoma, which is likely a fibrohistiocytic tumor and not of neural differentiation.
- Perineuriomas are circumscribed tumors with a storiform, fasciculated or whorled architecture. Cells are elongated with bipolar processes and spindled wavy nuclei and are usually S100−, EMA+ and CD34+, and sometimes claudin-1+.

Management and Prognosis

- Excision is curative.
- Plexiform lesions in patients with neurofibromatosis are at risk for malignant transformation.

REFERENCES

Anderson JL, Gutmann DH. Neurofibromatosis type 1. *Handb Clin Neurol.* 2015;132:75-86.

Campos MS, Fontes A, Marocchio LS, et al. Clinicopathologic and immunohistochemical features of oral neurofibroma. *Acta Odontol Scand.* 2012;70:577-582.

Chrysomali E, Papanicolaou SI, Dekker NP, Regezi JA. Benign neural tumors of the oral cavity: a comparative immunohistochemical study. *Oral Surg Oral Med Oral Pathol Oral Radiol Endod.* 1997;84:381-390.

Deichler J, Martinez R, Niklander S, et al. Solitary intraosseous neurofibroma of the mandible. Apropos of a case. *Med Oral Patol Oral Cir Bucal.* 2011;16:e704-e707.

Fetsch JF, Laskin WB, Miettinen M. Nerve sheath myxoma: a clinicopathologic and immunohistochemical analysis of 57 morphologically distinctive, S-100 protein- and GFAP-positive, myxoid peripheral nerve sheath tumors with a predilection for the extremities and a high local recurrence rate. *Am J Surg Pathol.* 2005;29:1615-1624.

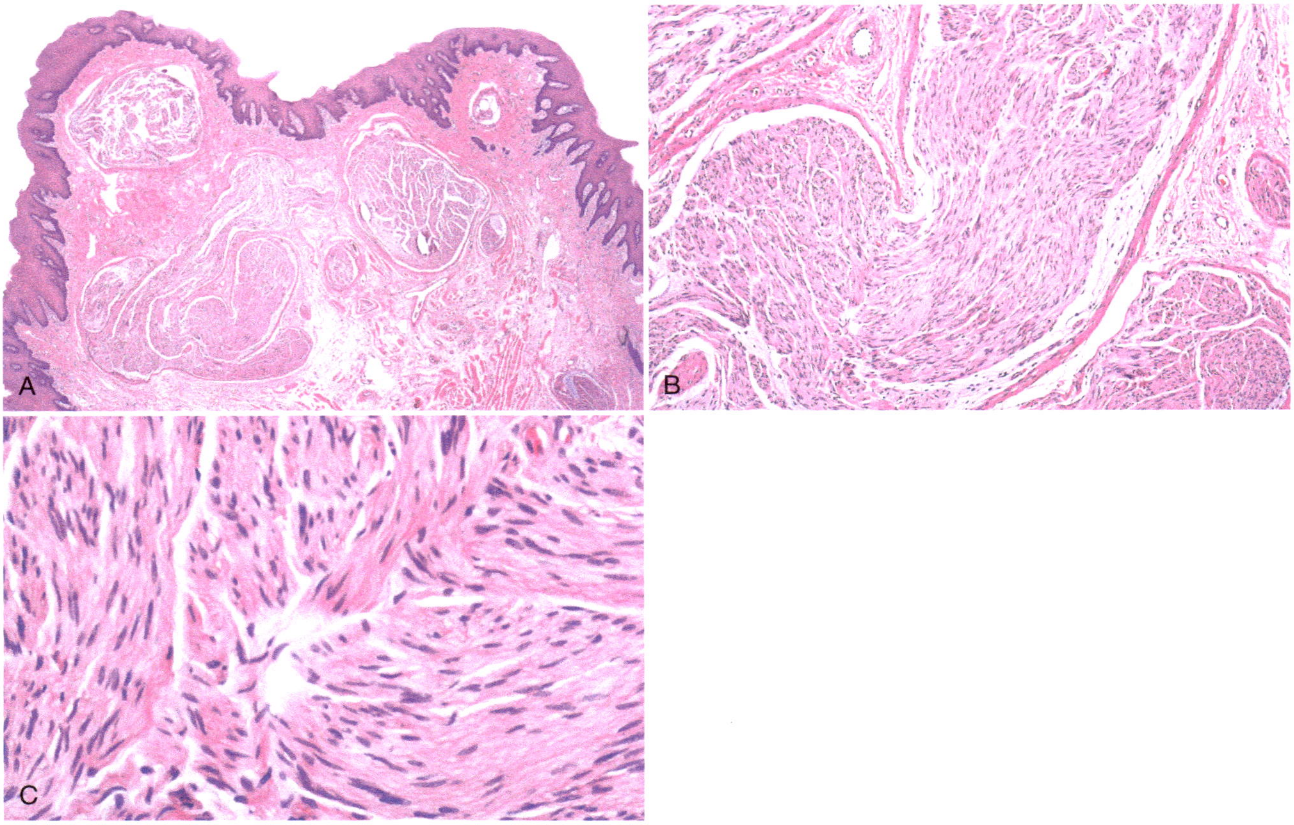

FIG 6.28 Mucosal neuroma (somewhat plexiform pattern) in a patient with MEN-2B. (A) Ropelike proliferation of nerve fibers of varying diameters in the lamina propria. (B) Nerve fibers show thickened perineurium. (C) Neurites and axons identified. *(A, Courtesy Dr. Carl Allen, The Ohio State University, Columbus, Ohio.)*

Hornick JL, Fletcher CD. Soft tissue perineurioma: clinicopathologic analysis of 81 cases including those with atypical histologic features. *Am J Surg Pathol.* 2005;29:845-858.

Lerman MA, Li CC, Woo SB. Dendritic cell neurofibroma with pseudorosettes: a clinicopathologic and immunohistochemical study of 5 intraoral cases. *Oral Surg Oral Med Oral Pathol Oral Radiol.* 2014;117:221-226.

MacIntosh RB, Shivapuja PK, Krzemien MB, Lee M. Multiple endocrine neoplasia type 2B: maxillofacial significance in 5 cases. *J Oral Maxillofac Surg.* 2014;72(2498):e1-e17.

Nishioka M, Aguirre RL, Ishikawa A, et al. Nerve sheath myxoma (neurothekeoma) arising in the oral cavity: histological and immunohistochemical features of 3 cases. *Oral Surg Oral Med Oral Pathol Oral Radiol Endod.* 2009;107:e28-e33.

Salla JT, Johann AC, Garcia BG, et al. Retrospective analysis of oral peripheral nerve sheath tumors in Brazilians. *Braz Oral Res.* 2009;23:43-48.

Zhou H, Coffin CM, Perkins SL, et al. Malignant peripheral nerve sheath tumor: a comparison of grade, immunophenotype, and cell cycle/growth activation marker expression in sporadic and neurofibromatosis 1-related lesions. *Am J Surg Pathol.* 2003;27:1337-1345.

SCHWANNOMA

Etiopathogenesis and Histopathologic Features

Schwannoma represents a neoplastic proliferation of Schwann cells and axons developing eccentrically on the surface of nerves. Most cases are sporadic and less than 5% are associated with neurofibromatosis type 2 (NF2), an autosomal dominant disorder associated with a mutation on chromosome 22; the most common tumor in that syndrome is the vestibular schwannoma.

- There is an encapsulated proliferation of spindled Schwann cells in fascicles in delicately collagenous stroma; the cells are elongated with indistinct cell borders, moderate amounts of eosinophilic cytoplasm, and spindle nuclei with dispersed chromatin and small nucleoli. Two patterns are recognized: the *Antoni type A pattern* exhibits areas of hypercellularity that contain Verocay bodies composed of palisaded nuclei and intervening eosinophilic accumulation of cell processes; the *Antoni type B pattern* exhibits nondescript hypocellular areas (Fig. 6.29); hyalinized vessels are a common finding and degenerative changes may be present with some cytologic atypia; intramucosal axons are seen in 50% of cases.
- Tumor cells are S-100+ and GFAP+, axons are NFP+, and the capsule being composed of perineurial cells is EMA+; nuclei of Schwann cells are SOX10+.
- Ancient schwannomas show extensive degenerative changes such as hemorrhage, hyalinization, pseudocystic degeneration of the stroma, atypical spindle cells with large nuclei, foamy macrophages, and pseudorosettes, variable inflammation (Fig. 6.30).

Differential Diagnosis

- Solitary circumscribed neuromas show some palisading of nuclei but contain many neurites and tissue clefts.
- Some leiomyomas demonstrate Verocay body–like structures with nuclear palisading but are S-100–.

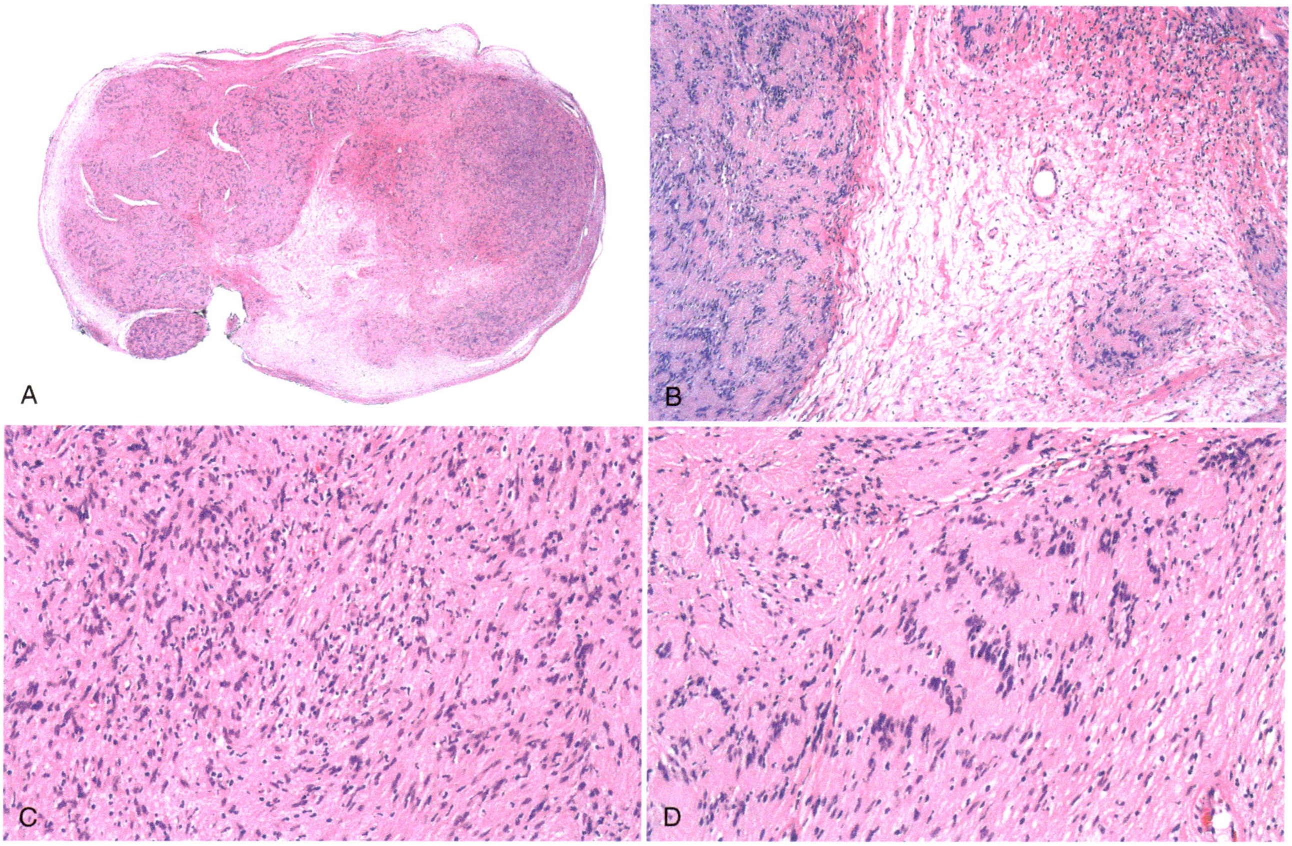

FIG 6.29 Schwannoma. (A) Encapsulated tumor. (B) Hypercellular areas with Verocay bodies of Antoni A pattern *(left)*, and hypocellular areas of Antoni B *(center)*. (C) Elongated spindle cells with only subtle palisading of nuclei. (D) Verocay bodies composed of palisaded nuclei and eosinophilic mass of cytoplasmic processes.

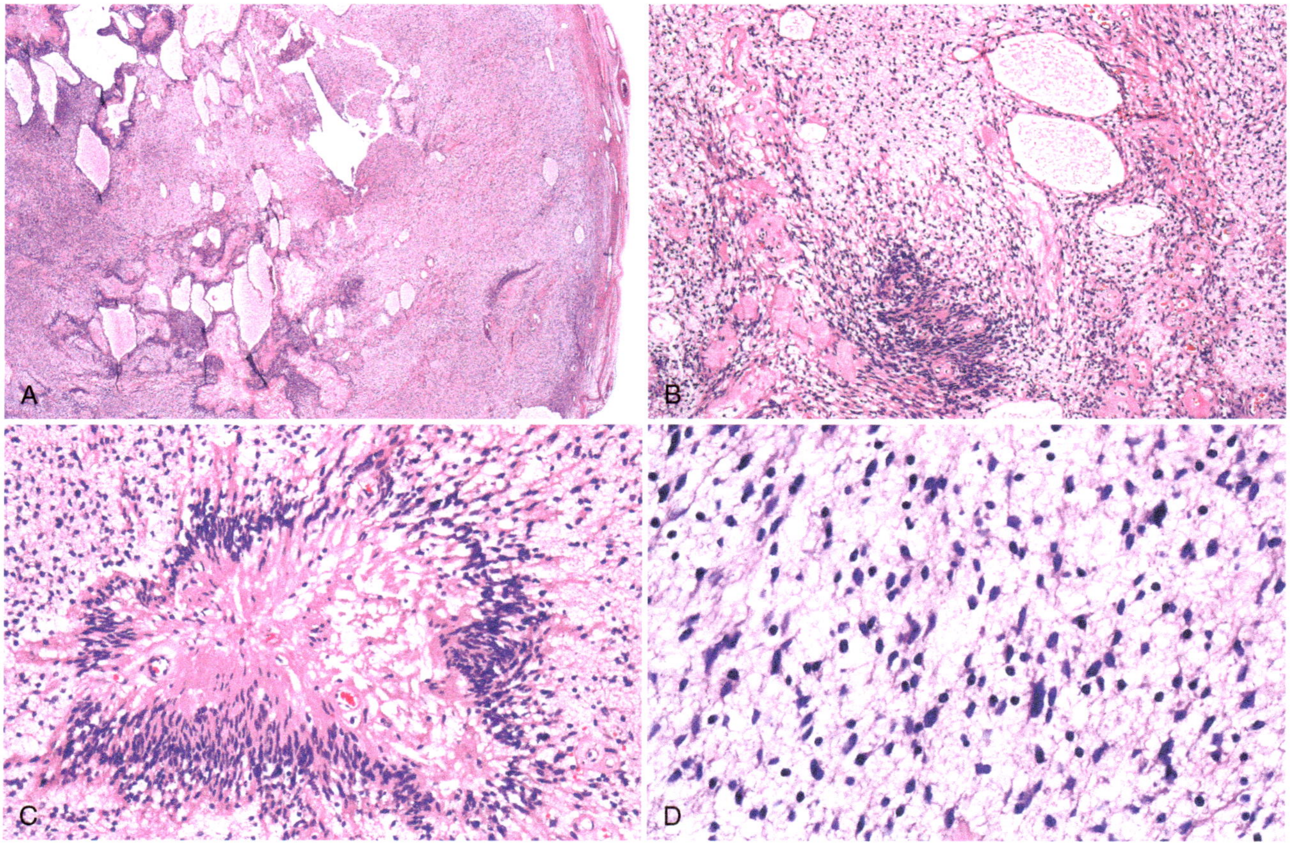

FIG 6.30 Ancient schwannoma. (A) Encapsulated tumor with marked edema and pseudocystic degeneration of the stroma. (B) Spindle cell proliferation with pseudocysts, perivascular hyalinization, chronic inflammation, and mostly Antoni type B tissue. (C) Palisading of nuclei forming unusual rosette-like structure. (D) Spindle cells with mild nuclear atypia.

REFERENCES

Berg JC, Scheithauer BW, Spinner RJ, et al. Plexiform schwannoma: a clinicopathologic overview with emphasis on the head and neck region. *Hum Pathol.* 2008;39:633-640.

Evans DG. Neurofibromatosis type 2. *Handb Clin Neurol.* 2015;132: 87-96.

Fletcher C, ed. *Diagnostic Histopathology of Tumors.* 3rd ed. New York: Churchill Livingstone; 2007.

Nascimento AF, Fletcher CD. The controversial nosology of benign nerve sheath tumors: neurofilament protein staining demonstrates intratumoral axons in many sporadic schwannomas. *Am J Surg Pathol.* 2007;31:1363-1370.

Rodriguez FJ, Folpe AL, Glennin C, et al. Pathology of peripheral nerve sheath tumors: Diagnostic overview and update on selected diagnostic problems. *Acta Neuropathol.* 2012;123:295-319.

Santos PP, Freitas VS, Pinto LP, et al. Clinicopathologic analysis of 7 cases of oral schwannoma and review of the literature. *Ann Diagn Pathol.* 2010;14:235-239.

SOLITARY CIRCUMSCRIBED NEUROMA (PALISADED ENCAPSULATED NEUROMA)

Etiopathogenesis and Histopathologic Features

Solitary circumscribed neuroma is likely a neoplastic proliferation of Schwann cells and neurites, possibly within a nerve.

- Lesions occur most commonly in the fifth decade and approximately 75% of lesions occur on the palatal mucosa or gingiva, with the lip mucosa being the second most common site.
- There is a circumscribed and sometimes partially encapsulated, unilobular, multilobular, or plexiform proliferation of Schwann cells, neurites, and fibroblasts in fascicles within a delicately collagenous stroma; cells are elongated with indistinct cell borders, moderate amounts of cytoplasm, and nuclei are plump, elongated and wavy with dispersed chromatin and inconspicuous nucleoli; subtle palisading of nuclei is characteristic and tissue clefts are a reliable feature (Figs. 6.31A–C and 6.32); some lesions are predominantly myxoid; epithelioid and vascular variants have been reported.
- Spindle cells are S-100+ and axons of neurites are NFP+ (Fig. 6.31D); EMA+, GLUT-1+, and claudin-1+ cells are present around the lobules.

Management and Prognosis

- Excision is curative and recurrence is rare.

REFERENCES

Argenyi ZB, Penick GD. Vascular variant of palisaded encapsulated neuroma. *J Cutan Pathol.* 1993;20:92-93.

Argenyi ZB, Cooper PH, Santa Cruz D. Plexiform and other unusual variants of palisaded encapsulated neuroma. *J Cutan Pathol.* 1993; 20:34-39.

Koutlas IG, Scheithauer BW. Palisaded encapsulated ("solitary circumscribed") neuroma of the oral cavity: a review of 55 cases. *Head Neck Pathol.* 2010;4:15-26.

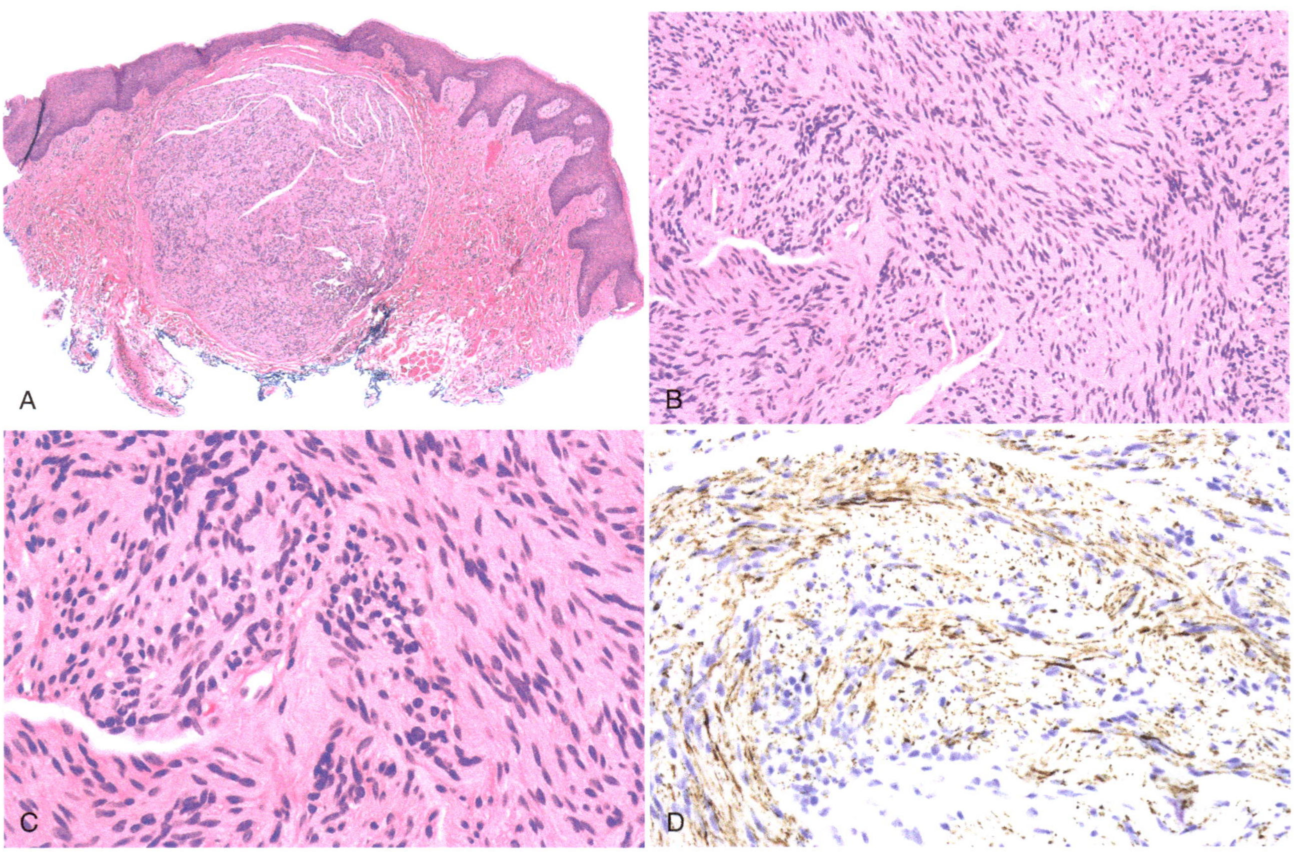

FIG 6.31 Solitary circumscribed neuroma. (A) Circumscribed proliferation of spindle cells. (B) Neurites and spindle cells present in short fascicles. (C) Spindle cells have tapered, elongated nuclei. (D) Neurofilament protein reveals the presence of numerous axons cut in various planes.

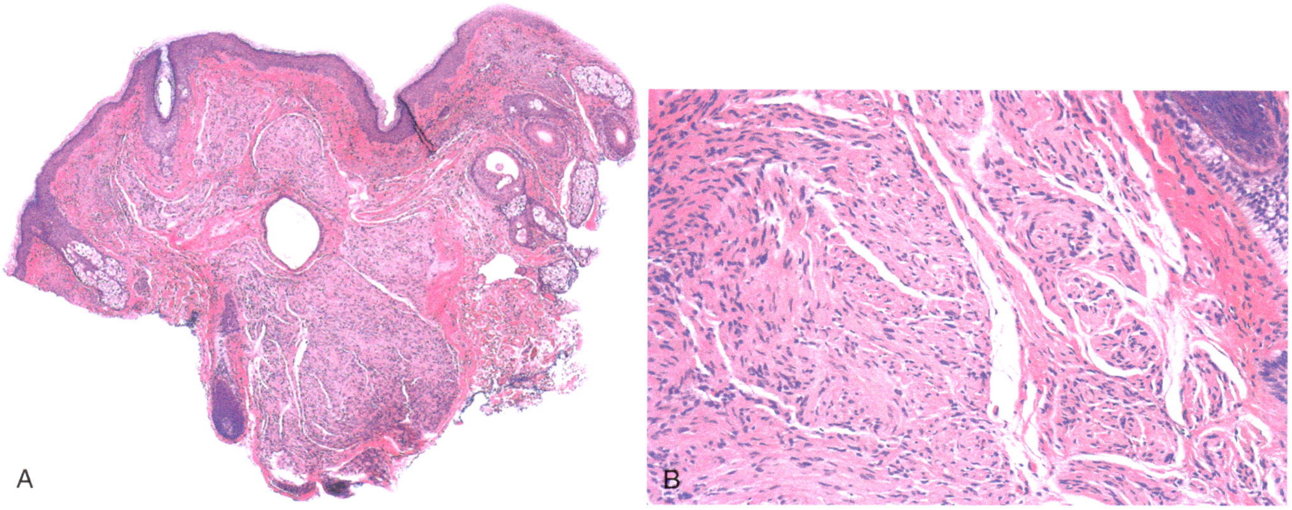

FIG 6.32 Solitary circumscribed neuroma. (A) Multilobular plexiform pattern. (B) Neurites and spindle cells with wavy nuclei and slight nuclear palisading.

Magnusson B. Palisaded encapsulated neuroma (solitary, circumscribed neuroma) of the oral mucosa. *Oral Surg Oral Med Oral Pathol Oral Radiol Endod*. 1996;83:302-304.

Tsang WY, Chan JK. Epithelioid variant of solitary circumscribed neuroma of the skin. *Histopathology*. 1992;20:439-441.

Granular Cell Tumor

Clinical Findings

- This occurs in adults, with a 2:1 female predilection; it presents as a firm mass, sometimes yellowish, beneath intact epithelium in the deep mucosa; it occurs most commonly on the tongue, buccal mucosa, and lips (Fig. 6.33).

Etiopathogenesis and Histopathologic Features

Granular cell tumor stains for neural markers and the cytoplasm is granular because of lysosomes. One theory of pathogenesis is that lysosomes are present to digest myelin, which has been noted to be present within the cytoplasm in ultrastructural studies.

- There is a nonencapsulated proliferation of cells with granular cytoplasm that sometimes contain eosinophilic globules; cells may be in sheets or nodules and often insinuate between skeletal muscle fibers; nuclei have dispersed chromatin and inconspicuous nucleoli without atypia or mitotic activity; the overlying epithelium may exhibit pseudoepitheliomatous hyperplasia (in 20%–30% of cases) or be atrophic (Figs. 6.34 and 6.35A–C).
- Cells demonstrate cytoplasmic and nuclear positivity for S-100, in addition to cytoplasmic positivity for CD68, PGP9.5, BCL2, caspase, calretinin, and myelin basic protein (Fig. 6.35D–E).
- Plexiform granular cell tumor is a variant; it forms fascicles and nodules that encase nerves, vessels, and skin adnexa.

Differential Diagnosis

- Congenital granular cell tumor exhibits arborizing small vessels, is S-100 negative, and occurs on the gingiva of neonates.
- Primitive polypoid nonneural granular cell tumor often has a collarette of epithelial cells around the tumor is S-100–, is NK1-C3+ and CD68+, sometimes neuron specific enolase (NSE)+, and may show nuclear atypia and mitotic activity; a desmoplastic variant exists.
- Granular cells may be seen focally in other tumors such as benign histiocytoma and leiomyoma, and may indicate degenerative change.

Management and Prognosis

- Excision is curative and malignant forms are rare.

REFERENCES

Agusti J, Martinez-Ciarpaglini C, Monteagudo C. Desmoplastic primitive nonneural granular cell tumor of the skin. *Am J Dermatopathol*. 2014; 36:e84-e86.

Aldabagh B, Azmi F, Vadmal M, et al. Plexiform pattern in cutaneous granular cell tumors. *J Cutan Pathol*. 2009;36:1174-1176.

Basile JR, Woo SB. Polypoid S-100-negative granular cell tumor of the oral cavity: a case report and review of literature. *Oral Surg Oral Med Oral Pathol Oral Radiol Endod*. 2003;96:70-76.

Brannon RB, Anand PM. Oral granular cell tumors: an analysis of 10 new pediatric and adolescent cases and a review of the literature. *J Clin Pediatr Dent*. 2004;29:69-74.

Chaudhry AP, Jacobs MS, SunderRaj M, et al. A clinico-pathologic study of 50 adult oral granular cell tumors. *J Oral Med*. 1984;39:97-103.

Fanburg-Smith JC, Meis-Kindblom JM, Fante R, Kindblom LG. Malignant granular cell tumor of soft tissue: diagnostic criteria and clinicopathologic correlation. *Am J Surg Pathol*. 1998;22:779-794.

Fine SW, Li M. Expression of calretinin and the alpha-subunit of inhibin in granular cell tumors. *Am J Clin Pathol*. 2003;119:259-264.

Lazar AJ, Fletcher CD. Primitive nonneural granular cell tumors of skin: clinicopathologic analysis of 13 cases. *Am J Surg Pathol*. 2005;29: 927-934.

Mahalingam M, LoPiccolo D, Byers HR. Expression of PGP 9.5 in granular cell nerve sheath tumors: an immunohistochemical study of six cases. *J Cutan Pathol*. 2001;28:282-286.

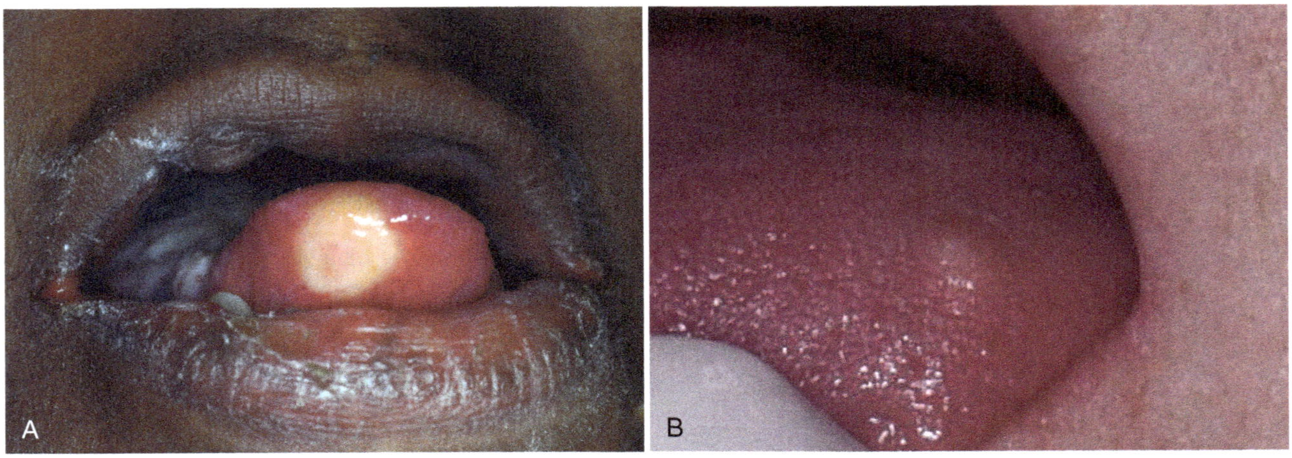

FIG 6.33 (A) Granular cell tumor on the ventral tongue with typical yellow color. (B) Granular cell tumor on the tongue dorsum.

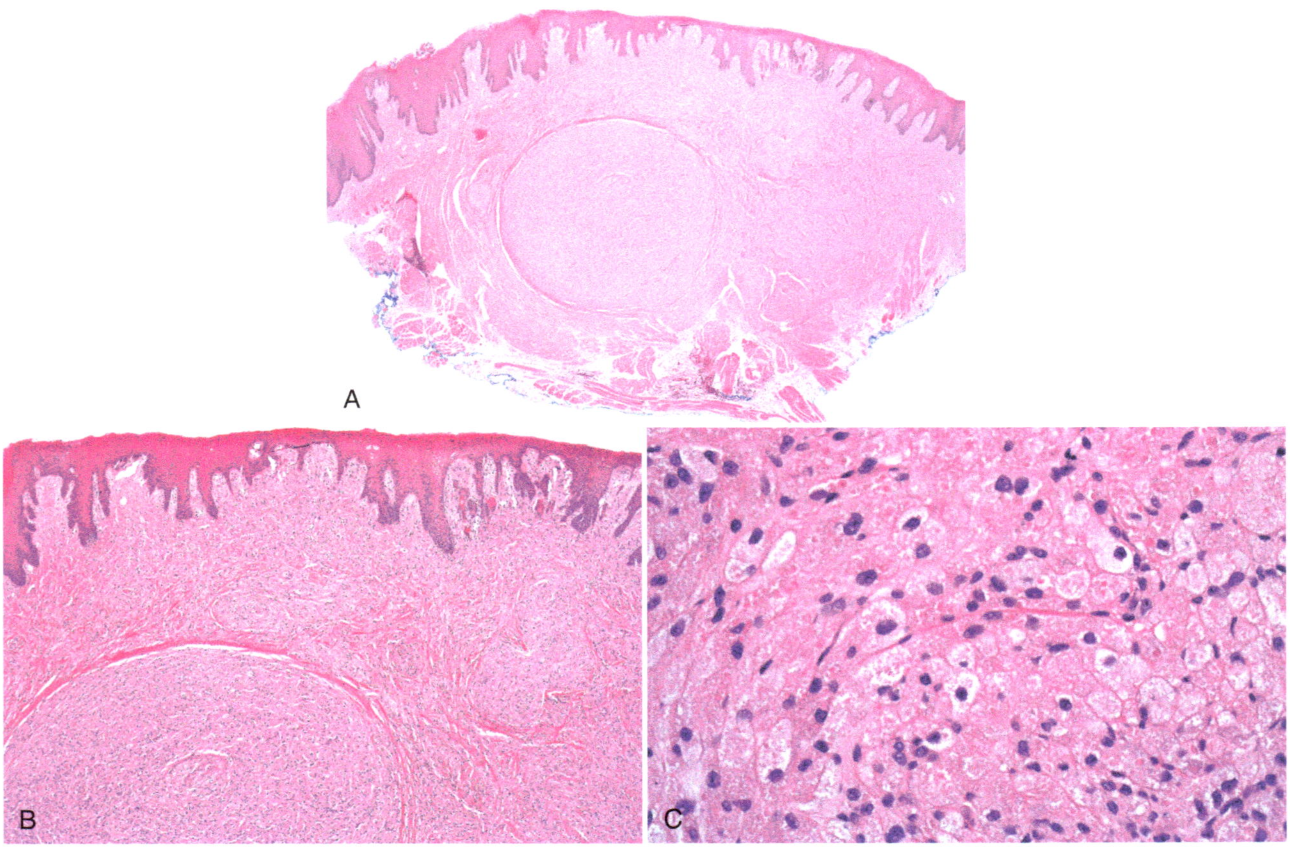

FIG 6.34 Granular cell tumor. (A) Nonencapsulated tumor with slightly nodular pattern extends into the underlying muscle. (B) Granular cells abut epithelium that exhibits slight pseudoepitheliomatous hyperplasia. (C) Cells have granular cytoplasm and benign nuclei.

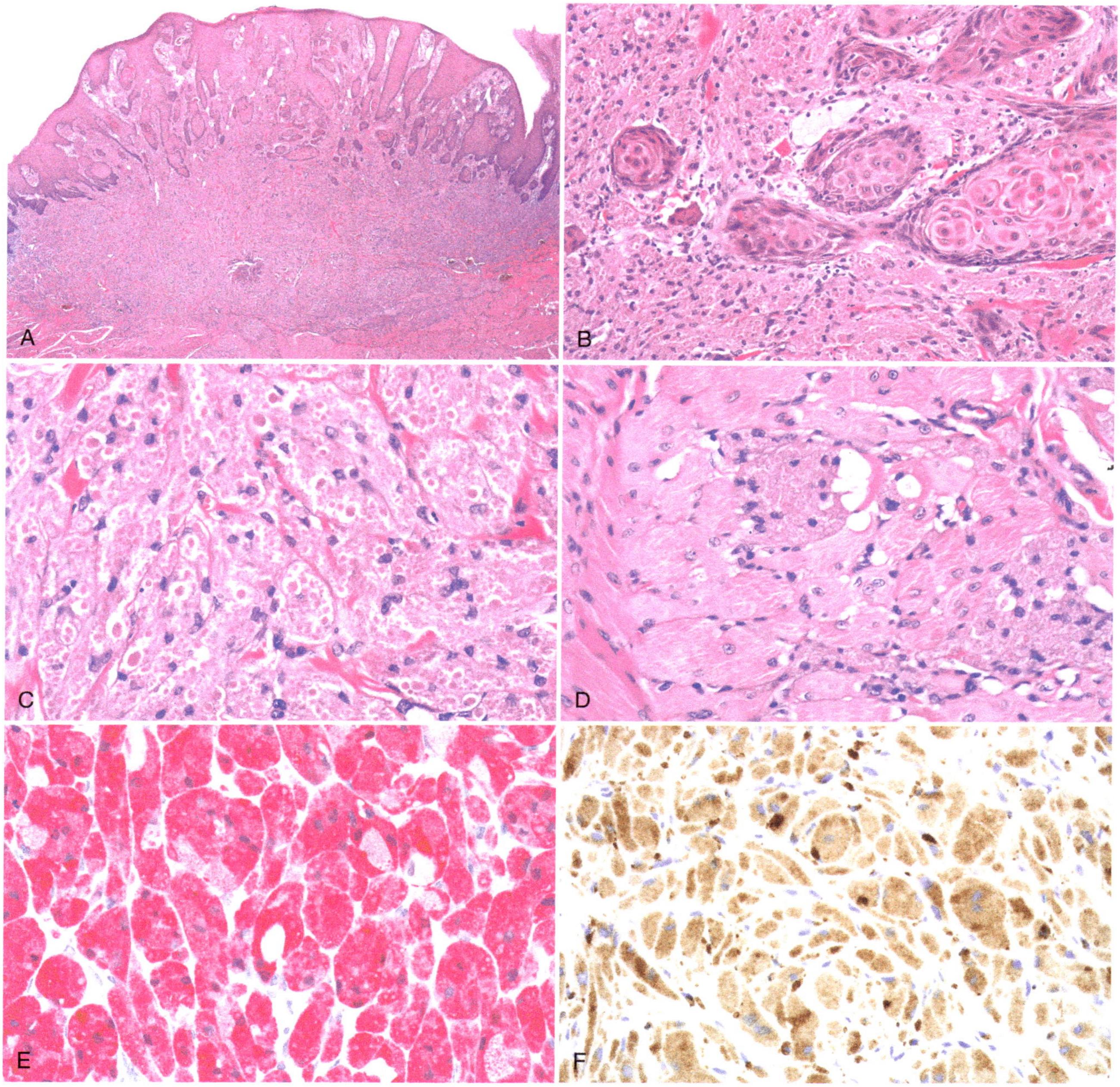

FIG 6.35 Granular cell tumor. (A) Marked pseudoepitheliomatous hyperplasia. (B) Epithelial islands exhibit cytologic atypia and dyskeratosis. (C) Granular cells with cytoplasmic eosinophilic globules. (D) Granular cells nestled between myocytes. (E) Cytoplasmic and nuclear positivity for S-100 protein. (F) Cytoplasmic positivity for CD68.

Nasser H, Danforth RD Jr, Sunbuli M, Dimitrijevic O. Malignant granular cell tumor: case report with a novel karyotype and review of the literature. *Ann Diagn Pathol.* 2010;14:273-278.

Ordonez NG, Mackay B. Granular cell tumor: a review of the pathology and histogenesis. *Ultrastruct Pathol.* 1999;23:207-222.

Muscle Tumors

ANGIOLEIOMYOMA (VASCULAR LEIOMYOMA) AND LEIOMYOMA

Clinical Findings

This presents in adults as a painless nodule, usually in the upper lip (50% of cases) of adults; the hard palatal mucosa is the second most common site (25% of cases) (Fig. 6.36).

Etiopathogenesis and Histopathologic Features

- This benign neoplasm shows differentiation toward smooth muscle.
- Angioleiomyoma (vascular leiomyoma): There is a discrete proliferation of spindle cells in a nodular configuration around a central endothelium-lined vascular channel; smooth muscle cells have indistinct borders, abundant pale, eosinophilic, vacuolated cytoplasm, and elongated, often blunt-ended, or cigar-shaped nuclei without mitotic activity or atypia (Figs. 6.37 and 6.38A).
- Leiomyoma: Spindled cells as noted above are present in sweeping fascicles but without a significant vascular component (Fig. 6.39A–B); granular cell and epithelioid variants have been reported.
- Spindle cells show cytoplasmic positivity for smooth muscle actin, muscle-specific actin, desmin, and h-caldesmon (Figs. 6.38B–C and 6.39C).

Differential Diagnosis

- Myofibroma has a chondroid-appearing stroma, and the spindle cells have less cytoplasm and may exhibit zoning phenomenon; it occurs in younger patients.
- Nodular fasciitis exhibits a proliferation of spindle cells in a myxoid/mucinous stroma with "tissue culture" appearance, often multinucleated giant cells, and a mixed inflammatory infiltrate.
- Leiomyosarcoma exhibits cytologic atypia, and high-grade lesions show pleomorphism, necrosis, and mitotic

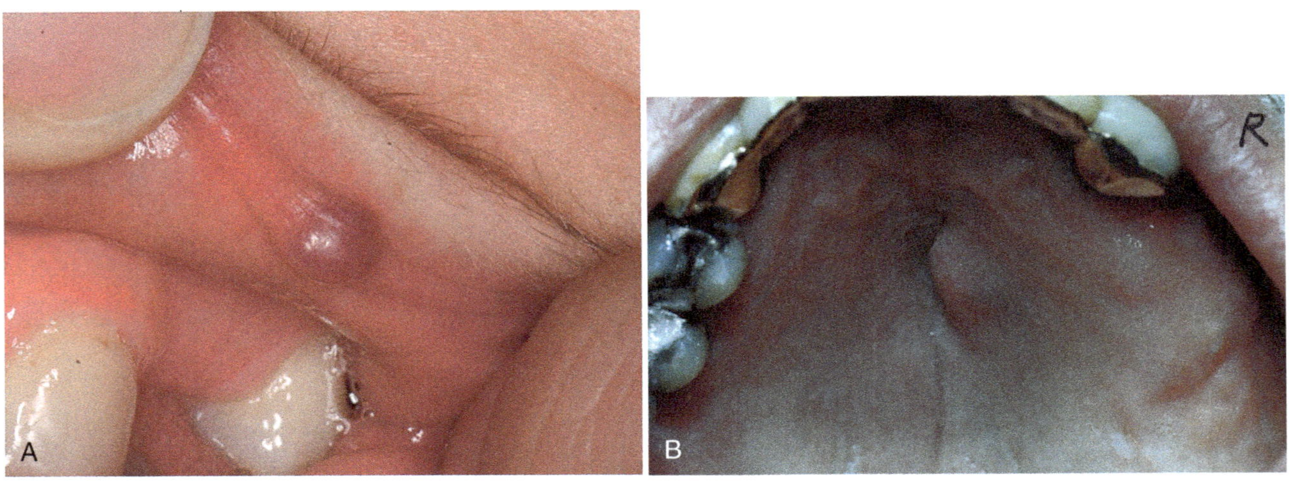

FIG 6.36 (A) Angioleiomyoma of the upper lip. (B) Angioleiomyoma of the hard palatal mucosa. *(Courtesy Dr. Sherwin Kershman, private practice, Houston, Tex.)*

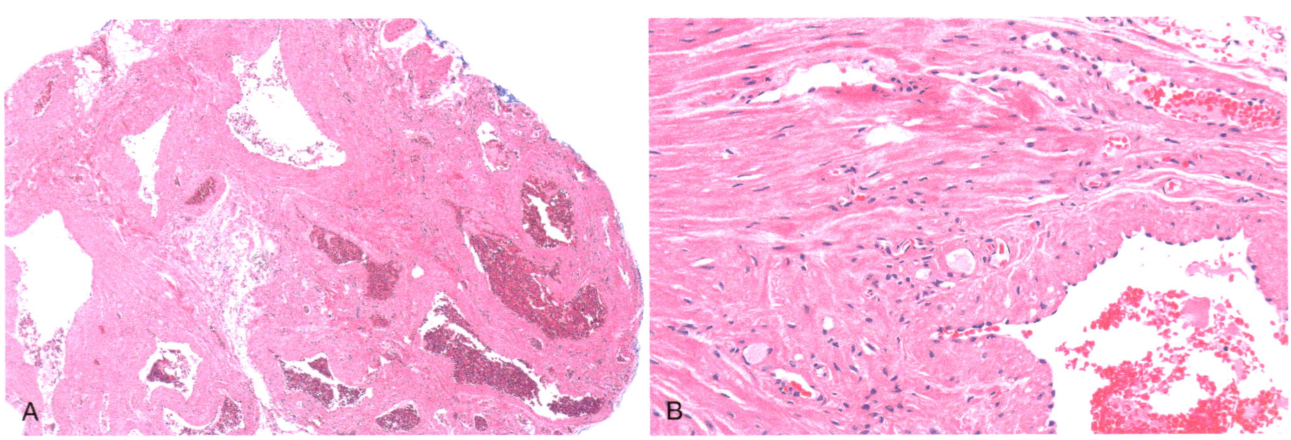

FIG 6.37 Angioleiomyoma. (A) Many dilated and congested vascular channels are present. (B) There is a proliferation of smooth muscle around vessels.

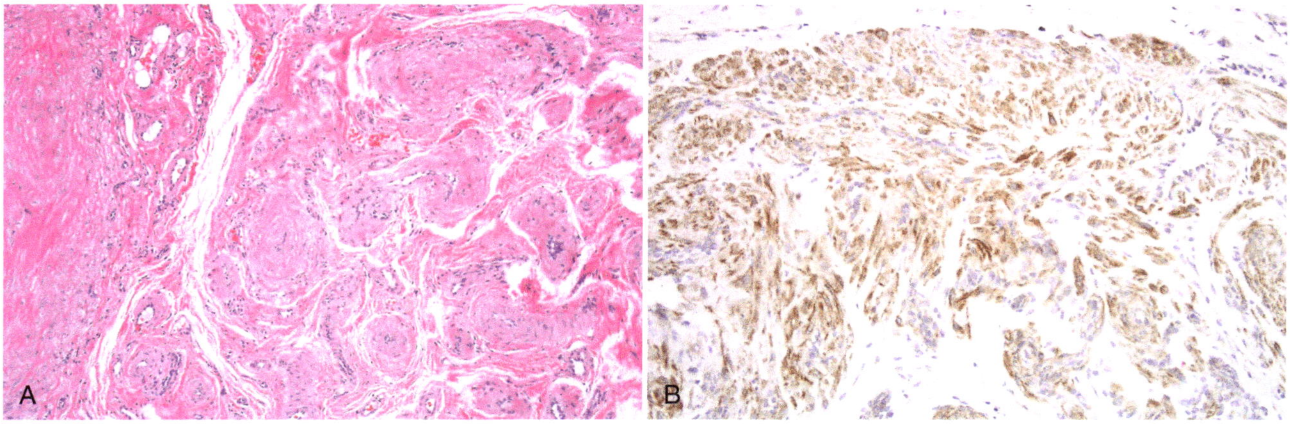

FIG 6.38 Angioleiomyoma. (A) Nodules of spindle cells around small vascular spaces. (B) Spindle cells are smooth muscle actin positive.

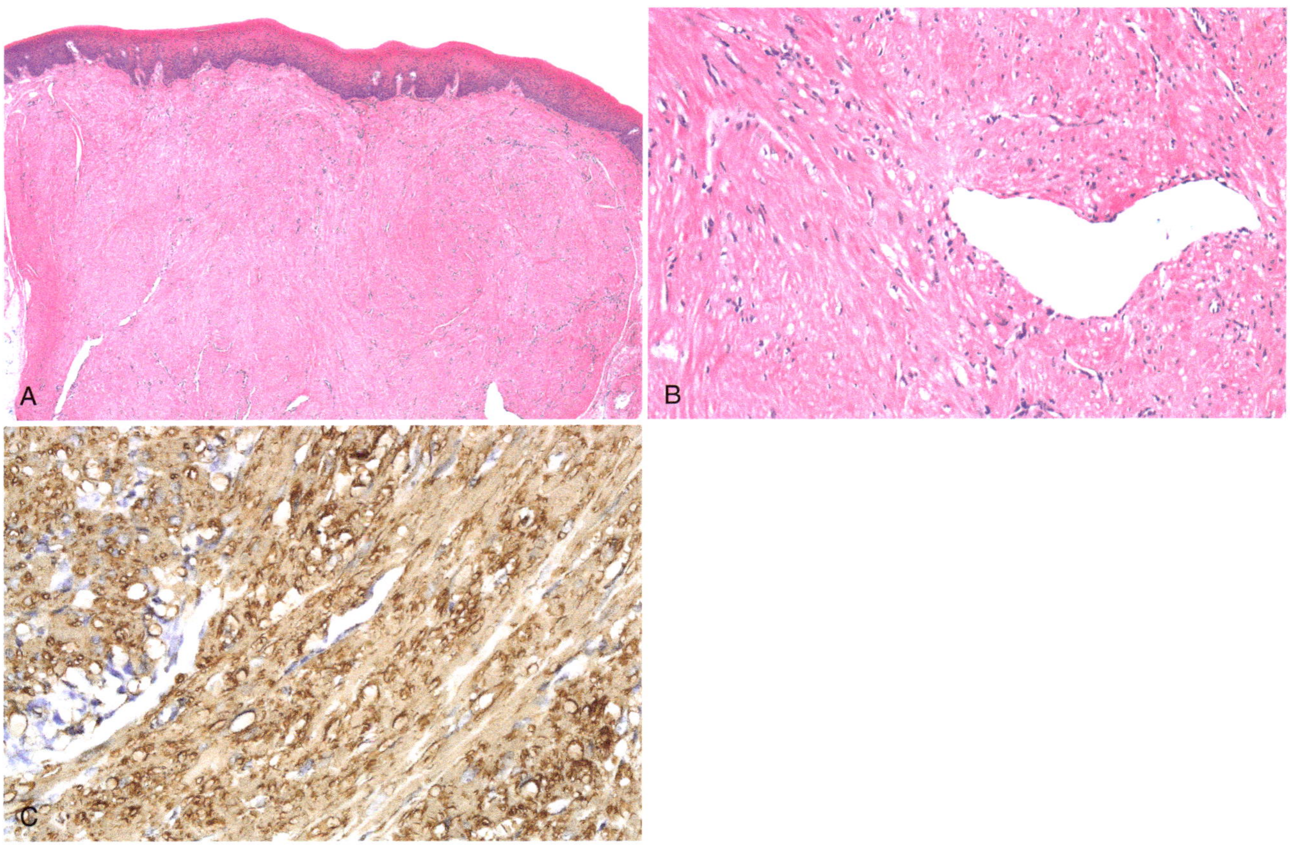

FIG 6.39 Leiomyoma. (A) Nonencapsulated spindle cell proliferation. (B) Spindle cells with abundant pale, vacuolated cytoplasm. (C) Spindle cells are smooth muscle actin positive.

activity; however, bland-appearing tumors with 1 to 5 mitotic figures/10 high power field should be considered tumors of uncertain malignant potential.

Management and Prognosis

- Excision is curative.

REFERENCES

Baden E, Doyle JL, Lederman DA. Leiomyoma of the oral cavity: a light microscopic and immunohistochemical study with review of the literature from 1884 to 1992. *Eur J Cancer B Oral Oncol.* 1994;30B:1-7.

Bhattacharyya I, Summerlin DJ, Cohen DM, et al. Granular cell leiomyoma of the oral cavity. *Oral Surg Oral Med Oral Pathol Oral Radiol Endod.* 2006;102:353-359.

Brooks JK, Nikitakis NG, Goodman NJ, Levy BA. Clinicopathologic characterization of oral angioleiomyomas. *Oral Surg Oral Med Oral Pathol Oral Radiol Endod.* 2002;94:221-227.

Dayan D, Nasrallah V, Vered M. Clinico-pathologic correlations of myofibroblastic tumors of the oral cavity: 1. Nodular fasciitis. *J Oral Pathol Med.* 2005;34:426-435.

Gaitan Cepeda LA, Quezada Rivera D, Tenorio Rocha F, et al. Vascular leiomyoma of the oral cavity. Clinical, histopathological and immunohistochemical characteristics. Presentation of five cases and review of the literature. *Med Oral Patol Oral Cir Bucal.* 2008;13:E483-E488.

Hornick JL, Fletcher CD. Criteria for malignancy in nonvisceral smooth muscle tumors. *Ann Diagn Pathol.* 2003;7:60-66.

Koutlas IG, Manivel JC. Epithelioid leiomyoma of the oral mucosa. *Oral Surg Oral Med Oral Pathol Oral Radiol Endod.* 1996;82:670-673.

ADULT RHABDOMYOMA

Unlike the more common cardiac rhabdomyoma, extracardiac rhabdomyoma is not associated with tuberous sclerosis. More than 90% of adult extracardiac rhabdomyoma occurs in the head and neck, especially in the larynx and pharynx. The adult form is more common and fetal types occur in children.

Clinical Findings

- This occurs in adults in the sixth to seventh decade with 3:1 male predilection.
- There is a nontender mass, usually in the deep mucosa in the tongue, larynx, or pharynx, causing obstructive symptoms; 3% to 5% are multifocal.

Etiopathogenesis and Histopathologic Features

This benign neoplasm shows differentiation toward skeletal muscle fibers.

- There is an encapsulated proliferation of large, polyhedral cells, with brightly eosinophilic cytoplasm that is granular or vacuolated, sometimes producing a "spider web" appearance with small peripheral or central nuclei and inconspicuous nucleoli (Fig. 6.40A–C); there is scant stroma with dilated vascular channels; cross-striations and rodlike inclusions can be seen with phosphotungstic acid-hematoxylin (Fig. 6.40D); cells contain abundant glycogen that is positive with periodic acid–Schiff stain and is diastase labile.
- Cells are positive for desmin, myoglobin, and muscle-specific actin; and less often for SMA.
- The fetal type occurs with a median age in the first decade and features spindle cells, primitive muscle cells resembling fetal myotubules, and rhabdomyoblast-like cells in a myxoid stroma.

Differential Diagnosis

- Granular cell tumor does not contain vacuolated cells and is S-100+.
- Hibernoma consists of uni- and multi-vacuolated cells that are S-100+.

Management and Prognosis

- Excision is the treatment of choice; recurrence rate is up to 40% mainly because of incomplete excision.

REFERENCES

Curatolo P, Bombardieri R, Jozwiak S. Tuberous sclerosis. *Lancet.* 2008; 372:657-668.

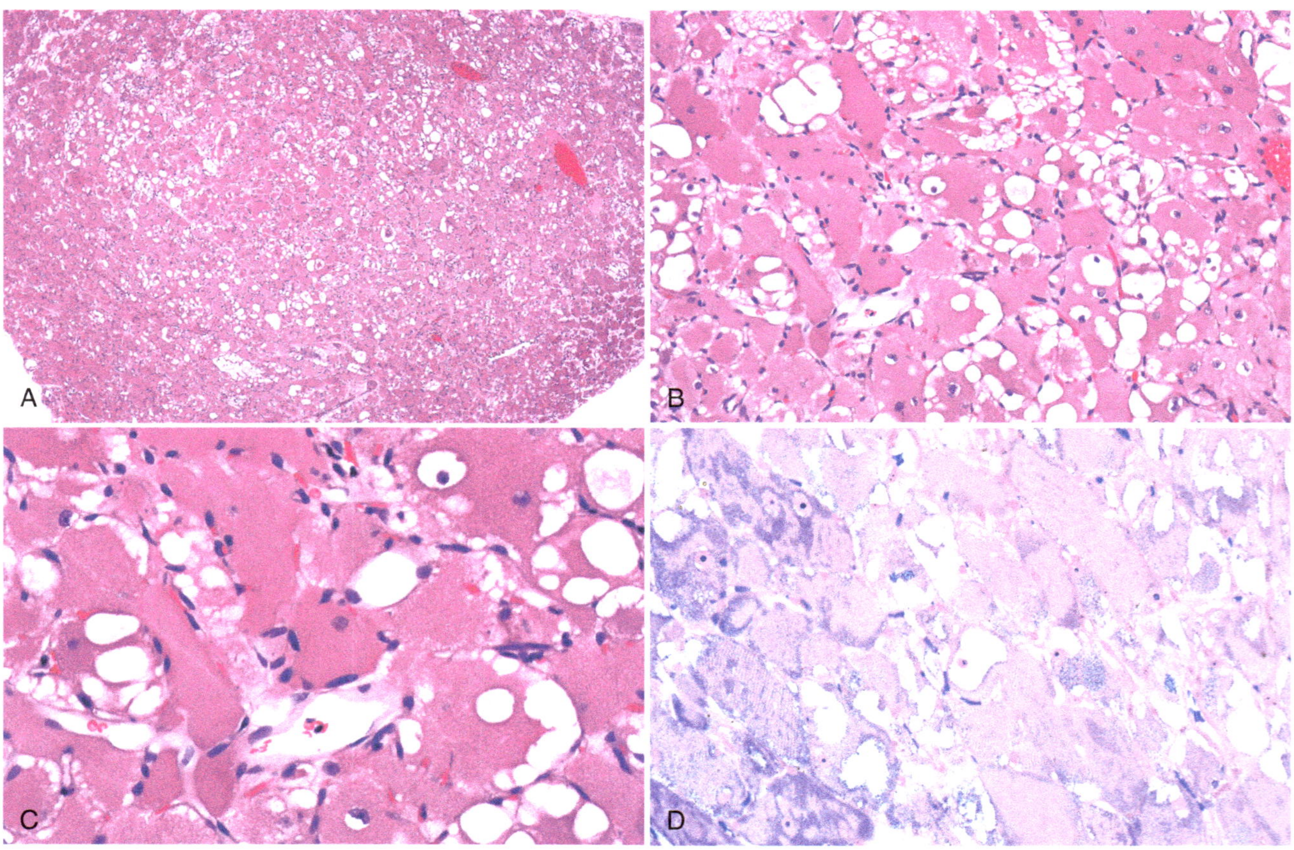

FIG 6.40 Rhabdomyoma. (A) Sheets of polyhedral cells with vacuolations. (B) Polyhedral cells with abundant eosinophilic cytoplasm and cytoplasmic vacuoles. (C) Cells have small nuclei with inconspicuous nucleoli, and cytoplasmic vacuoles. (D) Phosphotungstic acid stain showing striations.

de Trey LA, Schmid S, Huber GF. Multifocal adult rhabdomyoma of the head and neck manifestation in 7 locations and review of the literature. *Case Rep Otolaryngol.* 2013;2013:758416.
Hornick JL. *Practical Soft Tissue Pathology: A Diagnostic Approach.* Philadelphia: Elsevier; 2013.
Kapadia SB, Meis JM, Frisman DM, et al. Adult rhabdomyoma of the head and neck: a clinicopathologic and immunophenotypic study. *Hum Pathol.* 1993;24:608-617.
Kapadia SB, Meis JM, Frisman DM, et al. Fetal rhabdomyoma of the head and neck: a clinicopathologic and immunophenotypic study of 24 cases. *Hum Pathol.* 1993;24:754-765.
Papaspyrou G, Werner JA, Roessler M, et al. Adult rhabdomyoma in the parapharyngeal space: report of 2 cases and review of the literature. *Am J Otolaryngol.* 2011;32:240-246.
Parara E, Christopoulos P, Tosios K, et al. A swelling of the floor of the mouth. *Oral Surg Oral Med Oral Pathol Oral Radiol Endod.* 2010;109:12-16.

RHABDOMYOSARCOMA

Rhabdomyosarcoma is the most common soft tissue sarcoma in children (accounting for 5% to 10% of childhood malignancies).

Clinical Findings

- *Embryonal type:* this usually occurs in the first decade, often in patients younger than age 5; approximately 50% occur in the head and neck with the genitourinary tract being the next most common site; tumors present as a rapidly-growing mass in the cheek, buccal mucosa, or tongue.
- *Alveolar type:* this occurs in adolescents and young adults, usually involving extremities, but may also affect the paranasal sinuses, presenting as a rapidly-growing, infiltrative mass.

Etiopathogenesis and Histopathologic Features

Embryonal rhabdomyosarcoma is a malignant neoplasm that recapitulates embryonic striated muscle and includes botryoid, anaplastic, and spindle cell subtypes. Alveolar rhabdomyosarcoma has a poorer prognosis, and the majority exhibits chromosomal translocations t(2;13) or t(1;13), resulting in *PAX3-FOX01* and *PAX7-FOXO1* gene fusions.

- *Embryonal type:* there are stellate-shaped, spindle, and small ovoid-to-round cells with more compact cellular areas and less cellular myxoid areas; some cells are larger and elongated with eosinophilic cytoplasm and may show cross-striations; these are referred to as "strap" cells (Fig. 6.41A–D).
  - *Botryoid type:* this exhibits a multinodular growth pattern with similar cells but with a hypercellular area (cambium layer) just beneath the epithelium.
  - *Anaplastic type:* this consists of anaplastic cells with atypical, hyperchromatic, and pleomorphic nuclei often with bizarre mitotic figures.
  - *Spindle cell type:* this consists of spindle cells with rhabdomyoblastic or smooth muscle features in a storiform or fasciculated pattern.
  - *Alveolar type:* small round blue cells are arranged in a nested or alveolar pattern; tumor cells lie detached in the center of the alveolar spaces and others cling to fibrous septa; cells have little cytoplasm and hyperchromatic nuclei; giant tumor cells with rhabdomyoblastic differentiation are often noted (Fig. 6.42); the solid type has little fibrovascular stroma, and the third pattern is mixed embryonal-alveolar.
- Tumor cells show cytoplasmic positivity for desmin and muscle-specific actin and nuclear positivity for myogenin (more reliable) and MYOD1 (see Fig. 6.41E–F); myogenin, AP2β, NOS-1, and HMGA2 together as a panel may act as surrogates of fusion status.

Differential Diagnosis

- Lymphoma, neuroblastoma, primitive neuroectodermal tumor, and other small blue cell tumors must be ruled out with immunohistochemical studies.

Management and Prognosis

- Surgical excision is the treatment of choice with adjuvant radiotherapy as needed; new protocols that include chemotherapy have improved 5-year survival to 70%.
- Prognosis is dependent on stage, histologic type (embryonal tumors have better prognosis than alveolar or anaplastic types), age (patients younger than 10 years old fare better), and site (orbital and head and neck nonparameningeal tumors have better outcomes).

REFERENCES

Hicks J, Flaitz C. Rhabdomyosarcoma of the head and neck in children. *Oral Oncol.* 2002;38:450-459.
Hornick JL. *Practical Soft Tissue Pathology: A Diagnostic Approach.* Philadelphia: Elsevier; 2013.
Hostein I, Andraud-Fregeville M, Guillou L, et al. Rhabdomyosarcoma: value of myogenin expression analysis and molecular testing in diagnosing the alveolar subtype: an analysis of 109 paraffin-embedded specimens. *Cancer.* 2004;101:2817-2824.
Mehra S, de la Roza G, Tull J, et al. Detection of FOXO1 (FKHR) gene break-apart by fluorescence in situ hybridization in formalin-fixed, paraffin-embedded alveolar rhabdomyosarcomas and its clinicopathologic correlation. *Diagn Mol Pathol.* 2008;17:14-20.
Raney RB, Maurer HM, Anderson JR, et al. The Intergroup Rhabdomyosarcoma Study Group (IRSG): major lessons from the IRS-I through IRS-IV studies as background for the current IRS-V treatment protocols. *Sarcoma.* 2001;5:9-15.

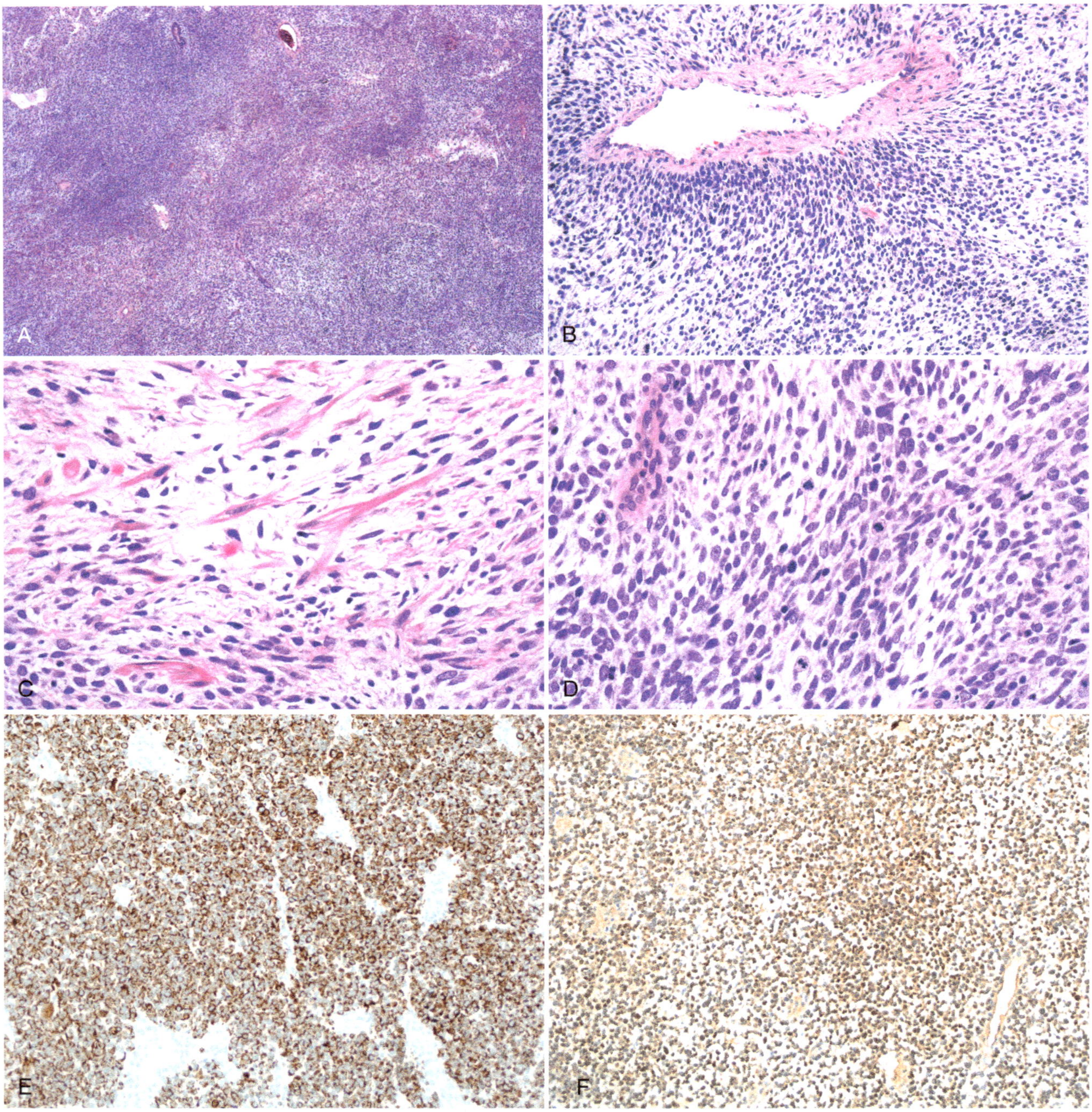

FIG 6.41 Embryonal rhabdomyosarcoma. (A) Cellular tumor with myxoid areas. (B) Cellular perivascular aggregates of tumor cells is a helpful sign. (C) More differentiated tumor cells are polygonal or elongated with eosinophilic cytoplasm. (D) More cellular area with mitotic figures. (E) Tumor cells are desmin+. (F) Tumor cells show nuclear positivity for MYOD1.

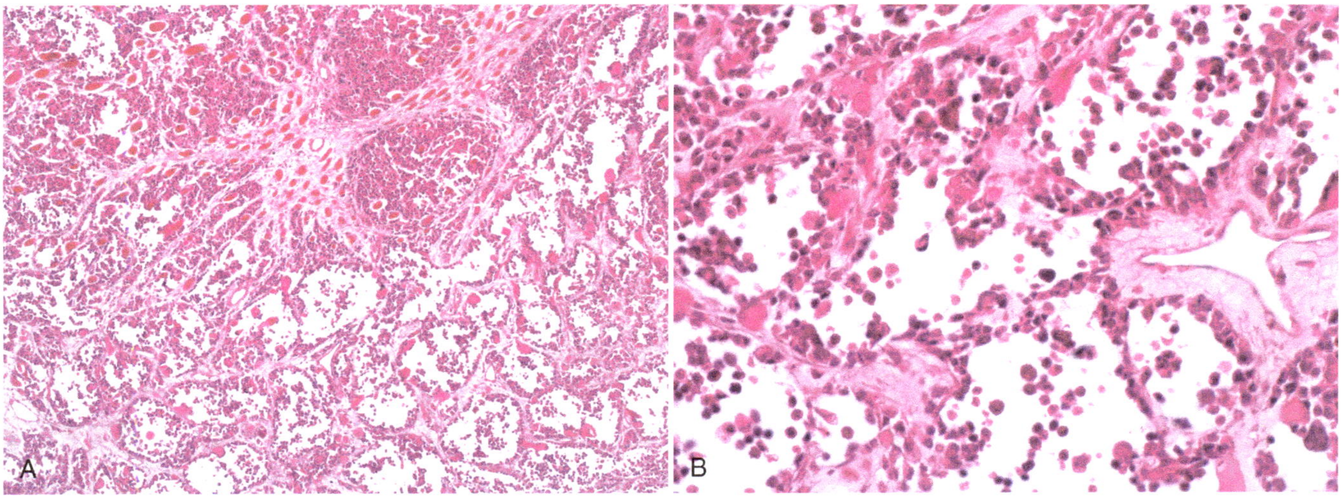

FIG 6.42 Alveolar rhabdomyosarcoma. (A) Small round blue cells are present in an alveolar pattern with detached tumor cells in the center. (B) Cells are round with atypical nuclei and multinucleated tumor cells are present.

Myofibroblastic Tumors

MYOFIBROMA AND MYOPERICYTOMA

Solitary myofibroma is more common than myofibromatosis (multifocal disease), which tends to occur in infants and children; the most common site of involvement is the head and neck.

Clinical Findings

- *Myofibroma* is most frequent in the first to third decades of life with a male predominance and presents as a fleshy, firm, rapidly-growing mass often involving the tongue, buccal mucosa, and gingiva; it may cause resorption of the underlying bone and one-third are primary intraosseous tumors (Fig. 6.43).
- *Myofibromatosis* is most frequent in the first and second year of life with 75% of cases being congenital (infantile type); mortality rate with visceral involvement is more than 70%.

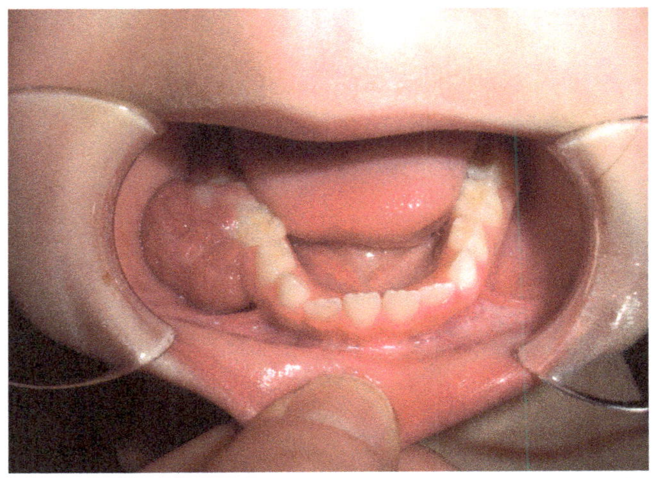

FIG 6.43 Myofibroma of the right mandibular gingiva and sulcus. *(Courtesy Dr. Bonnie Padwa, Harvard School of Dental Medicine, Boston, MA.)*

Etiopathogenesis and Histopathologic Features

Myofibroma, myofibromatosis, myopericytoma, and glomangiopericytoma are neoplasms that exhibit perivascular myoid differentiation.

- Myofibroma: there is a discrete nonencapsulated, nodular or multi-nodular, infiltrative, biphasic proliferation of spindle cells that form interlacing fascicles with "zoning" phenomenon; cells in the center are round-to-polygonal and associated with dilated vessels, and these are surrounded by less cellular areas composed of whorls of spindle cells (myoid nodules) at the periphery; the spindle cells have abundant eosinophilic cytoplasm and elongated, tapered, vesicular nuclei, and small nucleoli; this arrangement is sometimes reversed and sometimes myoid nodules are not prominent and tumors have a more monotonous appearance; mitoses are not uncommon and the stroma is slightly pseudochondroid; degenerative changes or necrosis and myxoid changes are seen in up to 60% of cases (Fig. 6.44).
- Myopericytoma: this is a discrete nodule composed of plump spindle cells arranged around vessels in a concentric layer; subtle myofibroblastic proliferation is noted at the periphery, surrounding small slitlike vessels appearing somewhat hemangiopericytoid (Fig. 6.45A–D).
- Spindle cells show positivity for smooth muscle actin and often h-caldesmon (Fig. 6.45E–F).

Differential Diagnosis

- Fibromatosis (extraabdominal desmoid tumor) is more uniform in appearance, with long sweeping fascicles, is more densely collagenous, and almost always shows nuclear positivity for β-catenin.
- Leiomyoma does not exhibit the "zoning" or myxochondroid stroma and has a more uniform fasciculated pattern; cells have more eosinophilic cytoplasm and

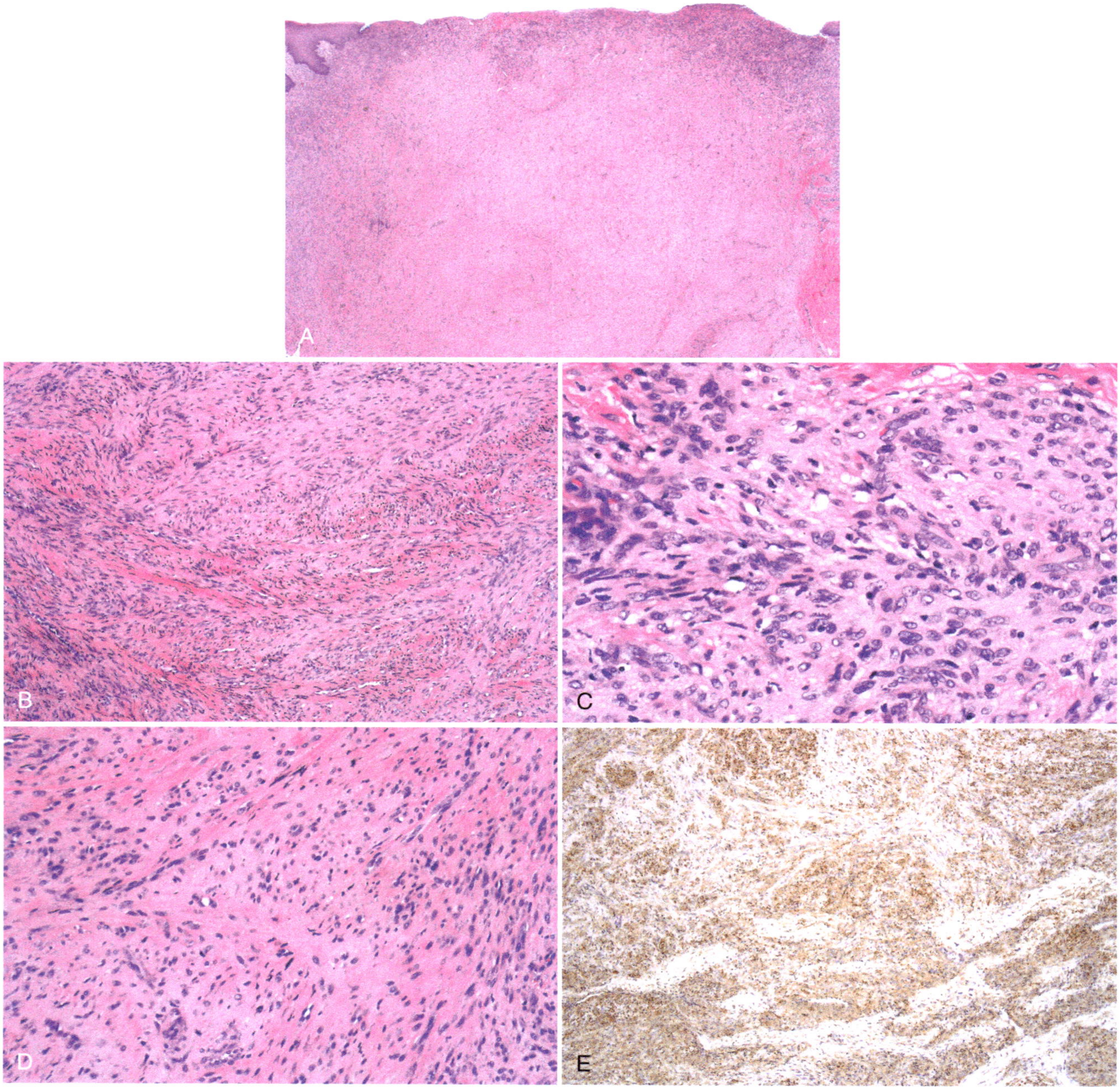

FIG 6.44 Myofibroma. (A) Spindle cell proliferation with overlying ulcer. (B) Tumor forms short fascicles. (C) Hypercellular areas; spindle cells have benign nuclei. (D) Less cellular areas with pseudochondroid stroma. (E) Cells are positive for smooth muscle actin.

nuclei are plumper; tumor cells are often positive for desmin.

- Nodular fasciitis has mucinous stroma with a "tissue culture" appearance, many inflammatory cells, and hemorrhage (see later).
- Solitary fibrous tumor has hypercellular and hypocellular areas and is CD34+.
- Monophasic synovial sarcoma consists of a cellular proliferation of spindle cells in a fasciculated, herringbone pattern; the spindle cells have scant cytoplasm and elongated, hyperchromatic nuclei with dispersed chromatin and small nucleoli that are overlapping because of high cellularity, and mitotic figures are readily identified (Fig. 6.46); cells often show cytoplasmic positivity for CD99, and are negative for desmin and CD34, with reliable nuclear positivity for transducin-like enhancer of split 1 (TLE-1); in the biphasic form, glandular structures are composed of cuboidal cells with the same nuclear morphology as spindle cells and are positive for keratin and EMA; they exhibit t(X;18)(p11;q11) translocation.

Management and Prognosis

- Wide surgical excision is the treatment of choice; approximately 15% to 30% of myofibromas recur, although this could be because of incomplete removal,

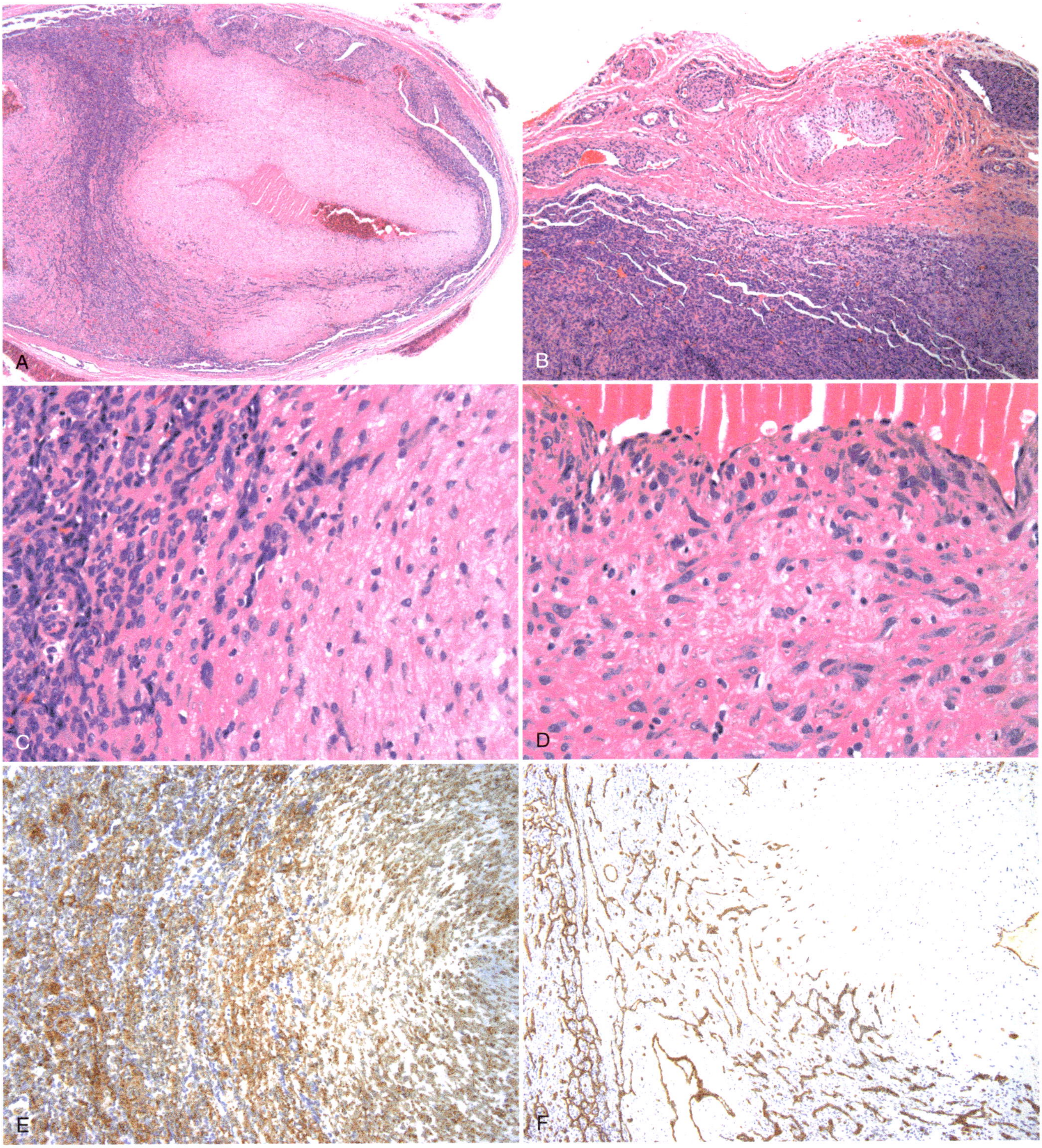

FIG 6.45 Myopericytoma. (A) Pale spindle cell proliferation around vessels with more cellular areas at the periphery. (B) Spindle cell proliferation around smaller vessels at the periphery. (C) Spindle cells with abundant pale cytoplasm and those with less cytoplasm associated with small vessels. (D) Myoid cells are spindled with abundant pale cytoplasm and large slightly pleomorphic nuclei. (E) Strong cytoplasmic positivity for smooth muscle actin. (F) CD31 highlights numerous small vessels within the cellular areas.

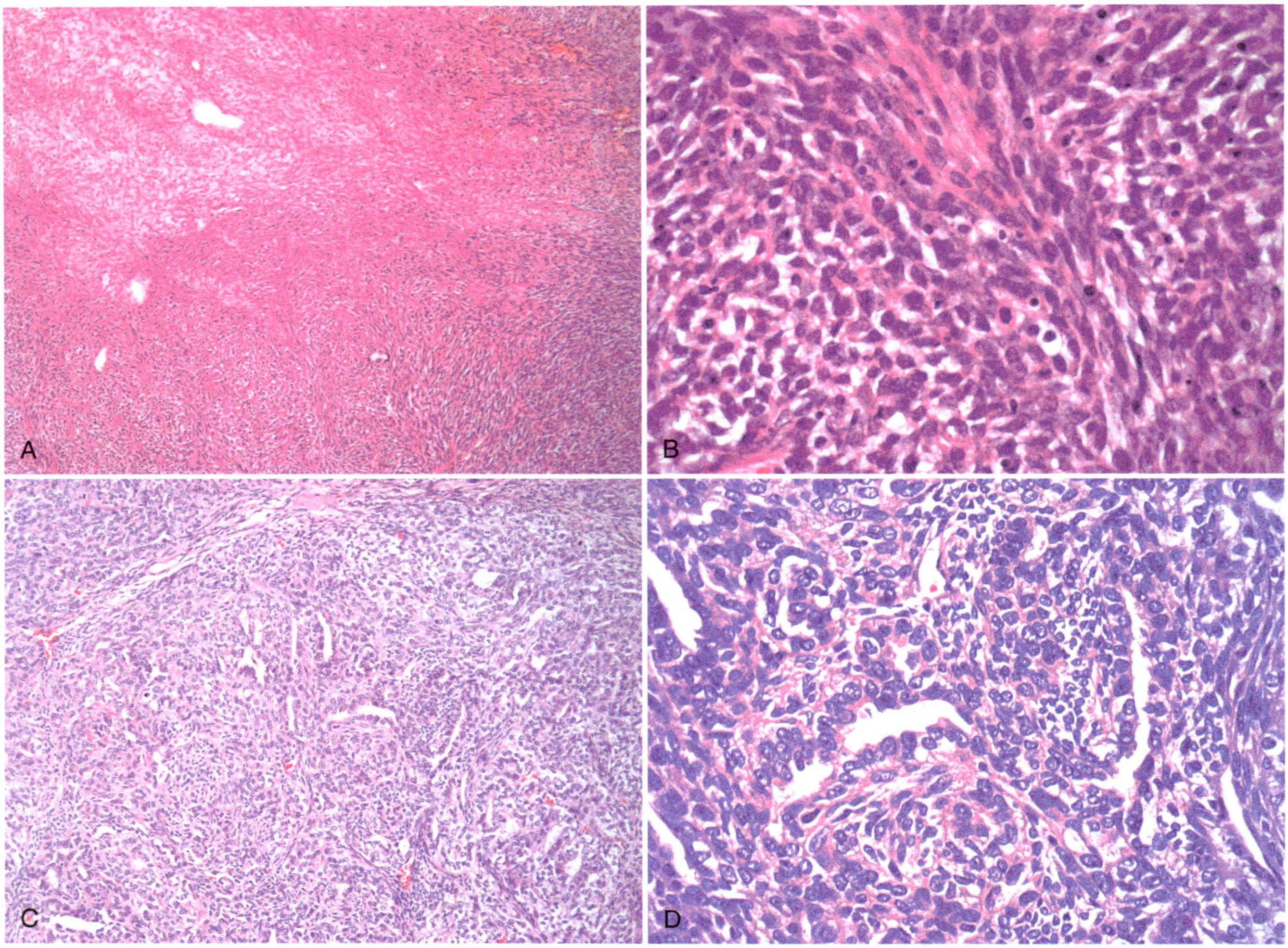

FIG 6.46 Biphasic synovial sarcoma. (A) Cellular fascicles of spindle cells. (B) Cells have high nuclear-cytoplasmic ratio and hyperchromatic nuclei. (C) Ductal structures are present in the biphasic variant. (D) Ductal structures are lined by low cuboidal cells.

and there have been rare reports of clinical tumor regression.

REFERENCES

Abramowicz S, Simon LE, Kozakewich HP, et al. Myofibromas of the jaws in children. *J Oral Maxillofac Surg.* 2012;70:1880-1884.

Beck JC, Devaney KO, Weatherly RA, et al. Pediatric myofibromatosis of the head and neck. *Arch Otolaryngol Head Neck Surg.* 1999;125:39-44.

Dayan D, Nasrallah V, Vered M. Clinico-pathologic correlations of myofibroblastic tumors of the oral cavity: 1. Nodular fasciitis. *J Oral Pathol Med.* 2005;34:426-435.

Foss RD, Ellis GL. Myofibromas and myofibromatosis of the oral region: a clinicopathologic analysis of 79 cases. *Oral Surg Oral Med Oral Pathol Oral Radiol Endod.* 2000;89:57-65.

Hornick JL. *Practical Soft Tissue Pathology: A Diagnostic Approach.* Philadelphia: Elsevier; 2013.

Jones AC, Freedman PD, Kerpel SM. Oral myofibromas: a report of 13 cases and review of the literature. *J Oral Maxillofac Surg.* 1994;52:870-875.

Montgomery E, Speight PM, Fisher C. Myofibromas presenting in the oral cavity: a series of 9 cases. *Oral Surg Oral Med Oral Pathol Oral Radiol Endod.* 2000;89:343-348.

Vered M, Allon I, Buchner A, Dayan D. Clinico-pathologic correlations of myofibroblastic tumors of the oral cavity. II. Myofibroma and myofibromatosis of the oral soft tissues. *J Oral Pathol Med.* 2007;36:304-314.

NODULAR FASCIITIS

Clinical Findings

- This occurs in the third and fourth decades of life and the buccal mucosa is the most common site affected; it presents as a firm, rapidly growing fleshy mass.

Etiopathogenesis and Histopathologic Features

- The identification of the MYH9-USP6 fusion gene has confirmed that this is a clonal neoplastic disorder.
- There is a discrete and often infiltrative proliferation of spindle cells, slightly fasciculated, and slightly storiform, with a "tissue culture" or "feathery" appearance in a myxoid/mucinous stroma often with many inflammatory cells and variable numbers of multinucleated giant cells; normal mitoses are often noted and pseudocystic spaces may be present; the cellular form has less mucinous stroma and fibrotic form is densely collagenous (Fig. 6.47).
- Spindle cells are SMA+ and calponin+, but desmin-, h-caldesmon- and smooth muscle myosin-.

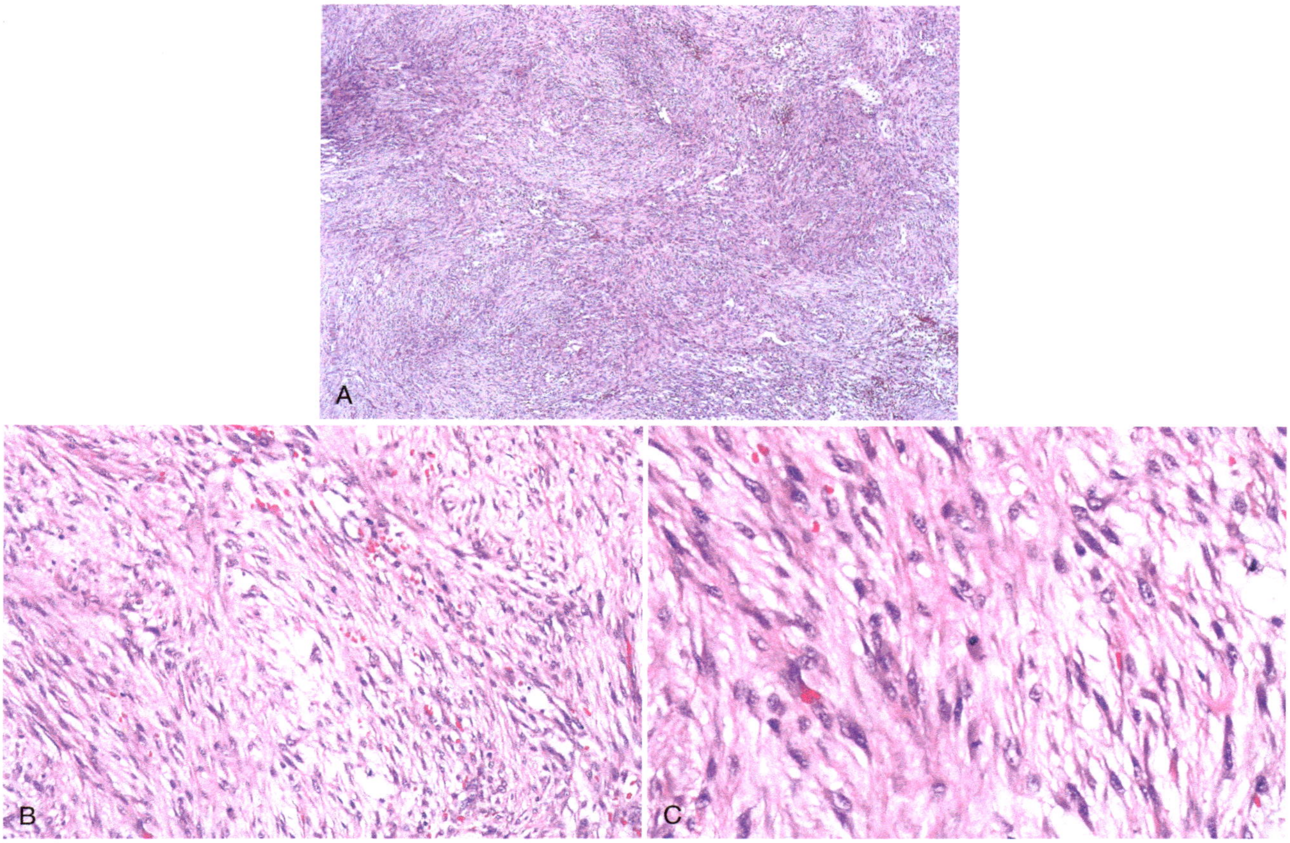

FIG 6.47 Nodular fasciitis. (A) Cellular proliferation of spindled myofibroblasts with chronic inflammation and fresh hemorrhage. (B) Fasciculated arrangement of myofibroblasts with a "feathery" appearance and many mitotic figures. (C) Cells show slight variation in shape and size (reactive atypia), and normal mitoses are frequent.

Differential Diagnosis

- Myofibroma, leiomyoma and other benign and malignant spindle cell tumors are ruled out based on the pattern and immunohistochemical findings.

Management and Prognosis

- Excision is the treatment of choice; these tumors do not tend to recur even if incompletely excised and spontaneous regression has been reported.

REFERENCES

Erickson-Johnson MR, Chou MM, Evers BR, et al. Nodular fasciitis: a novel model of transient neoplasia induced by MYH9-USP6 gene fusion. *Lab Invest.* 2011;91:1427-1433.

Morgen EK, Carter P, Weinreb I, et al. Immunohistochemistry in nodular fasciitis of the head and neck. *Pathology.* 2013;45:432-433.

Weinreb I, Shaw AJ, Perez-Ordonez B, et al. Nodular fasciitis of the head and neck region: a clinicopathologic description in a series of 30 cases. *J Cutan Pathol.* 2009;36:1168-1173.

7 ULCERATIVE AND INFLAMMATORY CONDITIONS

CHAPTER CONTENTS

Ulcerative Conditions

RECURRENT APHTHOUS ULCERS AND TRAUMATIC ULCERS

Most cases of *recurrent aphthous ulcers* are idiopathic; however, aphthous-like lesions are seen in Behçet disease, Crohn disease (often linear in the sulcus), hematinic deficiencies, some hypersensitivity reactions (such as to food or sodium lauryl sulfate found in toothpaste), cyclic neutropenia, and HIV infection. Complex aphthosis is often used to describe lesions associated with syndromes affecting the skin. Ulcers in children may be part of periodic fever, aphthosis, pharyngitis, and adenopathy (PFAPA) syndrome. Trauma and stress bring on episodes in susceptible individuals. Minor aphthous ulcers do not tend to be biopsied, owing to the typical history and presentation, whereas major ulcers are biopsied to rule out vesiculobullous disease or infections. Chemotherapy-induced ulcerations are much larger and diffuse, resolve predictably over 1 to 2 weeks, and are not aphthous ulcers. New therapies such as mammalian target of rapamycin (mTOR) inhibitors may cause severe aphthous-like ulcers that heal on withdrawal of drug.

Traumatic ulcers are caused by trauma, usually on the buccal mucosa, tongue, and lower lip (that are sites of morsicatio mucosae oris), and are indistinguishable histologically from recurrent aphthous ulcers. They also occur secondarily on lesions that protrude (eg, fibromas and gingival nodules).

Clinical Findings

- *Idiopathic aphthous ulcers:* Onset usually occurs in the second and third decades of life with a 2:1 female predilection, and lesions diminish in severity with age. Ulcers are episodic or continuous, single or multiple, and occur almost exclusively on the nonkeratinized mucosa. They are sharply demarcated and painful, with a yellow fibrin membrane with surrounding erythema.
- Four clinical types are recognized:
  - *Minor* ulcers are the most common, are smaller than 1 cm in size, and last 1 to 2 weeks.
  - *Major* ulcers are the least common, are larger than 1 cm in size, last for weeks or months, and often are associated with scarring. This form is often seen in HIV/AIDS.
  - *Herpetiform* ulcers are uncommon and number more than 10 ulcers (<1 cm) at each episode.
  - *Severe* aphthous ulcers present as continuous minor aphthous ulcerations (Fig. 7.1A–C).
- Aphthous-like ulcers associated with systemic disease may occur on the keratinized mucosa. Those associated with chemotherapy (such as mTOR inhibitors) regress on completion or discontinuation of therapy (Fig. 7.1D). Those associated with medications tend to occur in older individuals.
- Traumatic ulcers have a history of trauma or identifiable cause of trauma (such as a sharp cusp or broken tooth). They are often seen on protuberant areas, such as fibromas, gingival nodules, or exostoses (Fig. 7.1E–F).
- New international diagnostic criteria based on a point system have been established for Behçet disease with high sensitivity. Oral aphthous-like ulcers, genital ulcers, and eye lesions are the most important and consistent findings.

Etiopathogenesis and Histopathologic Features

Most cases of recurrent aphthae have a strong family history of recurrent aphthae, and some human leukocyte

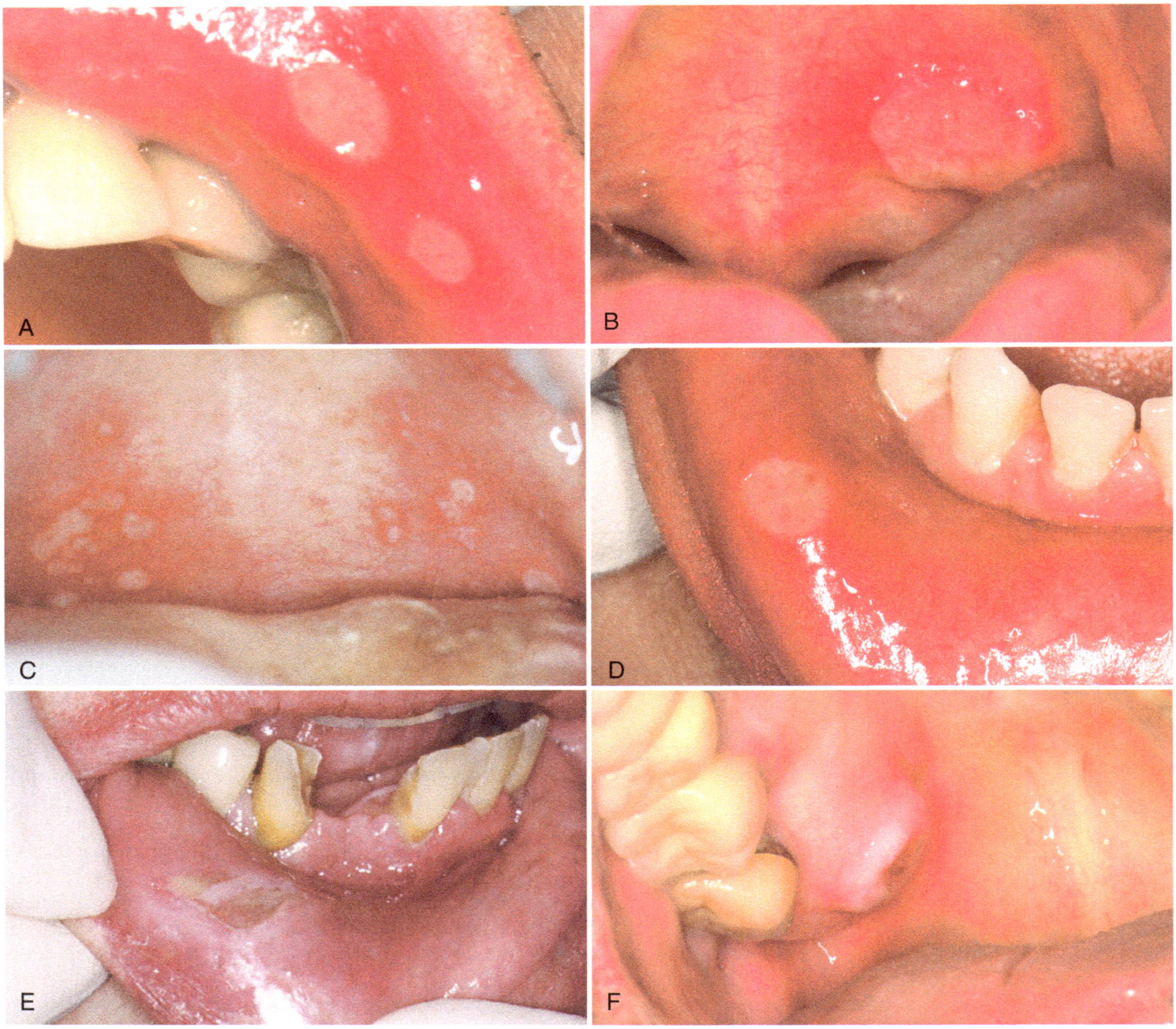

FIG 7.1 (A) Recurrent minor aphthous ulcers on the left upper lip mucosa. (B) Recurrent major aphthous ulcer on the left soft palate. (C) Recurrent herpetiform aphthous ulcers on the soft palate. (D) Ulcer caused by mammalian target of rapamycin inhibitor. (E) Traumatic ulcer caused by a broken tooth. (F) Traumatic ulcer on palatal exostosis.

antigen A haplotypes have been identified. Tumor necrosis factor (TNF)-α plays an important role in etiopathogenesis.

- Ulcers consist of a fibrin membrane with enmeshed neutrophils and underlying granulation tissue with acute and chronic inflammatory cells confined to the lamina propria and sometimes involving superficial skeletal muscle fibers. The adjacent epithelium exhibits spongiotic pustules and reactive atypia such as basal cell hyperplasia, nuclear hyperchromasia, and slight pleomorphism. Traumatic ulcers often show adjacent parakeratosis and surface bacterial colonies (Fig. 7.2).
- Healing ulcers or the edge of ulcers demonstrate subepithelial fibrin deposition, spongiotic pustules, reactive epithelial atypia, and often intraepithelial and subepithelial hemorrhage (Fig. 7.3).
- Spread of inflammation to underlying muscle results in myositis and, if chronic, traumatic ulcerative granuloma with eosinophilia (see later).

Differential Diagnosis

- The epithelium adjacent to the ulcer should be evaluated for herpes simplex virus cytopathic effect, and the connective tissue should be searched for cytomegalovirus and fungi in immunocompromised patients.
- Neutropenic ulcers have scarce neutrophils (Fig. 7.4).

Management and Prognosis

- Topical steroid therapy and topical analgesia are effective for minor aphthae, though idiopathic aphthous ulcers are episodic and will recur. Aphthous major and severe and/or continuous aphthous ulcers usually require systemic therapy (see Appendix A). TNF-α

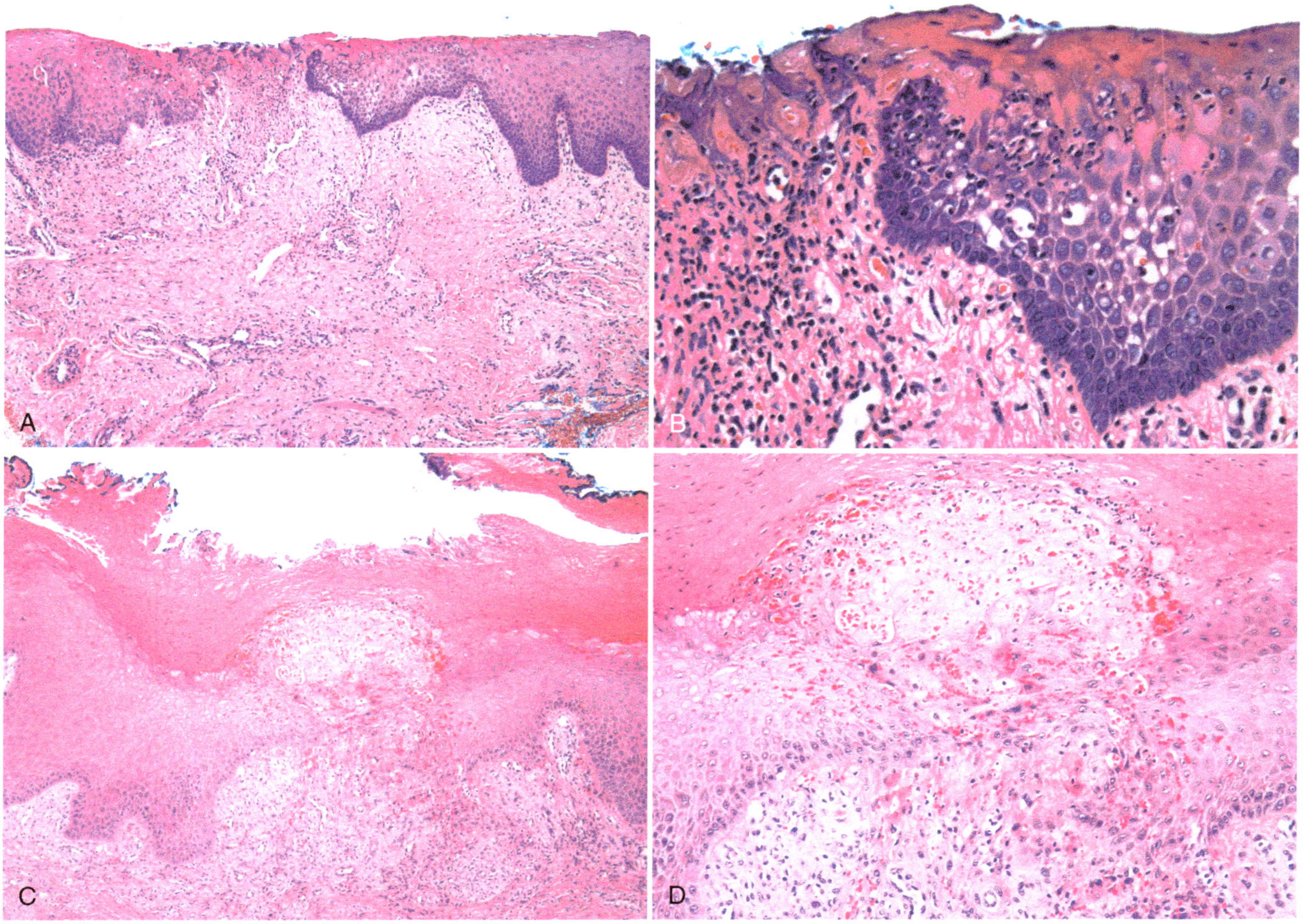

FIG 7.2 (A, B) Aphthous ulcer. (A) Ulcer composed of fibrin with inflammation involving only the superficial lamina propria. (B) The epithelium exhibits spongiosis, hemorrhage, neutrophilic exocytosis, and spongiotic pustules. (C, D) Traumatic ulcer. (C) Fibrin membrane with underlying granulation tissue and acute and chronic inflammation. Note adjacent traumatic parakeratosis with surface bacterial colonization. (D) Acanthosis, many spongiotic pustules, intraepithelial hemorrhage, and reactive epithelial atypia.

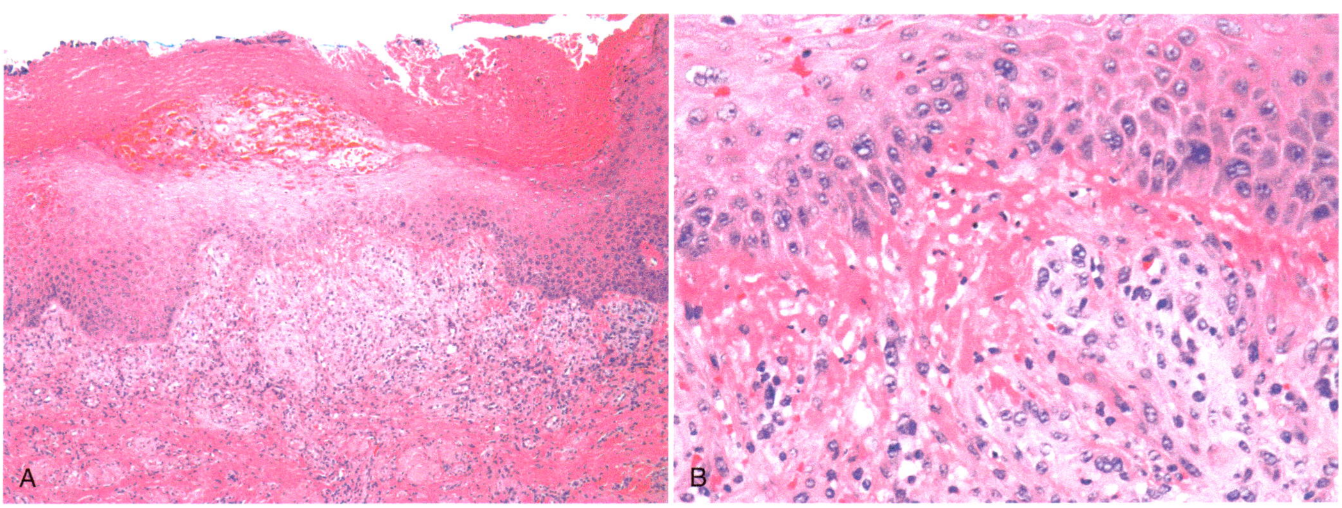

FIG 7.3 Edge of an ulcer. (A) Oral mucosa with intact epithelium, traumatic parakeratosis, intraepithelial hemorrhage, subepithelial fibrin deposition, and granulation tissue. (B) Subepithelial fibrin deposition with intraepithelial hemorrhage and reactive epithelial atypia.

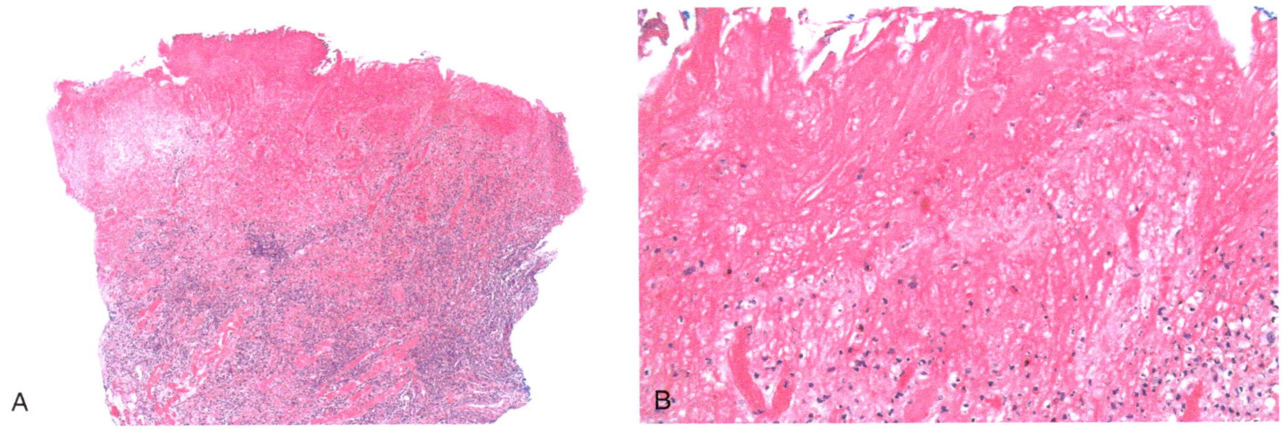

FIG 7.4 Neutropenic ulcer. (A) Fibrin membrane with underlying granulation tissue. (B) Paucity of neutrophils within fibrin meshwork.

inhibitors are useful for lesions resistant to other systemic therapy.

- For systemic conditions presenting with aphthous-like ulcers, careful history taking and work-up are important.
- Adenotonsillectomy may be effective in some patients with PFAPA syndrome.

REFERENCES

Albanidou-Farmaki E, Deligiannidis A, Markopoulos AK, et al. HLA haplotypes in recurrent aphthous stomatitis: a mode of inheritance? *Int J Immunogenet.* 2008;35:427-432.

Burton MJ, Pollard AJ, Ramsden JD. Tonsillectomy for periodic fever, aphthous stomatitis, pharyngitis and cervical adenitis syndrome (PFAPA). *Cochrane Database Syst Rev.* 2010;(9):CD008669.

Davatchi F, Abdollahi BS, Chams-Davatchi C, et al. Validation of the revised International Criteria for Behcet's Disease (ICBD) in Iran. *Clin Rheumatol.* 2015;34:315-320.

Feder HM, Salazar JC. A clinical review of 105 patients with PFAPA (a periodic fever syndrome). *Acta Paediatr.* 2010;99:178-184.

Martins F, de Oliveira MA, Wang Q, et al. A review of oral toxicity associated with mTOR inhibitor therapy in cancer patients. *Oral Oncol.* 2013;49:293-298.

Mendes D, Correia M, Barbedo M, et al. Behçet's disease—a contemporary review. *J Autoimmun.* 2009;32:178-188.

Sand FL, Thomsen SF. Efficacy and safety of TNF-α inhibitors in refractory primary complex aphthosis: a patient series and overview of the literature. *J Dermatolog Treat.* 2013;24:444-446.

Scully C. Aphthous ulceration. *N Engl J Med.* 2006;355:165-172.

Zadik Y, Findler M, Maly A, et al. A 78-year old woman with bilateral tongue necrosis. *Oral Surg Oral Med Oral Pathol Oral Radiol Endod.* 2011;111:15-19.

TRAUMATIC ULCERATIVE GRANULOMA WITH STROMAL EOSINOPHILS, EOSINOPHILIC ULCER OF TONGUE

These chronic traumatic ulcers with myositis have bimodal peaks of occurrence.

Clinical Findings

- *Adult form:* This occurs as a sharply punched-out ulcer, often with a white, keratotic rim, commonly on the lateral tongue, present for weeks, with or without pain, and raising the suspicion for malignancy. Any site with underlying muscle may be involved (Fig. 7.5A–C). Synchronous bilateral lesions or metachronous lesions may occur.
- *Infantile form (Riga-Fede disease):* This occurs in the first year of life when newly erupted incisors traumatize the ventral tongue or lip mucosa (see Fig. 7.5D).

Etiopathogenesis and Histopathologic Features

Traumatic ulcerative granuloma is secondary to deeply penetrating inflammation involving the underlying skeletal muscle and is most often associated with trauma, but it may also be seen in traumatized chronic ulcerative conditions, such as aphthous ulcers.

- There is an ulcer with acute and chronic inflammation that penetrates into the muscle with separation and degeneration of muscle fibers (sometimes with a "checkerboard" pattern), proliferation of histiocyte-like mononuclear cells, and many eosinophils (Figs. 7.6 and 7.7A–C). Eosinophils may be sparse, depending on the stage of the ulcer.
- Mononuclear cells are CD68+ and CD163+, and scattered factor XIIIa+ cells may be seen (see Fig. 7.7D).
- A few CD30+ cells are seen in up to 50% of cases.

Differential Diagnosis

- Diffuse, large B-cell lymphoma consists of sheets of large atypical cells that are CD20+. It is unclear if previously reported cases of atypical histiocytic granuloma may represent such lymphomas.
- Epstein-Barr virus–associated mucocutaneous ulcers contain many CD30+ and Epstein-Barr virus–encoded RNA-positive B cells; atypical Hodgkin-like cells; and Reed-Sternberg–like cells (see Chapter 4).

Management and Prognosis

- Lesions may heal after biopsy; otherwise, topical steroids, intralesional steroid injections, or complete excisions are indicated (see Appendix A).
- Recurrence is common, especially if the patient has a flabby or enlarged tongue (eg, older patients who wear lower full dentures or who have lost teeth in the posterior mandible).

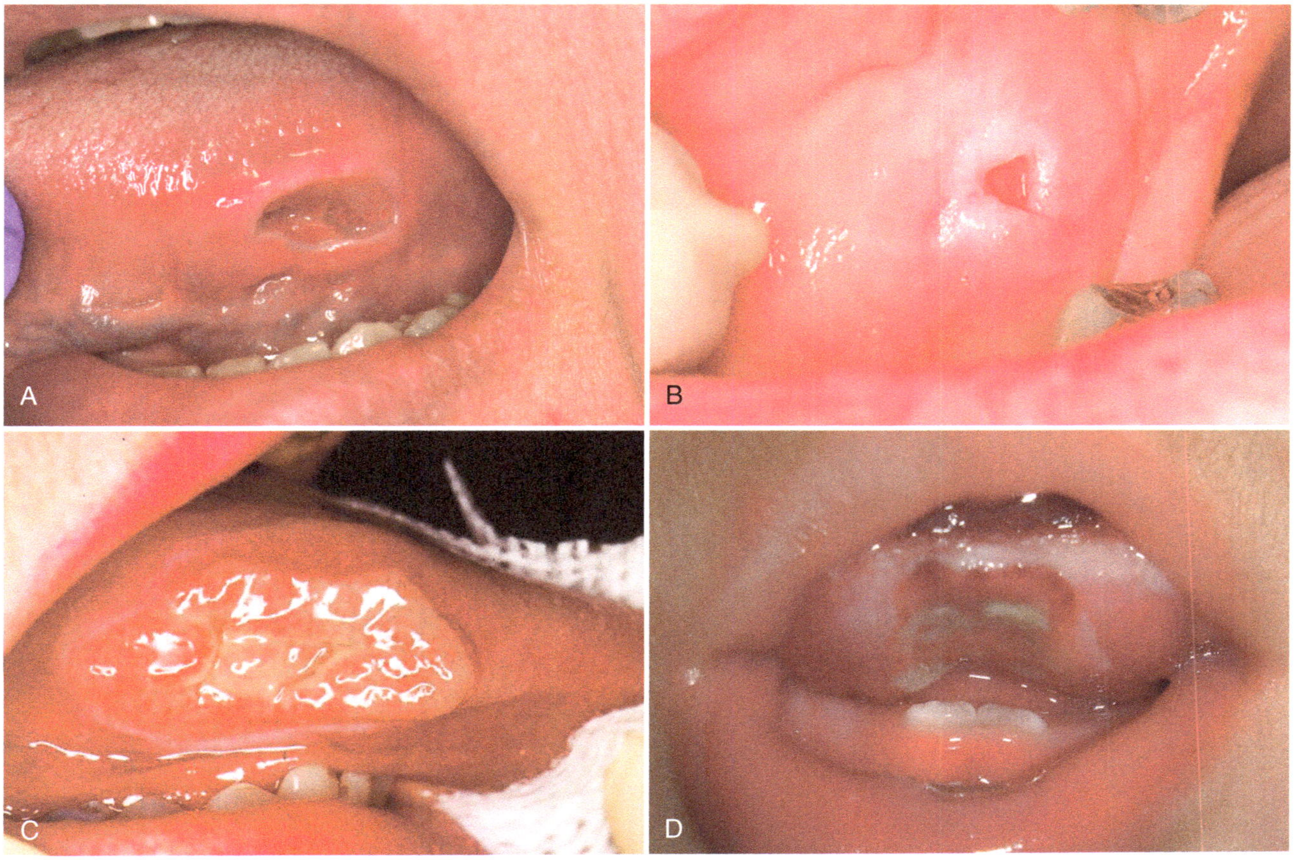

FIG 7.5 Traumatic ulcerative granuloma. (A) Punched-out deep ulcer of ventral tongue. (B) Punched-out ulcer of buccal mucosa with surrounding keratosis. (C) Slightly raised large ulcer that developed after a seizure and trauma to the tongue. (D) Ulcer resulting from trauma from teeth in an infant. *(Courtesy Dr. Ons Al-Khadra, Jeddah, Kingdom of Saudi Arabia.)*

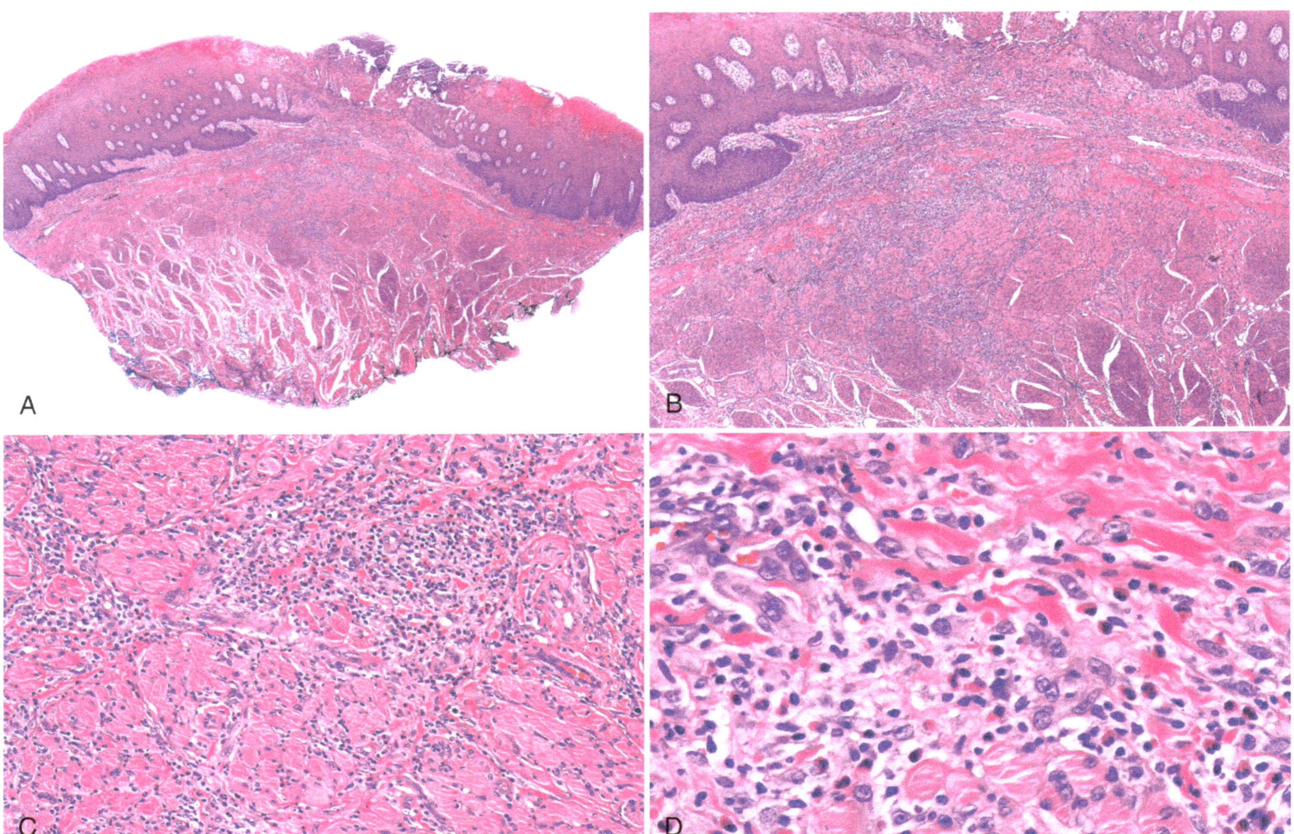

FIG 7.6 Traumatic ulcerative granuloma. (A) Oral mucosa with parakeratosis and penetrating inflammation. (B) Muscle infiltrated by inflammatory cells. (C) Myocyte degeneration and inflammation. (D) Many eosinophils and histiocyte-like mononuclear cells.

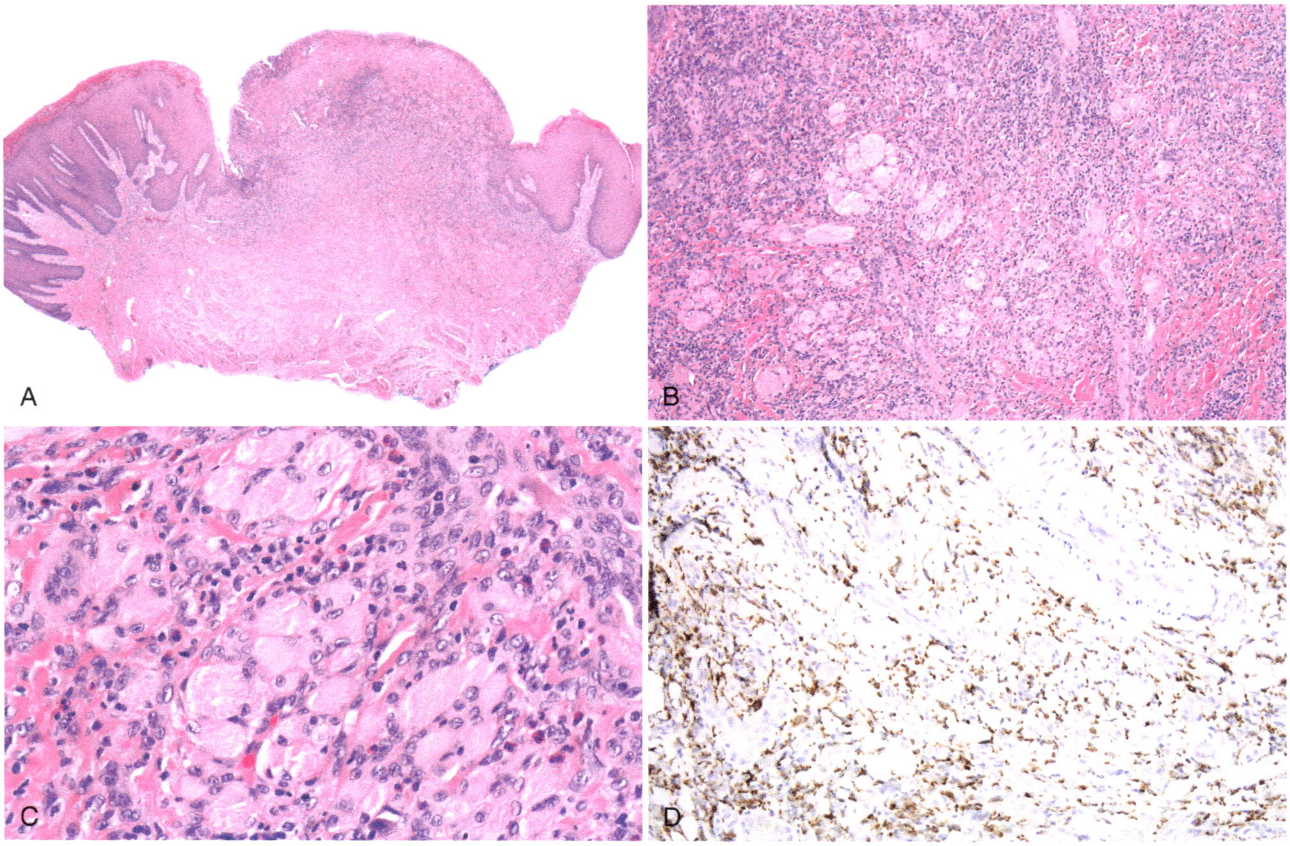

FIG 7.7 Traumatic ulcerative granuloma. (A) Oral mucosa with overlying frictional parakeratosis, ulceration, and penetrating inflammation. (B) Inflammation leading to fragmentation of skeletal muscle fibers with a checkerboard pattern. (C) Muscle fibers surrounded by histiocyte-like mononuclear cells and eosinophils. (D) Histiocyte-like cells around muscle fibers are CD68+.

REFERENCES

Alobeid B, Pan LX, Milligan L, et al. Eosinophil-rich CD30+ lymphoproliferative disorder of the oral mucosa: a form of "traumatic eosinophilic granuloma." *Am J Clin Pathol.* 2004;121:43-50.

del Río E, Sánchez Yus E, Requena L, et al. Oral pseudolymphoma: a report of two cases. *J Cutan Pathol.* 1997;24:51-55.

Dojcinov SD, Venkataraman G, Raffeld M, et al. EBV positive mucocutaneous ulcer—a study of 26 cases associated with various sources of immunosuppression. *Am J Surg Pathol.* 2010;34:405-417.

El-Mofty SK, Wick MR, Miller AS. Eosinophilic ulcer of the oral mucosa. *Oral Surg Oral Med Oral Pathol.* 1993;75:716-722.

Eversole LR, Leider AS, Jacobsen PL, Kidd PM. Atypical histiocytic granuloma. *Cancer.* 1985;55:1722-1729.

Salisbury CL, Budnick SD, Li S. T-cell receptor gene rearrangement and CD30 immunoreactivity in traumatic ulcerative granuloma with stromal eosinophilia of the oral cavity. *Am J Clin Pathol.* 2009;132:722-727.

Shen WR, Chang JY, Wu YC, et al. Oral traumatic ulcerative granuloma with stromal eosinophilia: a clinicopathological study of 34 cases. *J Formos Med Assoc.* 2015;114:881-885.

Contact and Inflammatory Conditions

NONSPECIFIC IRRITANT CONTACT STOMATITIS

Clinical Findings

- This presents as a whitish plaque with or without ulceration with an erythematous background and a history of exposure to a contactant.

Etiopathogenesis and Histopathologic Features

Irritation by contactants stronger than alcoholic mouth rinses or in longer contact with the mucosa (such as acrylates or substances applied by patients) leads to more severe changes in the epithelium than simple surface coagulation (discussed in Chapter 10). Stronger irritants (eg, aspirin) lead to necrosis, erosion, and ulceration.

- There is acanthosis with variable spongiosis and leukocyte (especially neutrophilic) exocytosis. Ulceration may be present (Figs. 7.8 and 7.9). Some lesions show coagulation of superficial keratinocytes with reactive keratinocytic atypia and karyorrhexis (see Fig. 7.10).

Differential Diagnosis

- The presence of a large number of eosinophils in the epithelium suggests a hypersensitivity reaction.
- Contact stomatitis caused by restorations or cinnamic aldehyde–containing products results in lichenoid reactions with peri- and paravascular lymphocytic infiltrates (see Chapter 8).

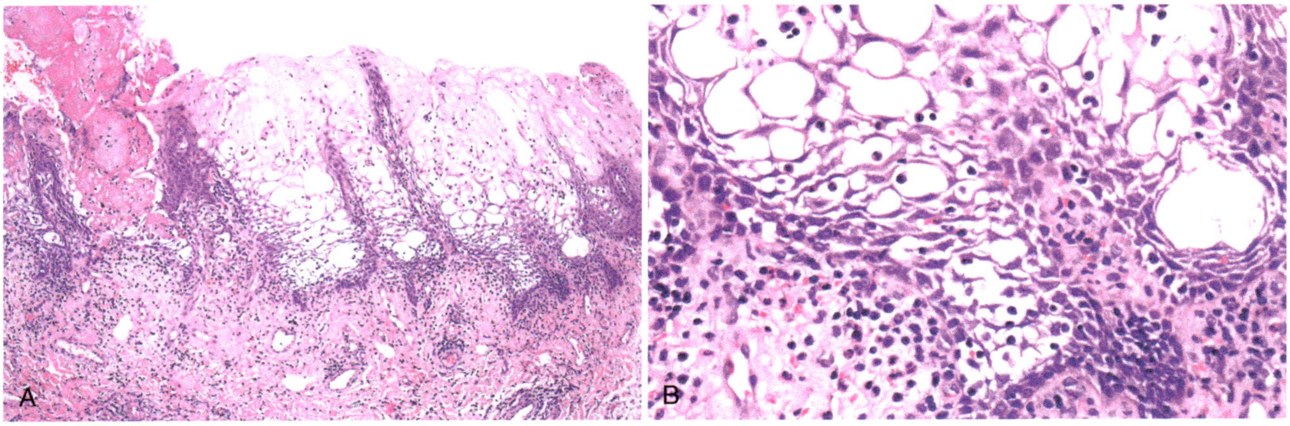

FIG 7.8 Irritant contact stomatitis. (A) Oral mucosa exhibiting ulceration, acanthosis, and spongiosis. (B) Marked spongiosis and leukocyte exocytosis with mild reactive epithelial atypia.

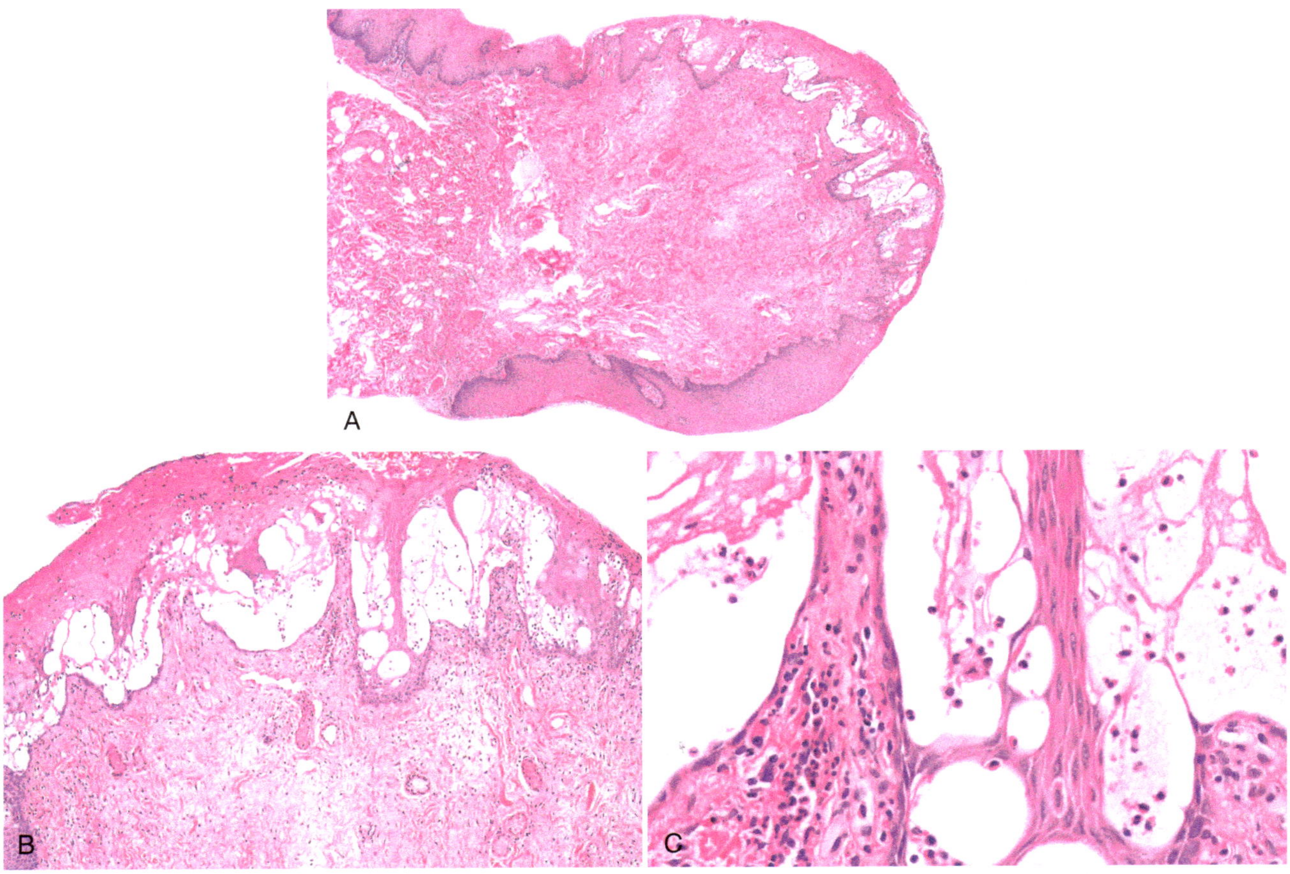

FIG 7.9 Fibroma with irritant contact stomatitis. (A) Fibroma with ulceration and marked spongiosis. (B) Ulceration and marked spongiosis resulting in intraepithelial blistering. (C) Marked spongiosis and leukocyte exocytosis.

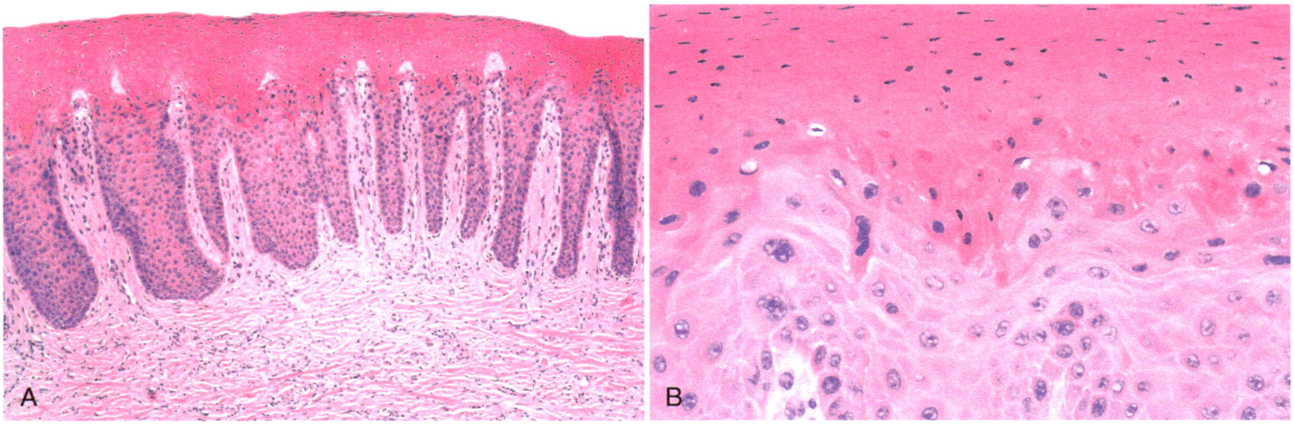

FIG 7.10 Irritant contact stomatitis. (A) Parakeratosis and coagulation of superficial keratinocytes. (B) Coagulated superficial keratinocytes with reactive epithelial atypia and nuclear pyknosis.

Management and Prognosis

- Avoiding contact with the offending agent resolves lesions, and topical steroid therapy may be helpful (see Appendix A).

REFERENCES

Bagga S, Thomas BS, Bhat M. Garlic burn as self-inflicted mucosal injury—a case report and review of the literature. *Quintessence Int.* 2008;39:491-494.

Gilvetti C, Porter SR, Fedele S. Traumatic chemical oral ulceration: a case report and review of the literature. *Br Dent J.* 2010;208:297-300.

Kuttan NA, Narayana N, Moghadam BK. Desquamative stomatitis associated with routine use of oral health care products. *Gen Dent.* 2001;49:596-602.

LeSueur BW, Yiannias JA. Contact stomatitis. *Dermatol Clin.* 2003;21:105-114.

Sapir S, Bimstein E. Cholinsalicylate gel induced oral lesion: report of case. *J Clin Pediatr Dent.* 2000;24:103-106.

FRICTIONAL BLISTERS

Clinical Findings

- Blisters occur at sites of trauma, particularly on the nonkeratinized mandibular or maxillary sulci and/or vestibules traumatized by denture flanges.

Etiopathogenesis and Histopathologic Features

Traumatic shear forces separate the epithelium from the connective tissue.

- There is acanthosis with intraepithelial or subepithelial blistering and accumulation of serum or fibrin with variable inflammation and vascular ectasia (Figs. 7.11 and 7.12).
- Bright, eosinophilic pools of plasma ("plasma pooling") are further evidence of surface injury (Fig. 7.13).

Differential Diagnosis

- Lymphatic malformations or lymphangioma circumscriptum consists of endothelium-lined spaces that abut the epithelium.
- Mucous membrane pemphigoid does not usually exhibit marked epithelial hyperplasia and accumulation of fluid or fibrin.
- Superficial mucoceles exhibit subepithelial collections of mucin and muciphages.

Management and Prognosis

- Lesions resolve if the source of trauma is removed.

REFERENCE

Reibel J. Immunohistochemical demonstration of plasma protein in squamous epithelium of formalin-fixed, paraffin-embedded oral mucosa. *J Oral Pathol.* 1984;13:75-84.

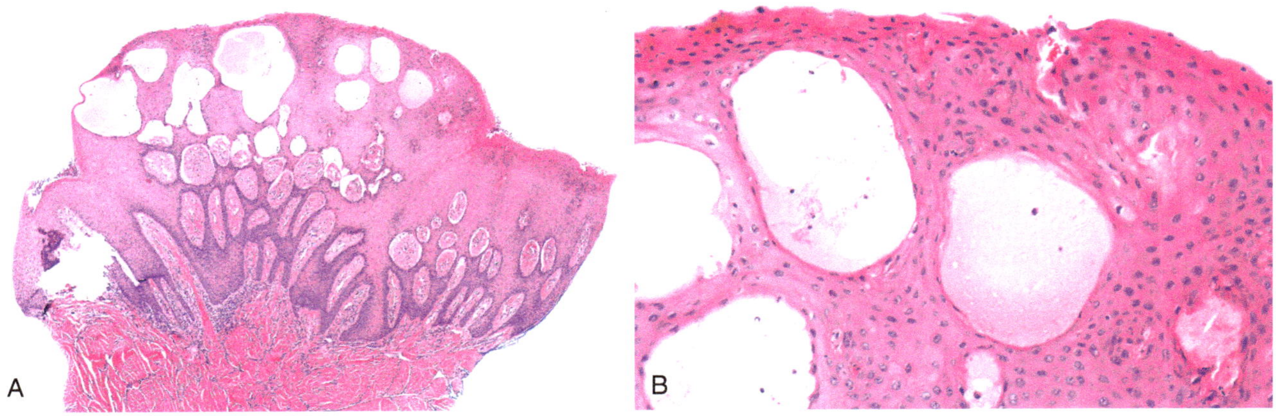

FIG 7.11 Frictional blister caused by denture. (A) Acanthosis with intraepithelial blisters. (B) Intraepithelial blisters filled with fluid.

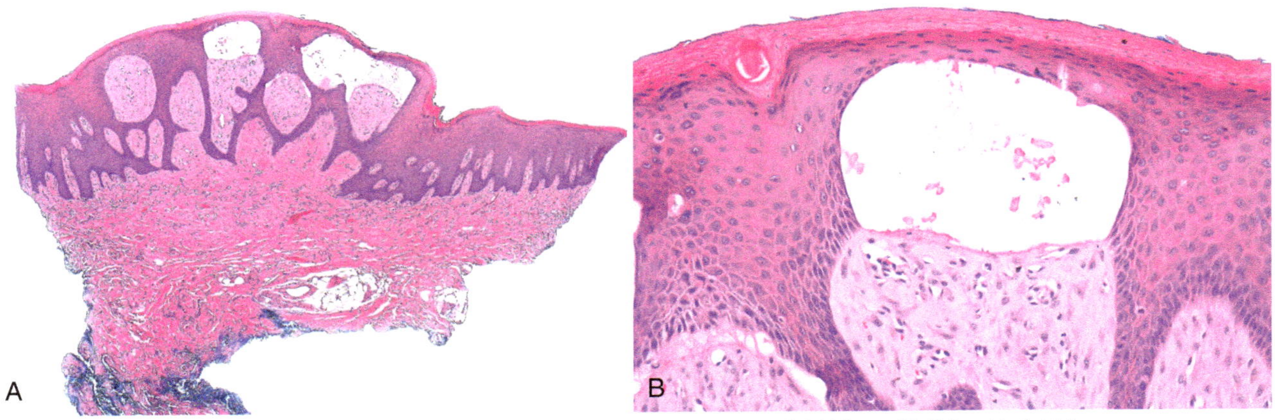

FIG 7.12 Frictional blister. (A) Parakeratosis, acanthosis, and superficial blister. (B) Subepithelial blister and underlying granulation tissue.

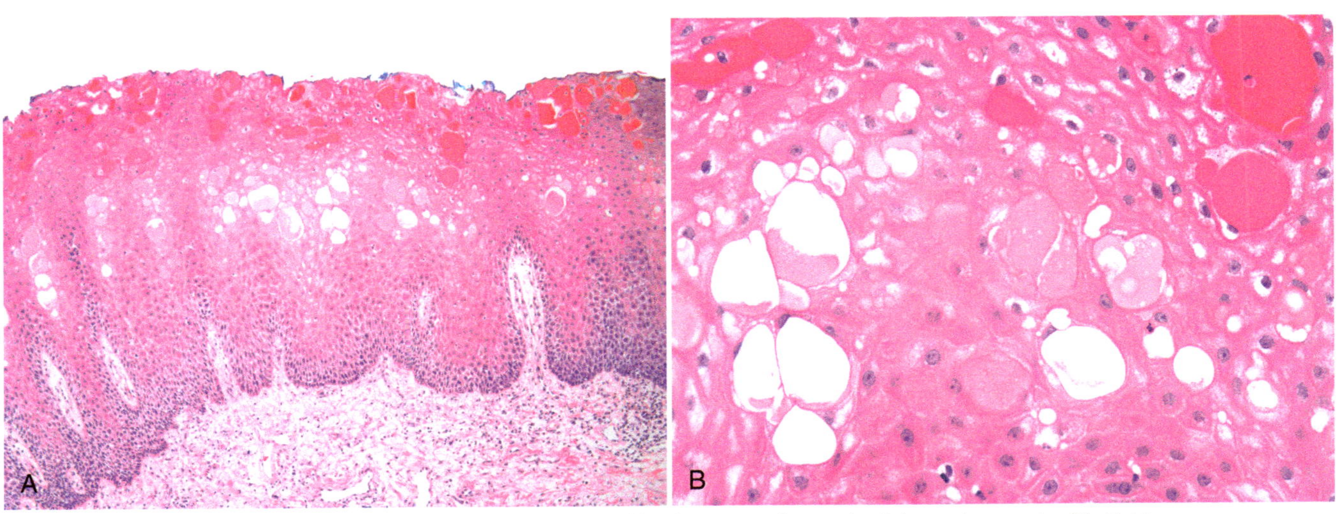

FIG 7.13 Plasma pooling. (A) Acanthosis with plasma pooling and mild reactive atypia. (B) Fluid accumulation between epithelial cells.

CHRONIC GINGIVITIS

Clinical Findings

- This is common at all ages, but in particular during adolescence and pregnancy because of hormonal influences. The gingiva is erythematous and tender and readily bleeds on brushing or eating (Fig. 7.14).

Etiopathogenesis and Histopathologic Features

Gingivitis and periodontitis result from production of inflammatory cytokines in response to plaque bacterial lipopolysaccharides.

- The gingiva loses its normal keratinization, and there is acanthosis with spongiosis and leukocyte exocytosis, as well as a plasma cell infiltrate (sometimes intense) in the lamina propria (Fig. 7.15). Plaque bacteria often are identified and commonly contain Actinomycetes but without surrounding neutrophils, and do not qualify for a diagnosis of actinomycosis (Fig. 7.16).

Differential Diagnosis

- Plasma cell gingivitis exhibits an intense polyclonal plasma cell infiltrate present in sheets.

Management and Prognosis

- Treatment is with dental scaling, root planing, and dental prophylaxis to remove plaque and reduce inflammation, in addition to maintenance of good oral hygiene.

REFERENCE

Wang PL, Ohura K. *Porphyromonas gingivalis* lipopolysaccharide signaling in gingival fibroblasts—CD14 and Toll-like receptors. *Crit Rev Oral Biol Med.* 2002;13:132-142.

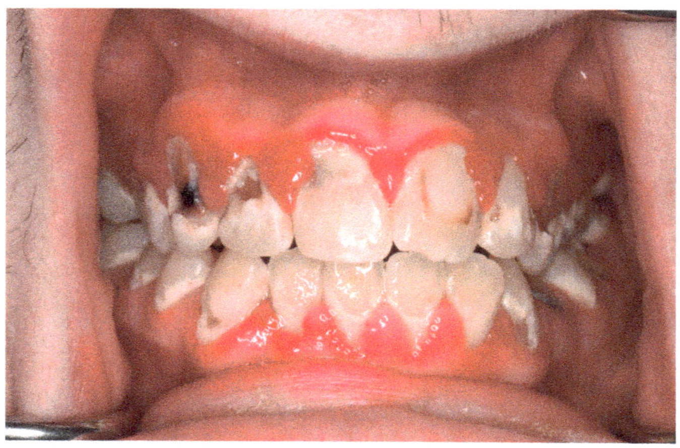

FIG 7.14 Chronic gingivitis with erythematous and edematous marginal gingiva with abundant dental plaque and many carious teeth. *(Courtesy Dr. Maria Dona, private practice, Andover, Mass.)*

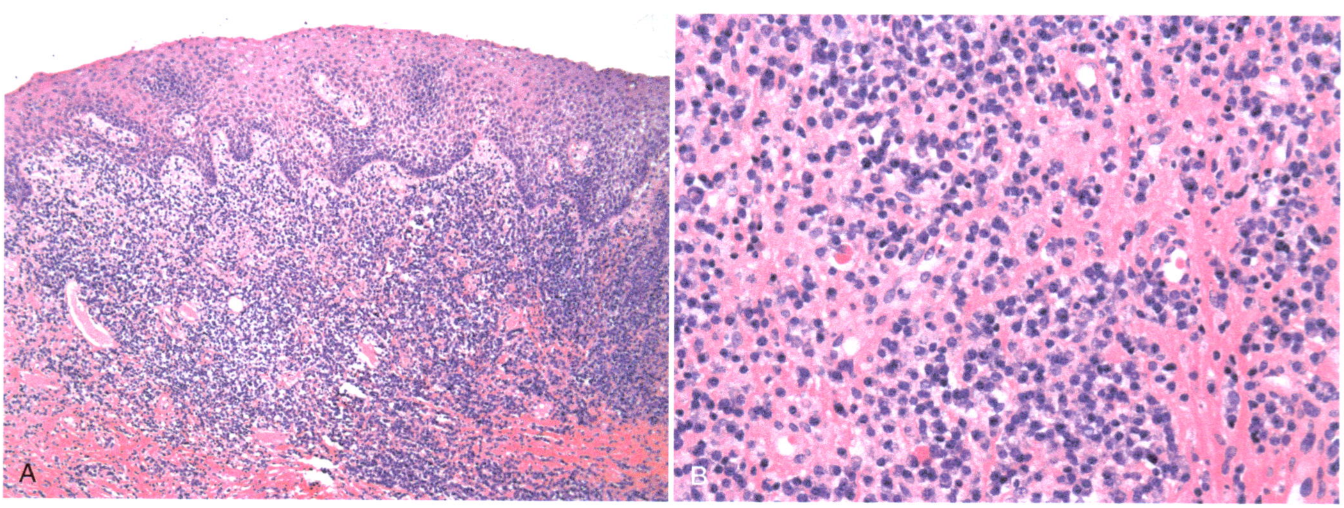

FIG 7.15 Chronic gingivitis. (A) Epithelium shows marked spongiosis and neutrophilic exocytosis. (B) Many plasma cells are present.

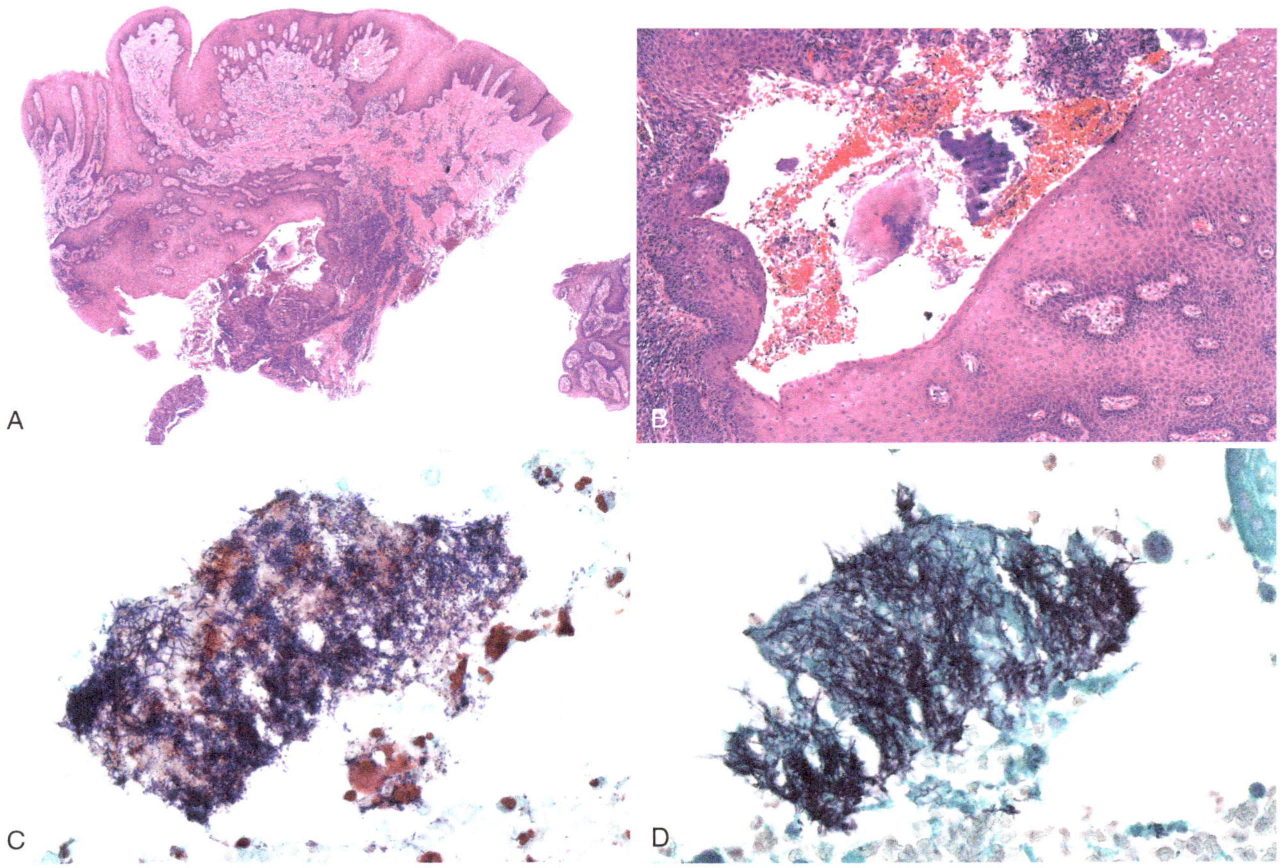

FIG 7.16 Chronic hyperplastic gingivitis. (A) Acanthosis and fibrous hyperplasia with chronic inflammation. (B) Dental plaque bacteria on the surface without a rim of neutrophils (Splendore-Hoeppli effect). (C) Dental plaque containing gram-positive filaments and cocci (Brown and Brenn stain). (D) Dental plaque containing argyrophilic filaments (methenamine silver stain).

FOREIGN BODY GINGIVITIS

Clinical Findings

- This occurs in the fifth and sixth decades of life. The gingiva is erythematous and tender. There may be a recent history of dental treatment, especially dental prophylaxis or placement of restorations, or a history of use of an abrasive toothpaste.

Etiopathogenesis

Foreign body gingivitis is a gingival reaction to iatrogenic implantation of foreign material. Energy-dispersive x-ray analysis confirms the presence of silver, tin, silica, aluminum, zinc, calcium, phosphorus, titanium, and barium from dental abrasives from professional polishing agents, toothpastes, and dental restorations, especially amalgam (see Chapter 9).

- There is acanthosis or epithelial atrophy and variable acute and chronic inflammation. Lichenoid or non-necrotizing granulomatous inflammation is present in 20% to 48% of cases. Fine granules of crystalline, refractile foreign material may be identified (Figs. 7.17 and 7.18).

Differential Diagnosis

- Granulomas in orofacial granulomatosis lack foreign material.
- Amalgam tattoos often show granulomatous inflammation related to larger fragments of amalgam, while smaller ones stain connective tissue fibers.

Management and Prognosis

- Surgery is usually necessary because, although topical steroids reduce inflammation and symptoms, the foreign material is not readily degradable.

REFERENCES

Gordon SC, Daley TD. Foreign body gingivitis: clinical and microscopic features of 61 cases. *Oral Surg Oral Med Oral Pathol Oral Radiol Endod.* 1997;83:562-570.

Gordon SC, Daley TD. Foreign body gingivitis: identification of the foreign material by energy-dispersive x-ray microanalysis. *Oral Surg Oral Med Oral Pathol Oral Radiol Endod.* 1997;83:571-576.

Koppang HS, Roushan A, Srafilzadeh A, et al. Foreign body gingival lesions: distribution, morphology, identification by x-ray energy dispersive analysis and possible origin of foreign material. *J Oral Pathol Med.* 2007;36:161-172.

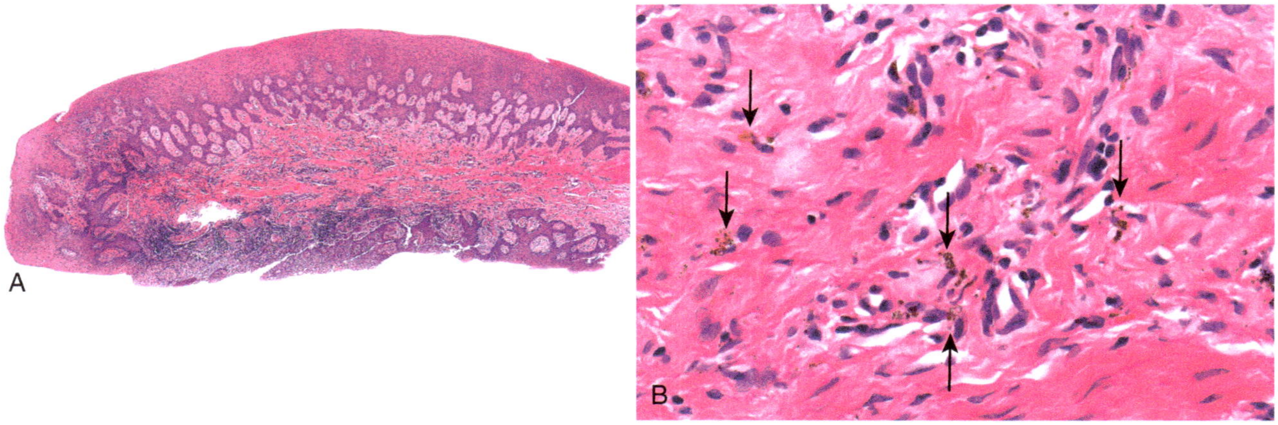

FIG 7.17 Foreign body gingivitis. (A) Oral mucosa with mild chronic inflammation. (B) Granules of foreign material, some of which are slightly crystalline *(arrows)*.

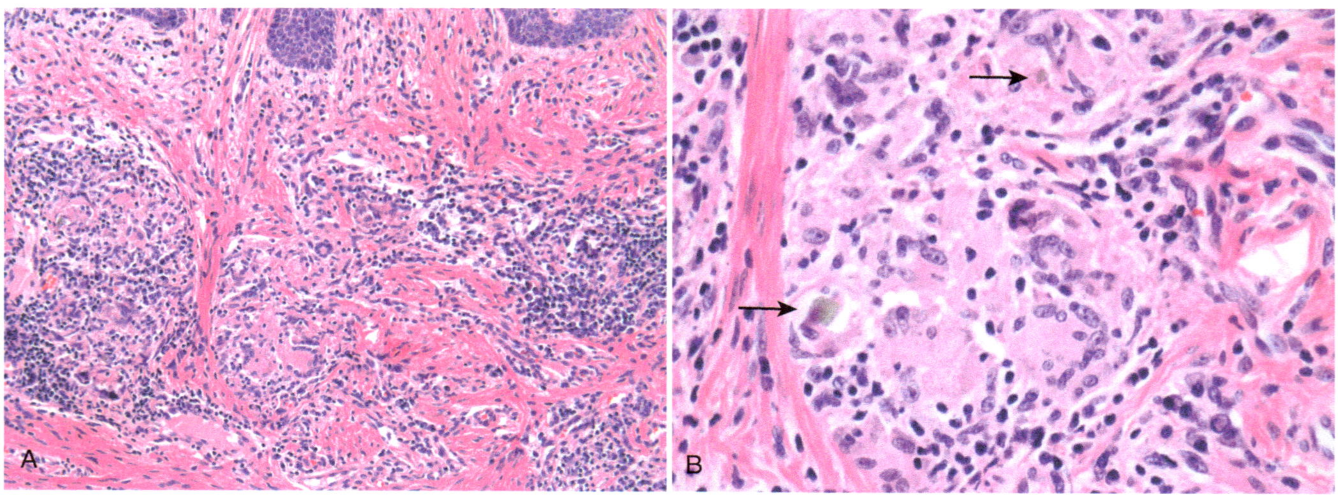

FIG 7.18 Foreign body gingivitis. (A) Non-necrotizing granulomas in the lamina propria. (B) Foreign material is present within the cytoplasm of giant cells *(arrows)*.

8 GRANULOMATOUS, IMMUNE-MEDIATED, AND AUTOIMMUNE CONDITIONS

CHAPTER CONTENTS

Granulomatous Inflammation

True granulomas are collections of activated macrophages with an epitheloid appearance with variable inflammation and often giant cells with a wide range of etiologies. Necrotizing granulomas are often seen in infectious processes and diseases of collagen degradation and necrobiosis. Table 8.1 lists the common noninfectious granulomatous processes affecting the oral cavity. Granulomas caused by infections are discussed in Chapter 4.

FOREIGN BODY GRANULOMAS

Clinical Findings

- A nondescript, painless, or painful papule or nodule occurs at sites of trauma or at sites of iatrogenically introduced substances (such as dermal fillers). The latter are much more common in women and located around the lips, and they are often yellow in color (Fig. 8.1).

Etiopathogenesis and Histopathologic Features

Extrinsic foreign material introduced accidentally (eg, glass) or intentionally (eg, sutures, dermal fillers) excites a foreign body response. Although generally resorbed, dermal fillers may migrate to sites distant from the original injection, such as the lips or oral cavity, or from the nasolabial fold. Foreign body granulomas also form as a reaction to endogenous substances, such as cholesterol (from degenerated red blood cells), keratin (ruptured epidermoid cyst), hair (ruptured hair follicle), and collagen (degenerated collagen in rheumatoid nodules).

- There is proliferation of macrophages and foreign body giant cells, usually non-necrotizing. Refractile or nonrefractile foreign material may be identified, such as fragments of hair (Fig. 8.2) or suture material (Fig. 8.3).
- Poly-L-lactic acid filler granulomas form circumscribed nodules containing refractile, fusiform, and geometric structures that often contain asteroid bodies within giant cells. A lymphocytic infiltrate is often present (Fig. 8.4).
- Calcium hydroxylapatite granulomas are present diffusely in the stroma, often infiltrating between skeletal muscle, and consist of gray-brown microspheres, 25 to 40 μm in diameter, that are nonrefractile. They stimulate endogenous collagen production and are resorbed within a few months, but they may cause a granulomatous response (Fig. 8.5).

TABLE 8.1 Types of Granulomatous Inflammation

Granulomatous Inflammation	Distinguishing Features
Foreign Body Granuloma	Refractile or nonrefractile foreign material is present, although this may not always be identified.
Intrinsic	Hair (ruptured hair follicle), cholesterol within cyst walls, and keratin from ruptured cysts or carcinomas
Extrinsic	Suture material, dermal filler, and amalgam are readily identified foreign materials
Infectious	
Bacterial infection (eg, *Bartonella henselae*)	Warthin-Starry stain
Mycobacterial infection (often necrotizing)	Acid-fast bacillus (Ziehl-Neelsen, Kinyoun, or Fite stain)
Spirochetal infection (eg, syphilitic gumma)	Warthin-Starry, Dieterle, or modified Steiner stain or immunostaining
Deep fungal infections	Methenamine silver or PAS stain; may see pseudoepitheliomatous hyperplasia
Others	
Sarcoidosis	Hilar lymphadenopathy, uveitis, lupus pernio, and elevated angiotensin-converting enzyme levels
Crohn disease	Gastrointestinal symptoms, positive endoscopic findings
Orofacial granulomatosis	Hypersensitivity to foods or related to Crohn disease
Wegener granulomatosis	Upper respiratory or renal findings, positive for antineutrophil cytoplasmic antibodies
Lichenoid granulomatous inflammation	History of contactant at the site
Palisaded granulomas (eg, rheumatoid nodule)	History of rheumatoid arthritis or necrobiotic disease

PAS, Periodic acid–Schiff.

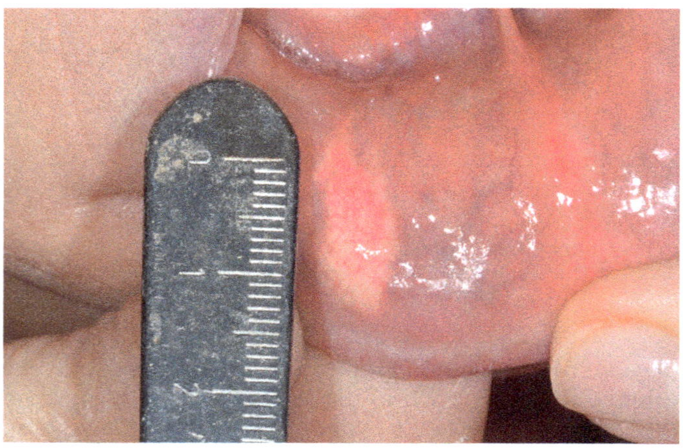

FIG 8.1 Dermal filler presenting as yellow plaque on lower lip mucosa, caused by calcium hydroxylapatite.

- Silicone granulomas are present diffusely within the stroma and consist of macrophages with bubbly cytoplasm with small- and medium-sized vacuoles (Fig. 8.6). Nonsilicone lipid granulomas exhibit leached-out foreign material in the form of vacuolated spaces that vary greatly in size, often associated with fibrosis (Fig. 8.7).
- Cholesterol granulomas are common in odontogenic cysts (see Chapter 14), and granulomas to keratin are often seen in keratinizing squamous cell carcinomas (see Chapter 11).

Differential Diagnosis

- Hyaluronic acid fillers appear as amorphous, basophilic pools of ground substance that stain for Alcian blue and colloidal iron. They generally do not incite a foreign body reaction but may show mild fibrosis (Fig. 8.8).

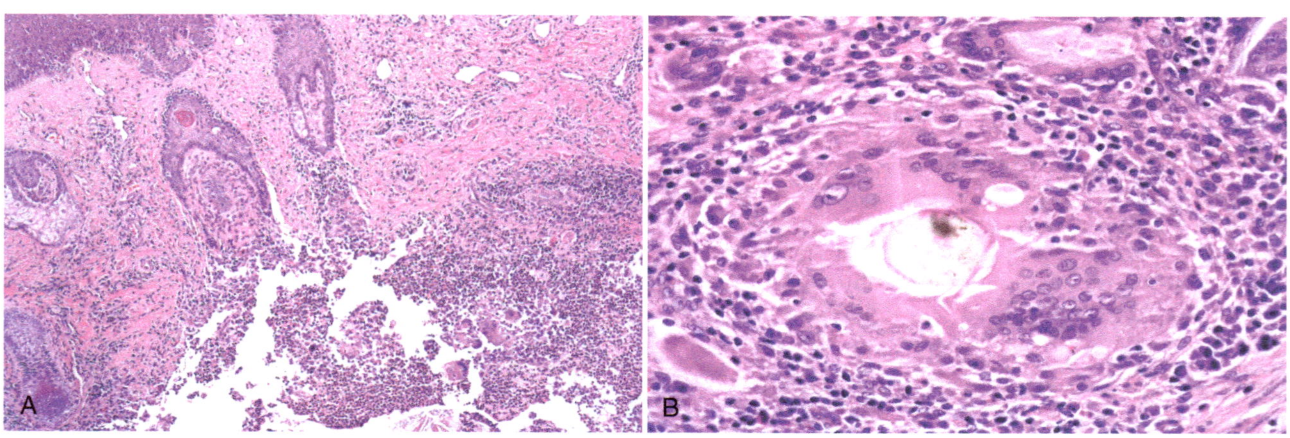

FIG 8.2 Ruptured hair follicle. (A) Granulomatous inflammation within the dermis with abscess. (B) Fragment of hair surrounded by foreign body giant cells.

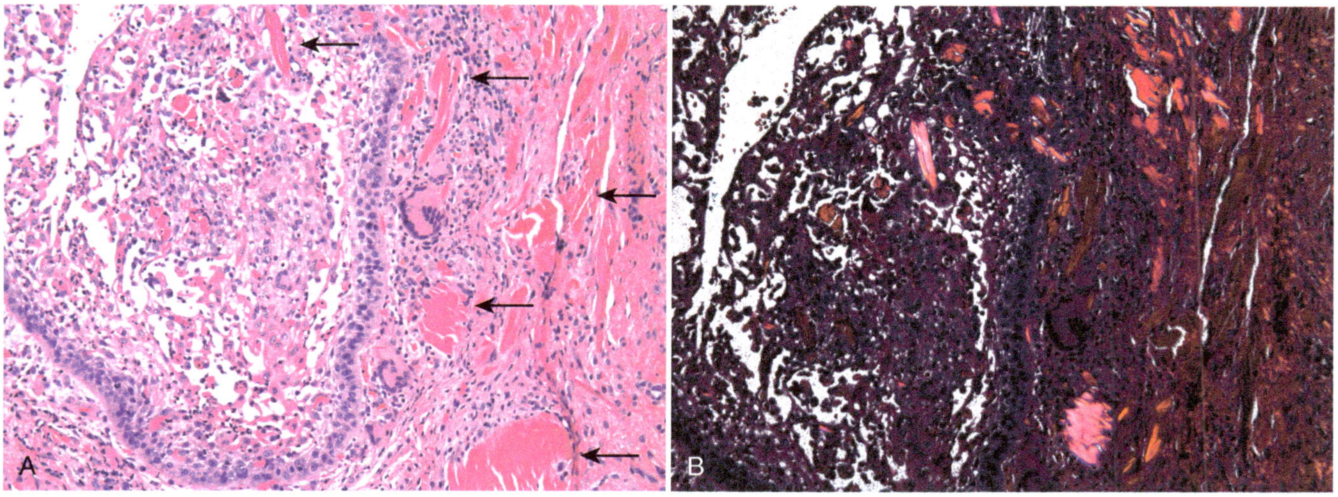

FIG 8.3 Suture granuloma (from chromic gut). (A) Amorphous eosinophilic fragments of suture material (*arrows*) within the stroma and being exteriorized by epithelium ingrowth that is inflamed. Note foreign body giant cell reaction. (B) Refractile fragments of suture in the stroma and within the epithelium.

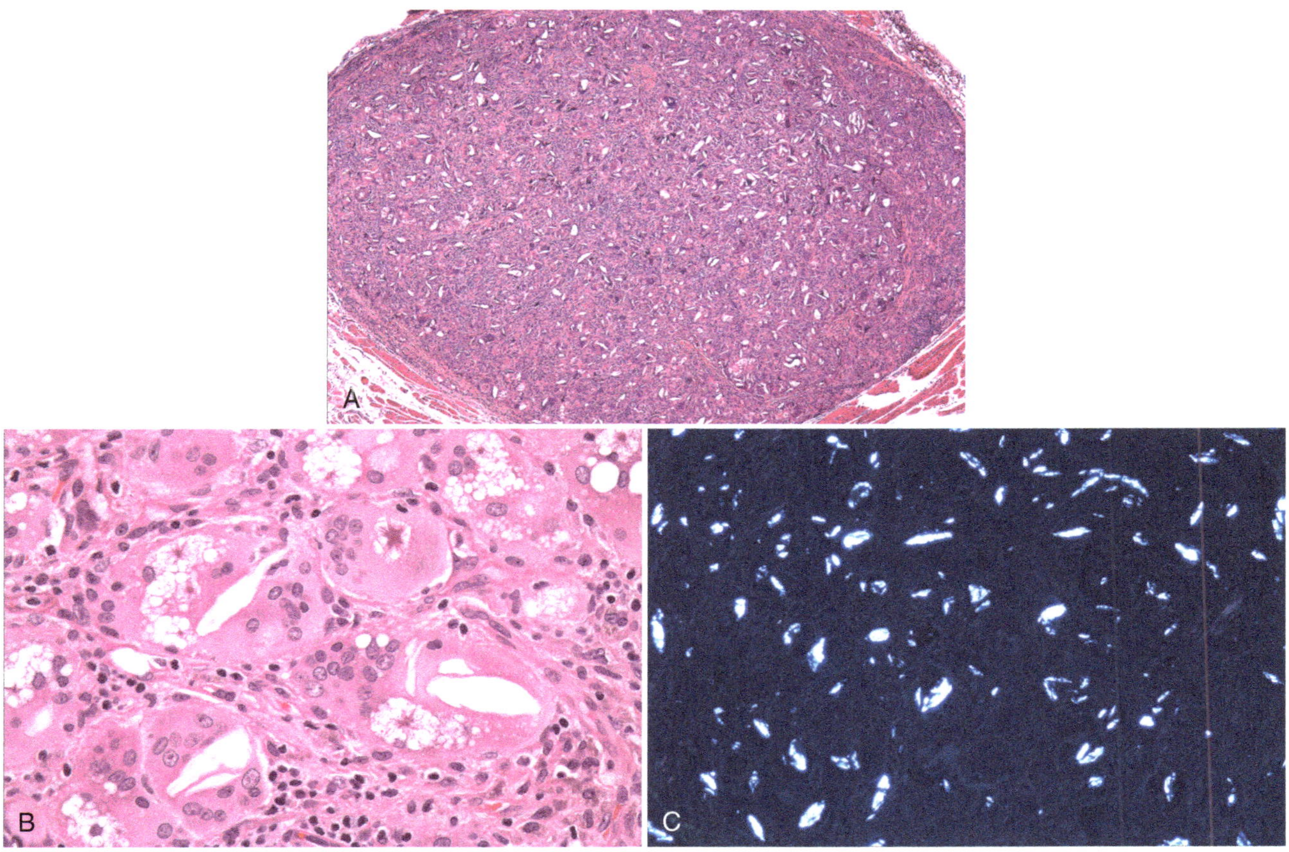

FIG 8.4 Poly-l-lactic acid granuloma. (A) Circumscribed nodule consists of multinucleated giant cells and fusiform clefts. (B) Multinucleated giant cells with bubbly cytoplasm, fusiform clefts, and asteroid bodies. (C) Poly-L-lactic acid is refractile.

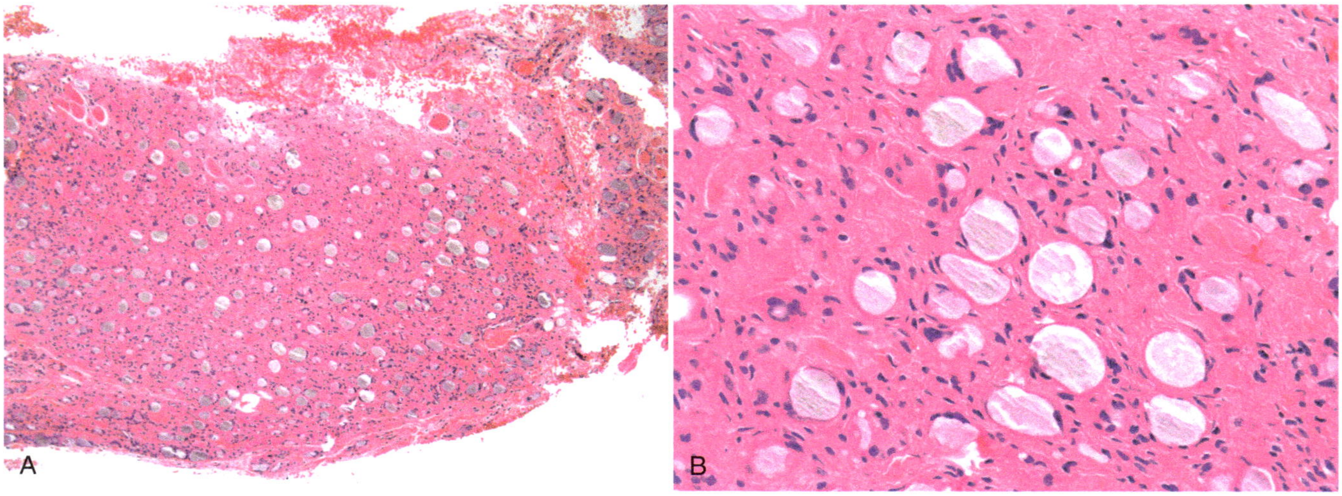

FIG 8.5 Calcium hydroxylapatite filler. (A) Uniform, round particulate material with many multinucleated foreign body giant cells located between muscle fibers. (B) Nonrefractile gray-mauve round particles within multinucleated foreign body giant cells.

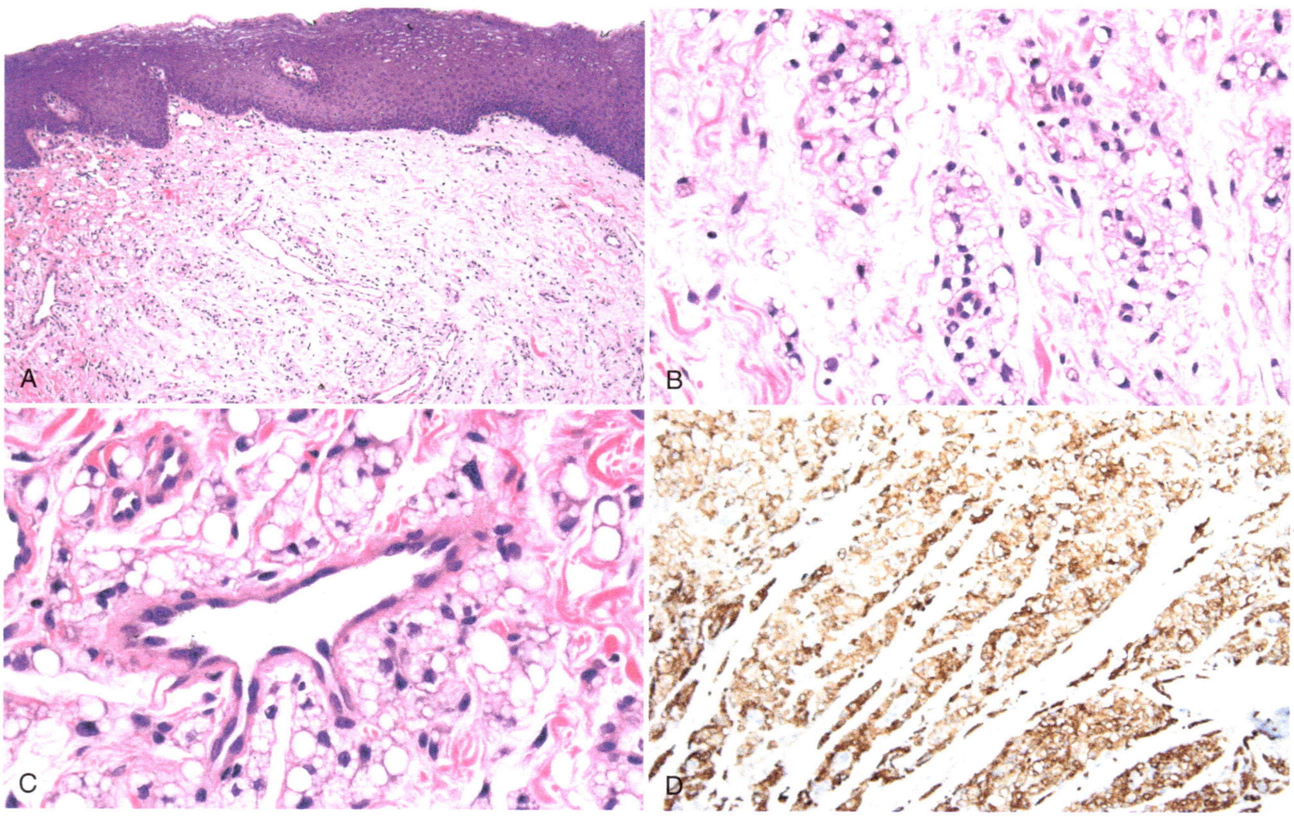

FIG 8.6 Silicone granuloma. (A) Many vacuolated cells in the lamina propria. (B) Macrophages containing vacuoles of varying sizes. (C) Macrophages with bubbly vesicular cytoplasm and slight reactive nuclear atypia. (D) Macrophages are CD68+.

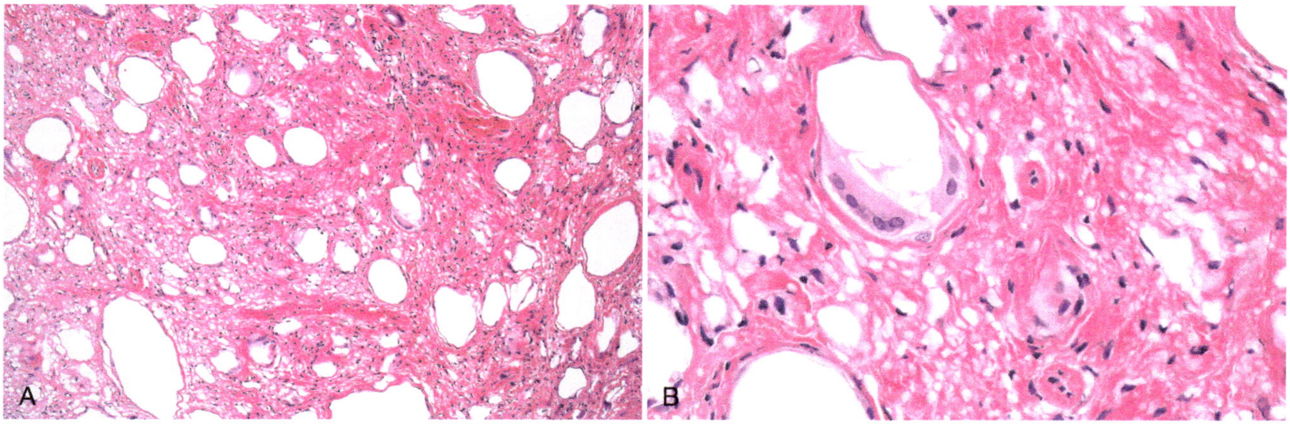

FIG 8.7 Lipid granuloma. (A) Leached-out lipid material forming vacuolated spaces of varying sizes, with fibrosis. (B) Lipid vacuoles of varying sizes and foreign body giant cells.

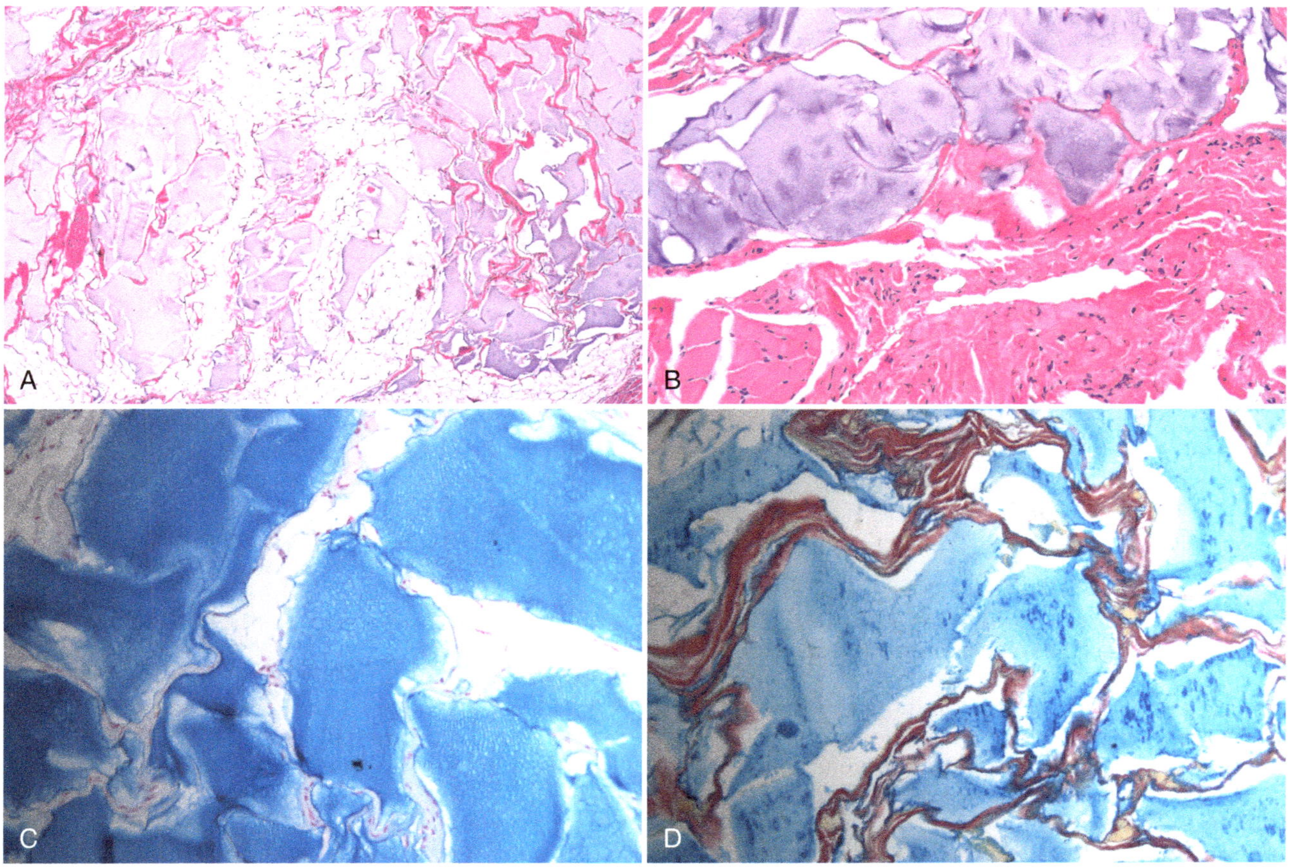

FIG 8.8 Hyaluronic acid filler. (A) Pools of inert amorphous basophilic material within fat. (B) Mild fibrosis without foreign body reaction or inflammation around the filler. (C) Positive Alcian blue stain. (D) Positive colloidal iron stain.

- Palisaded granulomas of granuloma annulare and rheumatoid arthritis are rarely encountered intraorally.
- Atypical lipomatous tumor may resemble a silicone granuloma, but the latter is positive for macrophage markers.

Management and Prognosis

- Excision is curative.

REFERENCES

Ficarra G, Mosqueda-Taylor A, Carlos R. Silicone granuloma of the facial tissues: a report of seven cases. *Oral Surg Oral Med Oral Pathol Oral Radiol Endod.* 2002;94:65-73.

Jham BC, Nikitakis NG, Scheper MA, et al. Granulomatous foreign-body reaction involving oral and perioral tissues after injection of biomaterials: a series of 7 cases and review of the literature. *J Oral Maxillofac Surg.* 2009;67:280-285.

Kato K, Segami N, Fukuda H, Minato H. Rheumatoid nodule in the lower lip of a patient with rheumatoid arthritis: a novel case report and review of literature. *J Oral Maxillofac Surg.* 2014;72:1532.e1-e5.

Lombardi T, Samson J, Plantier F, et al. Oral granulomas after injection of cosmetic fillers: histopathologic and clinical study of 11 cases. *J Oral Path Med.* 2004;33:115-120.

Narins RS, Coleman WP 3rd, Glogau RG. Recommendations and treatment options for nodules and other filler complications. *Dermatol Surg.* 2009;35(suppl 2):1667-1671.

Requena L, Requena C, Christensen L, et al. Adverse reactions to injectable soft tissue fillers [published erratum appears in *J Am Acad Dermatol.* 2011;64:1178]. *J Am Acad Dermatol.* 2011;64:1-34, quiz 35–36.

Sage RJ, Chaffins ML, Kouba DJ. Granulomatous foreign body reaction to hyaluronic acid: report of a case after melolabial fold augmentation and review of management. *Dermatol Surg.* 2009;35(suppl 2):1696-1700.

Shahrabi-Farahani S, Lerman MA, Noonan V, Kabani S, Woo SB. Granulomatous foreign body reaction to dermal cosmetic fillers with intraoral migration. *Oral Surg Oral Med Oral Pathol Oral Radiol.* 2014;117:105-110.

Shahrabi Farahani S, Sexton J, Stone JD, et al. Lip nodules caused by hyaluronic acid filler injection: report of three cases. *Head Neck Pathol.* 2012;6:16-20.

OROFACIAL GRANULOMATOSIS AND ORAL MANIFESTATION OF CROHN DISEASE

Clinical Features

- This generally affects young adults with a high prevalence in the United Kingdom. The lips show diffuse or localized rubbery swelling that does not remit (unlike angioedema). The tissues feel tight and are sensitive (Fig. 8.9A–B).
- Patients may also show concomitant swelling of the gingiva, and long-standing cases show cobblestoning and fissuring of the mucosa from edema. Some cases have a staghorn appearance of the distal portion of the submandibular duct (Fig. 8.9C).
- Melkersson-Rosenthal syndrome, in addition to the lip swelling, exhibits fissured tongue and facial palsy. The inclusion of a fissured tongue (a fairly common condition) in this triad has been questioned.
- Crohn disease: In addition to the features noted above, there may also be papular folds of tissue in the maxillary and mandibular sulci, aphthous-like ulcers (often linear), gastrointestinal symptoms, and thickened and erythematous appearance of perivermilion skin (see Fig. 8.9D). Oral findings precede the diagnosis of intestinal disease in 50% of cases. Some patients may also present with pyostomatitis vegetans (see later). The younger the patient who presents with orofacial granulomatosis, the more likely she or he is to develop Crohn disease.

Etiopathogenesis and Histopathologic Features

Orofacial granulomatosis is a hypersensitivity reaction, and most patients are atopic and/or have oral allergy syndrome. It is often associated with sensitivity to phenolic compounds that are found in flavorings such as cinnamaldehyde and in preservatives such as benzoates. Crohn disease is thought to be an inflammatory response, possibly to intestinal microbes in genetically susceptible hosts (eg, polymorphisms in the *NOD2/CARD15* genes). However, these polymorphisms have not been identified in patients with orofacial granulomatosis.

- This condition is characterized by non-necrotizing granulomas that may be subtle in early disease (Fig. 8.10) or more florid in later disease. Granulomas of Crohn disease often contain eosinophils and may occur in salivary glands (Figs. 8.11 and 8.12). Edema and chronic inflammation alone are not sufficient for the diagnosis, and multiple levels should be performed through the block, if necessary, to locate granulomas.

Differential Diagnosis

- Infectious granulomatous processes must be ruled out with histochemical stains (see Chapter 4).
- Granulomas of sarcoidosis are non-necrotizing, compact, and well-demarcated or "naked" (Fig. 8.13). Patients are often black and have hilar lymphadenopathy, pulmonary symptoms, uveitis, and lupus pernio. Elevated levels of angiotensin-converting enzyme (produced by the granulomas) may or may not be present and are not specific for the disease. Oral lesions take the form of gingival hyperplasia, nodules, and ulcers. Labial salivary gland biopsies are positive for disease in up to 33% of cases, but the chances of a positive biopsy are higher using fluorodeoxyglucose–positron emission tomography scan–guided biopsy.
- Lesions reported as being orofacial granulomatosis-like after organ (especially liver) transplantation in children likely represent a different entity.

Management and Prognosis

- Patients with orofacial granulomatosis should be patch-tested to determine if hypersensitivity to foods and other substances exists. Elimination diet is beneficial in 50% to 80% of patients, with 23% exhibiting complete resolution.
- Topical, intralesional, and systemic corticosteroid therapy controls disease in many patients, but relapse is common. Minocycline, thalidomide, mycophenolate mofetil, and tumor necrosis factor-α inhibitors show variable success in managing this condition.
- Gastrointestinal evaluation for Crohn disease is indicated if there are intestinal symptoms or if these symptoms develop.

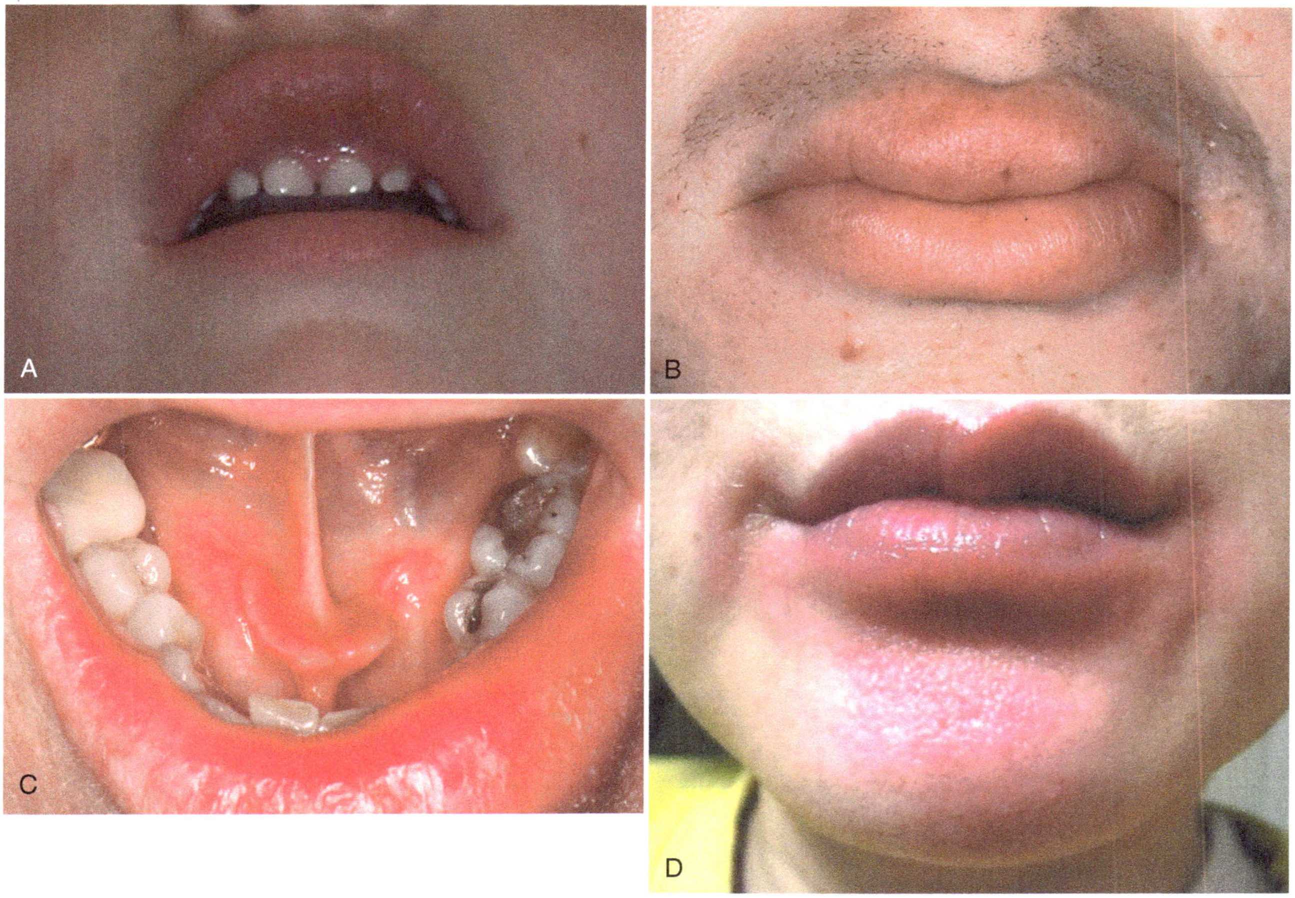

FIG 8.9 (A) Orofacial granulomatosis: a child with lip swelling and fissures but without gastrointestinal symptoms. (B) Orofacial granulomatosis: lip swelling without gastrointestinal symptoms or signs after a 15-year follow-up. (C) Orofacial granulomatosis: staghorn appearance of tissue around excretory salivary duct. (D) Crohn disease: typical "orange peel" appearance and thickening of the perivermilion skin as well as swollen lips. *(A, courtesy Dr. Bonnie Padwa, Children's Hospital Boston; D, Courtesy Dr. Jeffrey Stone, private practice, Lowell, Mass.)*

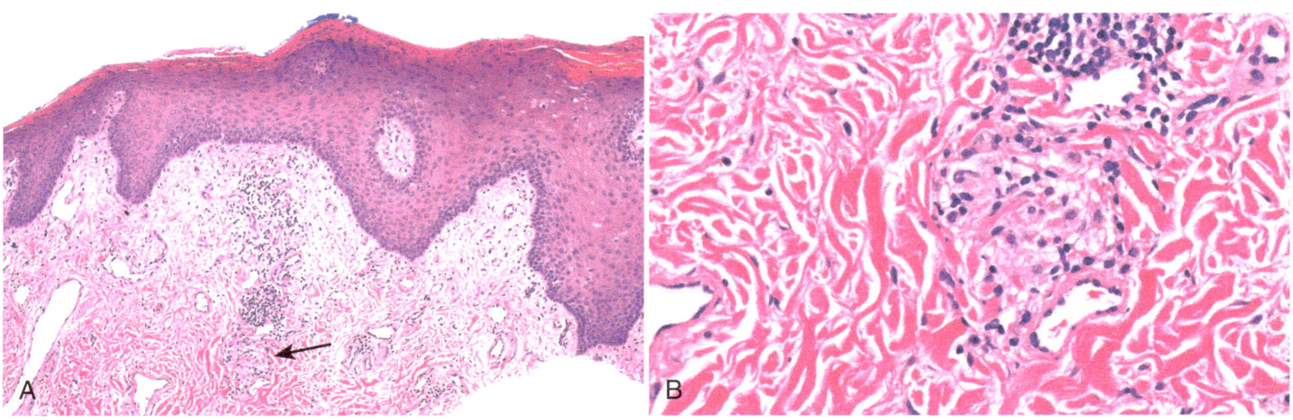

FIG 8.10 Orofacial granulomatosis. (A) The lamina propria is edematous and contains a subtle granuloma (*arrow*) and dilated vessels. (B) Subtle non-necrotizing granuloma around a vessel.

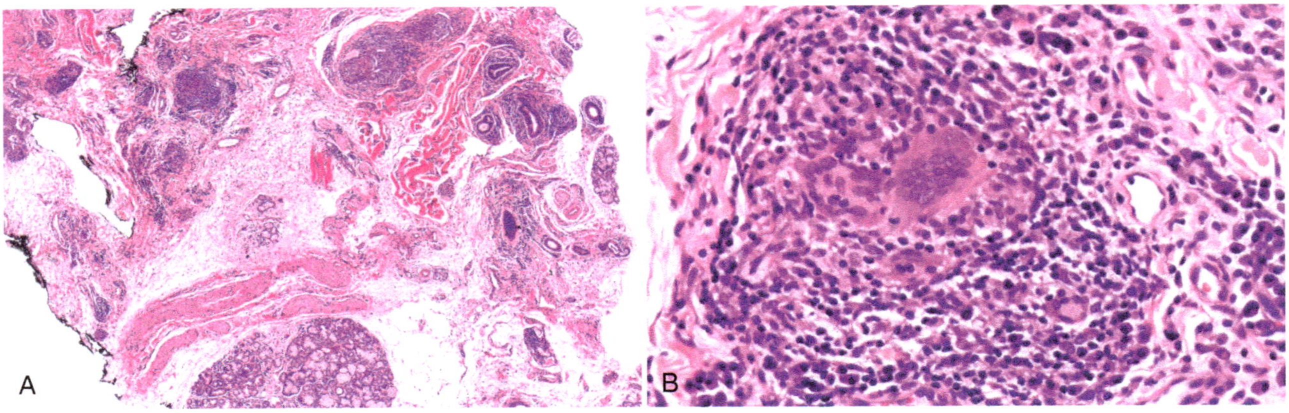

FIG 8.11 Crohn disease. (A) Many non-necrotizing granulomas within salivary glands of the lip. (B) Non-necrotizing granuloma with multinucleated giant cells and lymphocytes.

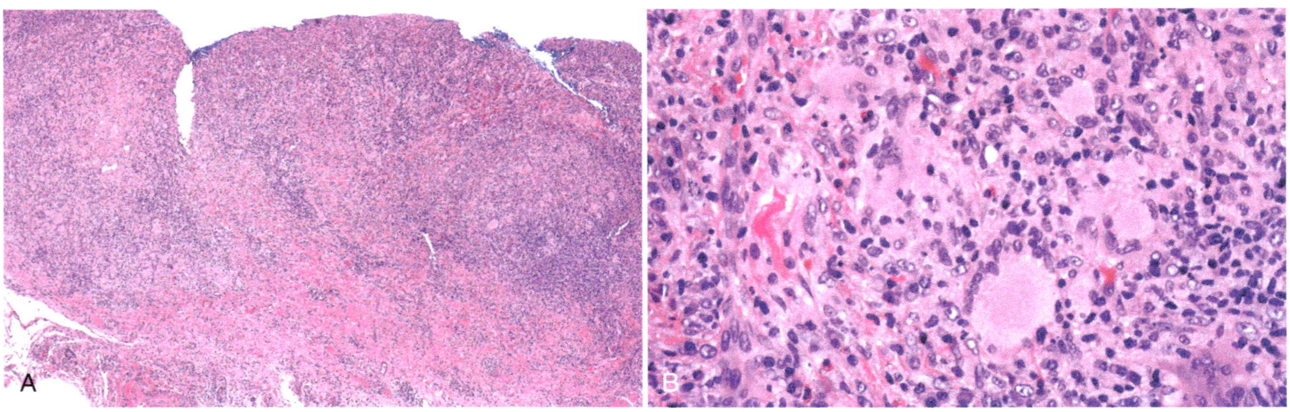

FIG 8.12 Crohn disease. (A) Diffuse granulomatous inflammation in the lamina propria with overlying ulceration. (B) Many eosinophils are noted within granulomas.

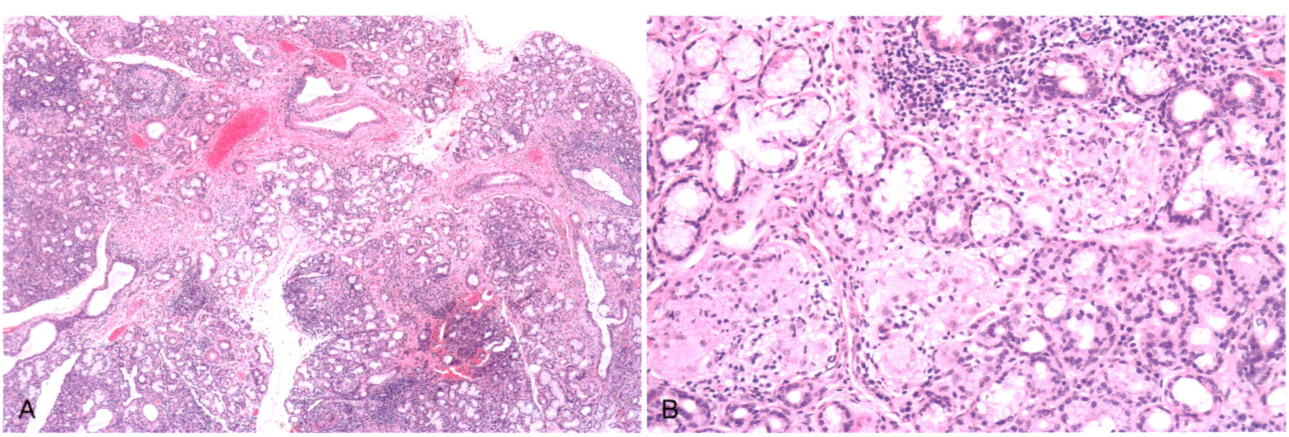

FIG 8.13 Sarcoidosis. (A) Minor salivary gland containing granulomas. (B) Non-necrotizing "naked" granulomas with multinucleated giant cells.

REFERENCES

Abraham C, Cho JH. Inflammatory bowel disease. *N Engl J Med.* 2009;361:2068-2078.

Al Johani KA, Moles DR, Hodgson TA, et al. Orofacial granulomatosis: clinical features and long-term outcome of therapy. *J Am Acad Dermatol.* 2010;62:611-620.

Bouaziz A, Le Scanff J, Chapelon-Abric C, et al. Oral involvement in sarcoidosis: report of 12 cases. *QJM.* 2012;105:755-767.

Campbell HE, Escudier MP, Milligan P, et al. Development of a low phenolic acid diet for the management of orofacial granulomatosis. *J Hum Nutr Diet.* 2013;26:527-537.

Campbell HE, Escudier MP, Patel P, et al. Review article: cinnamon- and benzoate-free diet as a primary treatment for orofacial granulomatosis. *Aliment Pharmacol Ther.* 2011;34:687-701.

Fedele S, Fung PPL, Bamashmous N, et al. Long-term effectiveness of intralesional triamcinolone acetonide therapy in orofacial granulomatosis: an observational cohort study. *Br J Dermatol.* 2014;170: 794-801.

Gale G, Östman S, Rekabdar E, et al. Characterisation of a Swedish cohort with orofacial granulomatosis with or without Crohn's disease. *Oral Dis.* 2015;21:e98-e104.

Grave B, McCullough M, Wiesenfeld D. Orofacial granulomatosis—a 20-year review. *Oral Dis.* 2009;15:46-51.

Harty S, Fleming P, Rowland M, et al. A prospective study of the oral manifestations of Crohn's disease. *Clin Gastroenterol Hepatol.* 2005;3:886-891.

Iannuzzi MC, Rybicki BA, Teirstein AS. Sarcoidosis. *N Engl J Med.* 2007;357:2153-2165.

Lourenco SV, Hussein TP, Bologna SB, et al. Oral manifestations of inflammatory bowel disease: a review based on the observation of six cases. *J Eur Acad Dermatol Venereol.* 2010;24:204-207.

O'Neill ID, Scully C. Biologics in oral medicine: oral Crohn's disease and orofacial granulomatosis. *Oral Dis.* 2012;18:633-638.

Patel P, Brostoff J, Campbell H, et al. Clinical evidence for allergy in orofacial granulomatosis and inflammatory bowel disease. *Clin Transl Allergy.* 2013;3:26.

Saalman R, Sundell S, Kullberg-Lindh C, et al. Long-standing oral mucosal lesions in solid organ-transplanted children - a novel clinical entity. *Transplantation.* 2010;89:606-611.

Tabak L, Agirbas E, Yilmazbayhan D, et al. The value of labial biopsy in the differentiation of sarcoidosis from tuberculosis. *Sarcoidosis Vasc Diffuse Lung Dis.* 2001;18:191-195.

Pyostomatitis Vegetans

This is not a granulomatous condition, but it is included here because of its association with Crohn disease (discussed above) and, more often, ulcerative colitis.

Clinical Findings

- This occurs in adults with a 3:1 female predilection and presents as shallow ulcers and erosions, miliary abscesses, and pustules on erythematous mucosa and as vegetations (Fig. 8.14). Folding and fissuring of the buccal mucosa occur.
- The most common associations are ulcerative colitis (approximately 70% of cases), Crohn disease (10–15% of cases), and liver disease, although some cases are idiopathic. Peripheral blood eosinophilia is present in 90% of cases.

Etiopathogenesis and Histologic Features

Pyostomatitis vegetans is the oral counterpart of pyodermatitis vegetans, and the etiology is unknown.

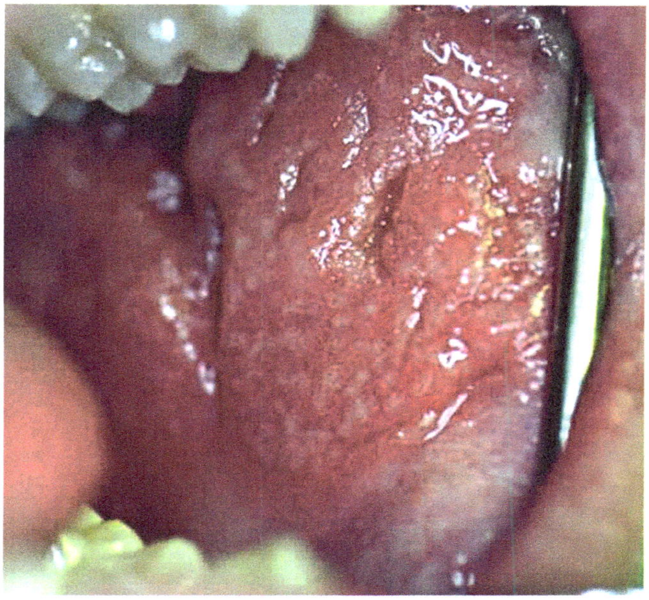

FIG 8.14 Pyostomatitis vegetans manifesting as punctuate pustules and linear ulcers. *(From Markiewicz M, Suresh L, Margarone J, et al. Pyostomatitis vegetans: a clinical marker of silent ulcerative colitis. J Oral Maxillofacial Surg. 2007;65:346–348.)*

- Acanthosis, spongiosis, and suprabasilar clefting with acantholysis are present. Neutrophilic and eosinophilic abscesses are noted within the clefts and in the connective tissue papillae (Fig. 8.15).
- Direct immunofluorescence studies for immunoglobulin G (IgG) and C3 are negative.

Differential Diagnosis

- Pemphigus vulgaris exhibits intercellular deposition of IgG on direct immunofluorescence studies.

Management and Prognosis

- Oral lesions respond well to topical steroids or tacrolimus (see Appendix A), in addition to systemic therapy for the underlying gastrointestinal disease.

REFERENCES

Gonzalez-Moles MA, Gil-Montoya JA, Ruiz-Avila I, et al. Pyostomatitis vegetans: dramatic clinical response to clobetasol propionate treatment in aqueous solution. *J Eur Acad Dermatol Venereol.* 2008; 22:252-253.

Hegarty AM, Barrett AW, Scully C. Pyostomatitis vegetans. *Clin Exp Dermatol.* 2004;29:1-7.

Ko HC, Jung DS, Jwa SW, et al. Two cases of pyodermatitis-pyostomatitis vegetans. *J Dermatol.* 2009;36:293-297.

Nico MM, Hussein TP, Aoki V, Lourenço SV. Pyostomatitis vegetans and its relation to inflammatory bowel disease, pyoderma gangrenosum, pyodermatitis vegetans, and pemphigus. *J Oral Pathol Med.* 2012;41:584-588.

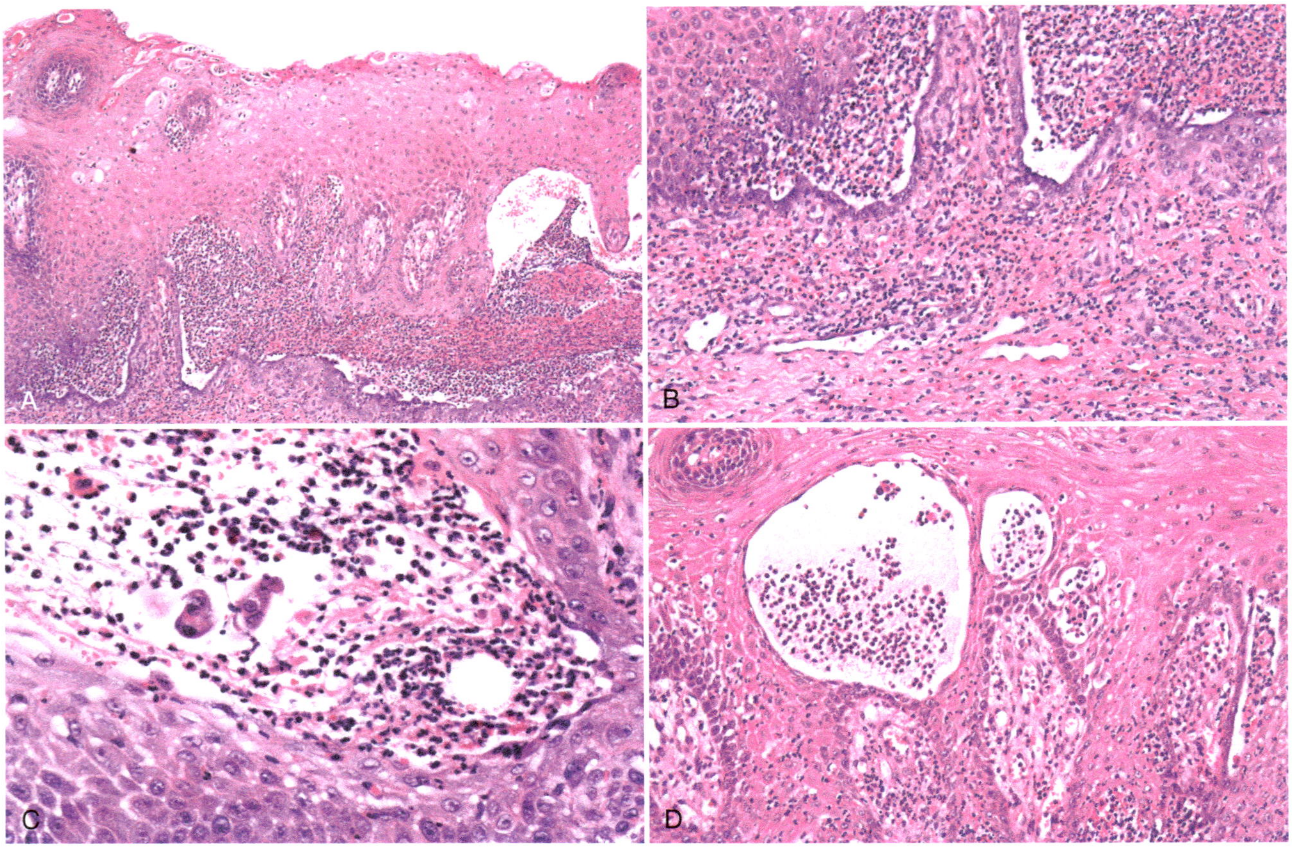

FIG 8.15 Pyostomatitis vegetans. (A) Acanthosis with suprabasilar clefting. (B) Suprabasilar clefting with eosinophils within cleft and in lamina propria. (C) Acantholytic cells and eosinophils within cleft. (D) Intraepithelial eosinophilic abscesses.

Immune-Mediated Conditions

BENIGN MIGRATORY GLOSSITIS (GEOGRAPHIC TONGUE, MIGRATORY STOMATITIS, ERYTHEMA AREATA MIGRANS)

Clinical Findings

- This occurs in 1% to 2% of the adult population, usually in the third decade of life, and with a 1.5:1 female predilection. It is a chronic relapsing-recurring condition.
- Well-demarcated, slightly depressed, erythematous depapillation of the tongue dorsum is noted, often surrounded by a raised, linear, arcuate or circinate white rim, although this rim is absent in resolving lesions (Fig. 8.16A–B). It is associated with a fissured tongue in 25% to 33% of cases. Some cases occur on the floor of the mouth, lip mucosa, or other oral sites (see Fig. 8.16C).
- There is an association with human leukocyte antigen (HLA)-Cw6 (which is also seen in psoriasis).

Etiopathogenesis and Histopathologic Features

There is a strong association with atopy (history of hay fever, eczema, asthma, or food intolerance), and some patients have concurrent psoriasis (especially pustular forms).

- There is loss of filiform papillae on the tongue dorsum with psoriasiform epithelial hyperplasia and often keratinocyte edema.
- Spongiosis and spongiotic pustules typically involve one-third to two-thirds of the thickness of the epithelium, which is a hallmark of the condition, although early or late lesions may show only superficial spongiotic pustules. A variable lymphocytic infiltrate is present, and there is vascular ectasia (Figs. 8.17 and 8.18).
- Stains for candidal hyphae are negative.

Differential Diagnosis

- Candidiasis exhibits psoriasiform epithelial hyperplasia and spongiotic pustules that are confined to the superficial two to three layers of keratinocytes. Candidal hyphae are identified with periodic acid–Schiff or methenamine silver stains.

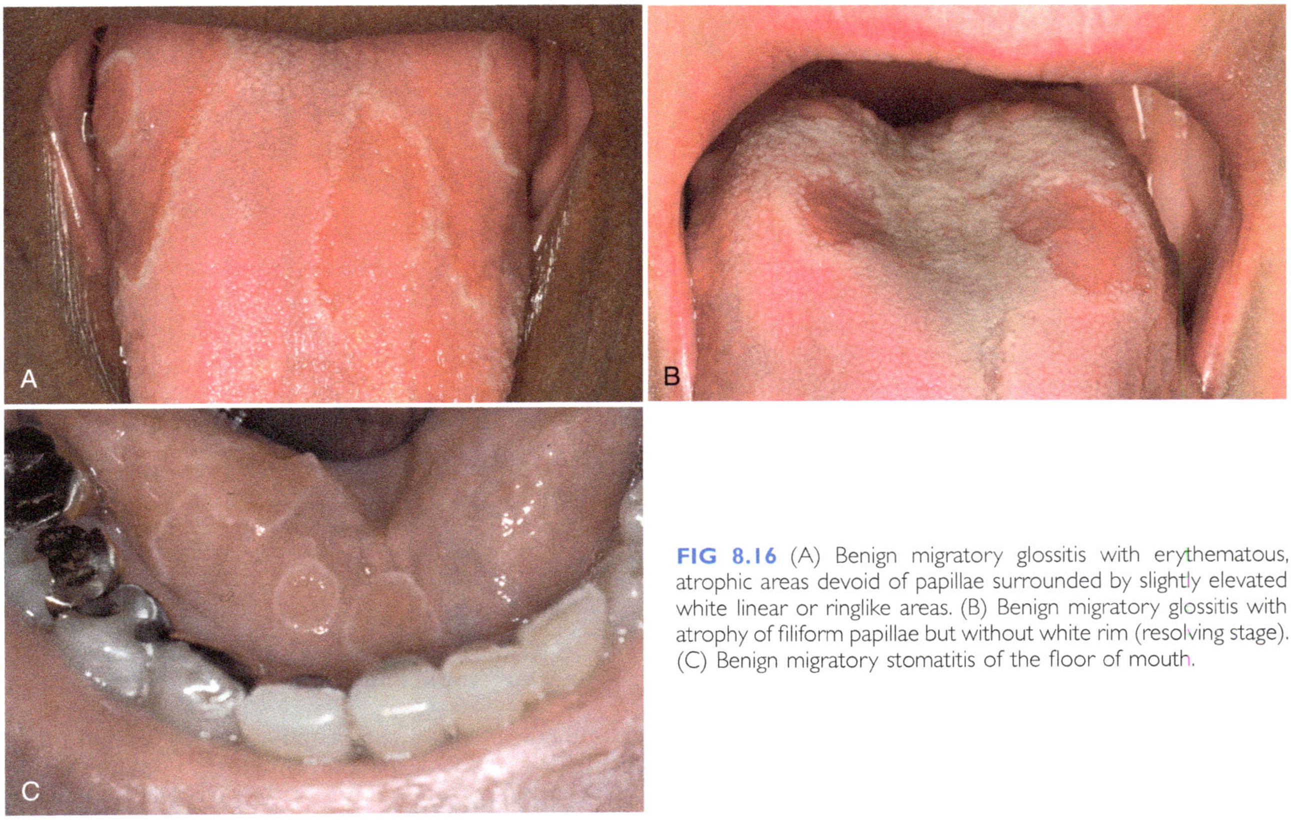

FIG 8.16 (A) Benign migratory glossitis with erythematous, atrophic areas devoid of papillae surrounded by slightly elevated white linear or ringlike areas. (B) Benign migratory glossitis with atrophy of filiform papillae but without white rim (resolving stage). (C) Benign migratory stomatitis of the floor of mouth.

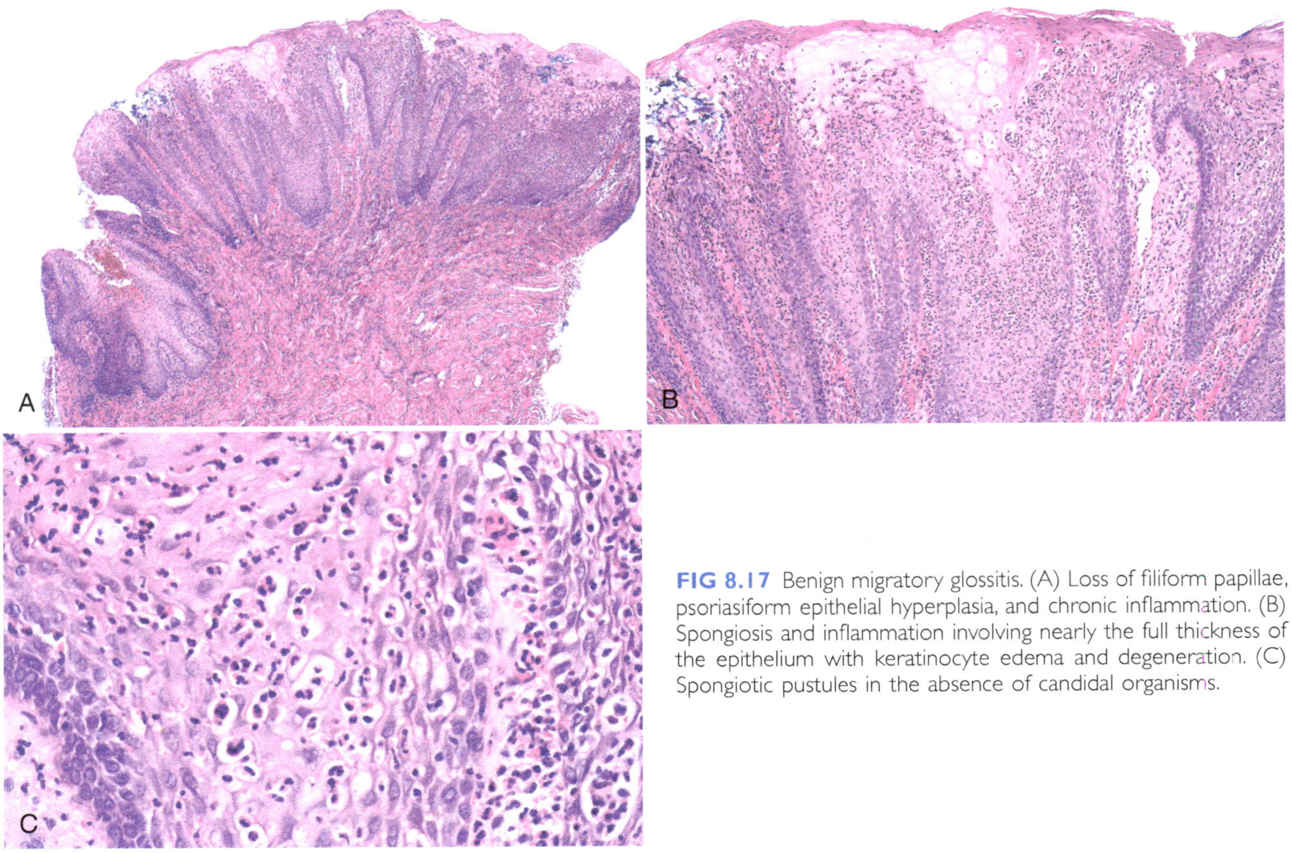

FIG 8.17 Benign migratory glossitis. (A) Loss of filiform papillae, psoriasiform epithelial hyperplasia, and chronic inflammation. (B) Spongiosis and inflammation involving nearly the full thickness of the epithelium with keratinocyte edema and degeneration. (C) Spongiotic pustules in the absence of candidal organisms.

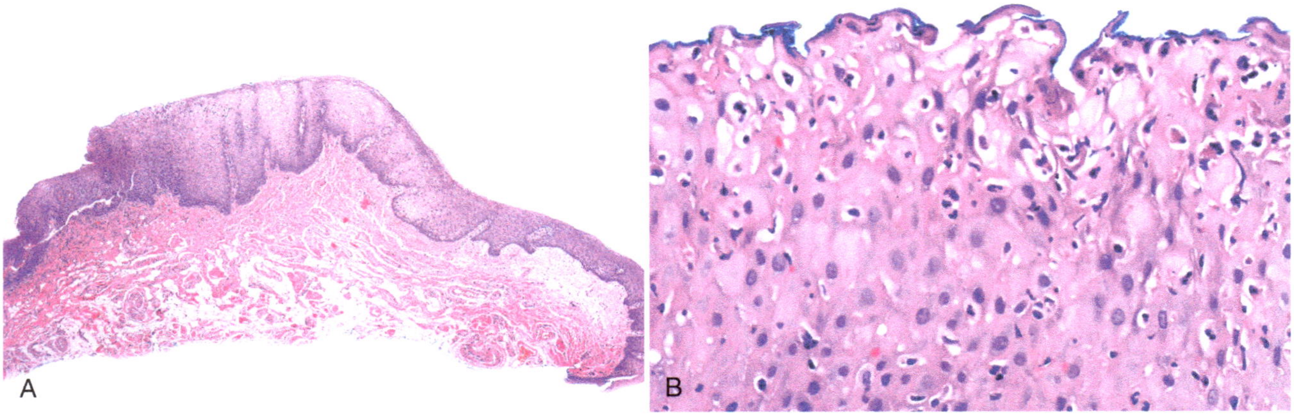

FIG 8.18 Benign migratory glossitis, likely evolving or resolving. (A) Mild acanthosis and focal inflammation. (B) Subtle spongiotic pustules.

- Spongiotic pustules are present at the edges of ulcers associated with fibrin deposition or in erosions.
- Spongiotic pustules may also be seen in irritant contact lesions (see Chapter 7).
- Oral psoriasis shares similar histopathologic features but is extremely rare.

Management and Prognosis

Management of pain and sensitivity is the primary goal because this is a chronic relapsing condition. This is achieved with viscous lidocaine and diphenhydramine used as a swish-and-spit preparation. Topical steroids are prescribed for severe cases (see Appendix A).

REFERENCES

Gonzaga HF, Torres EA, Alchorne MM, Gerbase-Delima M. Both psoriasis and benign migratory glossitis are associated with HLA-Cw6. *Br J Dermatol.* 1996;135:368-370.

Goregen M, Melikoglu M, Miloglu O, Erdem T. Predisposition of allergy in patients with benign migratory glossitis. *Oral Surg Oral Med Oral Pathol Oral Radiol Endod.* 2010;110:470-474.

Jainkittivong A, Langlais RP. Geographic tongue: clinical characteristics of 188 cases. *J Contemp Dent Pract.* 2005;6:123-135.

Marks R, Czarny D. Geographic tongue: sensitivity to the environment. *Oral Surg Oral Med Oral Pathol.* 1984;58:156-159.

Miloğlu O, Göregen M, Akgül HM, Acemoğlu H. The prevalence and risk factors associated with benign migratory glossitis lesions in 7619 Turkish dental outpatients. *Oral Surg Oral Med Oral Pathol Oral Radiol Endod.* 2009;107:e29-e33.

Zargari O. The prevalence and significance of fissured tongue and geographical tongue in psoriatic patients. *Clin Exp Dermatol.* 2006; 31:192-195.

CONTACT HYPERSENSITIVITY STOMATITIS

Clinical Findings

- This occurs in adult patients and has a female predilection. It presents as painful, erythematous, white or red-and-white lesions of the oral mucosa with symptoms coinciding with exposure.

Etiopathogenesis and Histopathologic Features

Contact hypersensitivity reactions in the mouth are a type IV hypersensitivity reaction similar to contact dermatitis. They are not to be confused with irritant contact stomatitis due to contact with a caustic agent. Some sources of these reactions include flavorings of dentifrices (especially cinnamic aldehyde and mint), dental filling materials (such as amalgams and crowns), and inadequately cured acrylic dentures (exposure to acrylic monomer, a rare phenomenon). Plasma cell gingivitis and lichenoid and granulomatous stomatitis are discussed later.

- There is spongiosis, acanthosis, variable chronic inflammation, and eosinophils in the lamina propria and epithelium (Fig. 8.19).

Differential Diagnosis

- Eosinophils and spongiosis may be seen in nonspecific inflammatory lesions.

Management and Prognosis

- Careful history-taking and patch-testing help to establish the diagnosis, and patients should avoid the inciting agent. Topical steroids help to resolve lesions (see Appendix A).

REFERENCES

Calapai G, Miroddi M, Mannucci C, et al. Oral adverse reactions due to cinnamon-flavoured chewing gums consumption. *Oral Dis.* 2014; 20:637-643.

Koutis D, Freeman S. Allergic contact stomatitis caused by acrylic monomer in a denture. *Australas J Dermatol.* 2001;42:203-206.

LeSueur BW, Yiannias JA. Contact stomatitis. *Dermatol Clin.* 2003;21:105-114.

Muris J, Goossens A, Gonçalo M, et al. Sensitization to palladium and nickel in Europe and the relationship with oral disease and dental alloys. *Contact Dermatitis.* 2015;72:286-296.

Tosti A, Piraccini BM, Peluso AM. Contact and irritant stomatitis. *Semin Cutan Med Surg.* 1997;16:314-319.

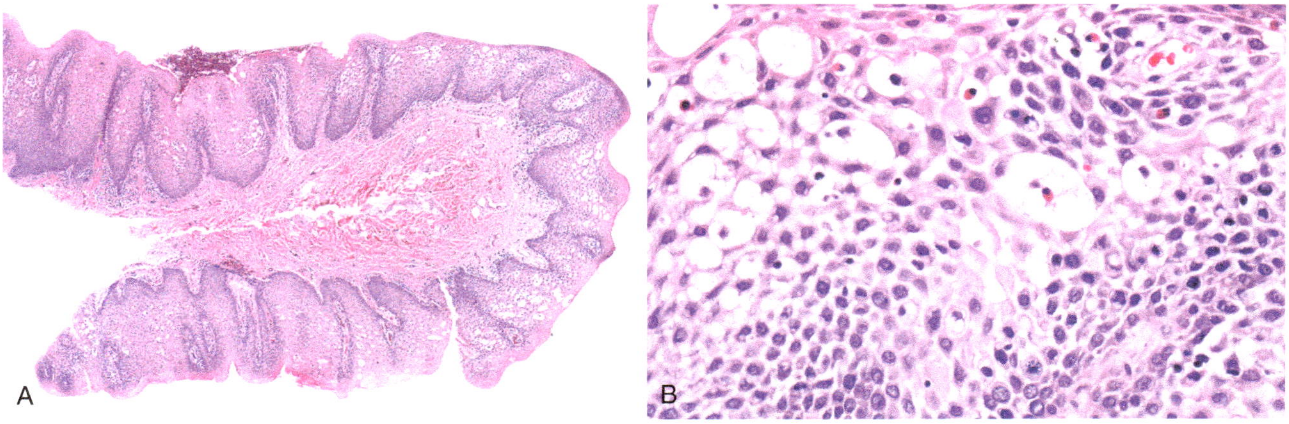

FIG 8.19 Hypersensitivity reaction. (A) Acanthosis, spongiosis, and a mild lymphocytic infiltrate in the lamina propria with eosinophils. (B) Eosinophils are present within spongiotic epithelium.

PLASMA CELL ORIFICIAL MUCOSITIS (PLASMA CELL STOMATITIS, MUCOUS MEMBRANE PLASMACYTOSIS)

Clinical Findings

- This occurs in adults, usually in the sixth decade of life, and presents as brightly erythematous, sometimes nodular gingival hyperplasia (Fig. 8.20). Other mucosal sites and the mucosa of the upper airway may be involved. Localized plaques and cobblestoning may be present, and fissuring of the corners of the mouth and swollen lips are often noted.

Etiopathogenesis and Histopathologic Features

Plasma cell mucositis represents a hypersensitivity reaction to contactants such as flavorings in chewing gum, candies, toothpaste, and mouthwash.

- There is loss of normal keratinization, acanthosis, spongiosis, leukocyte exocytosis, and an intense ("wall-to-wall") polyclonal plasma cell infiltrate within the lamina propria admixed with Russell bodies and lymphocytes (Fig. 8.21).

Differential Diagnosis

- Banal gingivitis and periodontitis are usually associated with pockets of plasma cells separated by dense fibrosis. Clinical findings are important in differentiating between these lesions.
- Plasmacytoma consists of a plasma cell proliferation with light chain restriction.

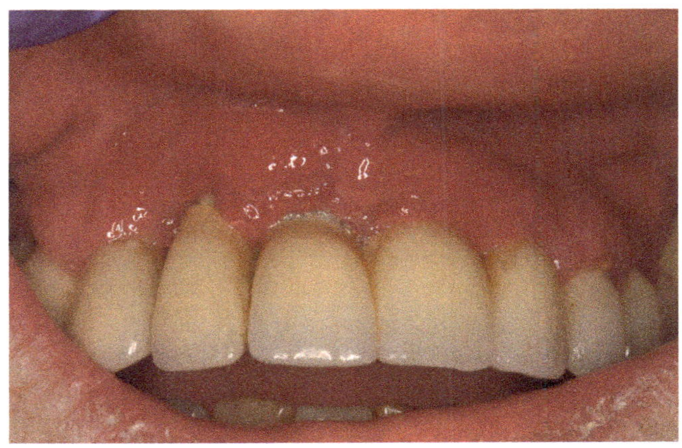

FIG 8.20 Plasma cell gingivitis manifesting as a nodular swelling and erythema of the maxillary facial gingiva.

Management and Prognosis

- Topical steroid therapy helps to resolve lesions, but these will recur if the contactant is not identified and avoided (see Appendix A).

REFERENCES

Anil S. Plasma cell gingivitis among herbal toothpaste users: a report of three cases. *J Contemp Dent Pract.* 2007;8:60-66.

Solomon LW, Wein RO, Rosenwald I, Laver N. Plasma cell mucositis of the oral cavity: report of a case and review of the literature. *Oral Surg Oral Med Oral Pathol Oral Radiol Endod.* 2008;106:853-860.

Timms MS, Sloan P. Association of supraglottic and gingival idiopathic plasmacytosis. *Oral Surg Oral Med Oral Pathol.* 1991;71:451-453.

White JW, Olsen KD, Banks PM. Plasma cell orificial mucositis: report of a case and review of the literature. *Arch Dermatol.* 1986;122:1321-1324.

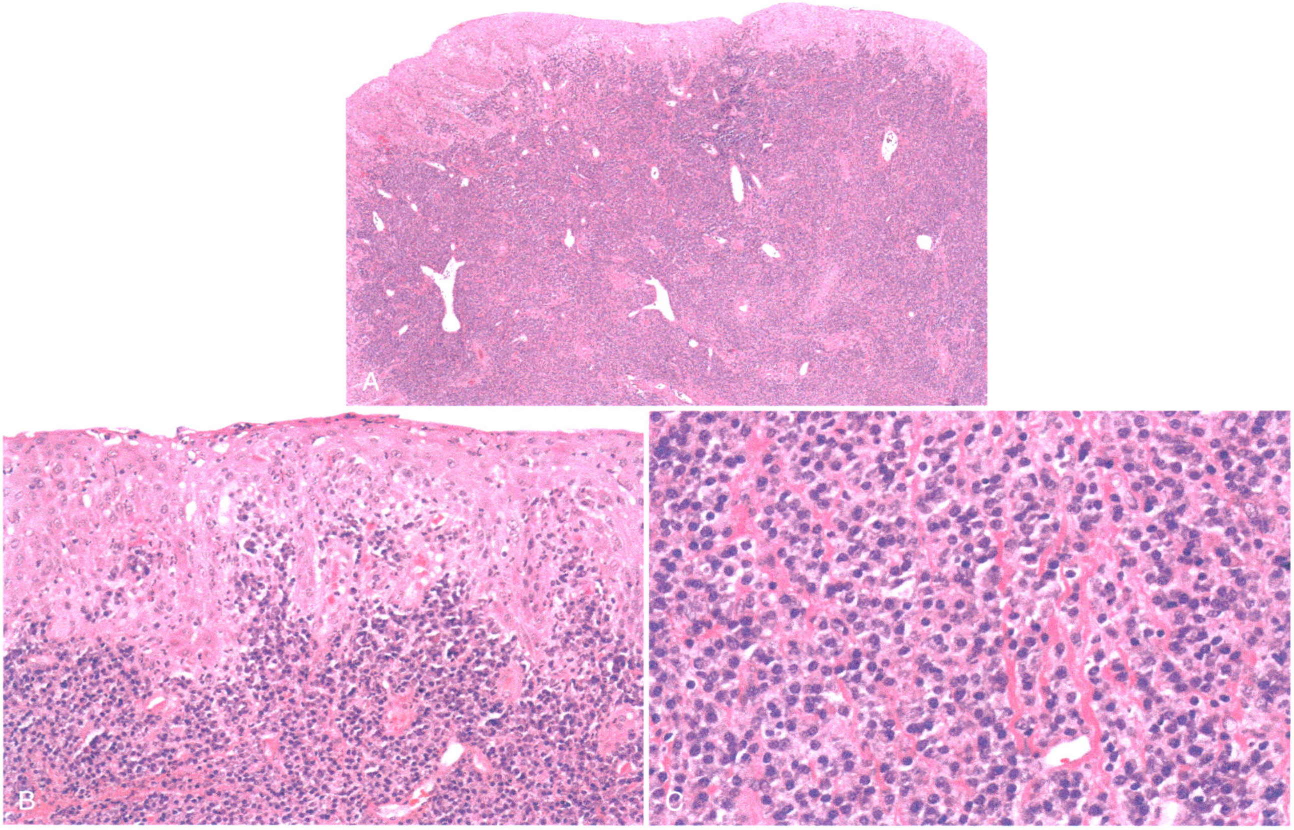

FIG 8.21 Plasma cell gingivitis. (A) Intense plasma cell infiltrate in the lamina propria, abutting the epithelium (from patient in Fig. 8.20). (B) There is loss of normal surface keratin, spongiosis, and neutrophilic exocytosis. (C) A dense polyclonal plasma cell infiltrate is present.

LICHEN PLANUS/LICHENOID MUCOSITIS

Although considered an autoimmune condition by some, the target antigen has yet to be identified. This pattern of tissue reaction is seen in many clinical situations, such as localized contact hypersensitivity reaction, idiopathic lichen planus, drug-induced lichenoid hypersensitivity reaction, oral lupus erythematosus, chronic oral graft-versus-host disease, hepatitis C virus infection, and sometimes even acute graft rejection.

Clinical Findings

- This occurs in 1% to 2% of middle-aged adults and with a 2–3:1 female predominance. Lesions are typically bilateral and symmetric.
- Three main presentations are noted, usually bilateral and often in combination:
  - *reticular/keratotic* (classic), where there are white striations or papules that are not usually painful, on the buccal mucosa, ventral and dorsal tongue, lip mucosa, and gingiva (Fig. 8.22A–B).
  - *erythematous/erosive,* where there are red, raw, sensitive, and painful areas of the mucosa, particularly on the gingiva, a condition referred to as *desquamative gingivitis* (see Fig. 8.22C–D) ruptured bullae/vesicles present in this fashion.
  - *ulcerative,* the most painful form, where yellow fibrin membranes are present (see Fig. 8.22A). Postinflammatory hyperpigmentation is noted in dark-skinned patients (see Fig. 8.22E). Lesions on the tongue result in atrophy of filiform papillae and may not be well reticulated (see Fig. 8.22F).
- Skin involvement is present in 10% to 15% of patients (see Fig. 8.22G). Genital-gingival planus and lichen planus are usually associated with the desquamative form of the condition, with buccal mucosa fibrosis occurring in a minority of patients. Cutaneous disease is associated with a higher incidence of HLA-DRB1*0101, and vulvovaginal-gingival syndrome may be associated with HLA-DQB1*0201. HLA-DR6 is seen in higher incidence in Italian patients with hepatitis C virus–associated lichen planus.
- Chronic graft-versus-host disease after allogeneic hematopoietic cell transplantation has a similar reticulated, erosive, and ulcerative appearance; however, the presence of white demarcated plaques (leukoplakia) should raise suspicion for leukoplakia or proliferative leukoplakia (see Fig. 8.22H).
- Granulomatous lichenoid mucositis tends to affect the upper lip mucosa as macular erythema, without reticulations of the buccal mucosa (see Fig. 8.22I).
- Demarcated white plaques that develop within lichen planus should always be biopsied. Well-demarcated,

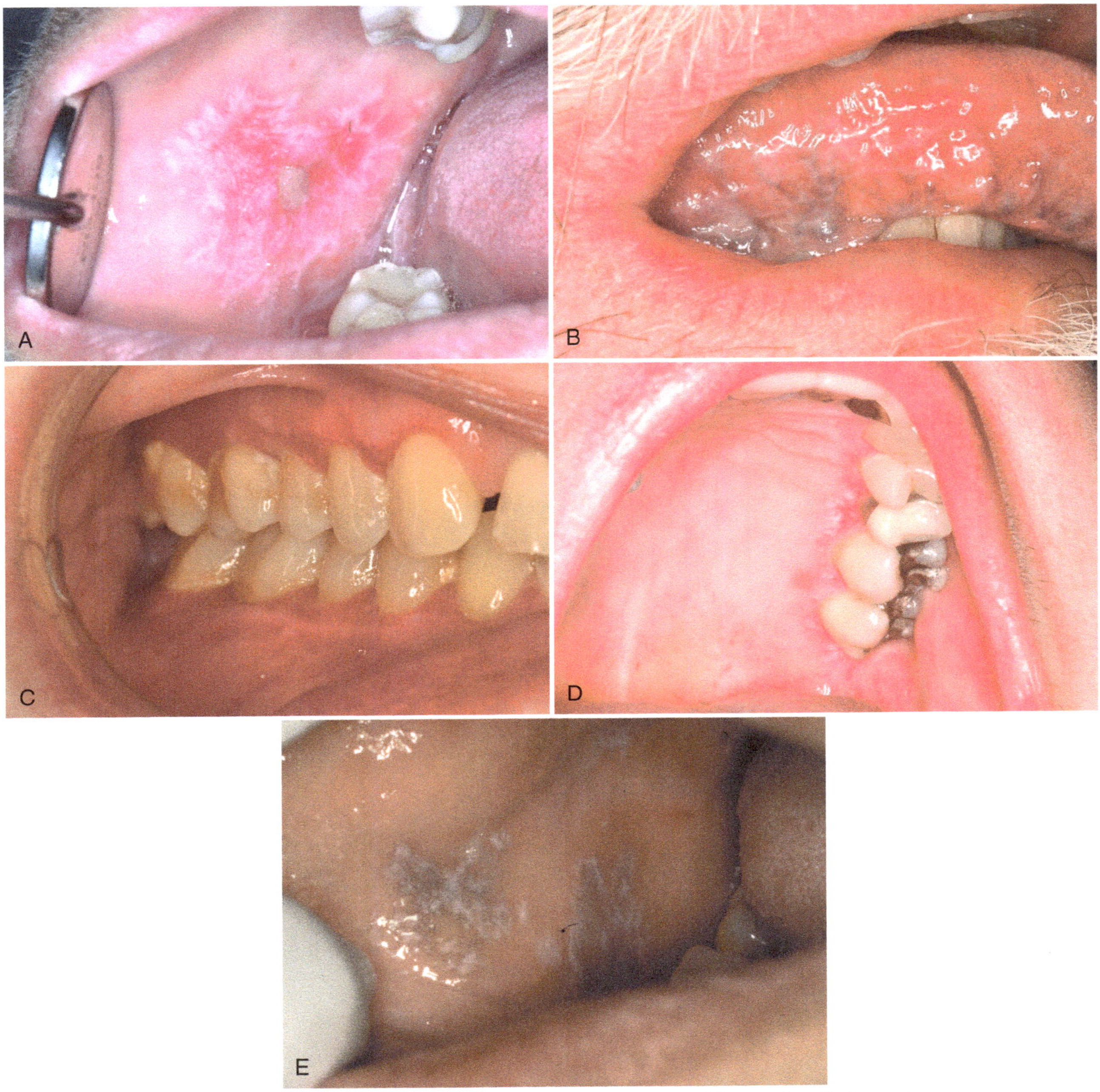

FIG 8.22 Lichen planus. (A) Reticulated, erythematous, and ulcerated (from yellow fibrin membrane) lesion. (B) Reticulated lichen planus of the ventral tongue. (C) Erythematous/erosive lichen planus presenting as diffuse desquamative gingivitis with faint reticulations on left posterior maxillary gingiva. (D) Same patient as in C with reticulated and erythematous areas of the palatal gingiva of posterior teeth. (E) Reticulatec lesion with associated postinflammatory hyperpigmentation.

Continued

unilateral white plaques, even if the histopathology shows "lichenoid mucositis," should be considered leukoplakia rather than plaque-type lichen planus, especially if at high-risk sites for dysplasia and carcinoma, such as the ventral tongue and the floor of the mouth (see Chapter 11).

Etiopathogenesis and Histopathologic Features

Lichen planus and lichenoid reactions are interface stomatitides and likely represent a final common pathway of tissue reaction. They are characterized *clinically* by reticulated or papular keratosis and variable erythema and ulceration resulting from T-cell destruction of the basal cells. Tumor necrosis factor-α plays an important role. It is not possible to distinguish by histopathology among idiopathic lichen planus, lichenoid hypersensitivity reactions related to medications (such as hydrochlorothiazide and other antihypertensive agents, carbamazepine, allopurinol, sulfasalazine, and some monoclonal antibodies), contact lichenoid reactions to dental amalgams, or lichen

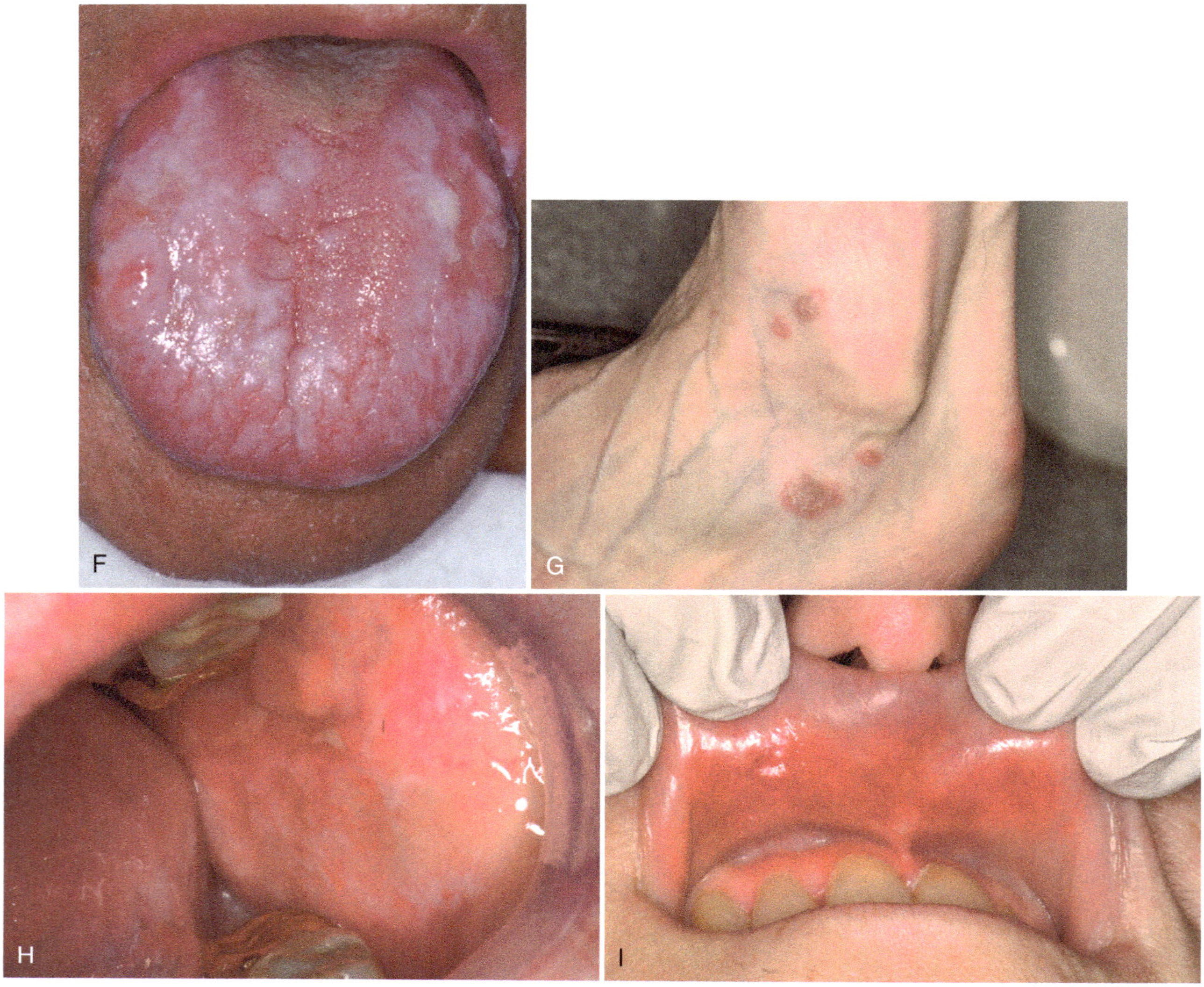

FIG 8.22, cont'd (F) Lichen planus on the tongue with nonreticulated, poorly demarcated keratotic areas, atrophy of filiform papillae, erythema, and ulceration on lateral aspects. The lips are also involved, as are other areas of the mouth. (G) Lichen planus of the skin of the foot. (H) Chronic graft-versus-host disease: reticulated, erythematous, and ulcerated lesions similar to idiopathic lichen planus. (I) Granulomatous lichenoid stomatitis: diffuse erythema of the upper lip mucosa.

planus associated with hepatitis C virus. The degree to which all histopathologic features are present depends on the stage of the lesion, whether the lesion has been treated, and the site of biopsy of these heterogeneous lesions, with the ulcerative areas being the least specific for the diagnosis.

- The two most important criteria are degeneration and loss (squamatization) of the basal cell layer and a lymphocytic band of variable thickness at the interface, often with blurring of the interface, although the interface may be accentuated with thickening of the basement membrane zone. Subepithelial clefting is a reliable artifact and is caused by lack of basal cell adhesion to the lamina propria rather than necessarily representing a clinical blister. Lesions may be parakeratotic or hyper(ortho)keratotic, and epithelium may be acanthotic or atrophic (Figs. 8.23–8.26).
- There is variable spongiosis, leukocyte exocytosis, colloid (Civatte or cytoid) body formation, sawtooth rete ridges, postinflammatory hypermelanosis, and increased numbers of Langerhans cells. Involvement of salivary ducts by inflammation may result in superficial mucoceles (Fig. 8.27).
- Plasma cells may be conspicuous in gingival lesions or if an ulcer is present. Eosinophils may be seen, and a hypersensitivity reaction should be considered if present in large numbers, especially if within the epithelium (Fig. 8.25B).
- Direct immunofluorescence studies show linear or shaggy fibrinogen deposition in a stalactite pattern at the basement membrane zone, as well as IgM positivity of colloid bodies and basement membrane zone (Fig. 8.28). Nonspecific granular (not linear) C3 deposition may be seen.
- A particular contact lichenoid hypersensitivity reaction is cinnamic aldehyde–associated lichenoid mucositis characterized by a dense lymphocytic infiltrate admixed with many macrophages at the interface and nodular peri- and paravascular lymphoid aggregates (these

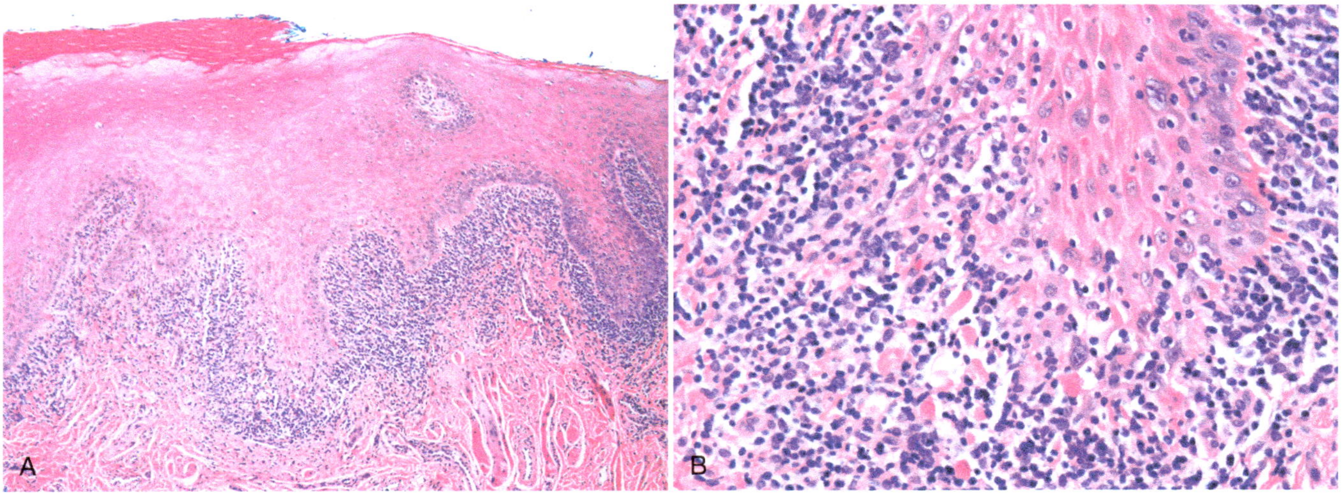

FIG 8.23 Lichen planus. (A) Parakeratosis, acanthosis, squamatized basal layer, thickened basement membrane zone, and lymphocytic band at the interface. (B) Squamatized basal cells with blurring of the interface and many colloid bodies.

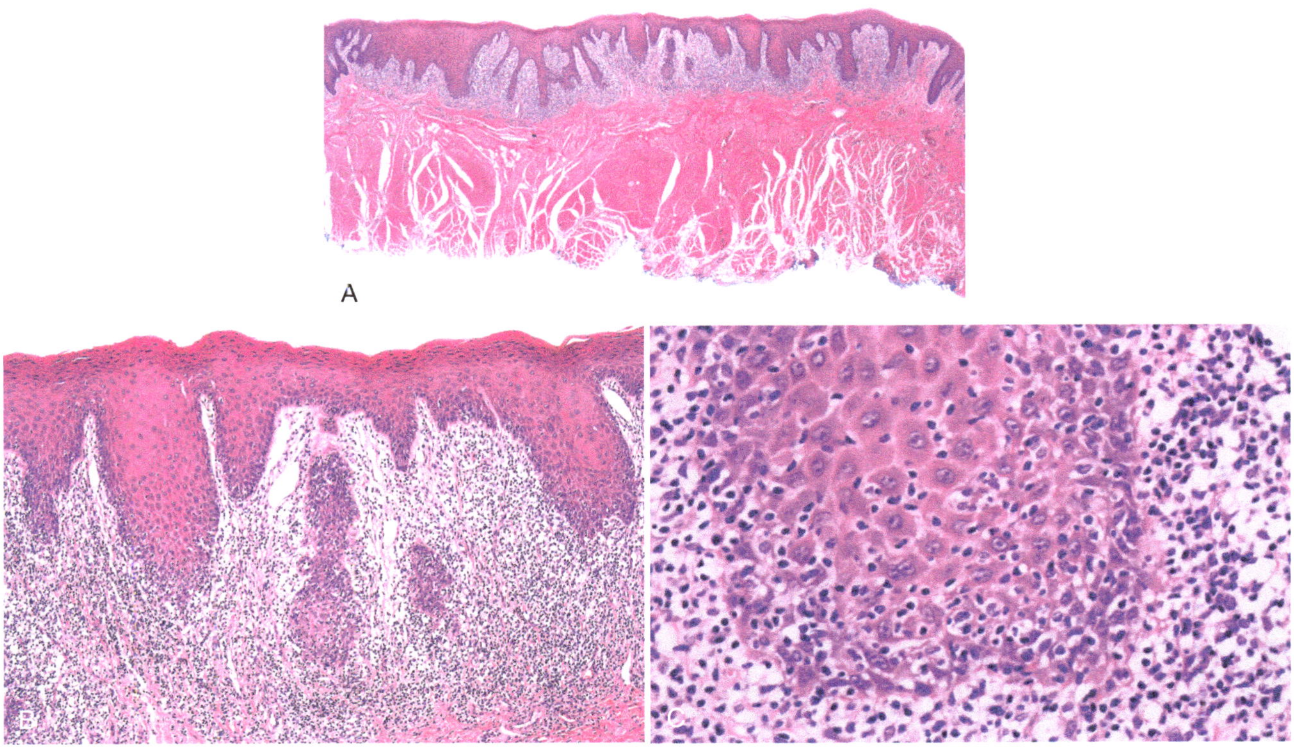

FIG 8.24 Lichen planus of tongue dorsum. (A) Atrophy of filiform papillae, acanthosis, tapered rete ridges, and a lymphocytic band. (B) Parakeratosis, leukocyte exocytosis, and lymphocytic band at the interface. (C) Squamatized (degenerated) basal cells without colloid bodies.

should not be interpreted as vasculitis). The keratin layer is often lost, and the basal cell layer may be intact or squamatized (Fig. 8.29). Other contactants are likely to cause a similar tissue reaction.

- Granulomatous lichenoid lesions (on the lip mucosa, especially the upper lip) exhibit many macrophages in the lamina propria, or even well-formed granulomas (Figs. 8.30 and 8.31). These are likely to represent contact hypersensitivity reactions, and a careful history-taking will help to elicit the offending agent. Etiopathogenetically, these are likely related to cinnamic aldehye–associated lichenoid mucositis.
- The terms *lichenoid stomatitis* and *mucositis* are often used if not all of the features are seen or if they are subtle. It is unclear if such lesions represent waxing or waning otherwise classic lichen planus or whether they may be a result of therapy (Fig. 8.32). Sometimes the phrase "lichenoid mucositis consistent with lichen

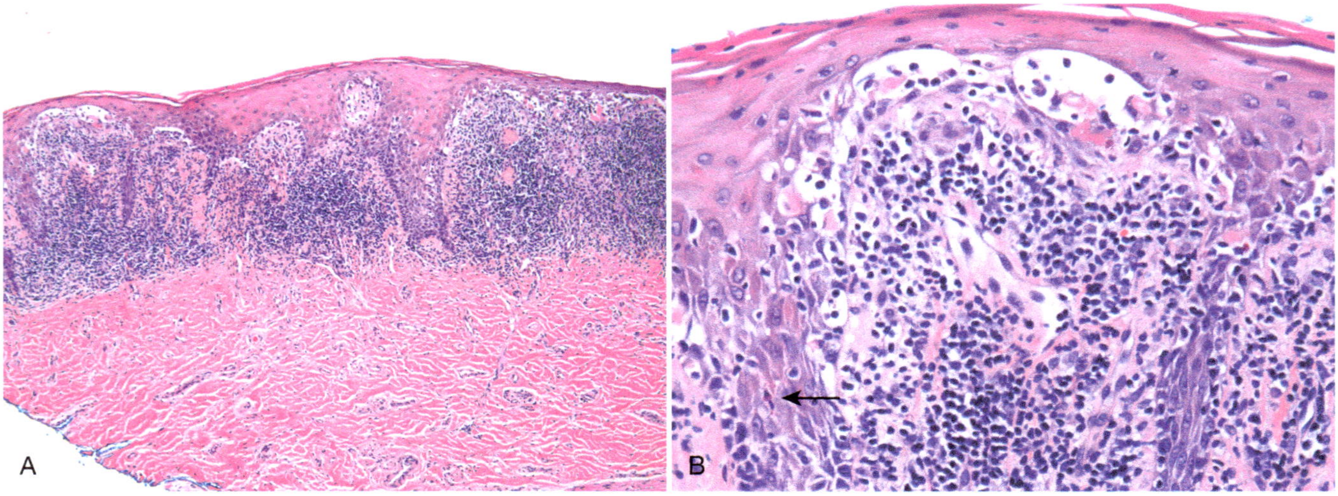

FIG 8.25 Gingival lichen planus, likely drug-induced. (A) Parakeratosis epithelial atrophy, saw-tooth rete ridges, subepithelial clefting, and lymphocytic infiltrate. (B) Epithelial atrophy, squamatization of basal cells with subepithelial clefting, many colloid bodies, and rare eosinophil in the epithelium (*arrow*).

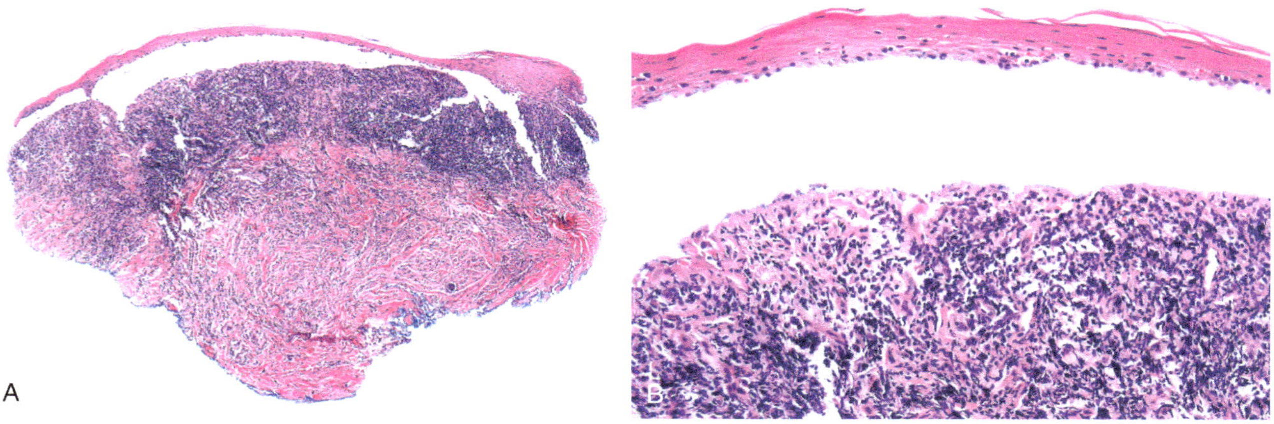

FIG 8.26 Gingival lichen planus. (A) Epithelial atrophy, subepithelial cleft, and lymphoplasmacytic band. (B) Squamatization of basal cells leads to subepithelial cleft.

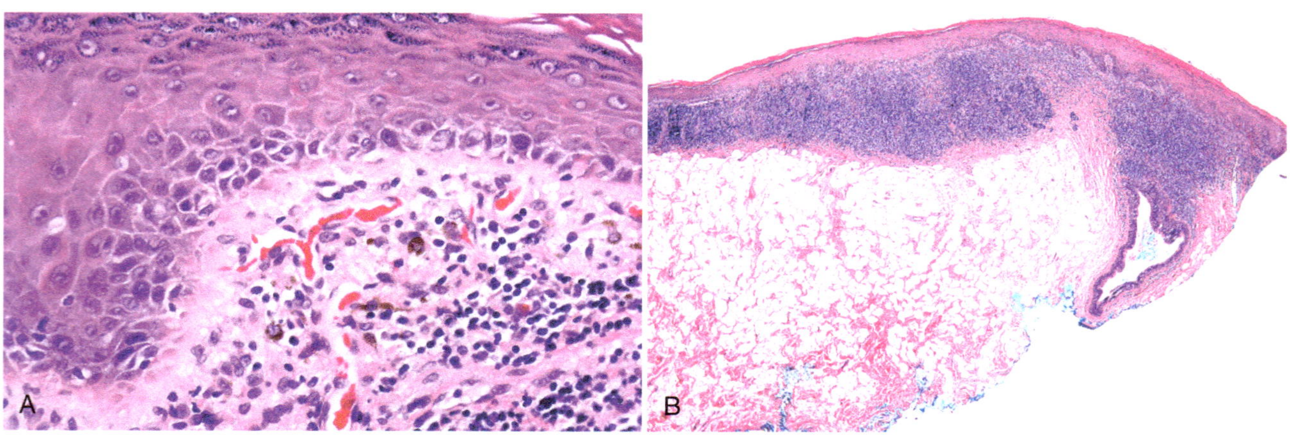

FIG 8.27 (A) Lichen planus with incontinent melanin and melanophages (postinflammatory hypermelanosis). (B) Lichen planus involving an excretory salivary duct.

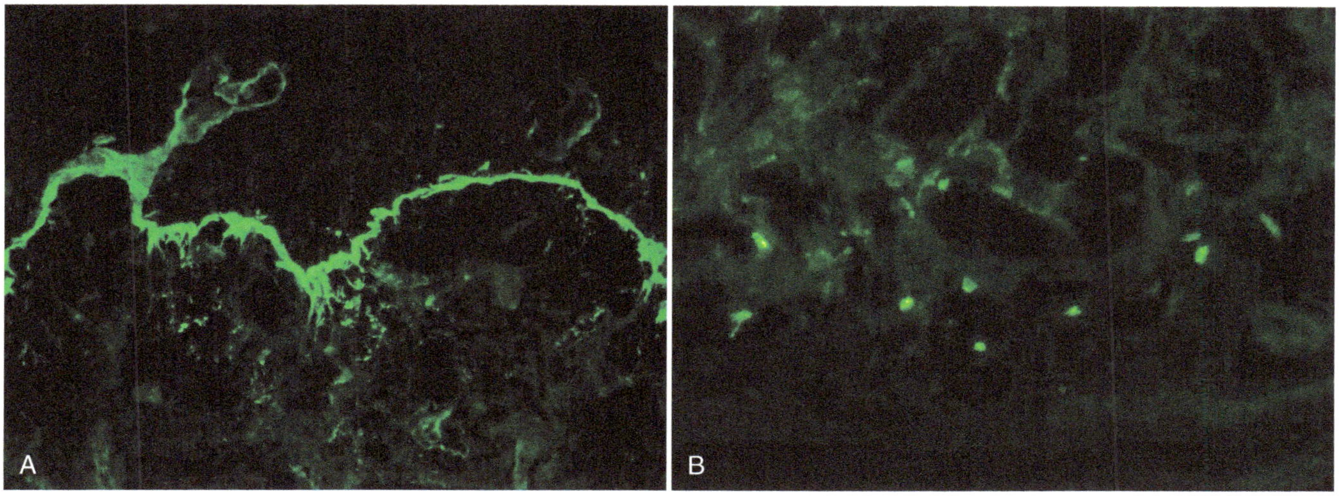

FIG 8.28 Lichen planus: direct immunofluorescence study. (A) Linear or shaggy deposits of fibrinogen at the basement membrane zone. (B) Immunoglobulin M staining of colloid bodies.

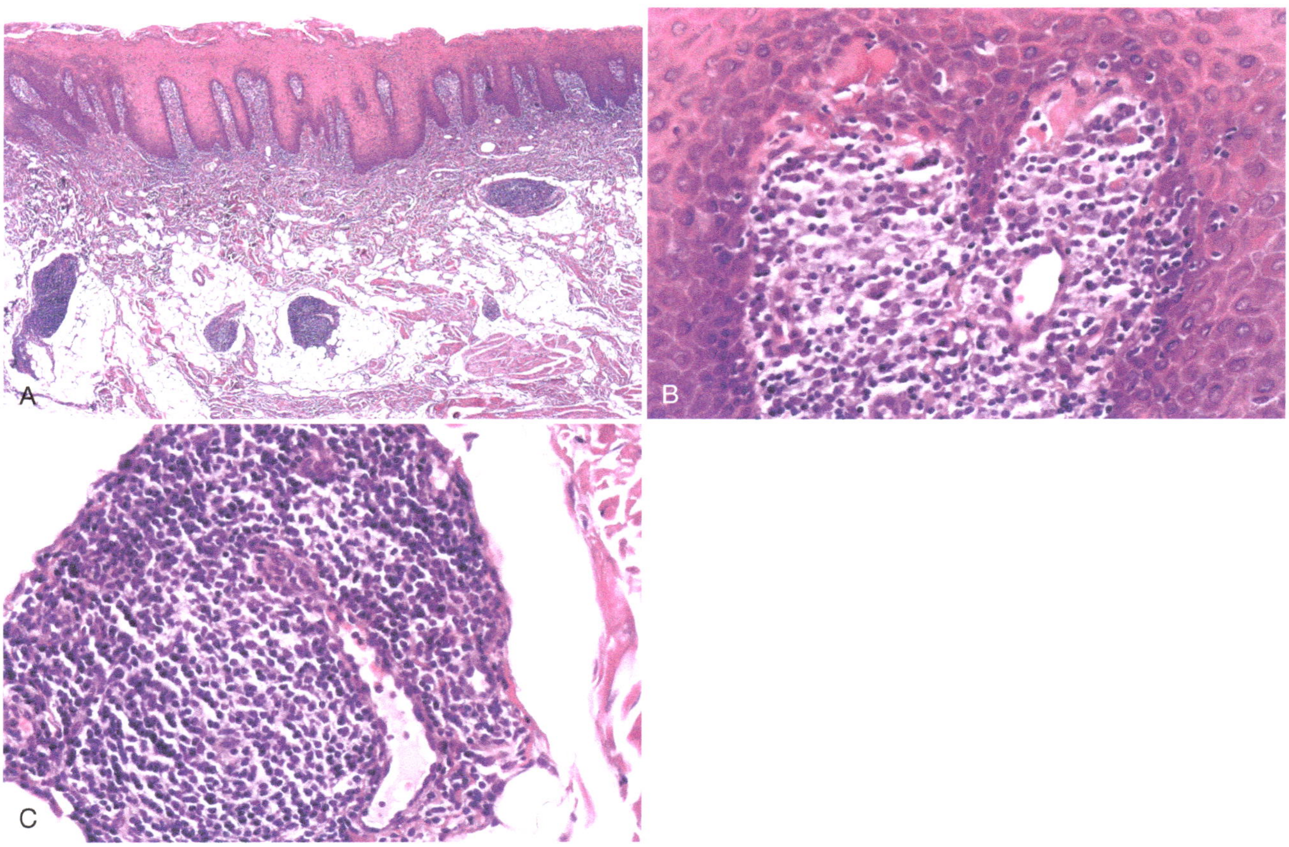

FIG 8.29 Cinnamic aldehyde–associated lichenoid mucositis. (A) Acanthosis, preservation of basal cells, with a mild lymphocytic band at the interface, and nodular peri- and paravascular lymphoid nodules. (B) Squamatized basal cells, colloid bodies, and lymphocytic infiltrate with many macrophages. (C) Peri- and paravascular lymphocytic infiltrate.

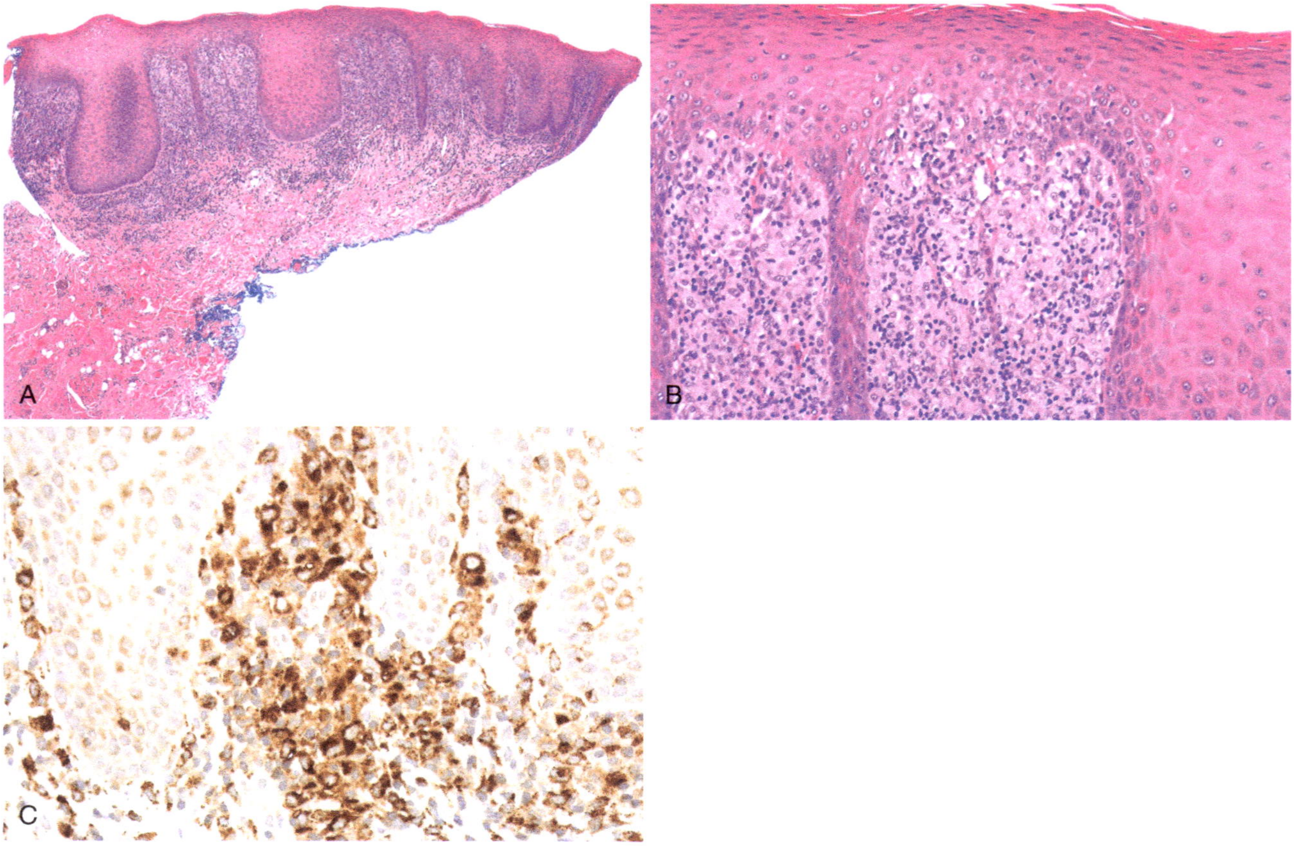

FIG 8.30 Lichenoid mucositis with prominent granulomatous inflammation. (A) Parakeratosis, acanthosis, and many macrophages and lymphocytes band at the interface. (B) Squamatized basal cells and sheets of activated macrophages in the lamina propria. (C) Macrophages are positive for CD68.

planus in the appropriate clinical context" is used because correlation with clinical findings is essential in arriving at the correct diagnosis.

Differential Diagnosis

- Epithelial dysplasia (and carcinoma) frequently exhibits a lymphocytic band at the interface (T-cell response to dysplastic keratinocytes) associated with hyperplasia (not loss) of the basal cell layer (see Chapter 11). Use of the term *lichenoid dysplasia* suggests dysplastic transformation of a preexisting lichen planus and should be avoided.
- Chronic graft-versus-host disease has muted features of lichen planus. The lymphocytic band is variable and may be sparse because of immunosuppression (Fig. 8.33). Patients with this condition have a high risk of developing oral dysplasia and squamous cell carcinoma as a result of prolonged immunosuppression, although high epithelial cell turnover due to mucosal injury may also be a contributing factor.
- Orofacial granulomatosis, unlike lichenoid and granulomatous mucositis, does not exhibit peri- and paravascular nodular lymphocytic infiltrates.
- Lupus erythematosus shows hydropic degeneration of basal cells, alternating epithelial atrophy and hyperplasia, a lymphocytic band at the interface, and linear IgG or other immunoglobulin at the interface on direct immunofluorescence (lupus band test).
- Mucous membrane pemphigoid exhibits preservation of the basal cells (see later).
- Chronic ulcerative stomatitis (a condition that histologically and clinically resembles erosive lichen planus) exhibits antibodies directed against δNp63α, an isoform of p63 in the nucleus of epithelial cells. Direct immunofluorescence studies using monkey esophagus show speckled nuclear staining. Indirect immunofluorescence using guinea pig esophagus demonstrates nuclear reactivity.
- Rare cases of lichen planus pemphigoides have been reported, possibly resulting from epitope spread.
- Lichen sclerosus et atrophicus is a white fibrotic area of the oral mucosa that exhibits marked hyalinization and sclerosis of the lamina propria and a lymphocytic band in the deep lamina propria.

Management and Prognosis

- Management of symptomatic lesions is with episodic topical anti-inflammatory therapy (see Appendix A). Systemic therapy includes prednisone, hydroxychloroquine, azathioprine, and tumor necrosis factor-α inhibitors. More recently, mycophenolate mofetil has also been efficacious.

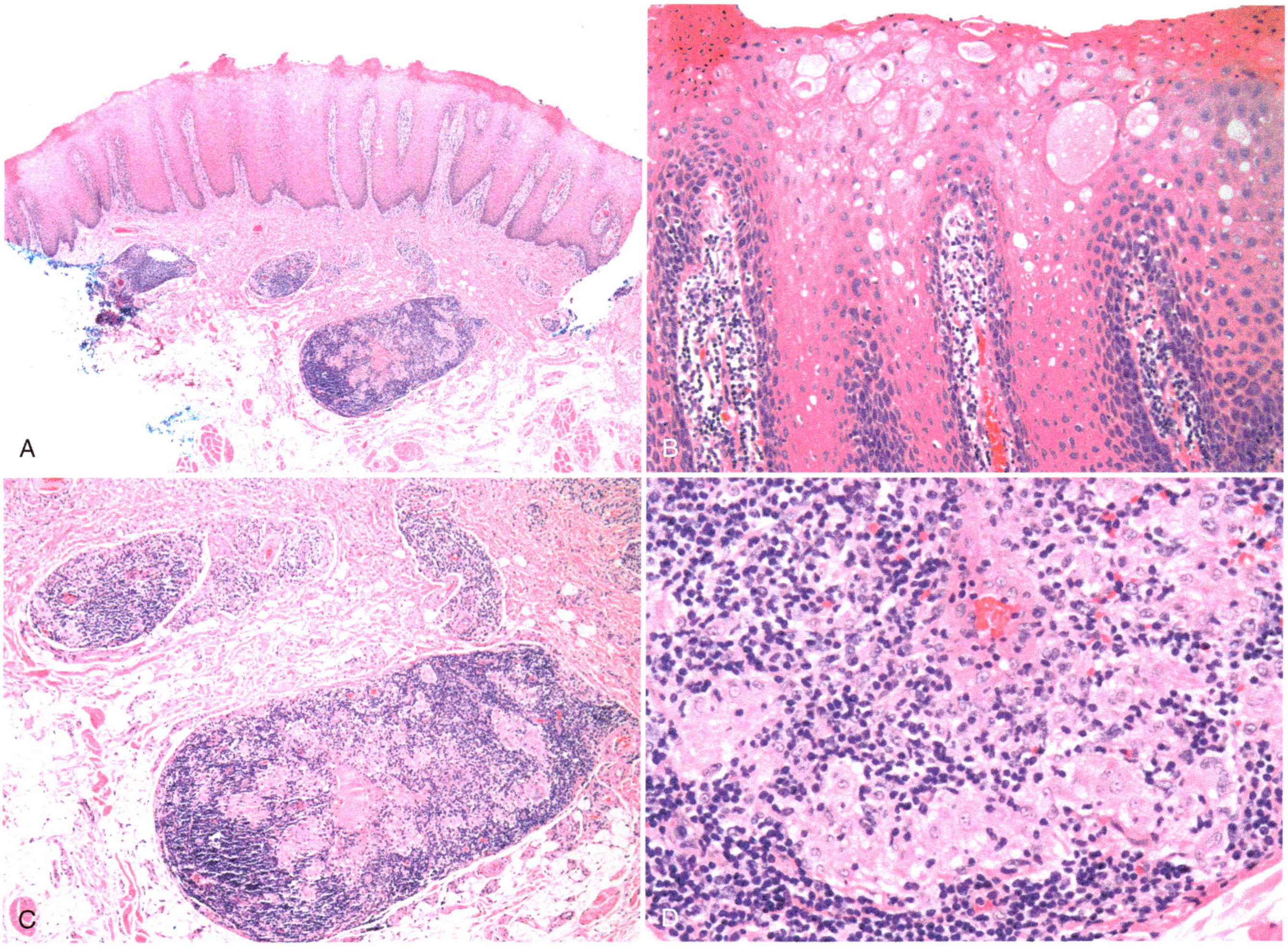

FIG 8.31 Lichenoid granulomatous mucositis of the upper lip mucosa from chronic contact with nicotine gum. (A) Parakeratosis, acanthosis, chronic inflammation, and peri- and paravascular lymphoid nodules. (B) Parakeratosis, plasma pooling, acanthosis, and chronic inflammation. (C) Peri- and paravascular lymphoid nodules with granulomas. (D) Non-necrotizing granulomatous inflammation.

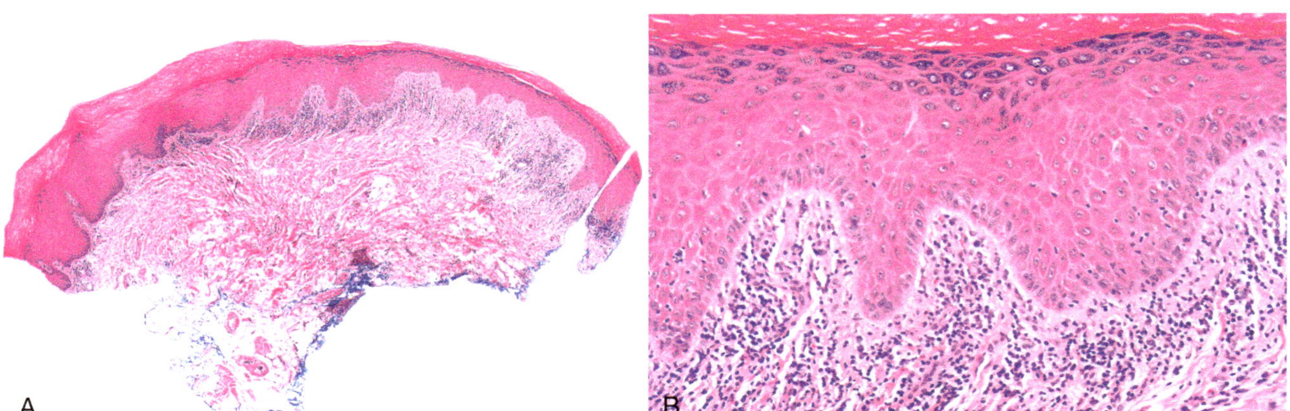

FIG 8.32 Lichenoid mucositis. (A) Hyperkeratosis of variable thickness, sawtooth rete ridges, and mild to moderate lymphocytic infiltrate; likely a waxing or waning lichen planus. (B) Mild leukocyte exocytosis, and a lymphocytic band at the interface.

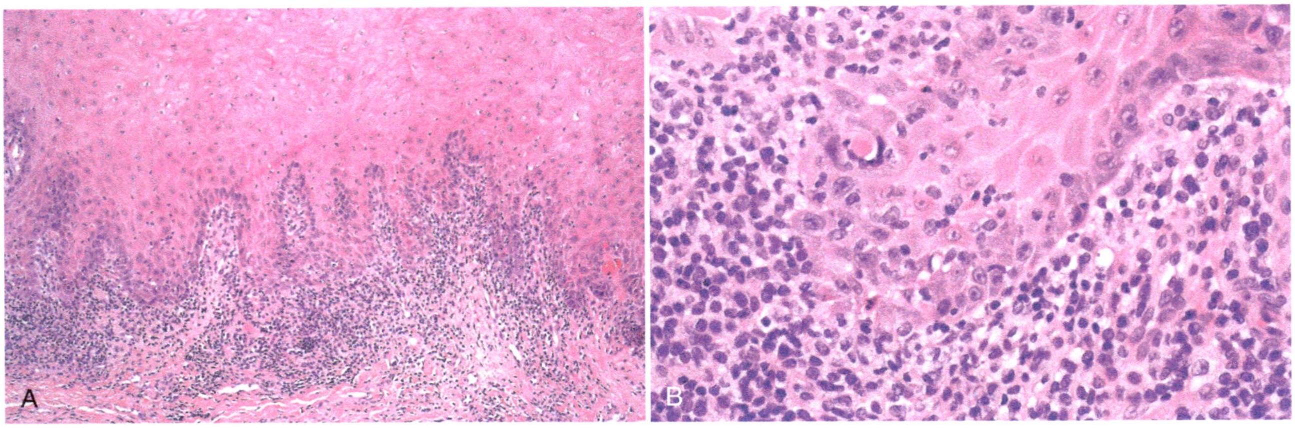

FIG 8.33 Chronic graft-versus-host disease. (A) Oral mucosa with bandlike lymphocytic infiltrate at interface. (B) Degeneration/squamatization of basal cells with colloid body and interface lymphocytic infiltrate.

- Changing putative triggering medications may not be helpful, because patients require control of systemic diseases and it is more practical to treat symptomatic oral disease.
- Replacing amalgam restorations in patients with demonstrated hypersensitivity to amalgams resolves lesions.
- Bona fide malignant transformation of lichen planus occurs in 0.1% to 1.0% of cases, with some researchers citing a much higher rate. Controversy regarding the frequency of malignant transformation revolves around two issues: (1) the concept of solitary, plaque-type lichen planus that may represent leukoplakia, which has a high risk for developing dysplasia and carcinoma; and (2) the use of the term *lichenoid dysplasia* for dysplastic leukoplakias.

REFERENCES

Al-Hashimi I, Schifter M, Lockhart PB, et al. Oral lichen planus and oral lichenoid lesions: diagnostic and therapeutic considerations. *Oral Surg Oral Med Oral Pathol Oral Radiol Endod.* 2007;103(suppl):S25. e1-e12.

Asarch A, Gottlieb AB, Lee J, et al. Lichen planus–like eruptions: an emerging side effect of tumor necrosis factor-alpha antagonists. *J Am Acad Dermatol.* 2009;61:104-111.

Azevedo RS, Romanach MJ, de Almeida OP, et al. Lichen sclerosus of the oral mucosa: clinicopathological features of six cases. *Int J Oral Maxillofac Surg.* 2009;38:855-860.

Carrozzo M, Brancatello F, Dametto E, et al. Hepatitis C virus–associated oral lichen planus: is the geographical heterogeneity related to HLA-DR6? *J Oral Pathol Med.* 2005;34:204-208.

Kimkong I, Hirankarn N, Nakkuntod J, Kitkumthorn N. Tumour necrosis factor-α gene polymorphisms and susceptibility to oral lichen planus. *Oral Dis.* 2011;17:206-209.

Kulthanan K, Jiamton S, Varothai S, et al. Direct immunofluorescence study in patients with lichen planus. *Int J Dermatol.* 2007;46: 1237-1241.

Lodi G, Scully C, Carrozzo M, et al. Current controversies in oral lichen planus: report of an international consensus meeting. Part 1. Viral infections and etiopathogenesis. *Oral Surg Oral Med Oral Pathol Oral Radiol Endod.* 2005;100:40-51.

Mawardi H, Elad S, Correa ME, et al. Oral epithelial dysplasia and squamous cell carcinoma following allogeneic hematopoietic stem cell transplantation: clinical presentation and treatment outcomes. *Bone Marrow Transplant.* 2011;46:884-891.

Qari H, Villasante C, Richert J, et al. The diagnostic challenges of separating chronic ulcerative stomatitis from oral lichen planus. *Oral Surg Oral Med Oral Pathol Oral Radiol.* 2015;120:622-627.

Sciubba JJ. Autoimmune oral mucosal diseases: clinical, etiologic, diagnostic, and treatment considerations. *Dent Clin North Am.* 2011;55: 89-103.

Scully C, Carrozzo M. Oral mucosal disease: lichen planus. *Br J Oral Maxillofac Surg.* 2008;46:15-21.

Setterfield JF, Neill S, Shirlaw PJ, et al. The vulvovaginal gingival syndrome: a severe subgroup of lichen planus with characteristic clinical features and a novel association with the class II HLA DQB1*0201 allele. *J Am Acad Dermatol.* 2006;55:98-113.

Solomon LW. Chronic ulcerative stomatitis. *Oral Dis.* 2008;14:383-389.

Sultan A, Stojanov IJ, Lerman MA, et al. Oral lichen planus pemphigoides: a series of four cases. *Oral Surg Oral Med Oral Pathol Oral Radiol.* 2015;120:58-68.

Thornhill MH, Sankar V, Xu XJ, et al. The role of histopathological characteristics in distinguishing amalgam-associated oral lichenoid reactions and oral lichen planus. *J Oral Pathol Med.* 2006;35: 233-240.

van der Meij EH, Mast H, van der Waal I. The possible premalignant character of oral lichen planus and oral lichenoid lesions: a prospective five-year follow-up study of 192 patients. *Oral Oncol.* 2007;43: 742-748.

Wee JS, Shirlaw PJ, Challacombe SJ, Setterfield JF. Efficacy of mycophenolate mofetil in severe mucocutaneous lichen planus: a retrospective review of 10 patients. *Br J Dermatol.* 2012;167:36-43.

ERYTHEMA MULTIFORME

Erythema multiforme is an acute, self-limited, inflammatory mucocutaneous disease that manifests on the skin. It often involves the oral, ocular, and genital mucosa. It is no longer considered within the spectrum of the necrolytic diseases, namely Stevens-Johnson syndrome and toxic epidermal necrolysis, that represent hypersensitivity reactions mainly to medications and have a different clinical presentation. These latter two will not be discussed here, because they are generally diagnosed on the basis of skin and not oral biopsies.

Clinical Findings

- This affects adults between 20 and 40 years of age; 20% of cases occur in children. There is a history of infection, especially herpes simplex virus infection or *Mycoplasma pneumoniae* infection, several days or weeks earlier.
- Patients develop pruritic red papules on the face, neck, and extremities that progress centripetally toward

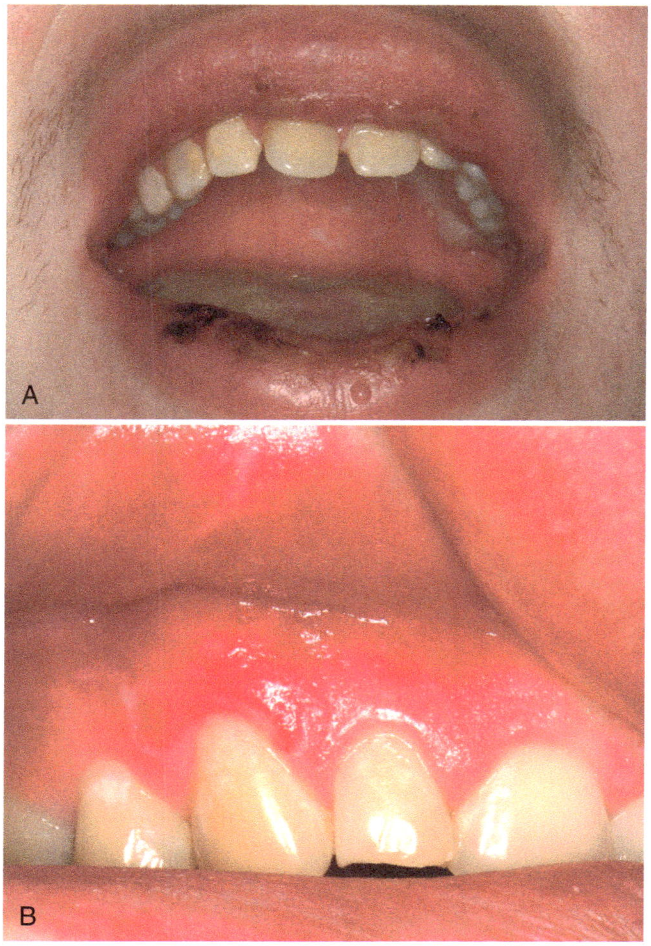

FIG 8.34 Recurrent oral erythema multiforme secondary to recurrent herpes simplex virus infection. (A) Ulcers of upper lip and palatal mucosa, and hemorrhagic crusts on lips. (B) Erythema and ulcers on the gingiva and lip mucosa. *(Courtesy Dr. Nathaniel Treister, Harvard School of Dental Medicine, Boston, Mass.)*

the trunk over days with postinflammatory hyperpigmentation. Ringlike "target" or "iris" lesions are typical.

- Oral lesions are noted in 25% to 70% of patients. There is diffuse, painful erythema and/or solitary and, more often, coalescent ulcers affecting the mucosa at multiple sites. Hemorrhagic crusts may be present on the vermilion (Fig. 8.34). Episodes may be single or recurrent.
- *Minor type:* Less than 10% of the skin is affected with little to no mucous membranes affected
- *Major type:* There is more extensive skin involvement with mucous membranes affected.
- *Chronic recurrent oral erythema multiforme:* This affects the oral mucosa only and not the skin.

Etiopathogenesis and Histopathologic Features

Erythema multiforme is a hypersensitivity reaction, mostly to herpes simplex virus (in at least 70% of cases) or *Mycoplasma pneumoniae* infection in children, although some of the latter cases have been classified as Stevens-Johnson syndrome or are considered a separate, distinct entity. Less often, cases result from reactions to nonsteroidal anti-inflammatory drugs, anticonvulsants, or benzoic acid.

- The epithelium exhibits spongiosis, leukocyte exocytosis, keratinocyte apoptosis and necrosis, hydropic degeneration of the basal cells, and sometimes subepithelial bulla formation, although these features vary depending on the stage of the lesion. The hallmark in skin biopsies is lymphocyte satellitosis around necrotic keratinocytes. A variable lymphohistiocytic infiltrate appears in the lamina propria and around vessels, and a variable number of eosinophils are present within the epithelium and in the lamina propria (Fig. 8.35). Often, however, the findings are nonspecific but rule out a primary autoimmune vesiculobullous disorder, and the diagnosis is made on the basis of clinical findings.
- Elevated serum IgM levels and high levels of IgG to herpes simplex virus are supportive of the etiopathogenesis, and negative IgG rules out herpes simplex virus as an etiologic agent. Because this is a hypersensitivity reaction to herpes simplex virus, cultures are usually negative for the virus, although shedding of the virus in damaged tissue may occur.

Differential Diagnosis

- Lichen planus and contact lichenoid hypersensitivity reactions may appear similar and are differentiated by the history and clinical findings.

Management and Prognosis

- Mild disease is managed with supportive care and systemic or topical analgesics for pain because the condition is self-limiting and resolves within a few weeks. More severe cases are usually managed with systemic and topical corticosteroids (see Appendix A) or other systemic immunosuppressive agents.
- Treatment with prophylactic acyclovir or valacyclovir prevents recurrent disease and helps to establish the diagnosis.

REFERENCES

Auquier-Dunant A, Mockenhaupt M, Naldi L, et al. Correlations between clinical patterns and causes of erythema multiforme majus, Stevens-Johnson syndrome, and toxic epidermal necrolysis: results of an international prospective study. *Arch Dermatol.* 2002;138:1019-1024.

Buchner A, Lozada F, Silverman S Jr. Histopathologic spectrum of oral erythema multiforme. *Oral Surg Oral Med Oral Pathol.* 1980;49:221-228.

Canavan TN, Mathes EF, Frieden I, Shinkai K. *Mycoplasma pneumoniae*–induced rash and mucositis as a syndrome distinct from Stevens-Johnson syndrome and erythema multiforme: a systematic review. *J Am Acad Dermatol.* 2015;72:239-245.

Farthing P, Bagan JV, Scully C. Mucosal disease series. Number IV. Erythema multiforme. *Oral Dis.* 2005;11:261-267.

Lewis MA, Lamey PJ, Forsyth A, Gall J. Recurrent erythema multiforme: a possible role of foodstuffs. *Br Dent J.* 1989;166:371-373.

Sanchis JM, Bagan JV, Gavalda C, et al. Erythema multiforme: diagnosis, clinical manifestations and treatment in a retrospective study of 22 patients. *J Oral Pathol Med.* 2010;39:747-752.

Sokumbi O, Wetter DA. Clinical features, diagnosis, and treatment of erythema multiforme: a review for the practicing dermatologist. *Int J Dermatol.* 2012;51:889-902.

Sun Y, Chan RK, Tan SH, Ng PP. Detection and genotyping of human herpes simplex viruses in cutaneous lesions of erythema multiforme by nested PCR. *J Med Virol.* 2003;71:423-428.

Wetter DA, Davis MD. Recurrent erythema multiforme: clinical characteristics, etiologic associations, and treatment in a series of 48 patients at Mayo Clinic, 2000 to 2007. *J Am Acad Dermatol.* 2010;62:45-53.

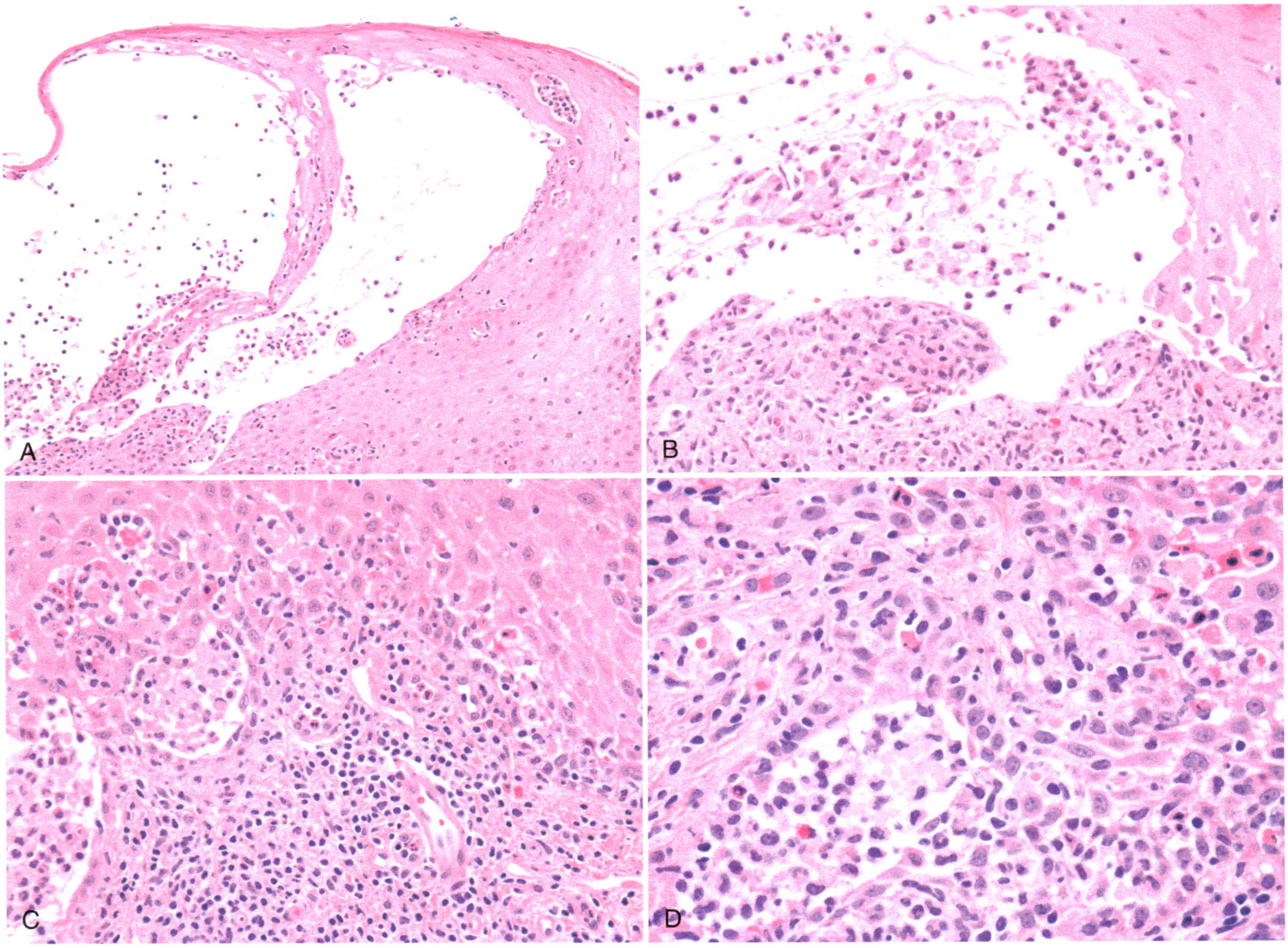

FIG 8.35 Recurrent oral erythema multiforme. (A) Subepithelial blister with many necrotic keratinocytes in the epithelium. (B) Subepithelial blister containing many necrotic keratinocytes and many monocytic cells. (C) Lymphocyte satellitosis composed of lymphocytes around necrotic keratinocytes present (*upper left*). (D) Degeneration of basal cells, necrotic keratinocytes, acute and chronic inflammation, and occasional eosinophils.

Autoimmune Conditions

The two autoimmune diseases that often present in the oral mucosa are mucous membrane pemphigoid (by far the more common) and pemphigus vulgaris. A common clinical presentation is desquamative gingivitis (generalized red, denuded gingiva), similar to lichen planus. Other autoimmune diseases, such as lupus erythematosus, linear IgA disease, and epidermolysis bullosa acquisita, rarely manifest in the mouth in the absence of skin lesions. Primary oral mucous membrane pemphigoid, unlike cicatricial pemphigoid, tends to run a benign course with little cicatrization and is limited to the oral mucous membranes without spread to other sites, such as the eye, skin, or genitalia.

MUCOUS MEMBRANE PEMPHIGOID

Mucous membrane pemphigoid is a subepithelial blistering disorder with autoantibodies directed against a number of antigens.

Clinical Findings

- This occurs in middle-aged females and presents as painful, bright red, denuded gingiva (desquamative gingivitis) that may bleed, usually on the buccal or facial aspect, sometimes with ulcers and a positive Nikolsky sign. Involvement of nongingival oral sites without gingival involvement occurs less frequently and almost never without involvement of the gingiva (Fig. 8.36A–C). Primary oral mucous membrane pemphigoid rarely causes scarring of the oral mucosa.

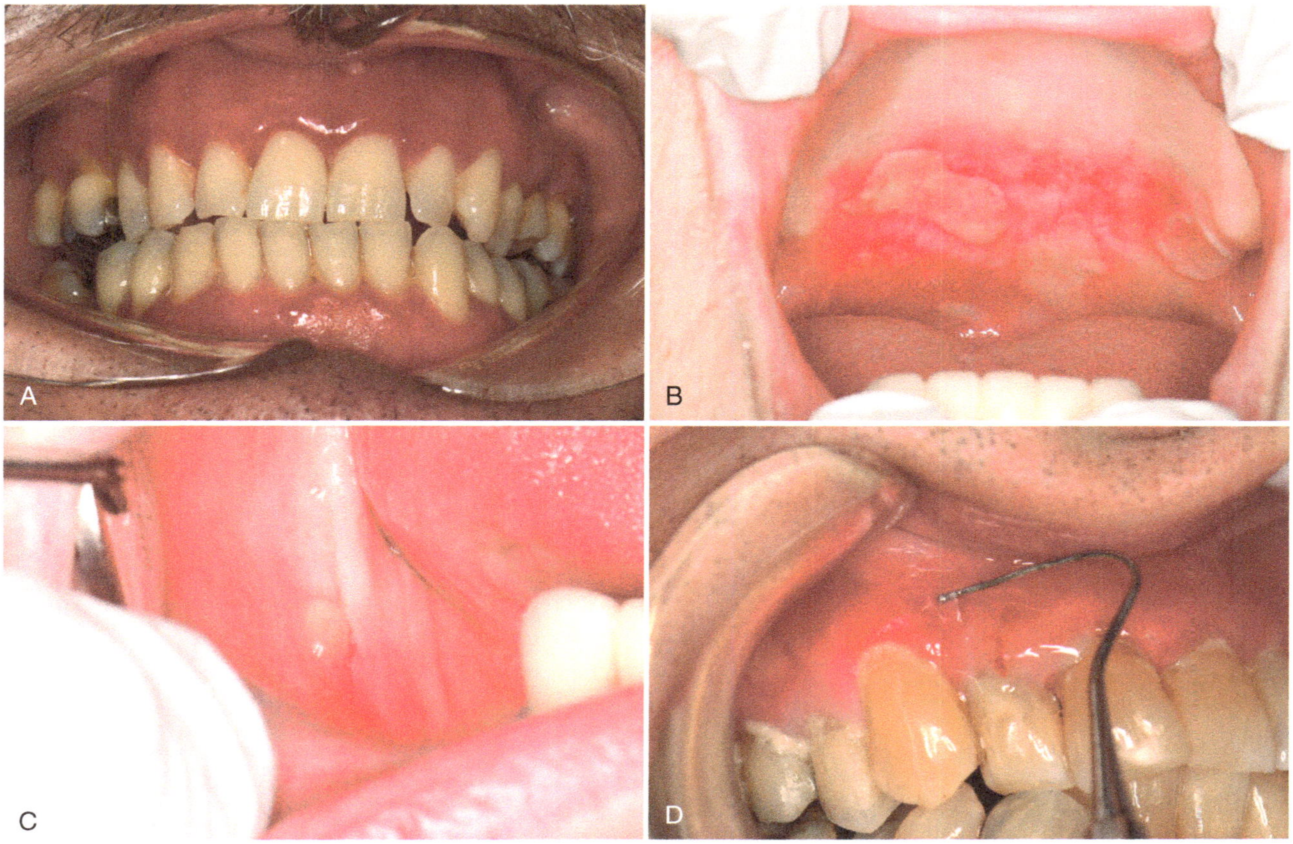

FIG 8.36 (A) Mucous membrane pemphigoid presenting as desquamative, diffusely erythematous gingival mucosa. (B) Mucous membrane pemphigoid affecting the hard and soft palatal mucosa with extensive ulcers/blisters, and erythema. (C) Same patient as in B, with a blister on the alveolar ridge mucosa. (D) Linear immunoglobulin A disease: desquamative and ulcerative gingivitis with delicate blister. Abundant plaque is present on teeth because it is painful to brush.

- Patients may report hoarseness (vocal cord involvement) and epistaxis (nasal mucosa involvement). Ocular cicatricial pemphigoid, if untreated, leads to symblepharon, scarring, and blindness, although it is uncommon to see patients with primary oral mucous membrane pemphigoid develop ocular lesions.
- Approximately 70% to 80% of all cases of desquamative gingivitis represent either mucous membrane pemphigoid or lichen planus. The rest represent hypersensitivity reactions or other autoimmune blistering diseases, such as pemphigus vulgaris, linear IgA disease, and others (see Fig. 8.36D).
- Oral and ocular pemphigoid are associated with increased frequency of HLA-DQB1*0301.
- Patients with only oral mucous membrane pemphigoid do not usually exhibit circulating antibodies.

Etiopathogenesis and Histopathologic Features

Primary mucosal disease generally involves BP180 (BPAg2 or type XVII collagen). It less often involves BP230 (BPAg1), laminin-332 (formerly laminin-5 or epiligrin), laminin-6, β_4 subunit of $\alpha_6\beta_4$ integrin, and a 120-kDa undefined epithelial antigen. Differential IgG and IgA recognition of targeted autoantigens is likely the cause of high variability in the clinical manifestations of the cutaneous, ocular, and mucous membrane pemphigoid group of diseases.

- Subepithelial clefting is noted with preservation of basal cells that protrude into the cleft. The epithelium may be acanthotic or atrophic and generally shows no to minimal spongiosis. Biopsies often show only detached fragments of epithelium with intact basal cells (Figs. 8.37 and 8.38). The lamina propria shows a variable lymphocytic infiltrate. Eosinophils are infrequently encountered, unlike in lesions of cutaneous pemphigoid.
- Direct immunofluorescence studies show linear IgG, C3, and/or IgA at the basement membrane zone (Fig. 8.39). Immunoreactants localize to the roof of the lesion in salt split-skin technique.

Differential Diagnosis

- Lichen planus shows subepithelial clefting resulting from degeneration or squamatization of basal cells, as well as colloid bodies and saw-tooth rete ridges, and a lymphocytic band at the interface.
- The presence of linear IgA on direct immunofluorescence should not be interpreted as primary linear IgA

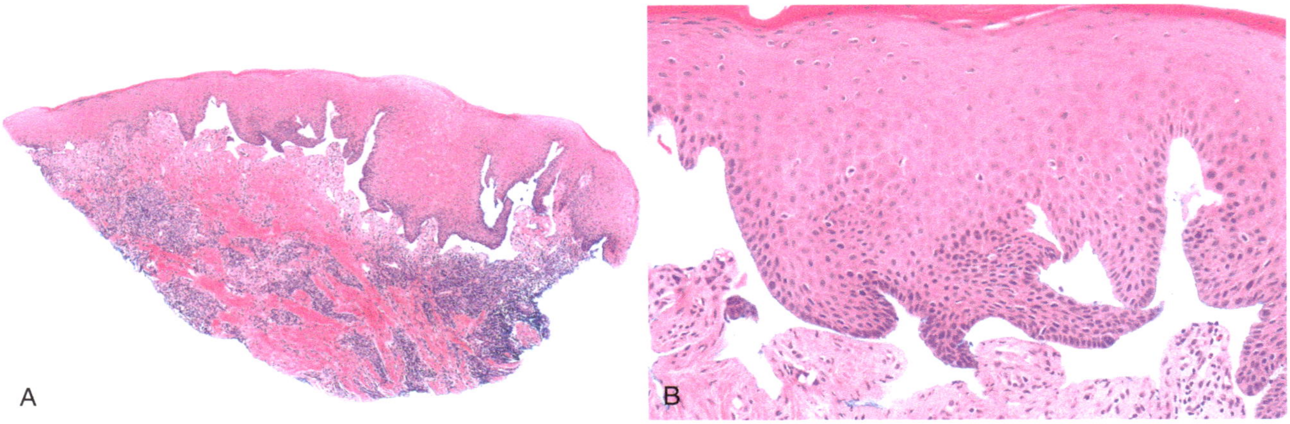

FIG 8.37 Mucous membrane pemphigoid. (A) Acanthosis with subepithelial cleft and a mild lymphocytic infiltrate. (B) Preservation of basal cells and little inflammation present.

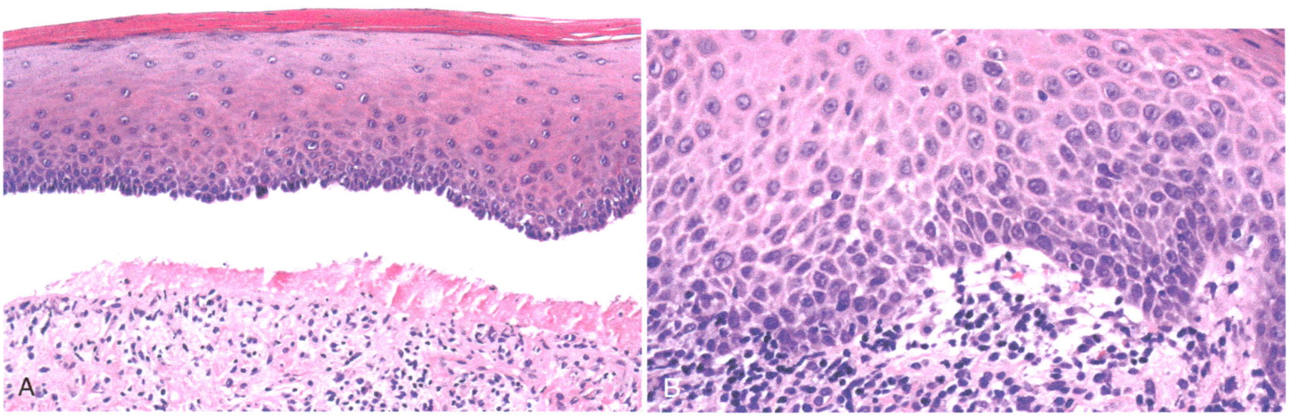

FIG 8.38 Mucous membrane pemphigoid. (A) Epithelial atrophy and sub-basal clefting with basal cells protruding into the cleft that contains fibrin. (B) Subtle subepithelial cleft with chronic inflammation. This biopsy was strongly positive for linear immunoglobulin G on direct immunofluorescence studies.

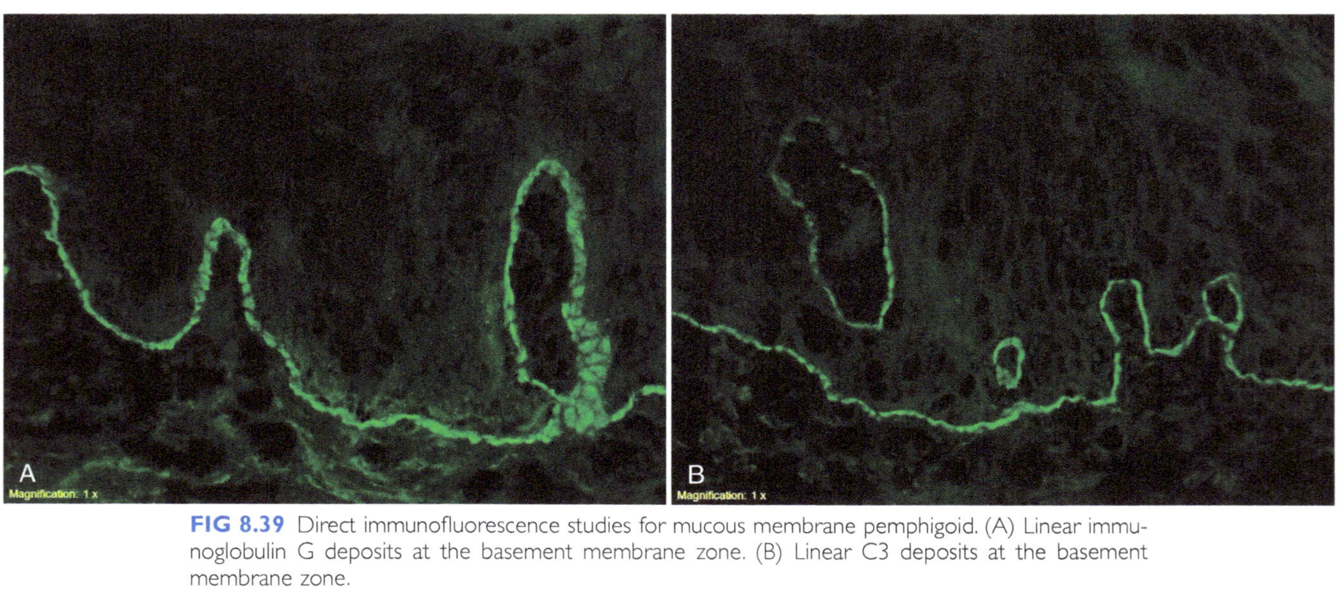

FIG 8.39 Direct immunofluorescence studies for mucous membrane pemphigoid. (A) Linear immunoglobulin G deposits at the basement membrane zone. (B) Linear C3 deposits at the basement membrane zone.

bullous disorder, unless there are typical skin lesions of linear IgA bullous dermatosis, bullous dermatosis of childhood, or dermatitis herpetiformis associated with celiac disease.

- Paraneoplastic pemphigoid may be seen as part of paraneoplastic autoimmune multiorgan syndrome (see later).
- Lichen planus pemphigoides occurs infrequently in long-standing cases of lichen planus because of epitope spread. This is a phenomenon whereby damage to the basement membrane zone exposes previously sequestered antigens that incite an autoimmune response in susceptible individuals.
- Angina bullosa hemorrhagica manifests with intact basal cells and hemorrhage within a subepithelial bulla and it exhibits a typical clinical history of waxing and waning hemorrhagic bullae, sometimes with a history of chronic steroid inhaler use (Fig. 8.40).

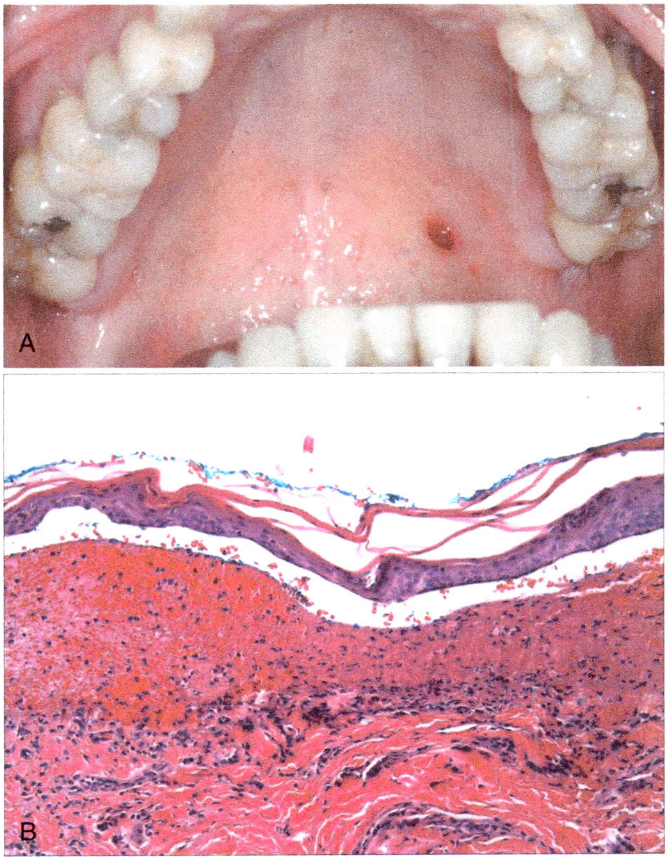

FIG 8.40 Angina bullosa hemorrhagica. (A) Blood-filled blister in the palatal mucosa. (B) Subepithelial cleft with abundant hemorrhage in the lamina propria from patient shown in A. *(Courtesy Dr. Mark Lerman, Tufts University School of Dental Medicine, Boston, Mass.)*

Management and Prognosis

- Topical steroids are the mainstay of treatment with or without up-front systemic steroid therapy to bring disease under control rapidly (see Appendix A). A soft plastic stent that covers the gingiva and is used to hold the steroid under occlusion is particularly helpful, although gauze may also be used to hold the steroid in place (Fig. 8.41). Patients should see an ophthalmologist and dermatologist to be evaluated for conjunctival, skin, and genital lesions.
- Other therapies include dapsone, nicotinamide and tetracycline in combination, mycophenolate mofetil, azathioprine, methotrexate, and biologic agents such as rituximab.

REFERENCES

Beguerie JR, Gonzalez S. Angina bullosa hemorrhagica: report of 11 cases. *Dermatol Reports*. 2014;6:5282.

Carrozzo M, Fasano ME, Broccoletti R, et al. HLA-DQB1 alleles in Italian patients with mucous membrane pemphigoid predominantly affecting the oral cavity. *Br J Dermatol*. 2001;145:805-808.

Chan LS, Ahmed AR, Anhalt GJ, et al. The first international consensus on mucous membrane pemphigoid: definition, diagnostic criteria, pathogenic factors, medical treatment, and prognostic indicators. *Arch Dermatol*. 2002;138:370-379.

Giuliani M, Favia GF, Lajolo C, Miani CM. Angina bullosa haemorrhagica: presentation of eight new cases and a review of the literature. *Oral Dis*. 2002;8:54-58.

Horvath B, Niedermeier A, Podstawa E, et al. IgA autoantibodies in the pemphigoids and linear IgA bullous dermatosis. *Exp Dermatol*. 2010;19:648-653.

Kharfi M, Khaled A, Karaa A, et al. Linear IgA bullous dermatosis: the more frequent bullous dermatosis of children. *Dermatol Online J*. 2010;16:2.

Knudson RM, Kalaaji AN, Bruce AJ. The management of mucous membrane pemphigoid and pemphigus. *Dermatol Ther*. 2010;23:268-280.

Leao JC, Ingafou M, Khan A, et al. Desquamative gingivitis: retrospective analysis of disease associations of a large cohort. *Oral Dis*. 2008;14:556-560.

Lo Russo L, Fierro G, Guiglia R, et al. Epidemiology of desquamative gingivitis: evaluation of 125 patients and review of the literature. *Int J Dermatol*. 2009;48:1049-1052.

Schmidt E, Zillikens D. Modern diagnosis of autoimmune blistering skin diseases. *Autoimmun Rev*. 2010;10:84-89.

Scully C, Lo Muzio L. Oral mucosal diseases: mucous membrane pemphigoid. *Br J Oral Maxillofac Surg*. 2008;46:358-366.

Sobjanek M, Sokolowska-Wojdylo M, Sztaba-Kania M, et al. Clinical and immunopathological heterogeneity of 22 cases of linear IgA bullous dermatosis. *J Eur Acad Dermatol Venereol*. 2008;22:1131.

Zakka LR, Keskin DB, Reche P, Ahmed AR. Relationship between target antigens and major histocompatibility complex (MHC) class II genes in producing two pathogenic antibodies simultaneously. *Clin Exp Immunol*. 2010;162:224-236.

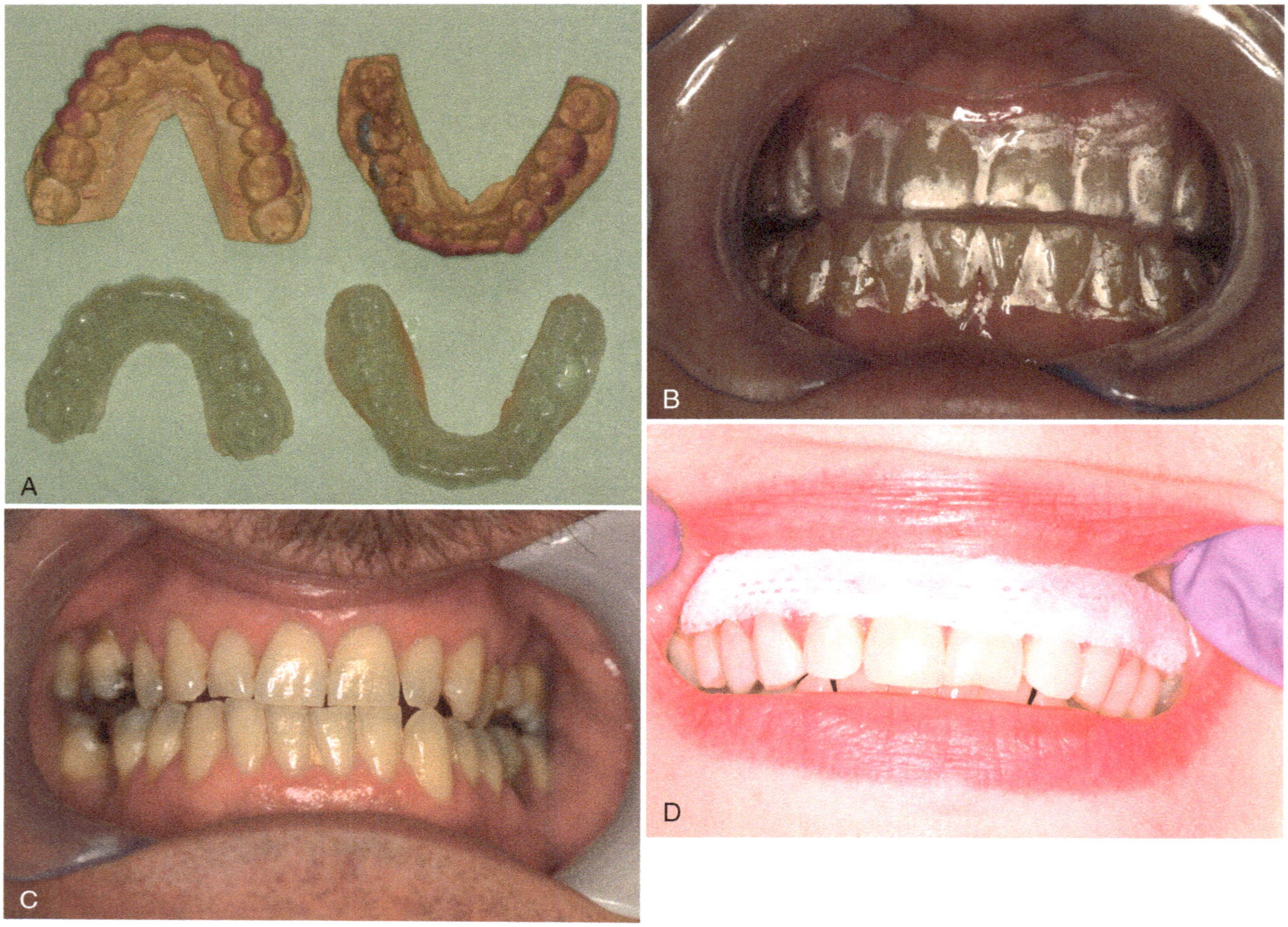

FIG 8.41 Treatment of mucous membrane pemphigoid using steroids placed in a stent. (A) A custom plastic stent is fabricated from molds of the teeth and gingiva. (B) Same patient as in Fig. 8.40A is wearing the stent. (C) Resolution of lesions after 4 weeks of topical steroid therapy. (D) Gauze may be used to hold the topical steroid against the gingiva.

PEMPHIGUS VULGARIS

Clinical Findings

- This occurs in middle-aged and older patients, often of Ashkenazi-Jewish descent. Painful ulcers and shallow erosions occur, characteristically on the hard and soft palates, and the necrotic blister roof appears as a pseudomembrane. Desquamative gingivitis is often present (Fig. 8.42A–D).
- Oral findings often precede skin findings (flaccid bullae and erosions) or may be the only manifestation (see Fig. 8.42E).
- Pemphigus may be induced by medications such as penicillamine and angiotensin-converting enzyme inhibitors.
- Patients with cutaneous disease usually demonstrate high serum levels of IgG, but this is not usually seen in patients with limited oral disease only.
- Susceptibility is associated with HLA-B38, HLA-DRB1*0402, and HLA-DRB1*0302, or HLA-B35, HLA-DRB1*0402, and HLA-DRB*0302 in Jewish patients and with HLA-DRB1*0402 and HLA-DQB1*0503 in white patients in the United States, while Asians may have an association with HLA-DRB1*0403 and HLA-DRB1*0406. Other putative associations may be a result of linkage disequilibrium.

Etiopathogenesis and Histopathologic Features

There are four main forms of pemphigus, namely pemphigus vulgaris, pemphigus foliaceous, IgA pemphigus, and paraneoplastic pemphigus (see later). Pemphigus vulgaris exhibits antibodies directed against desmoglein-3 present in the lower layers of the epithelium and therefore exhibits suprabasal clefting. Pemphigus vegetans is a vegetating variant of pemphigus vulgaris that occurs on the intertriginous areas, scalp and face, and may occur as part of healing of lesions. Pemphigus foliaceous (including fogo selvagem, the endemic form seen in parts of Brazil and North Africa) exhibits antibodies against desmoglein-1 present in the upper layers of the epithelium and therefore exhibits subcorneal clefting. Desmoglein-3 is more abundant in mucosa than desmoglein-1, and that is why pemphigus foliaceous seldom involves the mouth. Pemphigus erythematosus is a localized form of pemphigus foliaceus with features of lupus erythematosus, and 80% of patients test positive for antinuclear antibodies. IgA pemphigus rarely involves the oral mucosa and contains many

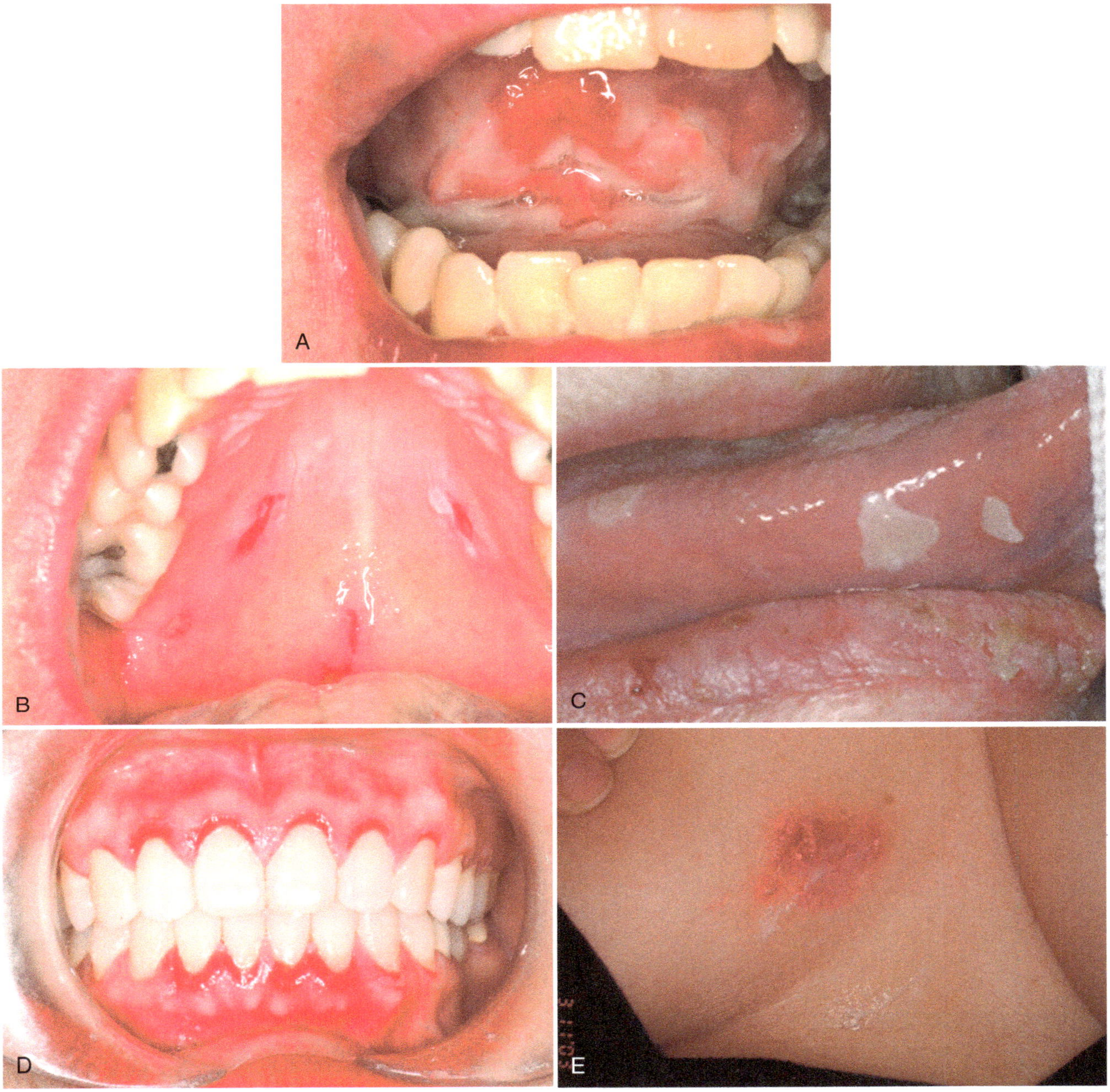

FIG 8.42 Pemphigus vulgaris. (A) Extensive ulcers of the floor of mouth and ventral tongue. (B) Same patient as in A with typical shallow erosions of the palatal mucosa from ruptured blisters. (C) Demarcated fibrin plaques or necrotic blister roof. (D) Multifocal areas of erosion from ruptured blisters. (E) Erosions on the skin and a small, fresh bulla.

neutrophils, while IgG/IgA pemphigus is associated with malignancy.

- There is suprabasilar clefting with rounded, acantholytic cells (Tzanck cells) within the cleft as well as intact basal cells. There is variable chronic inflammation in the lamina propria that may form villous-like structures capped by a few layers of epithelial cells (Figs. 8.43 and 8.44).
- Direct immunofluorescence shows intercellular deposition of IgG in a mesh- or netlike pattern (Fig. 8.45). Intercellular staining for IgA may also be seen, and up to two-thirds of patients show circulating IgA antibodies against desmoglein-3. Epitope spread may account for the production of antibodies against multiple antigens.
- Indirect immunofluorescence findings are seen in patients with more severe disease.

Differential Diagnosis

- Pyostomatitis vegetans shows acantholysis and eosinophilic abscesses that are negative on direct immunofluorescence studies, and patients may have inflammatory bowel disease.

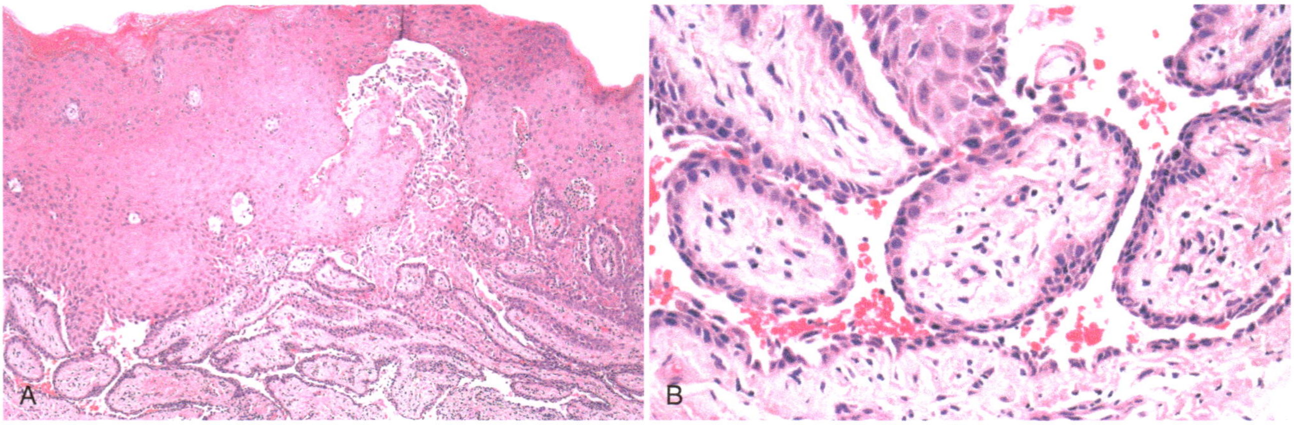

FIG 8.43 Pemphigus vulgaris. (A) Oral mucosa exhibiting suprabasilar clefting. (B) Rounded acantholytic cells are noted within the cleft, and villous-like connective papillae are rimmed by one to two layers of basal and parabasal keratinocytes.

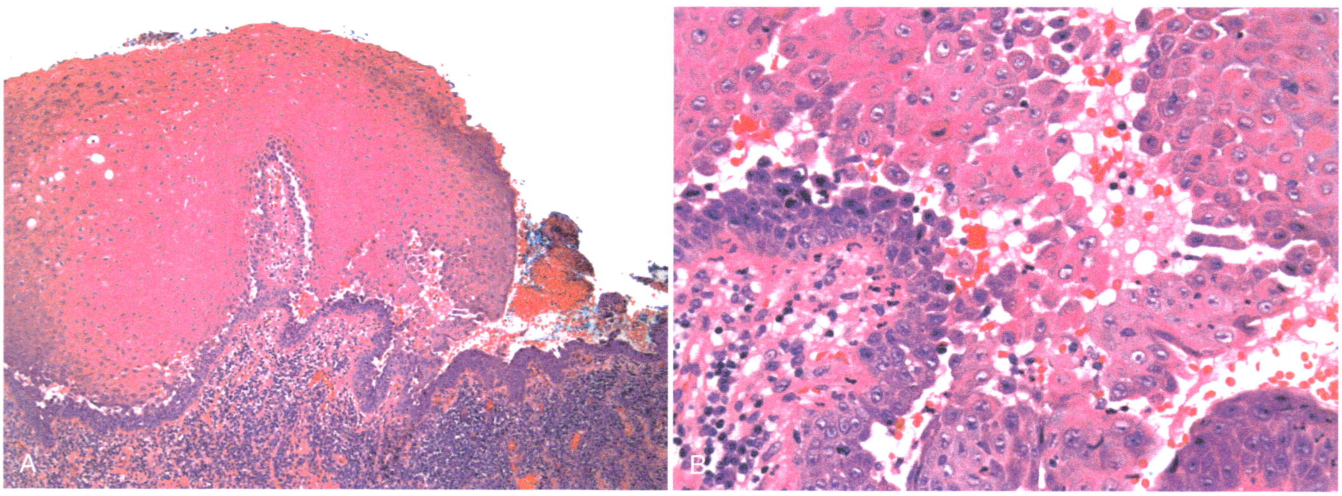

FIG 8.44 Pemphigus vulgaris. (A) Oral mucosa with acantholysis and villous-like projections of connective tissue covered by a few layers of epithelium (*center*). (B) Suprabasilar acantholysis with rounded, acantholytic cells.

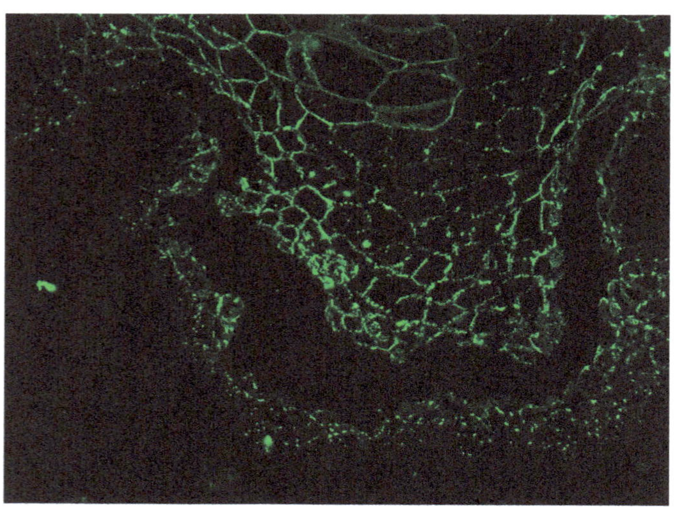

FIG 8.45 Pemphigus vulgaris: direct immunofluorescence shows intercellular deposition of immunoglobulin G in a mesh- or netlike pattern.

- Darier disease, warty dyskeratoma, and focal acantholytic dyskeratosis contain dyskeratotic cells and are negative on direct immunofluorescence. The clinical findings are also of dyskeratotic rather than bullosing disease.
- Pseudoacantholysis is seen as a suboptimal fixation artifact. Cells are not rounded, but rather are angulated (Fig. 8.46).

Management and Prognosis

- Oral disease may be successfully treated with topical steroids combined with systemic therapy to bring the disease under control (see Appendix A). Almost all patients with initial oral disease subsequently develop cutaneous disease.
- Mycophenolate mofetil as monotherapy or with prednisone, rituximab, and intravenous immunoglobulin therapy are effective and may lead to long-term remission.
- Circulating levels of IgG usually fall as patients respond to therapy.

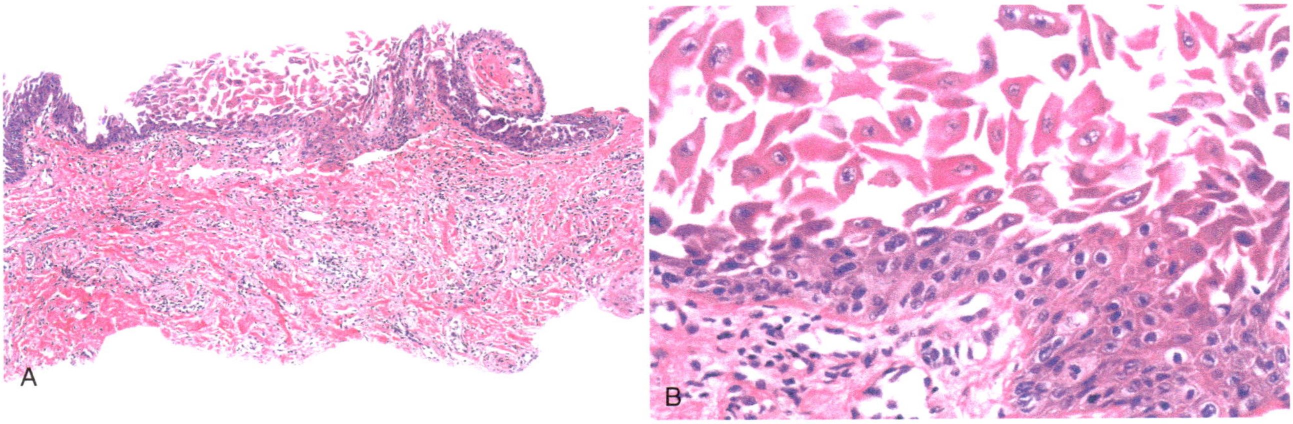

FIG 8.46 Suboptimal fixation artifact. (A) Mucosal lesion exhibiting pseudoacantholysis with suprabasilar clefting and villous-like connective tissue papillae. (B) Pseudoacantholytic cells are polyhedral and dyscohesive with degenerated nuclei exhibiting clumped chromatin.

REFERENCES

Aoki V, Rivitti EA, Diaz LA, Cooperative Group on Fogo Selvagem Research. Update on fogo selvagem, an endemic form of pemphigus foliaceus. *J Dermatol.* 2015;42:18-26.

Atzmony L, Hodak E, Gdalevich M, et al. Treatment of pemphigus vulgaris and pemphigus foliaceus: a systematic review and meta-analysis. *Am J Clin Dermatol.* 2014;15:503-515.

Baum S, Sakka N, Artsi O, et al. Diagnosis and classification of autoimmune blistering diseases. *Autoimmun Rev.* 2014;13:482-489.

McMillan R, Taylor J, Shephard M, et al. World Workshop on Oral Medicine VI: a systematic review of the treatment of mucocutaneous pemphigus vulgaris. *Oral Surg Oral Med Oral Pathol Oral Radiol.* 2015;120:132-142.e61.

Mentink LF, de Jong MC, Kloosterhuis GJ, et al. Coexistence of IgA antibodies to desmogleins 1 and 3 in pemphigus vulgaris, pemphigus foliaceus, and paraneoplastic pemphigus. *Br J Dermatol.* 2007;156:635-641.

Mignogna MD, Fortuna G, Leuci S, Ruoppo E. Oropharyngeal pemphigus vulgaris and clinical remission: a long-term, longitudinal study. *Am J Clin Dermatol.* 2010;11:137-145.

Porro AM, de Vasconcelos Nasser Caetano L, de Sena Nogueira Maehara L, Enokihara MM. Non-classical forms of pemphigus: pemphigus herpetiformis, IgA pemphigus, paraneoplastic pemphigus and IgG/IgA pemphigus. *An Bras Dermatol.* 2014;89:96-106.

Schmidt E, Zillikens D. Modern diagnosis of autoimmune blistering skin diseases. *Autoimmun Rev.* 2010;10:84-89.

Sciubba JJ. Autoimmune oral mucosal diseases: clinical, etiologic, diagnostic, and treatment considerations. *Dent Clin North Am.* 2011;55:89-103.

Sinha AA. The genetics of pemphigus. *Dermatol Clin.* 2011;29:381-391.

Strowd LC, Taylor SL, Jorizzo JL, Namazi MR. Therapeutic ladder for pemphigus vulgaris: emphasis on achieving complete remission. *J Am Acad Dermatol.* 2011;64:490-494.

Tsuruta D, Ishii N, Hamada T, et al. IgA pemphigus. *Clin Dermatol.* 2011;29:437-442.

PARANEOPLASTIC PEMPHIGUS (PARANEOPLASTIC AUTOIMMUNE MULTIORGAN SYNDROME)

Paraneoplastic pemphigus is a mucocutaneous manifestation of a paraneoplastic syndrome. Some have proposed that the term *paraneoplastic autoimmune multiorgan syndrome* may be more appropriate, because lesions may resemble pemphigus, pemphigoid, lichen planus, or erythema multiforme with multiorgan involvement. In particular, many patients exhibit bronchiolitis obliterans as well as involvement of other organs, such as the kidneys. Paraneoplastic pemphigus is associated with HLA-DRB1*03 in white patients and with Cw*14 in Chinese patients.

Clinical Findings

- This occurs in middle-aged men and presents as extensive painful ulcers and erosions of the oral cavity with hemorrhagic crusts on the lips, appearing similar to Stevens-Johnson syndrome (Fig. 8.47).
- Skin lesions are poikilodermic, lichenoid, or blistering and resemble pemphigus, pemphigoid, erythema multiforme, chronic graft-versus-host disease, and lichen planus. Biopsies are usually taken from the skin, owing to ease of access.
- This disorder is associated with non-Hodgkin lymphoma (40%), chronic lymphocytic leukemia (30%), Castleman disease (10%), thymoma (6%), sarcoma (6%), Waldenström macroglobulinemia (6%), and other malignancies.

Etiopathogenesis and Histopathologic Features

Two hypotheses regarding this disease have been postulated. One hypothesis suggests that autoantibodies produced against neoplastic cells cross-react with epithelial antigens. The other postulates that tumor cells either synthesize autoantibodies or produce cytokines that promote B-cell differentiation, promoting an autoimmune response. Autoantibodies are directed against periplakin and envoplakin, desmoplakin, desmoglein-1 and desmoglein-3, plectin, and a poorly characterized 170-kDa protein. Humoral-mediated tissue damage produces pemphigoid and pemphigus-like lesions, while cell-mediated damage produces lichenoid and chronic graft-versus-host disease–like findings.

- There is suprabasilar clefting with acantholysis, keratinocyte necrosis, and interface stomatitis with vacuolar

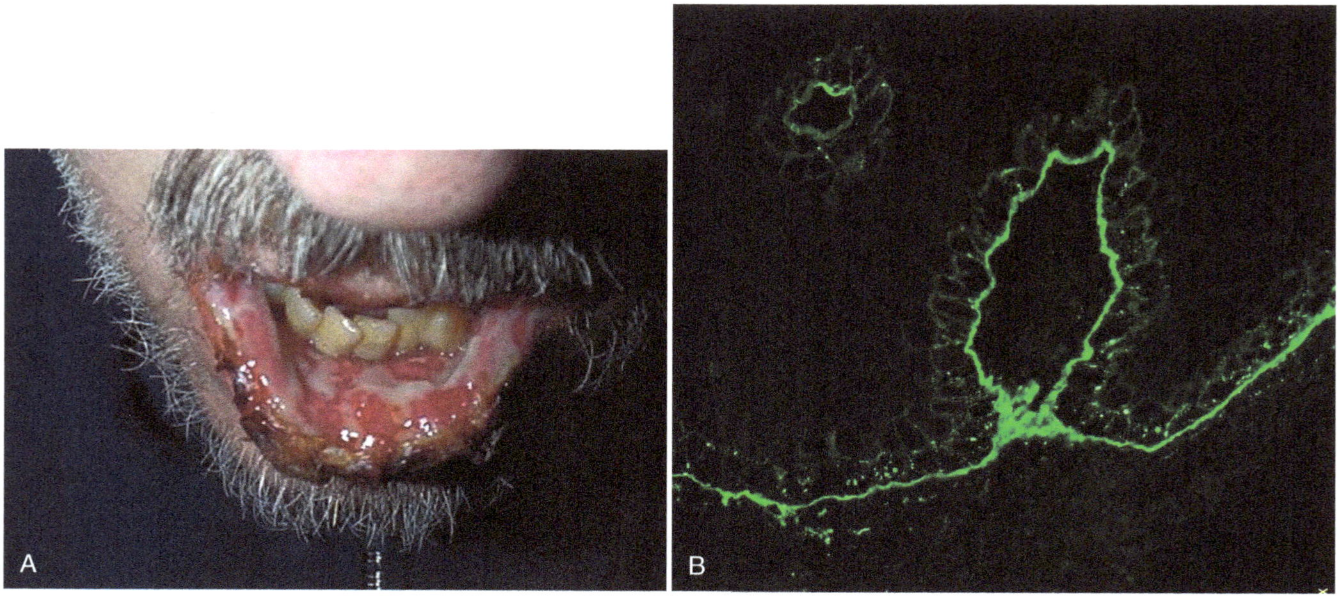

FIG 8.47 Paraneoplastic pemphigus. (A) Extensive ulcerations and crusting of the lips. (B) Direct immunofluorescence study showing deposition of immunoglobulin G in a linear pattern in the basement membrane zone as well as in a netlike pattern in intercellular spaces in the suprabasal cells. *(A, Courtesy Dr. Arturo Saavedra, Harvard Medical School, Boston, Mass.)*

degeneration of basal cells, subepithelial clefting, and a lichenoid lymphocytic band.
- Direct immunofluorescence shows intercellular, as well as linear and granular, subepithelial deposits of IgG and C3, and sometimes IgM (Fig 8.47B). Positive indirect immunofluorescence studies are noted using rat bladder epithelium.
- Identification of envoplakin and periplakin by immunoprecipitation is the most sensitive and specific test for this condition.

Management and Prognosis

- A search for and identification of underlying malignancy is of utmost importance, although treatment of the malignancy may not always halt progression of this severe mucocutaneous disorder.
- Resection of the tumor often leads to improvement of mucocutaneous disease, although pulmonary damage may be irreversible and respiratory failure is often the terminal event.
- Systemic therapy consists of high-dose prednisone, cyclophosphamide, cyclosporine, rituximab, intravenous immunoglobulin, and alemtuzumab.

REFERENCES

Allen CM, Camisa C. Paraneoplastic pemphigus: a review of the literature. *Oral Dis.* 2000;6:208-214.

Anhalt GJ. Paraneoplastic pemphigus. *J Invest Dermatol Symp Proc.* 2004;9:29-33.

Czernik A, Camilleri M, Pittelkow MR, Grando SA. Paraneoplastic autoimmune multiorgan syndrome: 20 years after. *Int J Dermatol.* 2011;50:905-914.

Kaplan I, Hodak E, Ackerman L, et al. Neoplasms associated with paraneoplastic pemphigus: a review with emphasis on non-hematologic malignancy and oral mucosal manifestations. *Oral Oncol.* 2004;40:553-562.

Nguyen VT, Ndoye A, Bassler KD, et al. Classification, clinical manifestations, and immunopathological mechanisms of the epithelial variant of paraneoplastic autoimmune multiorgan syndrome: a reappraisal of paraneoplastic pemphigus. *Arch Dermatol.* 2001;137:193-206.

Yan Z, Hua H, Gao Y. Paraneoplastic pemphigus characterized by polymorphic oral mucosal manifestations—report of two cases. *Quintessence Int.* 2010;41:689-694.

LUPUS ERYTHEMATOSUS

Discoid and systemic lupus erythematosus are commonly associated with oral lesions, although oral lesions of the subacute form have been reported.

Clinical Findings

- There is a 2:1 female predilection. Oral lesions rarely occur in the absence of skin lesions, which vary depending on the subtype, of which the three main ones are systemic, subacute, and discoid. A photodistributed "butterfly rash" on the malar region is typical for systemic lupus erythematosus, whereas scaly and atrophic plaques with follicular plugging, postinflammatory hyperpigmentation, and scarring are common in discoid lupus erythematosus (Fig. 8.48A–B). The subacute form of the disease results in annular plaques on the trunk and infrequently affects the face. Telangiectasia and Raynaud phenomenon are common.
- Oral disease presents as aphthous-like ulcers, reticulated and erythematous (lichenoid) lesions on the buccal mucosa, or erythematous macules and keratotic plaques on the palatal or lip mucosa. Up to 20% and 45% of patients with discoid and systemic lupus erythematosus, respectively, have oral lesions (see Fig. 8.48C–D).

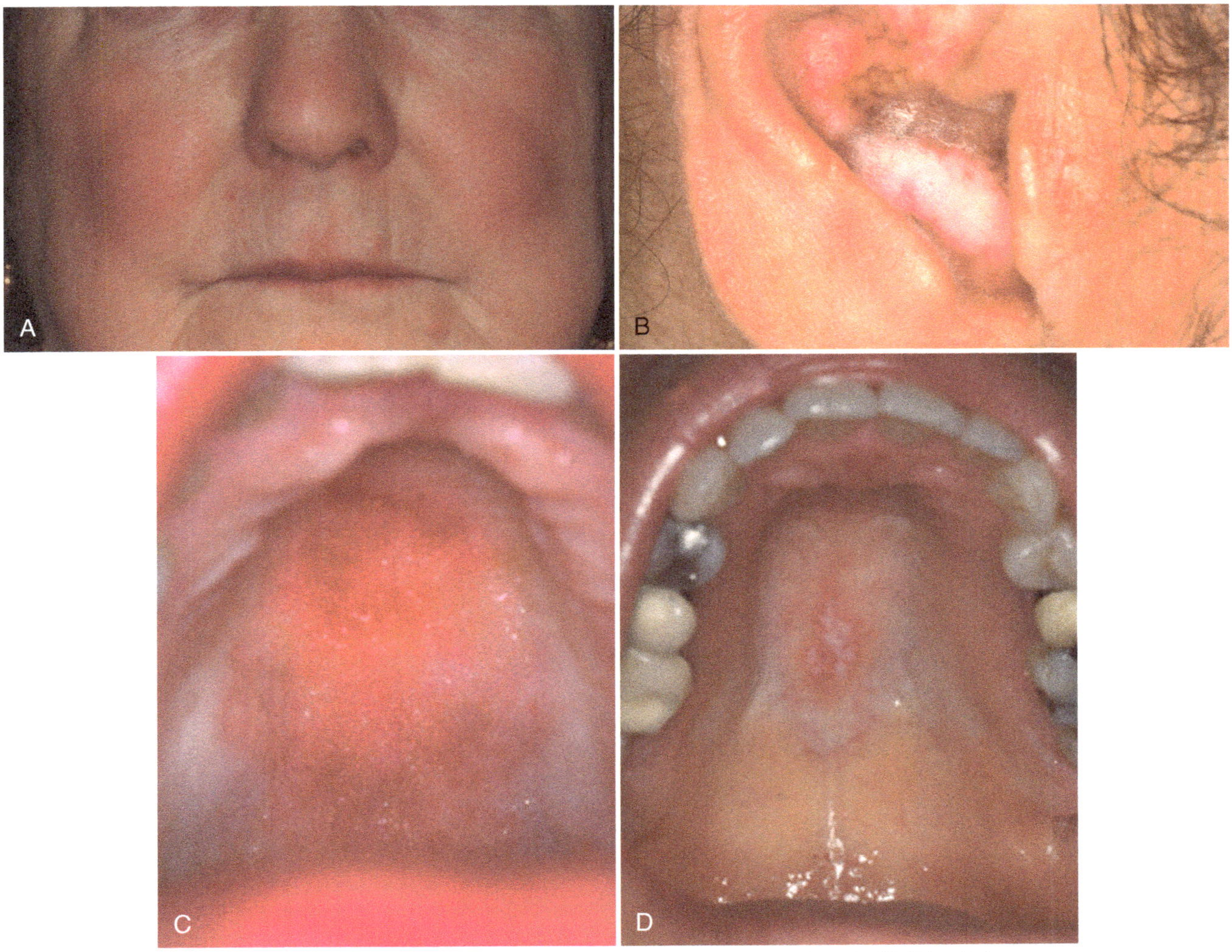

FIG 8.48 (A) Systemic lupus erythematosus: typical malar ("butterfly") rash. (B) Discoid lupus erythematosus: skin atrophy and hyperpigmentation of ear. (C) Oral lupus erythematosus: poorly demarcated erythema of the hard palatal mucosa with slight white reticulations (*right*), symmetric in distribution. (D) White plaque with surrounding erythema of the hard palatal mucosa, symmetric in distribution.

- Keratoconjunctivitis sicca may develop if there is concomitant Sjögren syndrome. Patients also may report fatigue, weight loss, alopecia, anemia and other hematologic abnormalities, photosensitivity, arthralgia, and arthritis.
- Circulating antinuclear antibodies such as anti-Smith, anti–double-stranded DNA, and antiribonucleoprotein are often noted in patients with systemic lupus erythematosus, whereas antibodies against Sjögren syndrome-A and Sjögren syndrome-B antigens are noted in patients with subacute lupus erythematosus. Patients with discoid lupus erythematosus do not usually produce such antibodies.

Etiopathogenesis and Histopathologic Features

Lupus erythematosus is the prototypical autoimmune disease that often shows multiorgan involvement, in particular involving the skin, musculoskeletal system, hematologic system, central nervous system, or kidneys. Discoid lupus erythematosus primarily affects the skin and mucosa.

- There is both acanthosis and atrophy of the epithelium with vacuolar degeneration of basal cells, a bandlike lymphocytic infiltrate at the interface, and deep perivascular and paravascular lymphocytic infiltrates. There is thickening of epithelial and vascular basement membranes and deposition of interstitial mucin (Fig 8.49).
- Direct immunofluorescence studies show a positive lupus band test or linear/granular deposition of IgG, IgM, or IgA at the basement membrane (lupus band test). A positive lupus band test from clinically normal skin is strongly predictive of systemic lupus erythematosus.

Differential Diagnosis

- Cinnamic aldehyde–associated or other contact stomatitis exhibits a lymphocytic band at the interface and

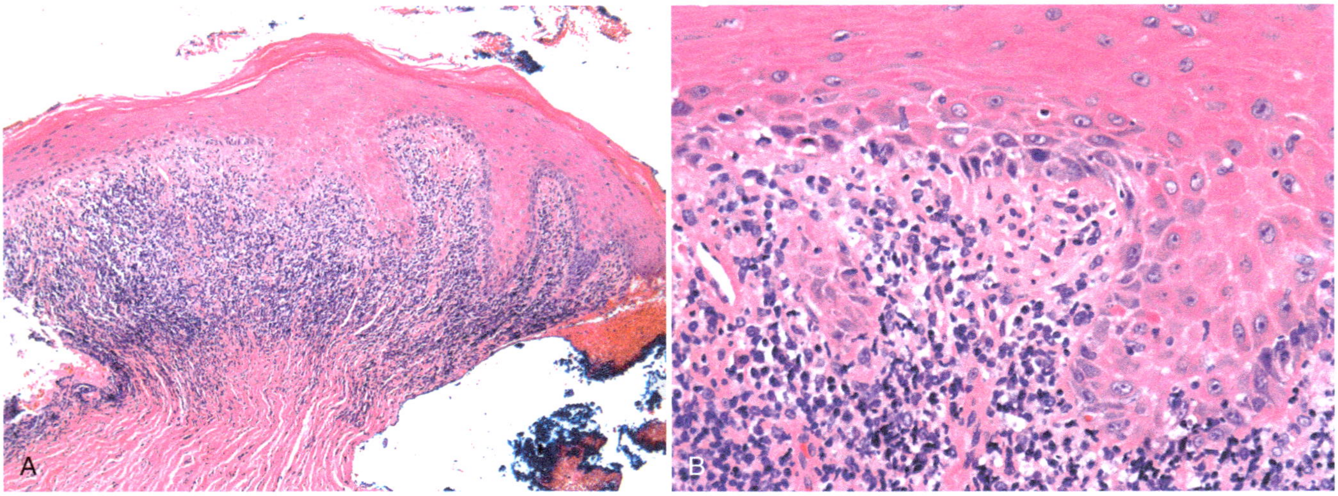

FIG 8.49 Oral lupus erythematosus. (A) Hyperkeratosis, alternating epithelial atrophy and acanthosis, and lymphocytic band at the interface. (B) Degeneration of the basal cells with apoptotic cells, thickened basement membrane, and lymphocytic band at the interface.

deep perivascular and paravascular infiltrates, but not usually hydropic degeneration of basal cells. The lupus band test is negative.
- Lichen planus does not show positive immunofluorescence for linear IgG.

Management and Prognosis

- Topical and/or systemic therapy is effective for mucosal lesions, depending on their severity (see Appendix A).

REFERENCES

Karjalainen TK, Tomich CE. A histopathologic study of oral mucosal lupus erythematosus. *Oral Surg Oral Med Oral Pathol.* 1989;67: 547-554.

Lopez-Labady J, Villarroel-Dorrego M, Gonzalez N, et al. Oral manifestations of systemic and cutaneous lupus erythematosus in a Venezuelan population. *J Oral Pathol Med.* 2007;36:524-527.

Lourenço SV, Nacagami Sotto M, Constantino Vilela MA, et al. Lupus erythematosus: clinical and histopathological study of oral manifestations and immunohistochemical profile of epithelial maturation. *J Cutan Pathol.* 2006;33:657-662.

Marques ER, Lourenço SV, Lima DM, Nico MM. Oral lesions in lupus erythematosus—cytokines profiles of inflammatory infiltrate. *J Cutan Pathol.* 2010;37:439-445.

Nico MM, Romiti R, Lourenço SV. Oral lesions in four cases of subacute cutaneous lupus erythematosus. *Acta Derm Venereol.* 2011;91: 436-439.

Nico MM, Vilela MA, Rivitti EA, Lourenço SV. Oral lesions in lupus erythematosus: correlation with cutaneous lesions. *Eur J Dermatol.* 2008;18:376-381.

Vera-Recabarren MA, García-Carrasco M, Ramos-Casals M, Herrero C. Cutaneous lupus erythematosus: clinical and immunological study of 308 patients stratified by gender. *Clin Exp Dermatol.* 2010;35: 729-735.

GRANULOMATOSIS WITH POLYANGIITIS (WEGENER GRANULOMATOSIS)

Granulomatosis with polyangiitis (formerly named *Wegener granulomatosis*) is a small-vessel necrotizing vasculitis (affecting mostly capillaries and venules) that represents one of three conditions which fall under the larger category of antineutrophil cytoplasmic antibody (ANCA)–associated vasculitis. The others are microscopic polyangiitis and eosinophilic granulomatosis with polyangiitis (formerly known as *Churg-Strauss disease*).

Clinical Findings

- The mean age of occurrence is in the seventh decade of life, with equal gender predilection. Oral findings are the first presentation in approximately 6% to 13% of patients. The limited form of the disease affects only the upper airways and oral cavity.
- The patient presents with hyperplastic gingiva that has a pebbly, granular, and erythematous appearance often with pinpoint hemorrhage ("strawberry gingivitis") (Fig. 8.50A). Painful, necrotic ulcers of the oral mucosa, in particular the hard palatal mucosa, fall under the clinical moniker *midline destructive disease* (Fig. 8.50B). Bone destruction leads to pain and mobility of teeth.
- This multisystem disorder may be associated with malaise, myalgia, weight loss, fevers and hematologic aberrations. Eye findings include scleritis, uveitis, and thrombosis of retinal vessels. Aural disease may manifest as otitis media. Cutaneous ulcers may be present, and the gastrointestinal tract, cardiovascular system, and central nervous system may also be affected.
- Nasal carriage of *Staphylococcus aureus* is associated with increased risk for relapse.
- This condition is associated with HLA-DPB1*15 in black patients and HLA-DPB*1501 in white patients.

Etiopathogenesis and Histopathologic Findings

Granulomatosis with polyangiitis is a small-vessel necrotizing vasculitis that in its full expression affects the upper respiratory tract and oral mucosa, lungs (small airway obstruction and alveolar capillaritis), and kidneys (necrotizing glomerulonephritis). ANCAs are directed against

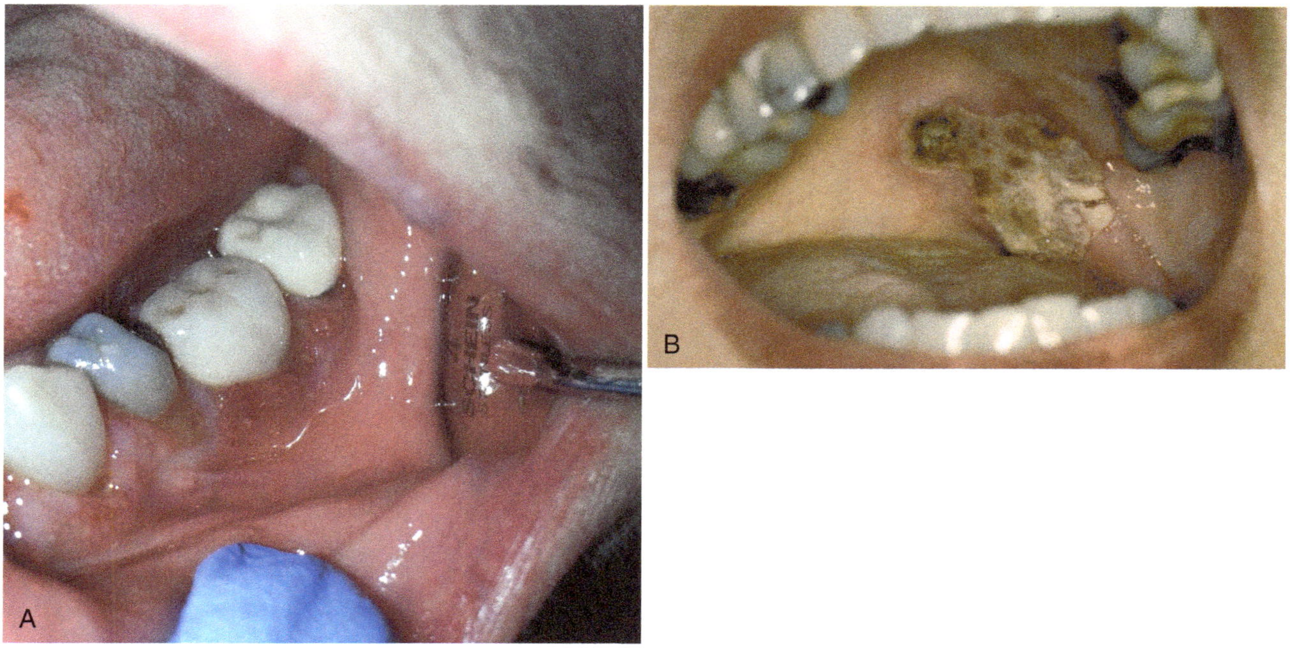

FIG 8.50 Granulomatosis with polyangiitis. (A) Hyperplastic gingival tissue with a granular, pebbly, hemorrhagic appearance. (B) Necrotic ulcer on palatal mucosa.

proteinase C (also known as *c-ANCA*) in 80% of cases and myeloperoxidase (also known as *p-ANCA*) in 20% of cases. Some patients also show antibodies against lysosome-associated membrane protein-1.

- The epithelium may exhibit pseudoepitheliomatous hyperplasia. There is edema of the lamina propria with a mixed inflammatory infiltrate composed of many neutrophils and microabscesses, lymphocytes, plasma cells, eosinophils, and multinucleated giant cells.
- Fresh hemorrhage is almost always present in the lamina propria. Vasculitis (characterized by fibrinoid necrosis of vessel walls, leukocytoclasis, and fibrin thrombi) may be difficult to identify.
- More advanced lesions exhibit irregular areas (geographic) of necrosis with surrounding palisading of macrophages forming palisaded granulomas (Fig. 8.51).
- Indirect immunofluorescence testing reveals the presence of cANCA in cytoplasmic pattern, or pANCA in a perinuclear pattern, with enzyme-linked immunosorbent assay positivity for antibodies against proteinase-3 and myeloperoxidase, respectively.

Differential Diagnosis

- Foreign body granuloma does not tend to show such intense inflammation and hemorrhage, and special stains should be used to rule out an infectious granulomatous disease.

Management and Prognosis

- High-dose prednisone and cyclophosphamide for several months is a mainstay of therapy. Methotrexate, azathioprine, and mycophenolate mofetil mitigate toxicity of prolonged cyclophosphamide use, and rituximab is useful for refractory cases.
- Surgical reconstruction may be necessary if there has been extensive tissue destruction.

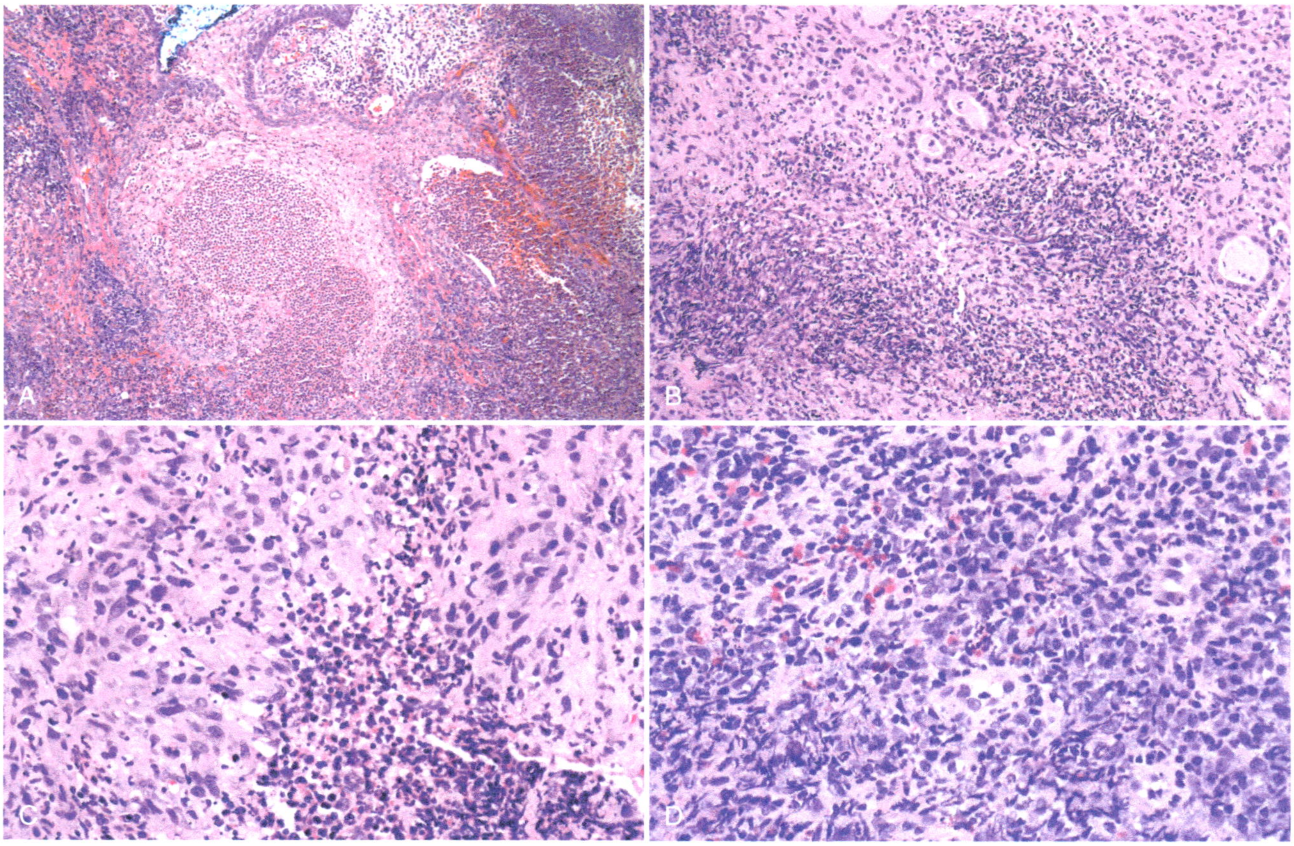

FIG 8.51 Granulomatosis with polyangiitis. (A) Pseudoepitheliomatous hyperplasia with many abscesses and fresh hemorrhage just beneath the epithelium. (B) Mixed inflammatory infiltrate with "geographic" necrosis. (C) Granulomatous inflammation adjacent to necrosis. (D) Acute and chronic inflammation with many eosinophils and nuclear debris.

REFERENCES

Almouhawis HA, Leao JC, Fedele S, Porter SR. Wegener's granulomatosis: a review of clinical features and an update in diagnosis and treatment. *J Oral Pathol Med*. 2013;42:507-516.

Chen M, Kallenberg CGM. The environment, geoepidemiology and ANCA-associated vasculitides. *Autoimmun Rev*. 2010;9:A293-A298.

Jennette JC, Falk RJ, Hu P, Xiao H. Pathogenesis of antineutrophil cytoplasmic autoantibody-associated small-vessel vasculitis. *Annu Rev Pathol*. 2013;8:139-160.

Lutalo PMK, D'Cruz DP. Diagnosis and classification of granulomatosis with polyangiitis (aka Wegener's granulomatosis). *J Autoimmun*. 2014;48–49:94-98.

Millet A, Pederzoli-Ribeil M, Guillevin L, et al. Antineutrophil cytoplasmic antibody-associated vasculitides: is it time to split up the group? *Ann Rheum Dis*. 2013;72:1273-1279.

Ponniah I, Shaheen A, Shankar KA, Kumaran MG. Wegener's granulomatosis: the current understanding. *Oral Surg Oral Med Oral Pathol Oral Radiol Endod*. 2005;100:265-270.

Rodrigo JP, Suarez C, Rinaldo A, et al. Idiopathic midline destructive disease: fact or fiction. *Oral Oncol*. 2005;41:340-348.

Stewart C, Cohen D, Bhattacharyya I, et al. Oral manifestations of Wegener's granulomatosis: a report of three cases and a literature review. *J Am Dent Assoc*. 2007;138:338-348, quiz 96, 98.

Stone JH, Merkel PA, Spiera R, et al. Rituximab versus cyclophosphamide for ANCA-associated vasculitis. *N Engl J Med*. 2010;363:221-232.

9 PIGMENTED LESIONS

CHAPTER CONTENTS

Exogenous Pigmentation

Amalgam tattoos are by far the most common form of exogenous pigmentation seen in the oral cavity. A distant second is graphite tattoo from implanted pencil lead.

AMALGAM TATTOO (FOCAL AGYROSIS)

Clinical Findings

- This occurs in adults as a nontender, localized lesion (usually <1 cm), or less commonly as a diffuse slate or blue-gray macule of the oral mucosa that is evenly pigmented.
- It often occurs on the gingiva adjacent to an amalgam restoration or crown, or around an apicoectomy (root apex surgery) scar after an amalgam retrofill (Fig. 9.1A–D); however, any mucosal site may be affected; larger particles may be evident on radiograph (Fig. 9.1E–F)

Etiopathogenesis and Histopathologic Features

Silver within amalgam restorations (a combination of silver, mercury, tin, and other metals) stains agyrophilic connective tissue fibers. It either leaches out of contacting amalgams or root canal fillings, or is traumatically implanted; the latter is the most often biopsied because it is not in direct contact with a restoration.

- Scarring and fibrosis are always present for traumatically implanted lesions with a variable lymphocytic infiltrate and may be the first clue that an amalgam tattoo is present (Figs. 9.2A–B and 9.4A).

Three patterns are recognized (Figs. 9.2–9.4):

- Fine golden-brown particles are deposited in a "beaded" pattern along connective tissue fibers, the basement membrane of the epithelium and blood vessels, perineurium and endomysium (Figs. 9.2C–D and 9.3)
- Golden-brown staining of connective tissue fibers occurs with or without particulate deposits (Figs. 9.2E and 9.4B)
- Larger particles are found within foreign body granulomas (Figs. 9.2B and 9.3B).
- Fine refractile crystalline foreign material likely represents fragments of dental cement placed with amalgams.

Differential Diagnosis

- Medication-induced pigmentation exhibits fine particles that align in linear fashion between collagen fibers, but they do not stain the fibers; usually they are Fontana-Masson and/or iron positive (see later).

Management and Prognosis

- No treatment is necessary although surgical or laser removal may be performed for cosmetic reasons.

REFERENCES

Buchner A. Amalgam tattoo (amalgam pigmentation) of the oral mucosa: clinical manifestations, diagnosis and treatment. *Refuat Hapeh Vehashinayim.* 2004;21:25-28, 92.

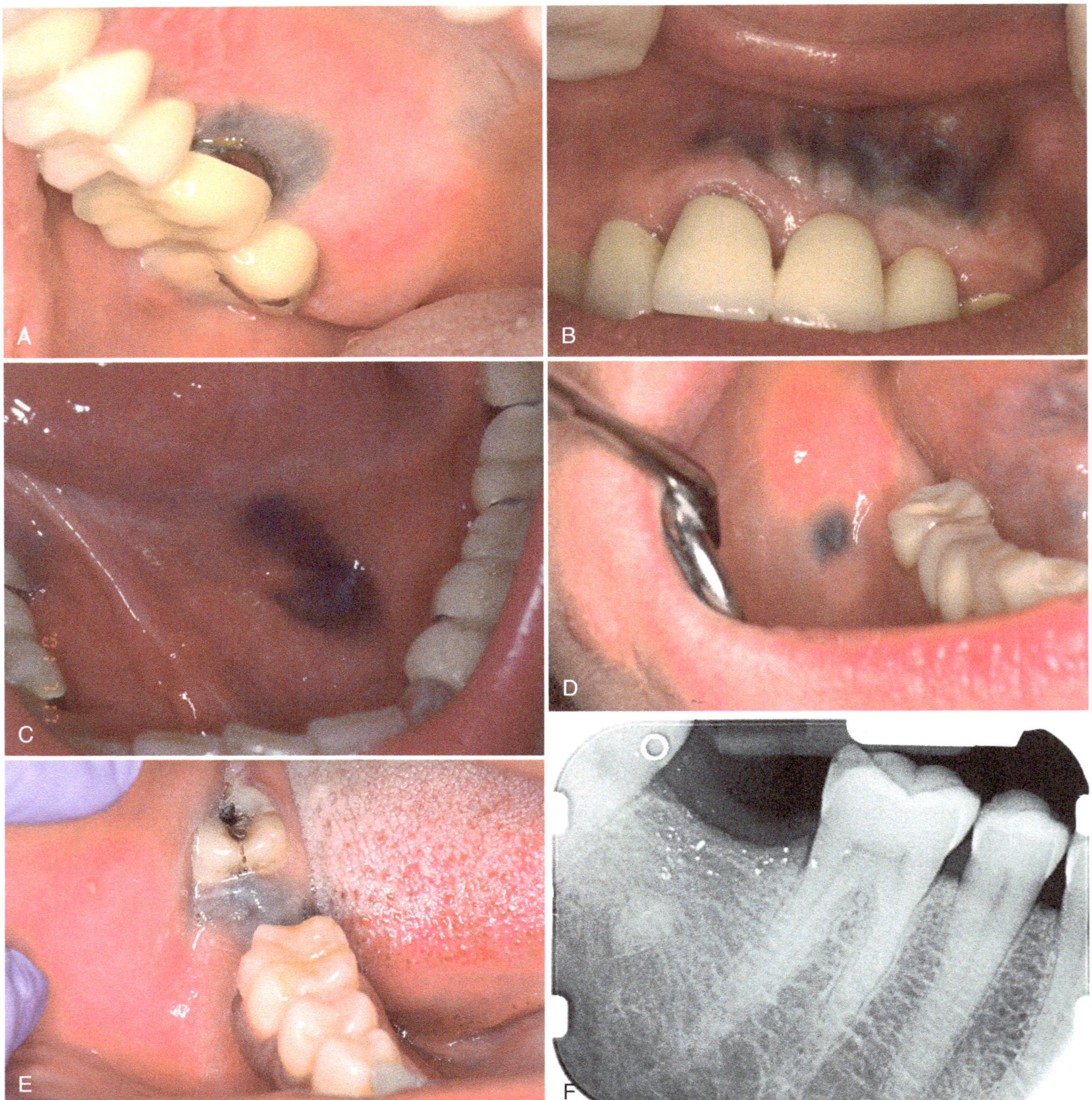

FIG 9.1 (A) Amalgam tattoo adjacent to a crown. (B) Amalgam tattoo related to apicoectomy (apical surgery) scar. (C) Amalgam tattoo on the floor of mouth. (D) Amalgam tattoo on the right buccal mucosa close to a crown. (E) Amalgam tattoo on the alveolar ridge after extraction. (F) Periapical radiograph of FIG 9.1E shows amalgam particles.

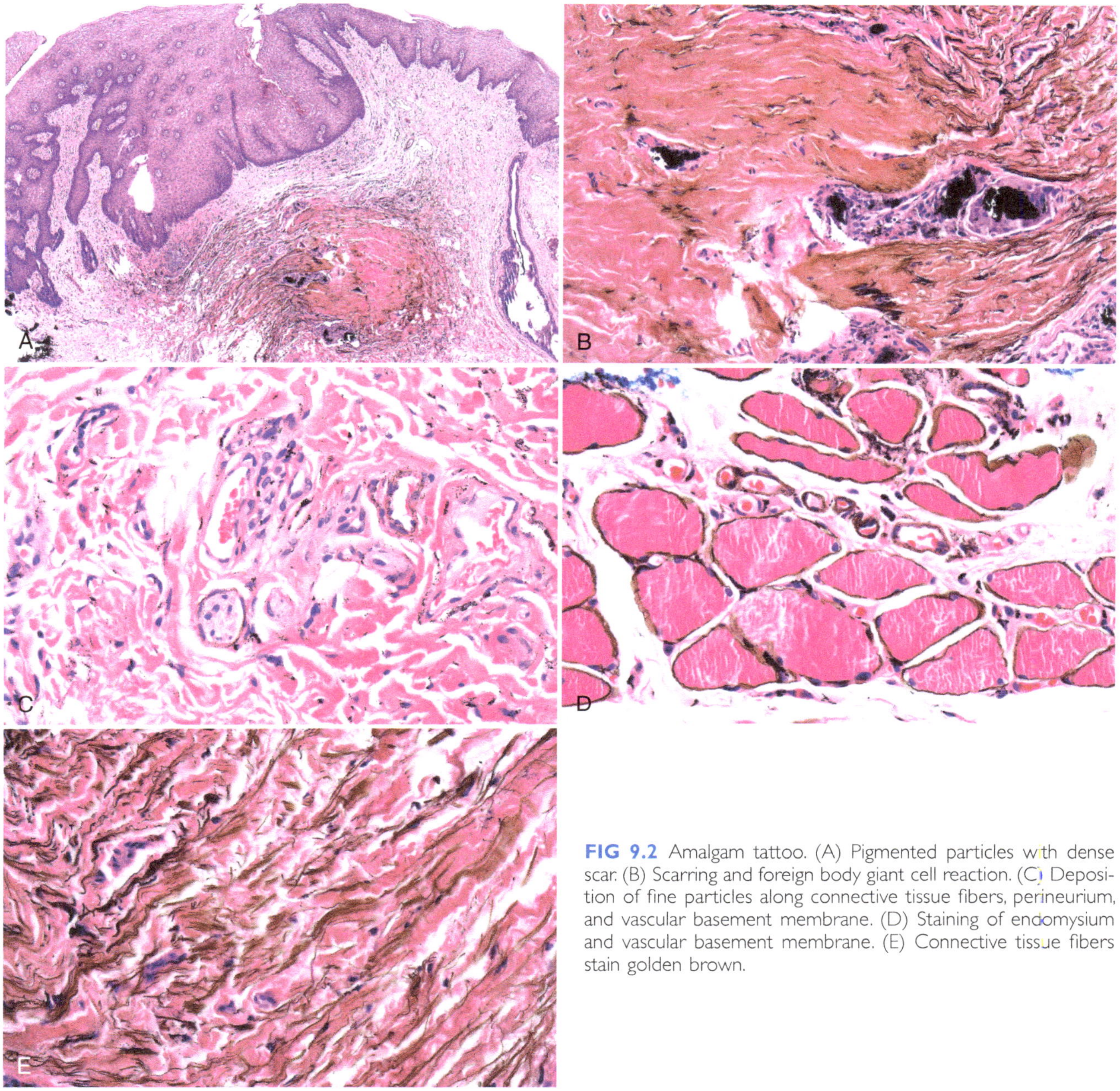

FIG 9.2 Amalgam tattoo. (A) Pigmented particles with dense scar. (B) Scarring and foreign body giant cell reaction. (C) Deposition of fine particles along connective tissue fibers, perineurium, and vascular basement membrane. (D) Staining of endomysium and vascular basement membrane. (E) Connective tissue fibers stain golden brown.

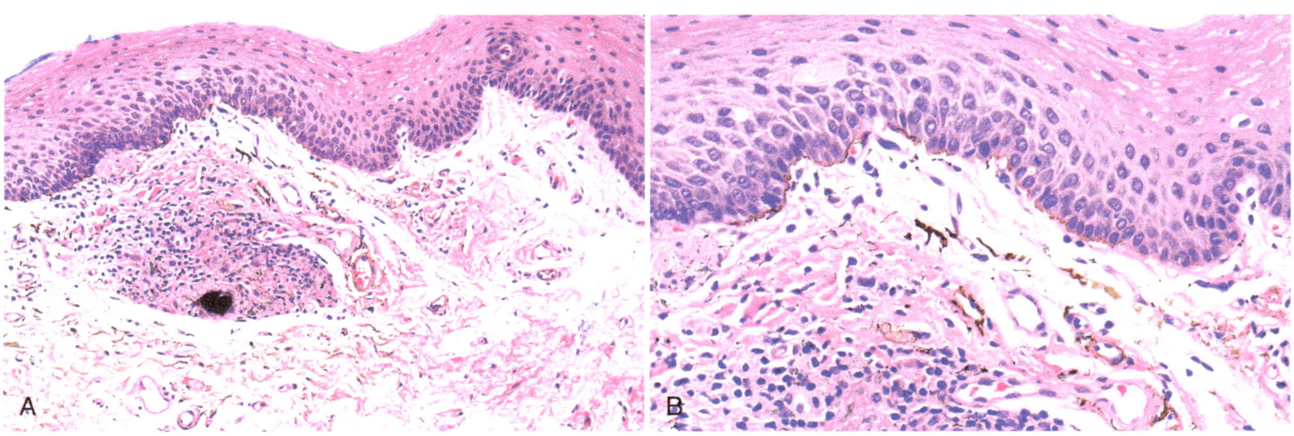

FIG 9.3 Amalgam tattoo. (A) Foreign body granuloma with coarse amalgam particles. (B) Staining of basement membrane of epithelium and capillaries.

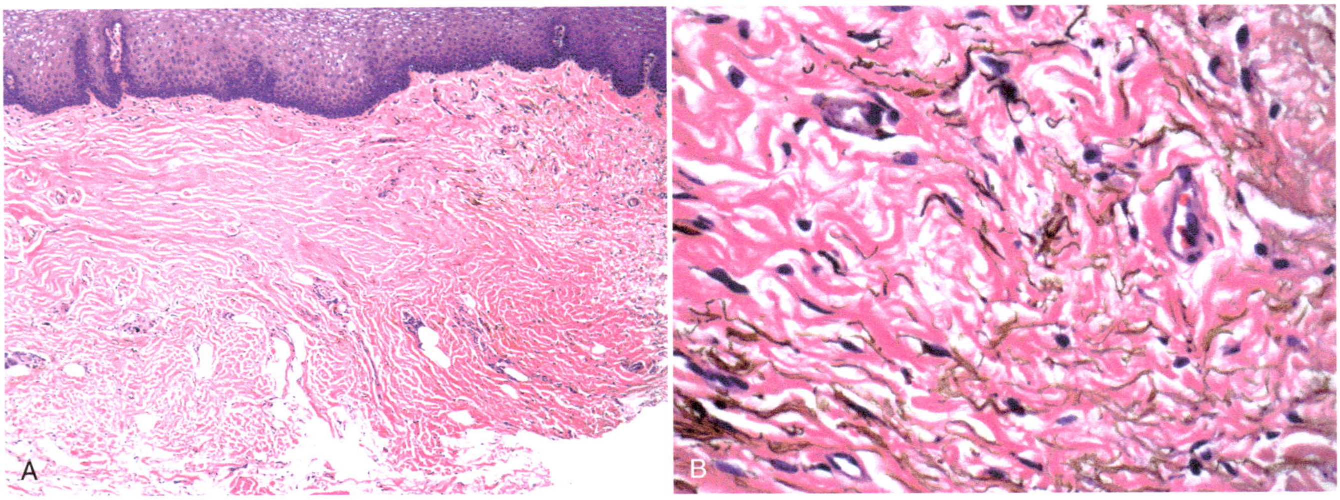

FIG 9.4 Subtle amalgam tattoo. (A) Focal scarring noted. (B) Golden-brown staining of connective tissue fibers.

Buchner A, Hansen LS. Amalgam pigmentation (amalgam tattoo) of the oral mucosa. A clinicopathologic study of 268 cases. *Oral Surg Oral Med Oral Pathol.* 1980;49:139-147.

Kanzaki T, Eto H, Miyazawa S. Electron microscopic x-ray microanalysis of metals deposited in oral mucosa. *J Dermatol.* 1992;19:487-492.

Koppang HS, Roushan A, Srafilzadeh A, et al. Foreign body gingival lesions: distribution, morphology, identification by X-ray energy dispersive analysis and possible origin of foreign material. *J Oral Pathol Med.* 2007;36:161-172.

Lau JC, Jackson-Boeters L, Daley TD, et al. Metallothionein in human gingival amalgam tattoos. *Arch Oral Biol.* 2001;46:1015-1020.

GRAPHITE AND OTHER FOREIGN BODY TATTOOS

Clinical Findings

- Localized gray-to-black, nontender macule or nodule occurs on any mucosal site but often on the palatal mucosa (eg, child who falls when running with a pencil held between the teeth, puncturing the palate) (Fig. 9.5A); other foreign material (eg, glass) may elicit inflammation and may be painful.
- Ritualistic tattooing of the skin and mouth (especially gingiva) is practiced in some cultures in the world (such as in Africa), as well as among incarcerated subjects; these are not usually biopsied (Fig. 9-5B)

Etiopathogenesis and Histopathologic Features

This is caused by traumatic implantation of pencil lead (graphite) or other material.

- Graphite takes the form of coarse black granules of nonrefractile, slightly geometric, foreign material, some of which lie within multinucleate giant cells of foreign body granulomas; there are no distinguishing features so the history of traumatic implantation is important (Fig. 9.6). There may be yellow birefringence under polarized light at the periphery of the particles.

Differential Diagnosis

- Unlike amalgam, graphite does not stain connective tissue fibers; it maintains birefringence after treatment with 10% ammonium sulfide, whereas amalgam may have weak birefringence that is quenched on treatment with ammonium sulfide.
- Other traumatically-implanted foreign bodies should be considered after a careful review of the history; dispersive spectroscopy may be employed to identify the foreign material.

Management and Prognosis

- No treatment is necessary although surgical or laser removal may be performed for cosmetic reasons.

REFERENCES

Daley TD, Gibson D. Practical applications of energy dispersive x-ray microanalysis in diagnostic oral pathology. *Oral Surg Oral Med Oral Pathol.* 1990;69:339-344.

Hussaini HM, Waddell JN, Girvan L, et al. Silver solder "tattoo," a novel form of oral pigmentation identified with the use of field emission scanning electron microscopy and electron dispersive spectrography. *Oral Surg Oral Med Oral Pathol Oral Radiol Endod.* 2011;112:e6-e10.

Peters E, Gardner DG. A method of distinguishing between amalgam and graphite in tissue. *Oral Surg Oral Med Oral Pathol.* 1986; 62:73-76.

Phillips GE, John V. Use of a subepithelial connective tissue graft to treat an area pigmented with graphite. *J Periodontol.* 2005;76:1572-1575.

Rawal SY, Burrell R, Hamidi CS, et al. Diffuse pigmentation of maxillary attached gingiva: four cases of the cultural practice of gingival tattoo. *J Periodontol.* 2007;78:170-176.

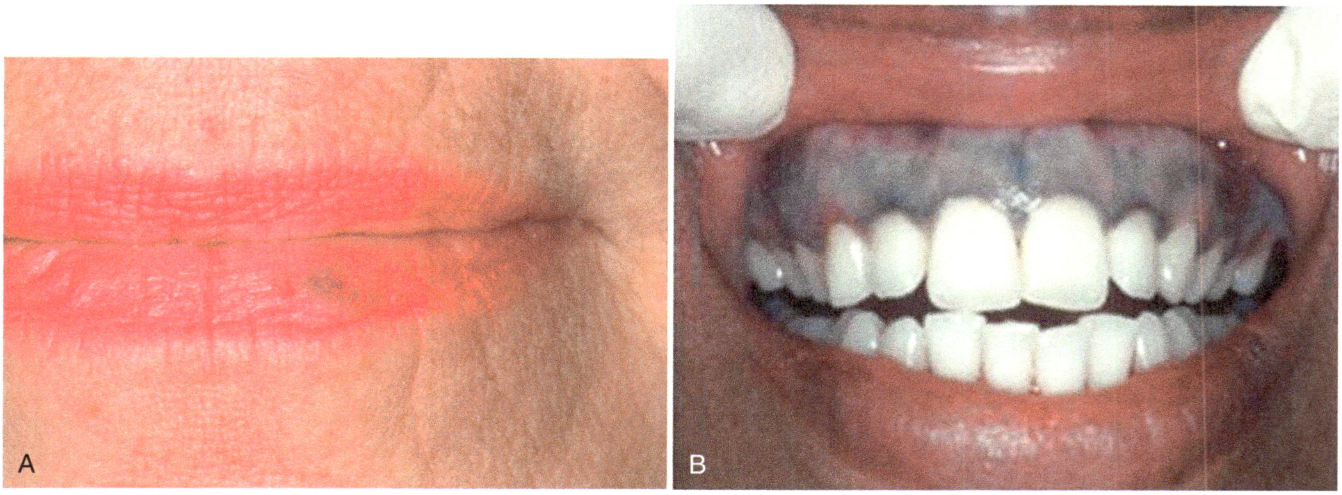

FIG 9.5 (A) Graphite tattoo on the left lower lip. (B) Ritualistic tattoo of the gingiva.

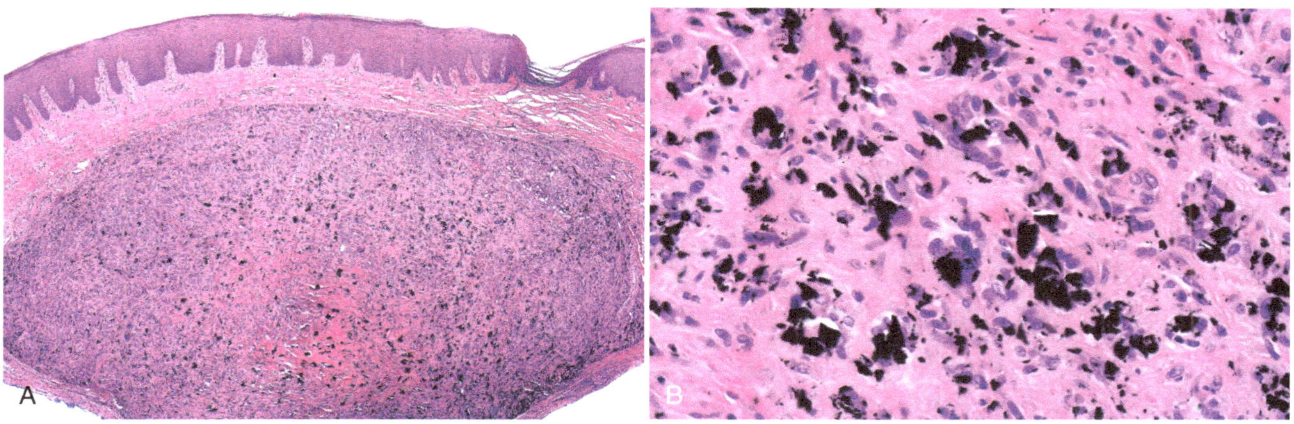

FIG 9.6 Graphite tattoo. (A) Granulomatous reaction and fibrosis. (B) Irregular, geometric, large and small, black particles with surrounding macrophages.

MEDICATION-INDUCED PIGMENTATION

Clinical Findings

- Diffuse, painless, symmetric, bluish-gray macular pigmentation of the hard palatal mucosa (may be subtle) is typical and there may be concomitant melanonychia and skin lesions (Fig. 9.7).
- Minocycline, antimalarial medications (such as mepacrine or quinacrine), imatinib, birth control pills, and clofazimine may give rise to this condition.
- Tetracycline and its analogues are taken up by teeth and bone, which appear brown; discoloration is visible through the oral mucosa.
- Rare instances of pigmentation caused by leaching of metals from a denture have been reported.

Etiopathogenesis and Histopathologic Features

Medication-induced pigmentation occurs through several mechanisms. Break-down products of antimalarial drugs, minocycline and imatinib chelate with iron or melanin and deposit within the lamina propria. Birth control pills lower cortisol level and increase levels of adrenocorticotrophic hormone (ACTH), leading to stimulation of melanocytes while the breakdown product of clofazamine is itself red. It is unclear why medication-associated pigment deposits exclusively on the hard palatal mucosa in the mouth.

- Particles are brown, uniformly spherical, only a few microns in diameter and align in linear fashion between collagen fibers, although this likely represents pigment within dendritic processes of macrophages or other dendritic cells (Fig. 9.8A–B).
- Particles stain with Prussian blue for iron and Fontana-Masson stain for melanin, although the degree of staining is variable (see Fig. 9.8C–D); they elicit no fibrosis or inflammation.
- Teeth and bone that are stained by tetracycline fluoresce under polarized light.

Differential Diagnosis

- Amalgam particles are not uniformly spherical, and they stain connective tissue fibers.
- Hemosiderin particles are larger, coarser, and more variable in size, and stain with Prussian blue stain (Fig. 9.9); there may be inflammation and hemorrhage present.

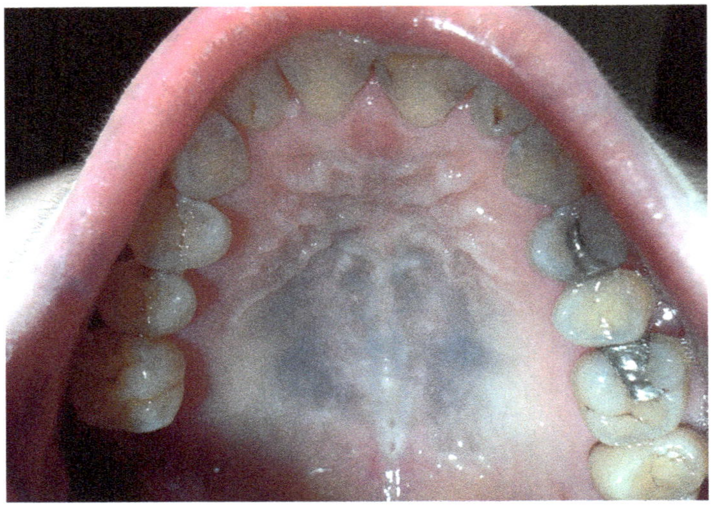

FIG 9.7 Imatinib-induced pigmentation of the palatal mucosa. *(Courtesy Dr. Paul Kuo, private practice, Brookline, Mass.)*

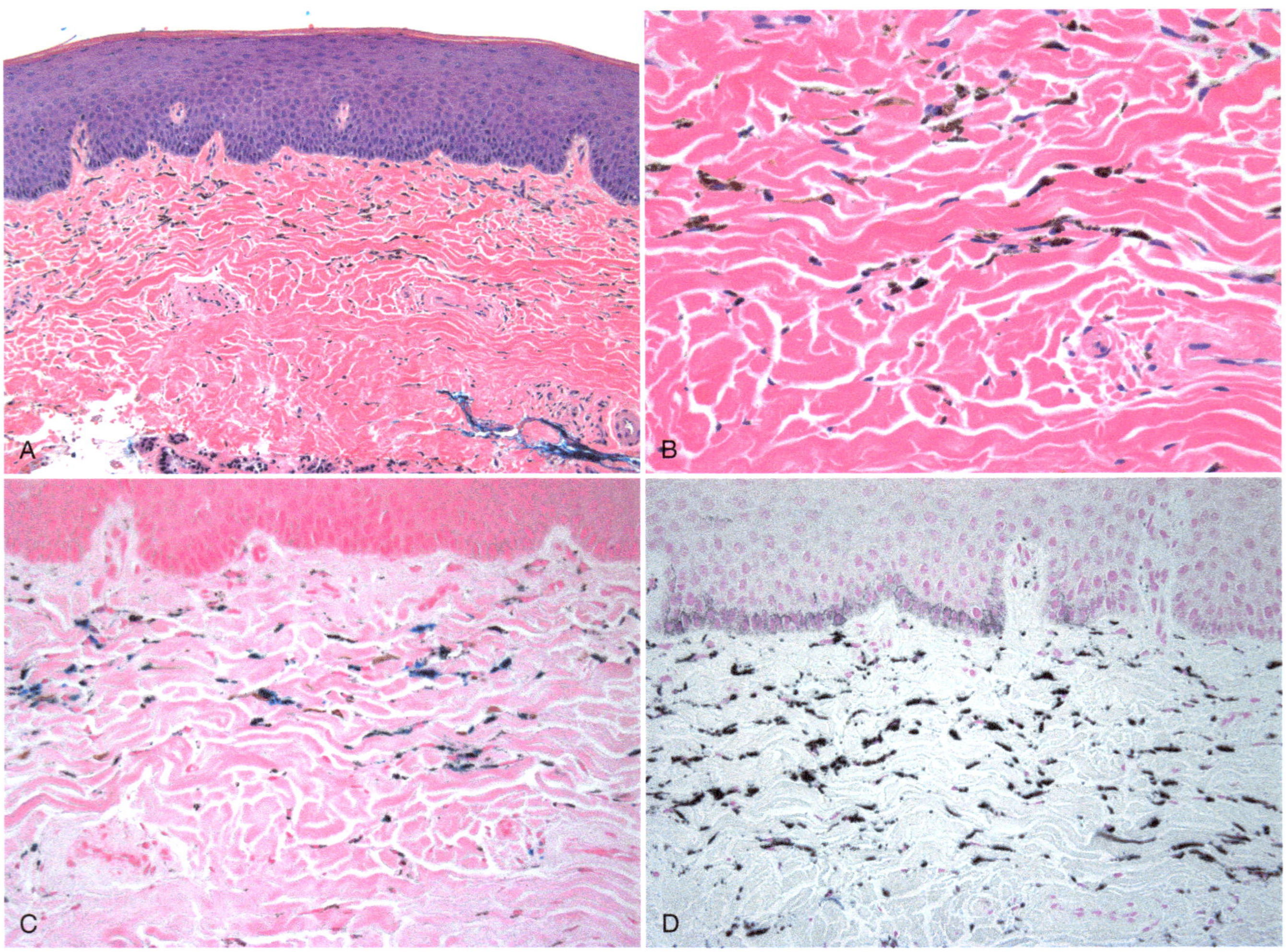

FIG 9.8 Quinacrine pigmentation. (A) Pigmented particles are noted in the lamina propria without tissue reaction. (B) Fine, spherical dark-brown pigment granules are present within macrophages or dendritic processes. (C) Granules stain for iron (Prussian blue stain). (D) Granules stain for melanin (Fontana-Masson stain).

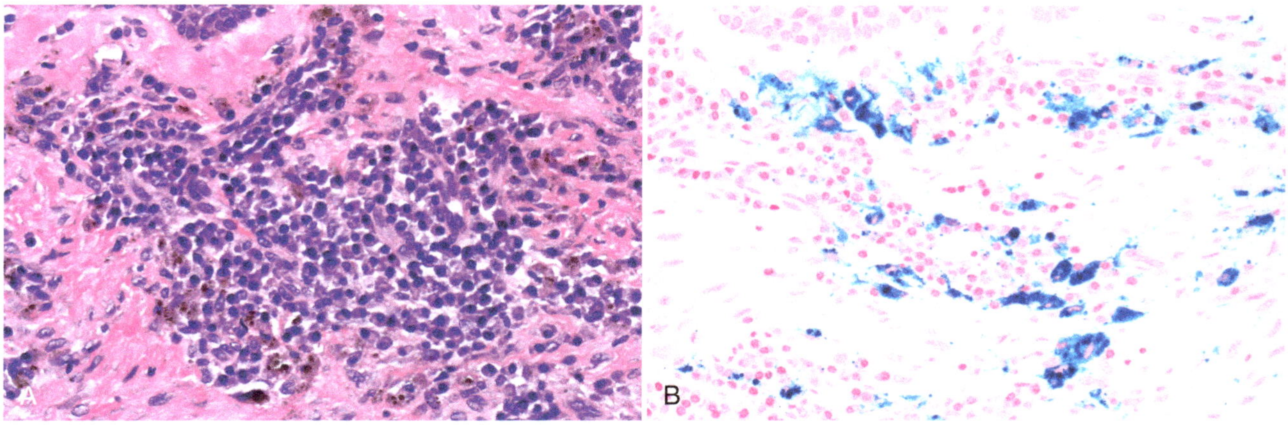

FIG 9.9 Hemosiderin deposits. (A) Coarse, irregular brown granules associated with many plasma cells. (B) Granules stain for iron (Prussian blue stain).

Melanotic macules exhibit melanophages in the lamina propria and melanin within basal cells.

- Blue nevus exhibits spindled melanocytes that react with MART-1 and HMB45 (see later).

Management and Prognosis

- No treatment is necessary.

REFERENCES

Cale AE, Freedman PD, Lumerman H. Pigmentation of the jawbones and teeth secondary to minocycline hydrochloride therapy. *J Periodontol.* 1988;59:112-114.

Kleinegger CL, Hammond HL, Finkelstein MW. Oral mucosal hyperpigmentation secondary to antimalarial drug therapy. *Oral Surg Oral Med Oral Pathol Oral Radiol Endod.* 2000;90:189-194.

Lerman MA, Karimbux N, Guze KA, Woo SB. Pigmentation of the hard palate. *Oral Surg Oral Med Oral Pathol Oral Radiol Endod.* 2009;107:8-12.

Li CC, Malik SM, Blaeser BF, et al. Mucosal pigmentation caused by imatinib: report of three cases. *Head Neck Pathol.* 2012;6:290-295.

Sloan P, Kujan O. Re: Martin TJM, Sharp I, Oral mucosal pigmentation secondary to treatment with mepacrine, with sparing of the denture bearing area (Br J Oral Maxillofac Surg 2004;42:351–3). *Br J Oral Maxillofac Surg.* 2005;43:268.

Treister NS, Magalnick D, Woo SB. Oral mucosal pigmentation secondary to minocycline therapy: report of two cases and a review of the literature. *Oral Surg Oral Med Oral Pathol Oral Radiol Endod.* 2004;97:718-725.

Melanocytic Pigmentation

Physiologic pigmentation is very common on the gingiva and elsewhere in the mouth in dark-skinned races and is generally bilaterally symmetric and evenly pigmented (Fig. 9.10A).

The two most common melanocytic lesions in the oral cavity are oral melanotic macule (comprising more than 80% of melanotic lesions) and postinflammatory hypermelanosis. Some melanotic macules are likely to represent end-stage postinflammatory hyperpigmentation. The less common melanoacanthosis is likely to represent an uncommon form of postinflammatory pigmentation. Smoker's melanosis are diffuse brown macules on the gingiva and may also represent postinflammatory hypermelanosis (Fig. 9.11).

ORAL MELANOTIC MACULE (LABIAL MELANOTIC MACULE)

Clinical Findings

- This occurs most frequently in the fifth decade with a 2–3 : 1 female predilection; rarely, macules may occur congenitally on the tongue sometimes associated with an epithelial choristoma.
- Discrete, usually solitary (sometimes multiple), tan-to-brown-to-black, painless macules are evenly pigmented, less than 1 cm, and occur frequently on the lower vermilion (labial melanotic macule, 33% of cases), gingiva and palatal, and mucosa, or buccal mucosa (see Fig. 9.10B–D).
- Multiple mapules are seen in patients with increased levels of ACTH, such as Addison disease, and in syndromes such as the Laugier-Hunziker syndrome (with melanonychia), neurofibromatosis, Peutz-Jeghers syndrome, McCune-Albright syndrome, Carney syndrome complex, LEOPARD (Lentigines, Electrocardiographic abnormalities, Ocular hypertelorism, Pulmonary stenosis, Abnormal genitalia, Retarded growth, Deafness) syndrome, and Bannayan-Ruvalcaba-Riley syndrome.

Etiopathogenesis and Histopathologic Features

Some solitary melanotic macules may represent postinflammatory hypermelanosis where the inflammatory infiltrate is no longer present, whereas others (especially multiple ones) may be idiopathic. It is unclear whether these resolve because it usually takes many months for postinflammatory hypermelanosis to resolve and most patients are not followed up after the diagnosis has been made. The fact that almost all solitary labial melanotic macules occur on the lower lip, a readily traumatized site, rather than the upper lip, supports this theory.

- There is mild acanthosis and increased melanin within basal cells in the absence of, or with minimal melanocytic hyperplasia, with melanin being most prominent in the lower half of the epithelium and at tips of rete ridges; incontinent melanin and melanophages are present in the lamina propria (Figs. 9.12 and 9.13).

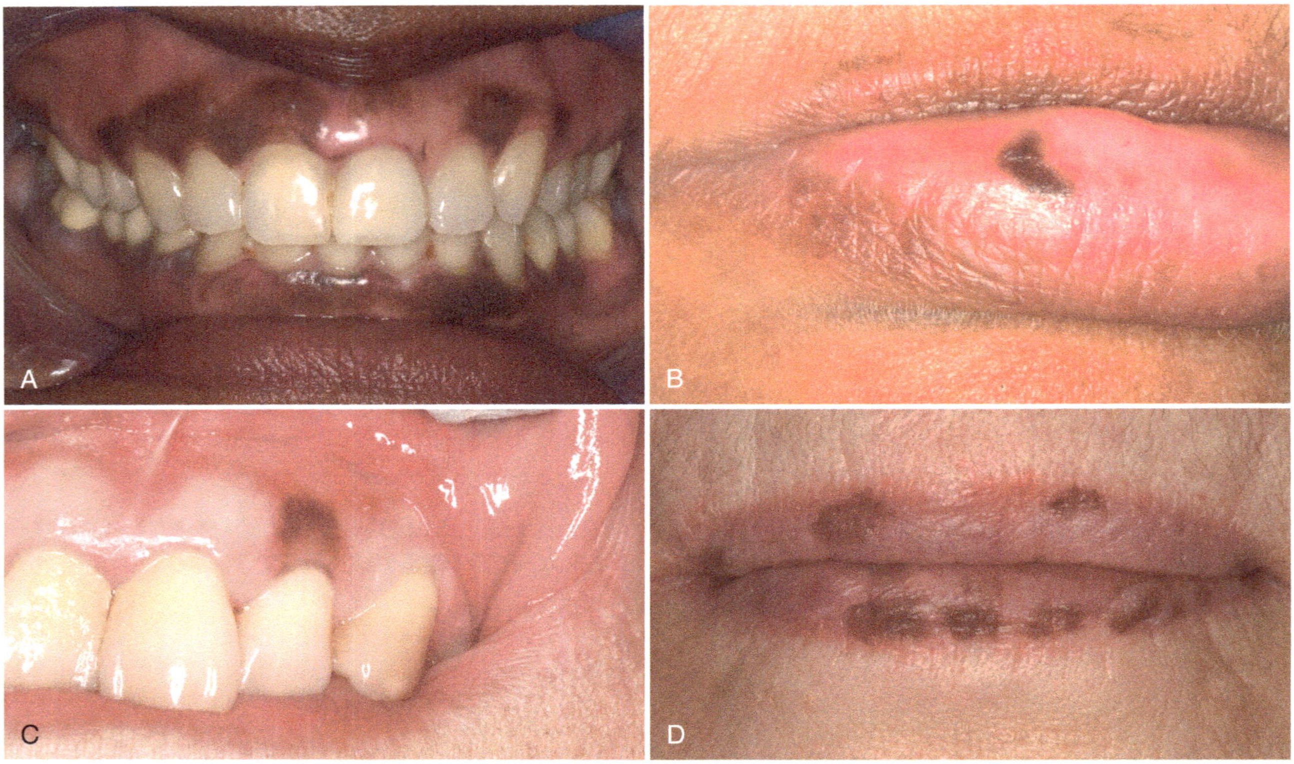

FIG 9.10 (A) Physiologic pigmentation of the gingiva. (B) Oral melanotic macule of the lower vermilion. (C) Oral melanotic macule of the gingiva. (D) Multiple oral melanotic macules, idiopathic.

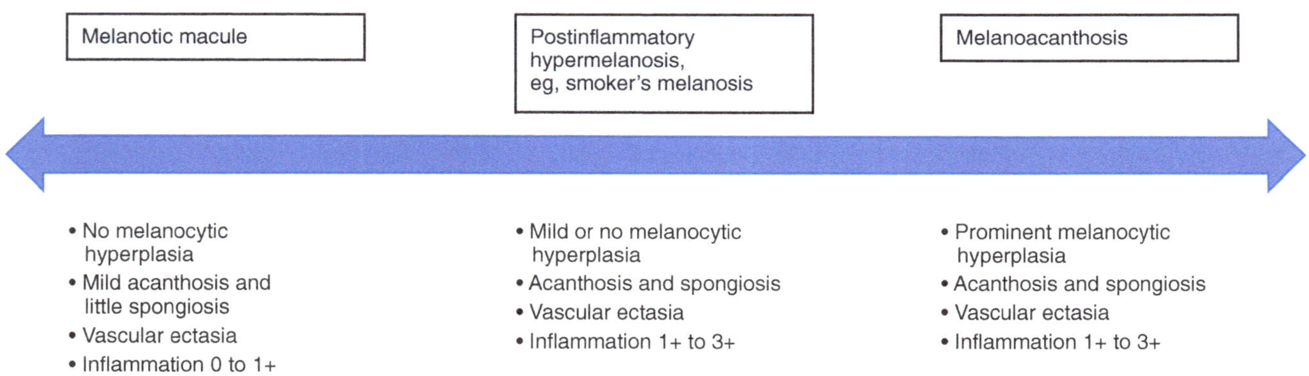

FIG 9.11 Possible relationship between melanotic macule, postinflammatory hypermelanosis, and melanoacanthosis.

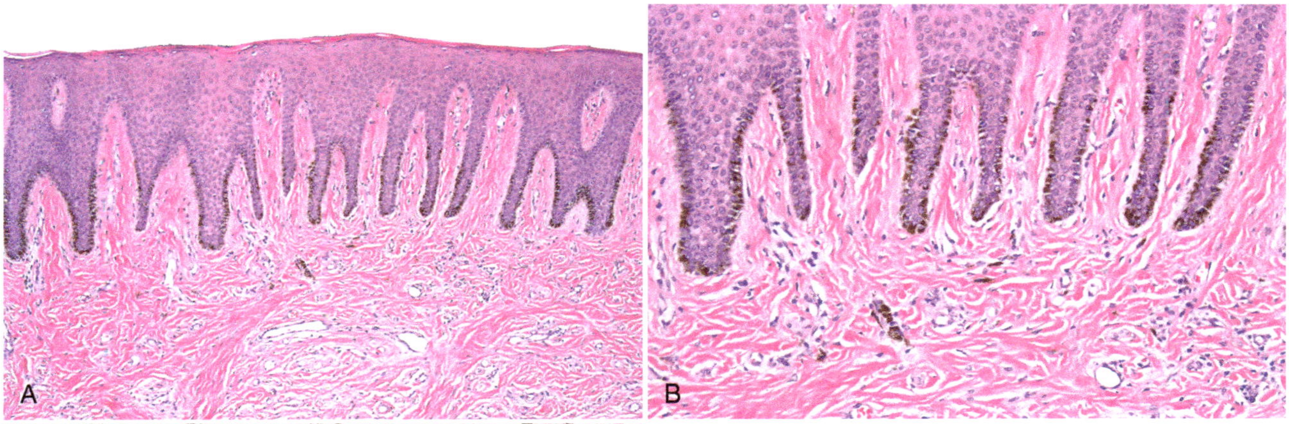

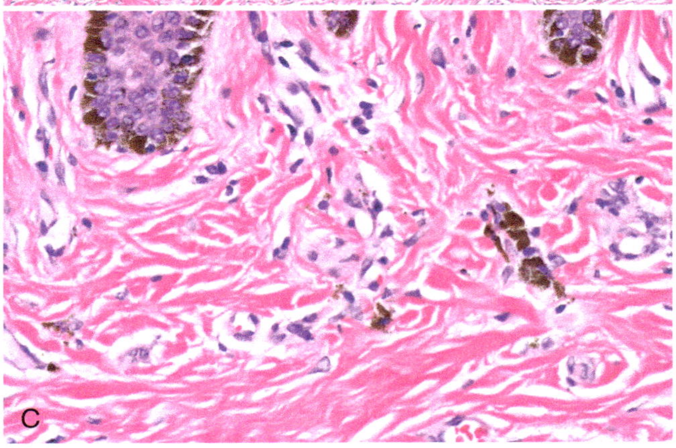

FIG 9.12 Oral melanotic macule of palatal mucosa. (A) Mild acanthosis and no inflammation. (B) Abundant melanin in basal cells at the lower half and tips of rete ridges without melanocytic hyperplasia. (C) Incontinent melanin and melanophages are noted in the lamina propria.

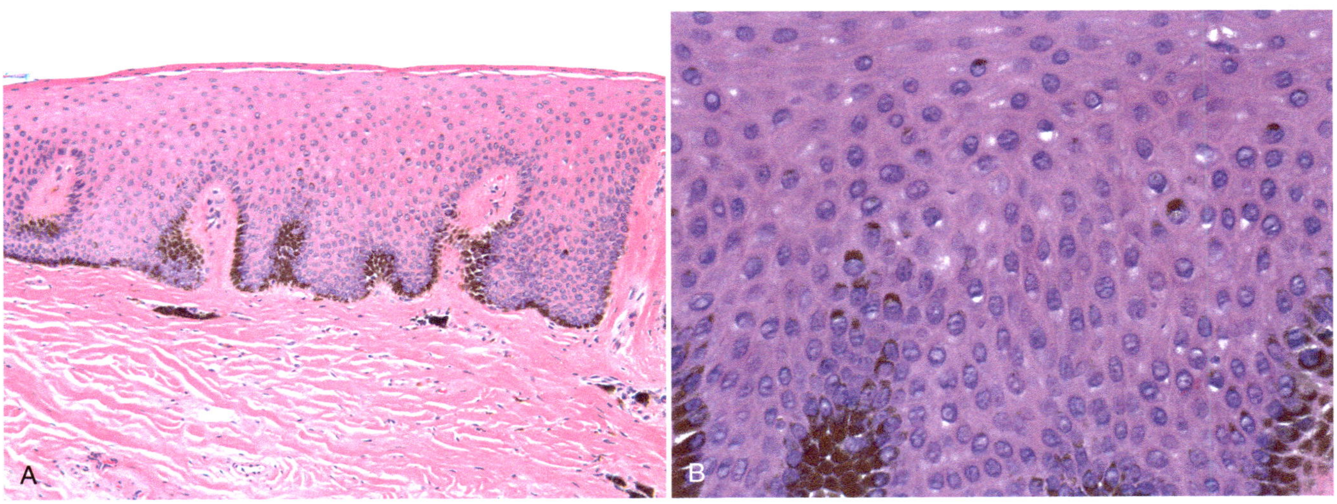

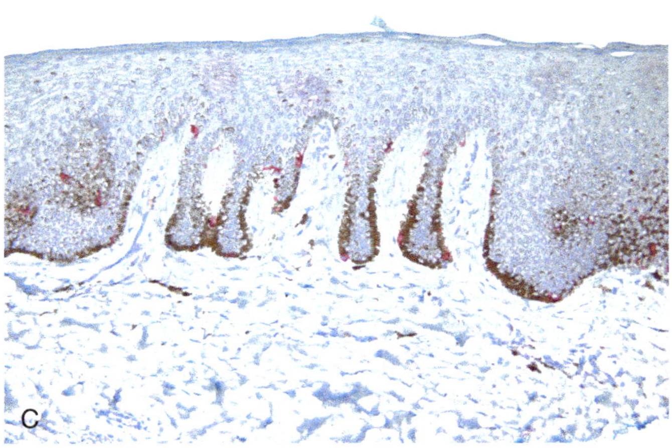

FIG 9.13 Melanotic macule. (A) Abundant melanin in basal cells at the tips of rete ridges. (B) Melanin within spinous cells forming a supranuclear cap. (C) Absence of melanocytic hyperplasia (Melan-A).

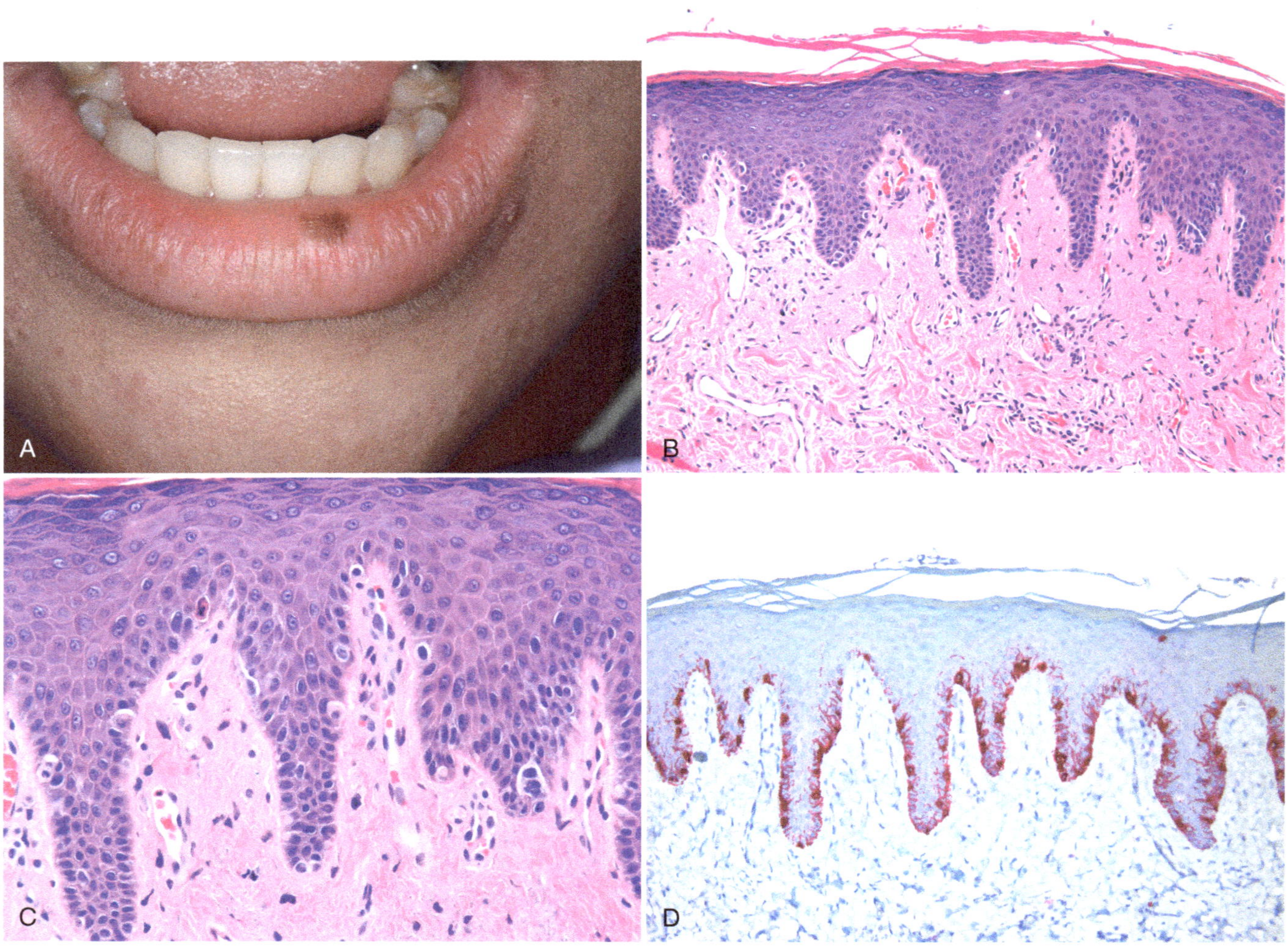

FIG 9.14 Lentigo simplex. (A) Brown macule on lower lip similar to melanotic macule, histology depicted in B–D. (B) Slight acanthosis with melanocytic hyperplasia, vascular ectasia, and mild chronic inflammation. (C) Melanocytic hyperplasia with slight reactive atypia. (D) Lentiginous melanocytic hyperplasia confined to the basal cell layer (Melan-A).

- Variable vascular ectasia is usually present with absent-to-mild lymphocytic infiltrate.

Differential Diagnosis

Postinflammatory hypermelanosis appears similar with obvious inflammation present and is often seen in interface stomatitides such as lichenoid stomatitis.

Melanoacanthosis shows acanthosis with dendritic melanocytes present throughout the thickness of the epithelium.

Lentigo exhibits benign melanocytic hyperplasia within the basal cell layer (Fig. 9.14).

Management and Prognosis

- No treatment is necessary although laser ablation may be helpful if there are cosmetic concerns.

REFERENCES

Buchner A, Merrell PW, Carpenter WM. Relative frequency of solitary melanocytic lesions of the oral mucosa. *J Oral Pathol Med.* 2004;33:550-557.

Curto-Barredo L, Vicente A, Rovira C, et al. Epidermal choristoma of the tongue mimicking a congenital melanotic macule. *Pediatr Dermatol.* 2015;32:536-538.

Dohil MA, Billman G, Pransky S, Eichenfield LF. The congenital lingual melanotic macule. *Arch Dermatol.* 2003;139:767-770.

Gupta G, Williams RE, Mackie RM. The labial melanotic macule: a review of 79 cases. *Br J Dermatol.* 1997;136:772-775.

Horvath A, Stratakis CA. Carney complex and lentiginosis. *Pigment Cell Melanoma Res.* 2009;22:580-587.

Kaugars GE, Heise AP, Riley WT, et al. Oral melanotic macules. A review of 353 cases. *Oral Surg Oral Med Oral Pathol.* 1993;76:59-61.

Mignogna MD, Lo Muzio L, Ruoppo E, et al. Oral manifestations of idiopathic lenticular mucocutaneous pigmentation (Laugier-Hunziker syndrome): a clinical, histopathological and ultrastructural review of 12 cases. *Oral Dis.* 1999;5:80-86.

Yago K, Tanaka Y, Asanami S. Laugier-Hunziker-Baran syndrome. *Oral Surg Oral Med Oral Pathol Oral Radiol Endod.* 2008;106:e20-e25.

POSTINFLAMMATORY HYPERMELANOSIS

Clinical Findings

- These are conditions leading to damage of the basal cell layer such as lichen planus or lichenoid stomatitis, ulcers, and other inflammatory conditions, and are much more common in dark-skinned races; it is likely that smoker's melanosis represents postinflammatory hypermelanosis.
- There is diffuse pigmentation of the mucosa in the area of the inflammatory condition although pigmentation may be discrete if the inflammation is localized (Fig. 9.15).

Etiopathogenesis and Histopathologic Features

Inflammatory lesions and, in particular, lichenoid lesions often result from destruction of melanin-containing basal cells, leading to release of melanin into the lamina propria, and/or increased production of melanin by melanocytes (sometimes with slight melanocytic hyperplasia) which are taken up by basal cells.

- Increased melanin pigment is present within basal cells with insignificant or mild benign melanocytic hyperplasia, and incontinent melanin, melanophages, and inflammation are noted in the lamina propria (Fig. 9.16); infrequently, there is benign melanocytic hyperplasia resembling early melanoacanthosis (Fig. 9.17).
- Variable inflammation is evident (eg, lichenoid mucositis or nonspecific chronic inflammation) (Fig. 9.18).

Differential Diagnosis

- There is likely overlap with melanoacanthosis if significant melanocytic hyperplasia is present.

Management and Prognosis

- No treatment is necessary; even with treatment of the underlying inflammatory condition with topical steroid therapy, it takes many months for the hyperpigmentation to fade.

REFERENCE

Calonje E, Brenn T, Lazar AJ, McKee PH, eds. *McKee's Pathology of the Skin*. ed 4. Philadelphia: Saunders; 2012.

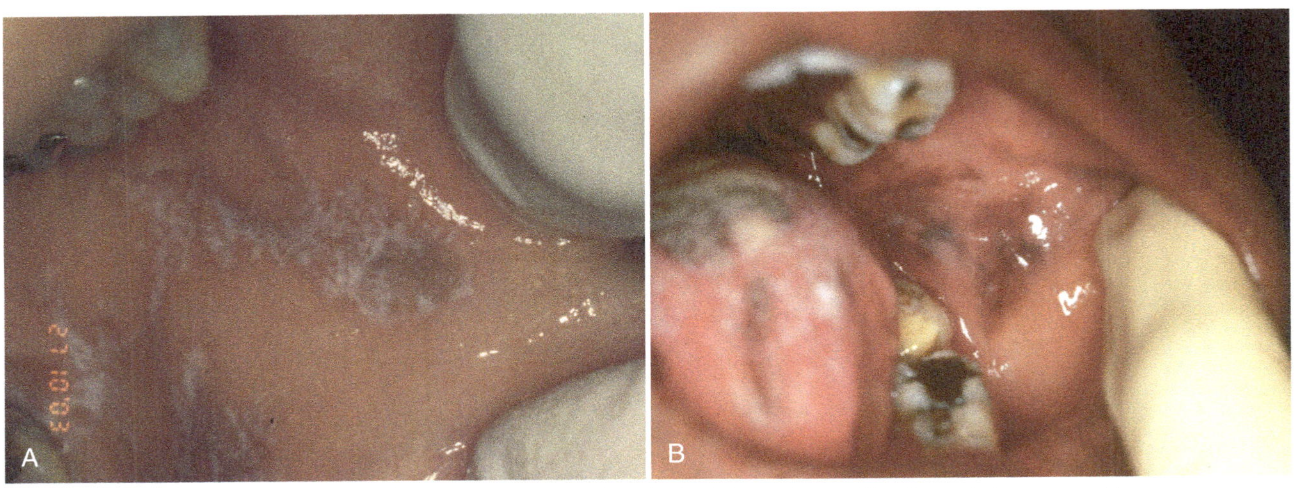

FIG 9.15 (A) Postinflammatory hypermelanosis in lichen planus. (B) Postradiation mucositis hypermelanosis.

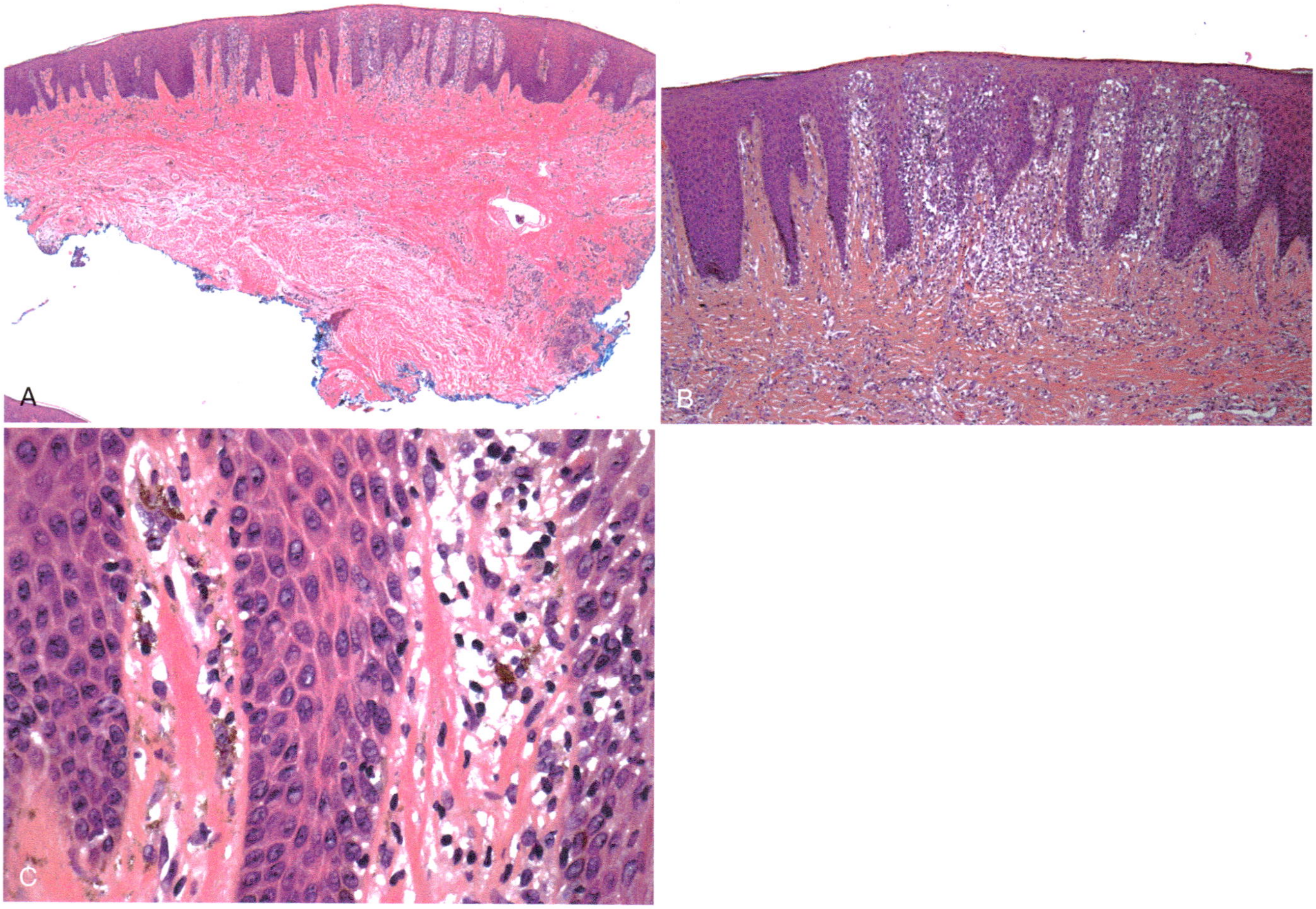

FIG 9.16 Oral melanotic macule of lower lip. (A) Multifocal areas exhibiting chronic inflammation at the interface. (B) Melanin within basal cells at tips of rete ridges *(left)* and chronic inflammation at the interface. (C) Melanin within basal cells and many melanophages and lymphocytes typical for postinflammatory hypermelanosis (right), much less inflammation on left.

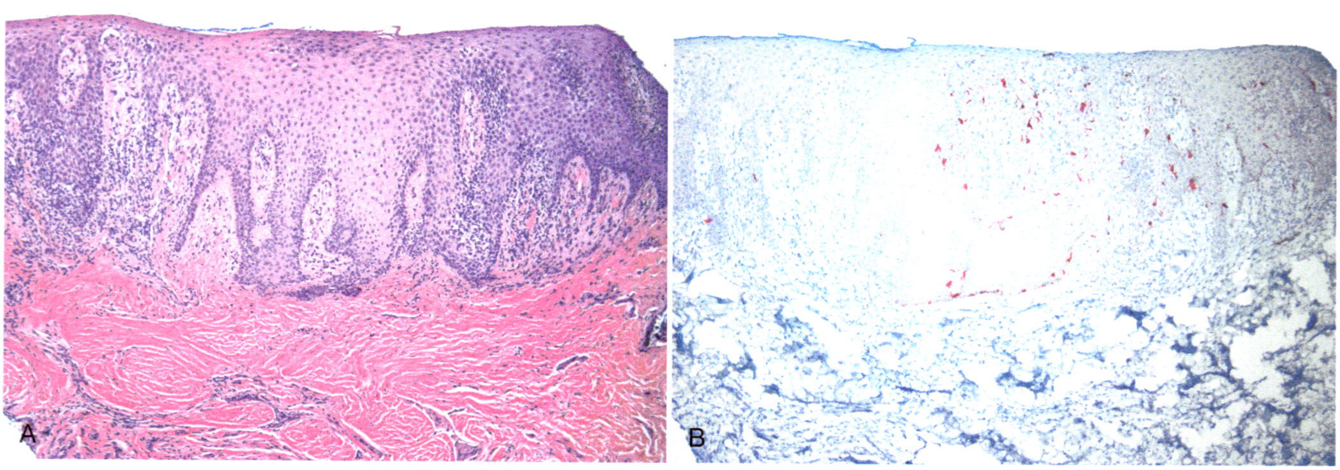

FIG 9.17 Postinflammatory hypermelanosis. (A) Acanthosis and focal spongiosis and chronic inflammation. (B) Benign melanocytic hyperplasia throughout the epithelium (Melan-A).

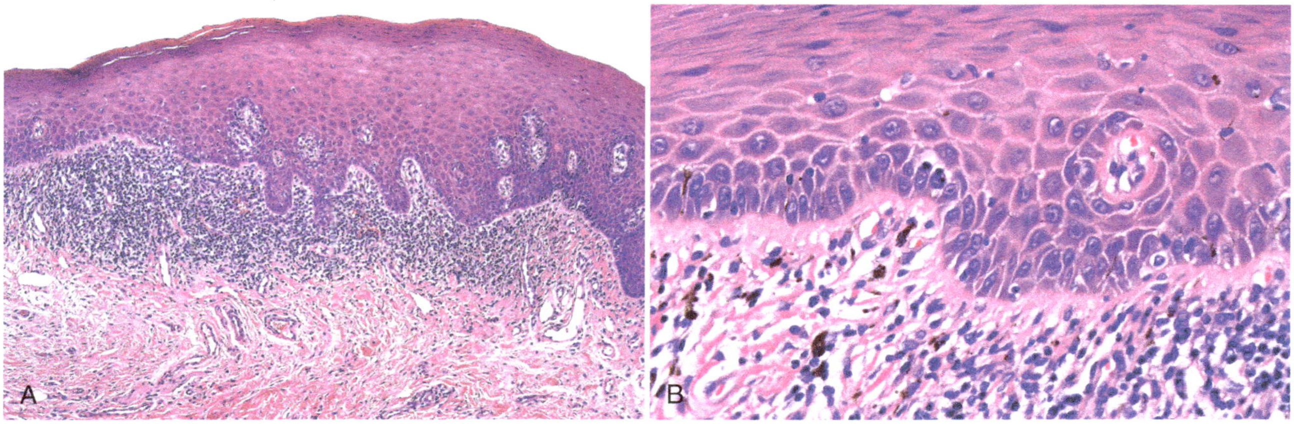

FIG 9.18 Lichenoid stomatitis. (A) Squamatization of basal cells and lymphocytic band at the interface. (B) Melanin pigment within melanocytes and mid-level dendritic processes in the epithelium and melanophages in lamina propria.

MELANOACANTHOSIS (MELANOACANTHOMA)

The term melanoacanthosis is preferable to melanoacanthoma because this is a macular lesion and not a tumor-like proliferation, and is clinically distinct from cutaneous melanoacanthoma that occurs in older Caucasian patients as plaques or nodules.

Clinical Findings

- It usually occurs in young, Black patients (80%), with a 3:1 female predilection, developing fairly rapidly within days to a few weeks as a painless, tan-brown macule that is usually solitary (80%) or multifocal and is often greater than 1 cm; the most common location is the buccal mucosa (50%), followed by the palatal mucosa and lips (Fig. 9.19).

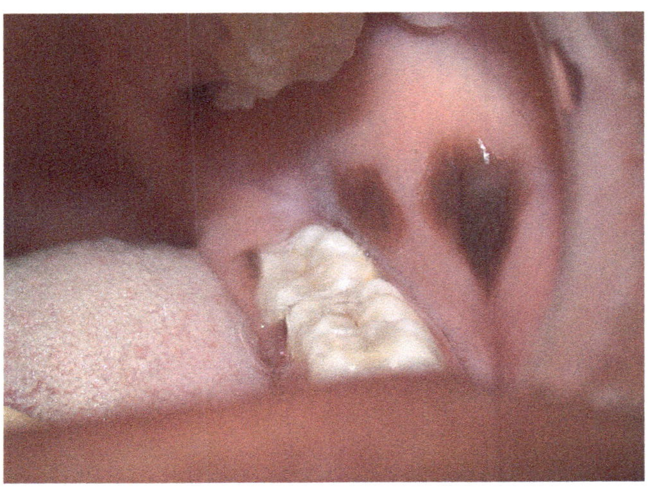

FIG 9.19 Melanoacanthosis of left buccal mucosa. *(Courtesy Dr. Bonnie Padwa, Harvard School of Dental Medicine, Boston, Mass.)*

Etiopathogenesis and Histopathologic Features

This condition likely represents one end of the spectrum of postinflammatory hypermelanosis, with the other end being the melanotic macule (see Fig. 9.11).

- There is acanthosis with proliferation of benign dendritic melanocytes located throughout the full thickness of the epithelium that exhibits spongiosis; there is increased melanin within basal cells with incontinent melanin, melanophages, and variable chronic inflammation in the lamina propria (Figs. 9.20A and 9.21A–C)
- Melanocytes positive for S-100 and Melan-A (see Figs. 9.20B and 9.21D)

Differential Diagnosis

- Lack of melanocytic atypia rules out an atypical melanocytic proliferation or melanoma-in-situ despite transmigration of melanocytes.

Management and Prognosis

- No treatment is necessary because lesions fade over time.

REFERENCES

Carlos-Bregni R, Contreras E, Netto AC, et al. Oral melanoacanthoma and oral melanotic macule: a report of 8 cases, review of the literature, and immunohistochemical analysis. *Med Oral Patol Oral Cir Bucal.* 2007;12:E374-E379.

Fatahzadeh M, Sirois DA. Multiple intraoral melanoacanthomas: a case report with unusual findings. *Oral Surg Oral Med Oral Pathol Oral Radiol Endod.* 2002;94:54-56.

Fornatora ML, Reich RF, Haber S, et al. Oral melanoacanthoma: a report of 10 cases, review of the literature, and immunohistochemical analysis for HMB-45 reactivity. *Am J Dermatopathol.* 2003; 25:12-15.

Goode RK, Crawford BE, Callihan MD, Neville BW. Oral melanoacanthoma. Review of the literature and report of ten cases. *Oral Surg Oral Med Oral Pathol.* 1983;56:622-628.

Tomich CE, Zunt SL. Melanoacanthosis (melanoacanthoma) of the oral mucosa. *J Dermatol Surg Oncol.* 1990;16:231-236.

Yarom N, Hirshberg A, Buchner A. Solitary and multifocal oral melanoacanthoma. *Int J Dermatol.* 2007;46:1232-1236.

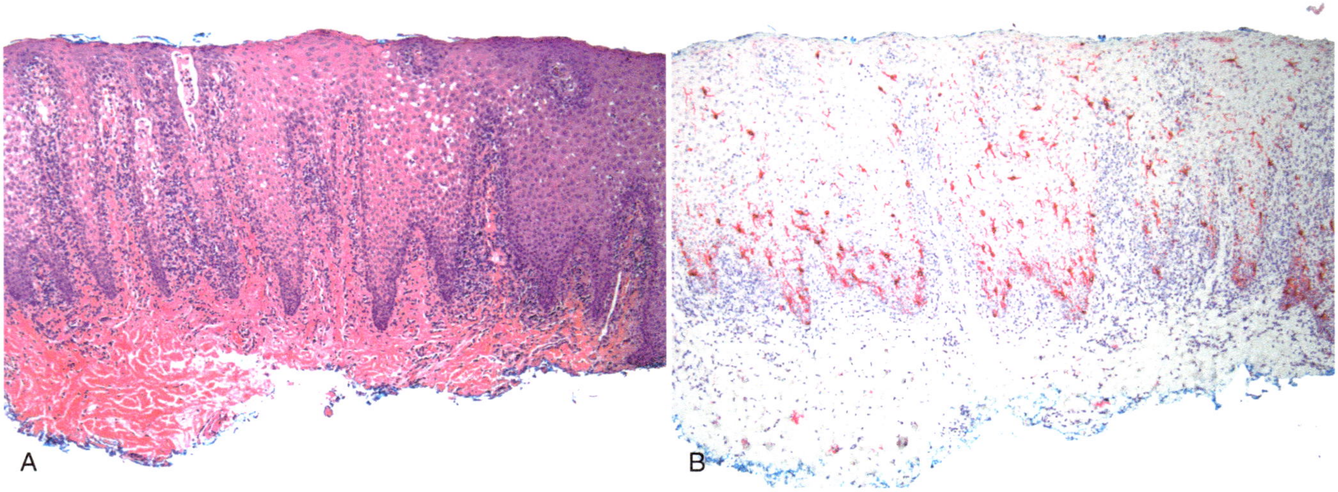

FIG 9.20 Melanoacanthosis. (A) Acanthosis, spongiosis, leukocyte exocytosis, and mild chronic inflammation. (B) Melanocytic hyperplasia throughout the thickness of the epithelium (Melan-A).

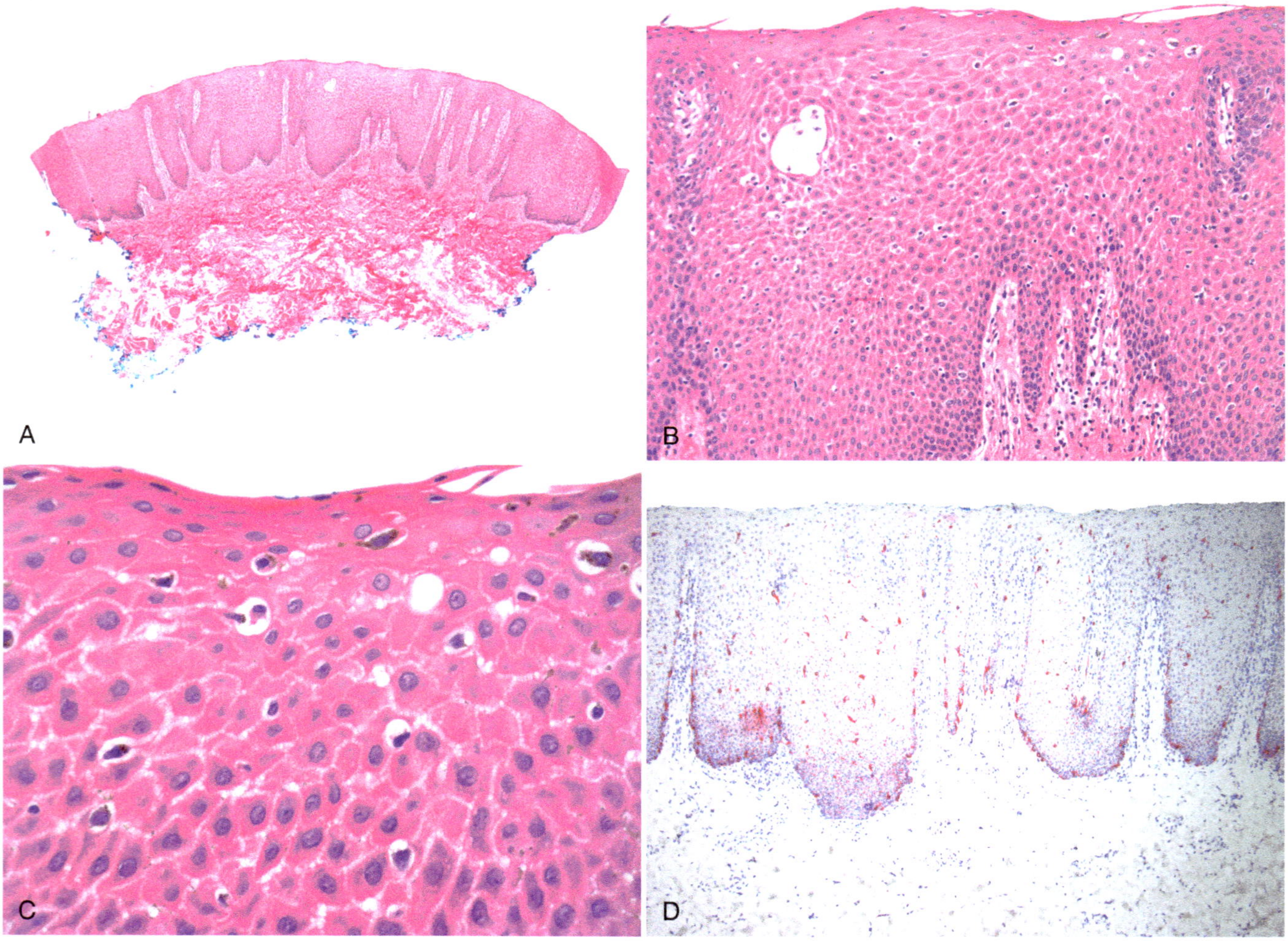

FIG 9.21 Melanoacanthosis. (A) Acanthosis and mild chronic inflammation. (B) Mild spongiosis with dendritic melanocytes throughout the epithelium, and scattered lymphocytes in the lamina propria. (C) Many melanin-laden dendritic melanocytes in the upper epithelium. (D) Melanocytic hyperplasia and transmigration through the epithelium (Melan-A).

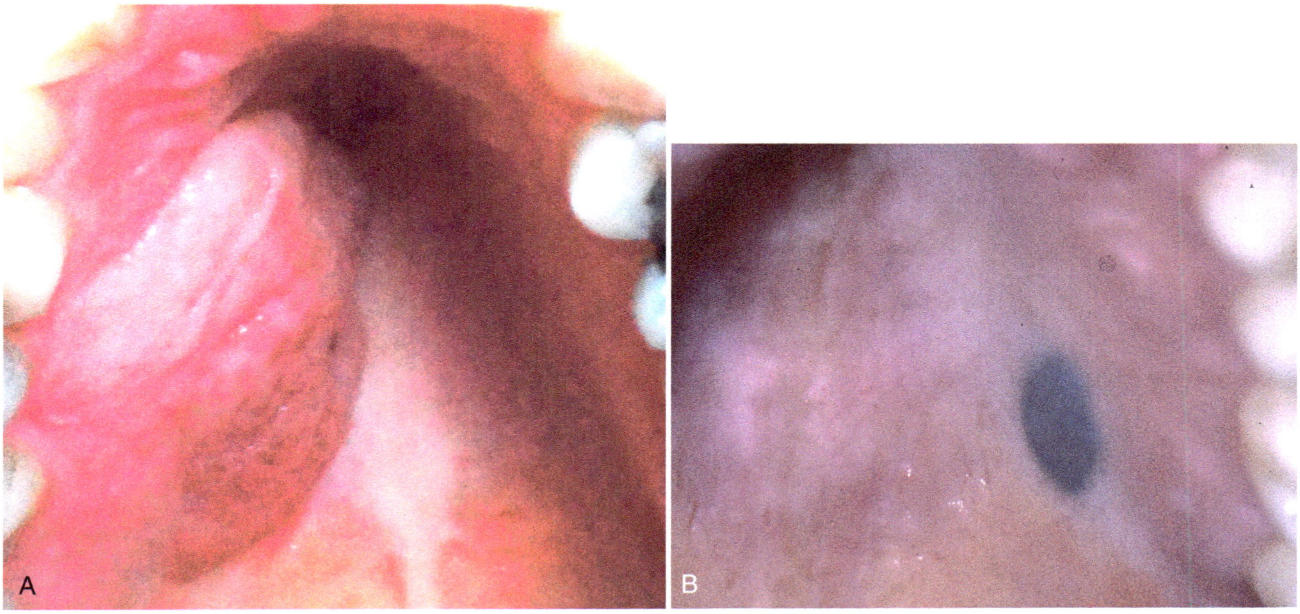

FIG 9.22 (A) Intramucosal melanocytic nevus of the palatal mucosa. (B) Blue nevus of the palate. *(A, Courtesy Dr. Robert Gilardetti, private practice, Wakefield, RI; B, Courtesy Dr. Sadru Kabani, private practice, Cambridge, Mass.)*

ORAL MELANOCYTIC NEVUS

Clinical Findings

- Most occur in the second to fourth decades of life and the most common site is the palatal mucosa (34–44%), with other sites being the mucobuccal fold, buccal mucosa, lip vermilion, and gingiva.
- As with cutaneous lesions, intramucosal, compound, and combined nevi tend to be plaques or nodules, and blue and junctional nevi are macules or plaques (Fig. 9.22).
- The frequency in the oral cavity is as follows: intramucosal nevus (64–80%), blue nevus (8–17%), and compound nevus (6–17%); junctional and combined nevi are uncommon.

Etiopathogenesis and Histopathologic Findings

Melanocytic nevi derive from melanocytes that originate from the neural crest. They are a heterogeneous group of lesions with molecular characteristics. Congenital cutaneous melanocytic nevi tend to harbor *NRAS* and to a lesser extent *BRAF* mutations, whereas *BRAF* mutations are noted in approximately 80% of acquired nevi as well as melanomas. As such, the *BRAF* mutation which activates the mitogen-activated protein kinase (MAPK) pathway that drives proliferation and is integral to development of acquired nevi is, in and of itself, not sufficient to confer malignancy within such nevi. Blue nevi exhibit *GNAQ* (and less often *GNA 11*) mutations while Spitz nevi exhibit *HRAS* mutation. Cutaneous melanocytic nevi undergo recognizable stages of initiation of growth, proliferation, senescence, and involution but it is not clear if oral lesions undergo the same process. Germline loss of function mutations in BAP1 have been noted in families with an increased incidence of uveal melanoma and nevi with spitzoid morphology.

- Intramucosal nevus: downward maturation is characteristic of this nevus as follows: nests and theques of epithelioid cells (type A) lie just beneath the epithelium with variable pigment content, although pigmentation is usually present close to the epithelium; cells have indistinct cell borders, moderate amounts of pale cytoplasm and nuclei with dispersed chromatin and inconspicuous nucleoli; nuclear pleomorphism is not uncommon; lymphocyte-like (type B) or neuroid spindle cells (type C) are present deeper in the lamina propria; slight and focal junctional activity is acceptable for intramucosal nevus (Figs. 9.23 and 9.24); prominent neurotization especially in deep portions of the lesion, and Wagner-Meissner bodies may be seen (Fig. 9.25).
- Junctional nevus: many nests of benign nevus cells are present in the basal layer only.
- Compound nevus: this is a combination of intramucosal and junctional nevus (Fig. 9.26)
- Blue nevus: the *common* type consists of a discrete proliferation of spindled nevus cells with variable melanin and benign nuclei exhibiting dispersed chromatin and small nucleoli, scattered within densely collagenous stroma; nevus cells are not present within the epithelium; the *epithelioid* variant consists of larger, ovoid cells with large central nucleoli; nonpigmented spindle cells are often HMB-45+, and may or may not be S-100+ (Figs. 9.27 and 9.28); the *plaque* type has features of both common and epithelioid blue nevus.
- Combined nevus: this exhibits the presence of two or more forms of nevi with the most common being intramucosal and blue nevi (Fig. 9.29)
- Rare cases of balloon cell and Spitz nevus have been reported.
    - Cells are positive for S-100 protein, melan-A, and occasionally for HMB45 (especially blue nevus)

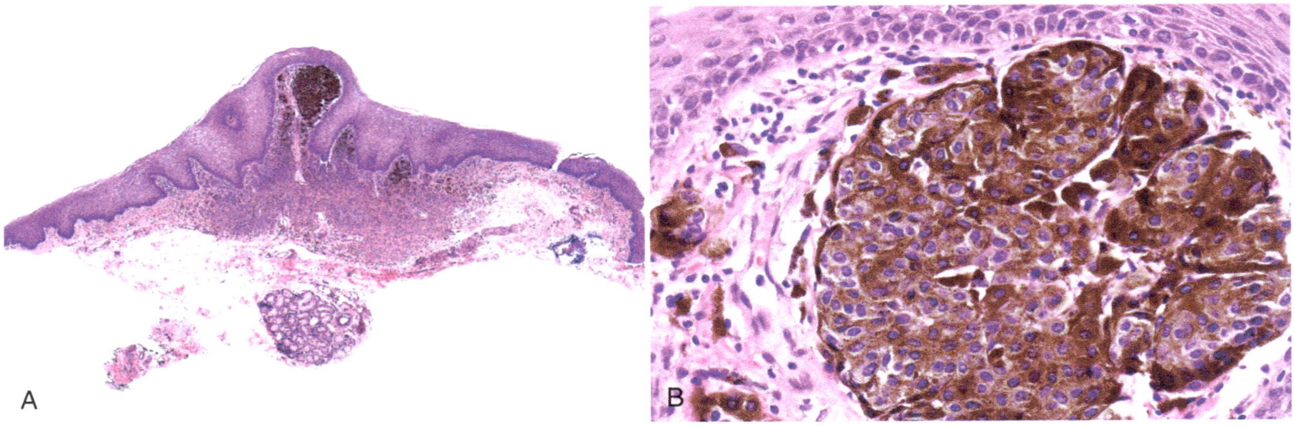

FIG 9.23 Intramucosal melanocytic nevus. (A) Nevus cells are heavily pigmented near the surface. (B) Nests of epithelioid pigmented melanocytic nevus cells.

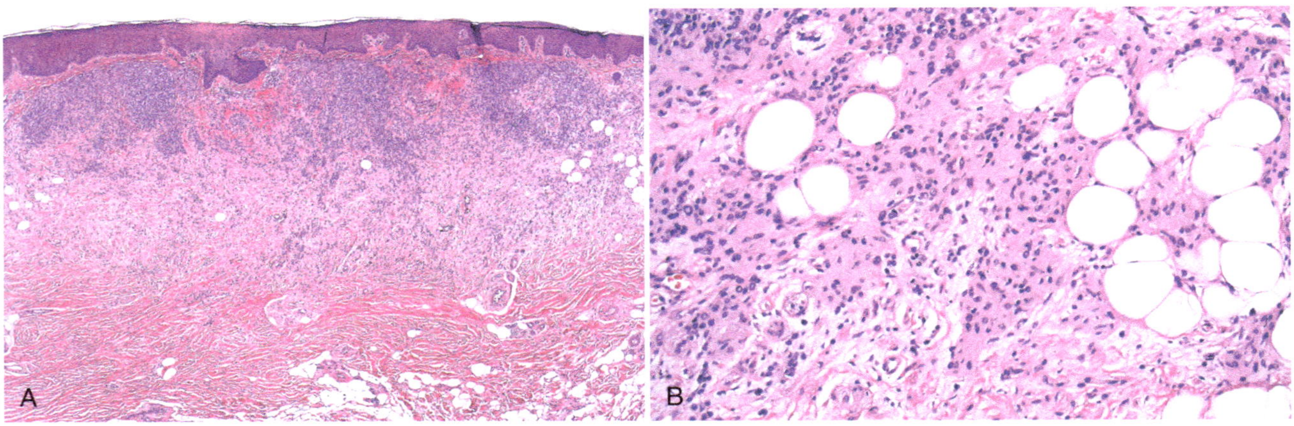

FIG 9.24 Intramucosal melanocytic nevus. (A) Grenz zone and superficial epithelioid and deeper spindle cells. (B) Lymphocyte-like (type B) cells *(top)* and spindled neuroid (type C) cells with mature lipocytes.

Differential Diagnosis

- Amalgam tattoo differs from blue nevus because of deposition of amalgam granules along connective tissue fibers and negativity for melanocytic markers.
- Medication-induced pigmentation exhibits small, spherical granules that stain for iron and are negative for melanocytic markers.
- If there is significant cytologic atypia (atypical lentiginous melanocytic proliferation), early malignant melanoma or melanoma-in-situ should be considered.

Management and Prognosis

- Excision is curative and positive margins do not require reexcision.

REFERENCES

Buchner A, Merrell PW, Carpenter WM. Relative frequency of solitary melanocytic lesions of the oral mucosa. *J Oral Pathol Med.* 2004;33:550-557.

Cohen Y, Goldenberg-Cohen N, Akrish S, et al. BRAF and GNAQ mutations in melanocytic tumors of the oral cavity. *Oral Surg Oral Med Oral Pathol Oral Radiol.* 2012;114:778-784.

Damm DD, White DK, Lyu PE, Puno P. Balloon cell nevus of the oral mucosa. *Oral Surg Oral Med Oral Pathol Oral Radiol Endod.* 2008; 105:755-757.

Ferreira L, Jham B, Assi R, et al. Oral melanocytic nevi: a clinicopathologic study of 100 cases. *Oral Surg Oral Med Oral Pathol Oral Radiol.* 2015;120:358-367.

Ficarra G, Hansen LS, Engebretsen S, Levin LS. Combined nevi of the oral mucosa. *Oral Surg Oral Med Oral Pathol.* 1987;63:196-201.

Fistarol SK, Itin PH. Plaque-type blue nevus of the oral cavity. *Dermatology.* 2005;211:224-233.

Li CC, Harrist TJ, Noonan VL, Woo SB. Intraoral Spitz nevus: case report and literature review. *Oral Surg Oral Med Oral Pathol Oral Radiol.* 2014;117:e320-e324.

Meleti M, Mooi WJ, Casparie MK, van der Waal I. Melanocytic nevi of the oral mucosa—no evidence of increased risk for oral malignant melanoma: an analysis of 119 cases. *Oral Oncol.* 2007;43: 976-981.

Ojha J, Akers JL, Akers JO, et al. Intraoral cellular blue nevus: report of a unique histopathologic entity and review of the literature. *Cutis.* 2007;80:189-192.

Pinto A, Raghavendra S, Lee R, et al. Epithelioid blue nevus of the oral mucosa: a rare histologic variant. *Oral Surg Oral Med Oral Pathol Oral Radiol Endod.* 2003;96:429-436.

Pollock PM, Harper UL, Hansen KS, et al. High frequency of BRAF mutations in nevi. *Nat Genet.* 2003;33:19-20.

Roh MR, Eliades P, Gupta S, Tsao H. Genetics of melanocytic nevi. *Pigment Cell Melanoma Res.* 2015;28:661-672.

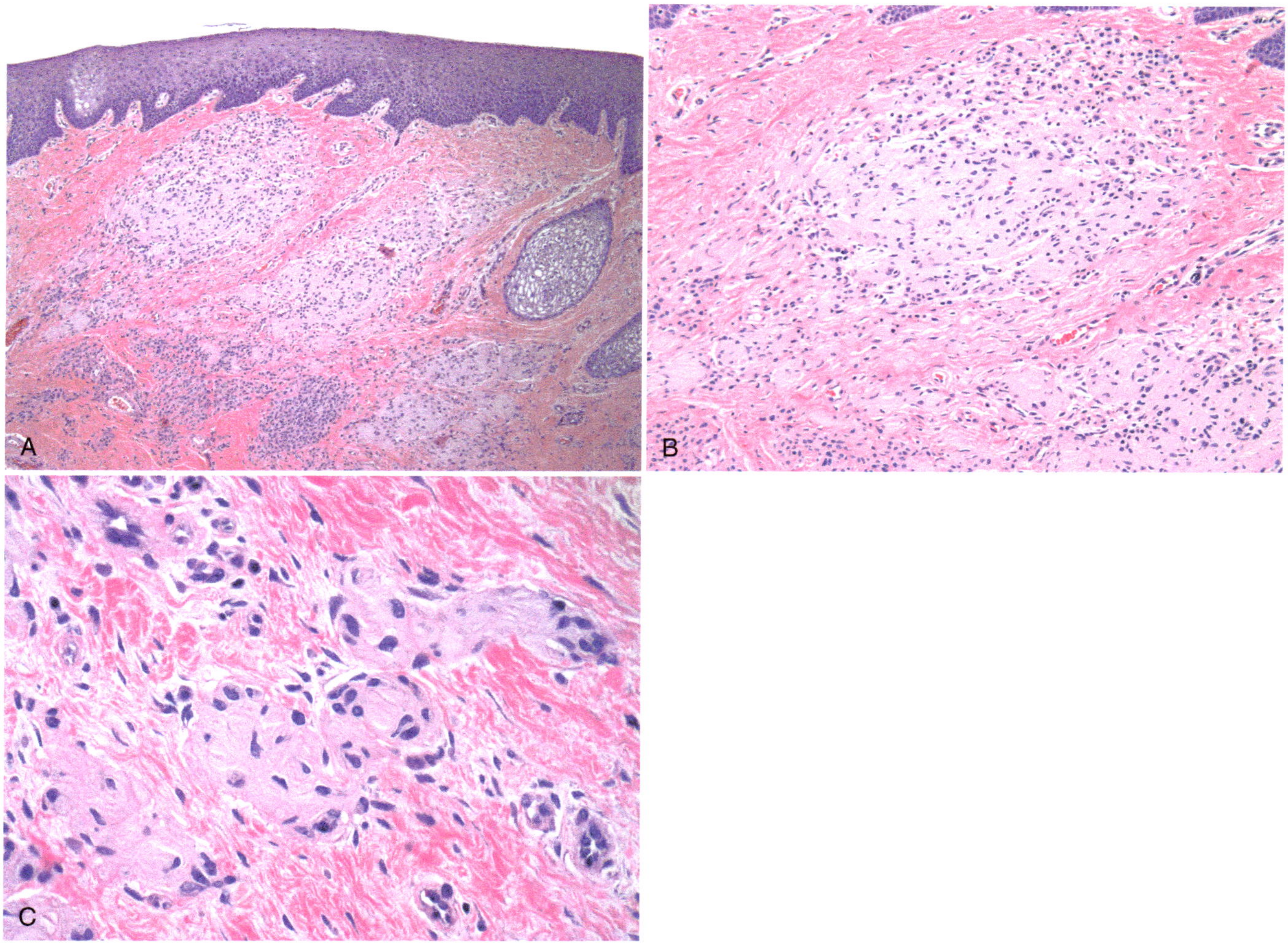

FIG 9.25 Unusual neurotized melanocytic nevus with superficial rather than deep neurotization. (A) Superficial nevus cells are pale and spindled and not nested; deeper cells are conventional epithelioid nevus cells. (B) Spindle cells have abundant pale cytoplasm. (C) Spindle nevus cells form neuroid structures.

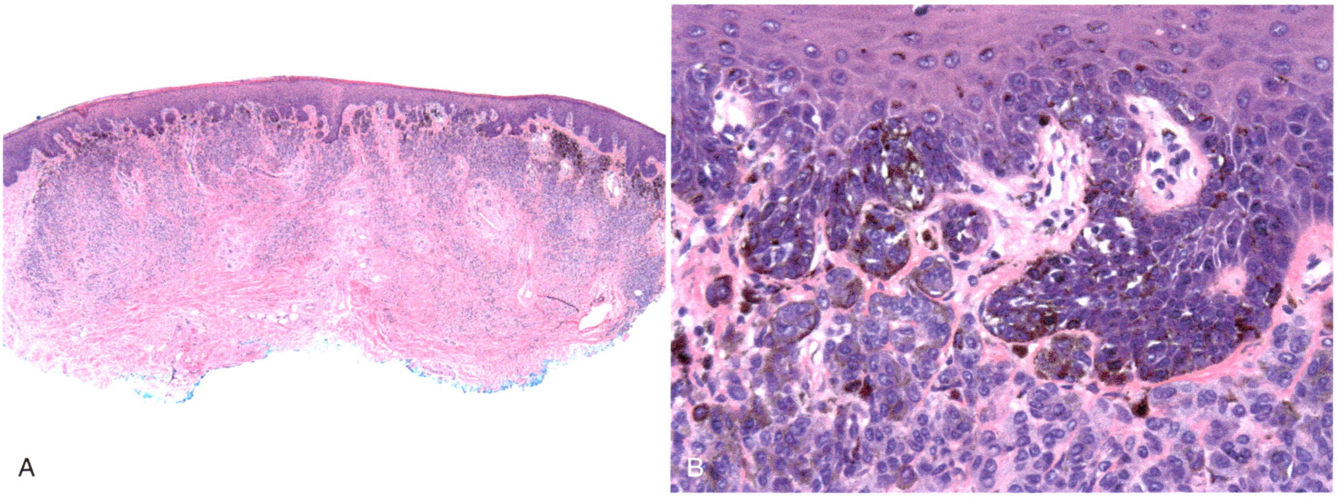

FIG 9.26 Compound melanocytic nevus. (A) Symmetric lesion with nevus cells abutting epithelium. (B) Subtle nesting of clusters of pigmented nevus cells at the basal cell layer.

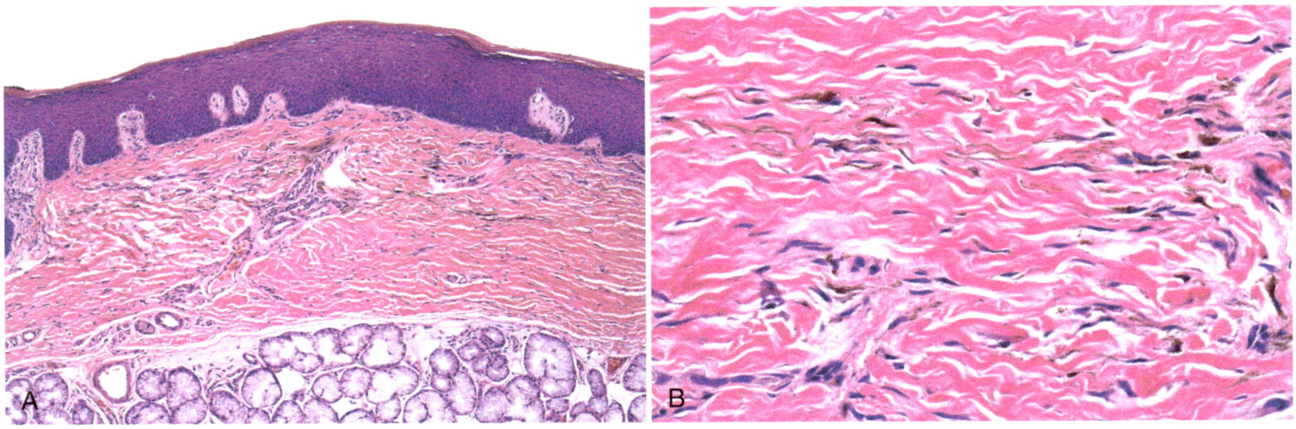

FIG 9.27 Blue nevus of palatal mucosa. (A) Subtly pigmented cellular area in the lamina propria. (B) Spindled pigmented dendritic melanocytes.

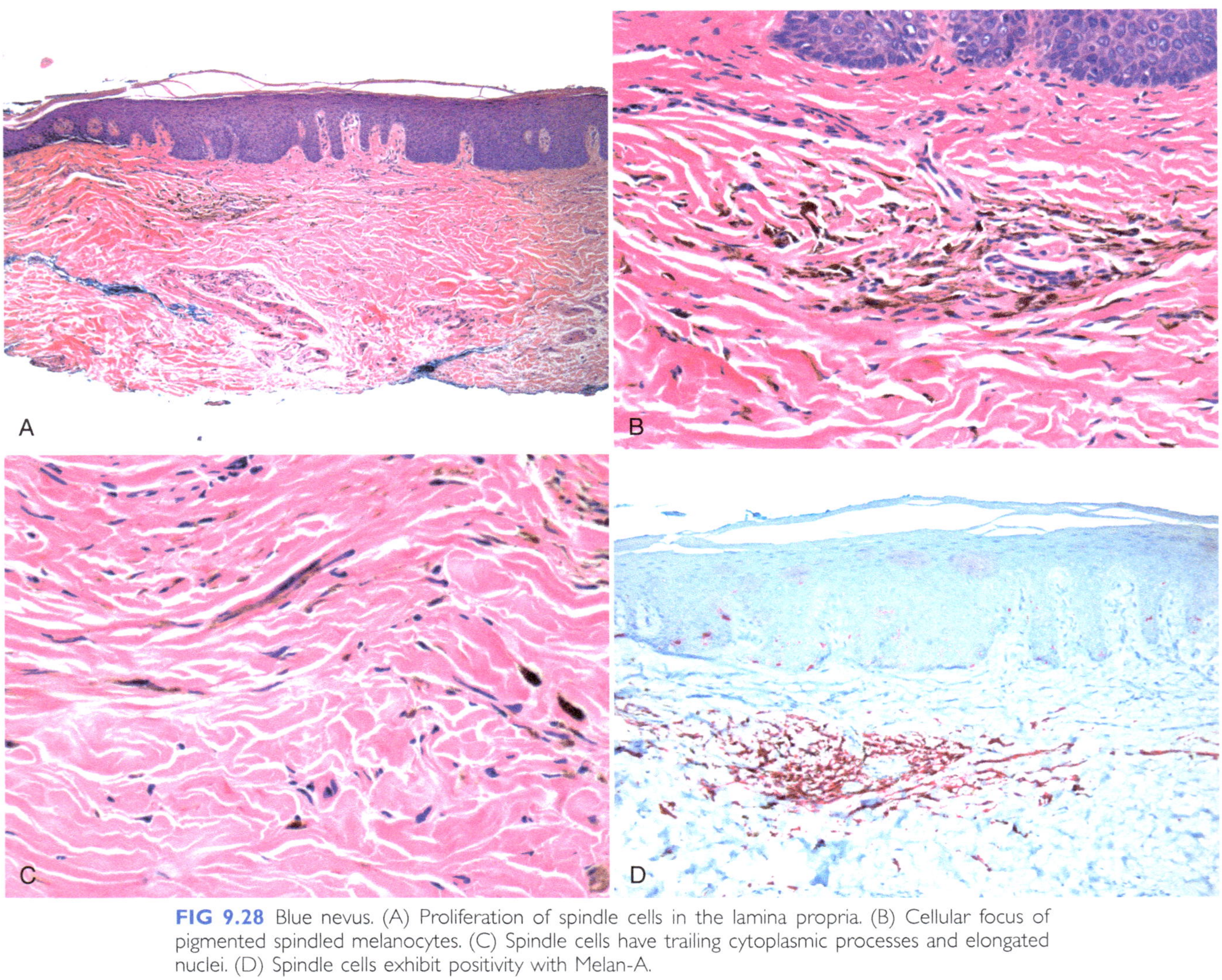

FIG 9.28 Blue nevus. (A) Proliferation of spindle cells in the lamina propria. (B) Cellular focus of pigmented spindled melanocytes. (C) Spindle cells have trailing cytoplasmic processes and elongated nuclei. (D) Spindle cells exhibit positivity with Melan-A.

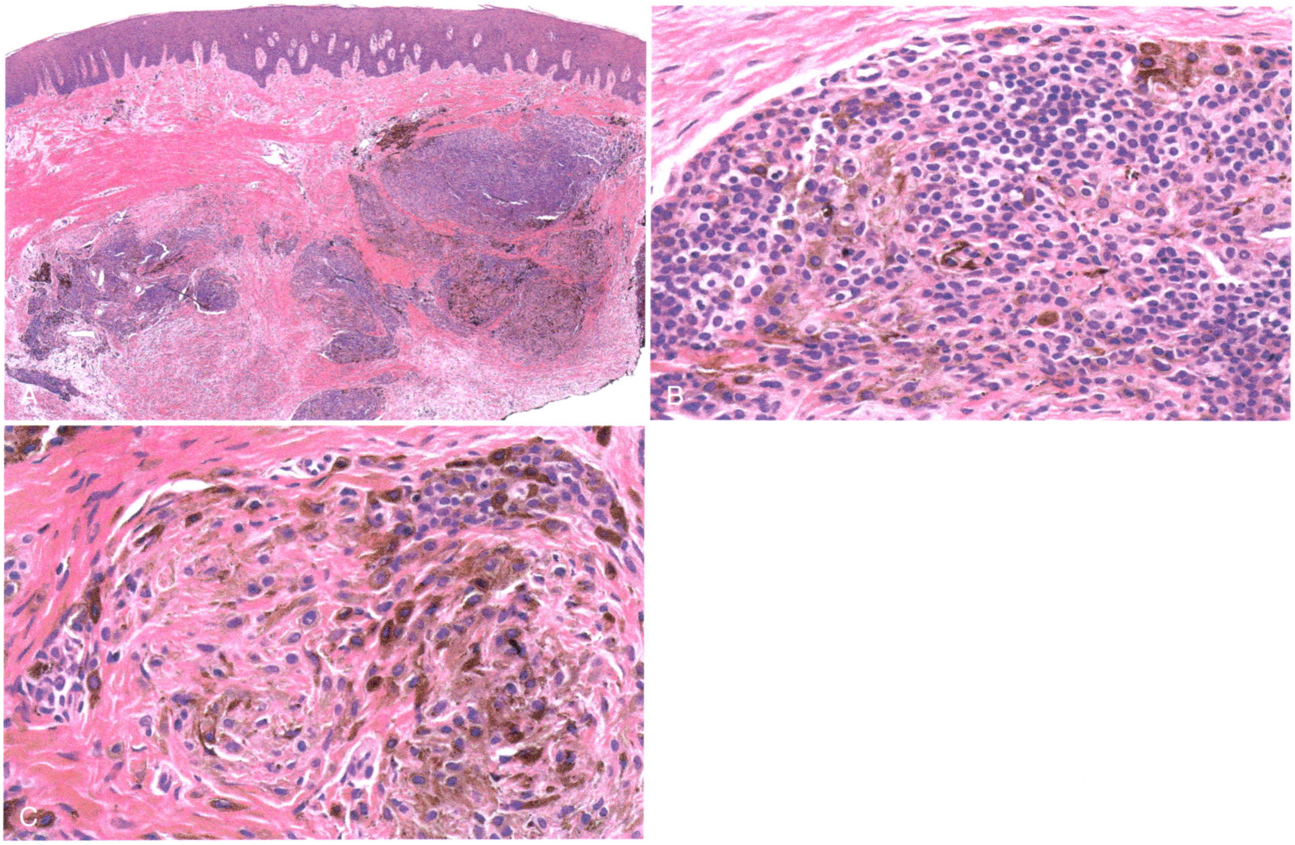

FIG 9.29 Combined melanocytic nevus. (A) Sheets of nevus cells and sclerosis without typical organization of intramucosal nevus. (B) Sheets of pigmented epithelioid cells. (C) Pigmented spindle and epithelioid cells.

Sun J, Morton TH Jr, Gown AM. Antibody HMB-45 identifies the cells of blue nevi. An immunohistochemical study on paraffin sections. *Am J Surg Pathol.* 1990;14:748-751.

Van Raamsdonk CD, Bezrookove V, Green G, et al. Frequent somatic mutations of GNAQ in uveal melanoma and blue naevi. *Nature.* 2009;457:599-602.

Wiesner T, Obenauf AC, Murali R, et al. Germline mutations of BAP1 predispose to melanocytic tumors. *Nat Genet.* 2011;43:1018-1021.

ORAL MELANOMA

Melanomas are divided into four main categories: melanoma on skin with chronic sun damage, melanoma on skin without chronic sun damage, acral melanoma, and mucosal melanoma. Mucosal melanoma of the head and neck constitute 1% to 3% of all melanomas, with primary oral melanoma constituting less than 1% of all melanomas. Mucosal melanomas are more common in Blacks and Japanese and these groups have a lower incidence of cutaneous melanoma. Oral melanomas do not arise within a preexisting melanocytic nevus but rather de novo, as atypical intraepithelial melanocytic proliferations. Most cases are diagnosed late. Breslow and Clark criteria for depth of invasion do not correlate with clinical behavior for oral melanoma.

Clinical Findings

- The mean age is in the seventh decade of life with a slight male predilection, and the most common sites are the palatal mucosa and maxillary gingiva (>70% of cases)
- An early lesion probably appears as a brown macule that spreads and becomes unevenly pigmented with irregular borders; as such all solitary pigmented macules >1 cm or with areas of irregular pigmentation, nodularity, or hemorrhage should be biopsied (Fig. 9.30).

Etiopathogenesis and Histopathologic Features

Cutaneous melanoma arises from stem cells that differentiate toward melanocytic nevi usually under the influence of *BRAF* mutation, and it is loss of senescence and other events that lead to the development of melanoma, many of which arise from preexisting nevi. However, oral melanomas are thought to arise de novo (likely from an atypical melanocytic proliferation) rather than from a preexisting melanocytic nevus and they behave in a similar fashion to acral melanomas. *BRAF* is strongly expressed in melanomas of non-sun-damaged skin (60% and greater), whereas mucosal melanomas are negative for *BRAF*, although many express c-kit (40% of mucosal tumors).

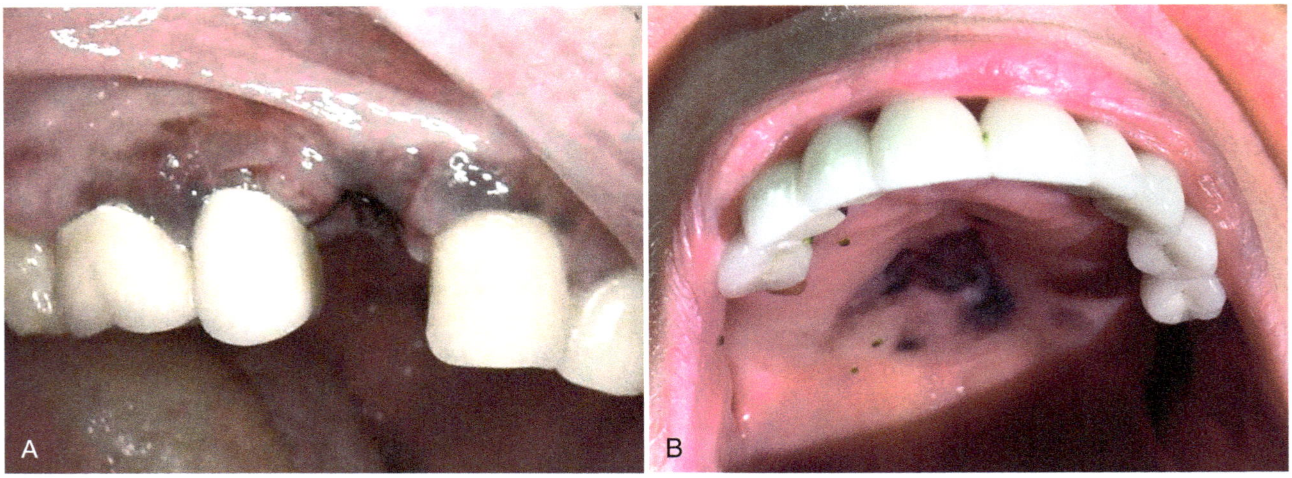

FIG 9.30 (A) Melanoma in situ of the maxillary gingiva presenting as irregular macular melanosis >1 cm. (B) Melanoma of the palatal mucosa with irregular borders, irregular pigmentation, and large size. *(Courtesy Dr. Gerald Fine, private practice, Brookline, Mass.)*

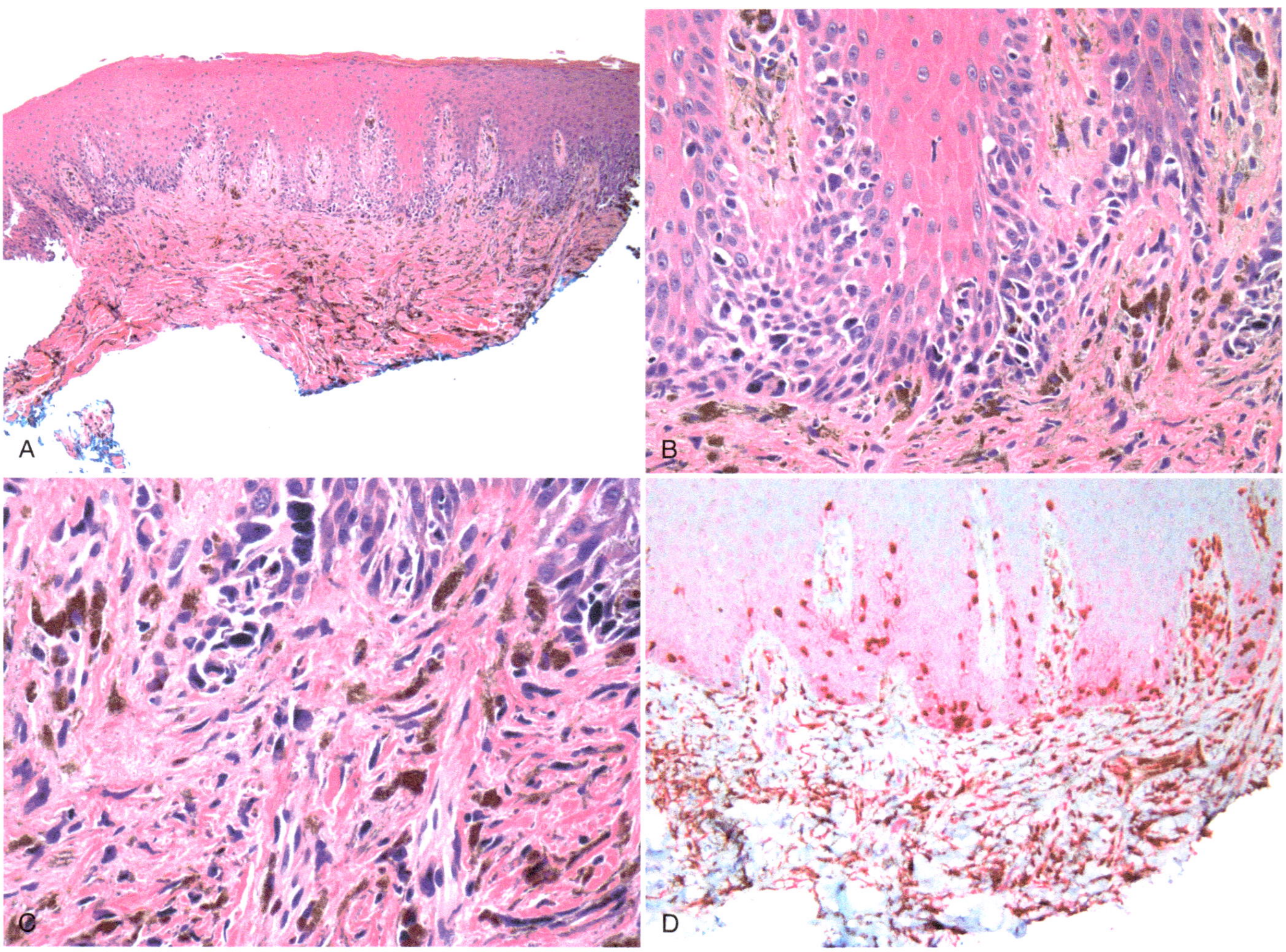

FIG 9.31 Melanoma arising from atypical melanocytic hyperplasia (from patient in Figure 30B). (A) Atypical melanocytic proliferation within the epithelium. (B) Atypical melanocytes with pleomorphic nuclei within the epithelium. (C) Atypical pigmented spindle melanocytes within the lamina propria. (D) Study for microphthalmic-associated transforming factor (MITF) is positive in melanocytes in both the epithelium and lamina propria.

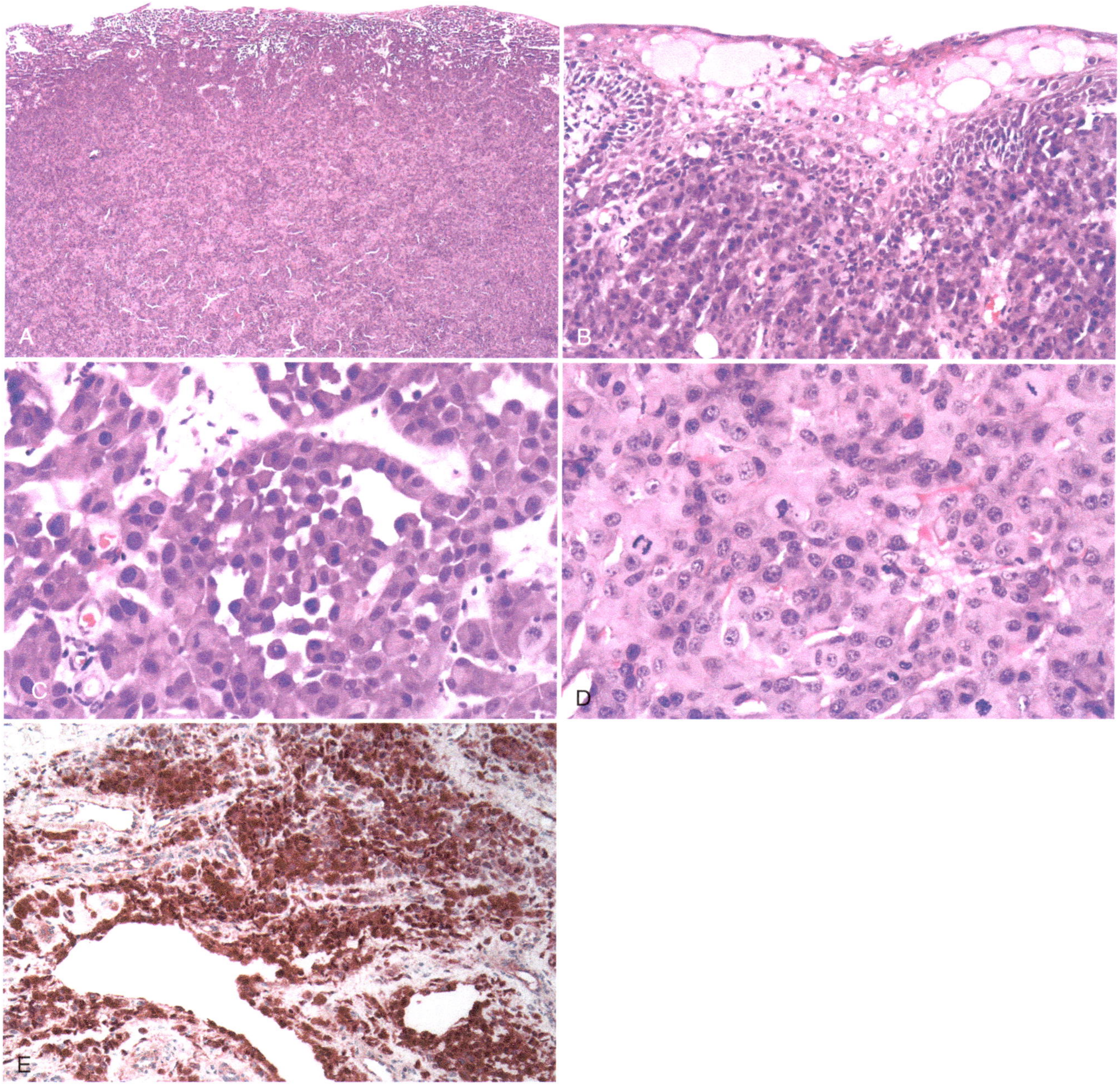

FIG 9.32 Amelanotic nodular melanoma. (A) Sheets of atypical melanocytes with overlying ulcer. (B) Atypical melanocytes within the epithelium. (C) Large polyhedral cells with eccentric nuclei and abundant cytoplasm without obvious melanin in a pseudoglandular pattern. (D) Sheets of epithelioid cells with many mitotic figures. (E) Tumor cells are S-100+.

- Atypical melanocytic hyperplasia or melanoma in situ (15% of cases, level I by Prasad et al., 2004): proliferation of atypical melanocytes within the epithelium either in lentiginous or pagetoid fashion; cells are pleomorphic with hyperchromatic nuclei and prominent nucleoli, and transmigration of atypical melanocytes through the epithelium is often seen (Fig. 9.31A–B); however, approximately 30% of cases do not exhibit an in situ component.
- Conventional melanoma: cells are present in sheets, an organoid/alveolar pattern, or a desmoplastic pattern; atypical spindled or epithelioid melanocytes are present within the lamina propria (level II) or invading bone and muscle (level III); epithelioid cells contain large nuclei, prominent nucleoli, and pseudoinclusions; up to 30% are amelanotic (see Figs. 9.31C and 9.32A–D)
- Desmoplastic melanomas consist of atypical spindle melanocytes with fibrosis and scarring and may have a better prognosis; rare cases exhibit osteo-cartilaginous differentiation.
- Sarcomatoid features, pseudopapillary architecture (cells amassing around vascular structures in necrotic tumors), undifferentiated cells (small, round blue

TABLE 9.1 Staging of Mucosal Melanoma (From the American Joint Committee on Cancer, 2010)

Primary Tumor			
T3	Mucosal disease		
T4a	Moderately advanced disease Tumor involving deep soft tissue, cartilage, bone, or overlying skin		
T4b	Very advanced disease Tumor involving brain, dura, skull base, lower cranial nerves (IX, X, XI, XII), masticator space, carotid artery, prevertebral space, or mediastinal structures		
N0	No regional node metastasis		
N1	Regional node metastasis present		
Stage	**T**	**N**	**M**
Stage III[a]	T3	N0	M0
Stage IVA	T4a	N0	M0
	T3–T4a	N1	M0
Stage IVB	T4b	Any N	M0
Stage IVC	Any T	Any N	M1

[a]No stages I and II because there is no T1 or T2 for the primary tumor.

cells), thickness greater than 5 mm, and vascular invasion are associated with poor survival

- Cells are positive for S-100 protein, HMB-45, Melan-A, and microphthalmia-associated transcription factor (MITF) and are keratin negative (see Figs. 9.31D and 9.32E)
- Expression of bcl-2, retention of p16, and loss of p53 may be correlated with improved survival
- In the new mucosal melanoma staging system, tumors are classified either as T3 (level I and II) or T4 (level III) only, without T1 and T2 tumors (Table 9.1); minimal stage is therfore III.

Differential Diagnosis

- Melanoma mimics many other malignancies. Poorly differentiated spindled and epithelioid malignancies are differentiated from melanoma based on positive identification of S-100 protein, HMB-45, Melan-A, and microphthalmia-associated transcription factor (MITF), and negativity for keratin.

Management and Prognosis

- Primary treatment may be with excision with clear margins or radiation but the recurrence rate is 50%; adjuvant radiotherapy reduces local relapse and metastases, but it may not improve survival; nodal and distant metastases occur in up to 50% and 65% of cases, respectively, and 5-year survival is 10% to 20% from distant metastases.
- Other therapies include combination chemotherapy, vaccines, interferon alpha, and targeted therapies including BRAF inhibitors (eg, vemurafenib), kit inhibitors (eg, imatinib), MEK inhibitors (eg, trametinib) and anti-CTLA4 agents (eg, ipilimumab).

REFERENCES

Barker BF, Carpenter WM, Daniels TE, et al. Oral mucosal melanomas: the WESTOP Banff workshop proceedings. Western Society of Teachers of Oral Pathology. *Oral Surg Oral Med Oral Pathol Oral Radiol Endod.* 1997;83:672-679.

Carvajal RD, Spencer SA, Lydiatt W. Mucosal melanoma: a clinically and biologically unique disease entity. *J Natl Compr Canc Netw.* 2012; 10:345-356.

Curtin JA, Busam K, Pinkel D, Bastian BC. Somatic activation of KIT in distinct subtypes of melanoma. *J Clin Oncol.* 2006;24:4340-4346.

Curtin JA, Fridlyand J, Kageshita T, et al. Distinct sets of genetic alterations in melanoma. *N Engl J Med.* 2005;353:2135-2147.

de Almeida LS, Requena L, Rutten A, et al. Desmoplastic malignant melanoma: a clinicopathologic analysis of 113 cases. *Am J Dermatopathol.* 2008;30:207-215.

Edge SB, Byrd DR, Compton CC, et al., eds. *AJCC Cancer Staging Manual.* ed 7. New York: Springer; 2010:97-100.

Eggermont AM, Spatz A, Robert C. Cutaneous melanoma. *Lancet.* 2014;383:816-827.

Kilpatrick SE, White WL, Browne JD. Desmoplastic malignant melanoma of the oral mucosa. An underrecognized diagnostic pitfall. *Cancer.* 1996;78:383-389.

Lourenco SV, Sangueza M, Sotto MN, et al. Primary oral mucosal melanoma: a series of 35 new cases from South America. *Am J Dermatopathol.* 2009;31:323-330.

Meleti M, Mooi WJ, van der Waal I. Oral malignant melanoma associated with pseudoepitheliomatous hyperplasia. Report of a case. *J Cutan Pathol.* 2006;33:331-333.

Meleti M, Leemans CR, de Bree R, et al. Head and neck mucosal melanoma: experience with 42 patients, with emphasis on the role of postoperative radiotherapy. *Head Neck.* 2008;30:1543-1551.

Mendenhall WM, Amdur RJ, Hinerman RW, et al. Head and neck mucosal melanoma. *Am J Clin Oncol.* 2005;28:626-630.

Prasad ML, Busam KJ, Patel SG, et al. Clinicopathologic differences in malignant melanoma arising in oral squamous and sinonasal respiratory mucosa of the upper aerodigestive tract. *Arch Pathol Lab Med.* 2003;127:997-1002.

Prasad ML, Patel SG, Huvos AG, et al. Primary mucosal melanoma of the head and neck: a proposal for microstaging localized, stage I (lymph node-negative) tumors. *Cancer.* 2004;100:1657-1664.

Prasad ML, Patel SG, Shah JP, et al. Prognostic significance of regulators of cell cycle and apoptosis, p16(INK4a), p53, and bcl-2 in primary mucosal melanomas of the head and neck. *Head Neck Pathol.* 2012;6:184-190.

Rapini RP, Golitz LE, Greer RO Jr, et al. Primary malignant melanoma of the oral cavity. A review of 177 cases. *Cancer.* 1985;55: 1543-1551.

Takata M, Murata H, Saida T. Molecular pathogenesis of malignant melanoma: a different perspective from the studies of melanocytic nevus and acral melanoma. *Pigment Cell Melanoma Res.* 2010;23: 64-71.

Umeda M, Komatsubara H, Shibuya Y, et al. Premalignant melanocytic dysplasia and malignant melanoma of the oral mucosa. *Oral Oncol.* 2002;38:714-722.

Vachtenheim J, Ondrusova L. Microphthalmia-associated transcription factor expression levels in melanoma cells contribute to cell invasion and proliferation. *Exp Dermatol.* 2015;24:481-484.

MELANOTIC NEUROECTODERMAL TUMOR OF INFANCY

Clinical Findings

- Most cases manifest in the first 6 months of life, more than 90% occur in the head and neck with a slight male predilection (1.5:1), and the maxilla is the most common site of involvement (60%) (Fig. 9.33); extra-oral cases (in the skull, brain, and testis) are more common in children older than 1 year.
- The tumor grows rapidly and presents as a radiolucency, often with extraosseous extension presenting as a brownish-red mass of the alveolar mucosa.

- High levels of vanillylmandelic acid (metabolic product of catecholamines) are noted in the urine.

Etiopathogenesis and Histopathologic Features

Melanotic neuroectodermal tumor of infancy shows differentiation toward neural crest tissues. More recently, the *BRAFV600E* mutation has been identified in some cases.

- The tumor is biphasic: larger, polygonal epithelioid cells with large nuclei and dispersed chromatin occur in islands, tubules or in an alveolar pattern; these cells contain melanin and are positive for HMB-45, PGP9.5, keratin, vimentin, and occasionally S-100 protein. These large cells surround smaller round-to-ovoid, poorly differentiated neuroblast-like cells with hyperchromatic nuclei and scant cytoplasm that stain for synaptophysin, chromogranin, and are positive for CD56; both populations are positive for neuron-specific enolase (Figs. 9.34 and 9.35), and these cells are readily identified on fine needle aspiration.
- Increased Ki67 fraction (usually seen in the neuroblast-like cells) and the presence of CD99 may correlate with poorer prognosis.
- Metastatic lesions usually contain neuroblast-like cells.

Differential Diagnosis

- The biphasic nature of the tumor and positivity for neural crest markers rules out other small blue cell tumors of childhood, such as neuroblastoma and rhabdomyosarcoma (which are myogenin positive and MyoD positive), and Ewing sarcoma/peripheral neuroectodermal tumor (which are CD99+); the presence of melanin is also not seen in other small blue cell tumors.

Management and Prognosis

- Surgical resection with a clear margin is the treatment of choice and the recurrence rate is 20%, with more than half of these being maxillary tumors and occurring within weeks of surgery; recurrence is also higher in those diagnosed before 2 months of age; some cases require radiotherapy and/or chemotherapy.
- Lymph node or distant metastases occur in 3% to 7% of cases.

REFERENCES

Barrett AW, Morgan M, Ramsay AD, et al. A clinicopathologic and immunohistochemical analysis of melanotic neuroectodermal tumor of infancy. *Oral Surg Oral Med Oral Pathol Oral Radiol Endod.* 2002;93:688-698.

Chaudhary A, Wakhlu A, Mittal N, et al. Melanotic neuroectodermal tumor of infancy: 2 decades of clinical experience with 18 patients. *J Oral Maxillofac Surg.* 2009;67:47-51.

Gochhait D, Dey P, Mitra S, Saikia UN. Fine-needle aspiration cytology of melanotic neuroectodermal tumor of infancy. *Diagn Cytopathol.* 2015;43:770-772.

Gomes CC, Diniz MG, de Menezes GH, et al. BRAFV600E Mutation in melanotic neuroectodermal tumor of infancy: toward personalized medicine? *Pediatrics.* 2015;136:e267-e269.

Kapadia SB, Frisman DM, Hitchcock CL, et al. Melanotic neuroectodermal tumor of infancy. Clinicopathological, immunohistochemical, and flow cytometric study. *Am J Surg Pathol.* 1993;17:566-573.

Kruse-Losler B, Gaertner C, Burger H, et al. Melanotic neuroectodermal tumor of infancy: systematic review of the literature and presentation of a case. *Oral Surg Oral Med Oral Pathol Oral Radiol Endod.* 2006;102:204-216.

Rachidi S, Sood AJ, Patel KG, et al. Melanotic neuroectodermal tumor of infancy: a systematic review. *J Oral Maxillofac Surg.* 2015;73:1946-1956.

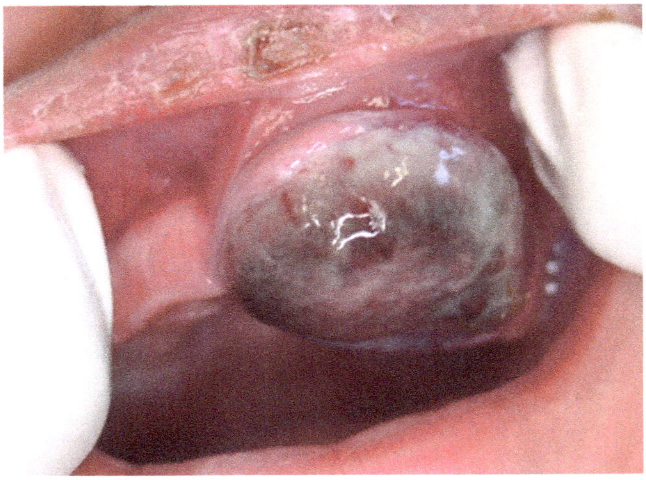

FIG 9.33 Melanotic neuroectodermal tumor of infancy: pigmented mass of the left maxillary alveolar ridge. *(From Gonçalves CF, Costa NL, Oliveira-Neto HH, et al. Melanotic neuroectodermal tumor of infancy: report of 2 cases. J Oral Maxillofac Surg. 2010;68:2344.)*

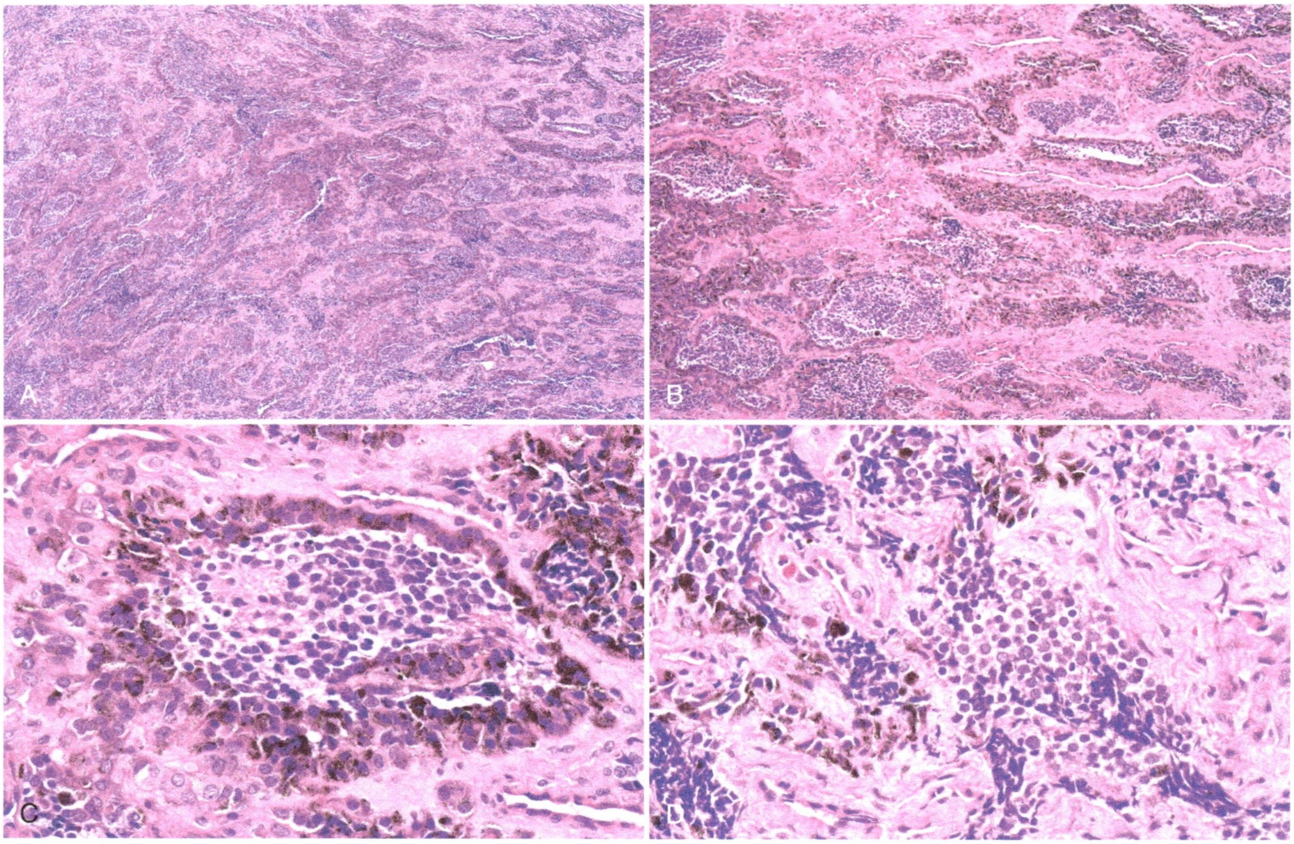

FIG 9.34 Melanotic neuroectodermal tumor of infancy. (A) Irregular islands of tumor cells with fibrous stroma. (B) Islands of biphasic tumor cells within fibrous stroma. (C) Larger epithelioid tumor cells with pale cytoplasm and large, pale nuclei containing dusty melanin surround smaller cells with dark nuclei. (D) Small cells with hyperchromatic nuclei juxtaposed against larger cells, some of which contain melanin.

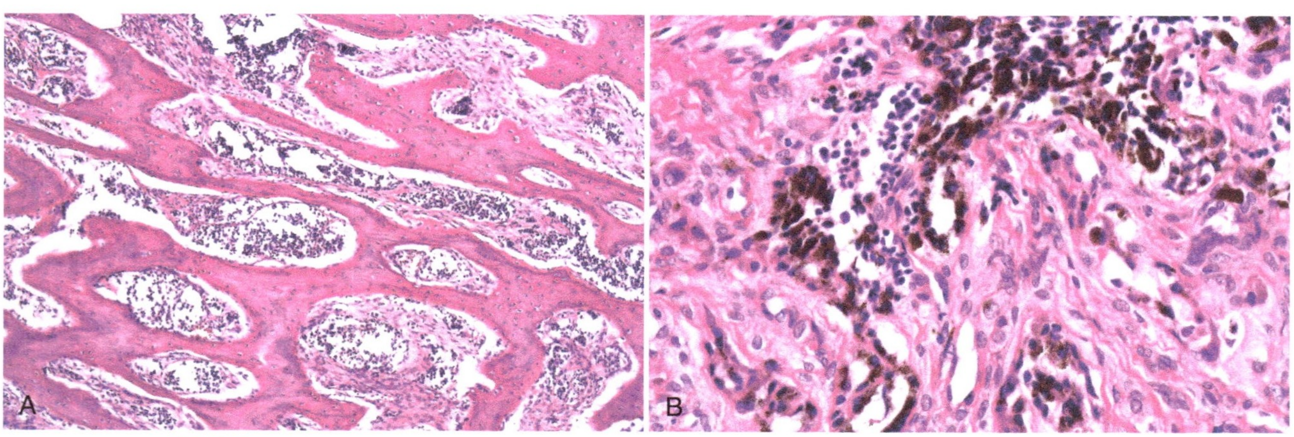

FIG 9.35 Melanotic neuroectodermal tumor of infancy. (A) Small blue cell tumor extensively infiltrates bone. (B) Biphasic population of darkly staining neuroblast-like cells and epithelioid cells containing melanin. *(A, Courtesy Dr. Harry Kozakewich, Harvard Medical School, Boston, Mass.)*

10 REACTIVE KERATOTIC LESIONS (NONLEUKOPLAKIAS)

CHAPTER CONTENTS

White keratotic mucosa lesions are some of the more commonly biopsied lesions and both benign and dysplastic lesions often pose a diagnostic challenge. Table 10.1 provides a list of mucosal conditions that are clinically white; these are discussed in this and other chapters. The term "leukoplakia" is not *any* white lesion, but rather a clinical term to denote a keratotic lesion that does not represent reactive keratosis or other known keratotic lesion, and has a high risk of developing dysplasia and carcinoma (see Chapter 11).

The oral mucosa appears white for several reasons:

- Presence of keratin in a normally nonkeratinized site (namely buccal and lip mucosa, ventral tongue, floor of mouth, and soft palate).
- Parakeratosis or hyper(ortho)keratosis in a normally keratinized site (hard palatal mucosa and attached gingiva); the tongue being normally parakeratinized is the only site that can show hyperparakeratosis.
- Degeneration and/or coagulation of superficial keratinocytes.
- Edema of keratinocytes.
- Alteration of the epithelial cells because of benign but abnormal keratin formation or aggregation (benign dyskeratotic disorders, see Chapter 2).
- Epithelial dysplasia (see Chapter 11).
- Nonepithelial changes such as underlying scarring and fibrosis.

Mild irritation of the oral mucosa leads to acanthosis, and keratinocyte damage that initially takes the form of keratinocyte edema, then degeneration of superficial keratinocytes, and in some cases spongiosis; there may be parakeratosis or in more chronic lesions, hyperkeratosis. In general, reactive keratotic lesions have poorly demarcated margins with keratosis tapering at the edges, whereas true leukoplakias, which are either dysplastic or represent keratoses of unknown significance, are white plaques with abrupt keratinization. Correlating the histopathologic and clinical findings is essential in arriving at an accurate diagnosis.

Leukoedema

This term should be reserved for the clinical presentation; the histopathologic feature is keratinocyte edema.

Clinical Findings

- This is present in up to 90% of the population and is more readily discerned in dark-skinned individuals.
- Delicate lacy, gray-white lines are present on the buccal mucosa or tongue (nonkeratinized site) that disappear with stretching (Fig. 10.1).

Etiopathogenesis and Histopathologic Features

Leukoedema usually results from mildly irritating substances (such as smoke from tobacco products or marijuana, caustic oral rinses, or toothpaste) in episodic contact with the mucosa. It is also associated with a minimally traumatic, parafunctional habit such as mucosal sucking.

- Acanthosis is always present and there is keratinocyte edema of superficial cells causing cells to be enlarged,

TABLE 10.1 Histologic Diagnoses for Maculopapular White Lesions

Developmental/Hereditary (see Chapter 2)
Cannon white sponge nevus
Hereditary benign intraepithelial dyskeratosis
Oral pachyonychia congenita
Darier disease
Reactive/Inflammatory
Chemical or Heat
Leukoedema
Dentifrice-associated desquamation
Smokeless tobacco lesion
Nicotinic stomatitis
Irritant contact stomatitis (see Chapter 7)
Frictional/Factitial
Morsicatio mucosae oris
Benign alveolar ridge keratosis (oral lichen simplex chronicus)
Frictional parakeratosis at the edge of traumatic ulcers
Other frictional/factitial keratoses
Retention Keratosis
Hairy tongue
Immune-Mediated or Autoimmune (see Chapter 8)
Lichenoid stomatitis, lichenoid hypersensitivity reaction, or lichen planus
Lupus erythematosus
Chronic graft-versus-host disease
Infectious (see Chapter 4)
Candidiasis
Hairy leukoplakia
Others (eg, geotrichosis)
Premalignant and Malignant (see Chapter 11)
Epithelial dysplasia
Carcinoma-in-situ
Atypical endophytic squamous proliferation
Verrucous hyperplasia
Squamous cell carcinoma
Verrucous carcinoma
Others
Warty dyskeratoma
Epidermolytic hyperkeratosis
Palifermin-induced keratosis
Fibrosis (Not Involving the Epithelium)
Submucous fibrosis (see Chapter 11)
Mucosal fibrosis in progressive systemic sclerosis

pale, and ballooned; anucleation may be caused by plane of section and/or nuclear degeneration; cell membranes have a compact "jigsaw puzzle" appearance and keratinocytes often exhibit perinuclear halos (but they do not represent koilocytes because the nuclei are not shrunken or hyperchromatic) (Fig. 10.2).
- Minimal to no keratin is noted, although parakeratin chevrons may be present, similar to smokeless tobacco lesions (Fig. 10.3). There is minimal to no inflammation in the lamina propria.

Differential Diagnosis

- Keratinocyte edema is seen in contact lesions and in association with frictional/factitial keratoses, although the latter will also show marked parakeratosis or hyperkeratosis.
- Hairy leukoplakia shows chromatin condensation against the nuclear membrane and Cowdry inclusion bodies, and are positive for Epstein-Barr virus (EBV).

Management and Prognosis

- No treatment is necessary for leukoedema, although patients should be educated about the causes and avoidance of the causative agent if appropriate.

REFERENCES

Axell T. Leukoedema—an epidemiologic study with special reference to the influence of tobacco habits. *Community Dent Oral Epidemiol.* 1981;9:142-146.

Canaan TJ, Meehan SC. Variations of structure and appearance of the oral mucosa. *Dent Clin North Am.* 2005;49:1-14.

Heyl T, Raubenheimer EJ. Sucking pads (sucking calluses) of the lips in neonates: a manifestation of transient leukoedema. *Pediatr Dermatol.* 1987;4:123-128.

Martin JL. Leukoedema: an epidemiological study in white and African Americans. *J Tenn Dent Assoc.* 1997;77:18-21.

Van Wyk CW, Ambrosio SC. Leukoedema: ultrastructural and histochemical observations. *J Oral Pathol.* 1983;12:319-329.

Versteeg PA, Slot DE, van der Velden U, van der Weijden GA. Effect of cannabis usage on the oral environment: a review. *Int J Dent Hyg.* 2008;6:315-320.

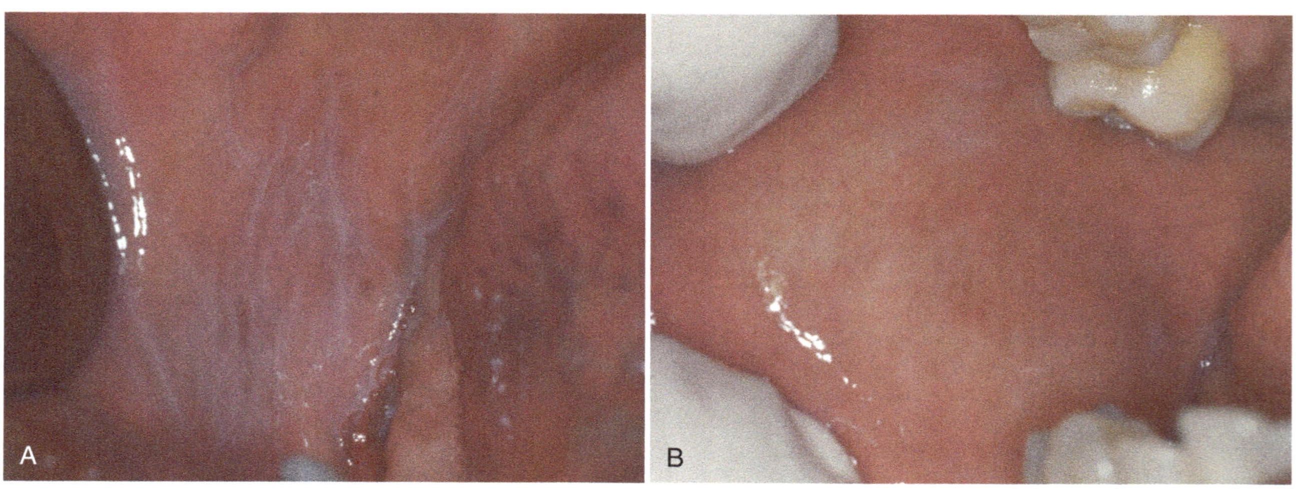

FIG 10.1 Leukoedema. (A) Grayish reticulations of the right buccal mucosa. (B) Stretching the mucosa of the patient in A causes the lesion to disappear.

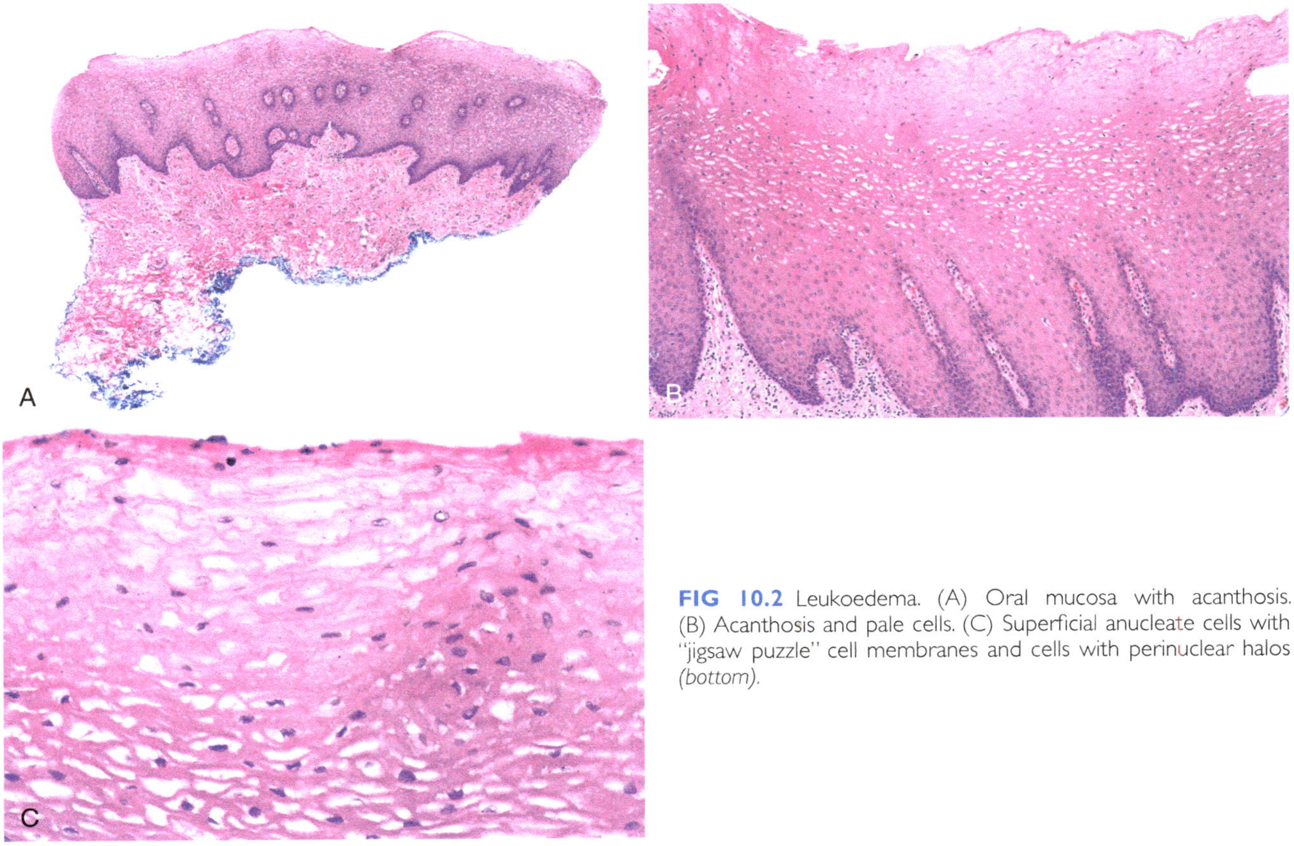

FIG 10.2 Leukoedema. (A) Oral mucosa with acanthosis. (B) Acanthosis and pale cells. (C) Superficial anucleate cells with "jigsaw puzzle" cell membranes and cells with perinuclear halos *(bottom)*.

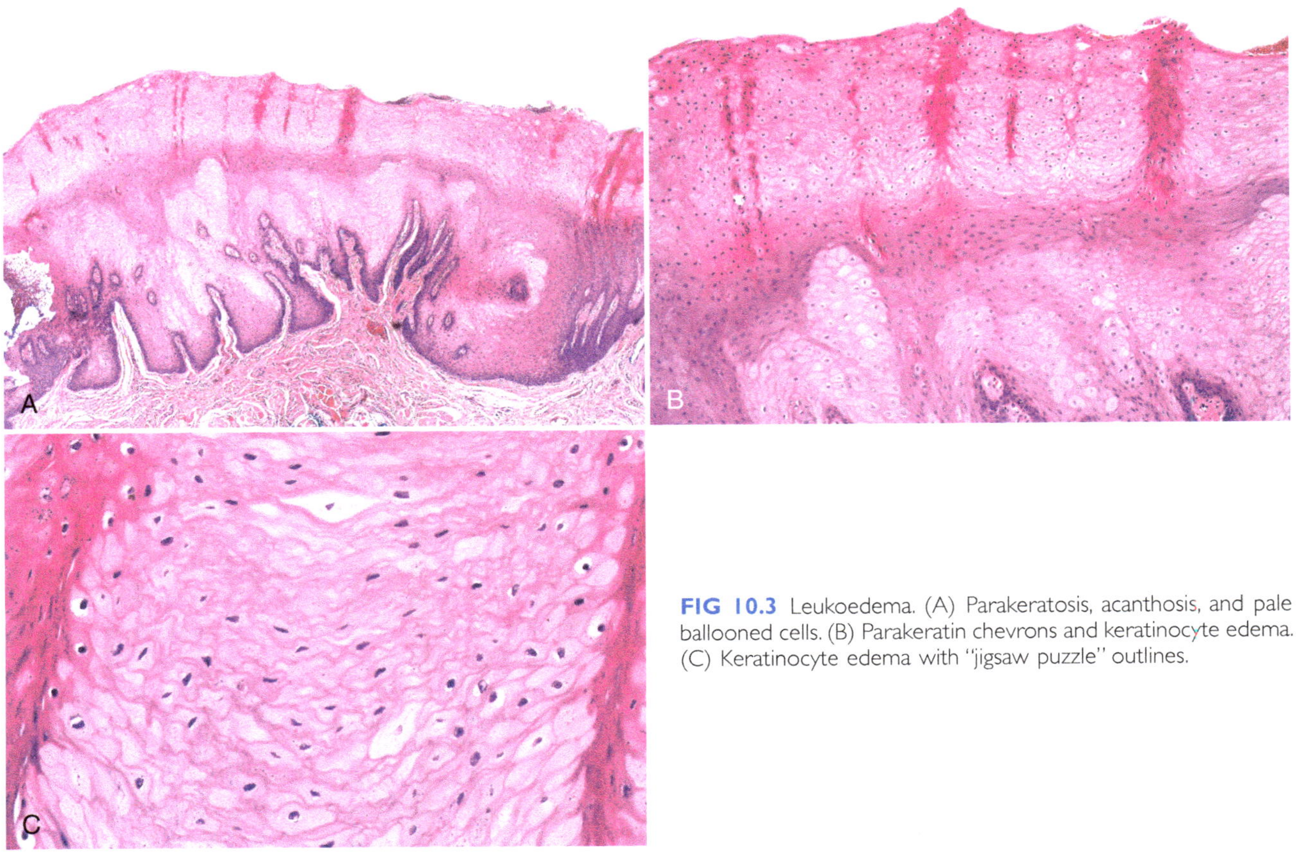

FIG 10.3 Leukoedema. (A) Parakeratosis, acanthosis, and pale ballooned cells. (B) Parakeratin chevrons and keratinocyte edema. (C) Keratinocyte edema with "jigsaw puzzle" outlines.

Contact Desquamation

Clinical Findings

- Painless, thready white tissue lies on the mucosa (usually nonkeratinized sites) which easily peels off, leaving normal mucosa (Fig. 10.4); surrounding leukoedema may be seen and patients may also exhibit contact desquamative cheilitis.

Etiopathogenesis and Histopathologic Features

This condition results from caustic mouth washes high in alcohol content, strong toothpastes, or other contactants that are irritants but not strong enough to cause necrosis and ulceration (as aspirin would).

- Strips of desquamated keratinocytes appear eosinophilic and degenerated or coagulated (Figs. 10.5 and 10.6).

Management

- Resolution occurs on discontinuation of use of dentifrice.

REFERENCES

Foti C, Romita P, Ficco D, et al. Allergic contact cheilitis to amine fluoride in a toothpaste. *Dermatitis.* 2014;25:209.

Francalanci S, Sertoli A, Giorgini S, et al. Multicentre study of allergic contact cheilitis from toothpastes. *Contact Dermatitis.* 2000;43:216-222.

Kowitz G, Jacobson J, Meng Z, Lucatorto F. The effects of tartar-control toothpaste on the oral soft tissues. *Oral Surg Oral Med Oral Pathol.* 1990;70:529-536.

Kuttan NA, Narayana N, Moghadam BK. Desquamative stomatitis associated with routine use of oral health care products. *Gen Dent.* 2001;49:596-602.

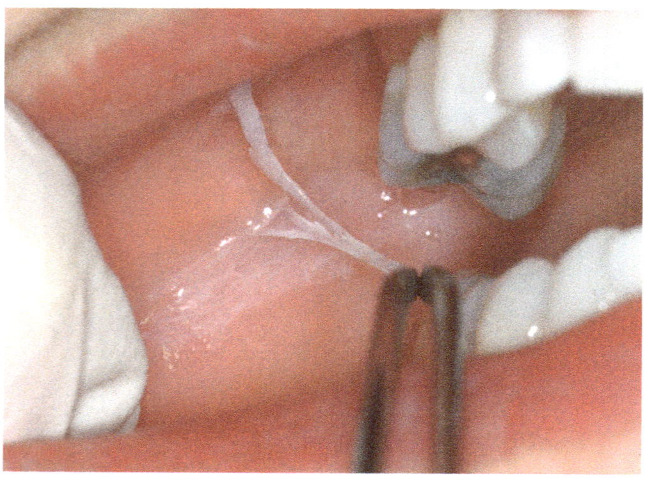

FIG 10.4 Dentifrice-induced desquamation: superficial keratinocytes are degenerated and peel off, leaving normal-appearing mucosa. Note the subtle leukoedema.

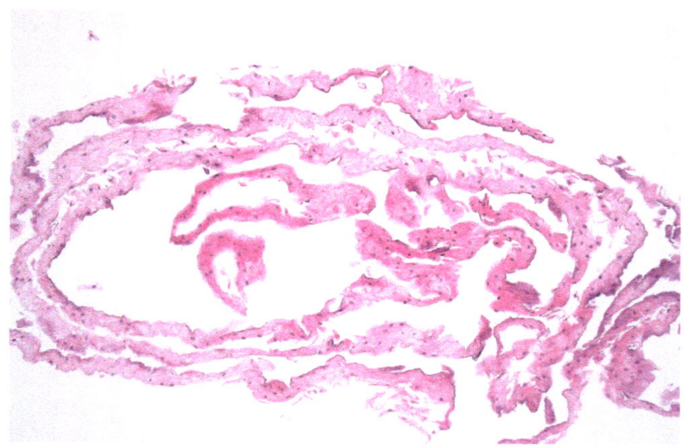

FIG 10.5 Dentifrice-induced desquamation: degenerated epithelium from patient shown in Fig. 10.4.

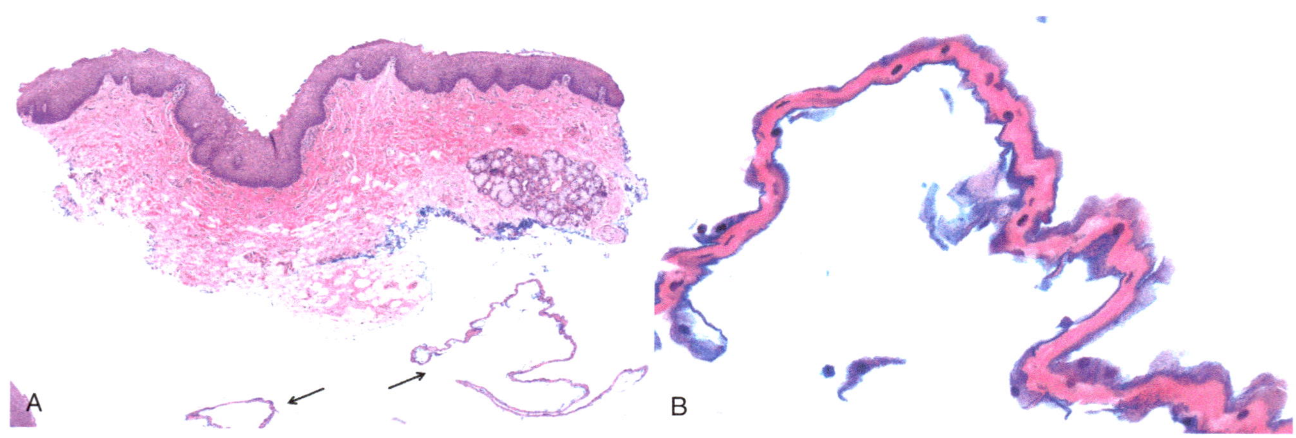

FIG 10.6 Dentifrice-induced contact desquamation. (A) Strips of epithelium *(arrows)* lie detached from the mucosa. (B) Ribbons of coagulated keratinocytes.

Frictional/Factitial Keratoses

The majority of parakeratotic and hyperkeratotic lesions in the oral cavity are reactive, frictional keratoses. Two histologically well-defined frictional keratoses in the oral cavity are morsicatio mucosae oris (generally on the nonkeratinized mucosa), and benign alveolar ridge keratosis (generally on the keratinized mucosa). The linea alba on the buccal mucosa is considered a variation of normal and represents either leukoedema or mild morsicatio mucosae oris (Fig. 10.7A).

MORSICATIO MUCOSAE ORIS (MORSICATIO BUCCARUM, PATHOMINIA MUCOSAE ORIS)

Clinical Findings

- These occur at any age; the most common locations lie close to the biting surfaces of the teeth, namely buccal mucosa, lateral/ventral tongue, and lower lip mucosa (rare on upper lip mucosa); more than 50% of patients are unaware of their habit (which may be nocturnal).
- Poorly demarcated papules and plaques often display a shaggy, macerated, sometimes papillary surface, and may be associated with areas of erythema and ulceration depending on the severity of the parafunctional chewing habit (Fig. 10.7B–D).
- Chronic irritation of the mucosa against an oral appliance or other hard foreign object results in similar findings.

Etiopathogenesis and Histologic Features

Parafunctional habits such as raking of the teeth, prosthesis, or other foreign object against the nonkeratinized mucosa result in these benign reactive keratotic lesions with distinctive histopathology. It is important that these lesions not be signed out as merely "parakeratosis or acanthosis" but as a frictional or reactive keratosis so that they do not get relegated to the category of leukoplakia (see Chapter 11).

- Linea alba shows leukoedema (Fig. 10.8).
- Classic lesions show mild to severe parakeratosis with fissures and clefts often rimmed by bacteria, but without inflammation; candidal hyphae are infrequently seen; parakeratosis diminishes toward the lateral edges, and there is acanthosis and keratinocyte edema (Figs. 10.9–10.11); ulcers may be present and long-standing lesions show hyperkeratosis similar to benign alveolar ridge keratosis (Fig. 10.12).
- Slight surface papillomatosis may be present and rete ridges are tapered; inflammation is usually absent unless an ulcer is present and there may be "plasma pooling" from trauma (Fig. 10.13).

Differential Diagnosis

- Hairy tongue is characterized by true hyperparakeratosis and hyperplastic filiform papillae composed of thick spires of parakeratin with many bacterial colonies (Figs. 10.14 and 10.15). This is a retention keratosis caused by dehydration and poor diet leading to retention of keratin rather than normal shedding. Lesions resolve on improved hydration and diet.
- Hairy leukoplakia usually shows sharp demarcation of the parakeratin from an underlying pale band of edematous keratinocytes, chromatin beading against the nuclear membrane, Cowdry inclusions, and presence of EBV in superficial keratinocytes.
- Any other papular/nodular lesion, such as a dysplasia or even a fibroma, may show overlying secondary frictional/factitial keratosis.

Management and Prognosis

- Use of barrier devices to prevent patients from habitually chewing the mucosa may or may not be helpful because patients may continue to rake the mucosa against the appliance.
- Lesions have no malignant potential and do not require further management.

REFERENCES

Glass LF, Maize JC. Morsicatio buccarum et labiorum (excessive cheek and lip biting). *Am J Dermatopathol.* 1991;13:271-274.

Hjorting-Hansen E, Holst E. Morsicatio mucosae oris and suctio mucosae oris. *Scand J Dent Res.* 1970;78:492-499.

Reichart PA, Philipsen HP. Betel chewer's mucosa—a review. *J Oral Pathol Med.* 1998;27:239-242.

Woo SB, Lin D. Morsicatio mucosae oris—a chronic oral frictional keratosis, not a leukoplakia. *J Oral Maxillofac Surg.* 2009;67:140-146.

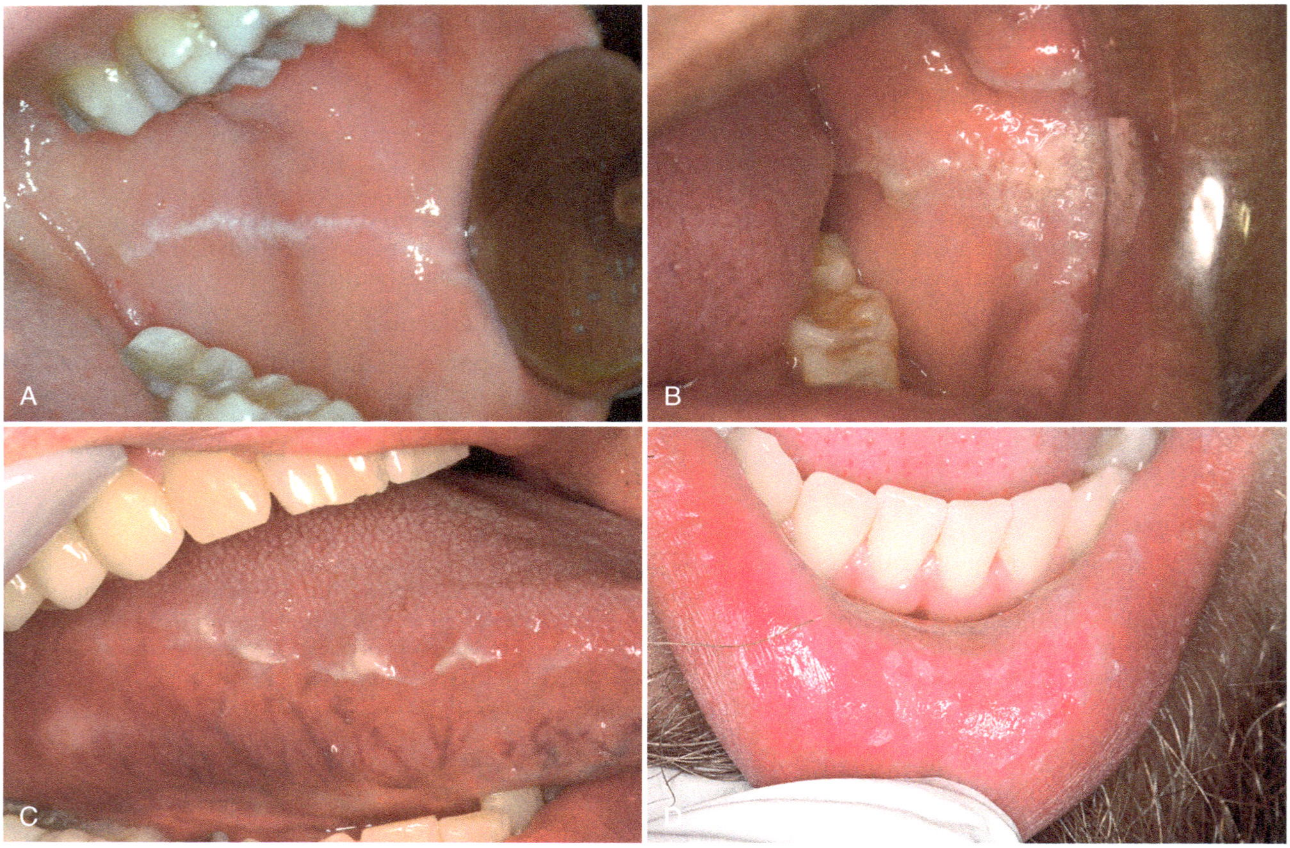

FIG 10.7 (A) Linea alba: keratotic linear lesion with fading margins. (B) Morsicatio mucosae oris: poorly demarcated yellowish-white, macerated plaque that fades into normal mucosa. (C) Morsicatio mucosae oris: white papules of right lateral tongue that fade into normal mucosa. (D) Morsicatio mucosae oris of lower lip mucosa with irregular macerated papules and plaques.

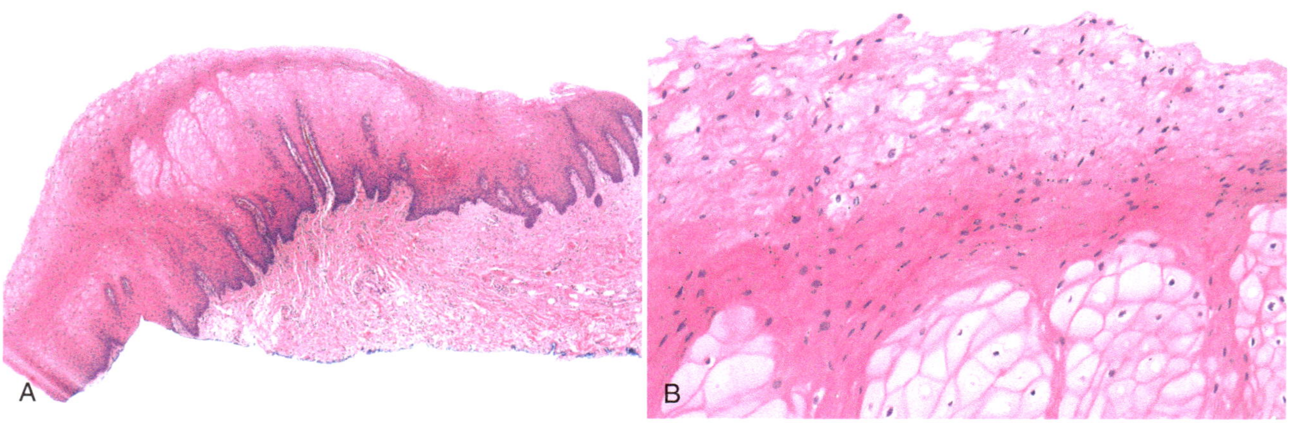

FIG 10.8 Linea alba. (A) Acanthosis and keratinocyte edema. (B) Anucleate superficial cells and keratinocyte edema.

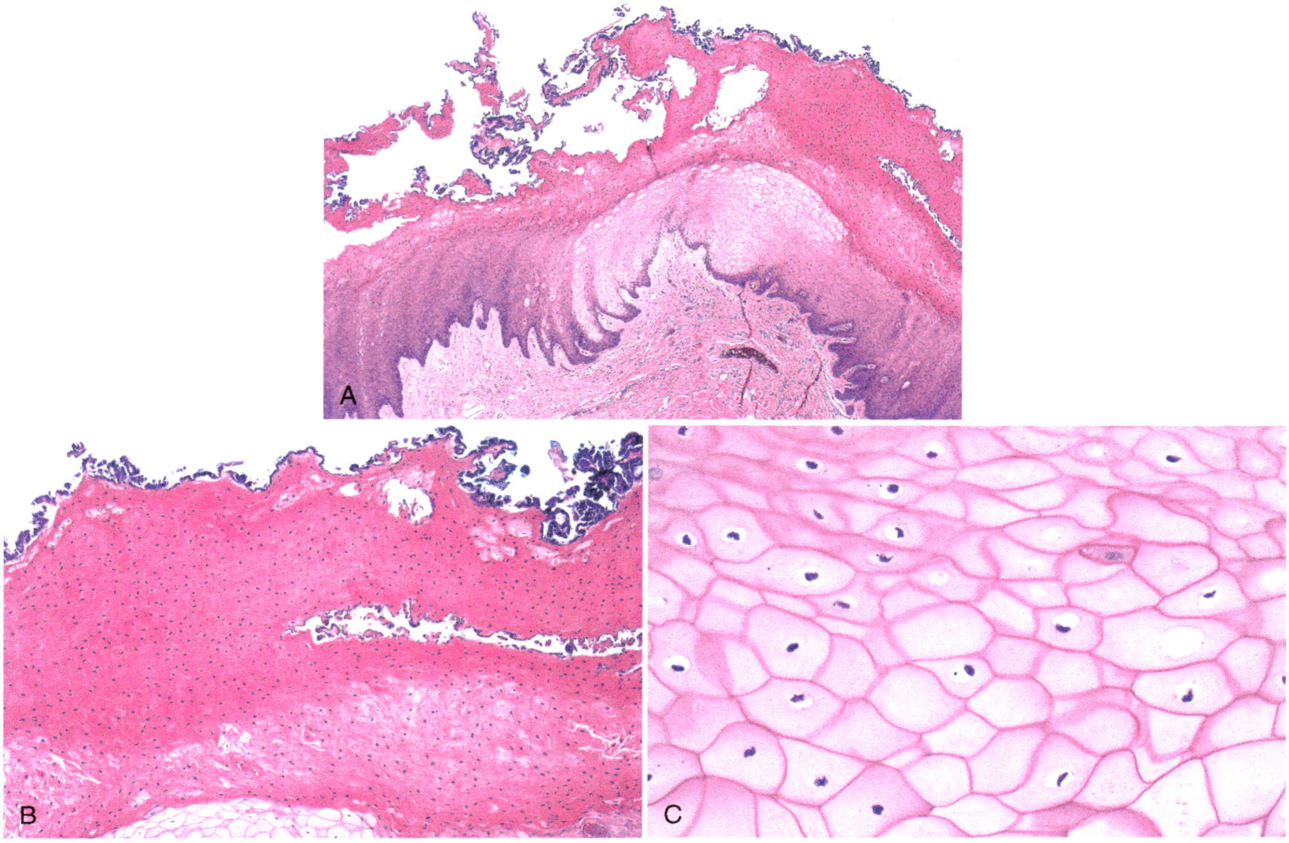

FIG 10.9 Morsicatio mucosae oris. (A) Marked parakeratosis with fissures and clefts rimmed by bacteria, and acanthosis. (B) Marked parakeratosis with bacterial colonization and no inflammation. (C) Prominent keratinocyte edema.

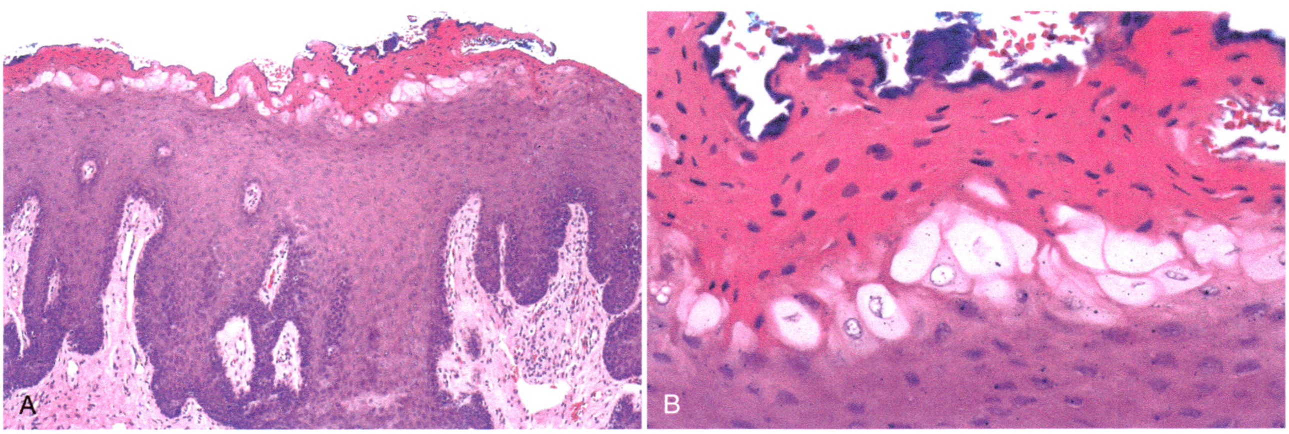

FIG 10.10 Morsicatio mucosae oris. (A) Tapering parakeratosis *(right)* and acanthosis. (B) Parakeratosis with bacterial colonies and keratinocyte edema.

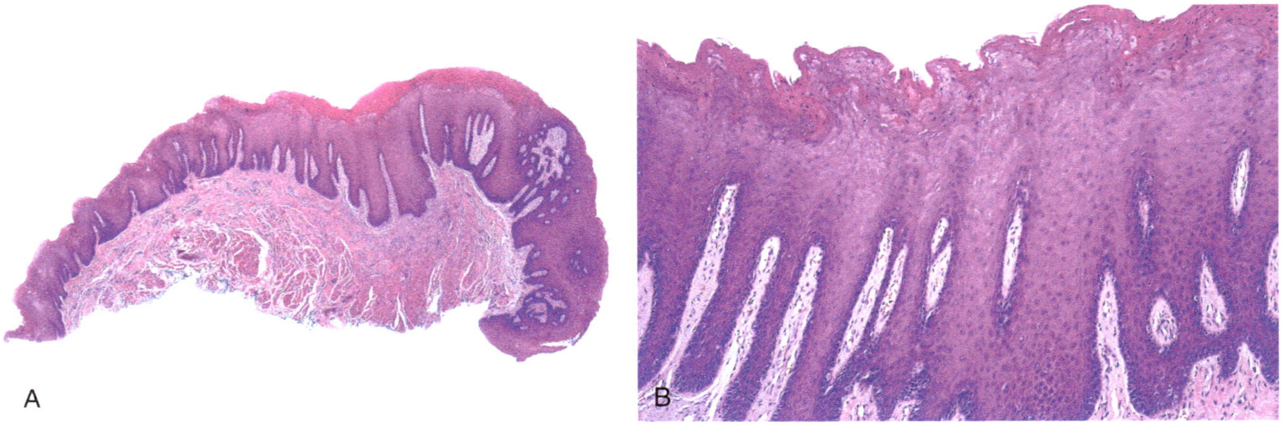

FIG 10.11 Morsicatio mucosae oris. (A) Parakeratosis that tapers toward the edges and acanthosis. (B) Lateral areas showing only mild parakeratosis with slight surface undulations.

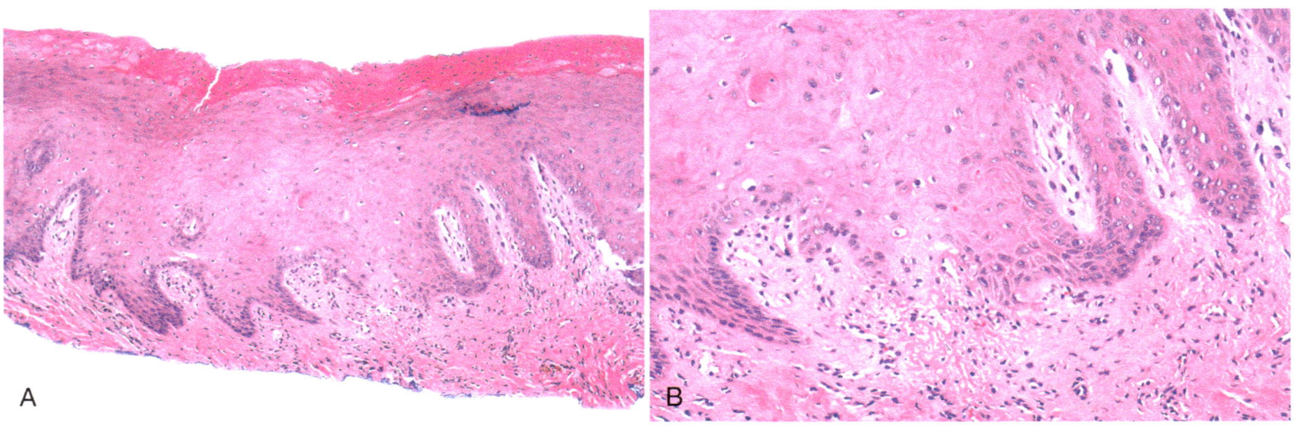

FIG 10.12 Morsicatio mucosae oris. (A) Parakeratosis and acanthosis. (B) Basal cell degeneration, subepithelial fibrin deposition, and mild chronic inflammation (edge of a traumatic ulcer).

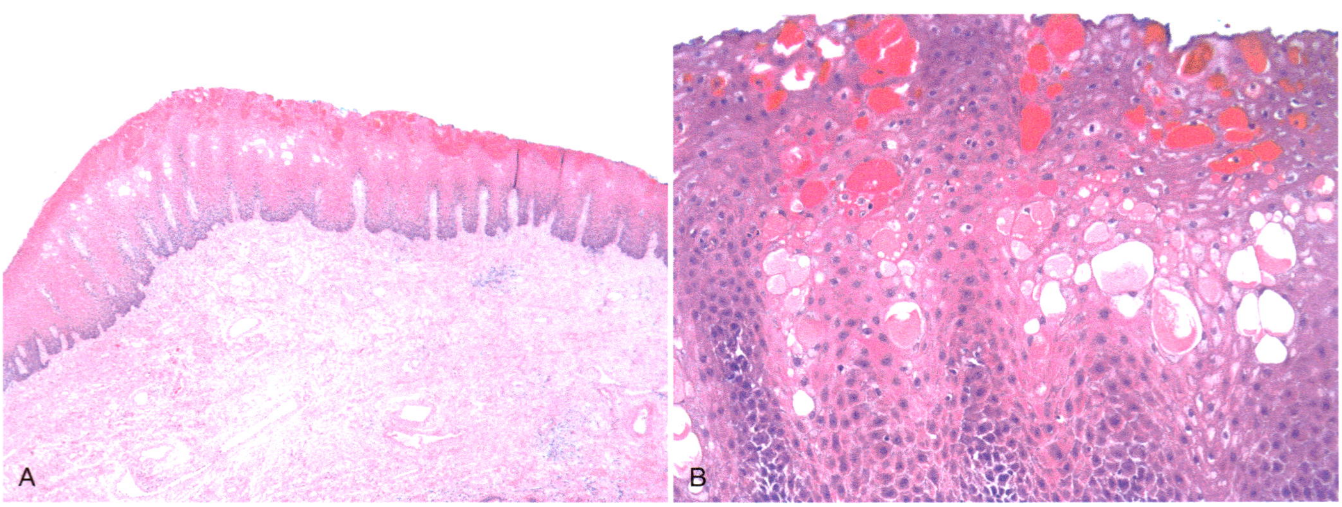

FIG 10.13 Morsicatio mucosae oris. (A) Acanthosis, plasma pooling, and mild chronic inflammation. (B) Plasma pooling between superficial keratinocytes.

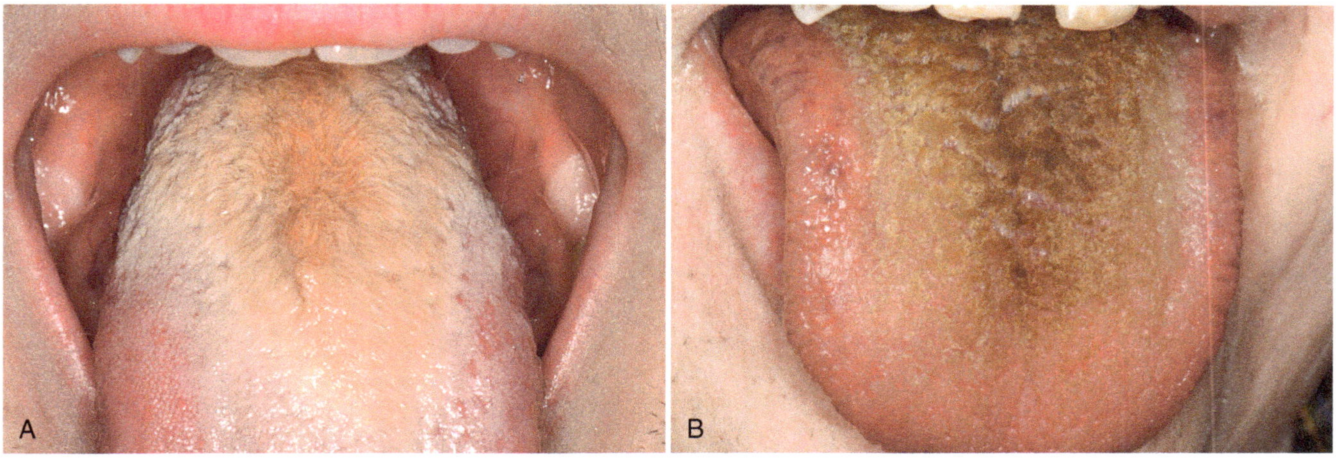

FIG 10.14 Hairy tongue. (A) Hairy dorsum of tongue (B) Brown-black hairy dorsum of tongue.

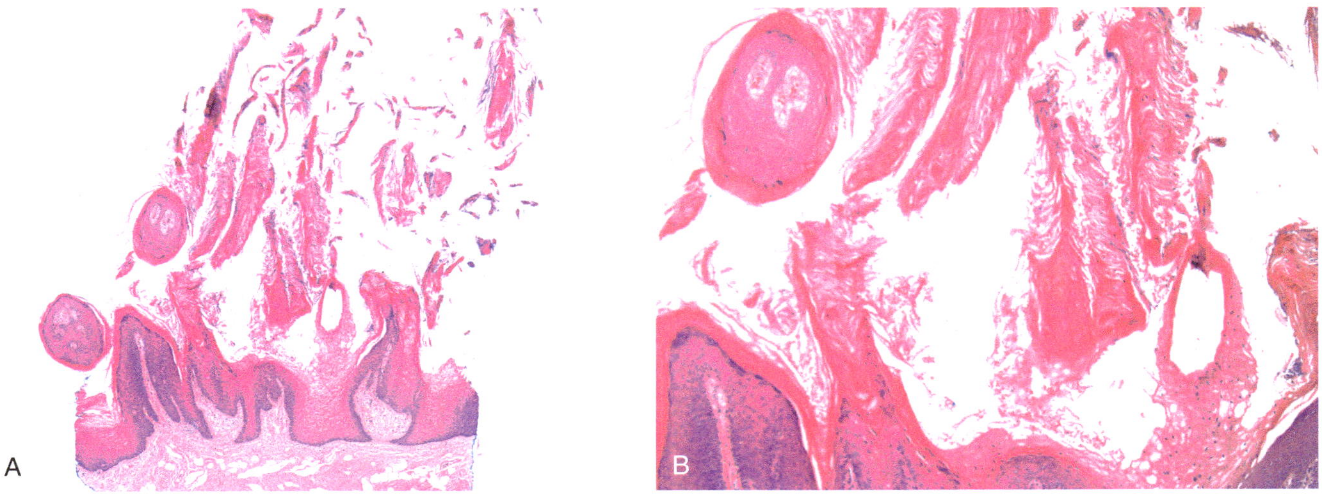

FIG 10.15 Hairy tongue. (A) Hyperplastic filiform papillae. (B) Spires of parakeratin with many bacterial colonies.

BENIGN ALVEOLAR RIDGE (FRICTIONAL) KERATOSIS (ORAL LICHEN SIMPLEX CHRONICUS)

Clinical Features

- This presents as a poorly demarcated, often rough white plaque of the keratinized mucosa of the retromolar pad, attached/keratinized gingiva, and hard palatal mucosa, particularly where teeth have been extracted (Fig. 10.16).

Etiopathogenesis and Histopathologic Features

This is the intraoral equivalent of lichen simplex chronicus of the skin, caused by local irritation and habitual picking of the skin. This oral condition is caused by the trauma of food being crushed against the gingiva or alveolar mucosa rather than by direct impingement of the teeth on mucosa.

- There is hyperkeratosis with wedge-shaped hypergranulosis usually with keratosis tapering at the edge of the lesion; the surface of the epithelium may be undulating or be significantly papillary, and there is acanthosis with tapered rete ridges and confluent rete ridges at the tips; parakeratosis is noted in recently traumatized lesions (Figs. 10.17–10.20).

Differential Diagnosis

- Dysplastic lesions generally show bulbous or drop-shaped rete ridges with significant cytologic atypia.

Management and Prognosis

- No treatment is necessary, and there is no malignant potential.

REFERENCES

Chi AC, Lambert PR 3rd, Pan Y, et al. Is alveolar ridge keratosis a true leukoplakia?: A clinicopathologic comparison of 2,153 lesions. *J Am Dent Assoc.* 2007;138:641-651.

Natarajan E, Woo SB. Benign alveolar ridge keratosis (oral lichen simplex chronicus): a distinct clinicopathologic entity. *J Am Acad Dermatol.* 2008;58:151-157.

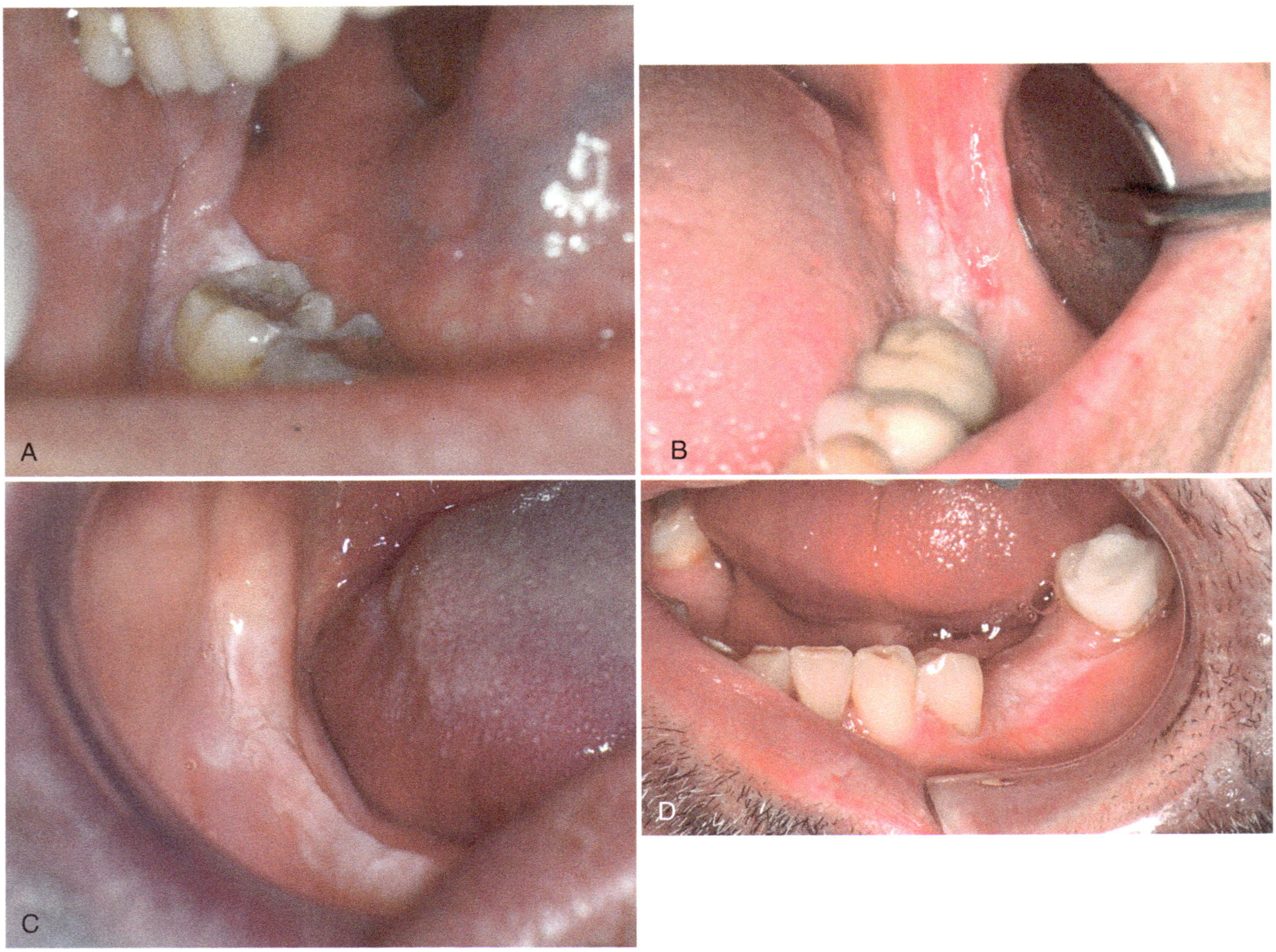

FIG 10.16 (A) Benign alveolar ridge keratosis of the right retromolar pad and linea alba of the buccal mucosa. (B) Benign alveolar ridge keratosis of the left retromolar pad with adjacent traumatic keratosis and erythema of the left buccal mucosa. (C) Benign alveolar ridge keratosis of the right edentulous mandible; poorly demarcated white lesion, which was bilateral under a denture. (D) Benign alveolar ridge keratosis of edentulous span. *(B, Courtesy Dr. Mary Grote, Beaver Dam, Wis.)*

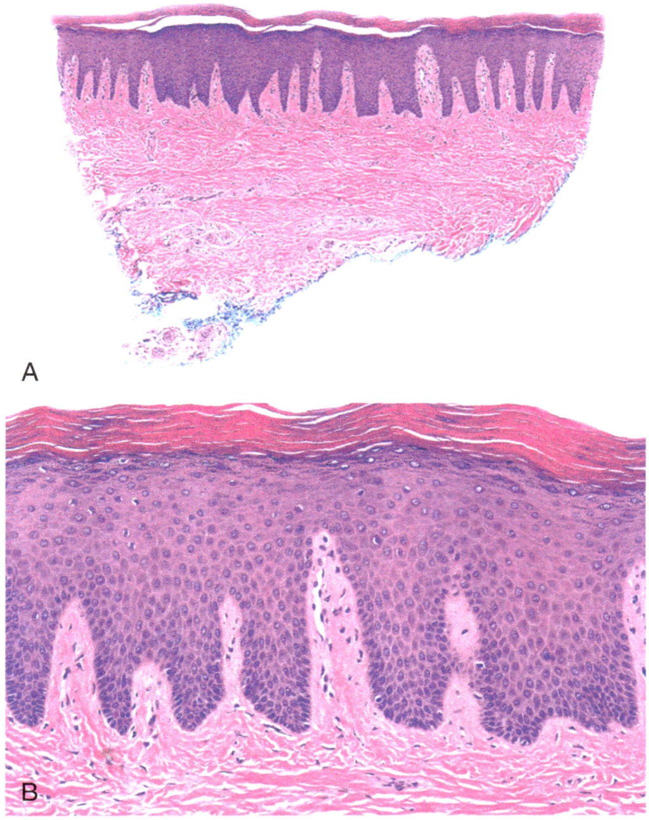

FIG 10.17 Benign alveolar ridge keratosis, mild. (A) Hyperkeratosis and long, tapered rete ridges. (B) Acanthosis without atypia.

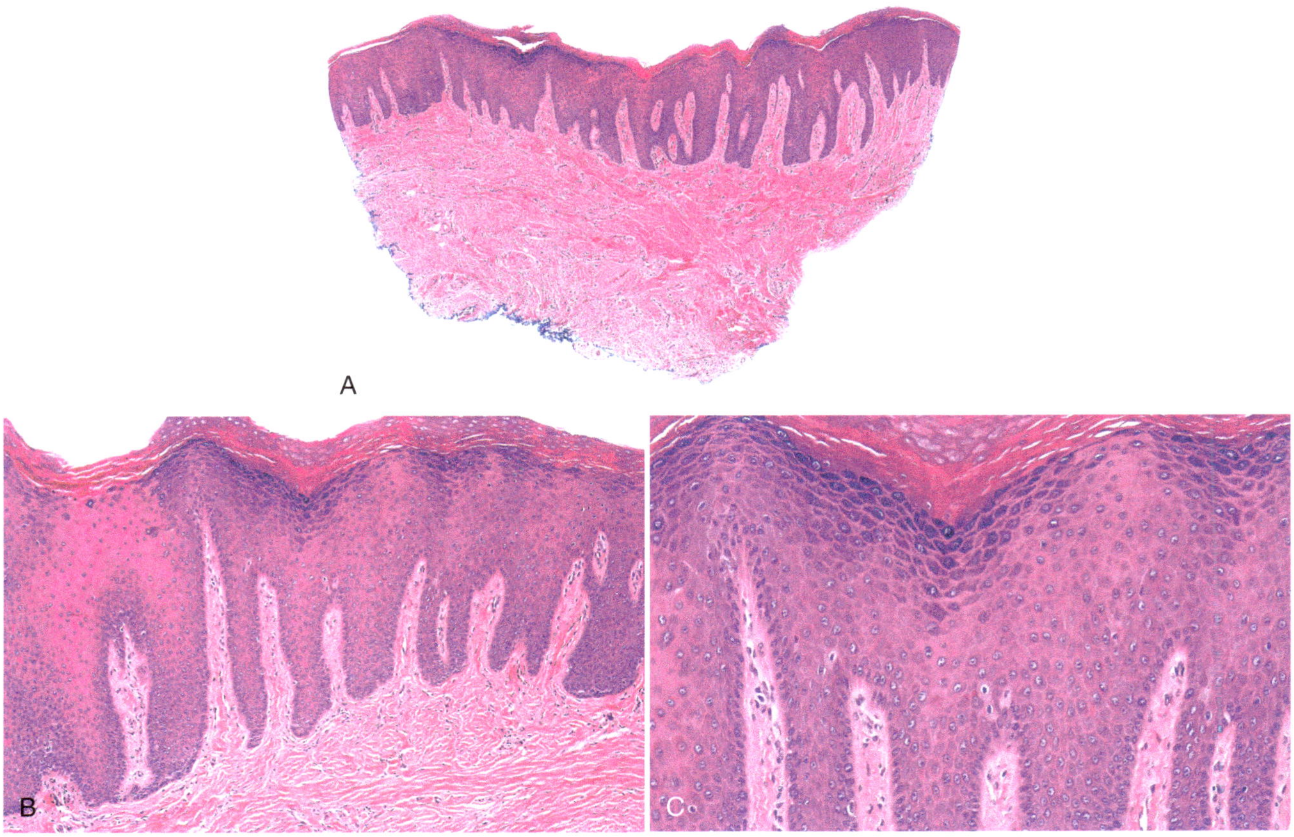

FIG 10.18 Benign alveolar ridge keratosis. (A) Tapering hyperkeratosis, undulating surface, and acanthosis. (B) Hyperkeratosis, wedge-shaped hypergranulosis, and tapered rete ridges. (C) Wedge-shaped hypergranulosis and no epithelial atypia.

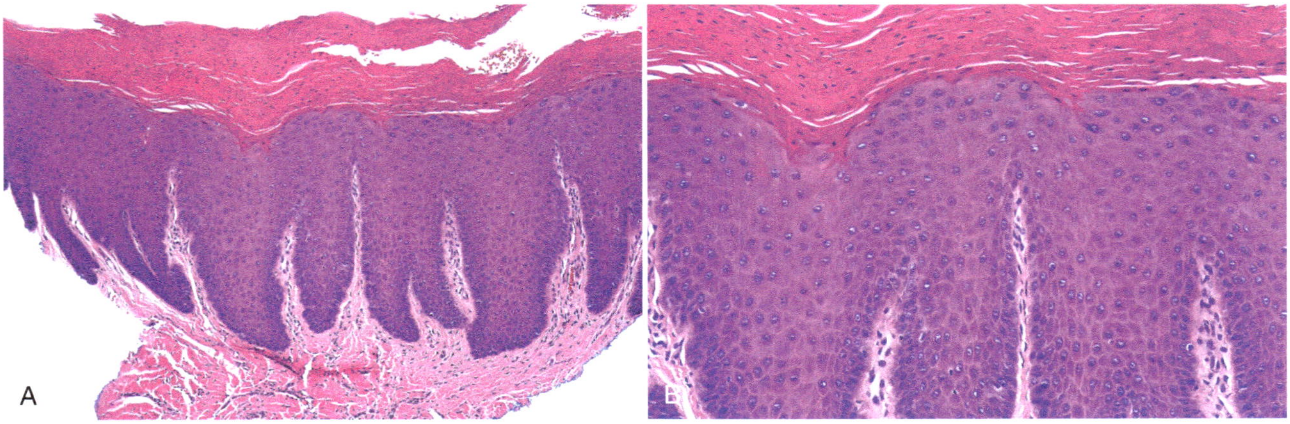

FIG 10.19 Benign alveolar ridge keratosis. (A) Parakeratosis and long, tapered rete ridges with mild vascular ectasia suggestive of previous inflammation. (B) Parakeratosis and acanthosis.

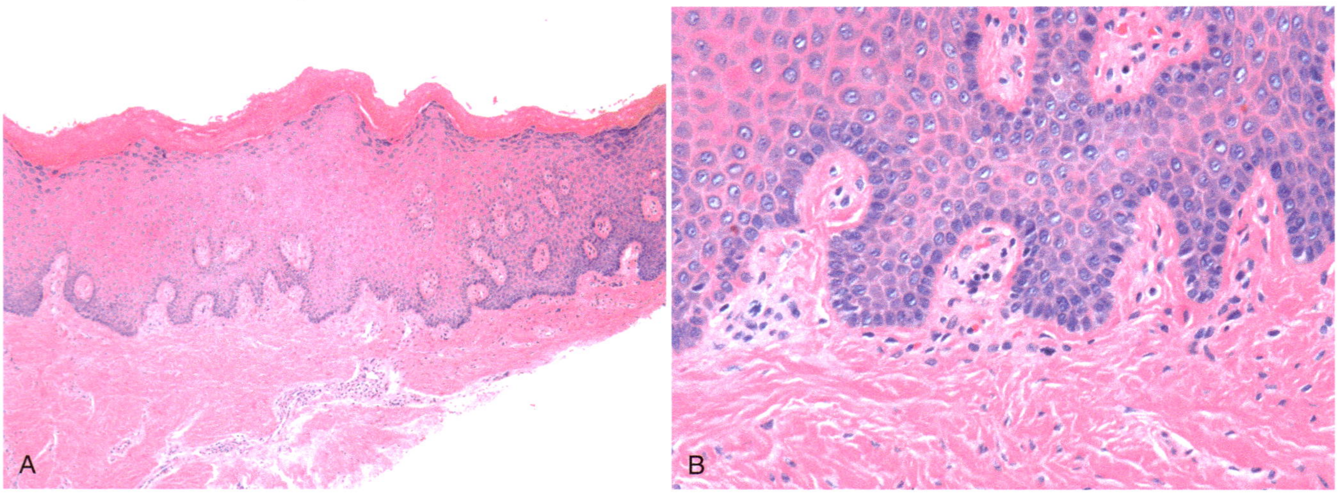

FIG 10.20 Benign alveolar ridge keratosis. (A) Parakeratosis and hyperkeratosis, surface undulations, acanthosis, and mild chronic inflammation. (B) There is no evidence of cytologic atypia or dysplasia.

OTHER BENIGN REACTIVE KERATOSES

Clinical Findings

- These are poorly demarcated white lesions present at sites of trauma.

Etiopathogenesis and Histopathologic Features

These keratotic lesions do not show the typical histopathologic features of well-defined, benign, reactive keratotic lesions, and may represent waxing or waning specific keratotic diseases such as morsicatio mucosae oris, benign alveolar ridge keratosis, lichen planus, or healing ulcers. When rendering a diagnosis, the phrase *reactive* or *likely reactive* should be added to *hyperkeratosis, parakeratosis, acanthosis,* and *chronic inflammation* because suggesting the etiology helps in patient management.

- Hyperkeratosis or parakeratosis diminishes at the periphery where it meets normal mucosa and there is acanthosis with tapered rete ridges; there is variable chronic inflammation and vascular ectasia (vertically oriented capillaries within the papillary lamina propria) often with mild reactive epithelial atypia; subepithelial fibrin is seen in areas of healing ulceration (Figs. 10.21 and 10.22).

Differential Diagnosis

- Early dysplasia must be differentiated from reactive atypia, especially if the clinical lesion is well demarcated and situated at a high-risk site for dysplasia and oral cancer.

Management and Prognosis

- Contact irritants should be removed and sharp teeth filed down; if the lesion persists, a re-biopsy should be performed.

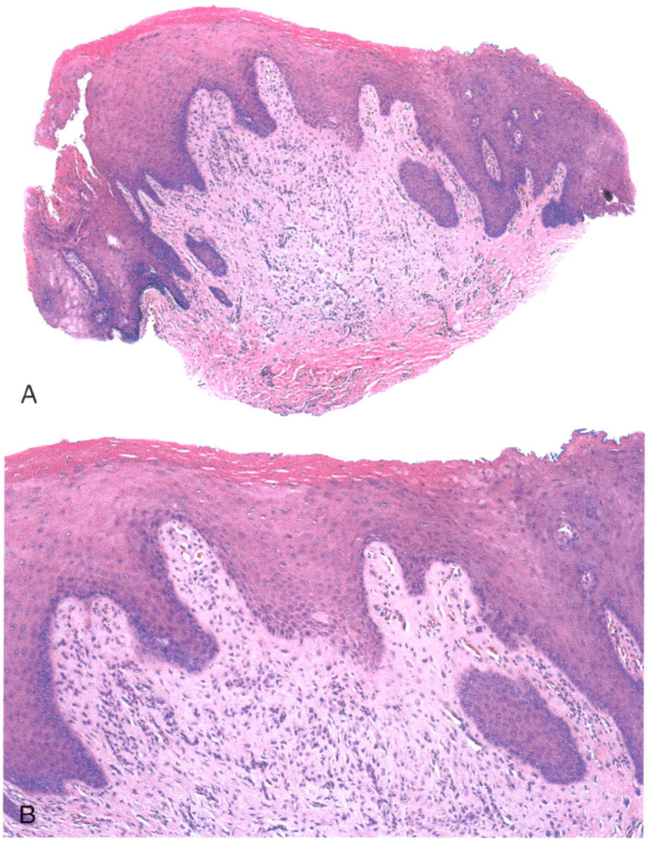

FIG 10.21 Reactive keratosis. (A) Hyperkeratosis that diminishes toward the right lateral edge. (B) Mild focal reactive atypia; this may be the edge of a healing ulcer because of focal squamatization of basal cells and presence of granulation tissue.

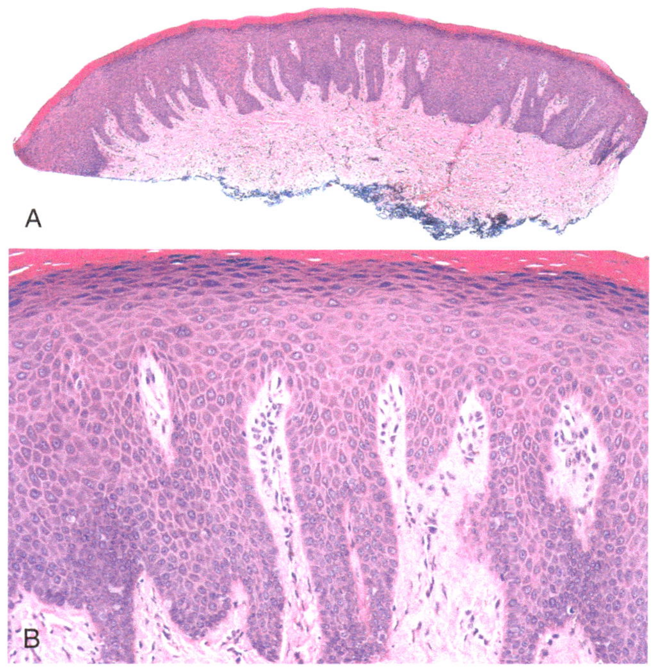

FIG 10.22 Reactive keratosis. (A) Hyperkeratosis and acanthosis forming tapered and confluent rete ridges. (B) Acanthosis with vertically oriented capillaries in the papillary lamina propria.

Tobacco-Related Lesions

SMOKELESS TOBACCO LESION (SMOKELESS TOBACCO KERATOSIS)

Smokeless tobacco is available in two forms for use in the mouth: cured, shredded, and flavored tobacco leaves called chewing tobacco, or snuff that can be moist or dry. Moist snuff (known as snus in Scandinavia) is finely cut or ground cured tobacco that is flavored and now available as preportion pouches similar to tea bags for convenience of use. Dry snuff, which is fermented, powdered tobacco used either in the mouth or inhaled, has substantially waned in popularity. These products vary in composition in different parts of the world depending on the tobacco species, fermentation, nicotine, and tobacco-specific nitrosamine content and pH. In general, snus is lower in carcinogenic tobacco–associated nitrosamines than American moist or dry snuff. Toombak from Ethiopia has the highest levels of nitrosamines and also high pH, which increases the rate of absorption of nicotine. Smokeless tobacco is called *shammah* in the Arabian Peninsula; gutka or paan used in South Asia is smokeless tobacco mixed with spices and areca nut.

Clinical Findings

- Early lesions are poorly demarcated, grayish-white, and edematous with wrinkles and parallel ridges and fissures in the area where the tobacco is placed, which is usually the mandibular vestibule between the gingiva and buccal mucosa; teeth may show brown staining, gingival recession, and root exposure; early lesions are reversible on stopping the habit (Fig. 10.23).
- More advanced lesions are dense, well-demarcated, keratotic plaques; these areas must be biopsied for evaluation of dysplasia, and the lesions are unlikely to be reversible and represent true leukoplakia.

Etiopathogenesis and Histopathologic Features

Smokeless tobacco lesions are caused by contact with caustic agents within the tobacco, and as such early lesions are a form of contact irritation that is reversible. However, long-standing lesions are essentially leukoplakias that result from carcinogens within the tobacco such as tobacco-associated nitrosamines (see Chapter 11). The risk of oral cancer associated with the use of smokeless tobacco is much lower compared with cigarette smoking.

- Early lesions: there is slight parakeratosis with prominent keratinocyte edema of superficial cells that characteristically stops abruptly; karyopyknosis is common and parakeratin "chevrons" often are seen, although this feature is not specific to this condition (see Leukoedema, earlier); acanthosis is present with minimal reactive atypia and variable chronic inflammation (Figs. 10.24A–B and 10.25).
- Amorphous amyloid-like eosinophilic deposits (likely altered collagen) that are not congophilic may be seen

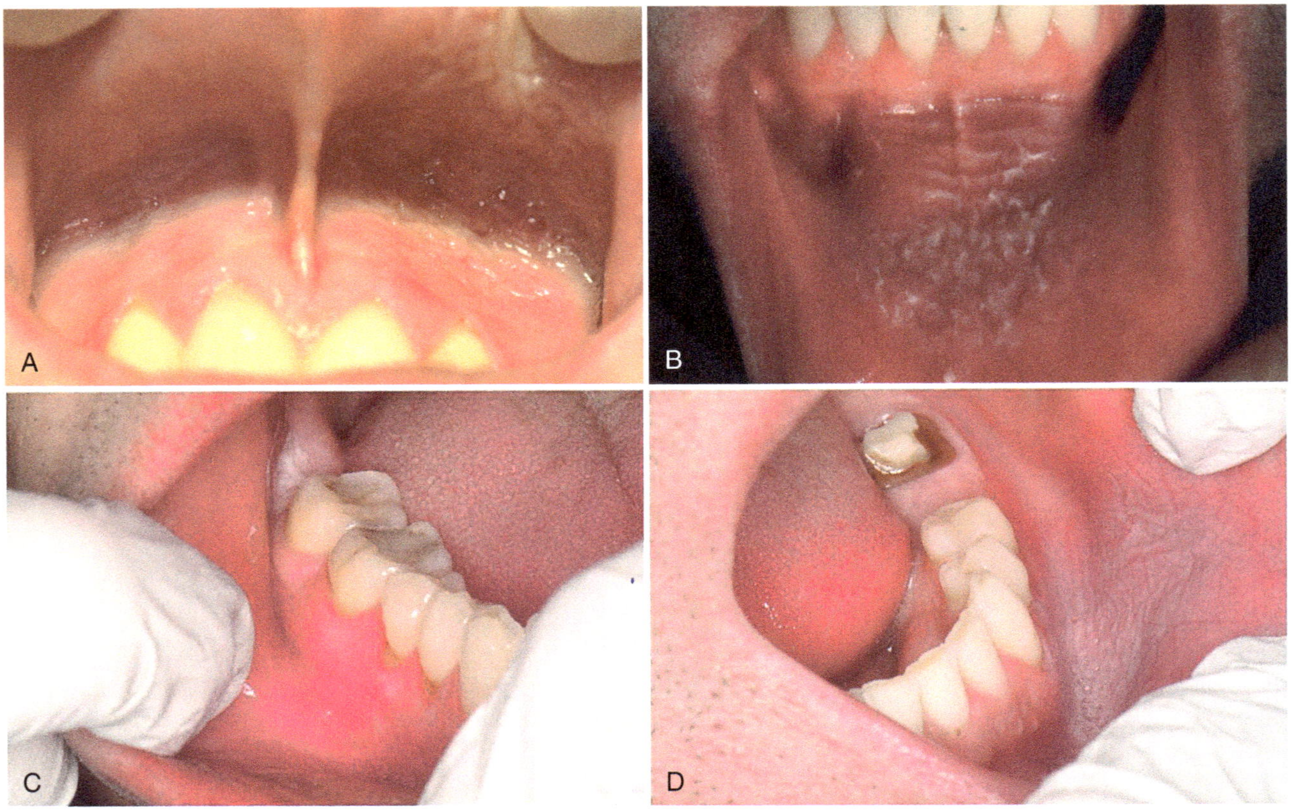

FIG 10.23 Smokeless tobacco lesion. (A) Typical wrinkled and ridged, poorly demarcated gray-white lesion of the vestibule where tobacco is placed. (B) Typical wrinkled and ridged, poorly demarcated gray-white lesion of the vestibule where tobacco is placed. (C) Mucosa appeared normal after cessation of habit for two weeks. (D) Same patient as in C who switched to placing tobacco on the left side for two weeks with gray, fissured, poorly demarcated edematous mucosa. *(B, Courtesy Dr. Sherwin Kershman, Houston, Tex.)*

in the lamina propria and within minor salivary gland parenchyma (see Figs. 10.24C and 10.26).
- Late lesions: these show parakeratosis or hyperkeratosis with or without atypia or dysplasia.

Differential Diagnosis

- Leukoedema may have similar histopathologic features but the edematous keratinocytes are not as well demarcated.

Management and Prognosis

- Early lesions generally resolve if the habit is discontinued.
- Hyperkeratotic lesions that are demarcated should be regularly evaluated for dysplasia or excised/ablated with discontinuation of the habit.

REFERENCES

Andersson G, Axell T, Larsson A. Histologic changes associated with the use of loose and portion-bag packed Swedish moist snuff: a comparative study. *J Oral Pathol Med.* 1989;18:491-497.

Daniels TE, Hansen LS, Greenspan JS, et al. Histopathology of smokeless tobacco lesions in professional baseball players. Associations with different types of tobacco. *Oral Surg Oral Med Oral Pathol.* 1992; 73:720-725.

Hirsch JM, Heyden G, Thilander H. A clinical, histomorphological and histochemical study on snuff-induced lesions of varying severity. *J Oral Pathol.* 1982;11:387-398.

Idris AM, Warnakulasuriya KA, Ibrahim YE, et al. Characterization of an amorphous deposit in the lamina propria in oral snuff users in the Sudan as collagen. *J Oral Pathol Med.* 1998;27:157-162.

Kallischnigg G, Weitkunat R, Lee PN. Systematic review of the relation between smokeless tobacco and non-neoplastic oral diseases in Europe and the United States. *BMC Oral Health.* 2008;8:13.

Rodu B, Jansson C. Smokeless tobacco and oral cancer: a review of the risks and determinants. *Crit Rev Oral Biol Med.* 2004;15:252-263.

Warnakulasuriya KA, Ralhan R. Clinical, pathological, cellular and molecular lesions caused by oral smokeless tobacco—a review. *J Oral Pathol Med.* 2007;36:63-77.

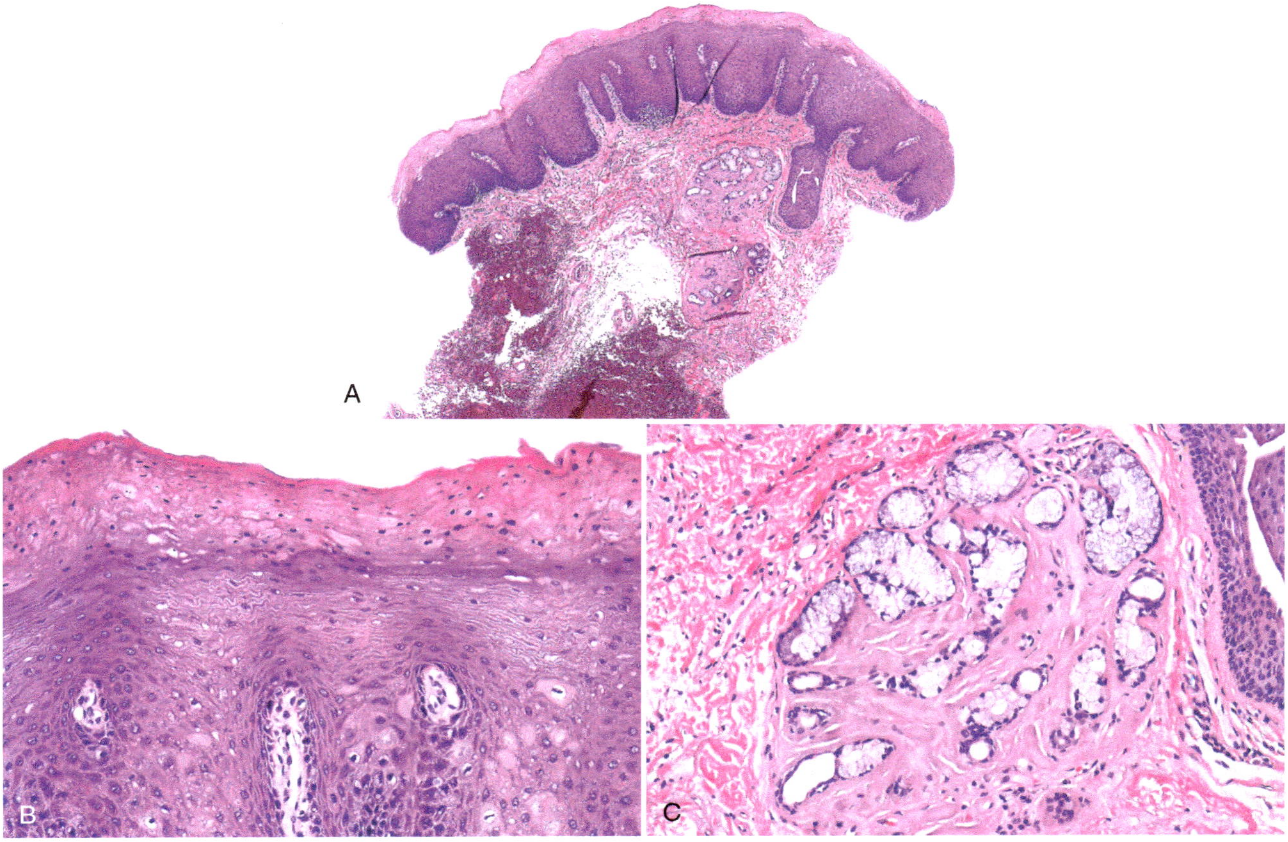

FIG 10.24 Smokeless tobacco lesion. (A) Oral mucosa with well-demarcated area of edematous superficial keratinocytes and salivary gland involvement. (B) Very thin layer of parakeratin on the surface and thick band of degenerated and anucleate keratinocytes. (C) Salivary glands containing amorphous amyloid-like material.

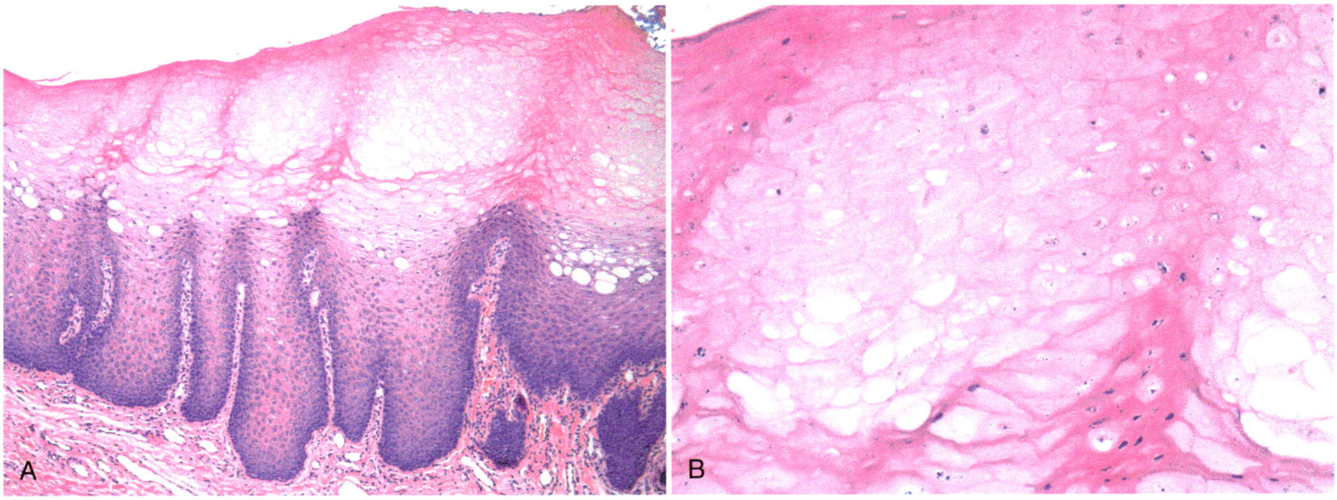

FIG 10.25 Smokeless tobacco lesion. (A) Oral mucosa with demarcated prominent band of degenerated keratinocytes, spongiosis, and parakeratin chevrons. (B) Edematous and degenerated keratinocytes with karyopyknosis and parakeratin chevrons.

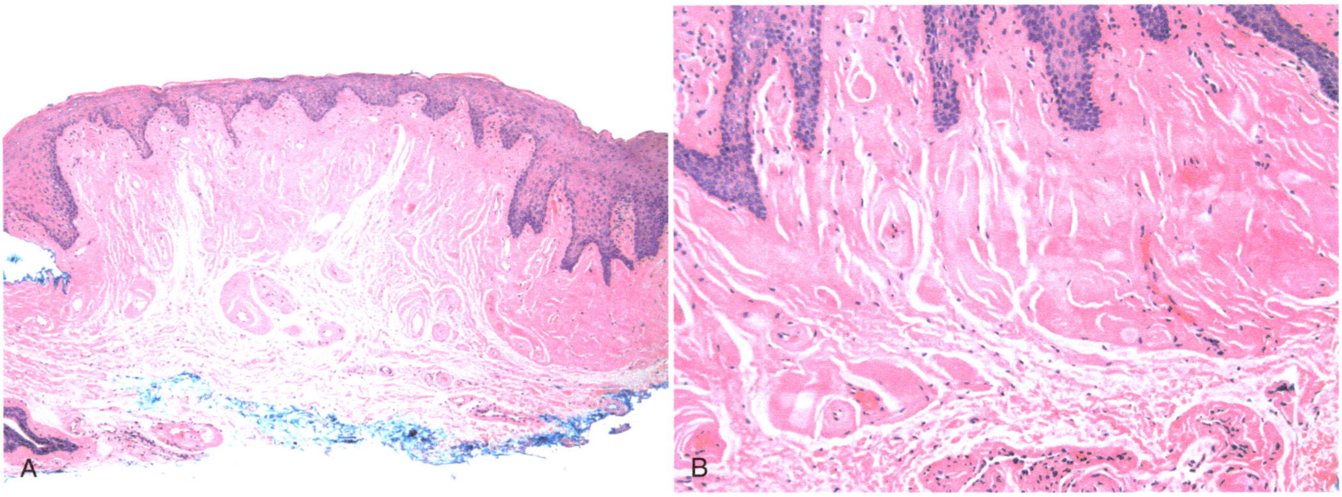

FIG 10.26 Smokeless tobacco lesion. (A) Thin layer of parakeratin, epithelial atrophy, and amorphous amyloid-like material. (B) Amorphous amyloid-like material within the lamina propria surrounding vessels.

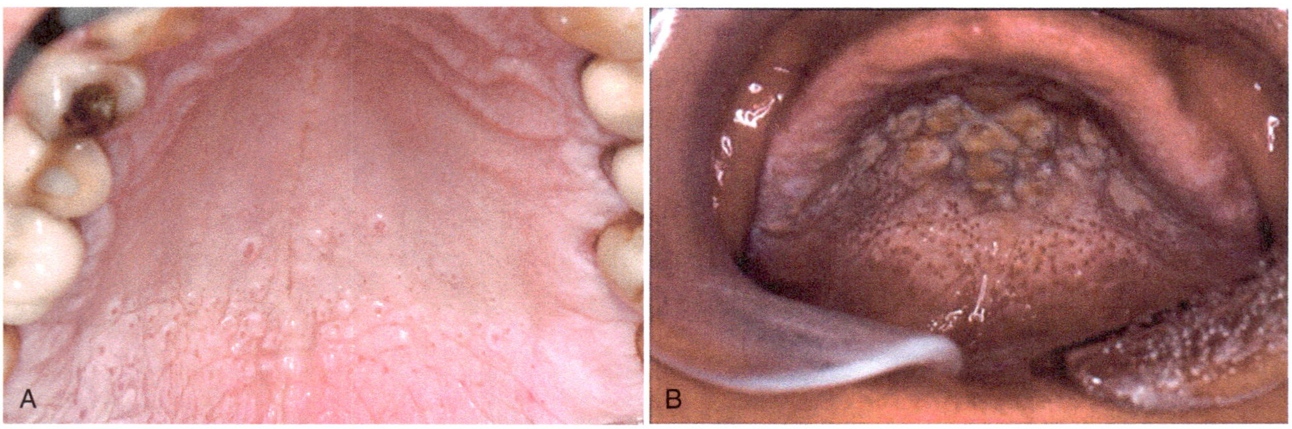

FIG 10.27 (A) Nicotinic stomatitis. (B) Severe nicotinic stomatitis from reverse smoking. *(A and B, Courtesy Dr. Linda Lee, Princess Margaret Hospital, Toronto, Ontario, Canada.)*

NICOTINIC STOMATITIS (STOMATITIS NICOTINA)

Clinical Findings

- This occurs in adults as symmetric, painless, or sensitive lesions involving the hard palatal mucosa and sometimes the soft palate; the mucosa has a white cast (variable in intensity depending on severity of disease) within which are scattered red punctate papules that represent the opening of excretory salivary ducts (Fig. 10.27A).

Etiopathogenesis and Histopathologic Features

This is a form of reactive keratosis caused by heat (not nicotine) usually from pipe smoking, although it may also occur in heavy cigarette smokers, "reverse smokers" (those who smoke with the lit end of the cigarette in their mouths), and those who frequently drink very hot beverages (Fig. 10.27B).

- There is hyperkeratosis or parakeratosis, acanthosis with or without reactive epithelial atypia, and variable chronic inflammation; there is squamous metaplasia of excretory salivary ducts and chronic sialodochitis (periductal inflammation) (Fig. 10.28).

Management and Prognosis

- Early mucosal changes are generally reversible on stopping the habit.
- Leukoplakias that develop require close follow-up and surveillance biopsies.

REFERENCES

dos Santos RB, Katz J. Nicotinic stomatitis: positive correlation with heat in maté tea drinks and smoking. *Quintessence Int.* 2009;40:537-540.

Ortiz GM, Pierce AM, Wilson DF. Palatal changes associated with reverse smoking in Filipino women. *Oral Dis.* 1996;2:232-237.

Reddy CR, Kameswari VR, Ramulu C, Reddy PG. Histopathological study of stomatitis nicotina. *Br J Cancer.* 1971;25:403-410.

Reddy CR, Raju MV, Ramulu C, Reddy PG. Changes in the ducts of the glands of the hard palatal mucosa in reverse smokers. *Cancer.* 1972;30:231-238.

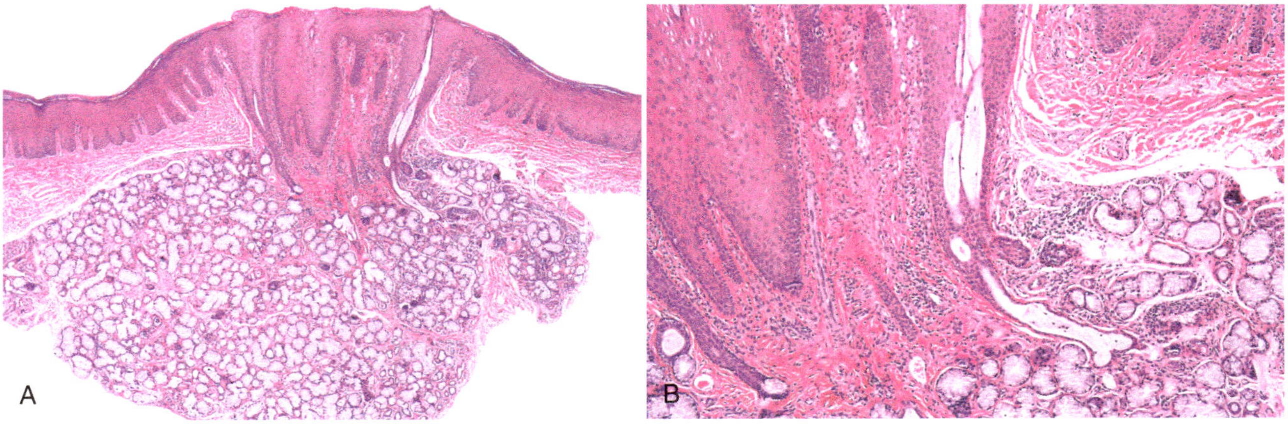

FIG 10.28 Nicotinic stomatitis. (A) Hyperkeratosis and squamous metaplasia of ducts forming a raised papule. (B) Periductal and parenchymal chronic inflammation of glands.

Warty Dyskeratoma (Focal Acantholytic Dyskeratosis, Isolated Darier Disease)

Unlike the reactive keratotic lesions described earlier that are generally diffuse, this is a solitary papular lesion. Some consider the intraoral lesion to be focal acantholytic dyskeratosis because it is almost always papular; only the nodular tumor-like lesions should be considered warty dyskeratoma.

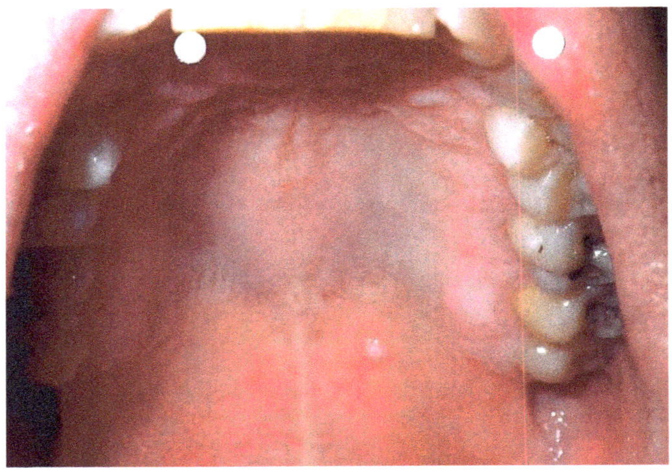

FIG 10.29 Keratotic papule on the hard palatal mucosa.

Clinical Findings

- This occurs usually in the fifth to seventh decade, with approximately 75% of cases occurring on the keratinized mucosa of the hard palate and gingiva; it presents as a solitary white, sometimes warty papule (Fig. 10.29).

Etiopathogenesis and Histopathologic Features

On the skin these may represent a follicular adnexal neoplasm. However, in the mouth the cause is unknown.

- There is umbilicated/crateriform parakeratosis and acanthosis forming elongated, slender rete ridges only a few cells wide at the crater base; there is suprabasilar acantholysis with villous-like projections of connective tissue papillae rimmed by basal cells; dyskeratotic cells with dark nuclei in the form of needle-shaped, slender grains are characteristic; *corps ronds* (round bodies) that are commonly seen in Darier disease are not usually prominent or even present; there is variable chronic inflammation and the adjacent epithelium exhibits papillomatosis (Fig. 10.30).

Differential Diagnoses

- Pemphigus shows acantholytic cells, no dyskeratosis, and positive direct immunofluorescence studies.
- Pyostomatitis vegetans shows suprabasilar clefting, no dyskeratosis, and many eosinophils.

Management and Prognosis

- Excision is curative.

REFERENCES

Allon I, Buchner A. Warty dyskeratoma/focal acantholytic dyskeratosis—an update on a rare oral lesion. *J Oral Pathol Med.* 2012;41:261-267.
Kaddu S, Dong H, Mayer G, et al. Warty dyskeratoma—"follicular dyskeratoma": analysis of clinicopathologic features of a distinctive follicular adnexal neoplasm. *J Am Acad Dermatol.* 2002;47:423-428.
Zunt SL, Tomich CE. Oral focal acantholytic dyskeratosis. *J Dermatol Surg Oncol.* 1990;16:510-515.

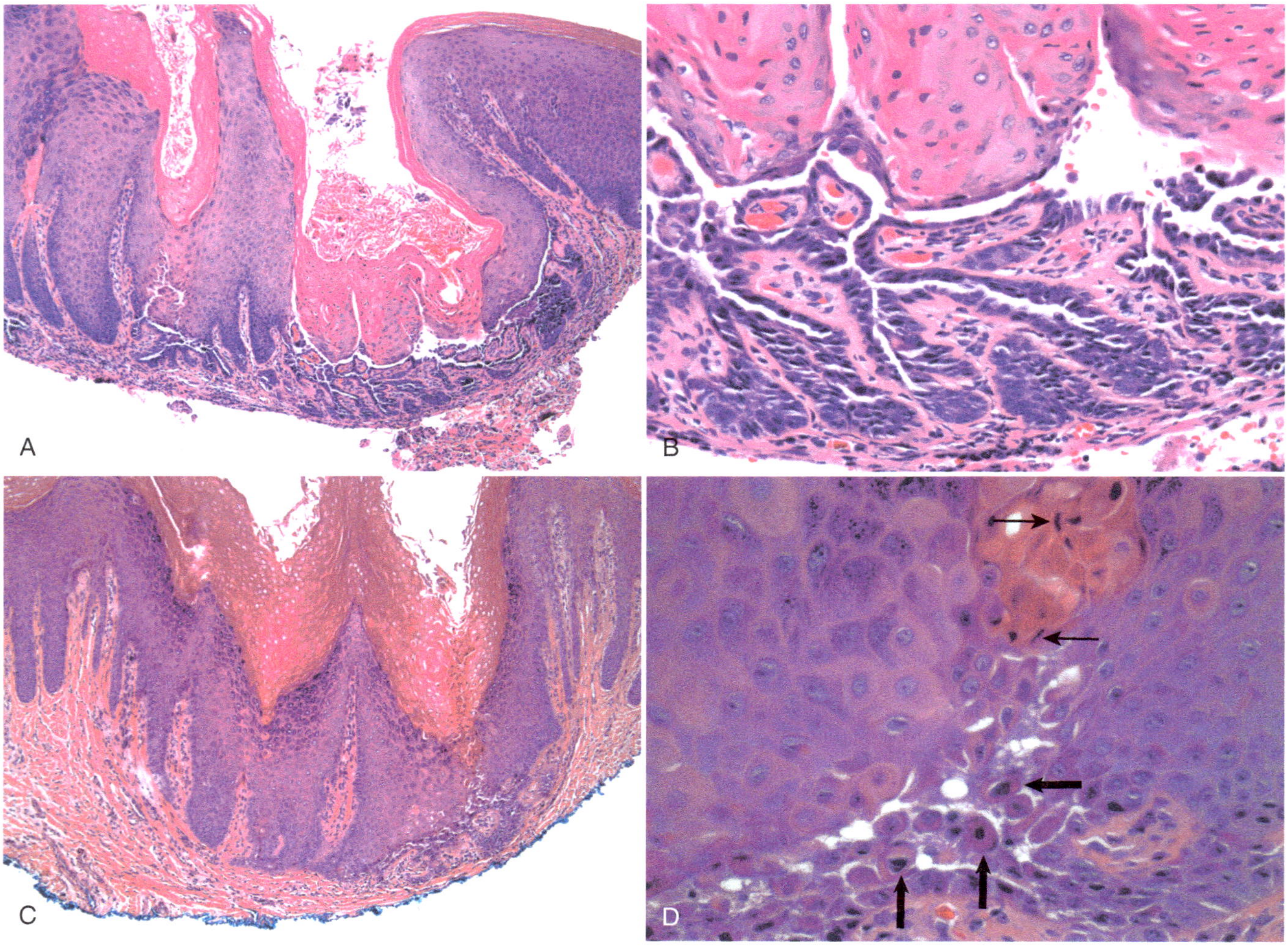

FIG 10.30 Warty dyskeratoma/focal acantholytic dyskeratosis. (A) Umbilicated lesion with parakeratosis, papillary acanthosis, and slender cords of cells at the crater base with suprabasal clefting. (B) Suprabasilar acantholysis with grains (eosinophilic cells with slender pyknotic nuclei). (C) Umbilicated parakeratosis and papillary acanthosis with subtle suprabasal acantholysis. (D) Corps ronds composed of large cell with eosinophilic cytoplasm and perinuclear halo *(thick arrows)* and slender grains with pyknotic nuclei *(thin arrows)*.

Epidermolytic Hyperkeratosis

Clinical Findings

- This is an uncommon finding in the oral cavity and appears as a white, warty area, usually on the gingiva.

Etiopathogenesis and Histopathologic Features

This is likely a reactive keratosis and may be seen as an incidental finding associated with other mucosal pathology.

- Hyperkeratosis and papillomatosis are present; superficial keratinocytes contain large keratohyaline granules and exhibit clear cytoplasm with eosinophilic globules; there is slight acanthosis with tapered rete ridges (Fig. 10.31).

Differential Diagnosis

- Benign alveolar ridge keratosis exhibits hyperkeratosis and wedge-shaped hypergranulosis with small keratohyaline granules.

Management and Prognosis

- Excision is curative.

REFERENCES

Brodsky G. Focal acantholytic dyskeratosis and epidermolytic hyperkeratosis of the oral mucosa adjacent to squamous cell carcinoma. *Oral Surg Oral Med Oral Pathol.* 1985;59:388-393.

Goette DK, Lapins NA. Epidermolytic hyperkeratosis as an incidental finding in normal oral mucosa. Report of two cases. *J Am Acad Dermatol.* 1984;10:246-249.

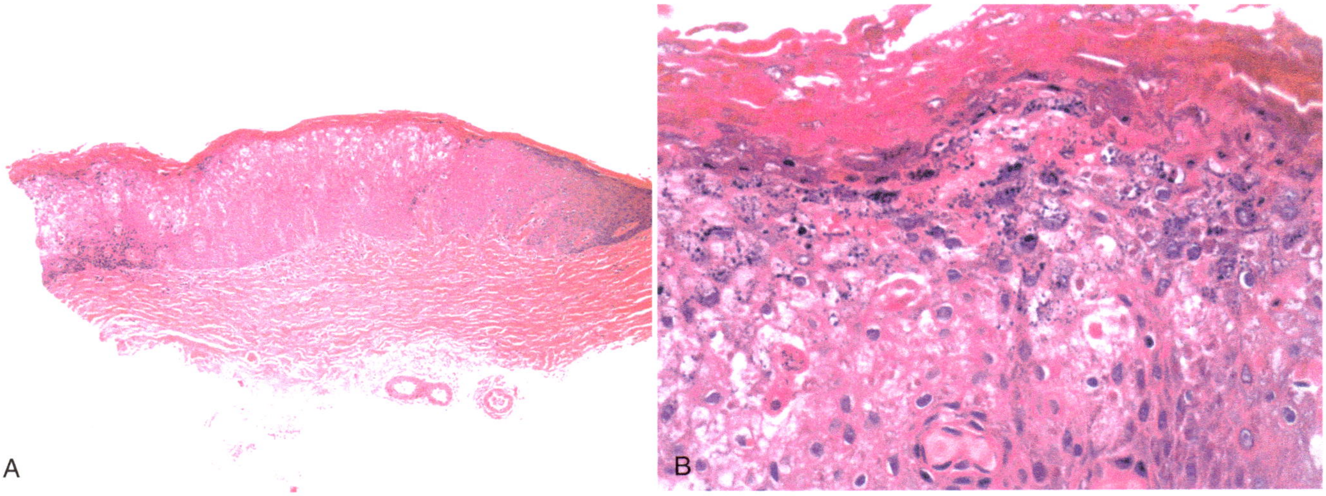

FIG 10.31 Epidermolytic hyperkeratosis. (A) Hyperkeratosis with clear cells and dyskeratotic cells in the upper half of the epithelium. (B) Hyperkeratosis, coarse keratohyaline granules, cytoplasmic clearing, and eosinophilic globules.

11 LEUKOPLAKIA, ERYTHROPLAKIA, ORAL DYSPLASIA, AND SQUAMOUS CELL CARCINOMA

CHAPTER CONTENTS

LEUKOPLAKIA, ERYTHROPLAKIA, AND DYSPLASIA

The term *oral dysplasia* is synonymous with *intraepithelial neoplasia* as used in the cervix. However, the terms *squamous intraepithelial neoplasia* and *oral intraepithelial neoplasia* are not universally accepted. The term *epithelial atypia* is sometimes used interchangeably with *epithelial dysplasia* and this may cause confusion. Reactive epithelial atypia should be reported as such, and epithelial atypia that is not within the spectrum of reactive change should be reported as either epithelial dysplasia, or that it is uncertain whether the atypia represents reactive change or dysplasia, understanding that it is sometimes extremely difficult to differentiate between the two. Reviewing clinical images is helpful in such instances.

According to the World Health Organization, leukoplakia is "a predominantly white plaque of questionable risk having excluded other known diseases or disorders that carry no increased risk for cancer." As such, it is not any white plaque but one that does not conform clinically or histopathologically to a defined disease (eg, primary candidiasis or lichen planus), cannot be attributed to reactive, frictional, or traumatic causes, and is highly associated with dysplasia and the development of cancer. It is a clinical term of exclusion and such lesions must always be biopsied. Leukoplakia is the most common precursor of invasive carcinoma.

Clinical Findings

- All forms of leukoplakia and erythroplakia are more often seen in older individuals.
- All lesions should be palpated to evaluate for firmness or induration, which may indicate the presence of an invasive carcinoma; the sites with the highest incidence of development of squamous cell carcinoma are the ventral tongue, floor of mouth, buccal mucosa, and gingiva; although the soft palate is an uncommon site for leukoplakia, it has a high prevalence of dysplasia or carcinoma when it does occur.

LOCALIZED LEUKOPLAKIA

Recent data show that of all leukoplakias, approximately 43% to 47% represent dysplasia, carcinoma-in-situ, or invasive carcinoma at the time of biopsy; the other 53% to 57% represent a keratosis of unknown significance; this higher prevalence of dysplasia (compared with 9% to 20% in older studies) is probably related to frictional and other reactive keratoses being included in older studies (Fig. 11.1).

Localized leukoplakia (at a single site) is more common in men, especially when it occurs on the ventral tongue and floor of mouth, and is strongly associated with smoking; two main clinical variants are identified:

- *Homogeneous leukoplakia* is a uniform white plaque, at least partially well-demarcated, with or without fissuring (Fig. 11.2A–B); these have a somewhat lower association with the development of dysplasia and invasive carcinoma. If not overtly dysplastic, lesions exhibit hyperkeratosis or parakeratosis, acanthosis, or atrophy, and when followed over time, up to 16% develop dysplasia or carcinoma.
- *Nonhomogeneous leukoplakia:* these plaques have a warty, rough, and verrucous character (verrucous leukoplakia), nodular areas, or red areas (erythroleukoplakia or speckled leukoplakia); nonhomogeneous leukoplakia has a higher frequency of developing into dysplasia or carcinoma; erythroleukoplakia (or speckled leukoplakia) is more likely to be misdiagnosed clinically as lichen planus because of its red and white character, although typical white reticulations are not present and it is often unilateral, with demarcation best seen around the white/keratotic areas of the lesion (see Figs. 11.2C–D and 11.3).
- *Verrucous leukoplakia* occurs frequently on the marginal gingiva or alveolar ridge mucosa (see Fig. 11.2E).

PROLIFERATIVE LEUKOPLAKIA

Proliferative leukoplakia is more common in women and is not strongly associated with smoking; it is persistent, recurs after removal, and progresses and spreads over decades to involve large areas of the mucosa. Over time, 60% to 100% of proliferative leukoplakias develop carcinoma. A hallmark of this condition is that repeated biopsies of early lesions show verrucous architecture with little to no evidence of cytologic dysplasia.

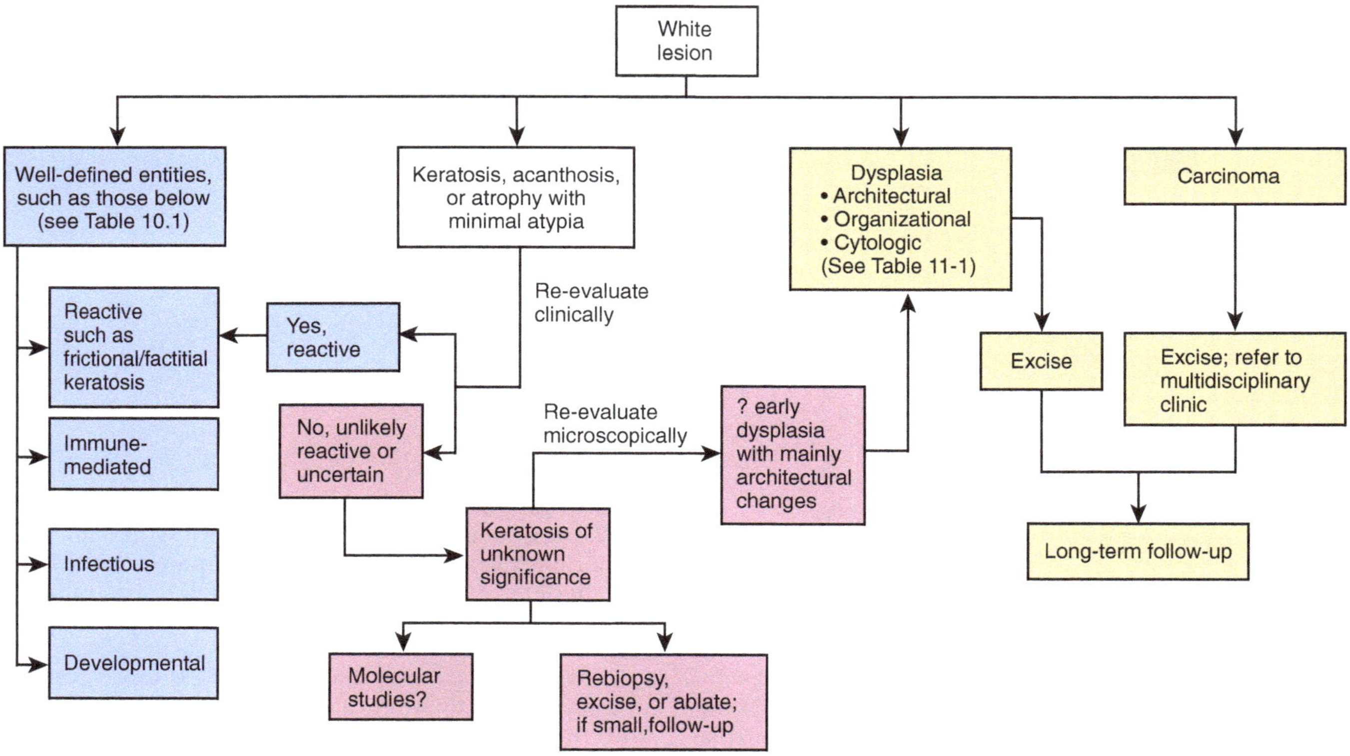

FIG 11.1 Algorithm for diagnosis of keratotic lesions

- Lesions are multifocal or a lesion may extensively affect a single site (such as the tongue dorsum) or contiguous sites (Fig. 11.4); the gingiva is frequently involved.
- Most cases are nonhomogeneous with fissuring and verrucous/nodular areas, and referred to as *proliferative verrucous leukoplakia* and although some areas may be well demarcated, others may not be; infrequently, erythroplakic areas may be present (Fig. 11.5).
- Proliferative erythroleukoplakia may resemble lichen planus because of bilaterality and multifocality, but reticulations are usually not seen, although trabecular keratotic bands may be encountered; demarcation and fissuring is almost always present around the keratotic areas.

ERYTHROPLAKIA

Of all erythroplakias, over 90% represent dysplasia, carcinoma-in-situ, or invasive carcinoma at the time of biopsy.

- Erythroplakia presents as a velvety, granular red plaque that is usually painless and may be indurated; it is much less common than leukoplakia (Fig. 11.6).

Etiopathogenesis and Histopathologic Features

Risk factors for localized leukoplakia (excluding the lip where lesions are usually related to actinic damage) are the same as for squamous cell carcinoma. These include cigarette smoking, excessive alcohol consumption, areca nut habit, history of cancer and cancer therapy, history of autoimmune disorder or prolonged immunosuppression, family history of cancer, human papillomavirus and age; risk factors for proliferative leukoplakia are less well defined.

Similar to precancerous lesions in other parts of the body that develop carcinoma over time, oral epithelial dysplasia is a result of genetic aberrations, with cumulative genetic and/or epigenetic events, and likely development of driver gene mutations leading to increasing severity of dysplasia and finally carcinoma. Aneuploidy has been shown to correlate with development of invasive carcinoma. Loss of heterozygosity in multiple chromosomes is also associated with progression of dysplasia to invasive carcinoma; these involve chromosomes 3p, 4p, 4q, 8p, 9p, 11q, and 17p. Some verrucous hyperplasias exhibit loss of heterozygosity involving 3p, 4q, 9p, and 11q. Overexpression of c-*erb*B-3 protein correlates with increased proliferative cell nuclear antigen labeling index as lesions progress from verrucous hyperplasia to verrucous carcinoma. Stabilizing mutations of *TP53* that inhibit degradation of p53 protein result in over-expression of this protein in some oral dysplasias.

Conventional parameters for dysplasia are based on cytologic features best seen at high power and that also are recognizable on cytopathology preparations harvested using a cyto-brush or other equivalent tool. However, gross architectural features noted on low power and organizational disarray noted on intermediate power are also important, and these may occur in the absence of, or with only minimal cytologic evidence of dysplasia. Some of these features belong in more than one category; for example, basal cell hyperplasia is both a cytologic and organizational feature of dysplasia. No single criterion for the diagnosis of dysplasia is sufficient for the diagnosis,

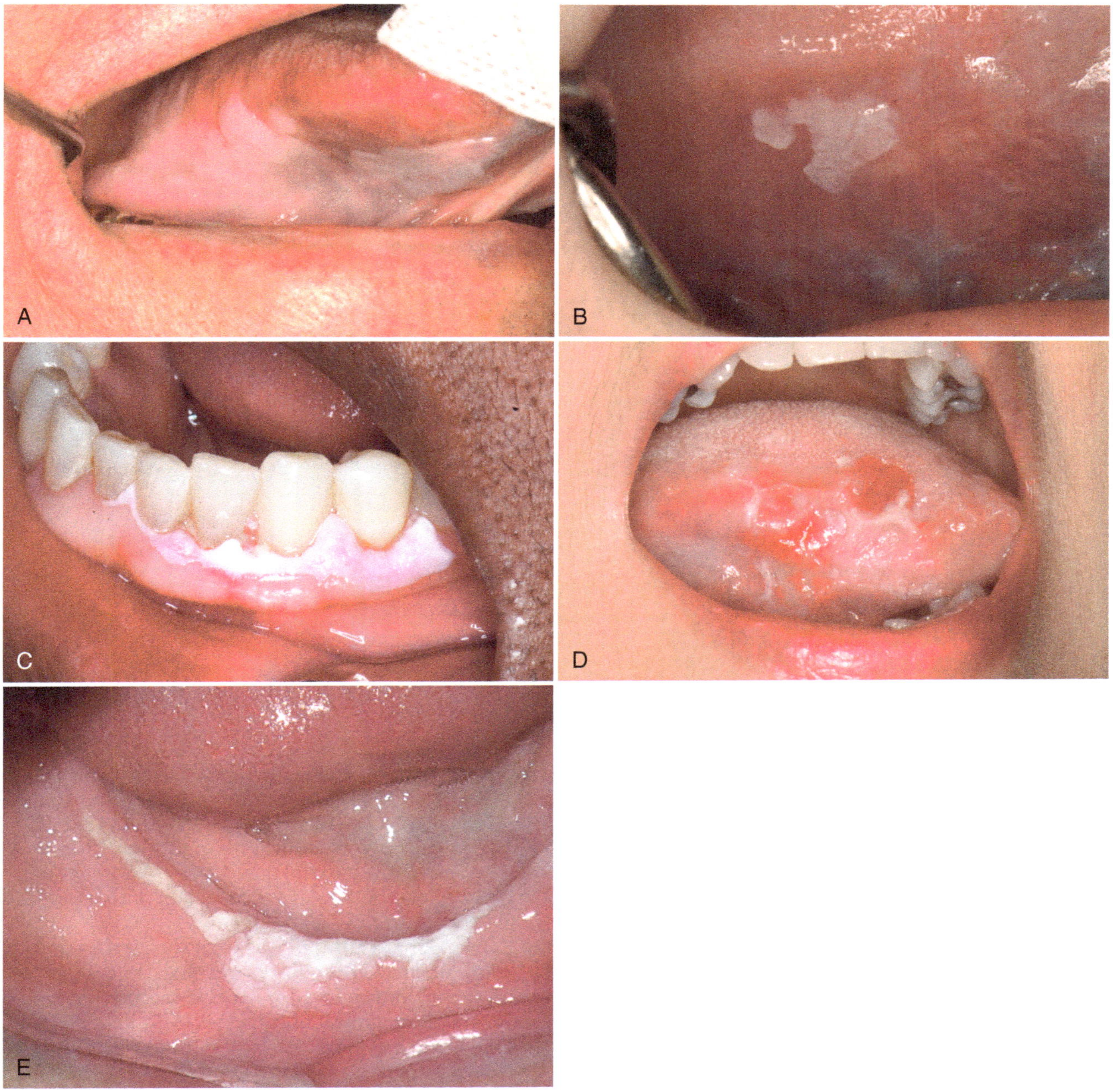

FIG 11.2 (A) Homogeneous leukoplakia: patient had been followed for years with multiple biopsies showing hyperkeratosis without dysplasia (keratosis of unknown significance), as the lesion gradually expanded to involve his entire right ventral tongue and part of the floor of mouth; note sharp demarcation. (B) Homogeneous leukoplakia: well-demarcated white plaque with slight fissuring; histologically, hyperkeratosis and acanthosis (keratosis of unknown significance). (C) Homogeneous leukoplakia, well-demarcated, of the mandibular gingiva; histologically dysplastic. (D) Erythroleukoplakia of the ventral tongue: histologically, a squamous cell carcinoma. (E) Verrucous leukoplakia of the mandibular alveolar ridge mucosa, well-demarcated, histologically dysplastic.

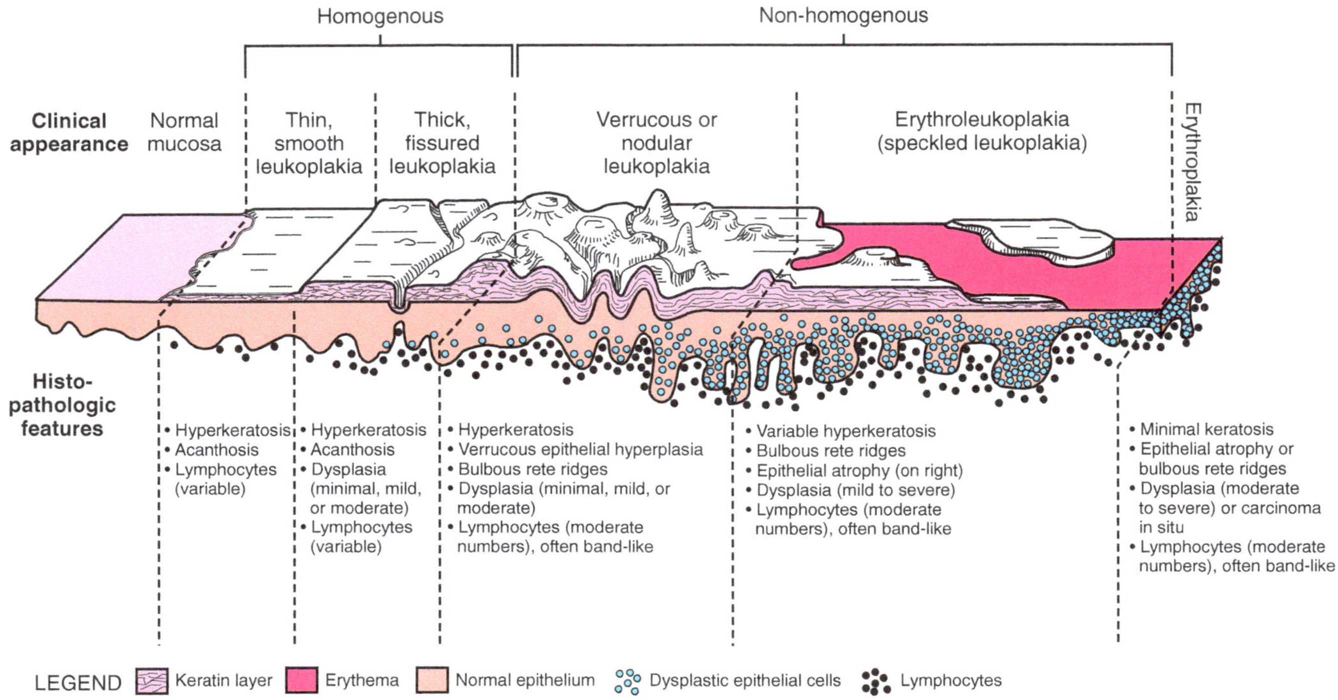

FIG 11.3 Representation of the clinical and corresponding histopathologic findings in leukoplakia. *(Modified from Bouquot JE, Gnepp DR. Laryngeal precancer: a review of the literature, commentary, and comparison with oral leukoplakia. Head Neck. 1991;13:488–497.)*

because many of the features of dysplasia may be seen as reactive atypia in inflamed epithelium, especially adjacent to ulcers. Correlation with clinical findings is of the utmost importance for accurate diagnosis when histopathologic features are equivocal for dysplasia. Cytologic features alone are insensitive for the diagnosis of oral dysplasia.

Finally, there is still no consensus as to how to best grade dysplasia; some use the traditional *mild*, *moderate* and *severe* grades depending on the thickness of the epithelium involved, whereas others use low grade and high grade. Each has its own merits and, in general, moderate and severe dysplasia (high grade dysplasia) show better inter-examiner reliability and consistency, and are generally associated with a higher incidence of, or shorter time to, development of carcinoma. However, neither system of grading dysplasia takes into account gross architectural features of dysplasia, such as verrucous hyperplasia, that are just as important.

ARCHITECTURAL EVIDENCE OF DYSPLASIA

Architectural features of dysplasia that occur in the absence of, or with minimal evidence of cytologic dysplasia are often observed in both localized verrucous leukoplakia and proliferative leukoplakia (Table 11.1). They may also occur with clear evidence of cytologic dysplasia.

- Bulky epithelial proliferation, especially if endophytic and without or with minimal leukocyte exocytosis or spongiosis (Figs. 11.7 and 11.8); many of these are thick plaques or masses clinically.
- Papillary or verrucous hyperplasia, broad-based, in an either exophytic and/or endophytic configuration and often also bulky (Figs. 11.9–11.12); this is characteristic for localized verrucous leukoplakia and for proliferative verrucous leukoplakia.
- Festooned, bulbous or drop-shaped rete ridges (Fig. 11.13).
- Sharp demarcation of the keratotic area from the adjacent normal epithelium and "skip" areas of normal mucosa sandwiched by hyperkeratotic, parakeratotic, or dysplastic epithelium (Figs. 11.14 and 11.15).
- Marked hyperkeratosis with epithelial atrophy (usually sharply demarcated) in the absence of inflammation not representing a specific disease entity (such as erosive or treated lichen planus) should be viewed with suspicion; not all dysplasias exhibit epithelial hyperplasia and the term *keratosis of unknown significance* has been used to refer to such lesions (Fig. 11.16).

ORGANIZATIONAL EVIDENCE OF DYSPLASIA

These changes show the abnormal relationship of dysplastic cells to each other within the epithelium.

- Dyscohesion, loss of normal upward maturation as a result of basal cell hyperplasia and as such, loss of normal stratification and polarization of spinous cells, crowding of basal cells, and increased mitotic activity beyond the basal and immediate parabasal cell layers (Table 11.1).

Text continued on p. 248

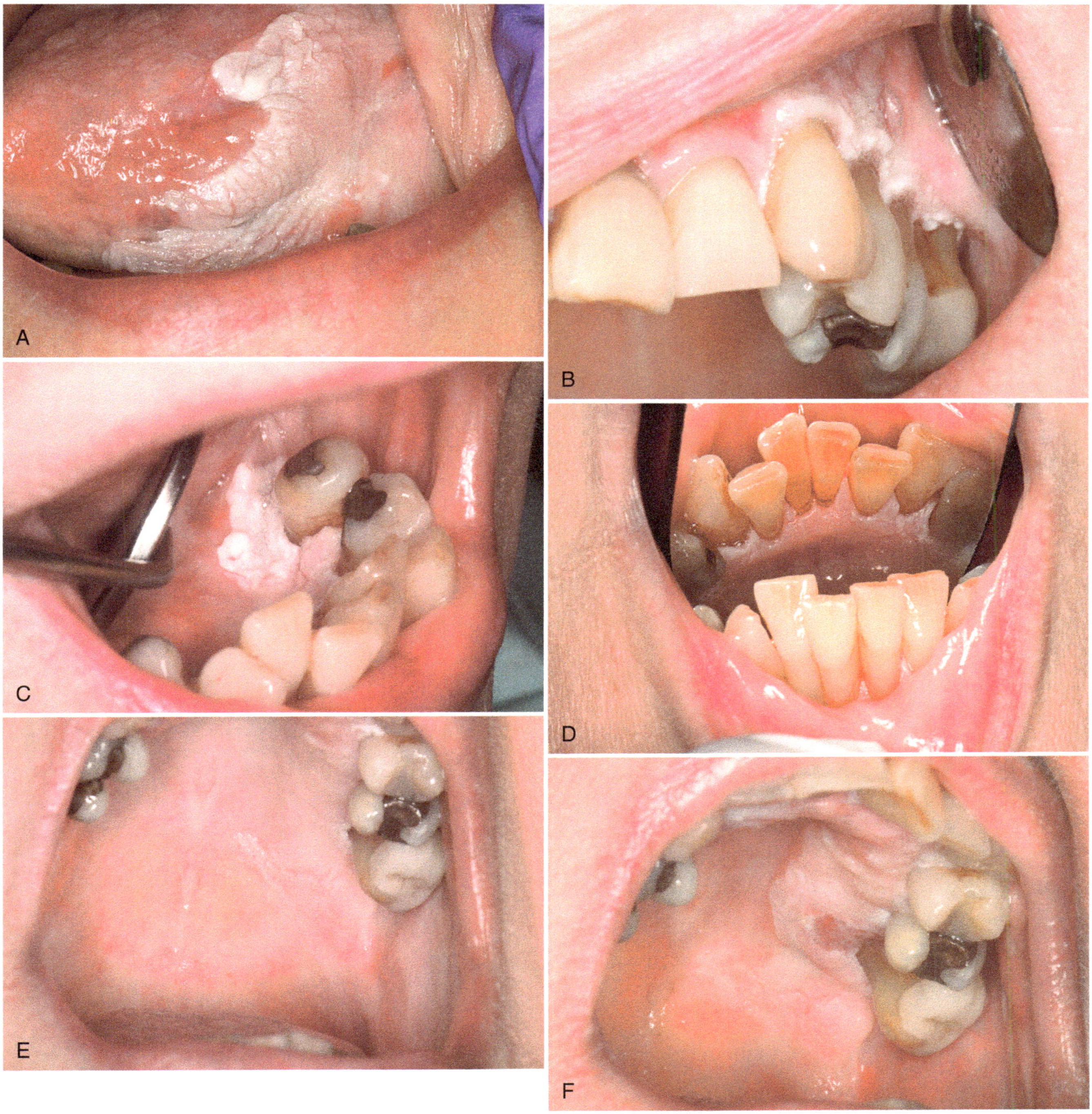

FIG 11.4 Proliferative leukoplakia, from one patient. (A) Ventral and dorsal tongue have fissured leukoplakia. (B) Maxillary gingiva has poorly demarcated keratosis. (C) Left mandibular lingual mucosa with demarcated leukoplakia. (D) Anterior lingual gingiva with poorly demarcated leukoplakia. (E) Hard palatal mucosa is only subtly keratotic. (F) Squamous cell carcinoma developed within this subtle leukoplakia.

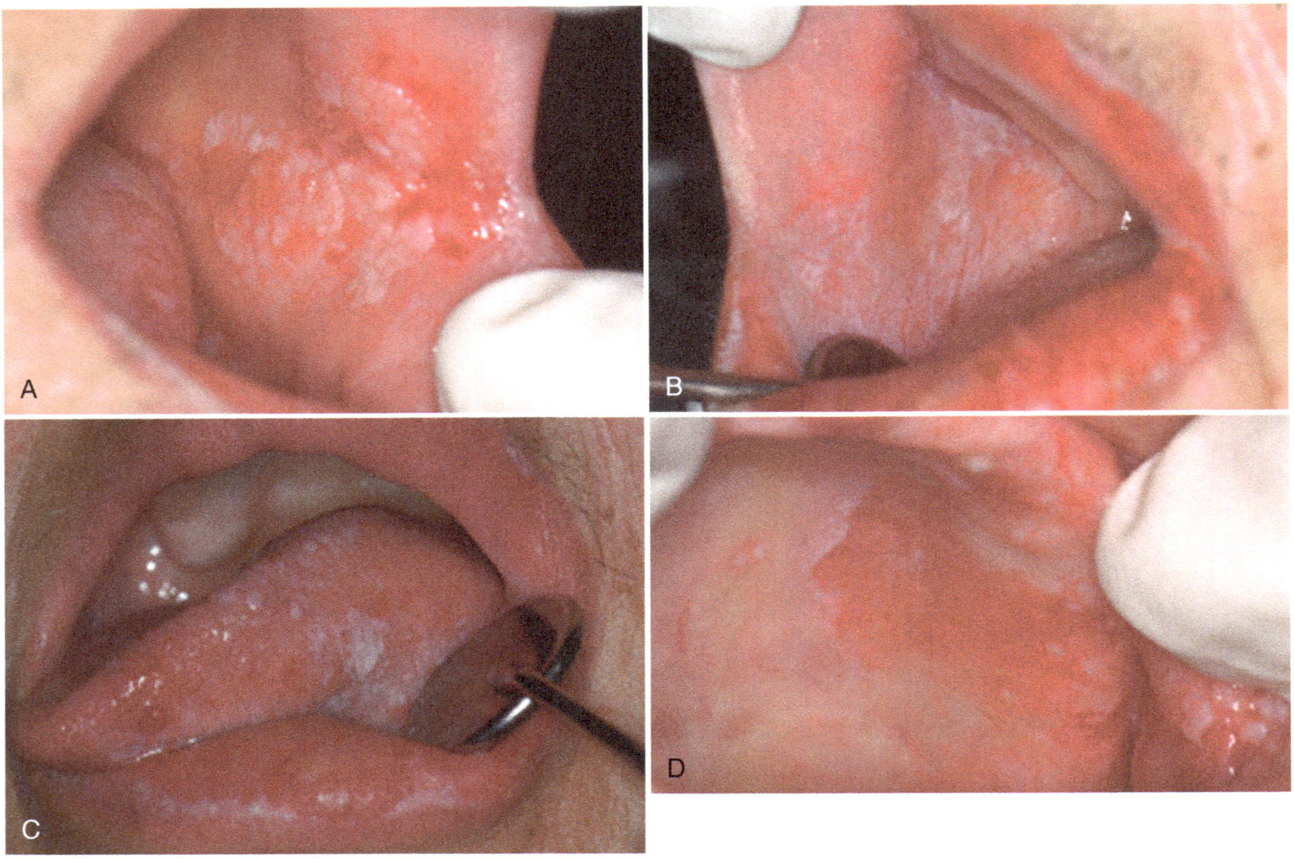

FIG 11.5 Proliferative erythroleukoplakia from one patient. (A) Red and white plaque on the left buccal mucosa; fissured white plaques are focally demarcated. (B) Red and white fissured plaque on the right buccal mucosa, not well demarcated. (C) Red and white fissured plaques on the ventral tongue and lower lip mucosa, not well demarcated. (D) Red and white plaques of the palatal mucosa. Patient developed invasive squamous cell carcinoma.

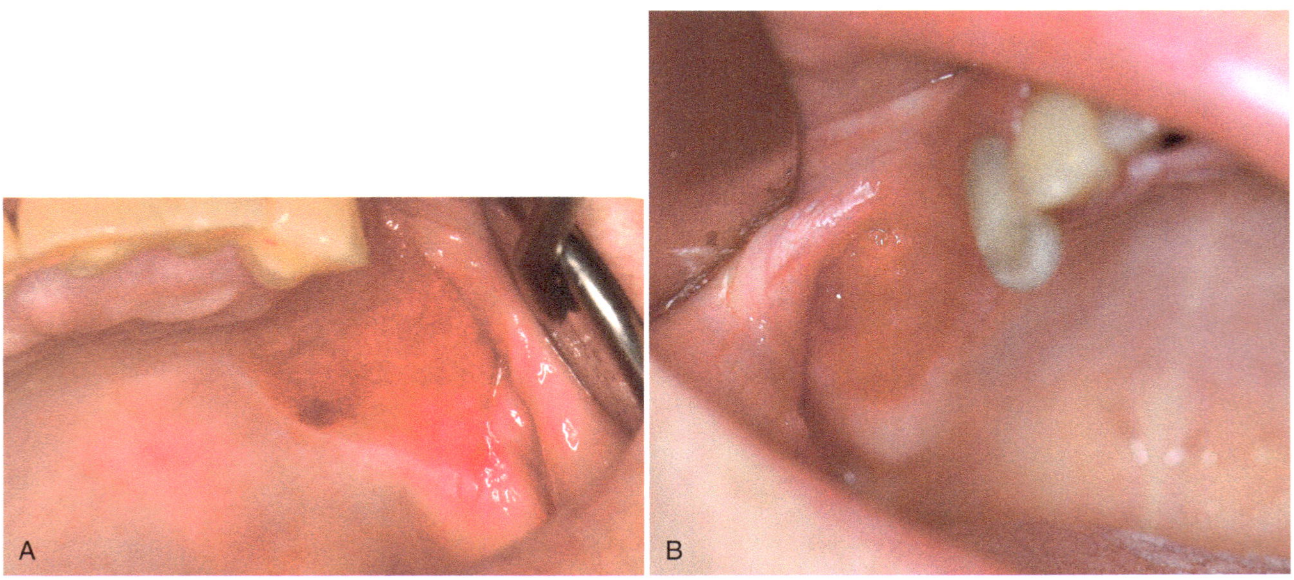

FIG 11.6 (A) Erythroplakia of the left palatal mucosa; histologically, carcinoma-in-situ. (B) Erythroplakia of the right maxillary alveolar ridge mucosa, histologically invasive carcinoma. *(B, Courtesy Dr. Carmine Colarusso, private practice, Gardner, Mass.)*

TABLE 11.1 Histopathologic Features of Dysplasia

Architectural features (best seen at low power)	• Bulky and/or endophytic proliferation • Verrucous or papillary epithelial proliferation • Bulbous or drop-shaped rete ridges • Sharply demarcated keratinization, usually multifocal with "skip" areas • Hyperkeratosis with atrophy in the absence of inflammation, usually sharply demarcated
Organizational features (best seen at intermediate power)	• Dyscohesion[a] • Basal cell hyperplasia leading to loss of normal stratification and polarity • Crowding of basal cells • Mitoses (even if normal-appearing) beyond the suprabasal keratinocytes
Cytologic features (those noted on exfoliative cytology and best seen at high power)	• Basal cell hyperplasia • Increased nuclear/cytoplasmic ratio • Variation in cell shape and size • Variation in nuclear shape and size • Coarse chromatin and prominent and/or multiple nucleoli • Hyperchromasia • Abnormal mitotic figures • Dyskeratosis and/or keratin pearl formation • Glassy appearance of cytoplasm • Multinucleate epithelial cells with increased nuclear-to-cytoplasmic ratio

[a]Dyscohesion is separation of epithelial cells unassociated with inflammation and as such is not spongiosis where cells show intercellular inflammation and edema.

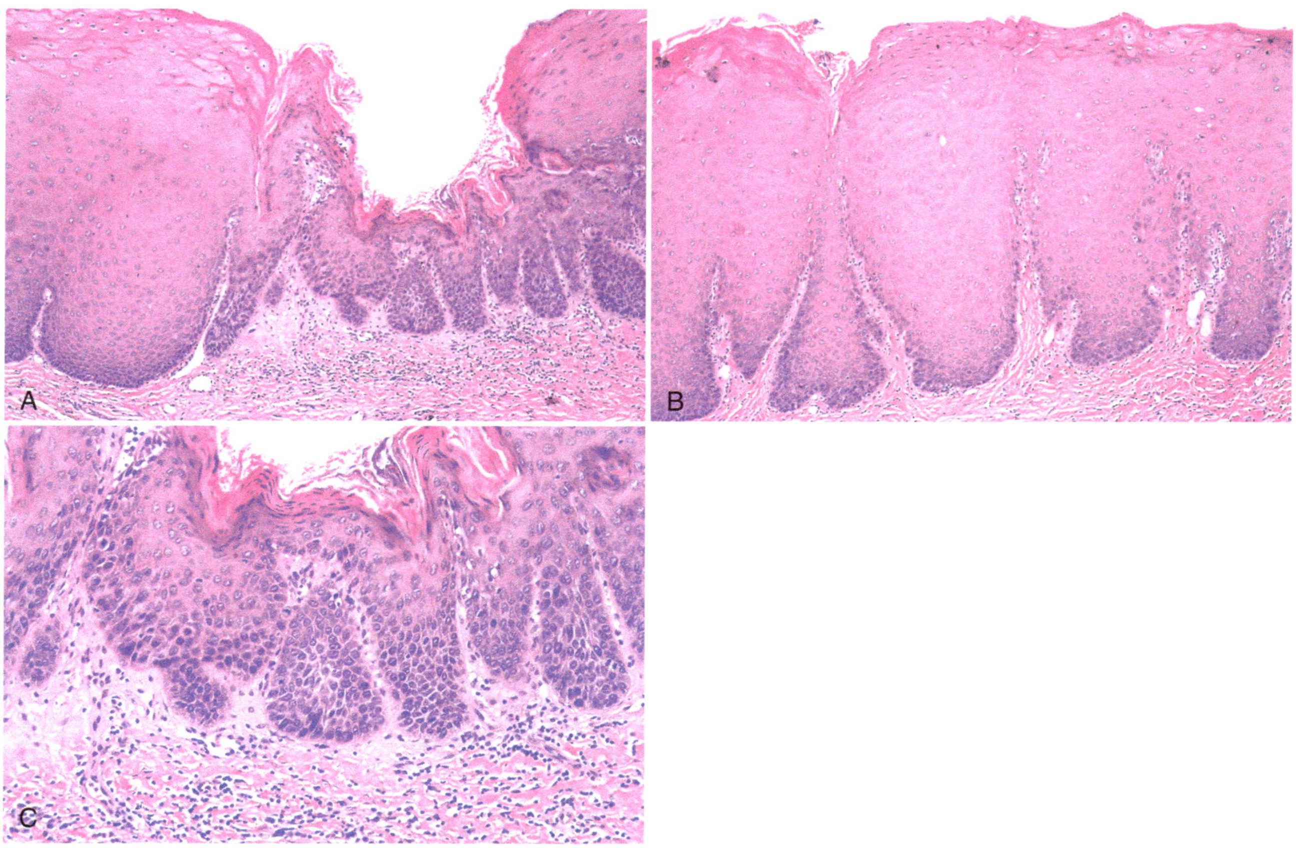

FIG 11.7 Bulky epithelial proliferation and cytologic dysplasia (floor of mouth). (A) Bulky epithelial proliferation with a central area of cytologic dysplasia. (B) Bulky epithelial proliferation with mild cytologic atypia, not reactive in nature. (C) Moderate epithelial dysplasia.

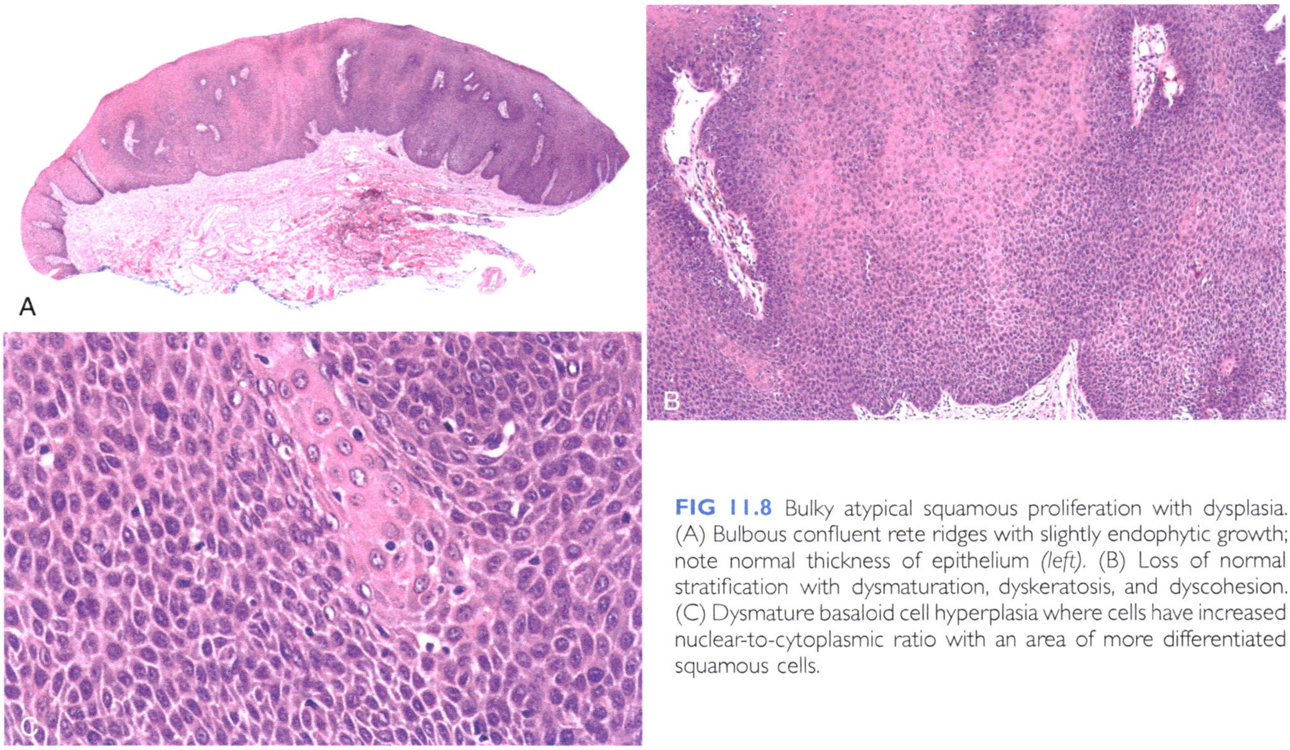

FIG 11.8 Bulky atypical squamous proliferation with dysplasia. (A) Bulbous confluent rete ridges with slightly endophytic growth; note normal thickness of epithelium *(left)*. (B) Loss of normal stratification with dysmaturation, dyskeratosis, and dyscohesion. (C) Dysmature basaloid cell hyperplasia where cells have increased nuclear-to-cytoplasmic ratio with an area of more differentiated squamous cells.

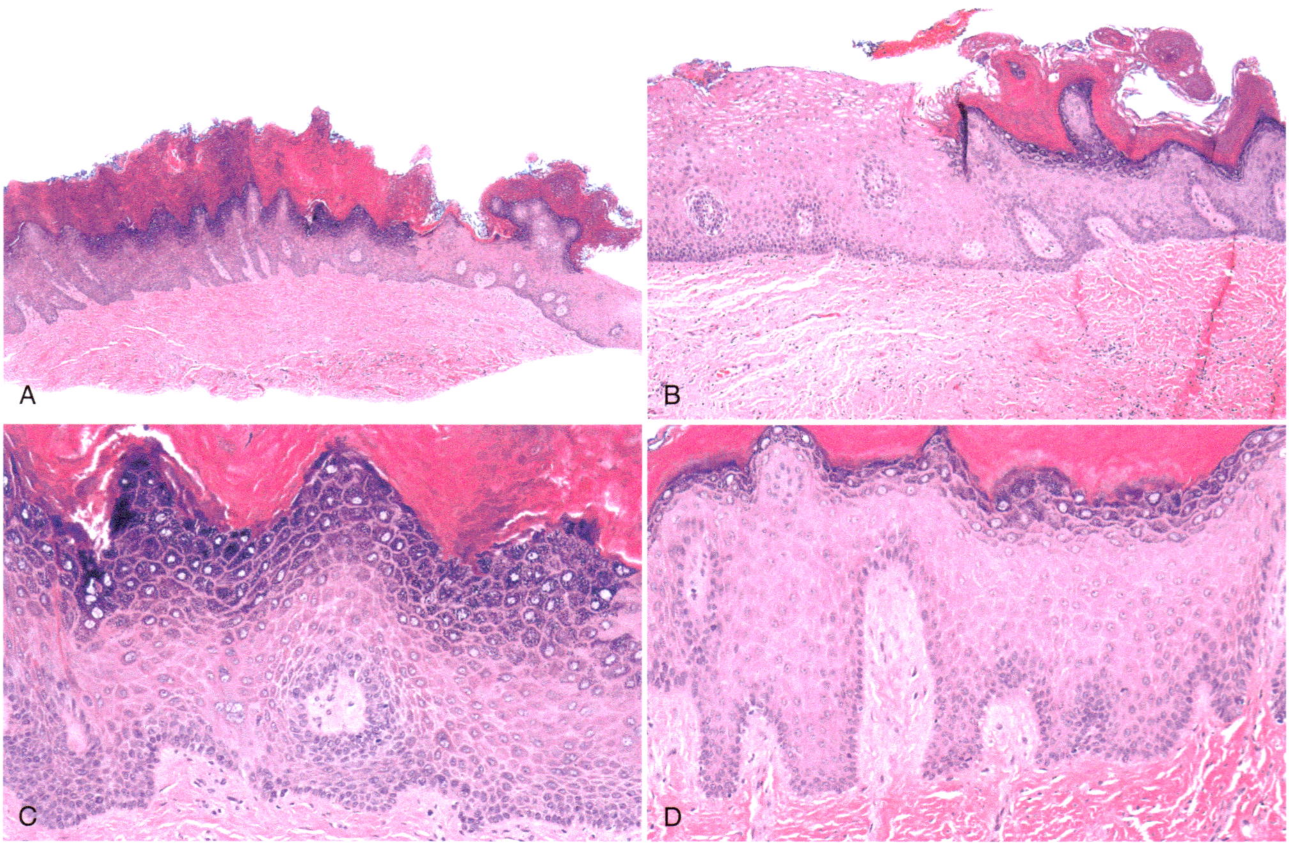

FIG 11.9 Verrucous hyperplasia with minimal to no dysplasia. (A) Hyperkeratosis, hypergranulosis, and verrucous epithelial proliferation showing sharp demarcation from surrounding normal epithelium *(right)*; note early, thinly keratotic area sandwiched by markedly hyperkeratotic areas. (B) Abrupt keratinization corresponding to sharp demarcation clinically. (C) Mild epithelial dysplasia. (D) A different site with verrucous architecture but no dysplasia or dysmaturation.

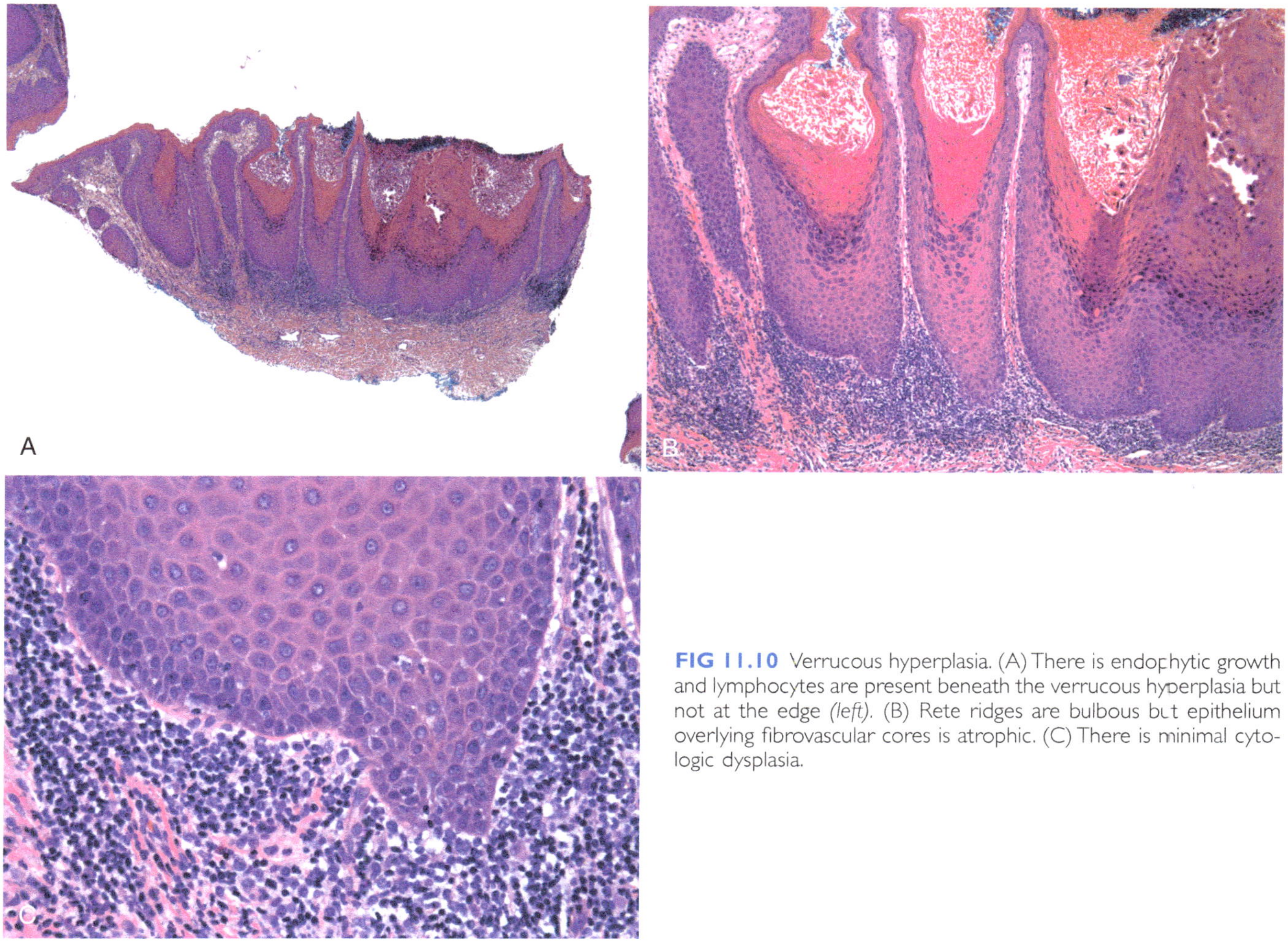

FIG 11.10 Verrucous hyperplasia. (A) There is endophytic growth and lymphocytes are present beneath the verrucous hyperplasia but not at the edge *(left)*. (B) Rete ridges are bulbous but epithelium overlying fibrovascular cores is atrophic. (C) There is minimal cytologic dysplasia.

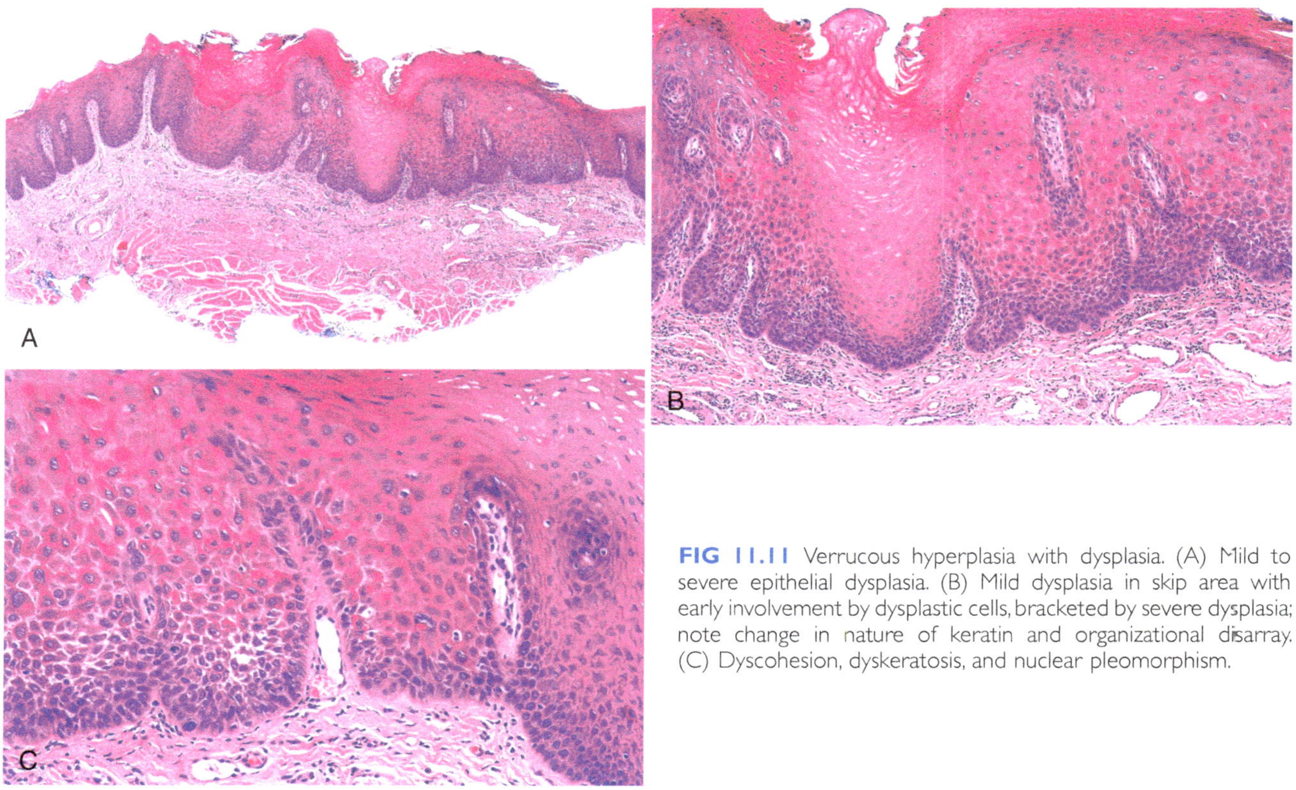

FIG 11.11 Verrucous hyperplasia with dysplasia. (A) Mild to severe epithelial dysplasia. (B) Mild dysplasia in skip area with early involvement by dysplastic cells, bracketed by severe dysplasia; note change in nature of keratin and organizational disarray. (C) Dyscohesion, dyskeratosis, and nuclear pleomorphism.

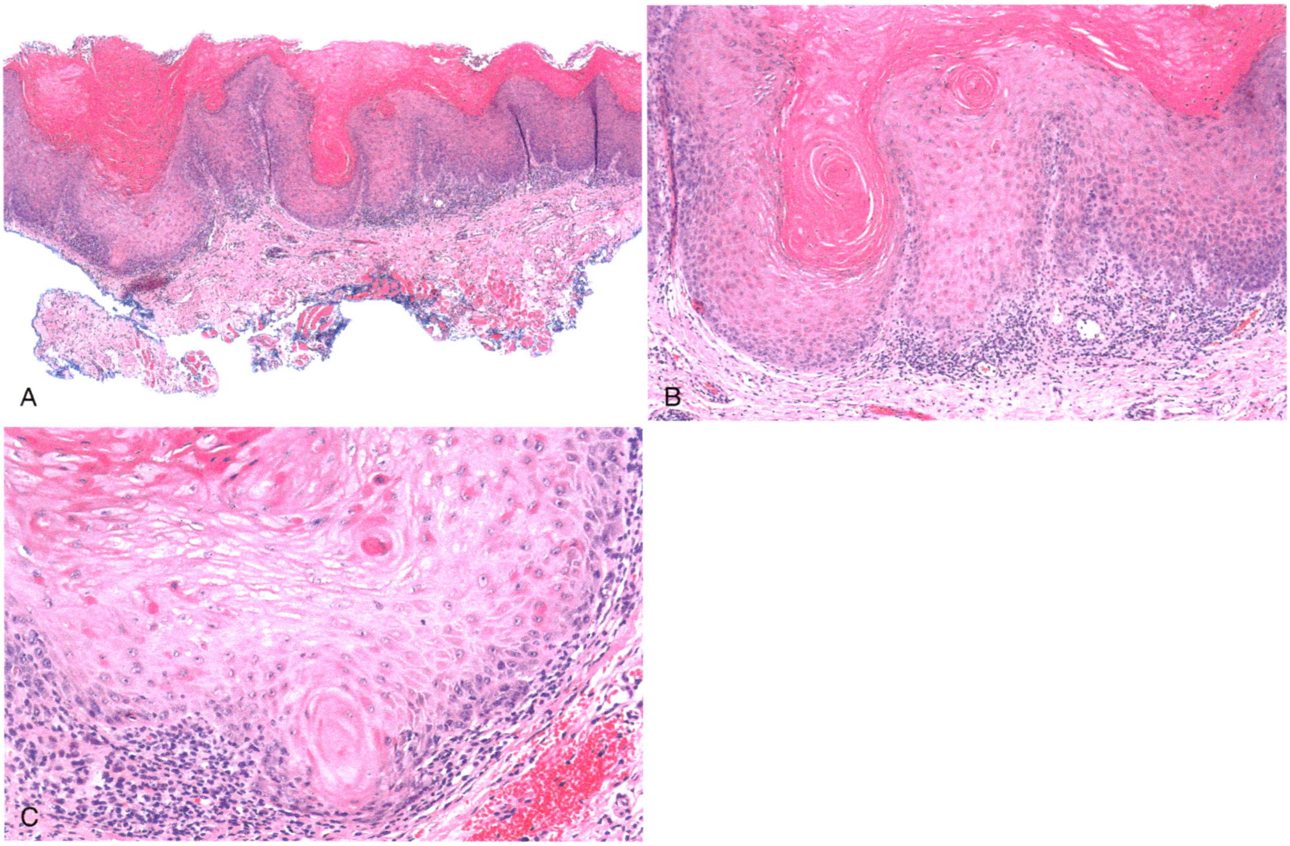

FIG 11.12 Verrucous hyperplasia with dysplasia. (A) Marked parakeratosis with papillary/verrucous epithelial hyperplasia and severe dysplasia with lymphocytic band at interface. (B) Severe dysplasia with dyskeratosis and lymphocytic band. (C) Keratin pearl at base of epithelium, dyskeratosis, and cells with glassy cytoplasm.

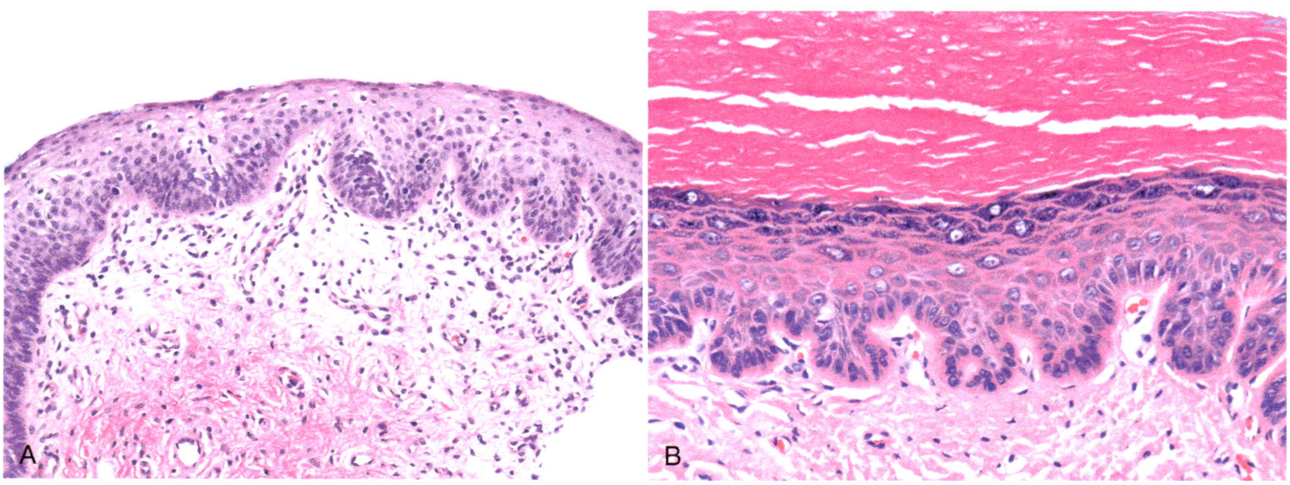

FIG 11.13 Festooned and drop-shaped rete ridges in dysplasia. (A) Festooned rete ridges with basal cell hyperplasia: mild to focally moderate dysplasia. (B) Drop-shaped rete ridges with basal cell hyperplasia and nuclear crowding involving half the thickness of the epithelium: moderate dysplasia.

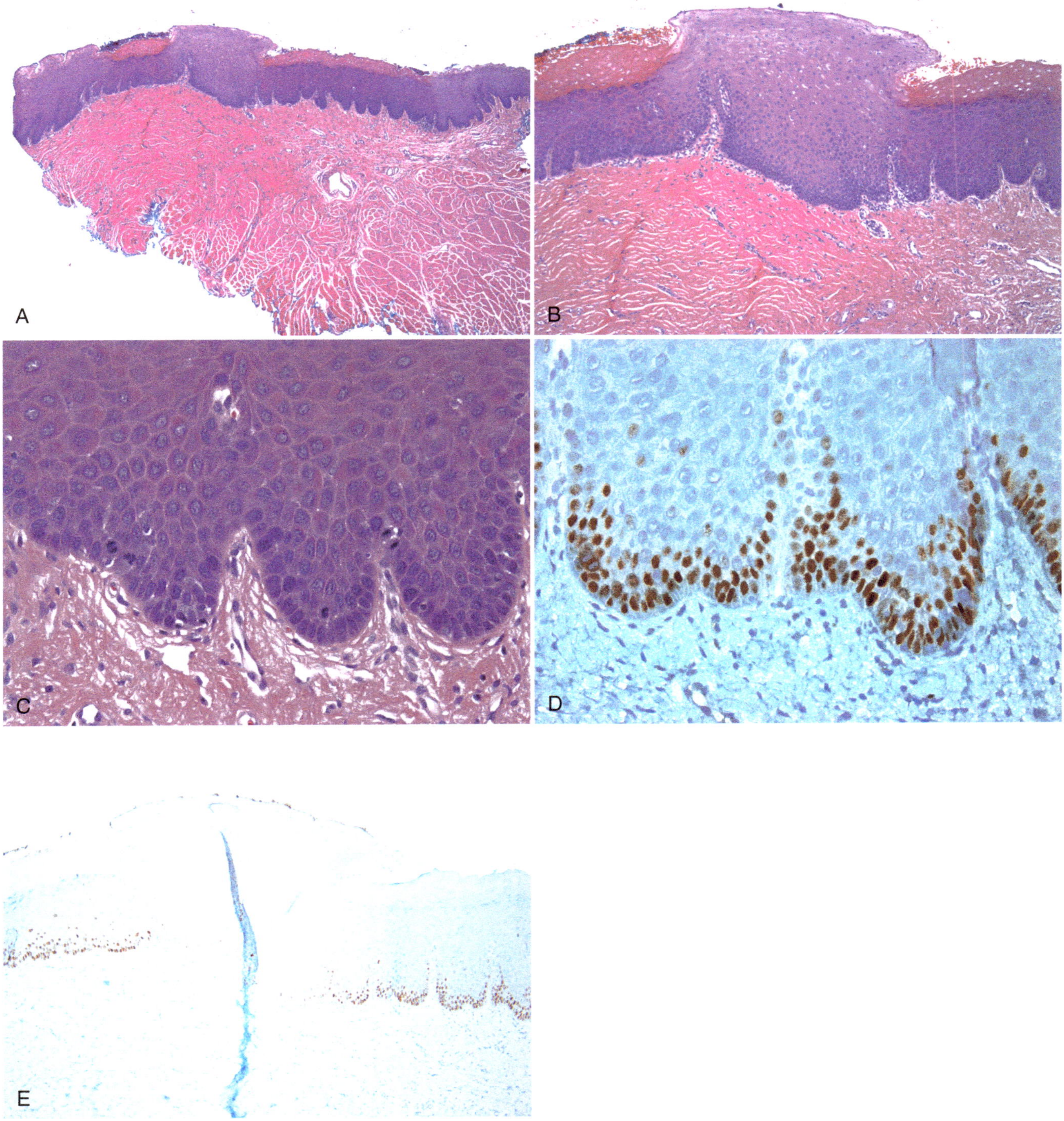

FIG 11.14 Hyperkeratosis with mild dysplasia. (A) Compact hyperkeratosis and several abrupt transitions to normal mucosa or skip lesions. (B) Transition from keratotic dysplasia to nonkeratotic area. (C) Mild dysplasia with basal cell hyperplasia and festooned rete ridges. (D) p53 is strongly positive within nuclei in a continuous band within the basal and suprabasal cells of the majority of rete ridges. (E) p53 is present only in scattered basal cell nuclei in the skip area.

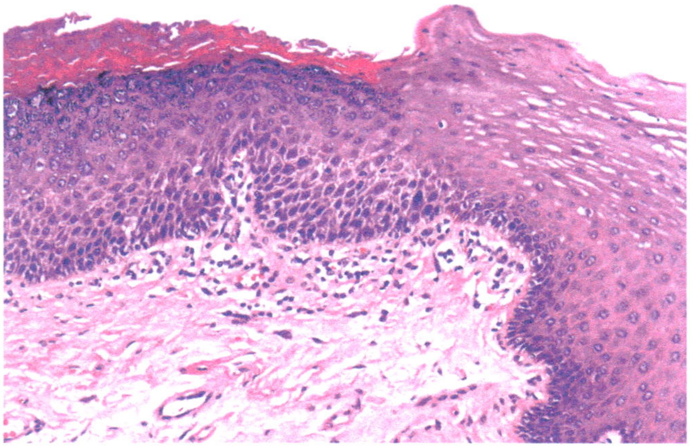

FIG 11.15 Hyperkeratosis with moderate epithelial dysplasia involving half the epithelium with abrupt transition between keratotic dysplasia with dyscohesive and pleomorphic cells and normal mucosa, corresponding to sharply demarcated clinical lesion.

CYTOLOGIC EVIDENCE OF DYSPLASIA

- Cytologic features are similar to those at other mucosal sites and are readily noted on exfoliative cytology (see Table 11.1); reactive epithelial atypia from inflammation may show the same features to a lesser degree.
- *Mild* dysplasia: less than one-third of the thickness of the epithelium is involved by dysplasia (Fig. 11.17).
- *Moderate* dysplasia: greater than one-third and less than two-thirds of the thickness of the epithelium is involved by dysplasia (Fig. 11.18).
- *Severe* dysplasia: greater than two-thirds but less than the full thickness of the epithelium is involved by dysplasia (Figs. 11.19 and 11.20).
- *Carcinoma-in-situ*: full thickness involvement of the epithelium is involved by dysplasia (Figs. 11.21 and 11.22).
- p53 nuclear positivity is often present in a fairly continuous and multilayered band at the lower half of rete ridges in dysplastic cells (see Fig. 11.14D–E).
- Low-grade dysplasia exhibits cells with fewer cytologic features of dysplasia while high grade dysplasia exhibits cells with a larger number of cytologic features of dysplasia regardless of the thickness of the epithelium, although from a practical perspective, the thicker the epithelium, the more features of dysplasia will be seen.

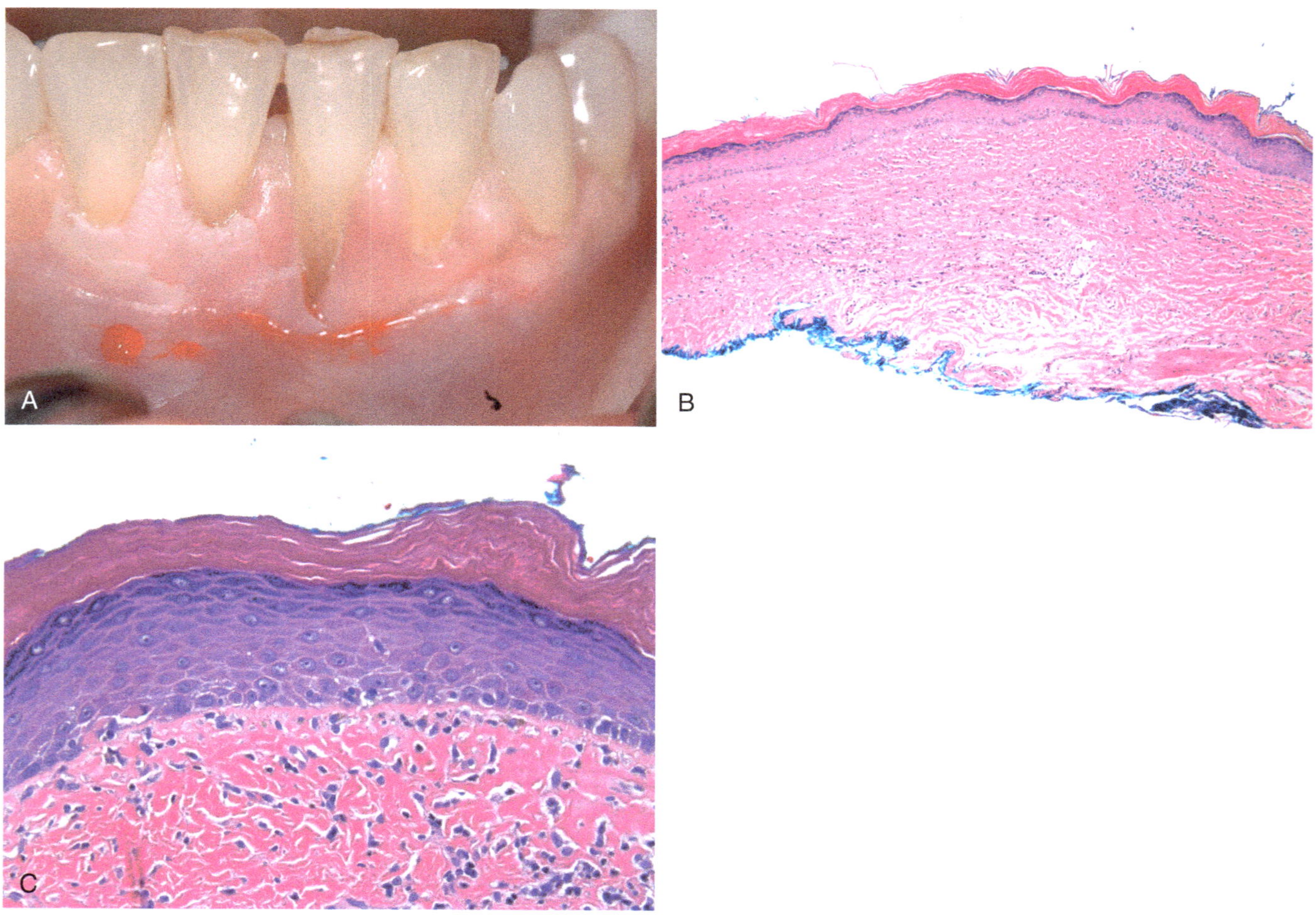

FIG 11.16 Keratosis of unknown significance from excision of an enlarging solitary gingival plaque. (A) Homogeneous, fissured gingival leukoplakia. (B) Marked hyperkeratosis and epithelial atrophy (from lesion in A). (C) Hyperkeratosis with no dysplasia.

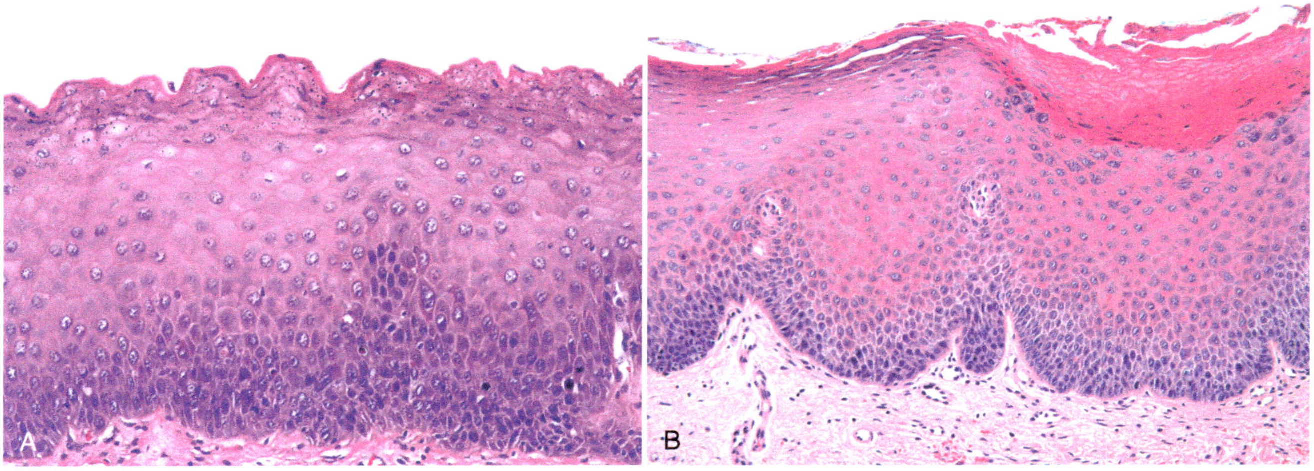

FIG 11.17 Mild epithelial dysplasia. (A) Parakeratosis, basal cell hyperplasia, and nuclear crowding involving less than one-third of the epithelium. (B) Parakeratosis, basal cell hyperplasia, mild pleomorphism, nuclear hyperchromasia, and festooned rete ridges involving less than one-third the thickness of the epithelium.

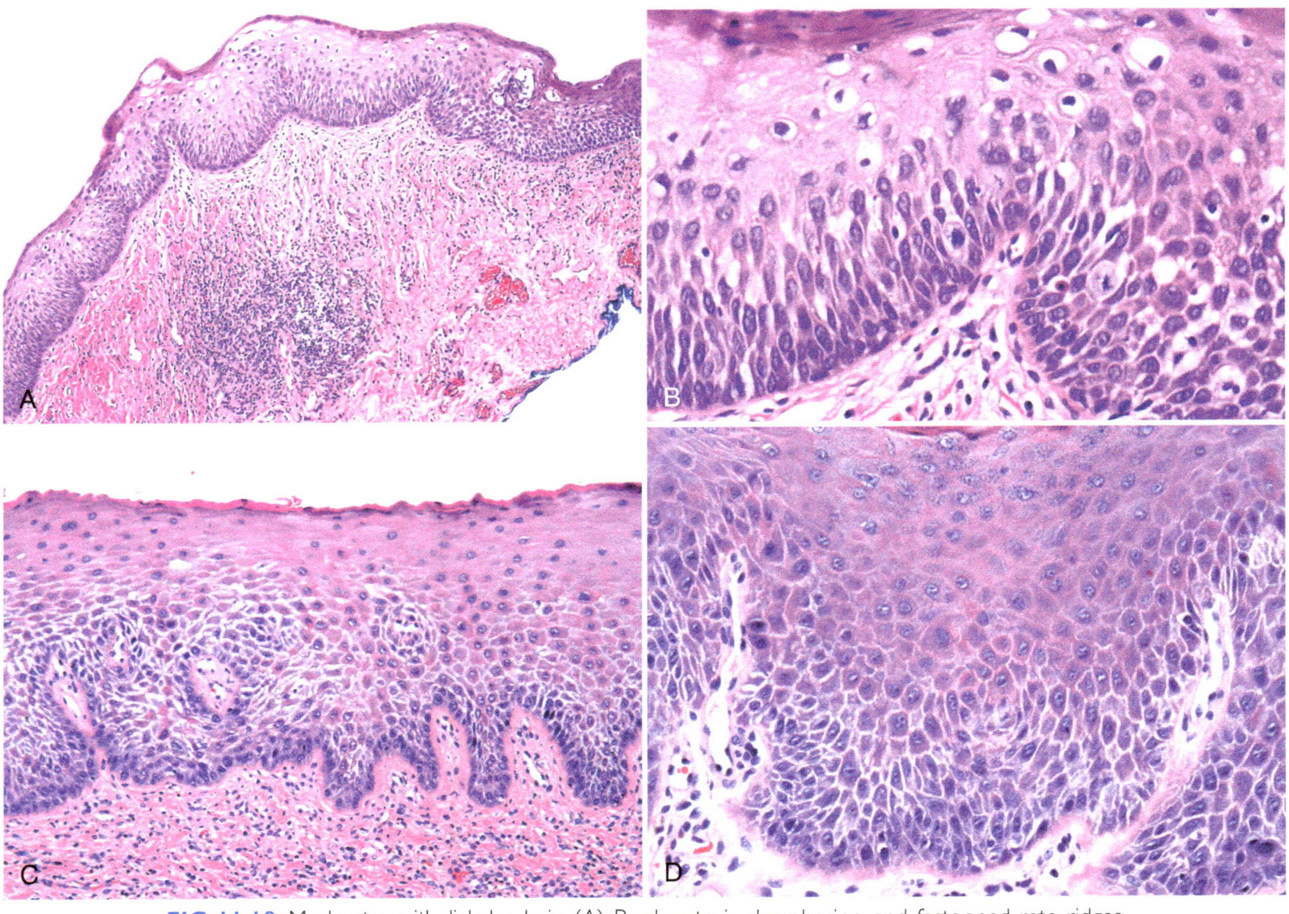

FIG 11.18 Moderate epithelial dysplasia. (A) Parakeratosis, dyscohesion, and festooned rete ridges. (B) Basal cell hyperplasia, suprabasal mitoses, and festooned rete ridges. (C) Dyscohesive cells and cells with hyperchromatic and pleomorphic nuclei. (D) Dyscohesion, basal cell hyperplasia, and pleomorphism involving half the epithelium; rete ridge is slightly bulbous.

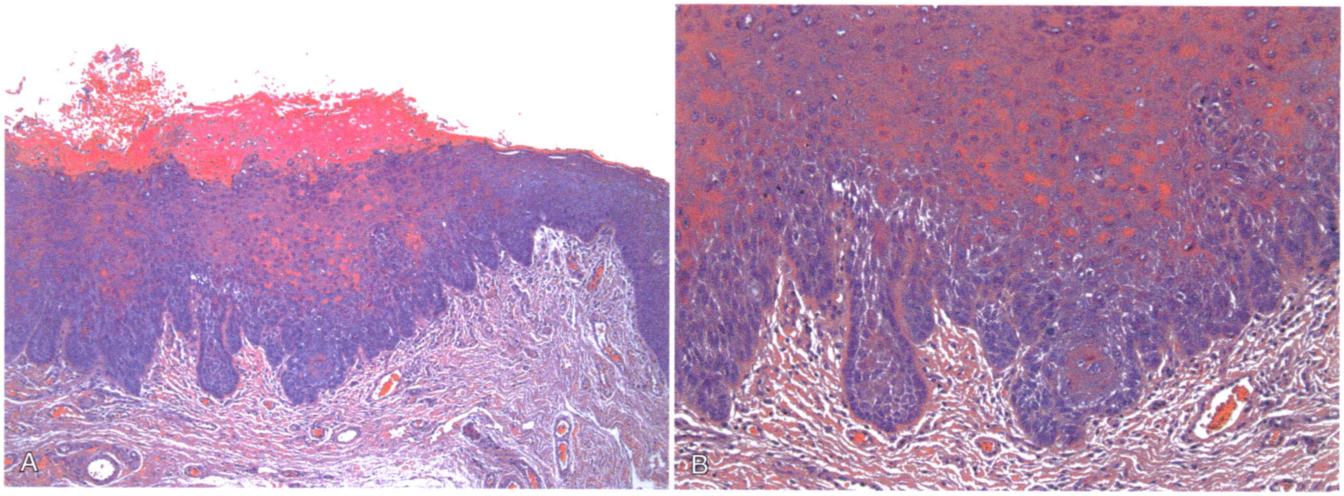

FIG 11.19 Severe epithelial dysplasia. (A) Dyscohesion, dyskeratosis, basal cell hyperplasia, and hyperchromasia. (B) Dyscohesion, dyskeratosis, basal cell hyperplasia, nuclear pleomorphism, hyperchromasia, and keratin pearl formation at the tip of a rete ridge.

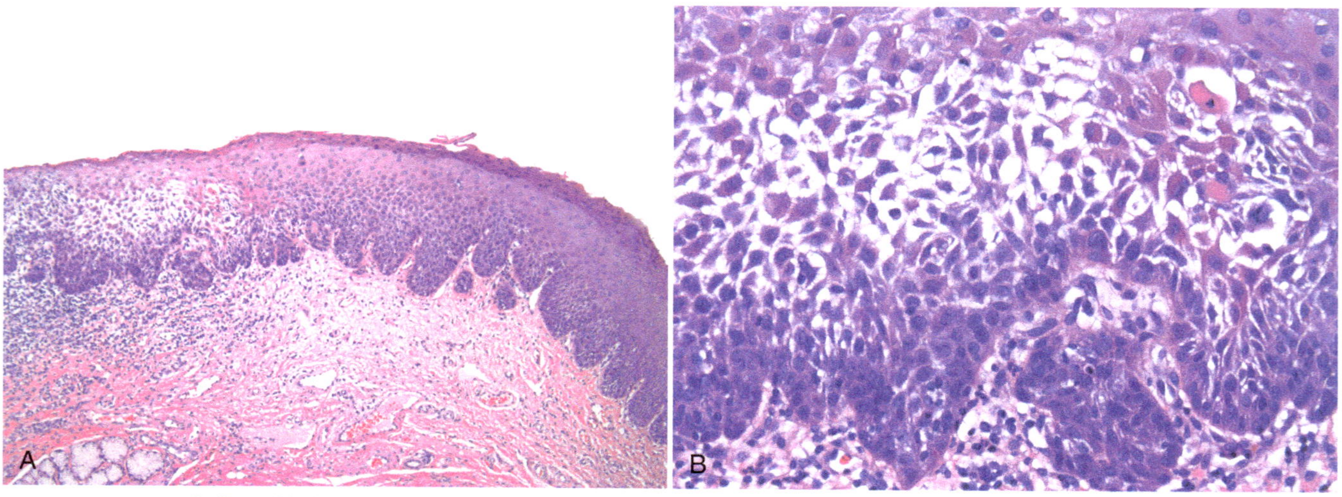

FIG 11.20 Severe dysplasia. (A) Moderate dysplasia is present on the *right* and severe dysplasia on the *left*. (B) Marked dyscohesion with pleomorphic and hyperchromatic cells and dyskeratosis.

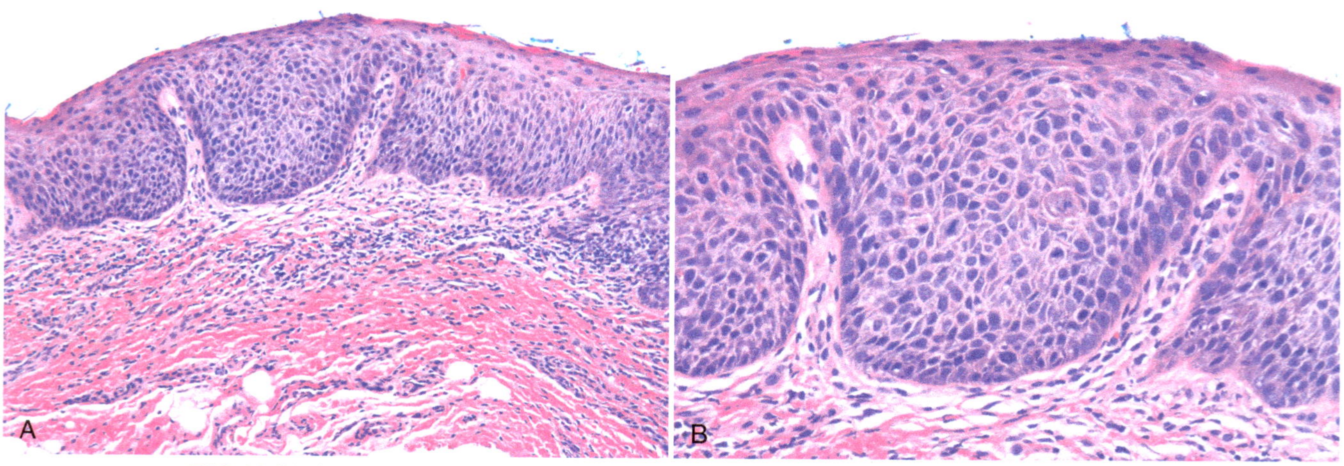

FIG 11.21 (A) Carcinoma-in-situ on the *left* with full thickness involvement of the epithelium and severe dysplasia on the *right* where the superficial two to three layers of keratinocytes are mature and still horizontally aligned. (B) Cells have pleomorphic nuclei throughout the epithelium and there are many high mitotic figures.

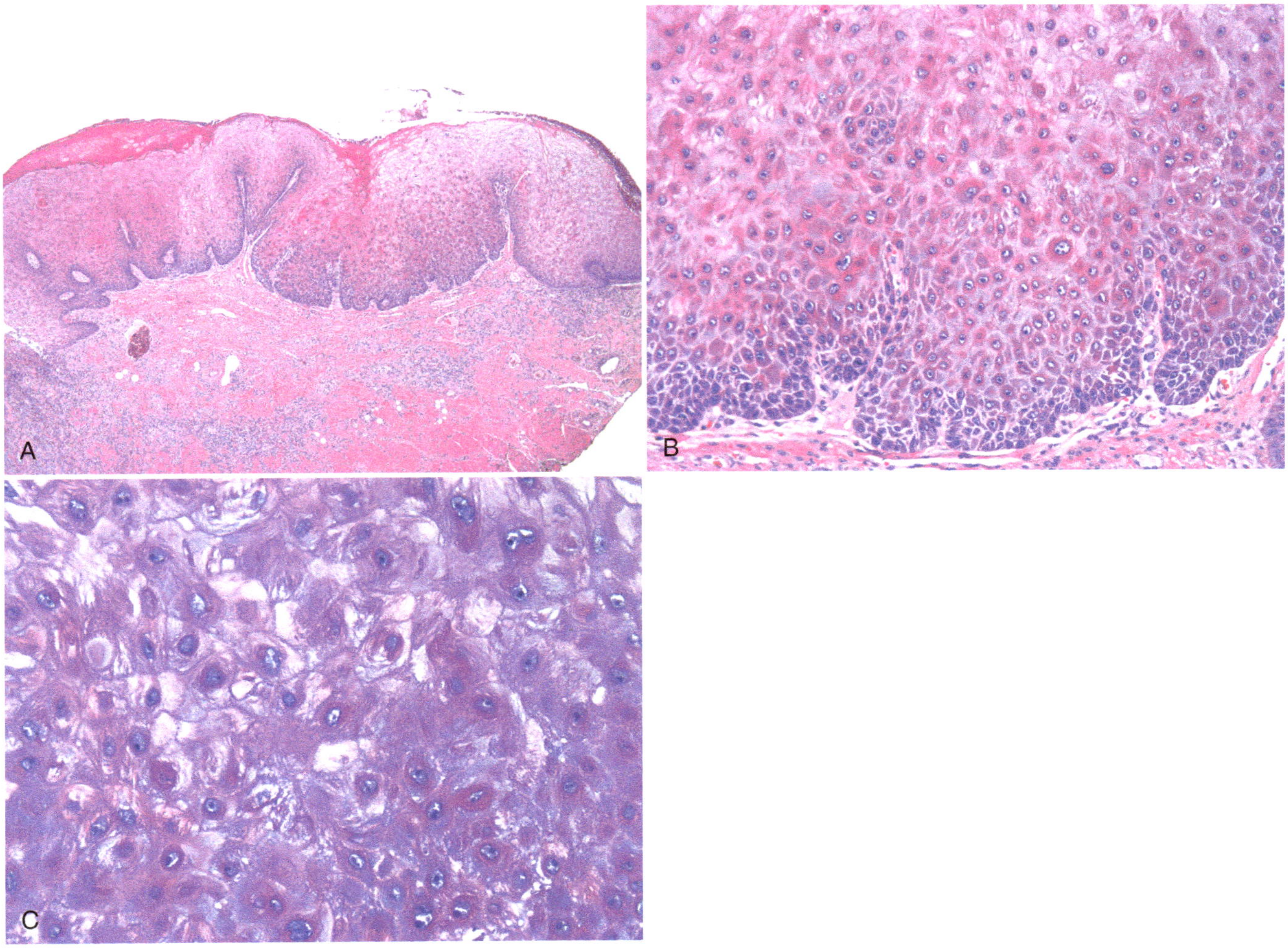

FIG 11.22 Carcinoma-in-situ. (A) Full thickness dysplasia with pale cells. (B) Pleomorphic cells with marked dyskeratosis, and many mitotic figures. (C) Cells have abundant, pale, glassy, slightly fibrillar cytoplasm and pleomorphic nuclei.

- The presence of a lymphocytic band at the interface is common and represents a T-cell response to dysplastic keratinocytes, similar to tumor-infiltrating lymphocytes or lymphocytic host response seen around invasive carcinoma; referring to this lymphocytic band as "lichenoid" is confusing and may cause the clinician to erroneously assume that the dysplasia arose within lichen planus.
- Involvement of ducts by dysplasia must be documented, because deep margins may not be free of dysplasia if deep portions of duct are involved; this feature is associated with an increased rate of local recurrence (Figs. 11.23 and 11.24).

Differential Diagnosis

- Reactive epithelial atypia is sometimes difficult to differentiate from true dysplasia, especially in the presence of reepithelialization and healing ulceration; if one cannot be sure, using the phrases *likely reactive* or *unsure if reactive* helps in patient management. Correlating the histopathology with the appearance of the lesions is always helpful.
- Lichen planus or lichenoid mucositis with reactive atypia tends to show squamatization of basal cells (instead of basal cell hyperplasia) and colloid body formation; multinucleate epithelial cells with finely dispersed chromatin and abundant cytoplasm are often seen in reactive lesions (Fig. 11.25); dysplastic multinucleated epithelial cells have little cytoplasm.
- Lesions of candidiasis may show significant reactive atypia; however, dysplastic epithelium is often colonized by *Candida*, but these dysplastic changes are still present after anti-fungal therapy.

Management and Prognosis

- Multiple biopsies should be performed for nonhomogeneous leukoplakia and proliferative leukoplakia.
- All dysplasias, including mild dysplasias (not reactive atypia) should be carefully followed or excised/ablated, depending on the clinical situation (eg, high-risk site with high-risk history); recurrence is common especially if margins are not free of dysplasia (including architectural features of dysplasia) or if keratosis is present at the margins.

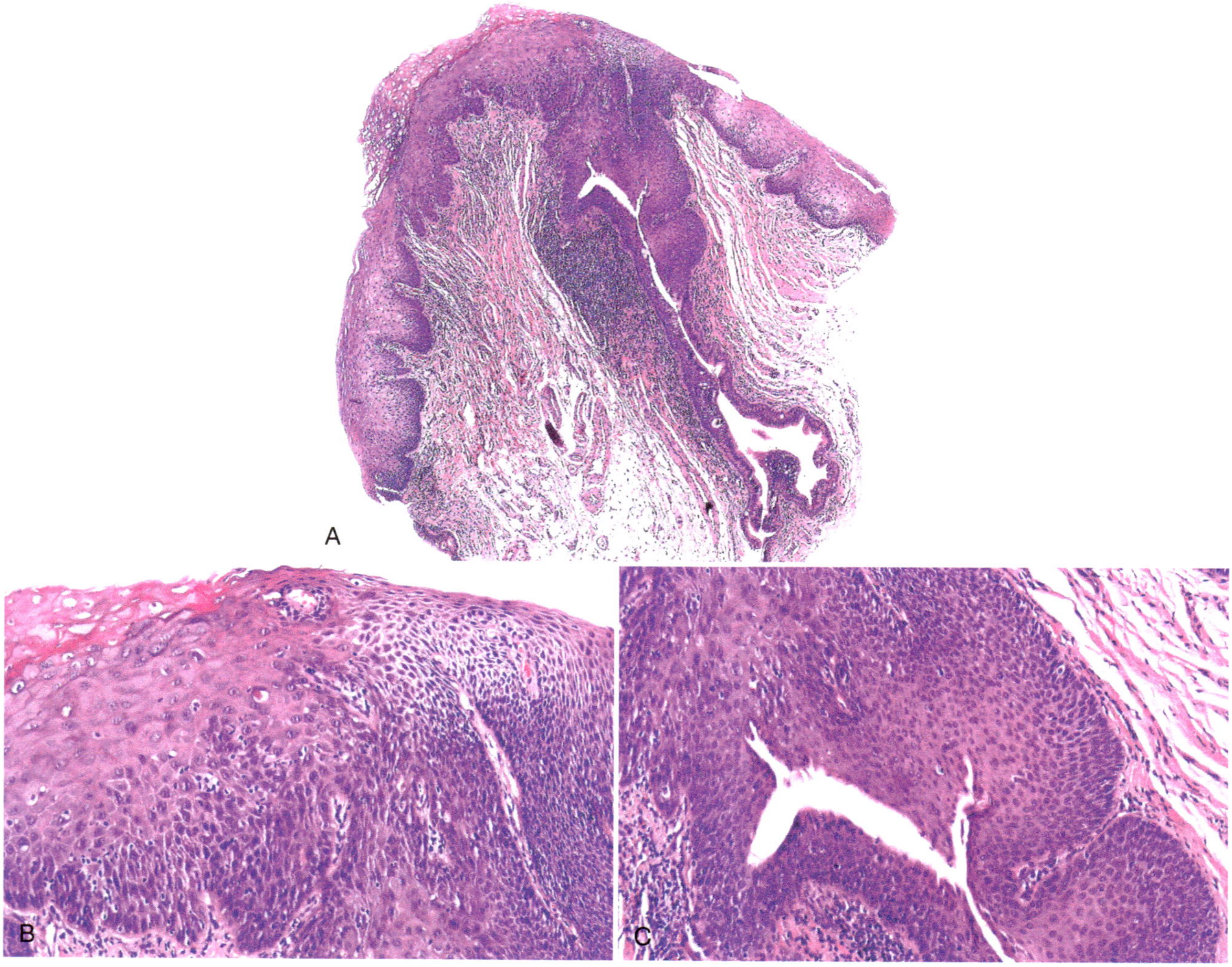

FIG 11.23 Moderate to severe epithelial dysplasia involving excretory duct. (A) Hyperkeratosis with dysplasia involving upper portion of the duct. (B) Surface exhibits dyscohesion, basal cell hyperplasia, and nuclear hyperchromasia. (C) Basal cell hyperplasia involving the duct.

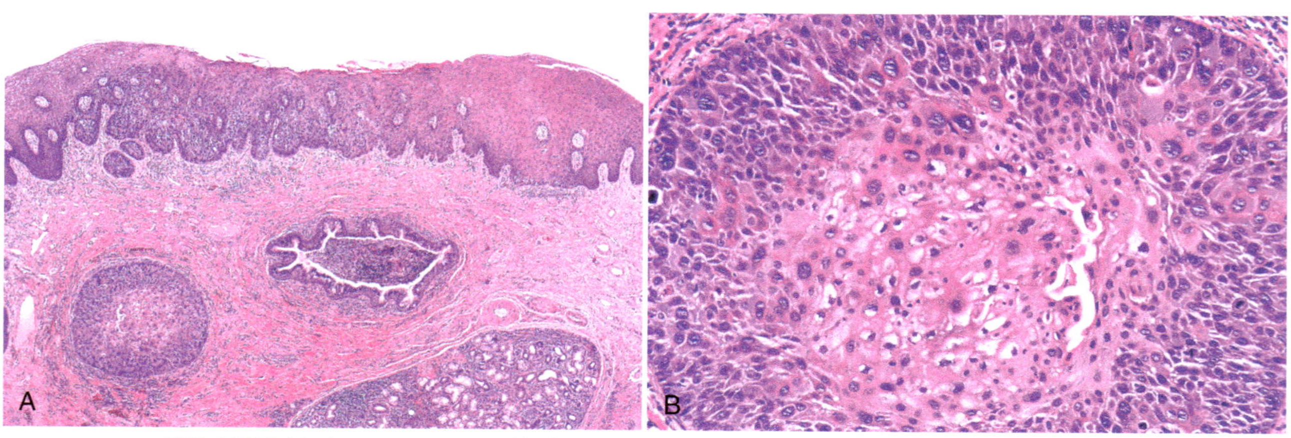

FIG 11.24 Moderate to severe epithelial dysplasia involving excretory duct. (A) The overlying epithelium exhibits dyscohesion and basal cell hyperplasia; one duct is involved by dysplasia. (B) Pleomorphic and dysplastic cells involve the full thickness of the duct.

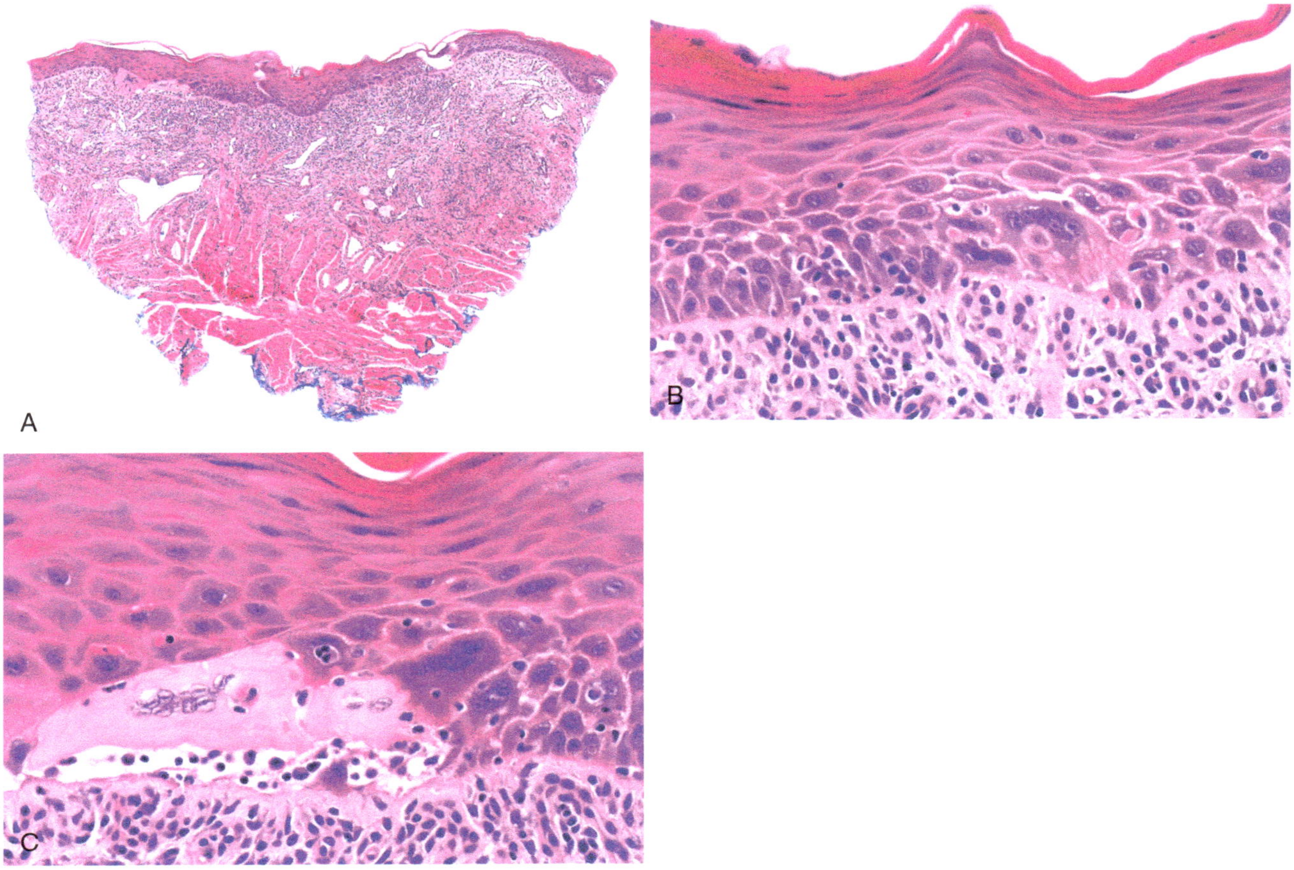

FIG 11.25 Lichenoid mucositis with reactive epithelial atypia. (A) Hyperkeratosis and lymphocytic band at the interface. (B) Squamatized basal cells, colloid bodies, and reactive epithelial atypia with multinucleate epithelial cells with abundant cytoplasm. (C) Squamous cells exhibit reactive atypia abutting the typical subbasal cleft.

- Photodynamic therapy has been shown to result in complete remission in 80% of cases.
- Recurrence after removal or progression of residual disease after incomplete removal occurs in up to 30% of cases and risk factors include large lesional size, involvement of margins, and poor accessibility for complete removal of the lesion; lesions on the gingiva and posterior tongue/floor of mouth are particularly prone to such recurrence.
- Rate of malignant transformation to invasive cancer is higher in leukoplakias that are >4 cm, and in cases exhibiting moderate to severe or high grade dysplasia; this occurs at a rate of 3% per year and rates of transformation depend largely on the length of follow-up; rate of malignant transformation in more recent literature is up to 18% at 5 years.
- Cases that are suspicious for dysplasia because of architectural abnormalities without cytologic evidence of dysplasia, location at high-risk sites, or sharp demarcation may be candidates for narrow excision or ablation, unless morbidity is unacceptable.
- Patients should receive life time follow-up not just because of recurrence but also because field cancerization places the patient at high risk for another primary site of dysplasia.

REFERENCES

Amagasa T, Yamashiro M, Uzawa N. Oral premalignant lesions: from a clinical perspective. *Int J Clin Oncol.* 2011;16:5-14.

Arduino PG, Surace A, Carbone M, et al. Outcome of oral dysplasia: a retrospective hospital-based study of 207 patients with a long follow-up. *J Oral Pathol Med.* 2009;38:540-544.

Bagan J, Scully C, Jimenez Y, Martorell M. Proliferative verrucous leukoplakia: a concise update. *Oral Dis.* 2010;16:328-332.

Barnes L, Eveson J, Reichart P, Sidransky D, eds. *Pathology and Genetics of Head and Neck Tumors.* Lyon, France: IARC Press; 2005.

Braakhuis BJ, Leemans CR, Brakenhoff RH. Expanding fields of genetically altered cells in head and neck squamous carcinogenesis. *Semin Cancer Biol.* 2005;15:113-120.

Brouns E, Baart J, Karagozoglu K, et al. Malignant transformation of oral leukoplakia in a well-defined cohort of 144 patients. *Oral Dis.* 2014;20:e19-e24.

Chainani-Wu N, Lee D, Madden E, et al. Clinical predictors of oral leukoplakia recurrence following CO2 laser vaporization. *J Craniomaxillofac Surg.* 2015;43:1875-1879.

Daley TD, Lovas JG, Peters E, et al. Salivary gland duct involvement in oral epithelial dysplasia and squamous cell carcinoma. *Oral Surg Oral Med Oral Pathol Oral Radiol Endod.* 1996;81:186-192.

Fleskens S, Slootweg P. Grading systems in head and neck dysplasia: their prognostic value, weaknesses and utility. *Head Neck Oncol.* 2009;1:11.

Gale N, Michaels L, Luzar B, et al. Current review on squamous intraepithelial lesions of the larynx. *Histopathology.* 2009;54:639-656.

Jeong WJ, Paik JH, Cho SW, et al. Excisional biopsy for management of lateral tongue leukoplakia. *J Oral Pathol Med.* 2012;41:384-388.

Jerjes W, Upile T, Hamdoon Z, et al. Photodynamic therapy outcome for oral dysplasia. *Lasers Surg Med.* 2011;43:192-199.

Kujan O, Oliver RJ, Khattab A, et al. Evaluation of a new binary system of grading oral epithelial dysplasia for prediction of malignant transformation. *Oral Oncol.* 2006;42:987-993.

Lee JJ, Hung HC, Cheng SJ, et al. Carcinoma and dysplasia in oral leukoplakias in Taiwan: prevalence and risk factors. *Oral Surg Oral Med Oral Pathol Oral Radiol Endod.* 2006;101:472-480.

Lingen MW, Pinto A, Mendes RA, et al. Genetics/epigenetics of oral premalignancy: current status and future research. *Oral Dis.* 2011;17(suppl 1):7-22.

Liu W, Wang YF, Zhou HW, et al. Malignant transformation of oral leukoplakia: a retrospective cohort study of 218 Chinese patients. *BMC Cancer.* 2010;10:685.

Napier SS, Speight PM. Natural history of potentially malignant oral lesions and conditions: an overview of the literature. *J Oral Pathol Med.* 2008;37:1-10.

Poh CF, Zhang L, Lam WL, et al. A high frequency of allelic loss in oral verrucous lesions may explain malignant risk. *Lab Invest.* 2001;81: 629-634.

Reichart PA, Philipsen HP. Oral erythroplakia—a review. *Oral Oncol.* 2005;41:551-561.

Sakurai K, Urade M, Takahashi Y, et al. Increased expression of c-erbB-3 protein and proliferating cell nuclear antigen during development of verrucous carcinoma of the oral mucosa. *Cancer.* 2000;89: 2597-2605.

Speight PM. Update on oral epithelial dysplasia and progression to cancer. *Head Neck Pathol.* 2007;1:61-66.

Sperandio M, Brown AL, Lock C, et al. Predictive value of dysplasia grading and DNA ploidy in malignant transformation of oral potentially malignant disorders. *Cancer Prev Res (Phila).* 2013;6:822-831.

Vogelstein B, Kinzler KW. The Path to Cancer –Three Strikes and You're Out. *N Engl J Med.* 2015;373:1895-1898.

Wang YP, Chen HM, Kuo RC, et al. Oral verrucous hyperplasia: histologic classification, prognosis, and clinical implications. *J Oral Pathol Med.* 2009;38:651-656.

Warnakulasuriya S, Reibel J, Bouquot J, Dabelsteen E. Oral epithelial dysplasia classification systems: predictive value, utility, weaknesses and scope for improvement. *J Oral Pathol Med.* 2008;37:127-133.

Woo SB, Grammer RL, Lerman MA. Keratosis of unknown significance and leukoplakia: a preliminary study. *Oral Surg Oral Med Oral Pathol Oral Radiol.* 2014;118:713-724.

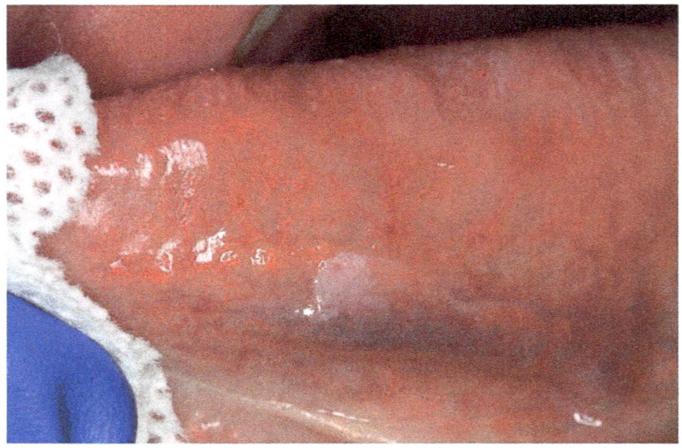

FIG 11.26 Human papillomavirus (HPV)–associated dysplastic leukoplakia on the left ventral tongue. *(Courtesy Dr. Thomas Sterio, private practice, Swampscott, Mass.)*

HUMAN PAPILLOMAVIRUS (HPV)–ASSOCIATED ORAL EPITHELIAL DYSPLASIA

This condition has a strong male predilection, similar to nasopharyngeal and tonsillar HPV-associated carcinoma. Although the precursor dysplastic lesion has not been identified in tonsillar carcinoma, likely because of the convoluted nature of the crypt epithelium, this HPV-driven oral condition presents as a leukoplakia and is easily identified by simple inspection of the oral mucosa. Older cases with similar histopathology have been referred to as "koilocytic dysplasia."

Clinical Findings

- This occurs most frequently in the seventh decade with a 5–6:1 male predilection; it is indistinguishable from other leukoplakias and presents as a well-demarcated white plaque, sometimes verrucous, usually on the ventral tongue and floor of mouth (Fig. 11.26).

Etiopathogenesis and Histopathologic Features

This particular type of dysplasia is associated with high-risk HPV types (mostly type 16), and it shares some features with Bowen disease. Transcriptionally active HPV produces E6 and E7 oncoproteins that inactivate p53 and pRb tumor-suppressor proteins, respectively, with the latter leading to overexpression of p16, the presence of which is highly correlated with HPV-associated squamous cell carcinoma of the tonsils and oropharynx; presence of p16 is now used as a surrogate marker for such cancers.

- There is bright compact parakeratosis, although hyperkeratosis may also be present, and papillary architecture is an infrequent finding; characteristically, there is full-thickness involvement of the epithelium by basaloid cells with high nuclear-to-cytoplasmic ratio as well as cells in varying stages of apoptosis, from karyorrhectic cells (similar to mitosoid bodies seen in Heck disease) to degenerated cells with pyknotic nuclei, to cytoid bodies; apoptotic cells are dyscohesive with surrounding halos; koilocytes may be present (Figs. 11.27A–B, 11.28, and 11.29A–C).
- A continuous band of p16 positivity within the nuclei and cytoplasm of keratinocytes is always present (see Fig. 11.27D).
- High-risk HPV types are identified in up to 80% of cases by in situ hybridization (see Figs. 11.27D and 11.29D), and most of these represent HPV-16.

Differential Diagnosis

- Heck disease also exhibits karyorrhectic cells (mitosoid bodies) but does not show significant atypia/dysplasia or continuous p16 positivity.
- Conventional carcinoma-in-situ does not show significant numbers of such apoptotic cells and is negative for p16 and high-risk HPV.
- Bowenoid papulosis may rarely occur in the mouth and presents as multiple papules clinically; bowenoid papulosis and Bowen disease of the skin may show p16 positivity but often not in a diffuse pattern, and often sparing the basal cells.

Management and Prognosis

- Excision with clear margins is treatment of choice; approximately 10% of cases develop squamous cell carcinoma.

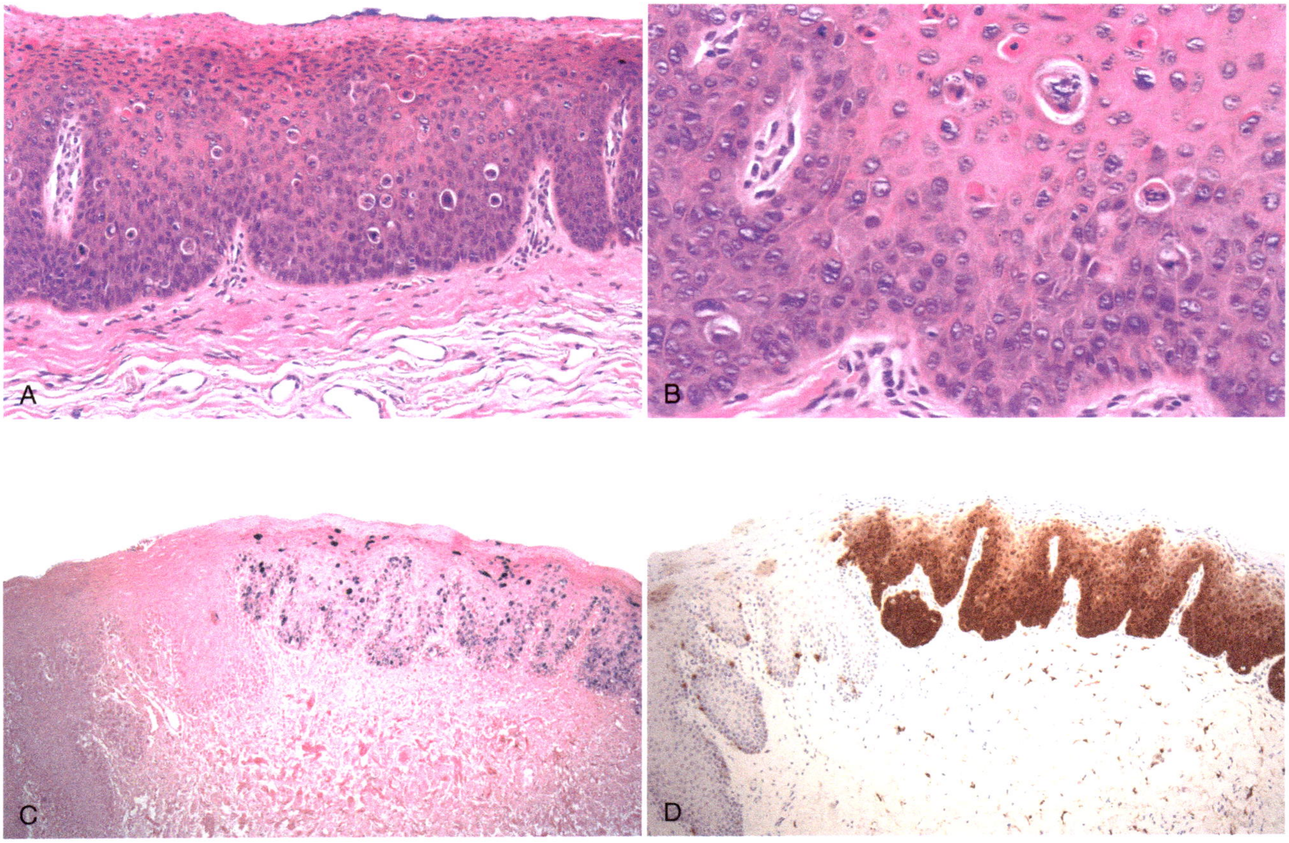

FIG 11.27 Human papillomavirus (HPV)–associated dysplasia. (A) Parakeratosis and many large, atypical cells exhibiting pericellular halos. (B) Karyorrhectic and apoptotic cells; adjacent cells show nuclear atypia and dysmaturation. (C) In situ hybridization is positive for high-risk HPV types; note abrupt transition to noninvolved epithelium that corresponds to clinical demarcation of lesion. (D) p16 positivity within most of the keratinocytes beneath the parakeratin in a pattern corresponding to the positive study for high-risk HPV in C.

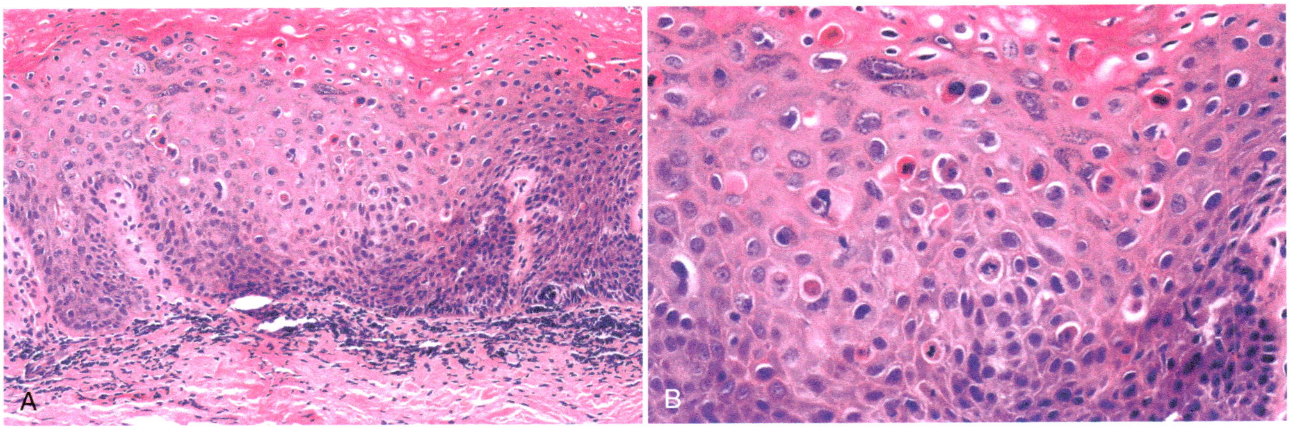

FIG 11.28 HPV-associated dysplasia. (A) Parakeratosis and full thickness involvement by dysplastic and apoptotic cells. (B) Koilocytes and karyorrhectic and apoptotic cells are present.

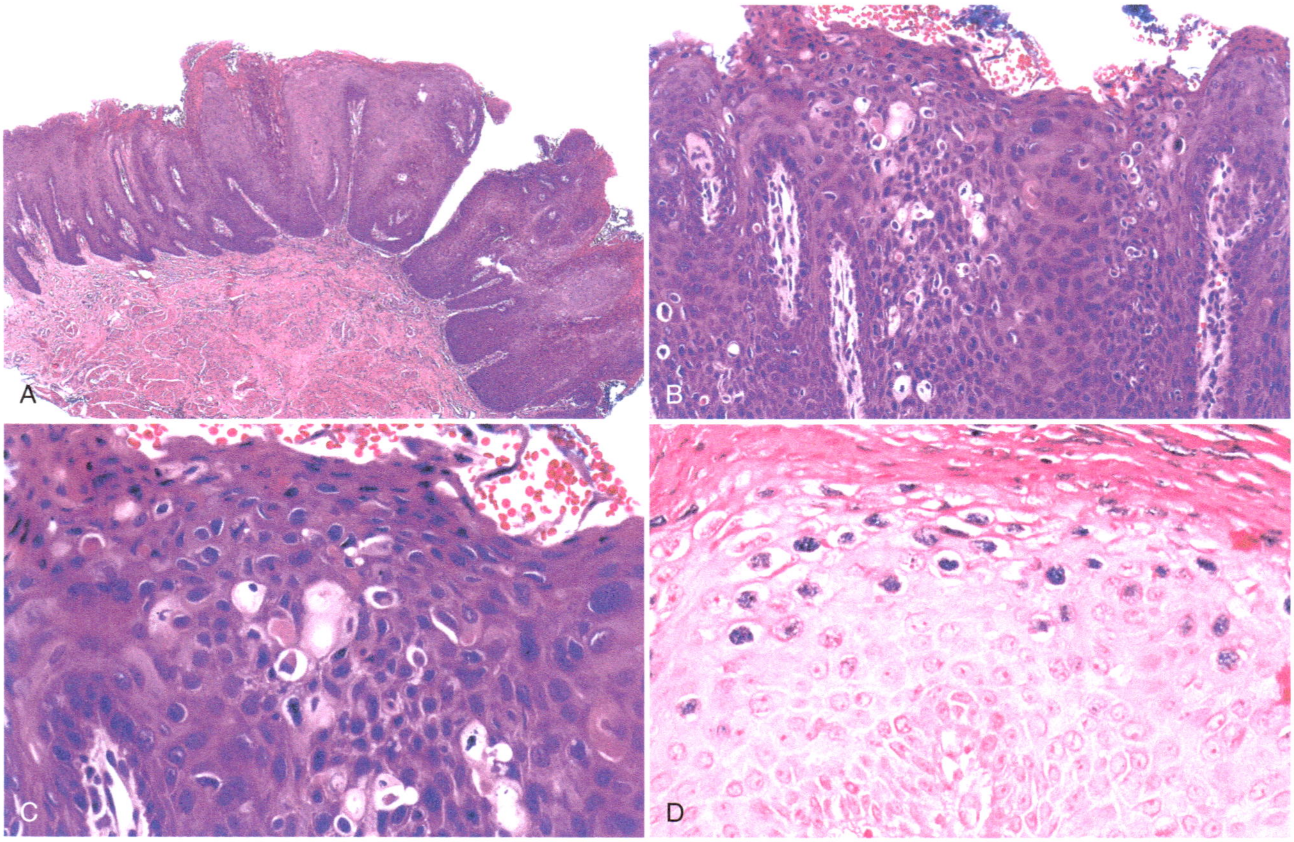

FIG 11.29 (A) Parakeratosis and papillary epithelial hyperplasia. (B) Many apoptotic cells are present. (C) Koilocytes, apoptotic and karyorrhectic cells are present. (D) In situ hybridization is positive for high-risk HPV.

REFERENCES

Daley T, Birek C, Wysocki GP. Oral bowenoid lesions: differential diagnosis and pathogenetic insights. *Oral Surg Oral Med Oral Pathol Oral Radiol Endod.* 2000;90:466-473.

Fornatora M, Jones AC, Kerpel S, Freedman P. Human papillomavirus-associated oral epithelial dysplasia (koilocytic dysplasia): an entity of unknown biologic potential. *Oral Surg Oral Med Oral Pathol Oral Radiol Endod.* 1996;82:47-56.

Harvey NT, Leecy T, Wood BA. Immunohistochemical staining for p16 is a useful adjunctive test in the diagnosis of Bowen's disease. *Pathology.* 2013;45:402-407.

Kazlouskaya V, Shustef E, Allam SH, Lal K, Elston D. Expression of p16 protein in lesional and perilesional condyloma acuminata and bowenoid papulosis: clinical significance and diagnostic implications. *J Am Acad Dermatol.* 2013;69:444-449.

Kratochvil FJ, Cioffi GA, Auclair PL, Rathbun WA. Virus-associated dysplasia (bowenoid papulosis?) of the oral cavity. *Oral Surg Oral Med Oral Pathol.* 1989;68:312-316.

McCord C, Xu J, Xu W, et al. Association of high-risk human papillomavirus infection with oral epithelial dysplasia. *Oral Surg Oral Med Oral Pathol.* 2013;115:541-549.

Rinaggio J, Glick M, Lambert WC. Oral bowenoid papulosis in an HIV-positive male. *Oral Surg Oral Med Oral Pathol Oral Radiol Endod.* 2006;101:328-332.

Woo SB, Cashman EC, Lerman MA. Human papillomavirus-associated oral intraepithelial neoplasia. *Mod Pathol.* 2013;26:1288-1297.

SUBMUCOUS FIBROSIS

Submucous fibrosis is a premalignant condition seen in areca nut and betel leaf chewers, a practice common in India, parts of South East Asia, and Taiwan. It is highly associated with the development of dysplasia and carcinoma.

Clinical Findings

- Patients report burning and increasing trismus, and there is diffuse, pale, marble-like, and keratotic areas on the buccal mucosa, soft palate, and tongue in patients who chew areca nut; late lesions have a taut, fibrotic, or typical "piano wire" feel to the mucosa from fibrous bands, and erythema and ulcers may be present; the teeth are characteristically stained reddish-brown; the appearance of a white plaque (leukoplakia) or red plaque (erythroplakia) usually precedes the development of squamous cell carcinoma (Fig. 11.30).
- Staging systems have been developed based on the presence of erythema and ulcers, pallor of the mucosa, and depapillation of the tongue, presence of fibrous bands, degree of interincisal opening, and the presence of leukoplakia, erythroplakia or squamous cell carcinoma.

Etiopathogenesis and Histopathologic Features

Areca nut contains abundant copper and flavonoids that act together to stabilize and enhance cross-linking of collagen resulting in fibrosis. Areca nut contains alkaloids, such as arecoline, that stimulate collagen synthesis and

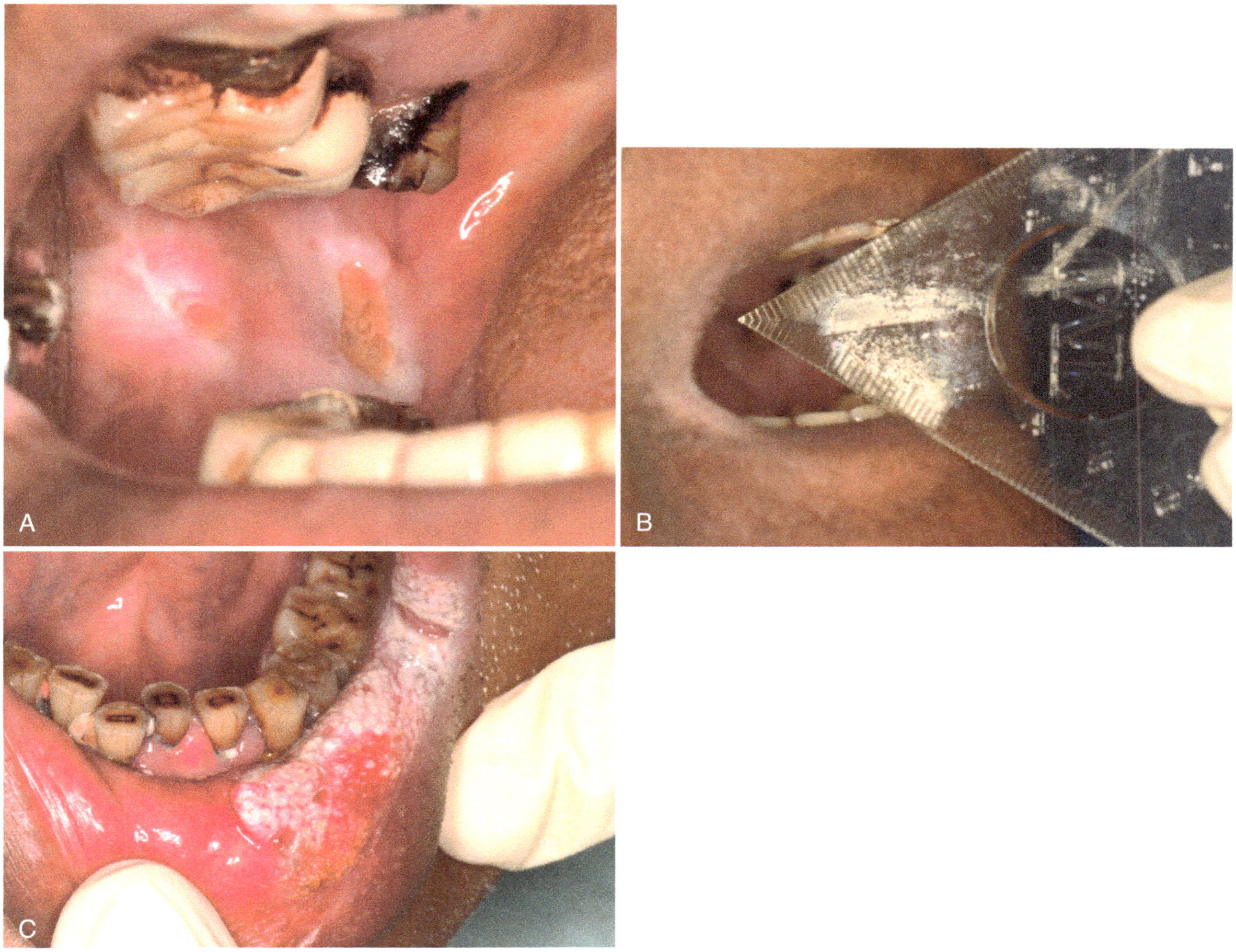

FIG 11.30 Submucous fibrosis. (A) Poorly demarcated white and ulcerated (yellow) areas on the buccal mucosa with brown staining of the teeth from areca nut chewing. (B) Same patient as in A; marked fibrosis leading to an interincisal opening of only 20 mm (normal 40–45 mm in males). (C) Squamous cell carcinoma arising from the buccal mucosa and extending onto the lower lip mucosa in a patient with submucous fibrosis; note the red-brown staining of teeth from this habit.

reduce collagen degradation, possibly through the transforming growth factor-β pathway; these alkaloids can be converted to carcinogenic nitrosamines. Areca nut products are constituents of gutka (a preparation of powdered tobacco, slaked lime, and spices) and paan (which includes slaked lime, spices, and sometimes tobacco wrapped in *Piper betle* leaf, also referred to as "betel leaf") that are chewed in many areas in India. Gutka use is associated with more rapid development of oral lesions.

- There is hyperkeratosis, epithelial atrophy, and diffuse fibrosis of varying severity in the lamina propria; the collagen becomes denser and more hyalinized with prolonged use (Fig. 11.31).
- Dysplasia and invasive squamous cell carcinoma develop in long-standing lesions (Fig. 11.32).

Differential Diagnosis

- Progressive systemic sclerosis appears similar, but the presence of anti-centromere and anti-Scl-70 antibodies and a negative history of areca nut use differentiate between the two.

Management and Prognosis

- Intralesional injections of corticosteroids, collagenase, hyaluronidase, and systemic treatment with pentoxifylline and interferon-γ have all been useful for the fibrosis; surgical excision of the scars with grafting helps to correct trismus temporarily.
- Patients should be followed closely because 7% to 13% of patients develop squamous cell carcinoma; of interest, patients who develop squamous cell carcinoma within submucous fibrosis tend to be younger males with smaller tumors and lower incidence of nodal metastasis or extracapsular spread.

REFERENCES

Alora Veedu R, Balan A, Sankar SP. A randomized double-blind, multiple-arm trial comparing the efficacy of submucosal injections of hyaluronidase, dexamethasone, and combination of

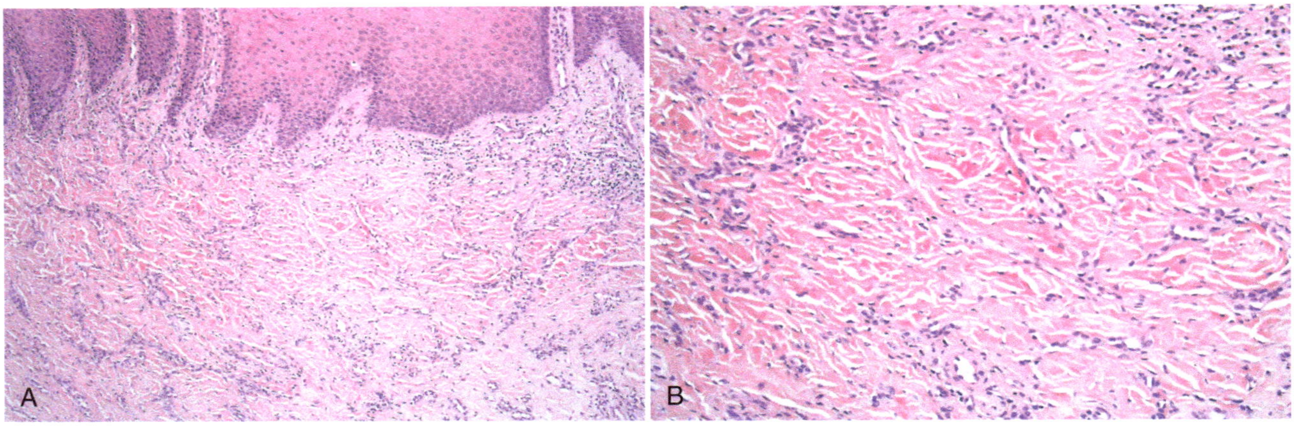

FIG 11.31 Submucous fibrosis. (A) Fibrosis of the lamina propria with mild chronic inflammation; epithelium has tapered rete ridges and does not exhibit dysplasia. (B) Moderately hyalinized collagen in the lamina propria and mild chronic inflammation.

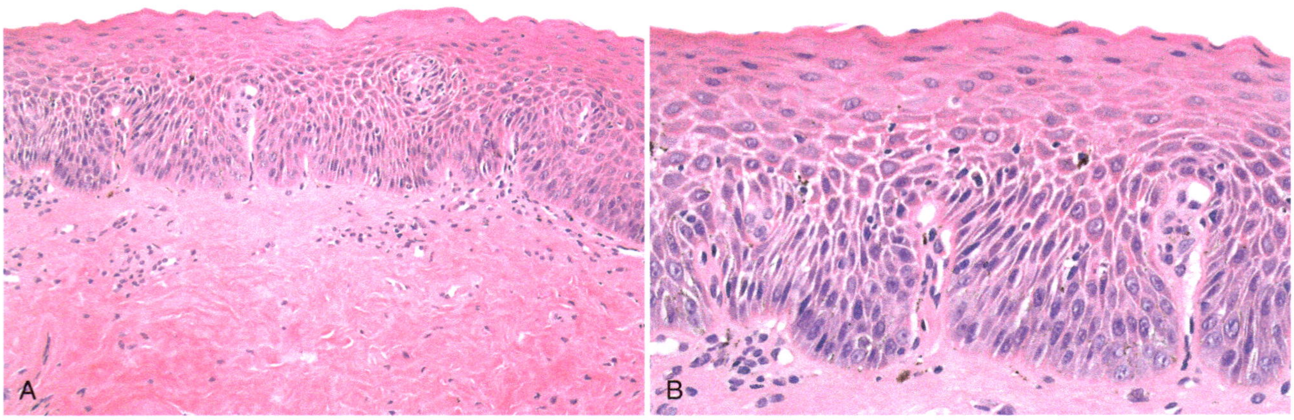

FIG 11.32 Submucous fibrosis with dysplasia. (A) The epithelium exhibits moderate dysplasia with basal cell hyperplasia, and marked fibrosis and stromal hyalinization in the lamina propria. (B) The epithelium exhibits basal cell hyperplasia, nuclear hyperchromasia, and bulbous rete ridges.

dexamethasone and hyaluronidase in the management of oral submucous fibrosis. *Oral Surg Oral Med Oral Pathol.* 2015;120:588-593, e1.

Arakeri G, Brennan PA. Oral submucous fibrosis: an overview of the aetiology, pathogenesis, classification, and principles of management. *Br J Oral Maxillofac Surg.* 2013;51:587-593.

Chaturvedi P, Vaishampayan SS, Nair S, et al. Oral squamous cell carcinoma arising in background of oral submucous fibrosis: a clinicopathologically distinct disease. *Head Neck.* 2013;35:1404-1409.

Javed F, Chotai M, Mehmood A, Almas K. Oral mucosal disorders associated with habitual gutka usage: a review. *Oral Surg Oral Med Oral Pathol Oral Radiol Endod.* 2010;109:857-864.

Kerr AR, Warnakulasuriya S, Mighell AJ, et al. A systematic review of medical interventions for oral submucous fibrosis and future research opportunities. *Oral Dis.* 2011;17(suppl 1):42-57.

Lee CH, Ko YC, Huang HL, et al. The precancer risk of betel quid chewing, tobacco use and alcohol consumption in oral leukoplakia and oral submucous fibrosis in southern Taiwan. *Br J Cancer.* 2003;88:366-372.

More CB, Das S, Patel H, et al. Proposed clinical classification for oral submucous fibrosis. *Oral Oncol.* 2012;48:200-202.

Pandya S, Chaudhary AK, Singh M, Mehrotra R. Correlation of histopathological diagnosis with habits and clinical findings in oral submucous fibrosis. *Head Neck Oncol.* 2009;1:10.

Tilakaratne WM, Klinikowski MF, Saku T, et al. Oral submucous fibrosis: review on aetiology and pathogenesis. *Oral Oncol.* 2006;42:561-568.

SQUAMOUS CELL CARCINOMA AND VARIANTS

Squamous cell carcinoma of the head and neck is the eighth most common malignancy in US males and in males in developing countries. Risk factors are similar to those for dysplasia and include cigarette smoking and other forms of tobacco use, excessive alcohol consumption, areca nut habit, history of cancer and cancer therapy, history of autoimmune disease and/or prolonged immunosuppression, family history of cancer, HPV and age, with tobacco and alcohol having synergistic activity. Cancers of the lip vermilion are caused by actinic damage. Approximately 70% and 40% of oral cavity and pharyngeal deaths are caused by smoking in high-income, and middle- and low-income countries, respectively. HPV infection is associated with base of tongue, oropharyngeal, and tonsillar carcinomas, and this form of cancer has increased in incidence within the US over the last 10 years. Patients with Plummer-Vinson syndrome (iron deficiency anemia, atrophic glossitis, and esophageal webs) are also predisposed to oral squamous cell carcinoma. Oral squamous cell carcinoma in younger adults may be associated with genetic disorders such as Fanconi anemia, Bloom syndrome, and dyskeratosis congenita.

Clinical Findings

- This affects older adults with a 2:1 male predilection; it often arises within preexisting leukoplakia, erythroplakia, or proliferative leukoplakia or may present as a nonhealing ulcer or mass (Fig. 11.33); the most common sites are the ventral tongue and floor of mouth and induration is always a present.
- Paresthesia, mobile teeth (if tumor invades the bone), and reduced mobility of soft tissues are signs of advanced disease (Fig. 11.34); only one-third of cases are diagnosed as localized tumors.

Etiopathogenesis and Histopathologic Features

Benzopyrenes and nitrosamines in cigarette smoke and tobacco products, and arecoline in areca nut are

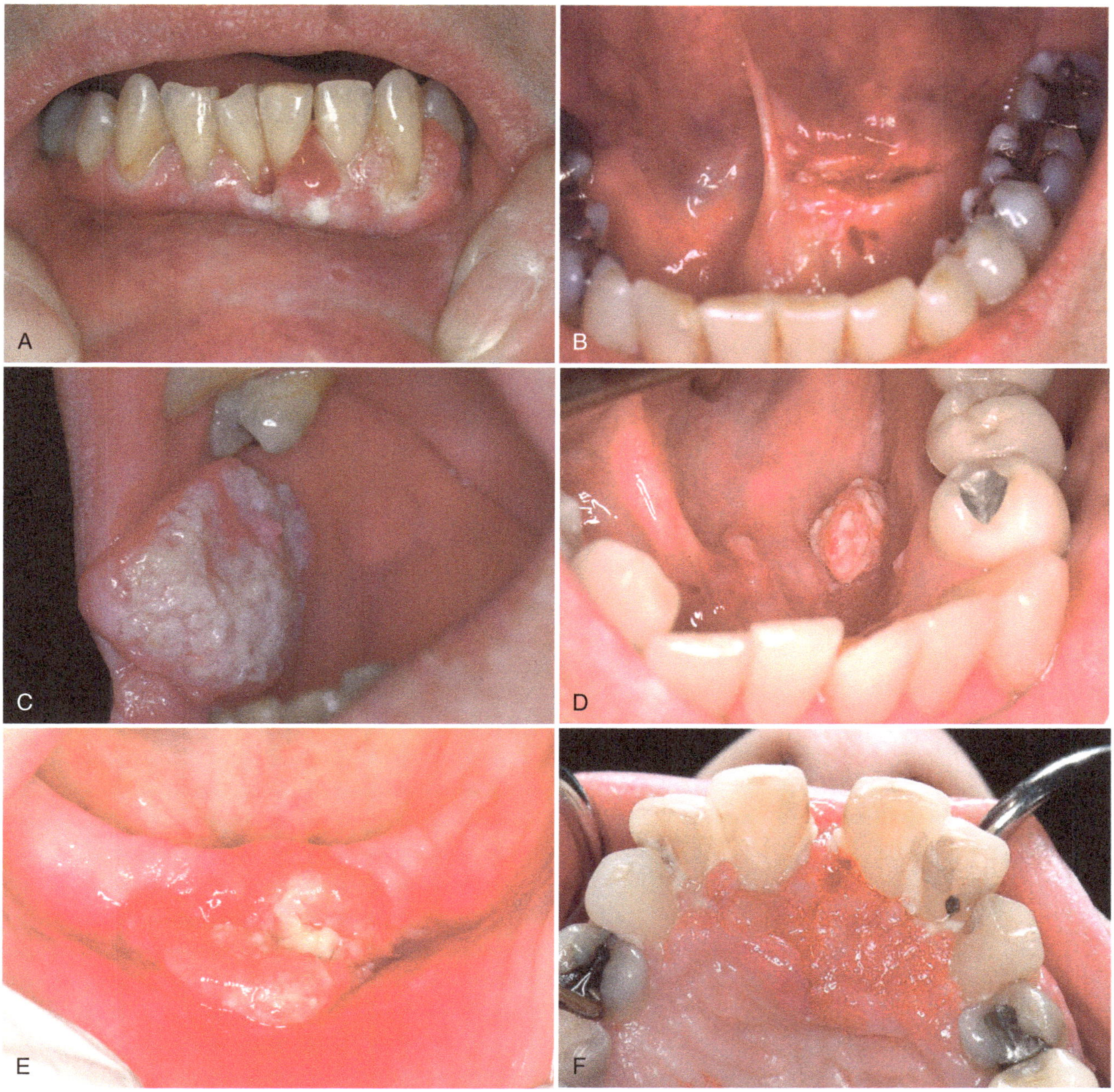

FIG 11.33 Squamous cell carcinoma. (A) Carcinoma arising in erythroleukoplakia. (B) Indurated ulcer in floor of mouth with background of faint leukoplakia *(anterior)*. (C) Mass in buccal mucosa. (D) Ulcerated carcinoma in an HIV-positive patient. (E) Carcinoma of the anterior mandibular vestibule causing poor fit of denture. (F) Pebbly mass of the hard palatal mucosa. *(Courtesy Dr. James Ubertalli, private practice, Hingham, Mass.)*

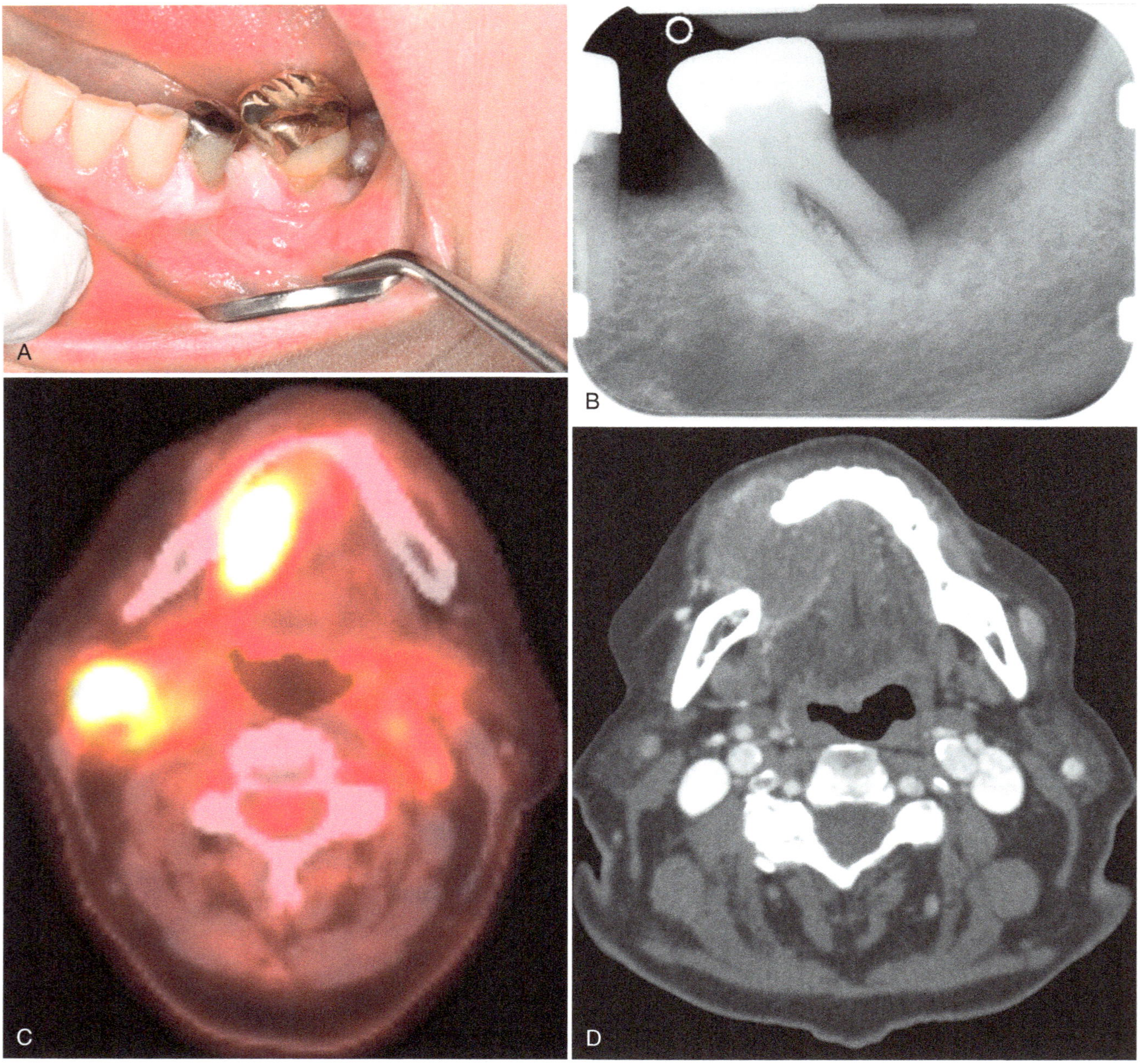

FIG 11.34 (A) Squamous cell carcinoma distal of molar *(right)* arising from gingival leukoplakia. (B) Periapical radiograph from patient in A exhibiting marked bone loss distal of molar. (C) Positron emission tomography–computed tomography (PET-CT) scan of a squamous cell carcinoma of the floor of mouth invading the mandible and with a positive level 2A node. (D) CT scan showing gingival carcinoma perforating both lingual and buccal cortical plates.

carcinogenic agents. There is enrichment for mutations in *TP53*, *CDKN2A*, *MLL2*, *CUL3*, *PIK3CA*, *NSD1*, and *NOTCH* with copy number increases in *EGFR*, *CCND1*, and *FGFR1*, and inactivating mutations in the Wnt/β-catenin signaling pathway. Approximately 90% of tumors overexpress EGFR and this together with aberrations in the FGFR and PI3K pathways are targets for therapy.

Several different histopathologic subtypes exist and distinct patterns of loss of heterozygosity in 3p, 4q, 8p, and 11p are noted for some subtypes, with a higher prevalence of loss of heterozygosity in more aggressive tumors. Of these subtypes, verrucous carcinoma does not tend to metastasize, whereas oropharyngeal HPV-associated carcinomas have a better prognosis, as compared with sarcomatoid carcinoma, which has a worse prognosis. Overall, the trend over the past several decades has been a decrease in the incidence of oral squamous cell carcinoma with improved 5-year survival at 60%, but there has been an upswing in incidence over the last 10 years, because of the increased incidence of HPV-associated oropharyngeal carcinomas.

CONVENTIONAL INFILTRATING SQUAMOUS CELL CARCINOMA

- Malignant epithelial cells arising from the surface epithelium invade the underlying lamina propria, as islands and cords of epithelial cells, and cytologic changes are similar to those for dysplasia; well-differentiated tumors produce abundant keratin and tumor cells exhibit less pleomorphism and are recognizably squamous, while poorly differentiated tumors are minimally-to-nonkeratinizing and pleomorphic; tumor cells may extensively involve underlying skeletal muscle, salivary gland, or invade the bone; a foreign body reaction is often seen around keratinaceous debris (Figs. 11.35–11.38); a rare clear cell variant is recognized.
- Desmoplasia, tumor-infiltrating lymphocytes, and eosinophils are often seen at the tumor front and may or may not correlate with prognosis; eosinophils are often present within tumor islands.
- The adjacent epithelium exhibits varying degrees of dysplasia and candidal infection is common (Fig. 11.39).
- Tumor thickness correlates with recurrence, nodal metastases, and survival, although this is somewhat site-specific; in general tumor thickness of >4 mm especially in the tongue is highly correlated with nodal metastasis, while this may be 2 mm for the floor of mouth.
- Pattern of invasion, poor lymphocytic host response, and lymphovascular, perineural (tumor cells in contact with at least 30% of the nerve fiber) and bone invasion correlate with local recurrence, metastases, and reduced survival (Fig. 11.40).

Management and Prognosis

- Intraoral and panoramic radiographs, and computed tomography (CT), magnetic resonance imaging (MRI), and positron emission tomography (PET) scans help delineate the extent of tumor and are important for clinical staging (cTNM) (Table 11.2).
- Stage I and II tumors are generally treated with en bloc resection with or without lymph node dissection.
- Stage III and IV tumors are treated with surgery with neck dissection, adjuvant, or primary radiation therapy with or without radiation sensitizers, and/or chemotherapy; cetuximab, a monoclonal antibody against epidermal growth factor receptor present in >90% of head and neck squamous cell carcinomas, has shown promise in improving disease control.
- Sentinel node biopsies are positive in 20% to 30% of clinically benign neck nodes and upstage tumors in 30% to 50% of cases; sensitivity and negative predictive value are 87% and 95%, respectively.
- Five-year survival is 83% with local disease, 55% with loco-regional disease, and 32% with distant metastases.
- Long-term follow-up is of utmost importance because second primary tumors occur in 7% to 33% of patients.

REFERENCES

Balasubramanian D, Ebrahimi A, Gupta R, et al. Tumour thickness as a predictor of nodal metastases in oral cancer: comparison between tongue and floor of mouth subsites. *Oral Oncol.* 2014;50:1165-11658.

Brandwein-Gensler M, Smith RV, Wang B, et al. Validation of the histologic risk model in a new cohort of patients with head and neck squamous cell carcinoma. *Am J Surg Pathol.* 2010;34:676-688.

Cancer Genome Atlas N. Comprehensive genomic characterization of head and neck squamous cell carcinomas. *Nature.* 2015;517:576-582.

Choi HR, Roberts DB, Johnigan RH, et al. Molecular and clinicopathologic comparisons of head and neck squamous carcinoma variants: common and distinctive features of biological significance. *Am J Surg Pathol.* 2004;28:1299-1310.

Edge SB, Byrd DR, Compton CC, et al., eds. Chapter 3: Lip and Oral Cavity. In: *AJCC Cancer Staging Manual.* 7th ed. New York: Springer; 2010:29-40.

El-Mofty SK. Histopathologic risk factors in oral and oropharyngeal squamous cell carcinoma variants: an update with special reference to HPV-related carcinomas. *Med Oral Patol Oral Cir Bucal.* 2014;19:e377-e385.

Haddad R, Annino D, Tishler RB. Multidisciplinary approach to cancer treatment: focus on head and neck cancer. *Dent Clin North Am.* 2008;52:1-17.

Huang SH, Hwang D, Lockwood G, et al. Predictive value of tumor thickness for cervical lymph-node involvement in squamous cell carcinoma of the oral cavity: a meta-analysis of reported studies. *Cancer.* 2009;115:1489-1497.

Li C, Woo S. Understanding the pathobiology of head and neck squamous cell carcinoma. *Curr Oral Health Rep.* 2014;1:196-203.

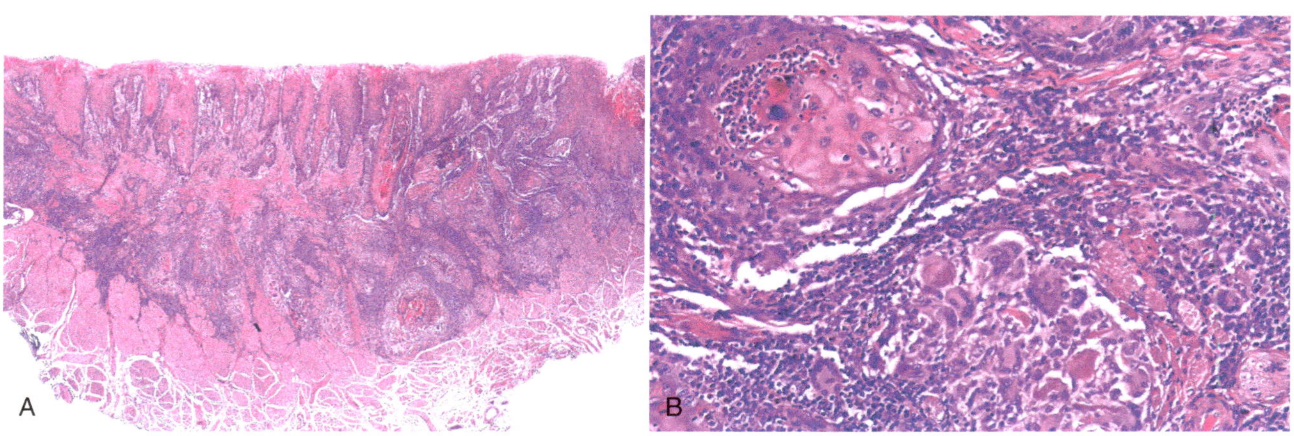

FIG 11.35 Keratinizing squamous cell carcinoma. (A) Tumor deeply infiltrates the tongue musculature. (B) Keratin pearl with intraepithelial microabscesses and foreign body reaction to keratin.

Martinez-Useros J, Garcia-Foncillas J. The challenge of blocking a wider family members of EGFR against head and neck squamous cell carcinomas. *Oral Oncol.* 2015;51:423-430.

Michikawa C, Uzawa N, Kayamori K, et al. Clinical significance of lymphatic and blood vessel invasion in oral tongue squamous cell carcinomas. *Oral Oncol.* 2012;48:320-324.

Pereira MC, Oliveira DT, Kowalski LP. The role of eosinophils and eosinophil cationic protein in oral cancer: a review. *Arch Oral Biol.* 2011;56:353-358.

Po Wing Yuen A, Lam KY, Lam LK, et al. Prognostic factors of clinically stage I and II oral tongue carcinoma—a comparative study of stage, thickness, shape, growth pattern, invasive front malignancy grading, Martinez-Gimeno score, and pathologic features. *Head Neck.* 2002;24:513-520.

Rogers SN, Brown JS, Woolgar JA, et al. Survival following primary surgery for oral cancer. *Oral Oncol.* 2009;45:201-211.

Roh J, Muelleman T, Tawfik O, Thomas SM. Perineural growth in head and neck squamous cell carcinoma: a review. *Oral Oncol.* 2015;51:16-23.

Rothenberg SM, Ellisen LW. The molecular pathogenesis of head and neck squamous cell carcinoma. *J Clin Invest.* 2012;122:1951-1957.

Scully C, Bagan J. Oral squamous cell carcinoma: overview of current understanding of aetiopathogenesis and clinical implications. *Oral Dis.* 2009;15:388-399.

Seiwert TY, Zuo Z, Keck MK, et al. Integrative and comparative genomic analysis of HPV-positive and HPV-negative head and neck squamous cell carcinomas. *Clin Cancer Res.* 2015;21:632-641.

Shah AA, Jeffus SK, Stelow EB. Squamous cell carcinoma variants of the upper aerodigestive tract: a comprehensive review with a focus on genetic alterations. *Arch Pathol Lab Med.* 2014;138:731-744.

Siegel RL, Miller KD, Jemal A. Cancer statistics, 2015. *CA Cancer J Clin.* 2015;65:5-29.

Torre LA, Bray F, Siegel RL, et al. Global cancer statistics, 2012. *CA Cancer J Clin.* 2015;65:87-108.

van Monsjou HS, Wreesmann VB, van den Brekel MW, Balm AJ. Head and neck squamous cell carcinoma in young patients. *Oral Oncol.* 2013;49:1097-1102.

Woolgar JA. Histopathological prognosticators in oral and oropharyngeal squamous cell carcinoma. *Oral Oncol.* 2006;42:229-239.

Yamauchi K, Kogashiwa Y, Nakamura T, et al. Diagnostic evaluation of sentinel lymph node biopsy in early head and neck squamous cell carcinoma: a meta-analysis. *Head Neck.* 2015;37:127-133.

Zhang L, Poh CF, Williams M, et al. Loss of heterozygosity (LOH) profiles—validated risk predictors for progression to oral cancer. *Cancer Prev Res (Phila).* 2012;5:1081-1089.

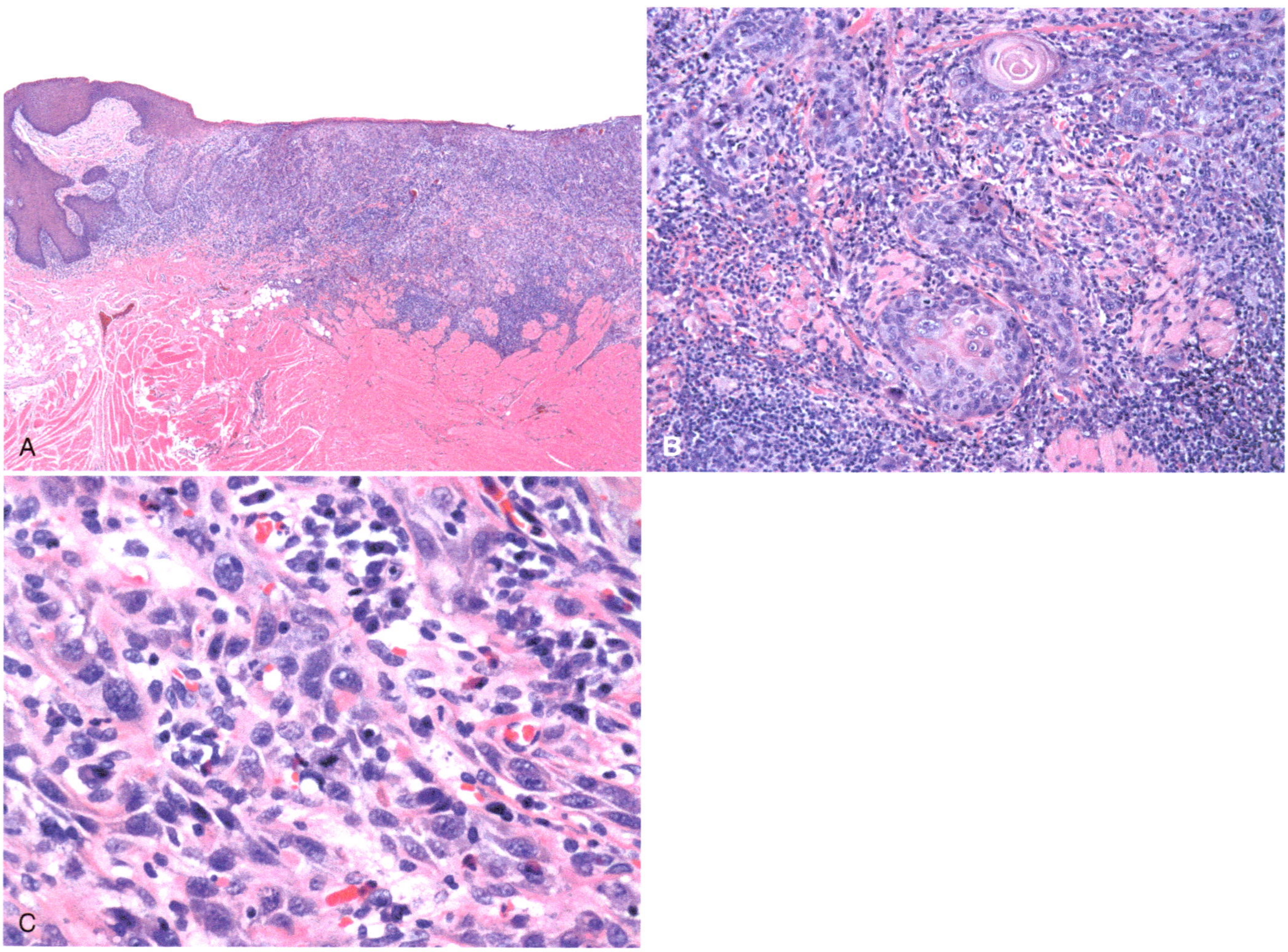

FIG 11.36 Minimally keratinizing squamous cell carcinoma. (A) The tumor infiltrates the skeletal muscle and there is a lymphocytic host response. (B) Tumor cells exhibit dyskeratosis and focal keratin pearl formation. (C) Tumor cells are less differentiated in this field and many eosinophils are present in the stroma and within tumor islands.

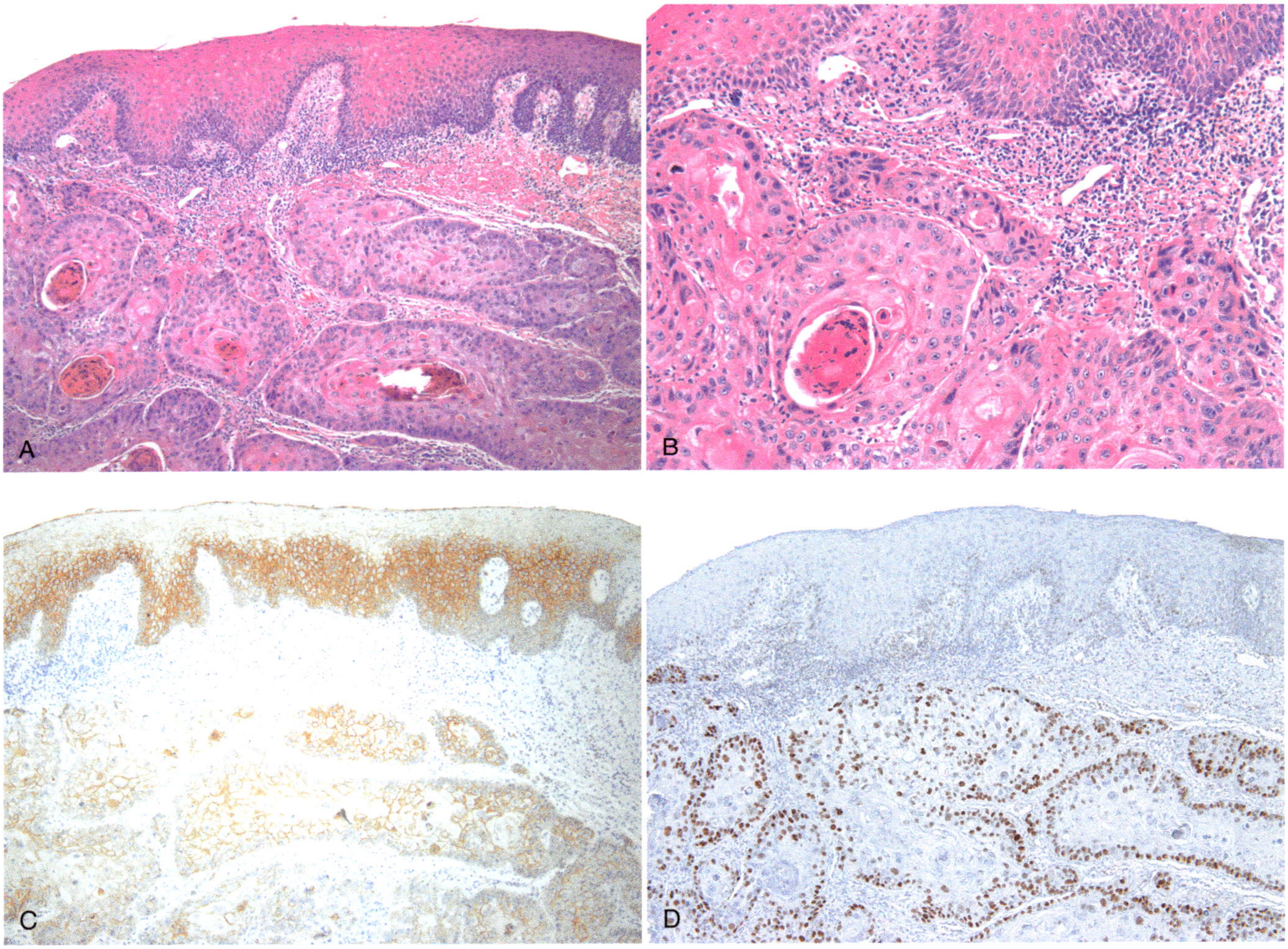

FIG 11.37 Keratinizing well-differentiated squamous cell carcinoma. (A) Tumor exhibits keratin pearl formation. (B) There is moderate pleomorphism and dyskeratosis. (C) The study for E-cadherin exhibits reduced membranous expression within the tumor cells. (D) The study for p53 is positive within the nuclei of tumor cells at the periphery of the tumor islands.

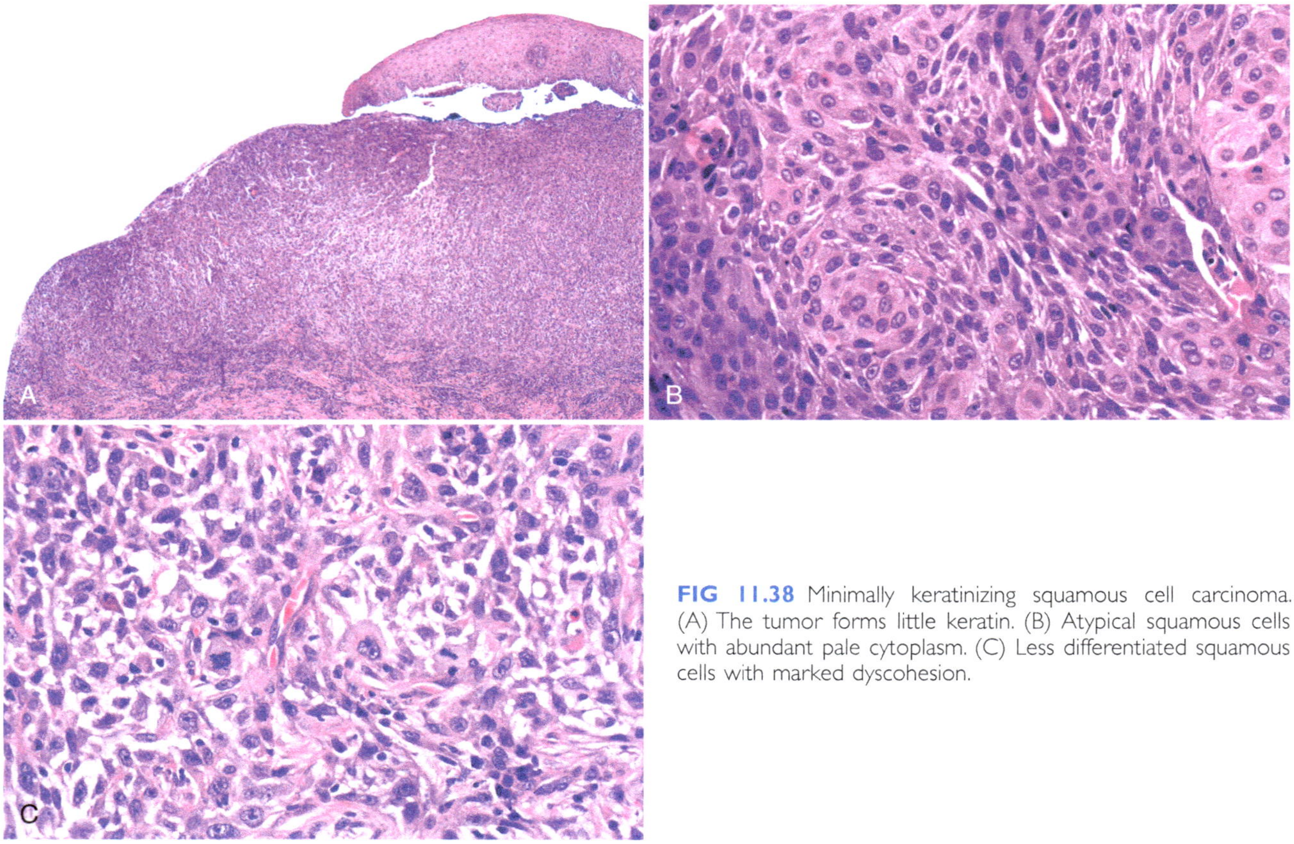

FIG 11.38 Minimally keratinizing squamous cell carcinoma. (A) The tumor forms little keratin. (B) Atypical squamous cells with abundant pale cytoplasm. (C) Less differentiated squamous cells with marked dyscohesion.

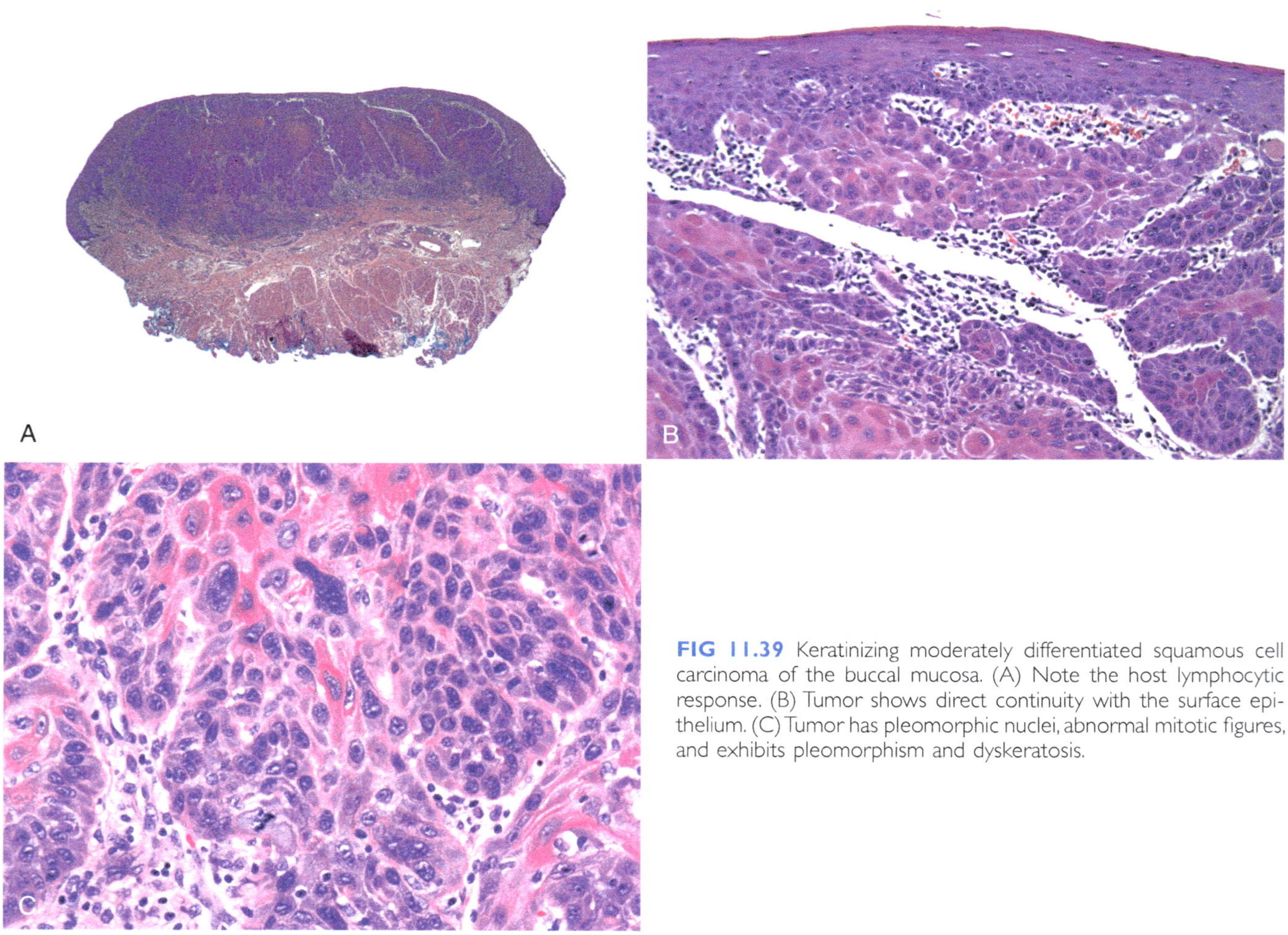

FIG 11.39 Keratinizing moderately differentiated squamous cell carcinoma of the buccal mucosa. (A) Note the host lymphocytic response. (B) Tumor shows direct continuity with the surface epithelium. (C) Tumor has pleomorphic nuclei, abnormal mitotic figures, and exhibits pleomorphism and dyskeratosis.

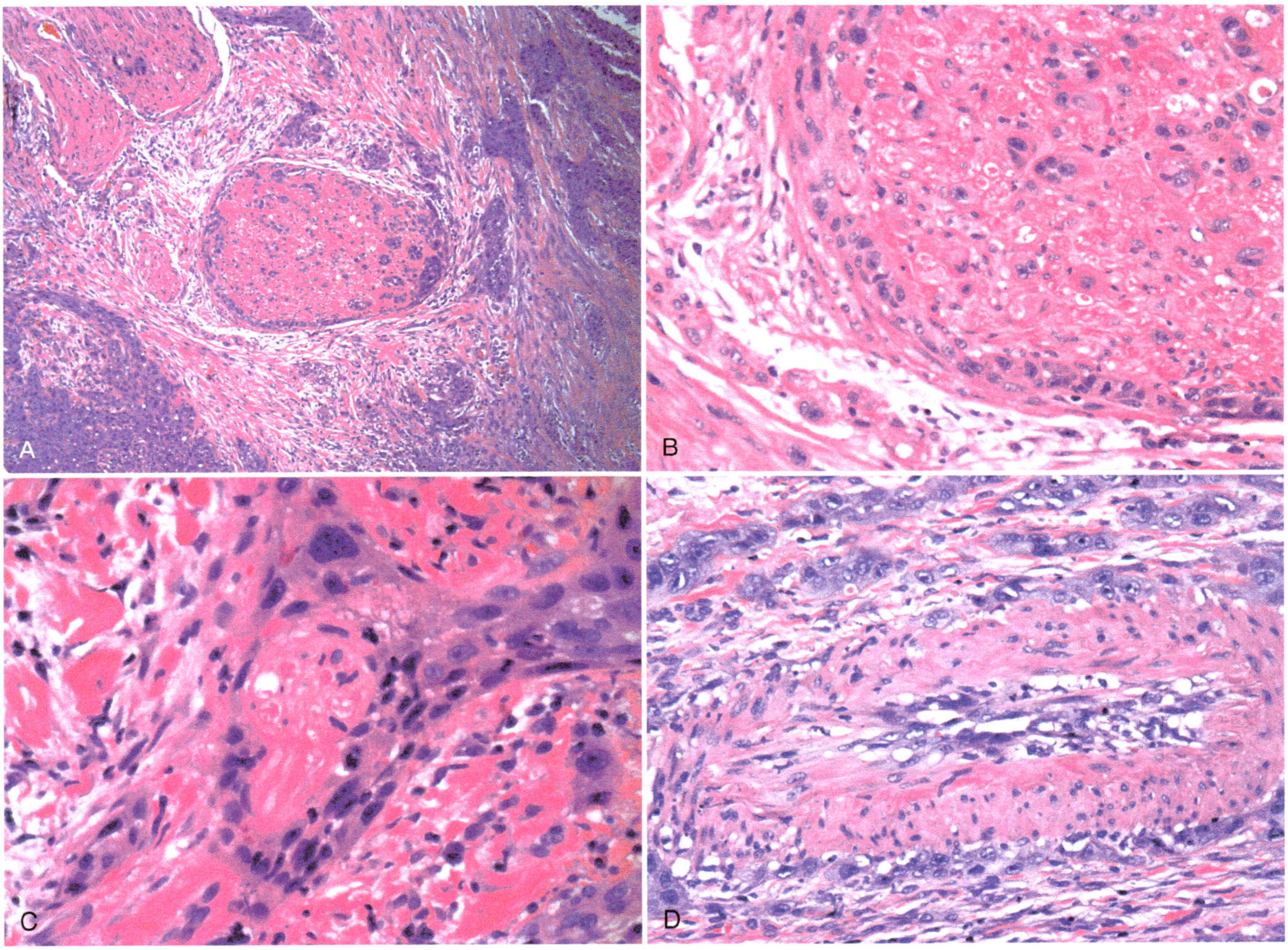

FIG 11.40 (A) Tumor exhibits peri- and intraneural invasion. (B) Tumor islands are present around and within this large nerve fiber. (C) Tumor exhibits perineural invasion. (D) Tumor cells infiltrate the wall of this vessel and are present within the lumen.

TABLE 11.2 Clinical Staging for Oral Cavity Lesions (Based on AJCC Cancer Staging Manual 2010)

Stage	T Stage	N Stage	M Stage
Stage 0	Tis	N0	M0
Stage I	T1	N0	M0
Stage II	T2	N0	M0
Stage III	T3	N0	M0
	T1	N1	M0
	T2	N1	M0
	T3	N1	M0
Stage IVA	T4a	N0	M0
	T4a	N1	M0
	T1	N2	M0
	T2	N2	N0
	T3	N2	M0
	T4a	N2	M0
Stage IVB	Any T	N3	M0
	T4b	Any N	M0
Stage IVC	Any T	Any N	M1

Tis: Carcinoma-in-situ
T1: Tumor ≤2 cm in greatest dimension
T2: Tumor >2 cm but ≤4 cm in greatest dimension
T3: Tumor >4 cm in greatest dimension
T4a: Moderately advanced disease
For lip: tumor invades through cortical bone, inferior alveolar nerve, floor of mouth, or skin of face (chin or nose)
For oral cavity: Tumor invades adjacent structures only (eg, into bone), into deep extrinsic muscles (eg, genioglossus, hyoglossus), maxillary sinus, skin of face
T4b: Very advanced local disease
Tumor invades masticator space, pterygoid plates, or skull case and/or encases internal carotid artery
N0: No regional node metastasis
N1: Metastasis to a single ipsilateral node, ≤3 cm in greatest dimension
N2a: Metastasis to a single ipsilateral node, >3 cm but ≤6 cm in greatest dimension
N2b: Metastases in multiple ipsilateral nodes ≤6 cm in greatest dimension
N2c: Metatases in bilateral or contralateral nodes ≤6 cm in greatest dimension
N3: Metastases in a lymph node >6 cm in greatest dimension
M0: No distant metastasis
M1: Distant metastasis

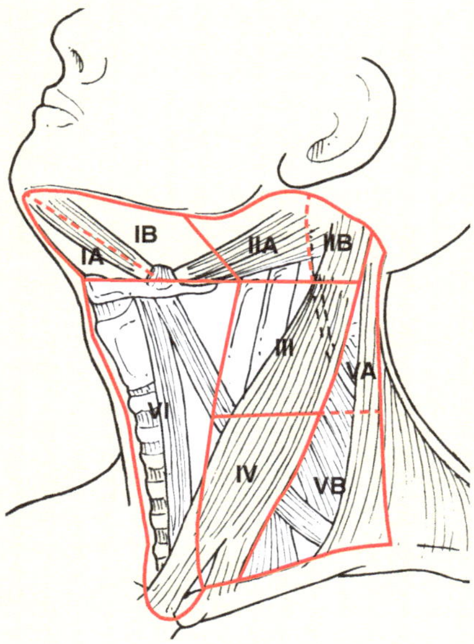

Pathologic staging (pTNM) from measurement of the unfixed tumor and evaluation of the microscopic pathology should also be reported.

VERRUCOUS CARCINOMA

This presents as a warty, exophytic lesion most commonly seen on the alveolar ridge mucosa, mandibular sulcus, or buccal mucosa, historically in patients who use smokeless tobacco but also in cigarette smokers (Fig. 11.41A). It must be borne in mind that all verrucous carcinomas began as small areas of leukoplakia or verrucous leukoplakia that histologically may have shown only hyperkeratosis or parakeratosis and verrucous epithelial hyperplasia in the beginning with minimal epithelial dysplasia. The difference between *verrucous hyperplasia* and *verrucous carcinoma* is that (1) verrucous hyperplasia is a mostly exophytic lesion whereas the latter also has an endophytic bluntly invasive component, (2) the degree of epithelial proliferation is more pronounced in verrucous carcinoma. This endophytic bluntly invasive pattern is the hallmark of this tumor and results in locally destructive disease but with little metastatic potential. One of the controversies in this diagnosis relates to what degree of epithelial atypia/dysplasia is acceptable for verrucous carcinoma before one uses the term "bluntly invasive papillary well-differentiated carcinoma." Loss of heterozygosity is frequently seen involving 3p, 4q, and 9p.

- There is a papillary exophytic and endophytic proliferation of squamous epithelium with marked parakeratosis and bulbous frondlike rete ridges with parakeratin plugging; hyperkeratosis is rarely prominent; these bulbous, frondlike rete ridges have smooth, rounded outlines and are present deep in the stroma on a broad, pushing front without single cell infiltration (blunt pattern of invasion); there is minimal cytologic atypia with mild basal cell hyperplasia and some mitotic activity but no anaplasia or marked pleomorphism; a lymphocytic host response is noted in at least half the cases and subbasal clefting may be seen at the interface (Figs. 11.42 and 11.43).

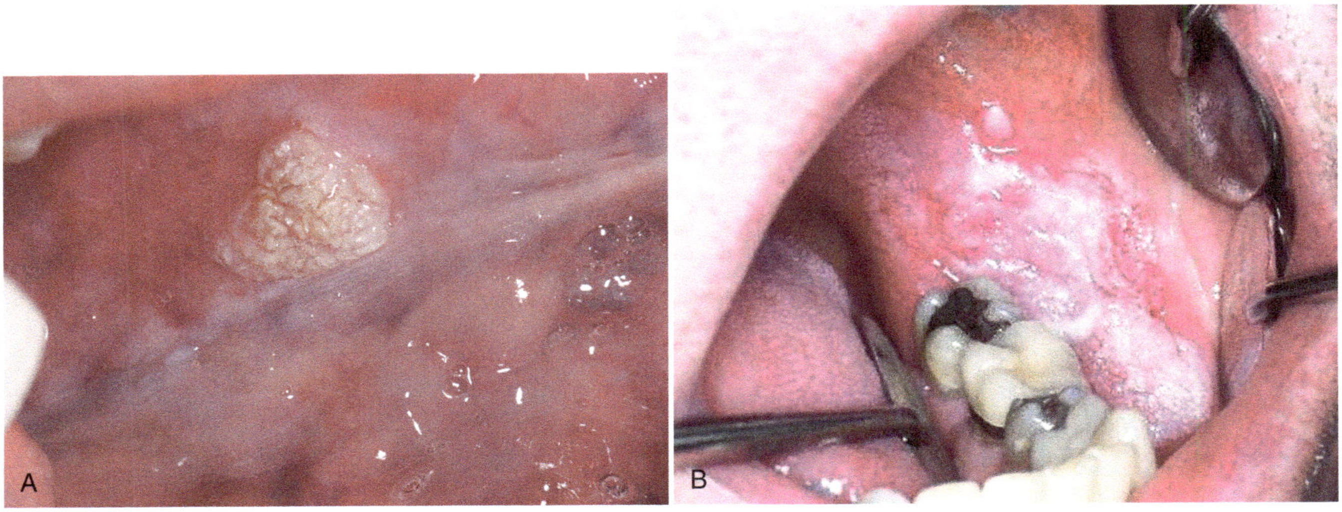

FIG 11.41 (A) Verrucous carcinoma presenting as a well-demarcated, rough, warty plaque on the ventral tongue. (B) Papillary squamous cell carcinoma of the buccal mucosa. *(A, Courtesy Dr. Dan Harris, private practice, Nashville, Tenn.)*

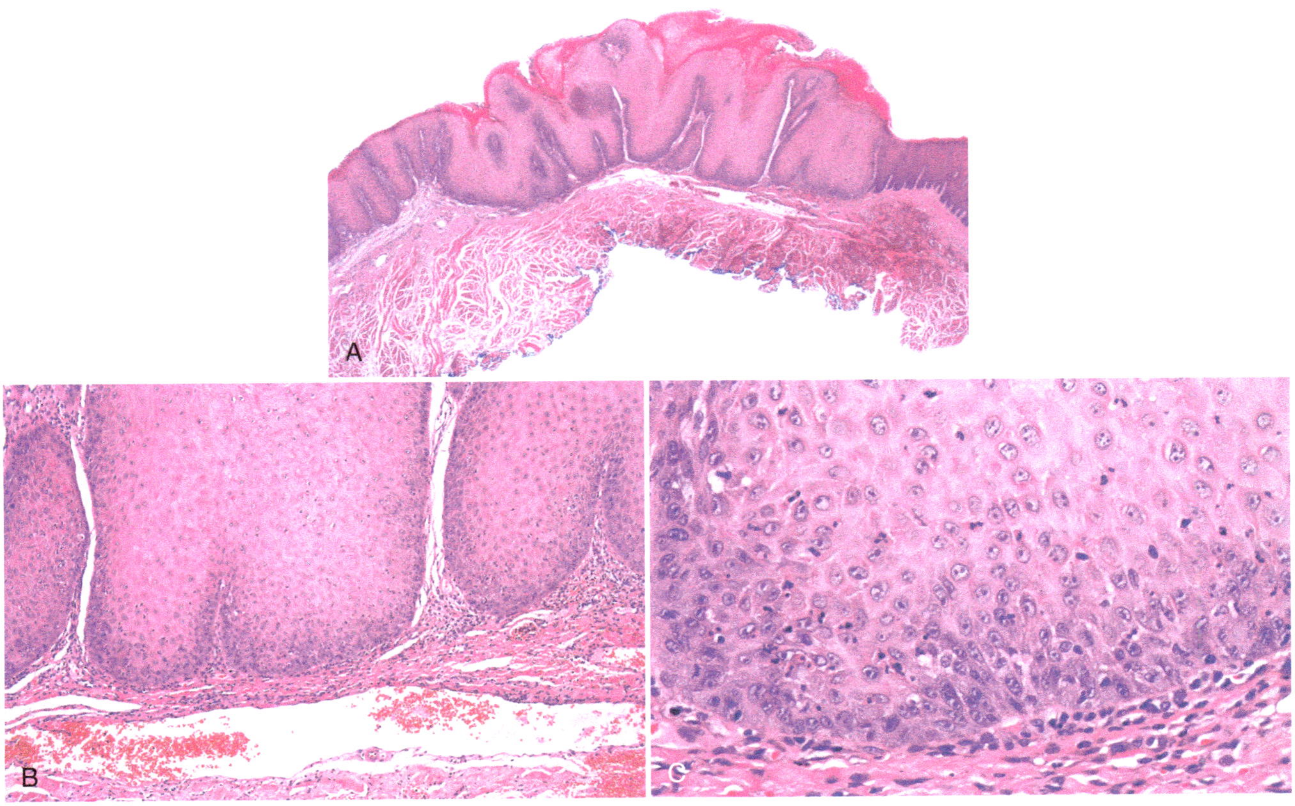

FIG 11.42 Verrucous carcinoma. (A) Exophytic and endophytic papillary proliferation of epithelium with parakeratin plugging and bulbous rete ridges; cells have pale cytoplasm, compared with normal mucosa. (B) Broad frondlike rete ridges with subepithelial cleft. (C) There is minimal cytologic atypia and cells have pale, glassy cytoplasm.

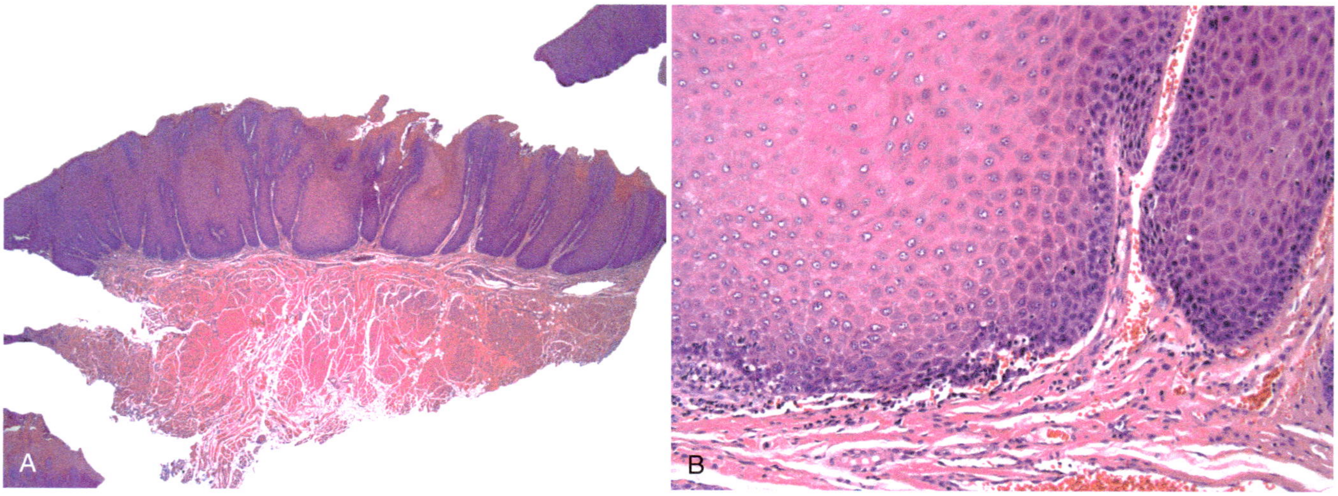

FIG 11.43 Verrucous carcinoma. (A) Bluntly invasive endophytic growth with parakeratin plugging, frondlike bulbous rete ridges; notice how closely the tumor lies to the skeletal muscle. (B) There is minimal cytologic atypia.

- A variant of this exists that has all the features of conventional verrucous carcinoma but in addition exhibits mild-to-moderate dysplasia but without infiltration of the stroma by small tumor islands or single cells; tumor cells are large with abundant cytoplasm, microabscesses often are noted at the tips of rete ridges and eosinophils often are noted within the deeply penetrating rete ridges; these have been referred to as verrucous carcinoma with mild dysplasia or papillary well-differentiated bluntly invasive squamous cell carcinoma (Figs. 11.44 and 11.45).
- Although some tumors harbor HPV, these are not usually the transcriptionally active high-risk type.
- Conventional squamous cell carcinoma may arise within verrucous carcinoma ("hybrid tumors") and these behave similarly to conventional squamous cell carcinoma (Fig. 11.46).
- β-Catenin is strongly expressed in a membranous fashion in verrucous carcinoma similar to normal epithelium, whereas this is lost in conventional squamous cell carcinoma; over-expression of c-*erb*B-3 protein has been correlated with increase in proliferative cell nuclear antigen labeling index as lesions progress from verrucous hyperplasia to verrucous carcinoma to squamous cell carcinoma.

Differential Diagnoses

- Giant condyloma acuminatum may appear similar, especially if traumatized and inflamed.

Management and Prognosis

- Wide excision is the treatment of choice and recurrence occurs in 6% of conventional verrucous carcinoma and in 19% of cases with dysplasia; the vast majority of tumors do not give rise to nodal metastases, even the ones with mild dysplasia; 5-year survival is 78% to 100% likely depending on diagnostic criteria. Tumors with concomitant squamous cell carcinoma show nodal metastases in 14% of cases and 36% die of disease.
- Radiation therapy alone is less successful than surgery and recurrence occurs in one-third of cases; anaplastic transformation is rare.

REFERENCES

del Pino M, Bleeker MC, Quint WG, et al. Comprehensive analysis of human papillomavirus prevalence and the potential role of low-risk types in verrucous carcinoma. *Mod Pathol.* 2012;25:1354-1363.

Devaney KO, Ferlito A, Rinaldo A, et al. Verrucous carcinoma (carcinoma cuniculatum) of the head and neck: what do we know now that we did not know a decade ago? *Eur Arch Otorhinolaryngol.* 2011;268:477-480.

Ferlito A, Devaney KO, Rinaldo A, Putzi MJ. Papillary squamous cell carcinoma versus verrucous squamous cell carcinoma of the head and neck. *Ann Otol Rhinol Laryngol.* 1999;108:318-322.

Huang SH, Lockwood G, Irish J, et al. Truths and myths about radiotherapy for verrucous carcinoma of larynx. *Int J Radiat Oncol Biol Phys.* 2009;73:1110-1115.

Koch BB, Trask DK, Hoffman HT, et al. National survey of head and neck verrucous carcinoma: patterns of presentation, care, and outcome. *Cancer.* 2001;92:110-1120.

Laxmidevi LB, Angadi PV, Pillai RK, Chandreshekar C. Aberrant beta-catenin expression in the histologic differentiation of oral squamous cell carcinoma and verrucous carcinoma: an immunohistochemical study. *J Oral Sci.* 2010;52:633-640.

McCoy JM, Waldron CA. Verrucous carcinoma of the oral cavity. *Oral Surg Oral Med Oral Pathol.* 1981;52:623-629.

Oliveira DT, de Moraes RV, Fiamengui Filho JF, et al. Oral verrucous carcinoma: a retrospective study in Sao Paulo Region, Brazil. *Clin Oral Investig.* 2006;10:205-209.

Patel KR, Chernock RD, Sinha P, et al. Verrucous carcinoma with dysplasia or minimal invasion: a variant of verrucous carcinoma with extremely favorable prognosis. *Head Neck Pathol.* 2015;9:65-73.

Patel KR, Chernock RD, Zhang TR, et al. Verrucous carcinomas of the head and neck, including those with associated squamous cell carcinoma, lack transcriptionally active high-risk human papillomavirus. *Hum Pathol.* 2013;44:2385-2392.

Poh CF, Zhang L, Lam WL, et al. A high frequency of allelic loss in oral verrucous lesions may explain malignant risk. *Lab Invest.* 2001;81:629-634.

Sakurai K, Urade M, Takahashi Y, et al. Increased expression of c-erbB-3 protein and proliferating cell nuclear antigen during development of verrucous carcinoma of the oral mucosa. *Cancer.* 2000;89:2597-2605.

Walvekar RR, Chaukar DA, Deshpande MS, et al. Verrucous carcinoma of the oral cavity: A clinical and pathological study of 101 cases. *Oral Oncol.* 2009;45:47-51.

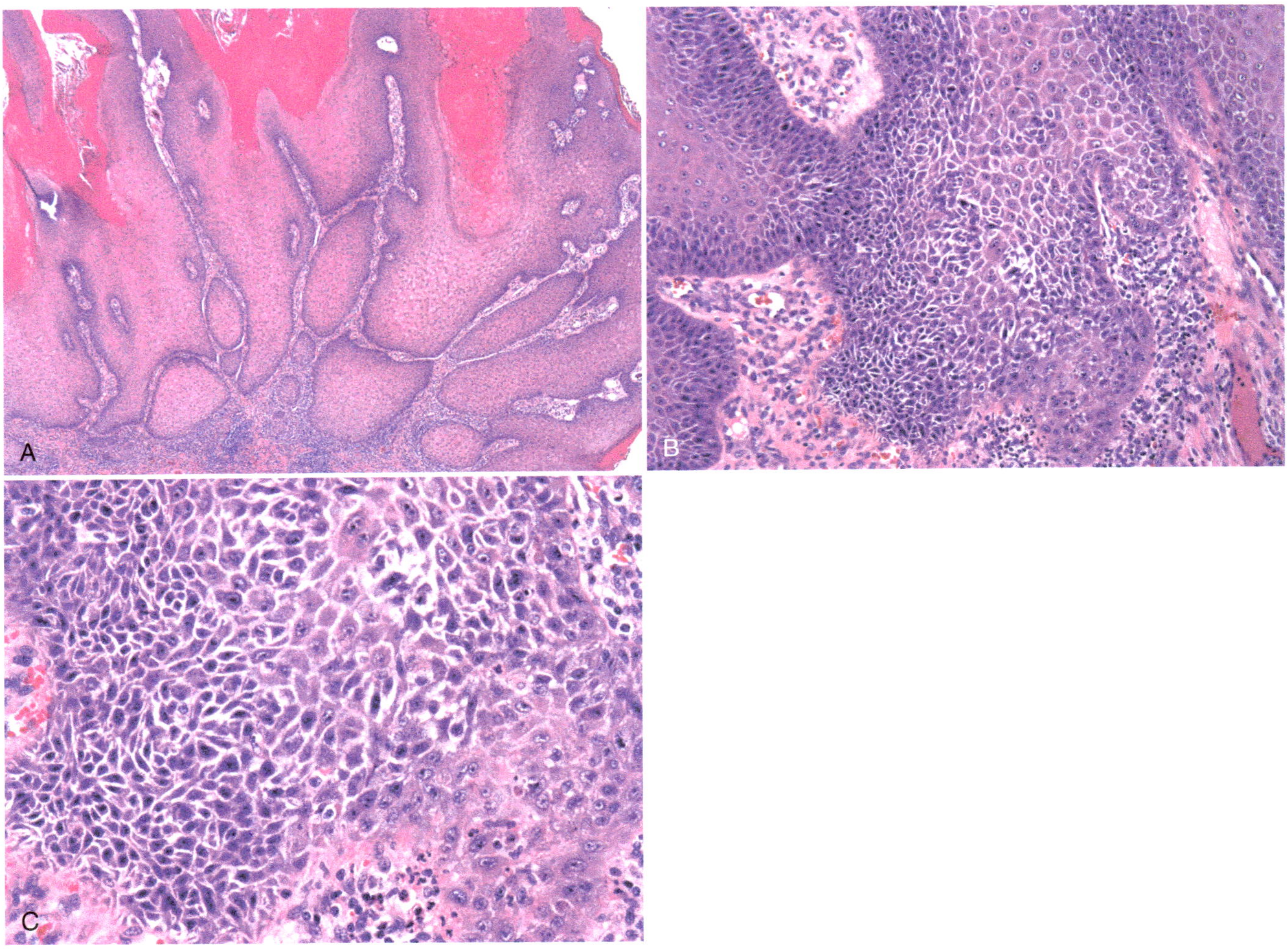

FIG 11.44 Verrucous carcinoma with dysplasia versus bluntly invasive papillary well-differentiated squamous cell carcinoma. (A) Bulky verrucous epithelial proliferation with marked parakeratosis, parakeratin plugging, and pale cells with glassy cytoplasm. (B) There is hyperchromasia and moderate cytologic atypia at the base of rete ridges. (C) There is basal cell hyperplasia, nuclear hyperchromasia, pleomorphism, and dyscohesion.

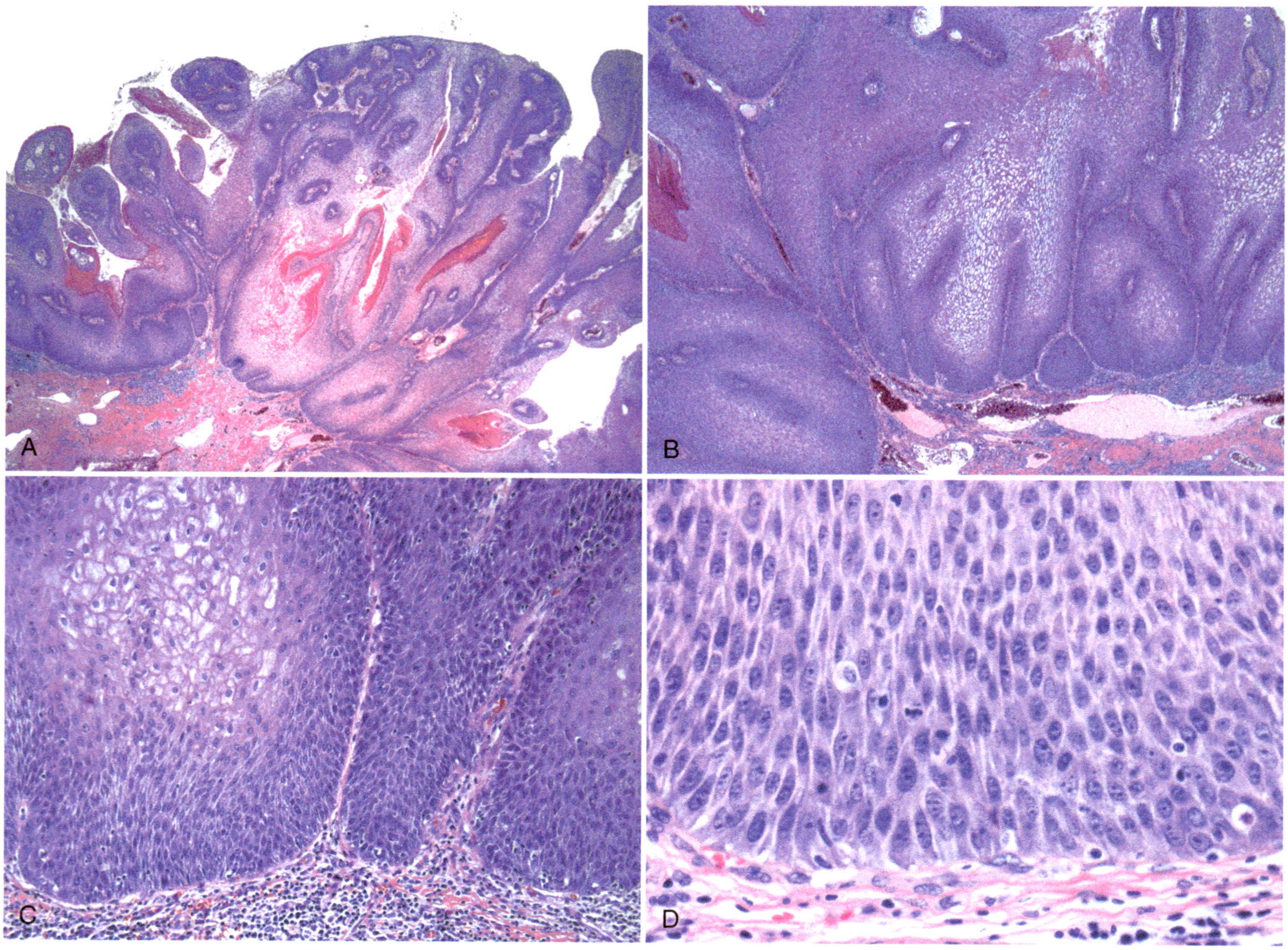

FIG 11.45 Verrucous carcinoma with dysplasia versus bluntly invasive papillary well-differentiated squamous cell carcinoma. (A) Papillary squamous proliferation forming bulbous rete ridges. (B) Deep epithelial extensions form bulbous rete ridges with hypercellularity and hyperchromasia. (C) There is moderate atypia characterized by basal cell hyperplasia but well-differentiated squamous cells are also noted. (D) Basal cell hyperplasia and mitotic figures are present.

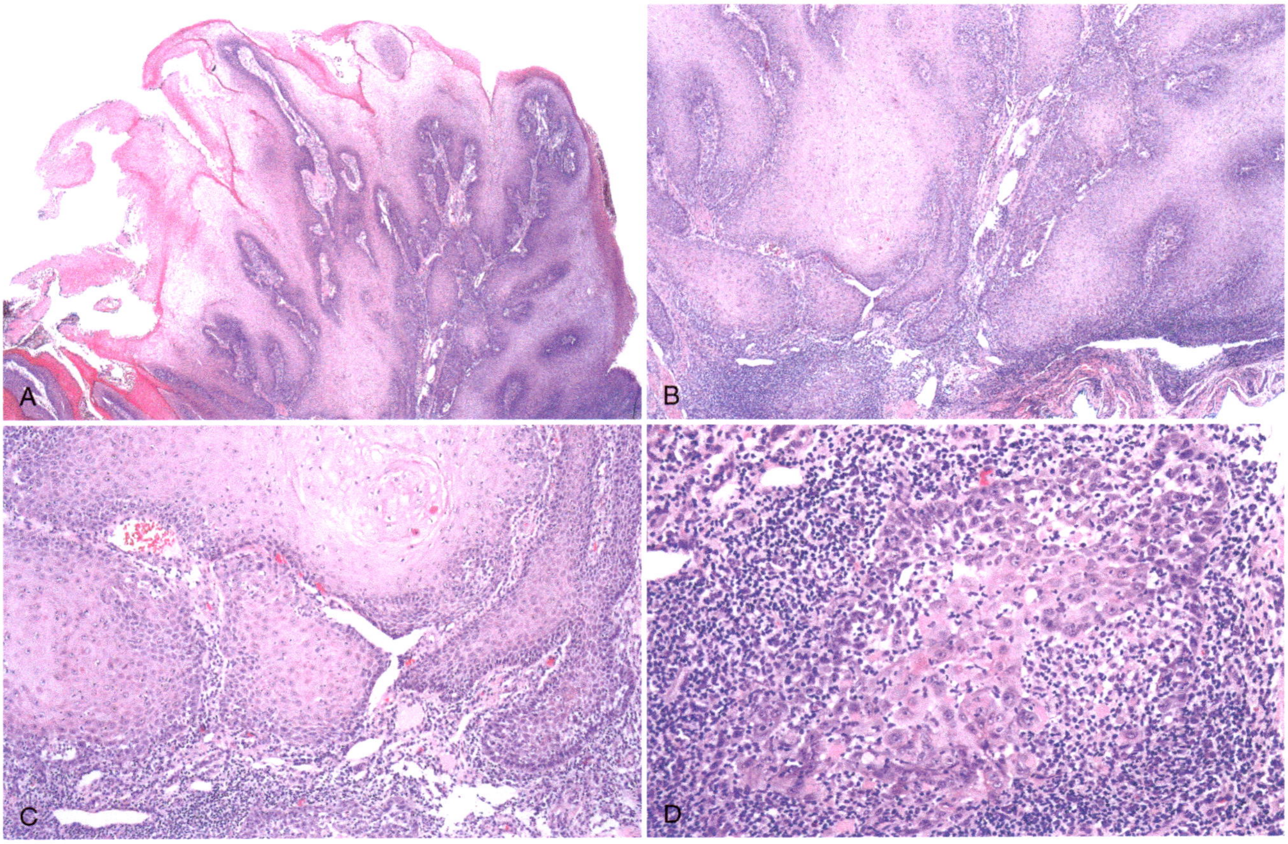

FIG 11.46 Verrucous carcinoma with focus of infiltrating squamous cell carcinoma versus papillary well-differentiated squamous cell carcinoma. (A) Low-power view bears resemblance to verrucous carcinoma with parakeratosis, bulbous rete ridges, and endophytic proliferation of pale epithelial cells. (B) Rete ridges are frond-like and cells are pale with glassy cytoplasm. (C) Base of rete ridges shows early keratin pearl formation and hyperchromasia with crowding of cells, and there is slight blurring of the epithelial–connective tissue interface. (D) One focus of atypical cells exhibits early microinvasive squamous cell carcinoma.

PAPILLARY SQUAMOUS CELL CARCINOMA

There are two forms of papillary squamous cell carcinoma, one that is more common in the oropharynx (including the palatine tonsil and base of tongue) and larynx, while the other, a less well-defined tumor, arises in the anterior oral cavity presenting as a warty mass that may or may not be keratotic (see Fig. 11.41B).

- Laryngeal and oropharyngeal papillary carcinoma: there is a papillary exophytic proliferation of squamous epithelium with in-situ full thickness dysplasia of the generally thin epithelium with approximately 40% of cases exhibiting stromal invasion; the exophytic component resembles a large, sessile papilloma with carcinoma-in-situ (Fig. 11.47); 68% to 76% are nonkeratinized; 34% to 75% are p16+ and approximately 50% are positive for HPV, even those that are p16–.
- Anterior oral cavity papillary carcinoma: these show an exophytic and endophytic squamous proliferation with variable amounts of keratin and cytologic atypia; often there are keratin pearls and microabscesses at the tips of rete ridges (Figs. 11.48 and 11.49).

Differential Diagnoses

- Verrucous carcinoma exhibits parakeratosis, bulbous frondlike rete ridges and insignificant to minimal epithelial atypia without blurring of the epithelium–connective tissue interface.
- Cuniculate carcinoma usually has a smooth rather than warty surface and complex, arborizing keratin-filled burrows in the connective tissue.

Prognosis

- In the laryngeal and oropharyngeal tumors, one-third exhibit recurrence, 16% to 31% exhibit nodal metastases, 3% distant metastases, and 20% died of their disease.

REFERENCES

Argyris PP, Kademani D, Pambuccian SE, et al. Comparison between p16 INK4A immunohistochemistry and human papillomavirus polymerase chain reaction assay in oral papillary squamous cell carcinoma. *J Oral Maxillofac Surg.* 2013;71:1676-1682.

Cobo F, Talavera P, Concha A. Review article: relationship of human papillomavirus with papillary squamous cell carcinoma of the upper aerodigestive tract: a review. *Int J Surg Pathol.* 2008;16:127-136.

Jo VY, Mills SE, Stoler MH, Stelow EB. Papillary squamous cell carcinoma of the head and neck: frequent association with human papillomavirus infection and invasive carcinoma. *Am J Surg Pathol.* 2009;33:1720-1724.

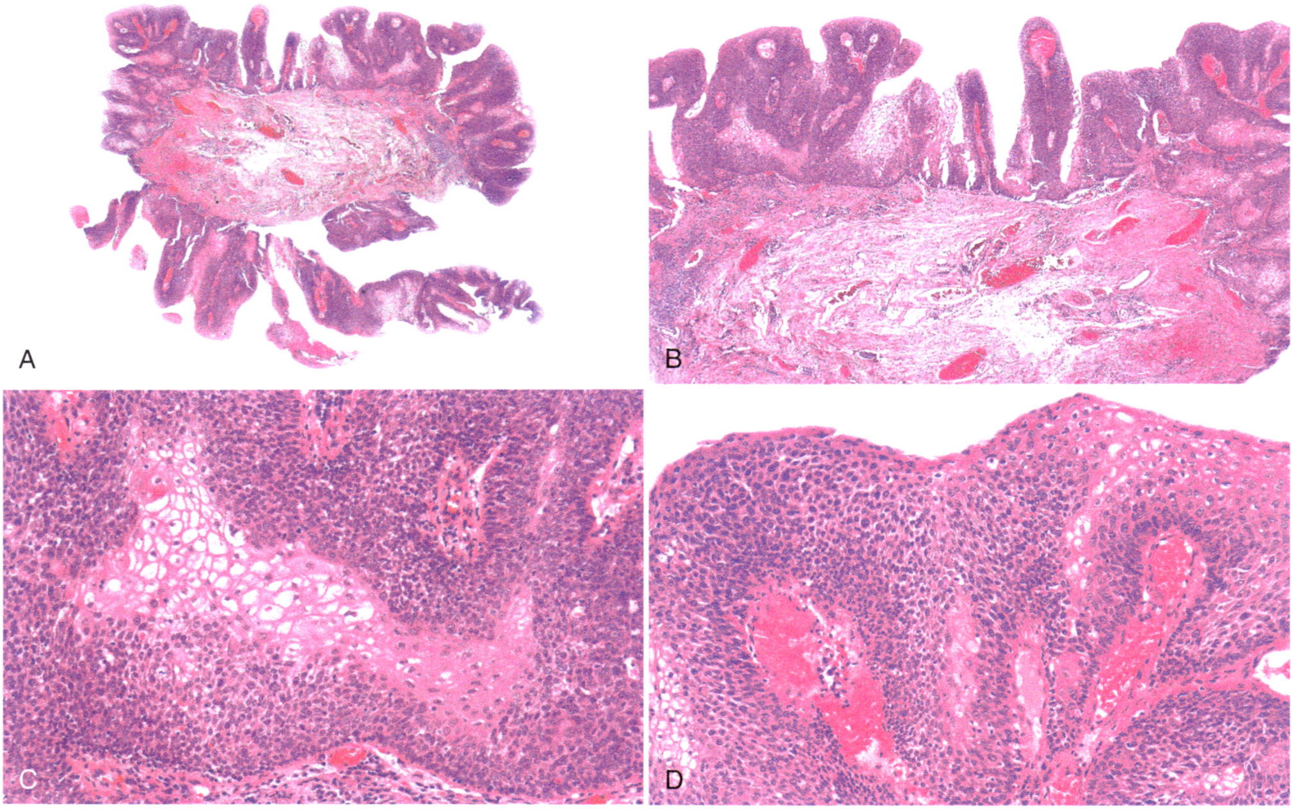

FIG 11.47 Oral papillary squamous cell carcinoma. (A) Broad-based papillary proliferation of dysplastic epithelium without surface keratin. (B) Papillary carcinoma-in-situ with insignificant surface keratin. (C) Dysplastic keratinocytes with foci of squamous cells. (D) Carcinoma-in-situ.

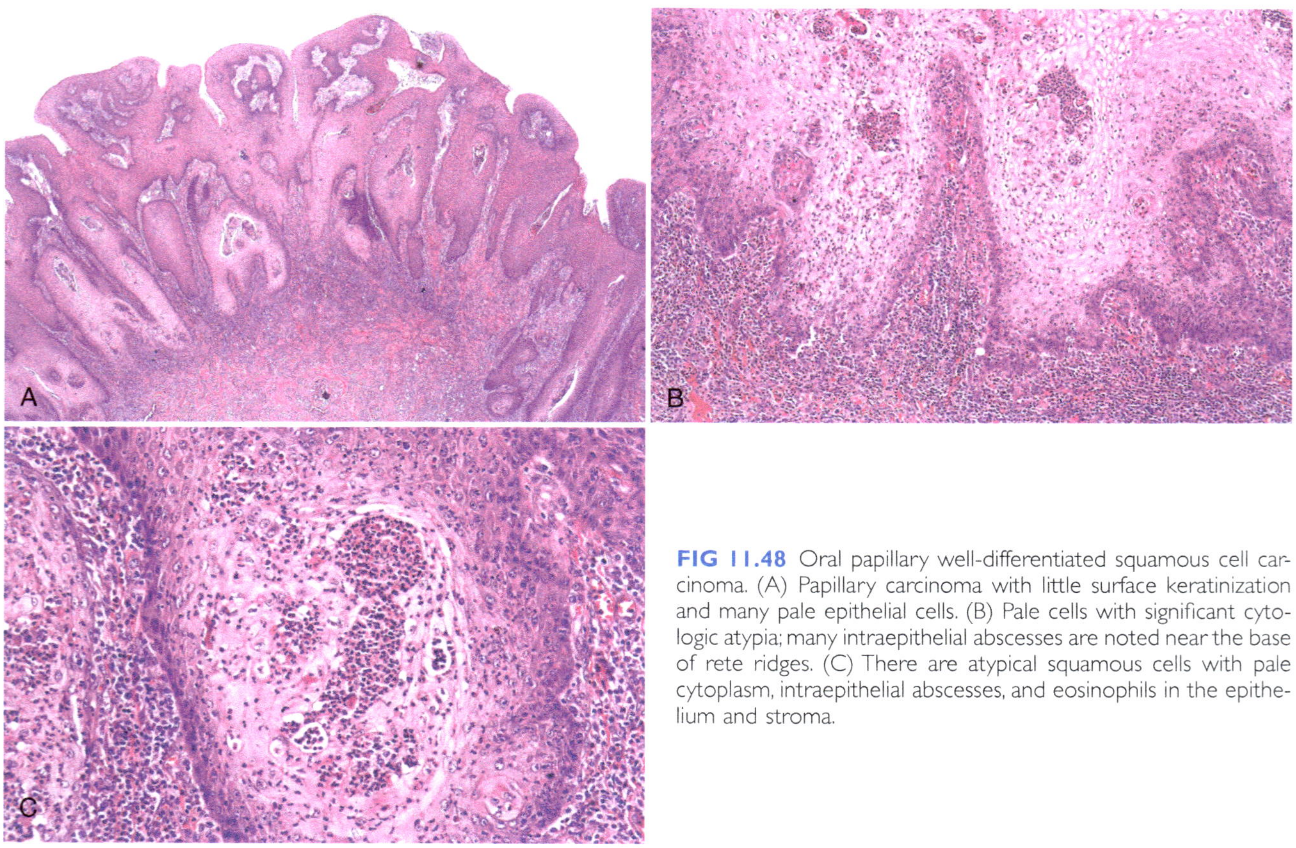

FIG 11.48 Oral papillary well-differentiated squamous cell carcinoma. (A) Papillary carcinoma with little surface keratinization and many pale epithelial cells. (B) Pale cells with significant cytologic atypia; many intraepithelial abscesses are noted near the base of rete ridges. (C) There are atypical squamous cells with pale cytoplasm, intraepithelial abscesses, and eosinophils in the epithelium and stroma.

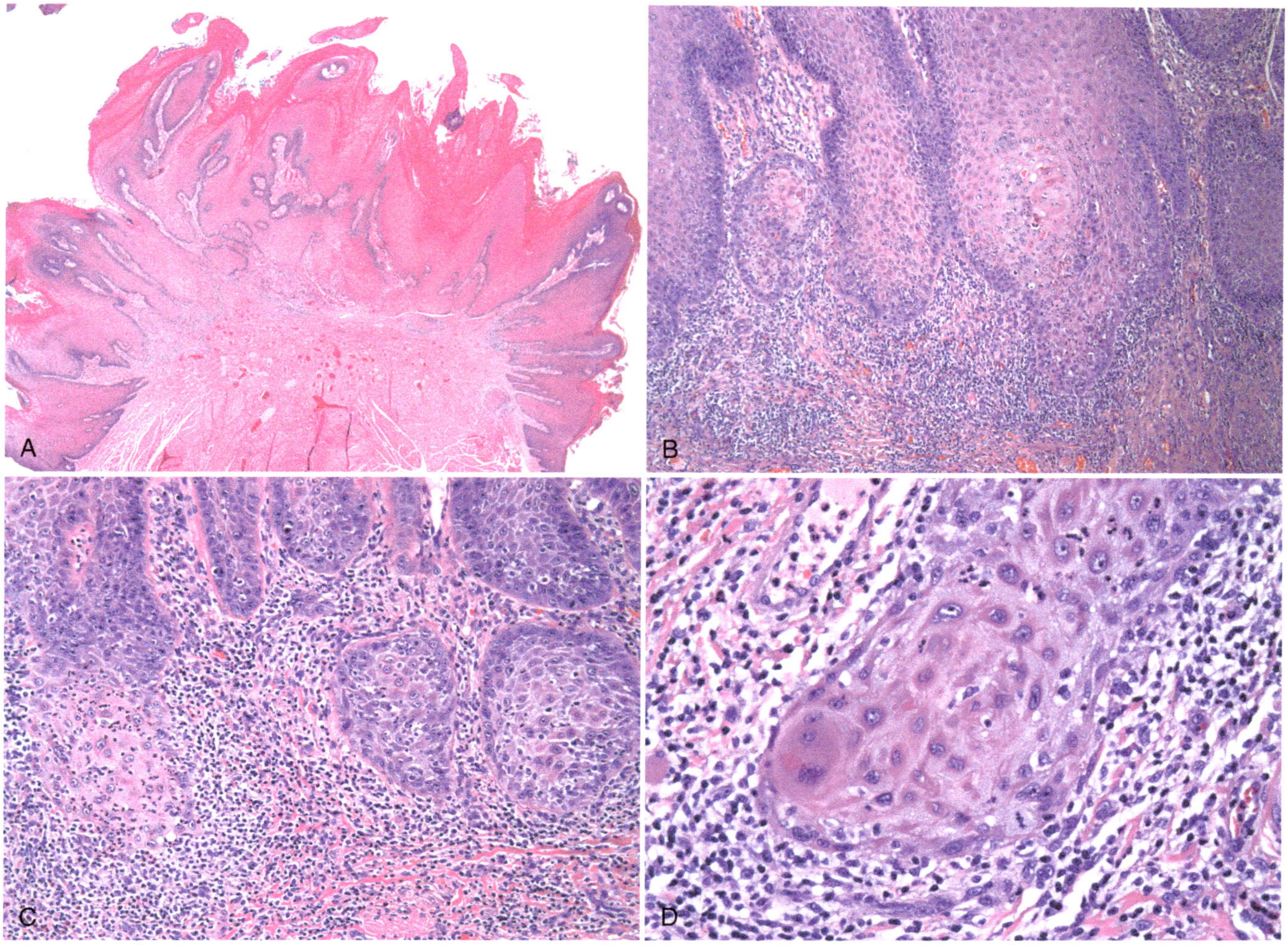

FIG 11.49 Papillary well-differentiated squamous cell carcinoma with stromal invasion. (A) Mostly exophytic papillary proliferation of squamous epithelium. (B) Tips of rete ridges show hypercellularity, dyskeratosis, and host lymphocytic response. (C) Some tumor islands are well demarcated from stroma, but there is blurring of the interface at some tips of rete ridges (*left*). (D) Keratin pearl at the tips of rete ridges often herald conventional invasion.

Mehrad M, Carpenter DH, Chernock RD, et al. Papillary squamous cell carcinoma of the head and neck: clinicopathologic and molecular features with special reference to human papillomavirus. *Am J Surg Pathol.* 2013;37:1349-1356.

Suarez PA, Adler-Storthz K, Luna MA, et al. Papillary squamous cell carcinomas of the upper aerodigestive tract: a clinicopathologic and molecular study. *Head Neck.* 2000;22:360-368.

Thompson LD, Wenig BM, Heffner DK, Gnepp DR. Exophytic and papillary squamous cell carcinomas of the larynx: a clinicopathologic series of 104 cases. *Otolaryngol Head Neck Surg.* 1999;120:718-724.

SARCOMATOID SQUAMOUS CELL CARCINOMA

Sarcomatoid squamous cell carcinoma is the most common spindle cell malignancy in the oral cavity and also occurs frequently in the larynx. This tumor frequently affects the buccal mucosa and vestibule, tongue, and alveolar mucosa; 90% of cases are polypoid and ulcerated (Fig. 11.50A); the tumor may be associated with a history of radiation in up to 10% of cases (see Fig. 11.50B).

- This is a biphasic polypoid tumor with both squamous epithelial and spindle cell/sarcomatoid elements; there is a proliferation of stellate-shaped and spindle cells with a fasciculated or storiform pattern; these tumor cells are generally pleomorphic or anaplastic with hyperchromatic nuclei, and mitotic figures frequently are encountered; this spindle cell population is often seen transitioning from a conventional keratinizing squamous cell carcinoma that is usually present at the edges of the tumor, and there is overlying epithelial dysplasia; osseous and cartilaginous metaplasia is present in <10% of cases (Figs. 11.51–11.53A–E).
- Spindle cells are positive for keratin (especially AE1/3, K6 and K14), epithelial membrane antigen (EMA), vimentin, smooth muscle actin (SMA), and p63, and negative for S-100 protein; keratin markers tend to be negative in the spindle cells, which are often p63+ (see Fig. 11.53F); a small percentage of lesions are negative for keratin, and differentiation from a true sarcoma (especially postradiation sarcoma) is difficult; EGF receptors are expressed only in 40% of spindle cells, as compared with >90% of cells in conventional squamous cell carcinoma.

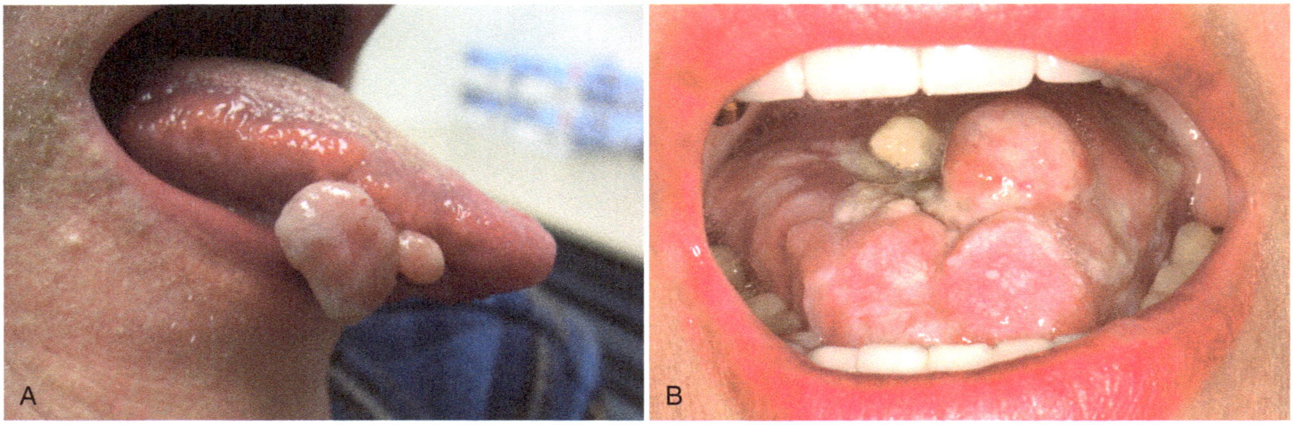

FIG 11.50 (A) Sarcomatoid squamous cell carcinoma of right tongue manifesting as a polypoid mass. (B) Sarcomatoid squamous cell carcinoma: tumor of the tongue dorsum in a patient previously irradiated for a squamous cell carcinoma of the left tongue. *(A, Courtesy Division of Dermatology, Brigham and Women's Hospital, Boston.)*

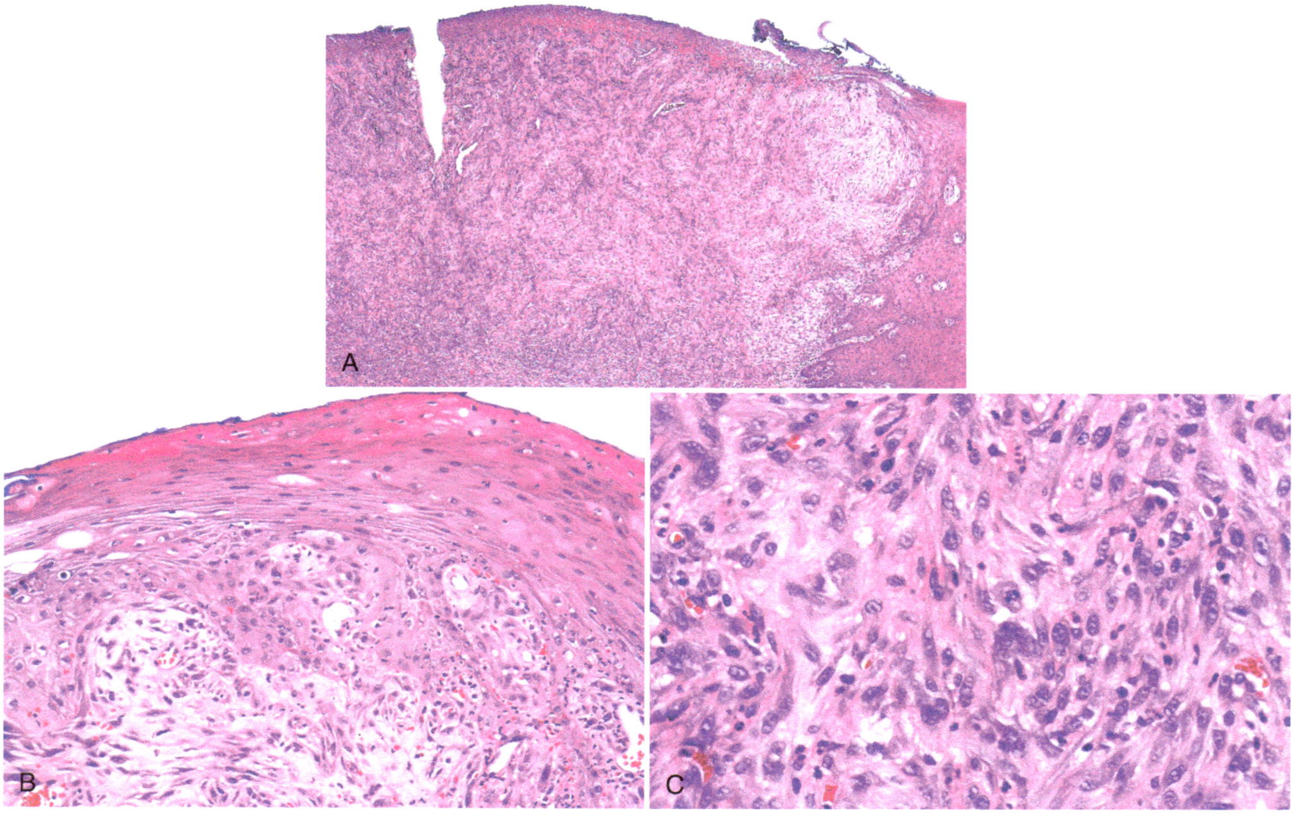

FIG 11.51 Sarcomatoid squamous cell carcinoma. (A) Spindle cell proliferation in short fascicles with storiform pattern, ulcerated. (B) Interface of invasive spindle cells and dysplastic surface epithelium. (C) Epithelioid and spindle cells with pleomorphic nuclei.

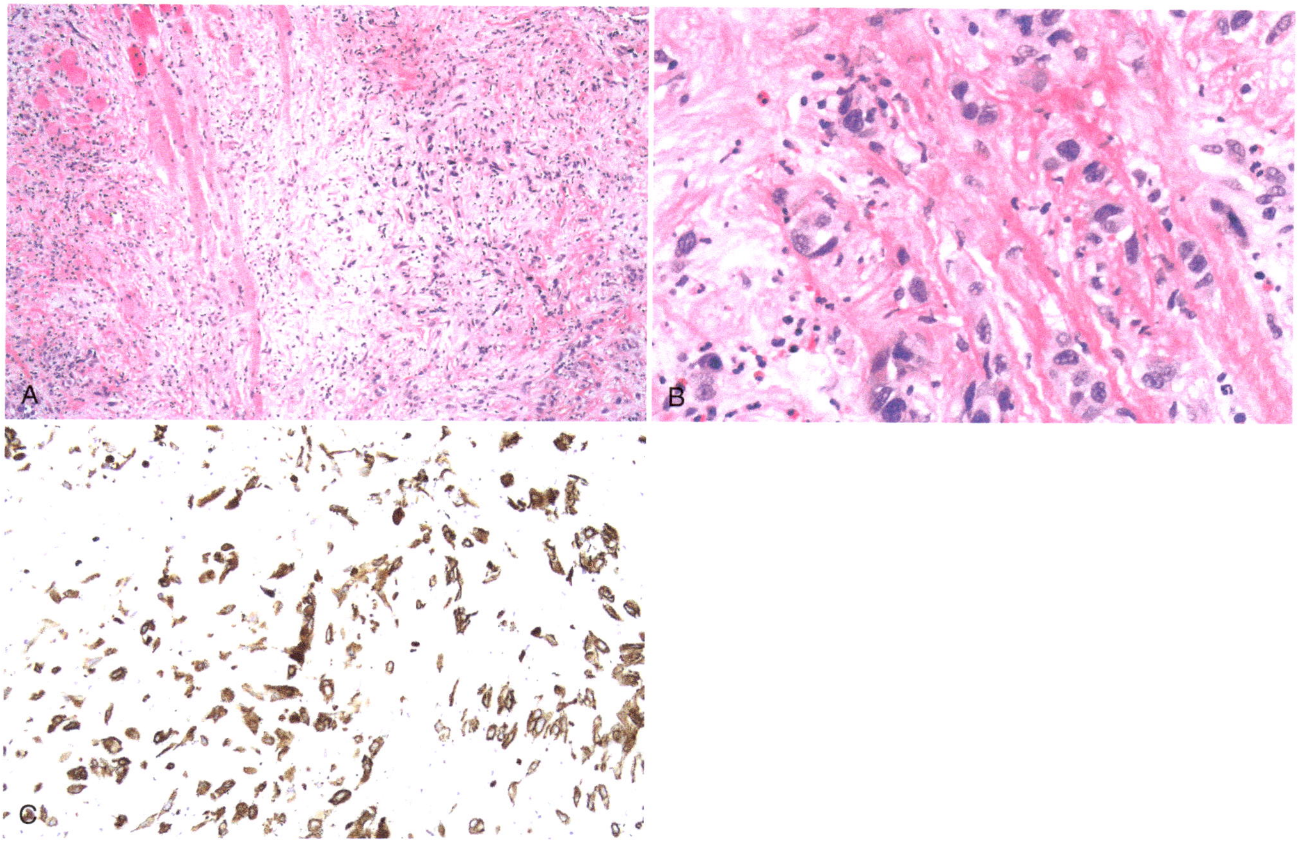

FIG 11.52 Sarcomatoid squamous cell carcinoma (from the patient in Fig. 11.50B). (A) Stellate-shaped and spindle cells infiltrating muscle. (B) Pleomorphic epithelioid cells. (C) Positivity for pankeratin within epithelioid and spindle cells.

Differential Diagnoses

- Nodular fasciitis has a "feathery" or tissue culture pattern with myxoid or edematous stroma, cells do not show significant atypia, and spindle cells are keratin-negative and SMA-positive (see Chapter 6).
- Desmoplastic melanoma is S-100- and SOX10+, may be HMB-45- and Melan-A-negative, and is keratin-negative.
- Spindle cell mesenchymal neoplasms will not have a conventional squamous cell carcinoma with keratin and vimentin-positive cells; myoepithelial carcinomas are positive for S-100 protein and calponin.
- Fibroblasts with radiation-induced atypia do not contain keratin and neither does radiation-induced fibrosarcoma; vessels in the irradiated field exhibit swollen endothelial cells and thickened intima (Fig. 11.54A–B).

Prognosis

- Recurrence occurs in 20% to 45% of cases and 20% develop nodal metastases; 5-year survival is 40%, with oral cavity and oropharyngeal lesions having a worse prognosis; some studies show that polypoid lesions have better prognosis compared with deeply infiltrating lesions.

REFERENCES

Bice TC, Tran V, Merkley MA, et al. Disease-specific survival with spindle cell carcinoma of the head and neck. *Otolaryngol Head Neck Surg.* 2015;153:973-980.

Chen YW, Tu HF, Wu TH, et al. Sarcomas and sarcomatoid tumor after radiotherapy of oral squamous cell carcinoma: analysis of 4 cases. *Oral Surg Oral Med Oral Pathol Oral Radiol Endod.* 2008;105:65-71.

Choi HR, Sturgis EM, Rosenthal DI, et al. Sarcomatoid carcinoma of the head and neck: molecular evidence for evolution and progression from conventional squamous cell carcinomas. *Am J Surg Pathol.* 2003; 27:1216-1220.

Ellis GL, Corio RL. Spindle cell carcinoma of the oral cavity. *Oral Surg Oral Med Oral Pathol.* 1980;50:523-534.

Ellis GL, Langloss JM, Heffner DK, Hyams VJ. Spindle-cell carcinoma of the aerodigestive tract. *Am J Surg Pathol.* 1987;11:335-342.

Lewis JS, Ritter JH, El-Mofty S. Alternative epithelial markers in sarcomatoid carcinomas of the head and neck, lung, and bladder-p63, MOC-31, and TTF-1. *Mod Pathol.* 2005;18:1471-1481.

Romanach MJ, Azevedo RS, Carlos R, de Almeida OP, Pires FR. Clinicopathological and immunohistochemical features of oral spindle cell carcinoma. *J Oral Pathol Med.* 2010;39:335-341.

Su HH, Chu ST, Hou YY, et al. Spindle cell carcinoma of the oral cavity and oropharynx: factors affecting outcome. *J Chin Med Assoc.* 2006; 69:478-483.

Thompson LD, Wieneke JA, Miettinen M, Heffner DK. Spindle cell (sarcomatoid) carcinomas of the larynx: a clinicopathologic study of 187 cases. *Am J Surg Pathol.* 2002;26:153-170.

Viswanathan S, Rahman K, Pallavi S, et al. Sarcomatoid (spindle cell) carcinoma of the head and neck mucosal region: a clinicopathologic review of 103 cases from a tertiary referral cancer centre. *Head Neck Pathol.* 2010;4:265-275.

Watson RF, Chernock RD, Zhang KH, et al. Epidermal growth factor receptor expression in spindle cell carcinomas of the head and neck. *Head Neck Pathol.* 2015;9:360-368.

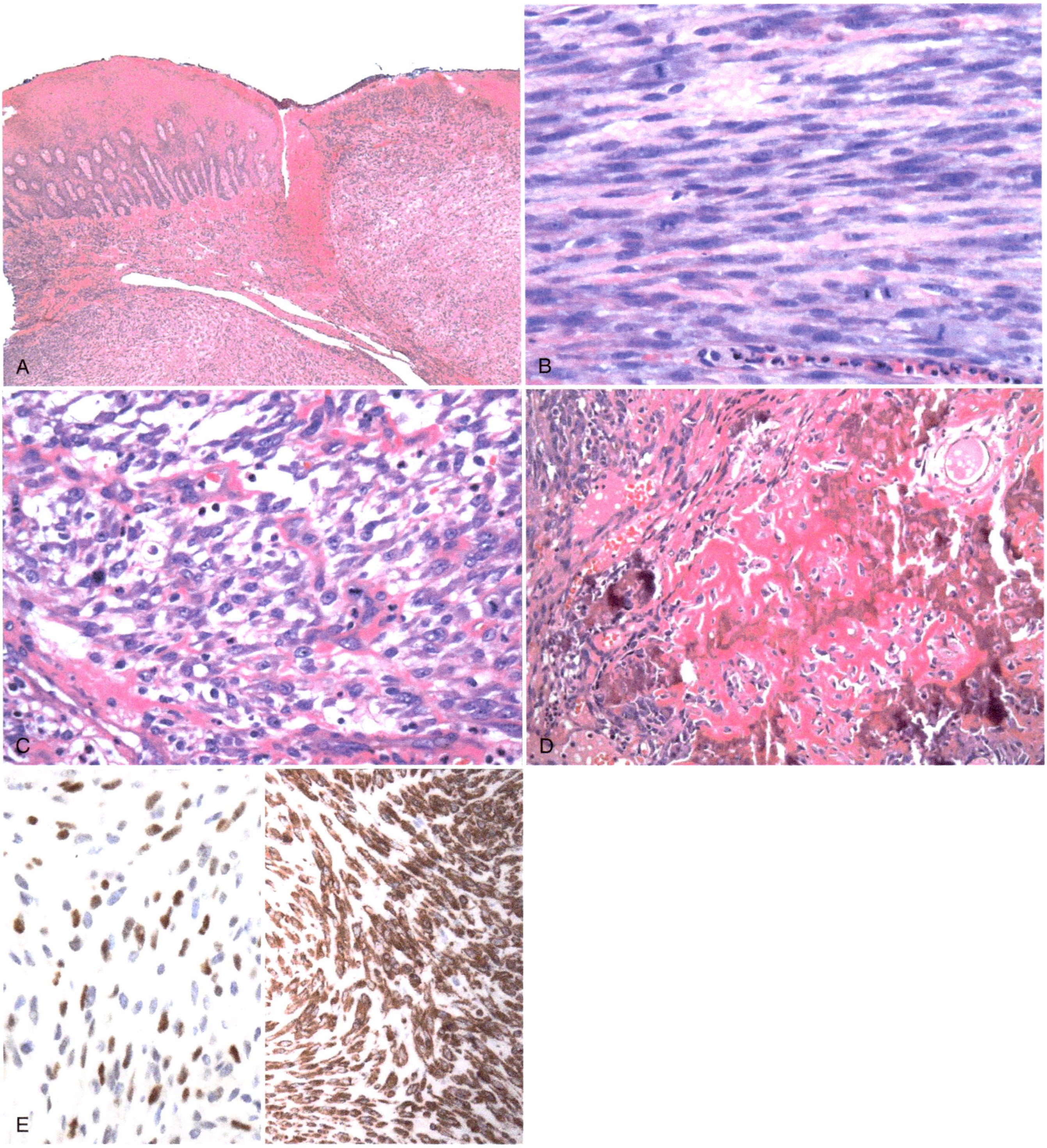

FIG 11.53 Sarcomatoid squamous cell carcinoma. (A) Spindle and epithelioid cell proliferation, ulcerated. (B) Spindle cells with nuclear atypia and many mitotic figures. (C) Epithelioid cells have large nuclei with prominent nucleoli. (D) Tumor exhibits deposition of osteoid. (E) Cells are positive for p63 *(left panel)* and vimentin *(right panel)*.

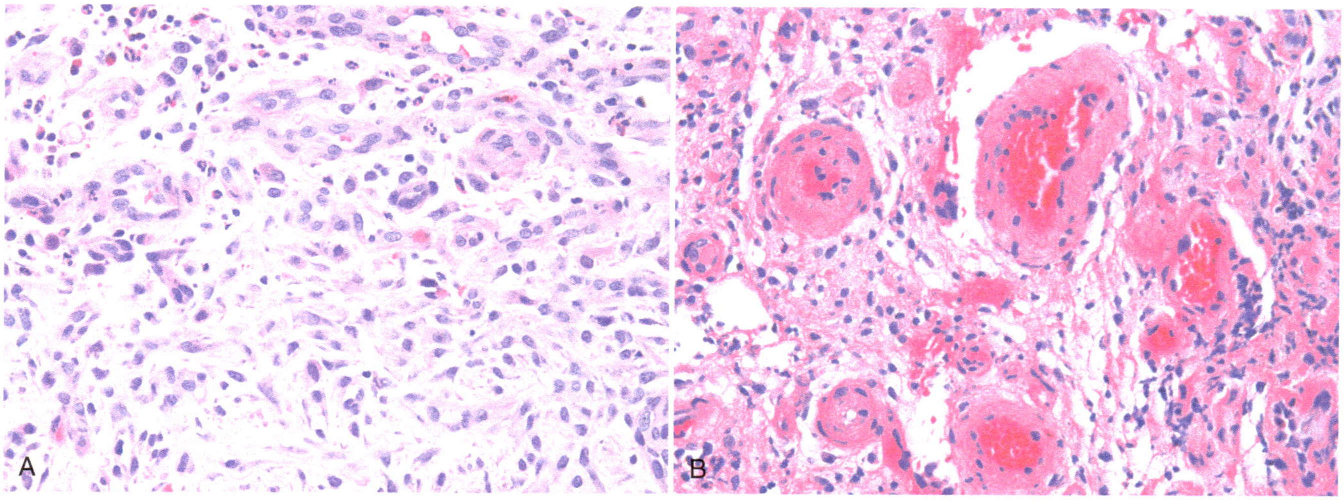

FIG 11.54 Postradiation changes. (A) Plump spindle and stellate fibroblasts and myofibroblast with slight nuclear pleomorphism; capillaries show swollen endothelial cells. (B) Vessels exhibit intimal fibrosis.

BASALOID SQUAMOUS CELL CARCINOMA

Most basaloid squamous cell carcinomas of the oropharynx (75% to 82%) as well as those of the base of tongue (76% of cases) are caused by high-risk HPV (mostly type 16). The term basaloid is controversial and many prefer the term "non- or minimally-keratinizing" for tumors of the oropharynx because the basaloid morphology is normal for tonsillar epithelium, although the term basaloid is still used for oral cavity lesions. Tumors with similar morphology in the oral cavity are generally not positive for HPV. They generally occur in the posterior oral cavity and base of tongue and are diagnosed at advanced stage with nodal involvement. HPV-associated oropharyngeal carcinoma has a better prognosis compared to non-HPV carcinoma, but the same may be true for oral cavity HPV-associated carcinoma. As such, HPV status should always be confirmed. HPV oncoprotein E7 inactivates pRb protein, resulting in overexpression of p16. As such, diffuse staining for p16 is a surrogate marker for HPV-driven carcinomas. Unlike conventional squamous cell carcinoma, HPV-associated carcinomas are usually p53–.

- The tumors are biphasic with a conventional squamous cell carcinoma and a nonkeratinizing basaloid cell proliferation; the latter is present as lobules of tumor often with comedonecrosis, or as interconnected trabeculae of cells with stromal hyalinosis often in the form of globules (HPV-driven tumors generally do not show such hyalinosis); tumor cells are basaloid with hyperchromatic nuclei, scant cytoplasm, indistinct cell borders, and many mitotic figures (Figs. 11.55 and 11.56); microcystic spaces are often present and these contain myxoid material that is periodic acid–Schiff (PAS) positive; a spindle cell variant has been identified.
- The study for p16 should be performed and if positive, in situ hybridization studies for high-risk HPV should be undertaken (Fig. 11.57); in situ hybridization using RNA probes may soon be commercially available.

Differential Diagnoses

- Many small cell (neuroendocrine) carcinomas of the oropharynx which also exhibit cells with dark hyperchromatic nuclei are p16+ and associated with high-risk HPV types; the tumors are also positive for synaptophysin, CD56, neuron-specific enolase (NSE) and high molecular weight keratins.
- HPV-associated carcinoma with adenoid cystic carcinoma-like features that are positive for p16 and high-risk HPV have been noted but mostly within the sinonasal tract; these tumors also contain mostly basaloid cells but are negative for *MYB* rearrangements unlike adenoid cystic carcinoma, which is positive for p63 in the abluminal and not luminal cells.

Prognosis

- Local recurrence occurred in 25% to 33% of patients and 5-year survival was 32% to 39%; 47% to 53% of patients died of disease; however, these studies did not evaluate for HPV status.

REFERENCES

Altrabulsi B, Carrizo F, Luna MA. Spindle basaloid squamous carcinoma of the upper aerodigestive tract: immunohistochemical and clinicopathological study of three cases. *Ann Diagn Pathol.* 2006;10:149-153.

Barnes L, MacMillan C, Ferlito A, et al. Basaloid squamous cell carcinoma of the head and neck: clinicopathological features and differential diagnosis. *Ann Otol Rhinol Laryngol.* 1996;105:75-82.

Begum S, Westra WH. Basaloid squamous cell carcinoma of the head and neck is a mixed variant that can be further resolved by HPV status. *Am J Surg Pathol.* 2008;32:1044-1050.

Bishop JA, Ogawa T, Stelow EB, et al. Human papillomavirus-related carcinoma with adenoid cystic-like features: a peculiar variant of head and neck cancer restricted to the sinonasal tract. *Am J Surg Pathol.* 2013;37:836-844.

Bishop JA, Westra WH. Human papillomavirus-related small cell carcinoma of the oropharynx. *Am J Surg Pathol.* 2011;35:1679-1684.

Chernock RD, Lewis JS Jr, Zhang Q, El-Mofty SK. Human papillomavirus-positive basaloid squamous cell carcinomas of the upper aerodigestive tract: a distinct clinicopathologic and molecular subtype of basaloid squamous cell carcinoma. *Hum Pathol.* 2010;41:1016-1023.

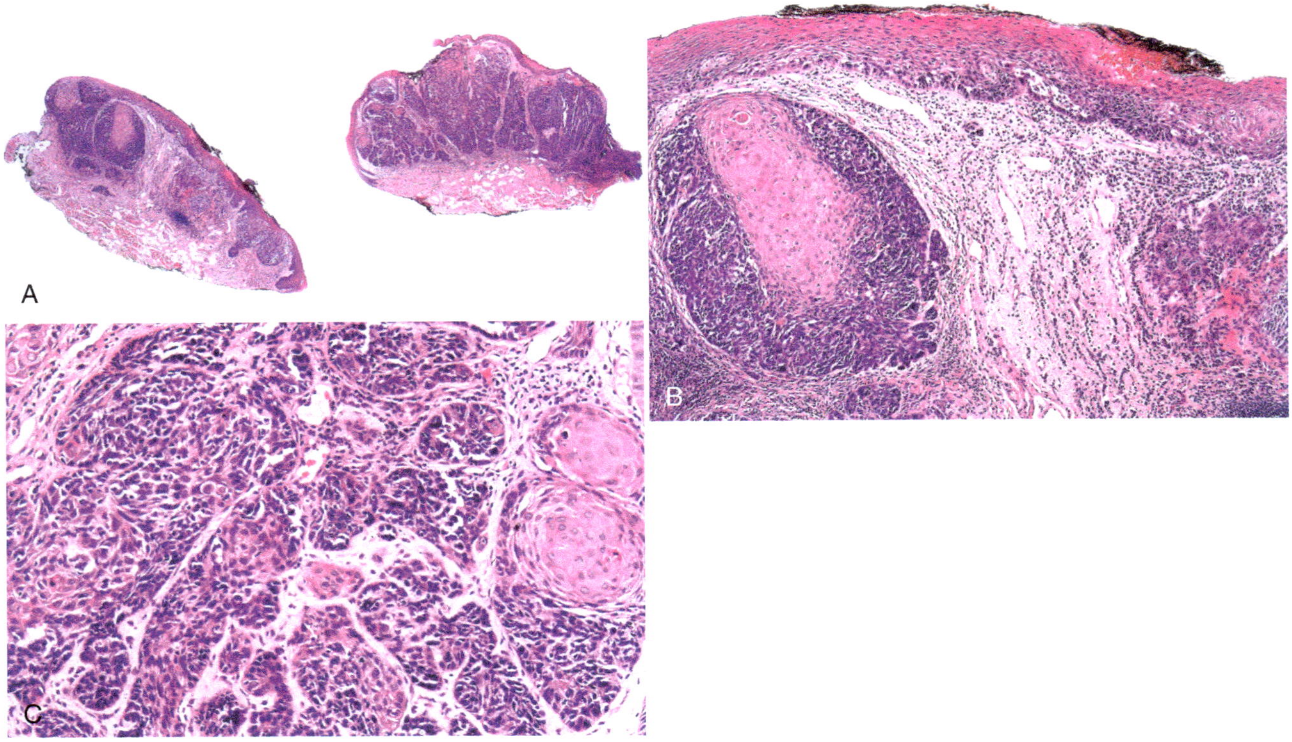

FIG 11.55 Basaloid squamous cell carcinoma. (A) Lobular proliferation of basaloid cells. (B) Basaloid and keratinizing squamous cells and overlying dysplasia. (C) Basaloid cells with hyperchromatic nuclei and squamous cells.

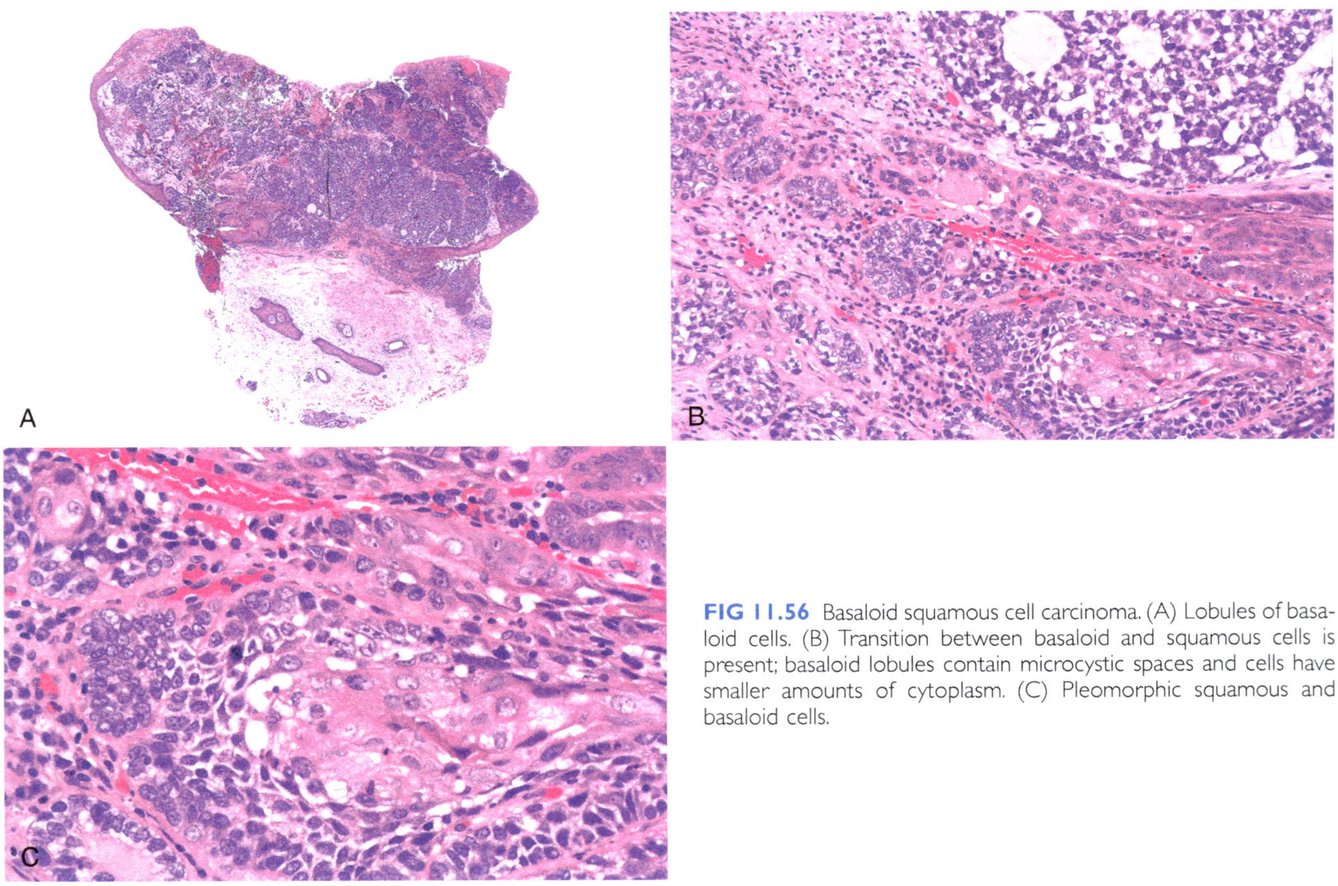

FIG 11.56 Basaloid squamous cell carcinoma. (A) Lobules of basaloid cells. (B) Transition between basaloid and squamous cells is present; basaloid lobules contain microcystic spaces and cells have smaller amounts of cytoplasm. (C) Pleomorphic squamous and basaloid cells.

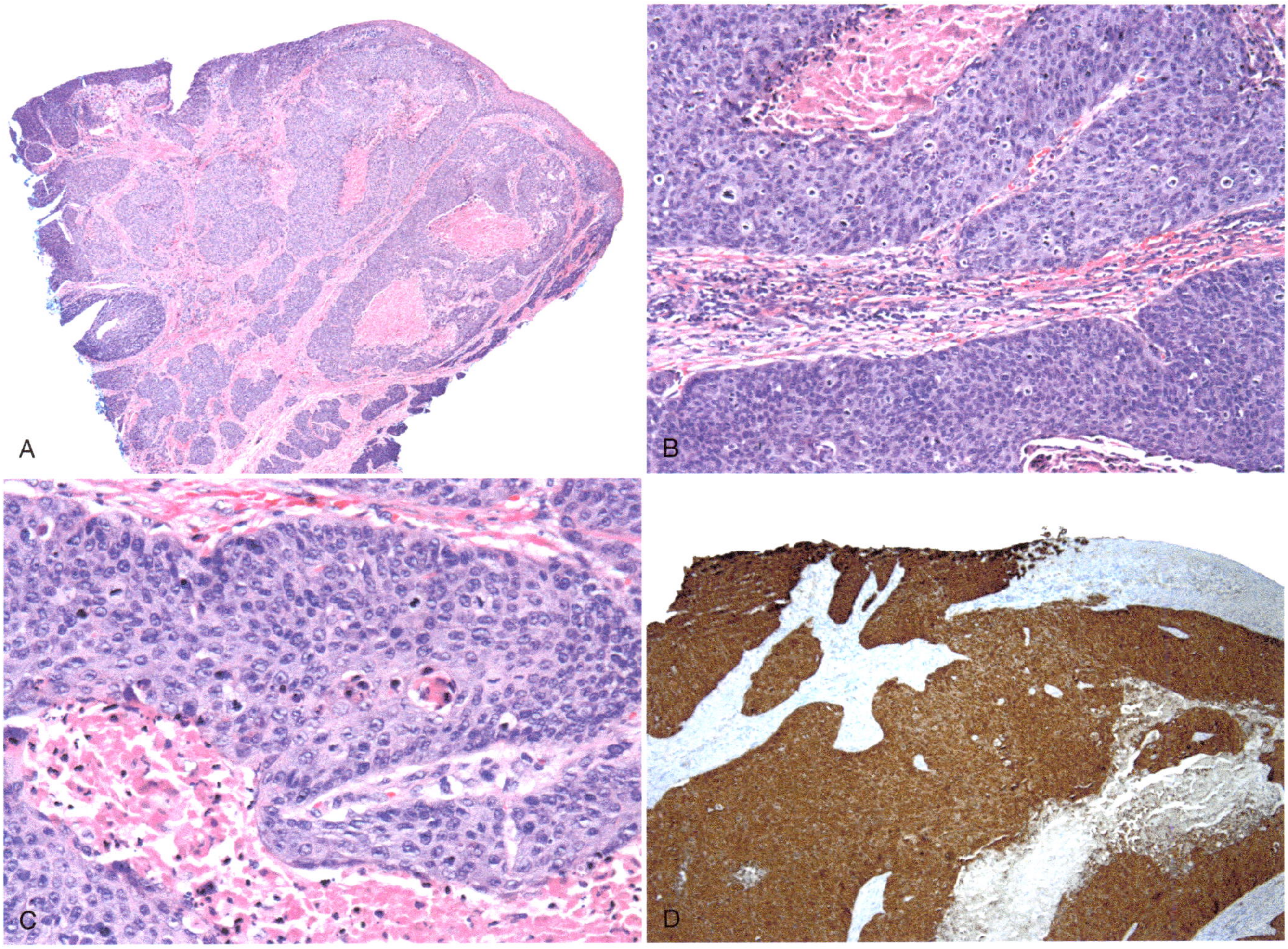

FIG 11.57 Human papillomavirus–associated squamous cell carcinoma of the oral cavity. (A) Tumor lobules with comedonecrosis; note the presence of carcinoma-in-situ on the left margin. (B) Hyperchromatic cells surround areas of necrosis. (C) Apoptotic cells and many mitotic figures are noted. (D) p16 is diffusely positive within the tumor cells and the precursor carcinoma-in-situ on the surface.

Emanuel P, Wang B, Wu M, Burstein DE. p63 Immunohistochemistry in the distinction of adenoid cystic carcinoma from basaloid squamous cell carcinoma. *Mod Pathol.* 2005;18:645-650.

Ereno C, Gaafar A, Garmendia M, et al. Basaloid squamous cell carcinoma of the head and neck: a clinicopathological and follow-up study of 40 cases and review of the literature. *Head Neck Pathol.* 2008;2:83-91.

Friedrich RE, Sperber C, Jakel T, et al. Basaloid lesions of oral squamous epithelial cells and their association with HPV infection and P16 expression. *Anticancer Res.* 2010;30:1605-1612.

Kraft S, Faquin WC, Krane JF. HPV-associated neuroendocrine carcinoma of the oropharynx: a rare new entity with potentially aggressive clinical behavior. *Am J Surg Pathol.* 2012;36:321-330.

Wain SL, Kier R, Vollmen RT, Bossen EH. Basaloid-squamous carcinoma of the tongue, hypopharynx, and larynx: report of 10 cases. *Hum Pathol.* 1986;17:1158-1166.

Yu GY, Gao Y, Peng X, et al. A clinicopathologic study on basaloid squamous cell carcinoma in the oral and maxillofacial region. *Int J Oral Maxillofac Surg.* 2008;37:1003-1008.

HUMAN PAPILLOMAVIRUS–ASSOCIATED NONKERATINIZING SQUAMOUS CELL CARCINOMA

Patients with this tumor are younger, have less tobacco exposure, and have more lifetime oral sex partners than those with conventional squamous cell carcinoma. This tumor occurs mostly in the tonsils and oropharynx, and is uncommon in the oral cavity; most are associated with HPV 16. HPV-driven oral cavity carcinoma has a prevalence of approximately 6% using high-risk HPV E6/E7 expression, with a much higher prevalence using polymerase chain reaction likely because of oversensitivity. Although most patients present with smaller tumors but stage III disease, they have a better prognosis than those with conventional squamous cell carcinoma, and deescalation trials are

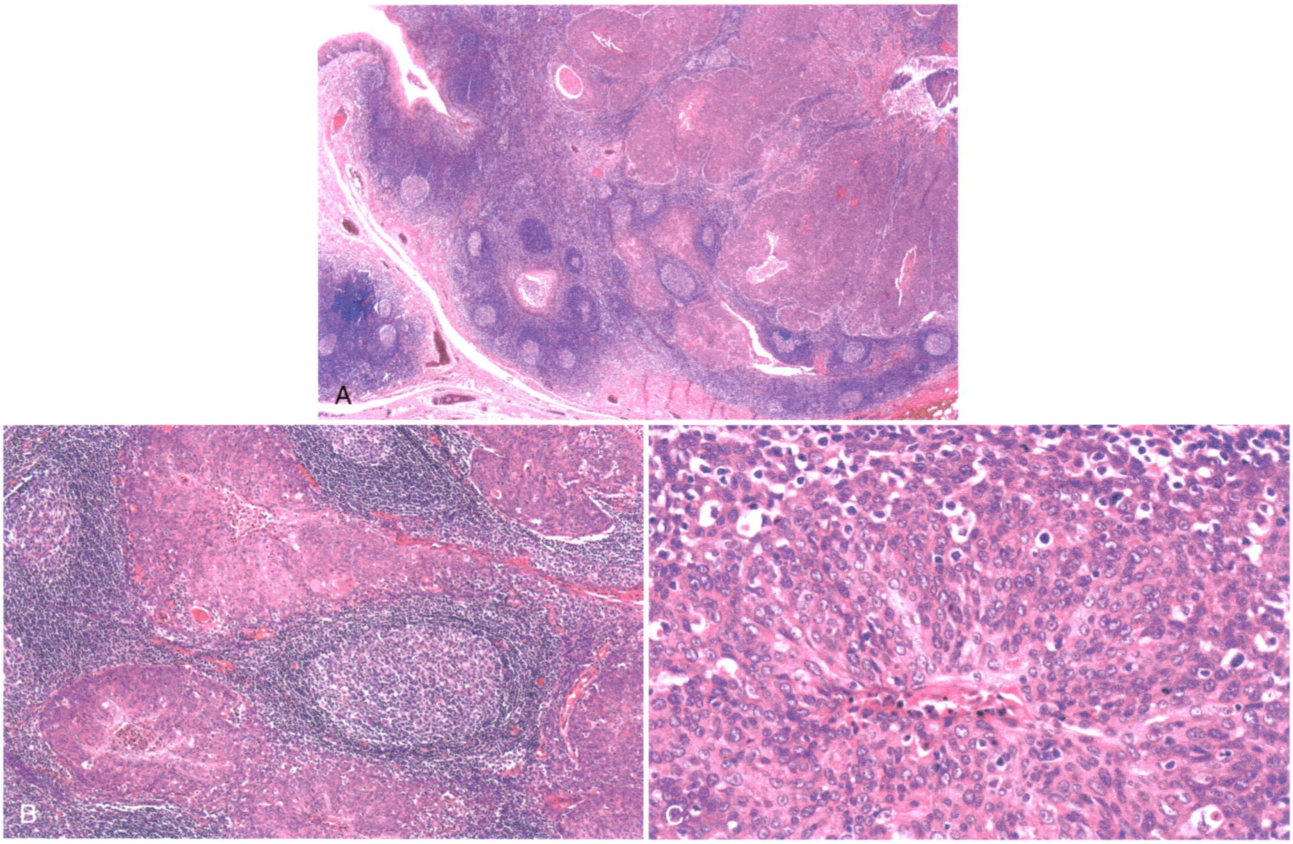

FIG 11.58 Human papillomavirus–associated carcinoma of the tonsil. (A) Trabeculae and ribbons of squamous cells within the tonsil. (B) Tumor contains pale cells and exhibits comedonecrosis. (C) Cells have abundant pale cytoplasm and ovoid nuclei with small nucleoli; mitotic figures are present and there is early necrosis. *(A, Courtesy Dr. Jeffrey Krane, Harvard Medical School, Boston.)*

currently being performed. The presence of p16 correlates with overall survival and those with antibodies against HPV early (E) proteins may also have a better prognosis.

HPV-associated E7 oncoprotein of HPV inactivates pRb tumor suppressor protein resulting in overexpression of p16, the presence of which is highly correlated with HPV-associated squamous cell carcinoma of the oropharynx, tonsils, and base of tongue. HPV-associated E6 protein degrades p53, which is rarely detected in such tumors. Mutations have been noted in *DDX3X*, *CYLD*, and *FGFR* as well as enrichment for PI3K pathway alterations and rarely *KRAS* mutations. This mutational profile differs considerably from that of non-HPV associated cancers.

- Tumors are typically nonkeratinizing with a lobular and trabecular pattern and often comedonecrosis similar to basaloid squamous cell carcinoma; however, tumors tend to be monophasic without a conventional squamous cell carcinoma; cells have ovoid or spindled morphology, indistinct cytoplasmic outlines, and small amounts of pale cytoplasm; nuclei are ovoid or spindled and hyperchromatic, have small nucleoli, and many mitoses and apoptotic cells are present (Figs. 11.58 and 11.59).
- A ciliated variant has been reported and it is unclear of the relationship of this variant and ciliated adenosquamous carcinoma, which is also HPV-positive.
- Tumors are diffusely p16+ and most harbor HPV 16, with -18, -31, 33, 45, 52, and 58 types less commonly expressed (see Figs. 11.36–11.38).
- Nodal metastases are usually present; conversely, carcinomas (often cystic) that are p16+ within cervical nodes usually represent metastases from occult primary tumors in the oropharynx or tonsil.

Prognosis

- When compared with non-HPV cancers, patients with HPV-related oropharyngeal carcinoma show lower risk of loco-regional relapse and dying of disease with 3-year survival at 57% versus 82%, respectively; 5-year survival ranges from 19% to 32% and 54% to 62%, respectively.

REFERENCES

Ang KK, Harris J, Wheeler R, et al. Human papillomavirus and survival of patients with oropharyngeal cancer. *N Engl J Med.* 2010; 363:24-35.

Ang KK, Sturgis EM. Human papillomavirus as a marker of the natural history and response to therapy of head and neck squamous cell carcinoma. *Semin Radiat Oncol.* 2012;22:128-142.

Bishop JA, Lewis JS Jr, Rocco JW, Faquin WC. HPV-related squamous cell carcinoma of the head and neck: An update on testing in routine pathology practice. *Semin Diagn Pathol.* 2015;32:344-351.

Bishop JA, Westra WH. Ciliated HPV-related carcinoma: a well-differentiated form of head and neck carcinoma that can be mistaken for a benign cyst. *Am J Surg Pathol.* 2015;39:1591-1595.

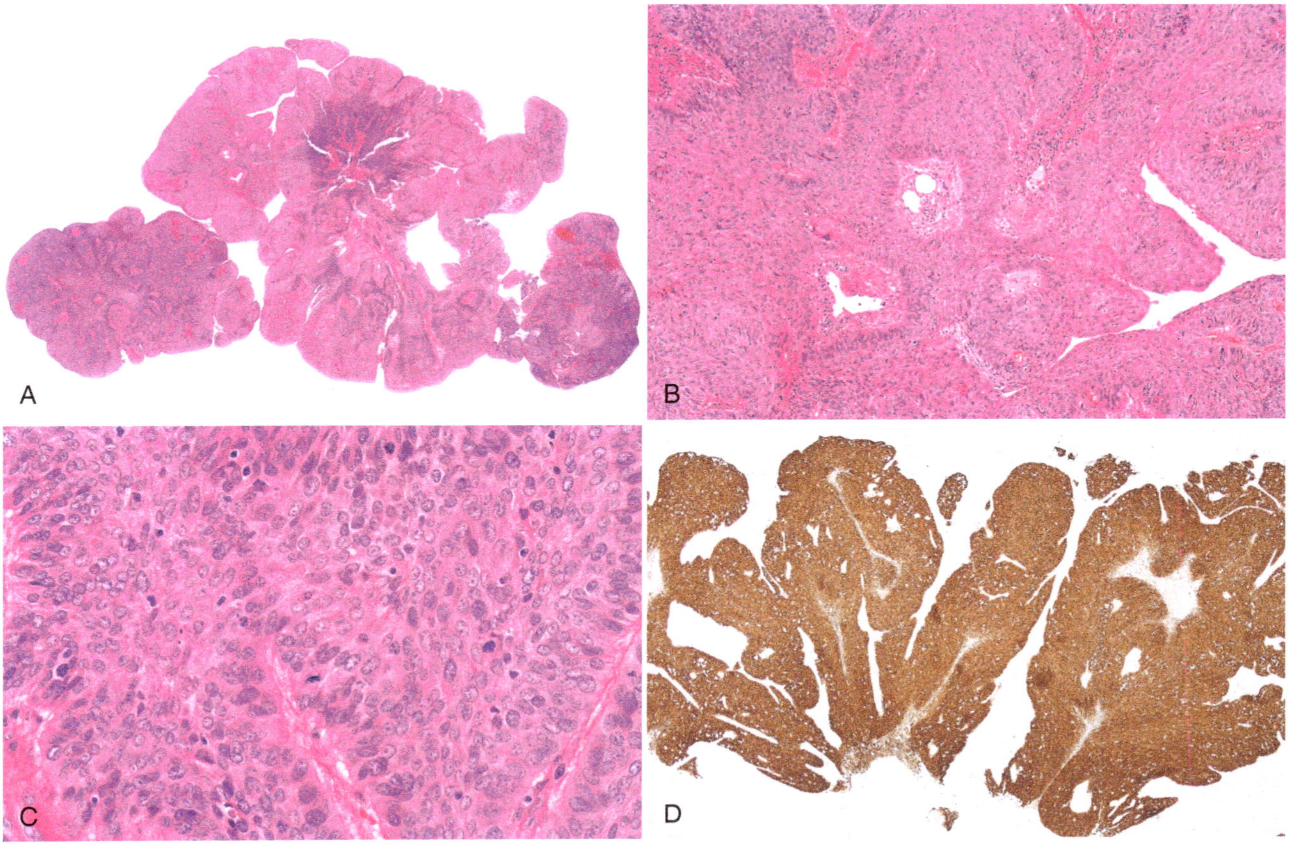

FIG 11.59 Human papillomavirus (HPV)-associated papillary squamous cell carcinoma. (A) Nonkeratinizing tumor in a papillary configuration. (B) Interlacing trabeculae of tumor cells. (C) Tumor cells have pale eosinophilic cytoplasm and ovoid nuclei with small nucleoli, and many mitotic figures are present. (D) Tumor shows strong p16 positivity.

Chernock RD. Morphologic features of conventional squamous cell carcinoma of the oropharynx: 'keratinizing' and 'nonkeratinizing' histologic types as the basis for a consistent classification system. *Head Neck Pathol.* 2012;6(suppl 1):S41-S47.

Chung CH, Bagheri A, D'Souza G. Epidemiology of oral human papillomavirus infection. *Oral Oncol.* 2014;50:364-369.

Dahlstrom KR, Anderson KS, Cheng JN, et al. HPV Serum antibodies as predictors of survival and disease progression in patients with HPV-positive squamous cell carcinoma of the oropharynx. *Clin Cancer Res.* 2015;21:2861-2869.

El-Mofty SK, Patil S. Human papillomavirus (HPV)-related oropharyngeal nonkeratinizing squamous cell carcinoma: characterization of a distinct phenotype. *Oral Surg Oral Med Oral Pathol Oral Radiol Endod.* 2006;101:339-345.

El-Mofty SK, Zhang MQ, Davila RM. Histologic identification of human papillomavirus (HPV)-related squamous cell carcinoma in cervical lymph nodes: a reliable predictor of the site of an occult head and neck primary carcinoma. *Head Neck Pathol.* 2008;2:163-168.

Fakhry C, Zhang Q, Nguyen-Tan PF, et al. Human papillomavirus and overall survival after progression of oropharyngeal squamous cell carcinoma. *J Clin Oncol.* 2014;32:3365-3373.

Hubbers CU, Akgul B. HPV and cancer of the oral cavity. *Virulence.* 2015;6:244-248.

Lewis JS Jr, Thorstad WL, Chernock RD, et al. p16 positive oropharyngeal squamous cell carcinoma: an entity with a favorable prognosis regardless of tumor HPV status. *Am J Surg Pathol.* 2010;34:1088-1096.

Lingen MW, Xiao W, Schmitt A, et al. Low etiologic fraction for high-risk human papillomavirus in oral cavity squamous cell carcinomas. *Oral Oncol.* 2013;49:1-8.

Saraiya M, Unger ER, Thompson TD, et al. US assessment of HPV types in cancers: implications for current and 9-valent HPV vaccines. *J Natl Cancer Inst.* 2015;107:djv086.

ADENOID (ACANTHOLYTIC) SQUAMOUS CELL CARCINOMA (PSEUDOGLANDULAR SQUAMOUS CELL CARCINOMA)

Approximately 80% of this tumor is located on the lip. Cutaneous lesions have shown a loss of at least one desmosomal cell adhesion protein, with the two most commonly lost being desmoglein and desmoplakin.

- A conventional squamous cell carcinoma is present but some tumor islands exhibit central acantholysis, imparting an adenoid, pseudoglandular, or alveolar appearance; these spaces are lined by pleomorphic tumor cells with a "hobnail" appearance suggestive of vascular spaces; tumor cells within the spaces are large and round with abundant eosinophilic cytoplasm and exhibit nuclear pleomorphism, dyskeratosis, and other features of malignancy (Figs. 11.60–11.62); sometimes, the adenoid spaces may be complex and sinusoidal in appearance.
- Cells are positive for keratin, EMA, CEA, p63, and often vimentin, and negative for CD31 and CD34.

Differential Diagnoses

- Adenosquamous cell carcinoma is a variant of squamous cell carcinoma that forms true ductal structures and often contains mucous cells.

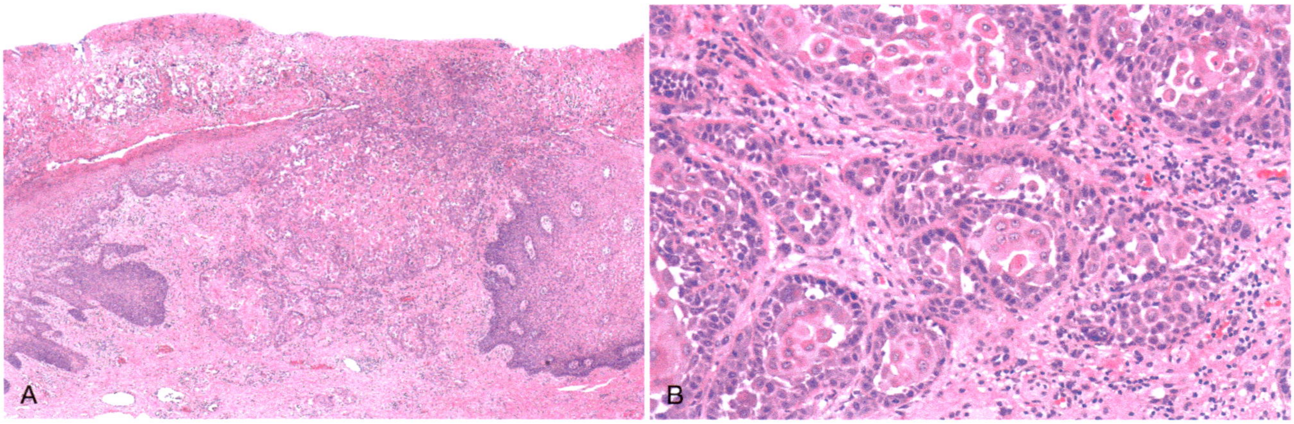

FIG 11.60 Minimally keratinizing adenoid (acantholytic) squamous cell carcinoma. (A) Infiltrating squamous cell carcinoma. (B) Pseudoglandular spaces contain acantholytic, dyskeratotic, and pleomorphic cells.

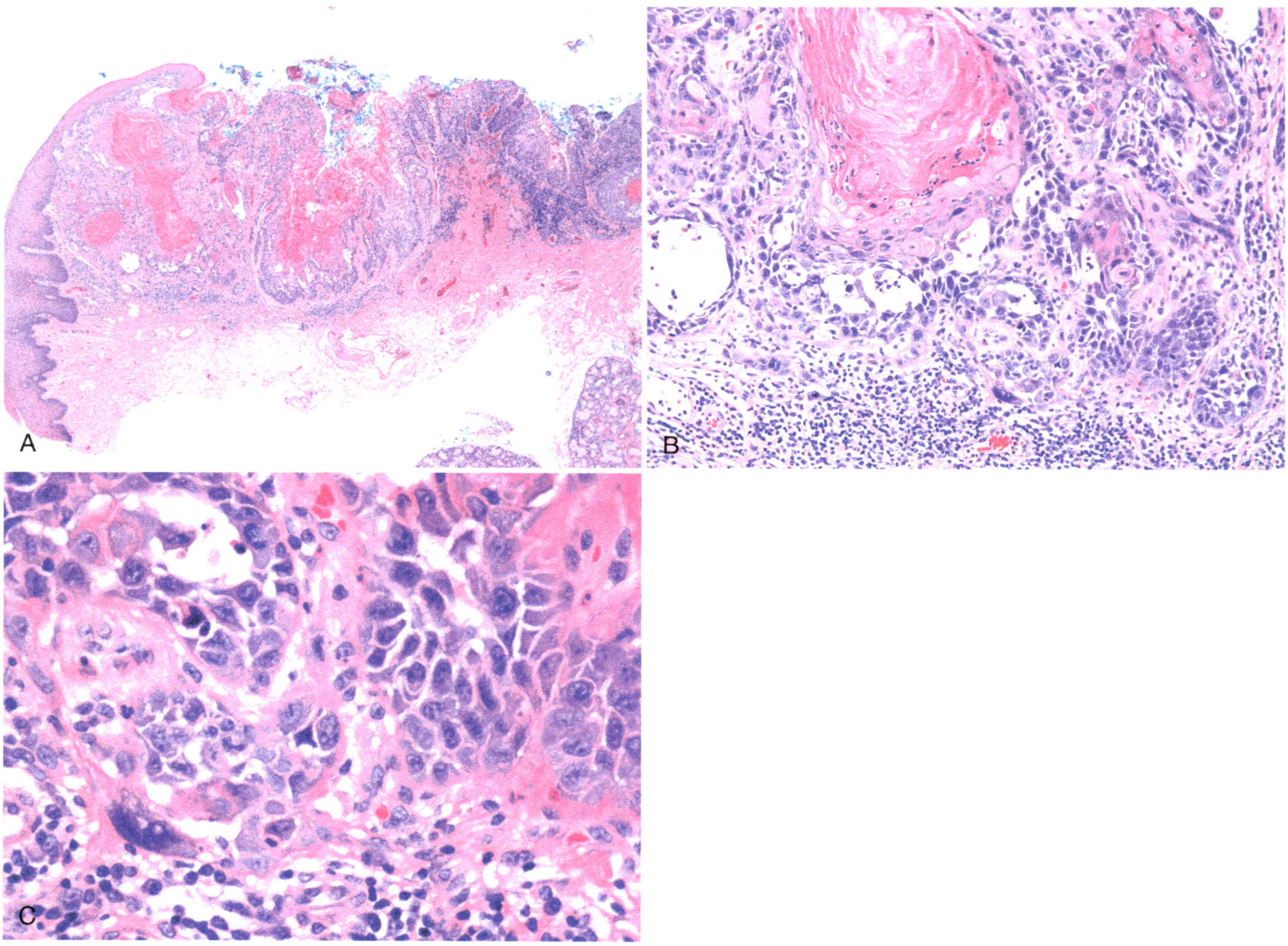

FIG 11.61 Keratinizing adenoid (acantholytic) squamous cell carcinoma. (A) Squamous cell carcinoma producing abundant keratin and pseudoglandular structures at the base of the tumor. (B) Acantholytic tumor cells float within spaces in the center of tumor islands, and a conventional squamous cell carcinoma is present. (C) Tumor cells are pleomorphic.

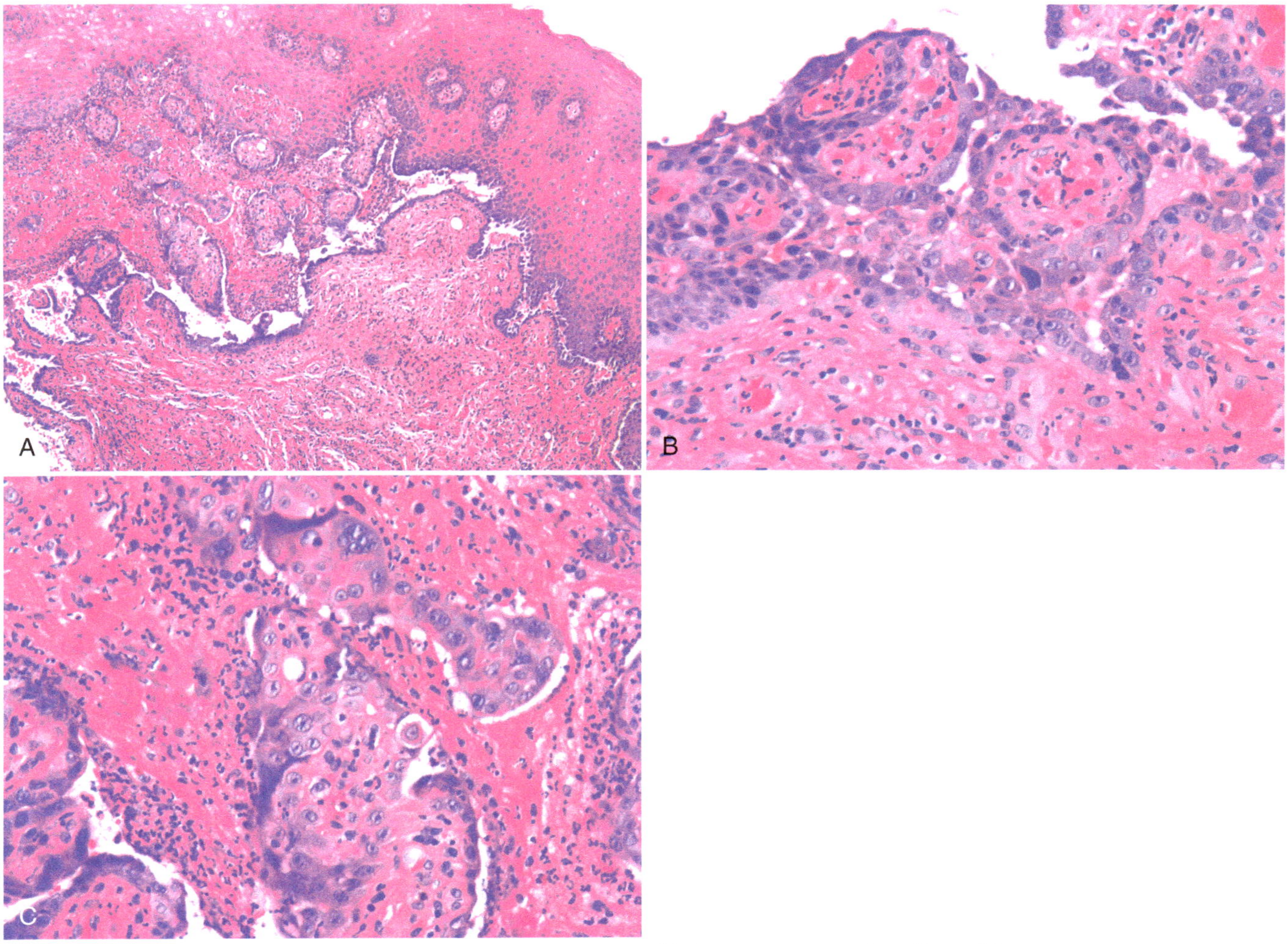

FIG 11.62 Acantholytic squamous cell carcinoma. (A) This tumor is pemphigus-like and forms suprabasilar clefts and papillary structures. (B) Tumor cells have pleomorphic, hyperchromatic nuclei. (C) Tumor cells within the tissue cleft exhibit pleomorphism and dyskeratosis.

- Adenocarcinomas of salivary gland or skin adnexal origin would not exhibit a conventional squamous cell carcinoma.
- True acantholytic lesions such as pemphigus vulgaris or focal acantholytic dermatosis exhibit acantholysis that is suprabasilar without significant cytologic atypia or invasive islands of tumor cells; these must be distinguished from acantholytic carcinoma-in-situ; direct immunofluorescence confirms the diagnosis in pemphigus vulgaris.

Prognosis

- Intraoral tumors may be more aggressive than those on sun-exposed skin; 11% of patients died of their disease in one study and all were intraoral tumors.

REFERENCES

Bunn B, Hunter K, Khurram SA, van Heerden WF. Adenoid dysplasia of the oral mucosa. *Oral Surg Oral Med Oral Pathol Oral Radiol.* 2014;118:586-592.

Ferlito A, Devaney KO, Milroy CM, et al. Mucosal adenoid squamous cell carcinoma of the head and neck. *Ann Otol Rhinol Laryngol.* 1996;105:409-413.

Gu X, Jiang R, Fowler MR. Acantholytic squamous cell carcinoma in upper aerodigestive tract: histopathology, immunohistochemical profile and epithelial mesenchymal transition phenotype change. *Head Neck Pathol.* 2012;6:438-444.

Jacoway JR, Nelson JF, Boyers RC. Adenoid squamous-cell carcinoma (adenoacanthoma of the oral labial mucosa). *Oral Surg Oral Med Oral Pathol.* 1971;32:444-449.

Jones AC, Freedman PD, Kerpel SM. Oral adenoid squamous cell carcinoma: a report of three cases and review of the literature. *J Oral Maxillofac Surg.* 1993;51:676-681.

Kusafuka K, Ebihara M, Ishiki H, et al. Primary adenoid squamous cell carcinoma of the oral cavity. *Pathol Int.* 2006;56:78-83.

O'Shea C, Fitzpatrick JE, Koch PJ. Desmosomal defects in acantholytic squamous cell carcinomas. *J Cutan Pathol.* 2014;41:873-879.

Papadopoulou E, Tosios KI, Nikitakis N, et al. Acantholytic squamous cell carcinoma of the gingiva: report of a case and review of the literature. *Oral Surg Oral Med Oral Pathol Oral Radiol Endod.* 2010;109:e67-e71.

ADENOSQUAMOUS CELL CARCINOMA

This is a tumor with features of both squamous cell carcinoma and adenocarcinoma. The most common location is the larynx, followed by the oropharynx, floor of mouth, and tongue and tonsils.

- There is a conventional infiltrating and usually keratinizing squamous cell carcinoma with overlying dysplasia; adenocarcinoma is usually noted within deep portions of the tumor with the formation of ductal structures containing mucous cells and exhibiting secretion of mucin; cells often exhibit intracytoplasmic vacuoles/lumina consistent with rudimentary duct formation (Figs. 11.63 and 11.64).
- Perineural invasion is seen in some cases and 16% of cases are associated with high-risk HPV and p16 positivity; a ciliated variant is also recognized with low-grade cytology.
- Mucous cells are highlighted with the mucicarmine stain and glandular structures are positive for CK7, CAM5.2, and CEA.

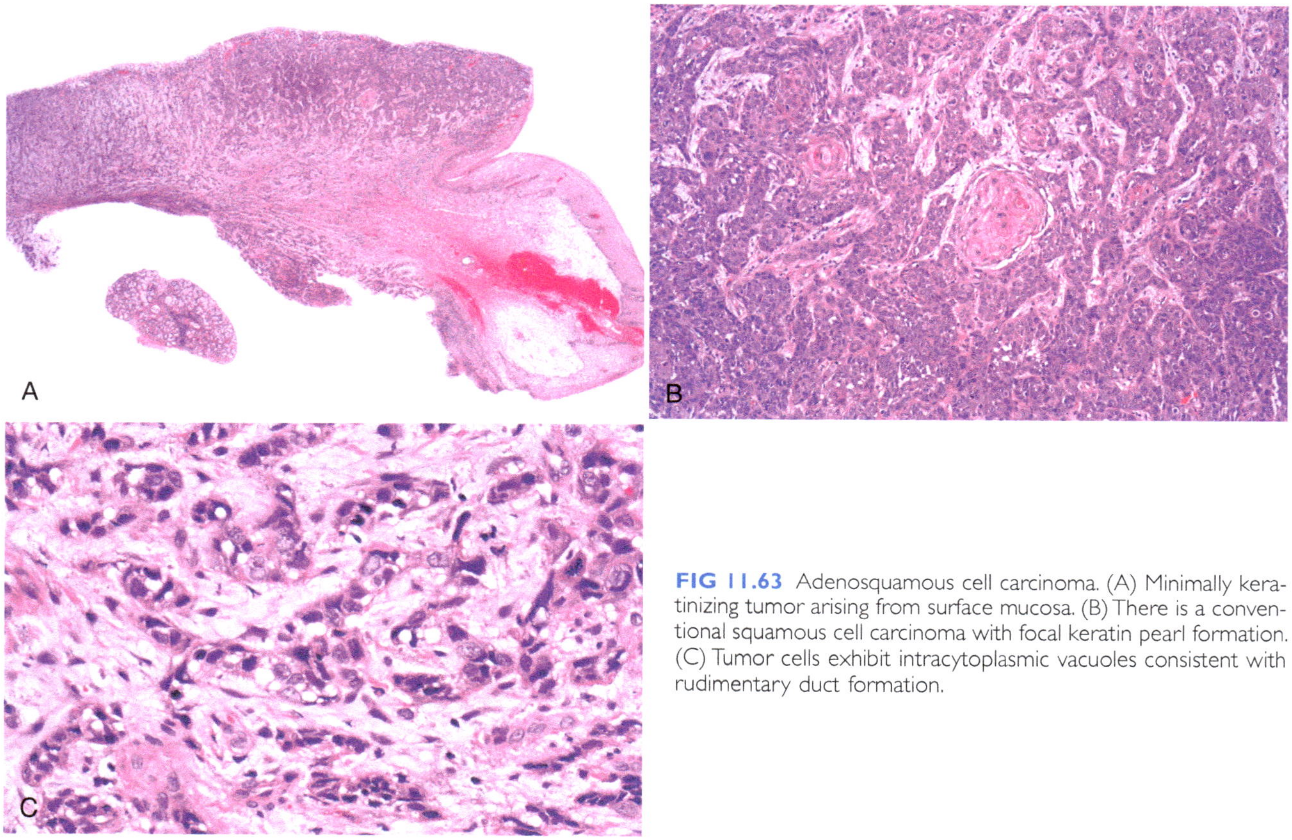

FIG 11.63 Adenosquamous cell carcinoma. (A) Minimally keratinizing tumor arising from surface mucosa. (B) There is a conventional squamous cell carcinoma with focal keratin pearl formation. (C) Tumor cells exhibit intracytoplasmic vacuoles consistent with rudimentary duct formation.

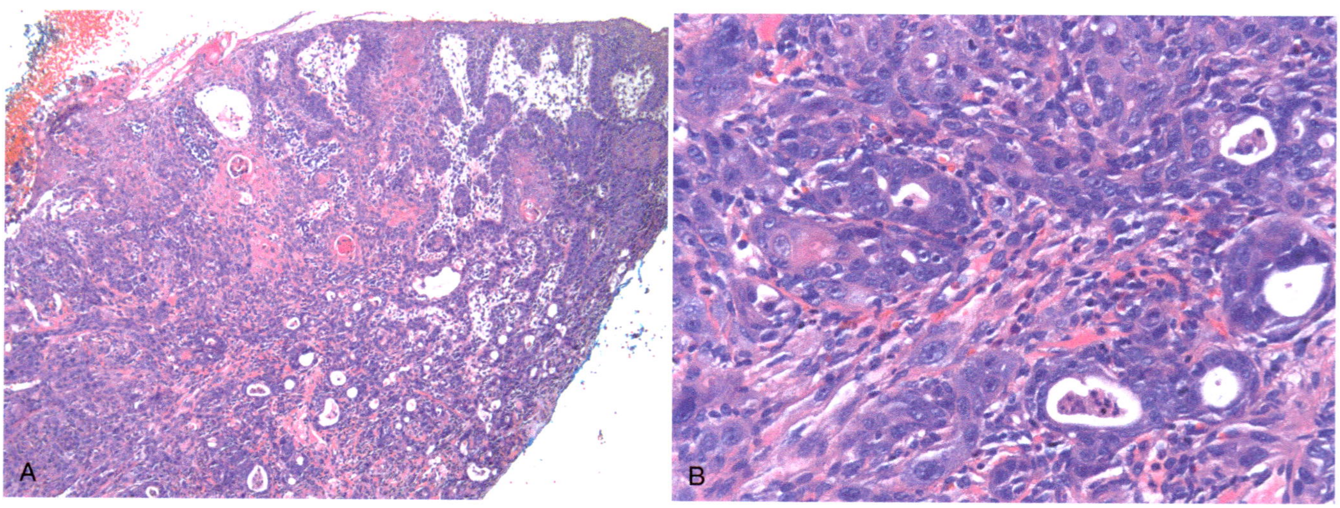

FIG 11.64 Adenosquamous cell carcinoma. (A) Keratinizing squamous cell carcinoma forming ductal structures. (B) Tumor cells form ducts and there is focal keratinization.

- This tumor is not associated with *MECT1-MAML2* fusion.

Differential Diagnoses

- Mucoepidermoid carcinoma shows less cytologic atypia (except for high-grade lesions), has recognizable epidermoid, mucous, and intermediate cell population, and keratinizing squamous cell carcinoma is not identified; it is strongly associated with *MECT1-MAML2* fusion.

Prognosis

- Local recurrence occurs in 46% of cases, 65% and 23% of cases have nodal or distant metastases, respectively, and 40% to 50% die of disease within 2 years; 5-year survival is 13%. A more recent study has shown 5-year disease-free survival to be 36%.

REFERENCES

Alos L, Castillo M, Nadal A, et al. Adenosquamous carcinoma of the head and neck: criteria for diagnosis in a study of 12 cases. *Histopathology*. 2004;44:570-579.

Gerughty RM, Hennigar GR, Brown FM. Adenosquamous carcinoma of the nasal, oral and laryngeal cavities. *Cancer*. 1968;6:1140-1155.

Kass JI, Lee SC, Abberbock S, Seethala RR, Duvvuri U. Adenosquamous carcinoma of the head and neck: Molecular analysis using CRTC-MAML FISH and survival comparison with paired conventional squamous cell carcinoma. *Laryngoscope*. 2015;125:E371-E376.

Keelawat S, Liu CZ, Roehm PC, Barnes L. Adenosquamous carcinoma of the upper aerodigestive tract: a clinicopathologic study of 12 cases and review of the literature. *Am J Otolaryngol*. 2002;23:160-168.

Masand RP, El-Mofty SK, Ma XJ, et al. Adenosquamous carcinoma of the head and neck: relationship to human papillomavirus and review of the literature. *Head Neck Pathol*. 2011;5:108-116.

Radkay-Gonzalez L, Faquin W, McHugh JB, et al. Ciliated adenosquamous carcinoma: expanding the phenotypic diversity of human papillomavirus-associated tumors. *Head Neck Pathol*. 2016;10:167-175.

Schick U, Pusztaszeri M, Betz M, et al. Adenosquamous carcinoma of the head and neck: report of 20 cases and review of the literature. *Oral Surg Oral Med Oral Pathol Oral Radiol*. 2013;116:313-320.

Scully C, Porter SR, Speight PM, et al. Adenosquamous carcinoma of the mouth: a rare variant of squamous cell carcinoma. *Int J Oral Maxillofac Surg*. 1999;28:125-128.

CUNICULATE CARCINOMA (CARCINOMA CUNICULATUM)

Lesions are most commonly reported on the plantar surface of the foot and some use this term interchangeably with verrucous carcinoma for skin and genital lesions, which leads to confusion. Most lesions in the mouth occur on the gingiva/alveolar ridge (58% of cases, with most being on the mandibular mucosa) and more than half show involvement of underlying bone. Importantly, the mucosal surface is usually smooth, unlike in verrucous carcinoma. A striking feature is the presence of numerous sinuses or deep invaginations that may exude foul-smelling keratinaceous material. The term "cuniculate" comes from the word "cuniculus" meaning rabbit burrow.

- The tumor consists of a well-differentiated squamous cell carcinoma with an endophytic growth pattern, composed of interconnected trabeculae of dysplastic tumor cells that are complex and arborizing and associated with cystic structures and burrows filled with keratin; connection with the surface epithelium may be difficult to identify (Fig. 11.65).
- Tumor cells are p53+ but negative for HPV.

Differential Diagnosis

- Verrucous carcinoma consists of an obviously verrucous exophytic and endophytic squamous cell carcinoma that is well differentiated with minimal cytologic atypia and forms frondlike bulbous rete ridges; plane of section may make it seem as if there are arborizing keratin cysts.
- Papillary well-differentiated bluntly invasive squamous cell carcinoma has a papillary and verrucous surface and may also exhibit keratin-filled burrows from plane of section.
- Keratocystic odontogenic tumor (odontogenic keratocyst) arising in the jaw bones may erode through the bone and present on the gingiva as a mass; this tends to present as a single large cyst within the jaw bones rather than as a solid tumor, although smaller microscopic satellite cysts may be present; carcinomatous transformation may lead to significant cytologic atypia and pleomorphism.
- Some squamous cell carcinomas may form one or two cystic structures that are not tortuous (Fig. 11.66).

Prognosis

- Most tumors behave indolently; one study showed 20% of cases with local recurrence and 20% with lymph node metastasis, but 5-year survival is 85% and most patients do not die of this disease.

REFERENCES

Allon D, Kaplan I, Manor R, Calderon S. Carcinoma cuniculatum of the jaw: a rare variant of oral carcinoma. *Oral Surg Oral Med Oral Pathol Oral Radiol Endod*. 2002;94:601-608.

Fonseca FP, Pontes HA, Pontes FS, et al. Oral carcinoma cuniculatum: two cases illustrative of a diagnostic challenge. *Oral Surg Oral Med Oral Pathol Oral Radiol*. 2013;116:457-463.

Kao GF, Graham JH, Helwig EB. Carcinoma cuniculatum (verrucous carcinoma of the skin): a clinicopathologic study of 46 cases with ultrastructural observations. *Cancer*. 1982;49:2395-2403.

Kruse AL, Graetz KW. Carcinoma cuniculatum: a rare entity in the oral cavity. *J Craniofac Surg*. 2009;20:1270-1272.

Kubik MJ, Rhatigan RM. Carcinoma cuniculatum: not a verrucous carcinoma. *J Cutan Pathol*. 2012;39:1083-1087.

McKee PH, Wilkinson JD, Black MM, Whimster IW. Carcinoma (epithelioma) cuniculatum: a clinico-pathological study of nineteen cases and review of the literature. *Histopathology*. 1981;5:425-436.

Padilla RJ, Murrah VA. Carcinoma cuniculatum of the oral mucosa: a potentially underdiagnosed entity in the absence of clinical correlation. *Oral Surg Oral Med Oral Pathol Oral Radiol*. 2014;118:684-693.

Pons Y, Kerrary S, Cox A, et al. Mandibular cuniculatum carcinoma: apropos of 3 cases and literature review. *Head Neck*. 2012;34:291-295.

Sun Y, Kuyama K, Burkhardt A, Yamamoto H. Clinicopathological evaluation of carcinoma cuniculatum: a variant of oral squamous cell carcinoma. *J Oral Pathol Med*. 2012;41:303-308.

Thavaraj S, Cobb A, Kalavrezos N, et al. Carcinoma cuniculatum arising in the tongue. *Head Neck Pathol*. 2012;6:130-134.

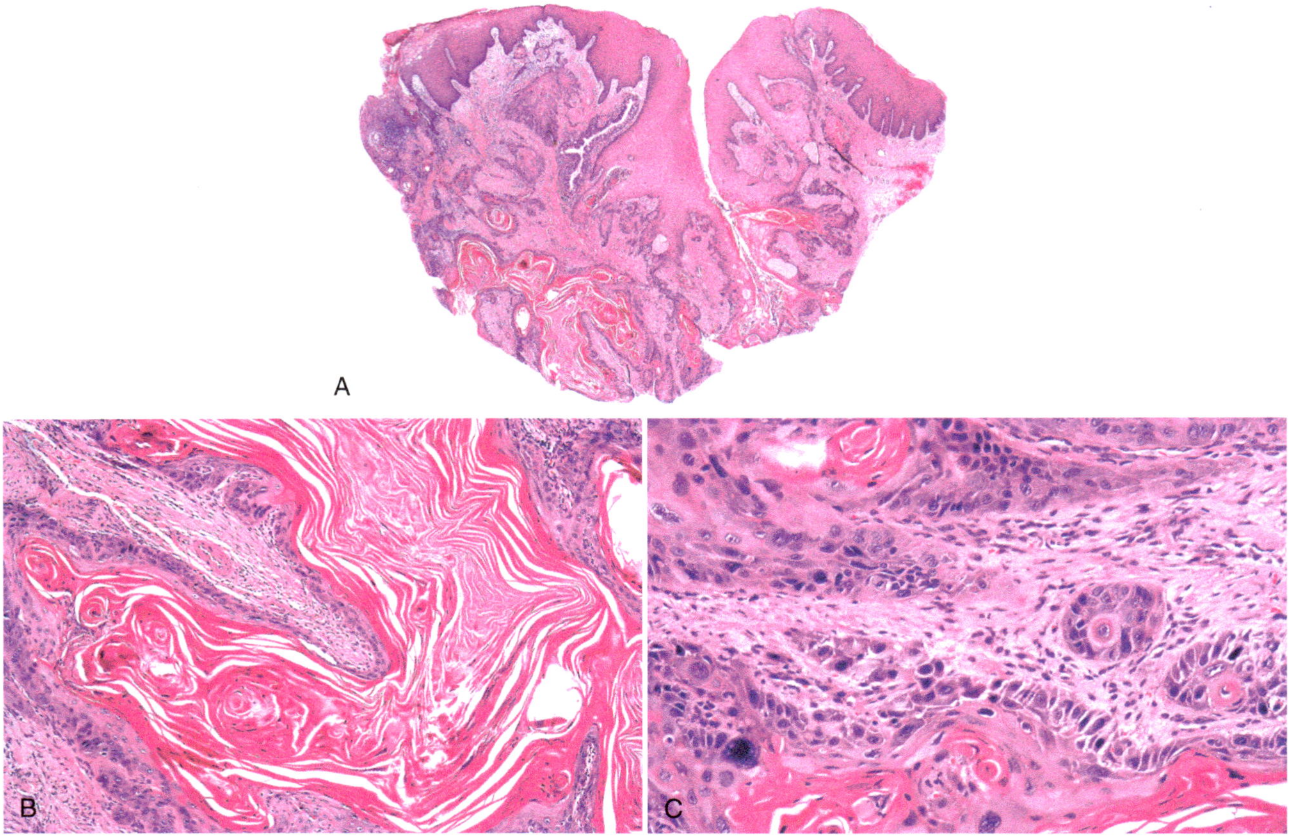

FIG 11.65 Cuniculate carcinoma. (A) Deeply ramifying, irregular cystic spaces filled with keratin; tumor arises from the surface which is usually smooth. (B) Keratin-filled spaces surrounded by dysplastic epithelium. (C) Pleomorphic tumor cells and stromal infiltration.

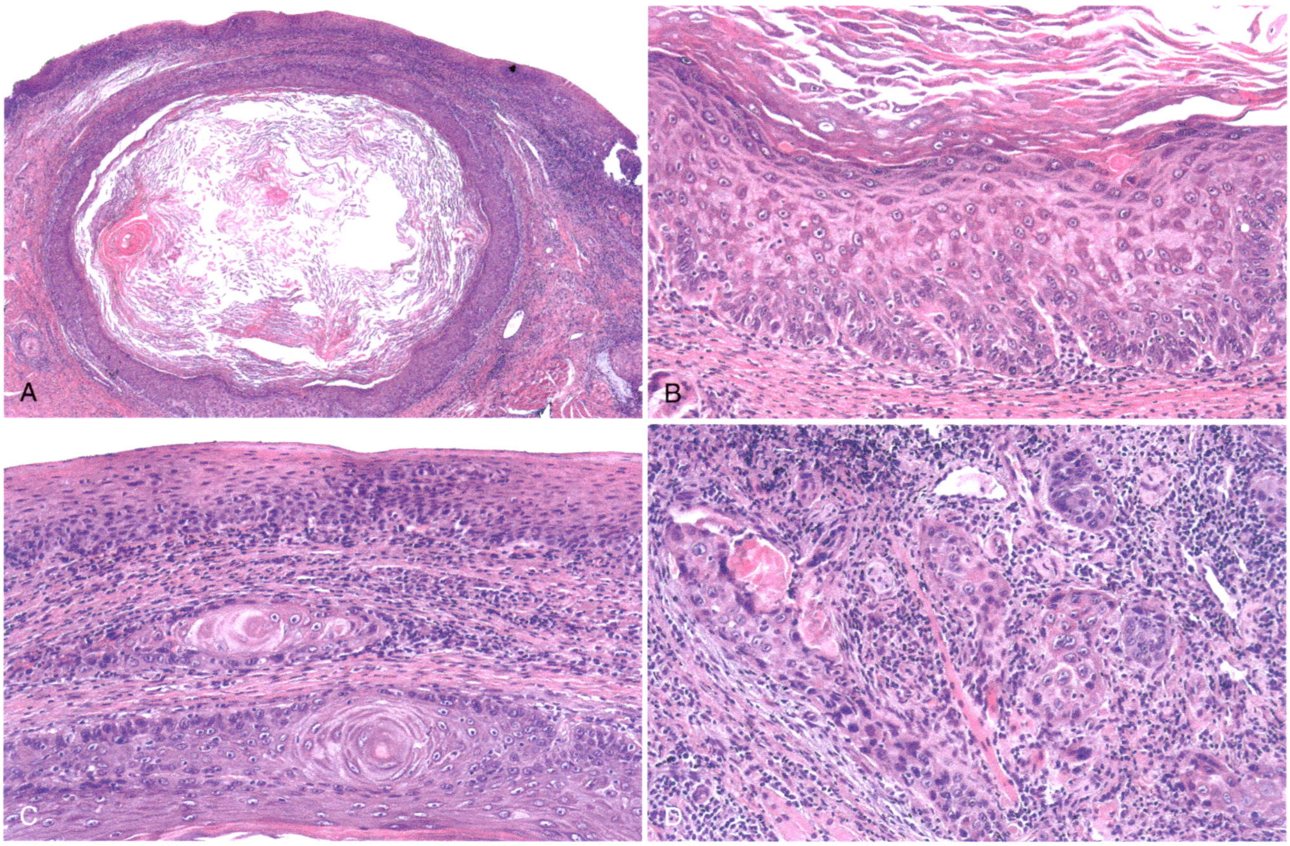

FIG 11.66 Cystic squamous cell carcinoma. (A) Keratin-filled cyst lined by dysplastic epithelium; note invasive islands of tumor cells at the *right* and *left* margins of image. (B) Cyst lining contains dyskeratotic, dysplastic cells. (C) The surface epithelium exhibits moderate dysplasia and islands of tumor cells infiltrate the stroma. (D) Conventional infiltrating squamous cell carcinoma is noted.

KERATOACANTHOMATOUS SQUAMOUS CELL CARCINOMA

This is still a controversial issue regarding nomenclature. The terms "well-differentiated squamous cell carcinoma, keratoacanthomatous pattern" and "keratoacanthoma" are often used interchangeably for skin lesions because although some tumors resolve, some do not and behave as cutaneous invasive carcinoma; perineural and lymphovascular invasion have also been reported and rare cases have metastasized. This is an uncommon condition within the oral cavity though they may be seen with some frequency on the lips and perivermilion skin. It presents as a nodule with central umbilication filled with yellowish, cheesy keratin (Fig. 11.67).

There are several clinical presentations, the most common of which is the solitary type (which may be giant) that occurs on sun-damaged skin and that tends to regress. Inherited forms such as the Ferguson-Smith type seen in the Scottish, or the eruptive Gryzbowski type manifest with multiple lesions, as well as those in Muir-Torre syndrome. One study showed that 98% of classic keratoacanthoma of the skin regressed after partial excision, while only 33% of keratoacanthomas with a squamous cell carcinoma pattern (with significant atypia/dysplasia) regressed. It is likely that not all keratoacanthomas behave the same way even on the skin, and that most mucosal ones do not tend to regress and may represent a different subtype.

- This is a well-differentiated squamous cell carcinoma that shows endophytic growth forming a cup-shaped depression filled with keratin with a "lip" around the tumor; there may be papillary projections of the tumor epithelium into this keratin-filled space that may not be well formed; lobules of tumor extend from the cavity into the stroma and tumor cells are large with abundant pale, "glassy" cytoplasm with variable pleomorphism and dyskeratosis; infiltration of muscle may be seen at the base (Figs. 11.68 and 11.69); oral lesions that

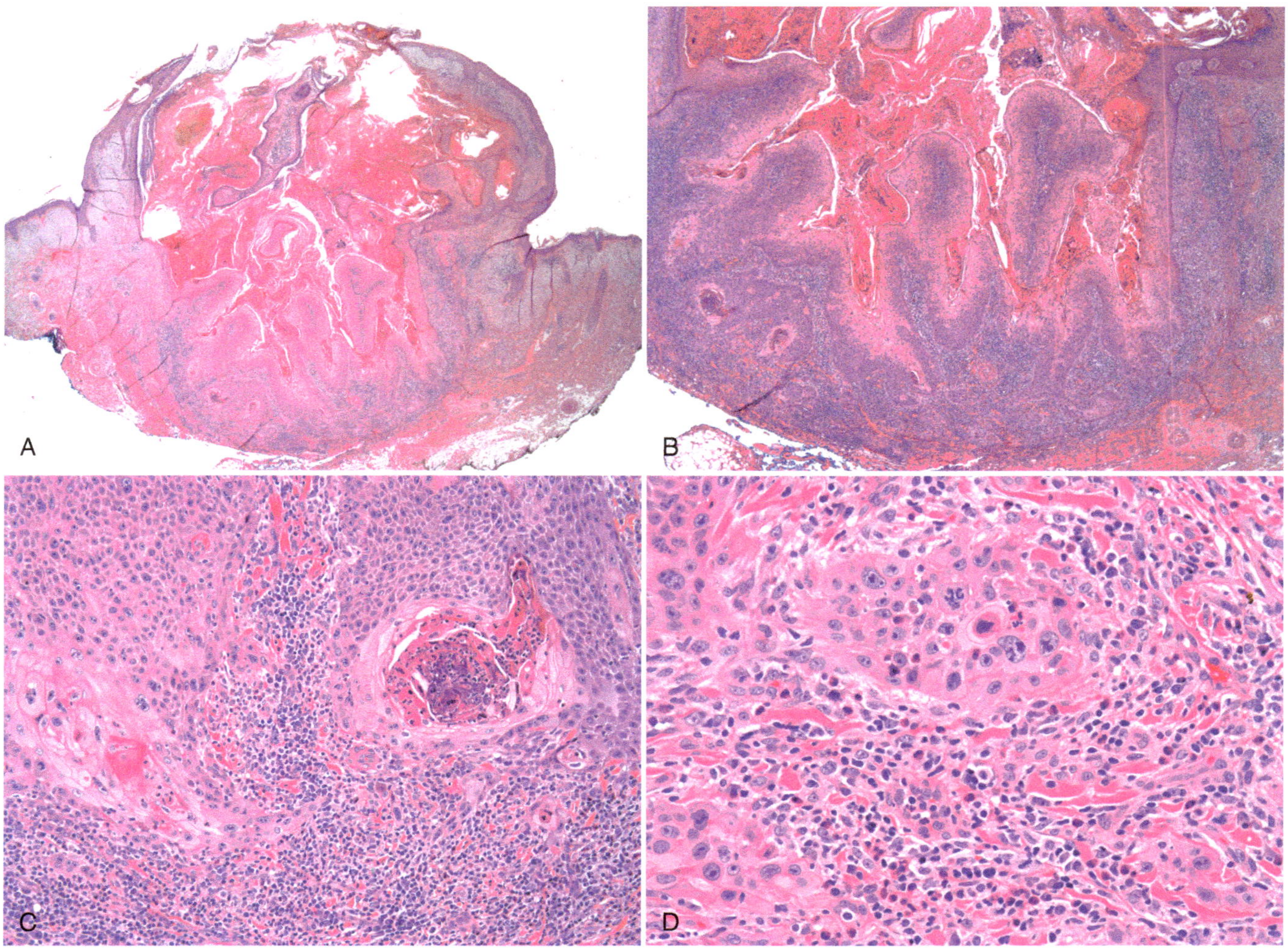

FIG 11.67 Well-differentiated squamous cell carcinoma, keratoacanthomatous pattern, of the lip. (A) Cup-shaped, umbilicated tumor with a central keratin-filled cavity into which papillary projections of epithelium project. (B) Cells with pale, glassy cytoplasm are present as well as darker basaloid cells, and invasion of the stroma is evident. (C) Keratin pearls with microabscesses are present at the tips of rete ridges, and there is stromal infiltration and a strong lymphocytic host response. (D) Tumor cells have pleomorphic nuclei and abnormal mitoses are noted, as well as many eosinophils in the stroma and within the epithelium.

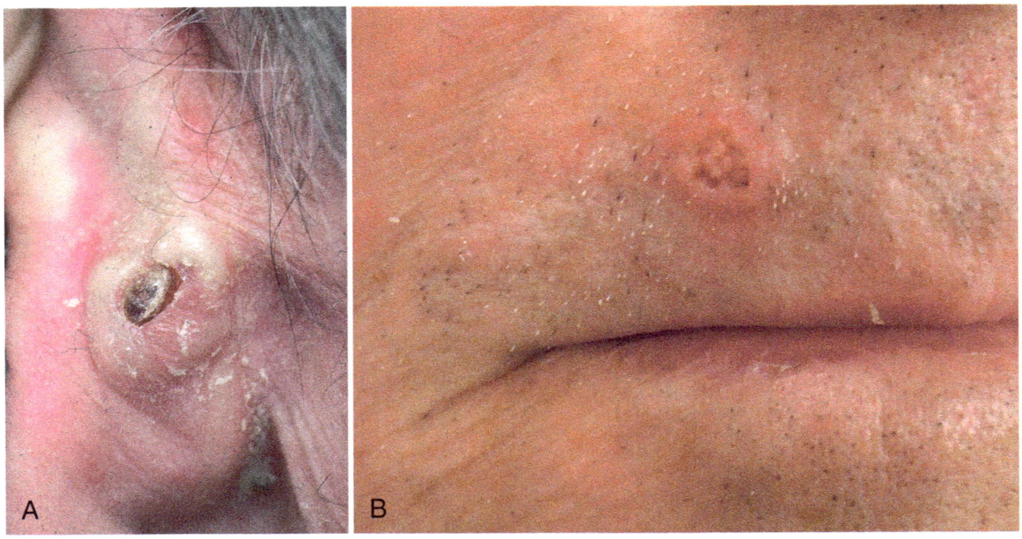

FIG 11.68 Keratoacanthoma of the skin. (A) Nodule with raised firm borders and central umbilication. (B) Nodule with central umbilication and yellow keratin. *(A, Courtesy Dr. Philip McKee; B, Courtesy Dr. Victor Neel, Boston.)*

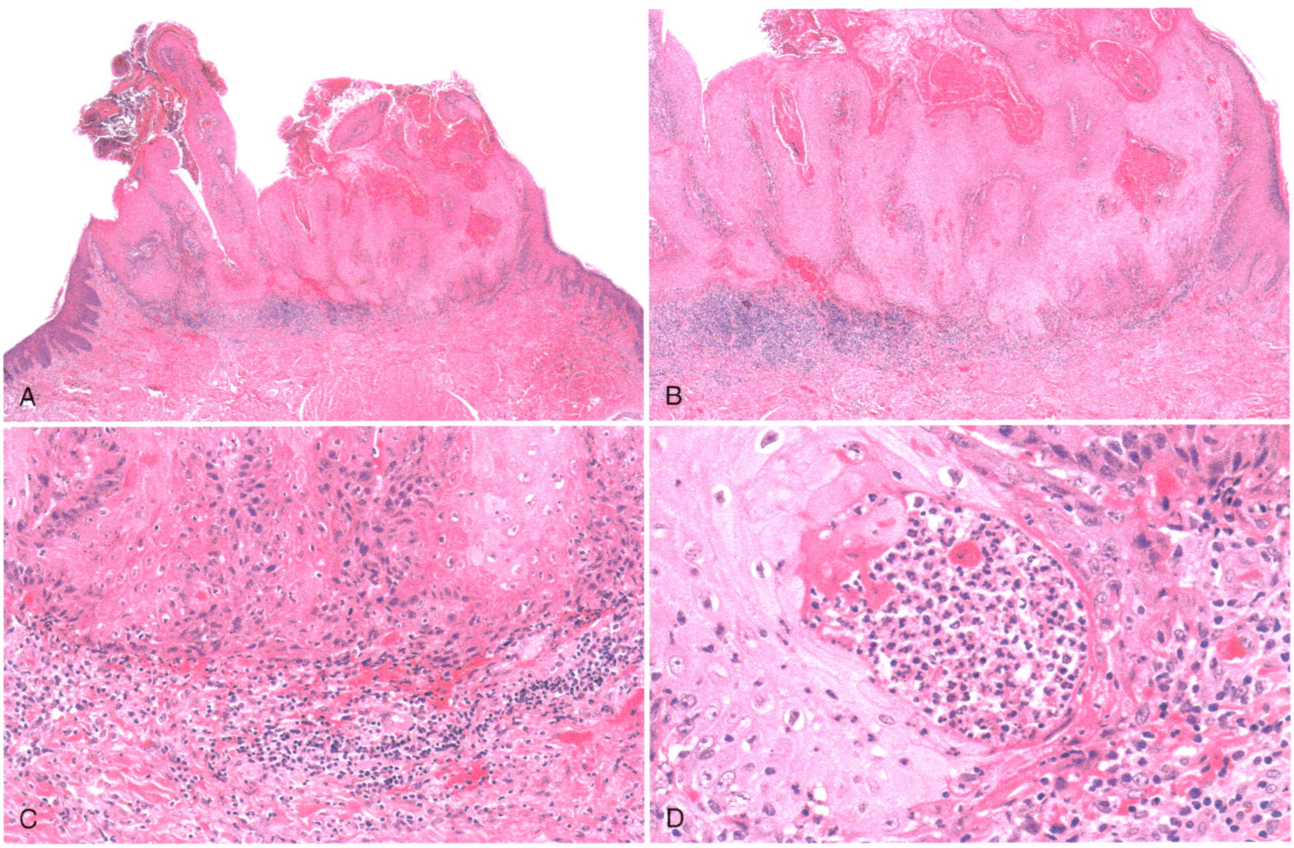

FIG 11.69 Well-differentiated squamous cell carcinoma, keratoacanthomatous pattern. (A) There is a papillary proliferation of pale squamous cells with endophytic, cupped morphology. (B) There are pale cells with a broad pushing front and a lymphocytic host response. (C) Cells have abundant, pale glassy cytoplasm and there is basal cell hyperplasia with hyperchromatic nuclei. (D) Dyskeratotic cells and microabscesses are present at tips of rete ridges.

present on the gingiva are difficult to orient and the central keratin-filled cavity may be difficult to discern.

Differential Diagnosis

- Pseudoepitheliomatous hyperplasia does not give rise to the bulky squamous proliferation seen in this tumor.

Prognosis

- These have a very good prognosis with little recurrence if an adequate lesion-free margin can be achieved.

REFERENCES

Beham A, Regauer S, Soyer HP, Beham-Schmid C. Keratoacanthoma: a clinically distinct variant of well differentiated squamous cell carcinoma. *Adv Anat Pathol.* 1998;5:269-280.

Habel G, O'Regan B, Eissing A, Khoury F, Donath K. Intra-oral keratoacanthoma: an eruptive variant and review of the literature. *Br Dent J.* 1991;170:336-339.

Karaa A, Khachemoune A. Keratoacanthoma: a tumor in search of a classification. *Int J Dermatol.* 2007;46:671-678.

Ko CJ. Keratoacanthoma: facts and controversies. *Clin Dermatol.* 2010;28:254-261.

Ko CJ, McNiff JM, Bosenberg M, Choate KA. Keratoacanthoma: clinical and histopathologic features of regression. *J Am Acad Dermatol.* 2012;67:1008-1012.

Misago N, Inoue T, Koba S, Narisawa Y. Keratoacanthoma and other types of squamous cell carcinoma with crateriform architecture: classification and identification. *J Dermatol.* 2013;40:443-452.

Takai T, Misago N, Murata Y. Natural course of keratoacanthoma and related lesions after partial biopsy: clinical analysis of 66 lesions. *J Dermatol.* 2015;42:353-362.

SQUAMOUS CELL CARCINOMA IN THE PEDIATRIC POPULATION

Less than 30 cases exist in the literature and most occur on the tongue or gingiva presenting as an exophytic mass, sometimes with a granular or papillary surface (Fig. 11.70). Some of these have been reported as keratoacanthomas.

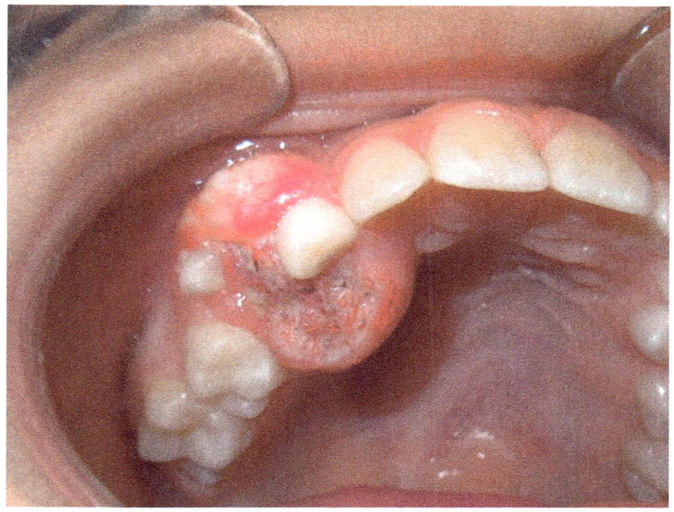

FIG 11.70 Carcinoma in a 9-year-old child presenting as a mass with a granular surface on the gingiva. *(Courtesy Dr. Bonnie Padwa, Children's Hospital, Boston.)*

- The lesions are very well-differentiated and most show cells with glassy cytoplasm similar to that seen in the keratoacanthomatous pattern of carcinoma, sometimes with umbilication; there is infiltration of the stroma by pleomorphic cells (Fig. 11.71).

Differential Diagnosis

- Pseudoepitheliomatous hyperplasia is the most common misdiagnosis primarily because of the well-differentiated nature of the epithelial cells, and the young age of the patient; however, the clinical appearance of a tumor together with the bulky epithelial proliferation would not support a diagnosis of benign hyperplasia.

Prognosis

- The prognosis is very good and most patients do not die of this disease if correctly diagnosed.

REFERENCES

Bill TJ, Reddy VR, Ries KL, et al. Adolescent gingival squamous cell carcinoma: Report of a case and review of the literature. *Oral Surg Oral Med Oral Pathol Oral Radiol Endod.* 2001;91:682-685.

Janette A, Pecaro B, Lonergan M, Lingen MW. Solitary intraoral keratoacanthoma: report of a case. *J Oral Maxillofac Surg.* 1996;54:1026-1030.

Stolk-Liefferink SA, Dumans AG, van der Meij EH, et al. Oral squamous cell carcinoma in children; review of an unusual entity. *Int J Pediatr Otorhinolaryngol.* 2008;72:127-131.

Woo VL, Kelsch RD, Su L, et al. Gingival squamous cell carcinoma in adolescence. *Oral Surg Oral Med Oral Pathol Oral Radiol Endod.* 2009;107:92-99.

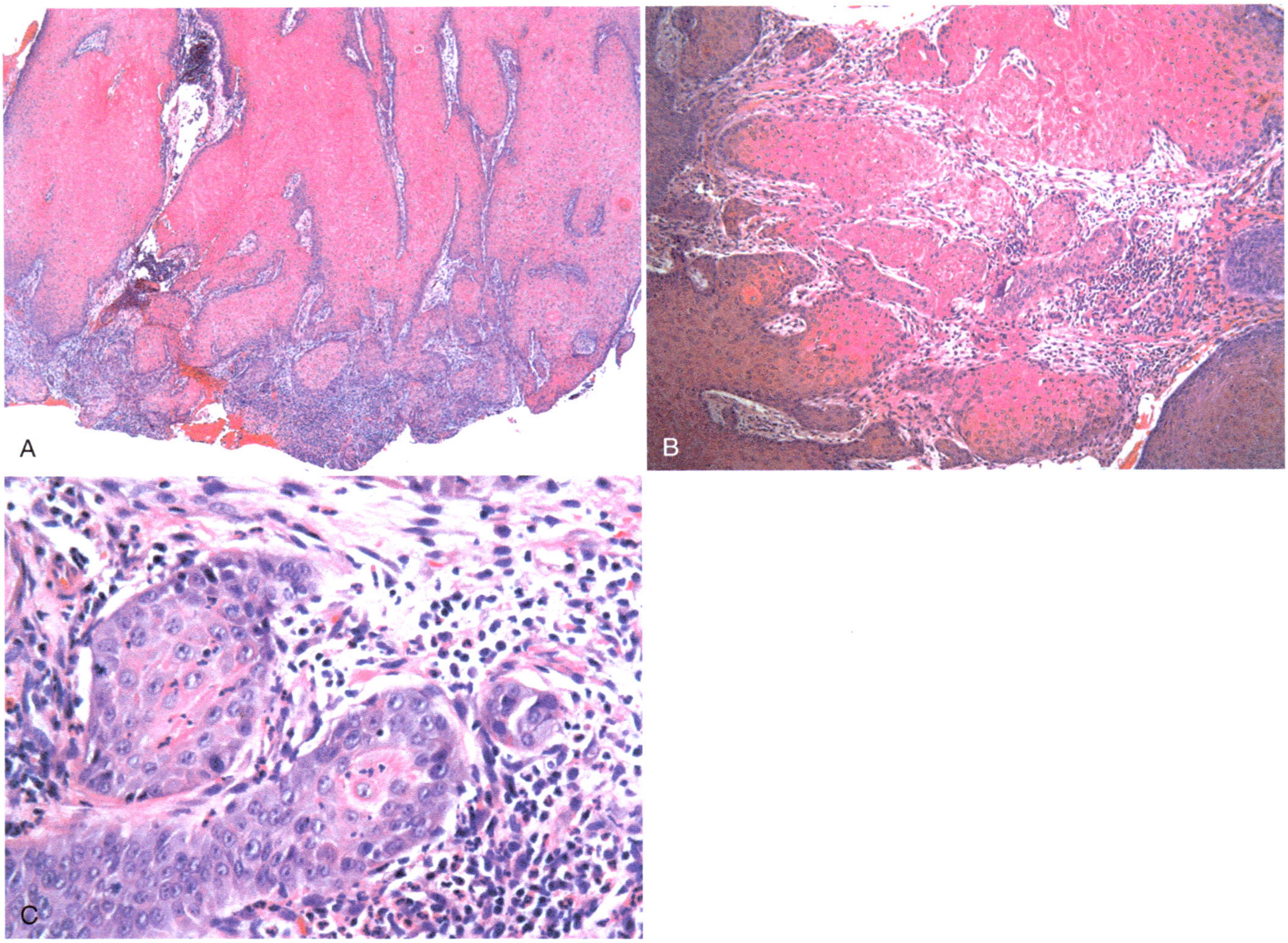

FIG 11.71 Well-differentiated squamous cell carcinoma. (A) Sheets of squamous cells with abundant, pink, glassy cytoplasm. (B) Tumor infiltrates the stroma as small islands of cells with many dyskeratotic cells. (C) Tumor cells exhibit moderate cytologic atypia.

12 INFLAMMATORY SALIVARY GLAND DISORDERS

CHAPTER CONTENTS

MUCOCELE (MUCOUS EXTRAVASATION PHENOMENON)

The term mucocele sometimes is used to include both extravasation and retention mucoceles. Here only the extravasation type is termed mucocele while the retention type is termed salivary duct cyst. They have different sites of occurrence, etiopathogenesis, and histopathology.

Clinical Findings

- Mucoceles are most common in the first three decades of life; they manifest as dome-shaped, bluish, sessile nodules most commonly located on the lower lip mucosa (70% to 90% of cases), ventral tongue (also referred to as ranula), buccal mucosa, and floor of mouth; they wax and wane and are usually painless (Fig. 12.1A–C); some resolve spontaneously.
- Superficial mucoceles are seen in patients with hyposalivation and mucosal disease and are most frequent on the palatal mucosa (especially in patients with chronic graft-versus-host disease); they are generally painless blisters or vesicles, <5 mm in diameter, often leading to a clinical misdiagnosis of herpes infection, which is almost always painful (see Fig. 12.1D).

Etiopathogenesis and Histopathologic Features

Mucoceles are pseudocysts that arise from trauma to the excretory salivary duct resulting in extravasation of mucin into the surrounding soft tissues. This becomes walled off by granulation tissue and eventually organized by fibrous tissue. Superficial mucoceles occur because of either salivary gland hypofunction (such as dehydration or chronic graft-versus-host disease) or mucosal disease causing inflammation around the ducts (such as chronic graft-versus-host disease or lichen planus).

- There is a cystlike cavity filled with mucin with muciphages and variable numbers of neutrophils, surrounded by condensed granulation tissue also containing muciphages; eosinophilic globular structures are sometimes present and can be prominent (referred to as myxoglobulosis) and they are mucicarmine-positive and represent condensations of mucin; a feeder duct exhibiting squamous metaplasia may be seen (Figs. 12.2–12.4).
- Mucin may be present diffusely in the connective tissue or within glandular parenchyma rather than in a cystlike space (Fig. 12.5); lesions not removed intact manifest as fragments of granulation tissue with muciphages and sometimes condensed mucin globules (Fig. 12.6); ventral tongue lesions tend not to have a thick wall of granulation tissue (Fig. 12.7).
- Minor salivary glands maintain their lobular architecture and exhibit variable degrees of obstructive changes, namely acinar atrophy, ductal dilatation with inspissated secretions, periductal hyalinization, interstitial fibrosis, and an interstitial lymphoplasmacytic infiltrate (Fig. 12.8).
- An organizing mucocele may consist of a solid mass of granulation tissue with muciphages without a mucin pool (Fig. 12.9); muciphages may have clear cytoplasm (Fig. 12.10).
- Papillary synovium–like areas are frequently seen (Fig. 12.11).

- Superficial mucoceles contain mucin pools that abut the overlying atrophic epithelium and are often surrounded by a collarette of epithelium that forms part of the wall of the mucocele (Figs. 12.12 and 12.13).

Differential Diagnosis

- An organizing mucocele with a predominance of clear cells may resemble salivary gland neoplasm such as a clear cell mucoepidermoid carcinoma or even clear cell carcinoma, but there is lack of stromal invasion by nests of neoplastic cells and the cells are keratin-negative, and CD68+.
- Periductal lymphocytic infiltrates are frequently seen in obstructive sialadenitis and should not be confused with autoimmune sialadenitis as seen in Sjögren syndrome, in which obstructive changes are minimal and the lymphocytic infiltrate is strikingly periductal, at least in early stages (see later).

Management

- Enucleation or excision of the mucoceles, sometimes with overlying mucosa (especially superficial mucoceles), and removal of damaged salivary glands in the vicinity is curative; recurrence rate is up to 8% after excision because of further damage of salivary glands.

REFERENCES

Bermejo A, Aguirre JM, Lopez P, Saez MR. Superficial mucocele: report of 4 cases. *Oral Surg Oral Med Oral Pathol Oral Radiol Endod.* 1999;88:469-472.

Campana F, Sibaud V, Chauvel A, et al. Recurrent superficial mucoceles associated with lichenoid disorders. *J Oral Maxillofac Surg.* 2006;64:1830-1833.

Chi AC, Haigney RJ 2nd, Spagnoli DB, et al. Papillary synovial metaplasia-like change in oral mucoceles: a rare and previously undescribed histopathologic variant of a common oral lesion. *Oral Surg Oral Med Oral Pathol Oral Radiol Endod.* 2010;109:268-273.

Chi AC, Lambert PR 3rd, Richardson MS, Neville BW. Oral mucoceles: a clinicopathologic review of 1,824 cases, including unusual variants. *J Oral Maxillofac Surg.* 2011;69:1086-1093.

Conceicao JG, Gurgel CA, Ramos EA, et al. Oral mucoceles: a clinical, histopathological and immunohistochemical study. *Acta Histochem.* 2014;116:40-47.

Jinbu Y, Kusama M, Itoh H, et al. Mucocele of the glands of Blandin-Nuhn: clinical and histopathologic analysis of 26 cases. *Oral Surg Oral Med Oral Pathol Oral Radiol Endod.* 2003;95:467-470.

Minguez-Martinez I, Bonet-Coloma C, Ata-Ali-Mahmud J, et al. Clinical characteristics, treatment, and evolution of 89 mucoceles in children. *J Oral Maxillofac Surg.* 2010;68:e2468-e2471.

Schulman JM, Jordan RC. Oral mucus extravasation phenomenon with myxoglobulosis. *J Cutan Pathol.* 2014;41:767-770.

Shah KA. Myxoglobulosis in oral extravasation mucocele: an entity? *Histopathology.* 2003;43:291-296.

Treister NS, Cook EF Jr, Antin J, et al. Clinical evaluation of oral chronic graft-versus-host disease. *Biol Blood Marrow Transplant.* 2008;14:110-115.

Text continued on p. 298

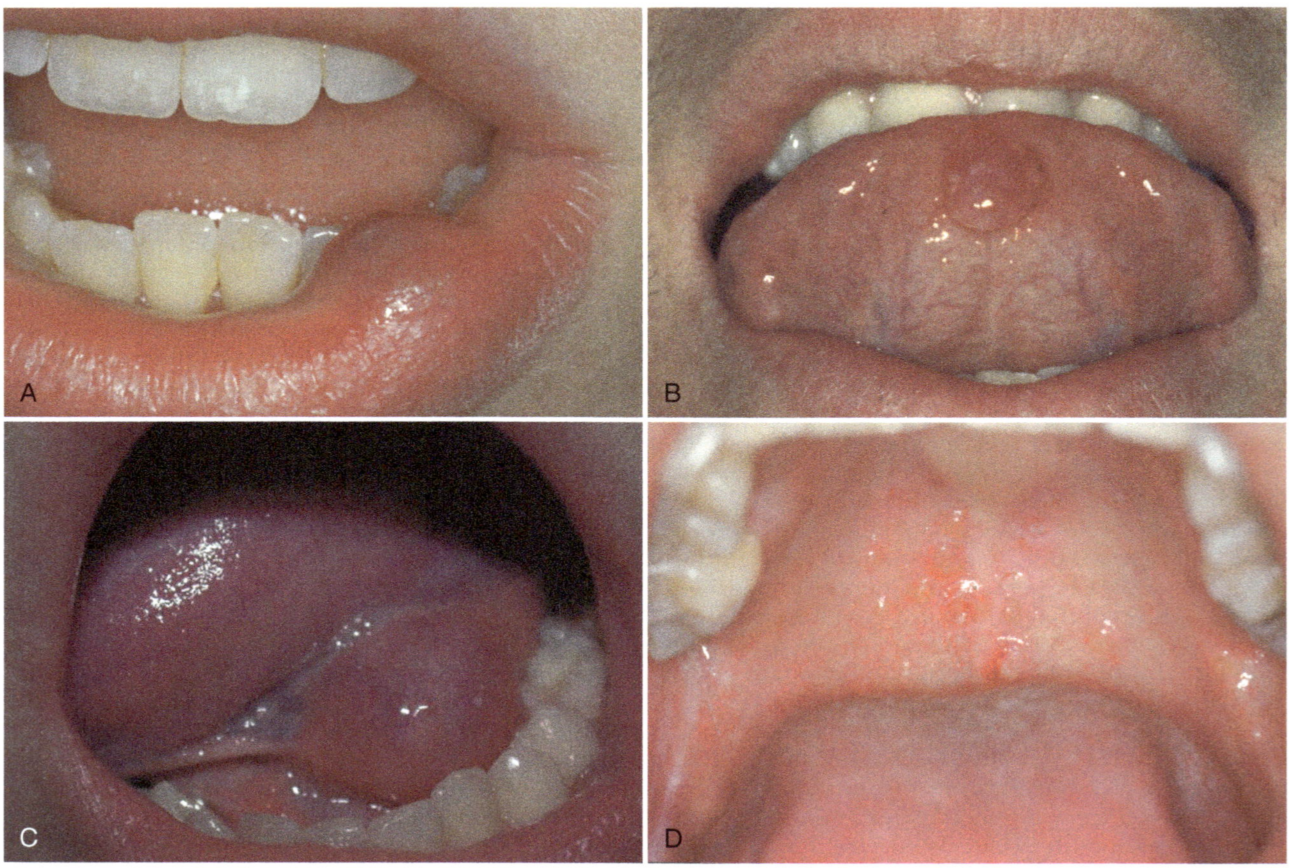

FIG 12.1 (A) Mucocele on lower lip. (B) Mucocele on ventral tongue. (C) Ranula (floor of mouth mucocele). (D) Superficial mucocele. *(C, Courtesy Dr. Bonnie Padwa, Harvard School of Dental Medicine, Boston.)*

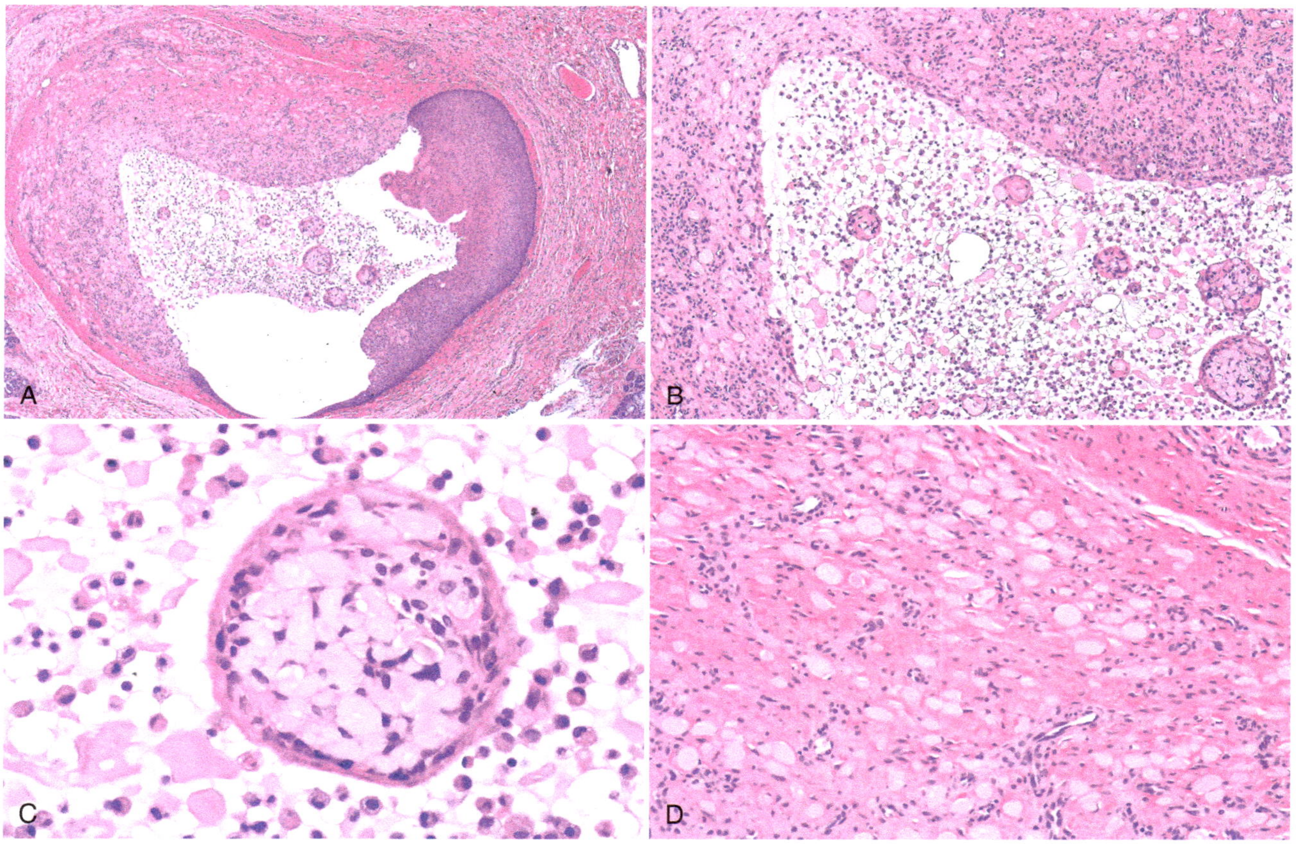

FIG 12.2 Mucocele with mucin globules. (A) Pool of mucin containing eosinophilic globules, surrounded by granulation tissue; part of the feeder duct is present. (B) Surrounding granulation tissue contains muciphages and mucin globules. (C) Hyaline mucin globules within mucin. (D) Condensed eosinophilic mucin globules in the connective tissue.

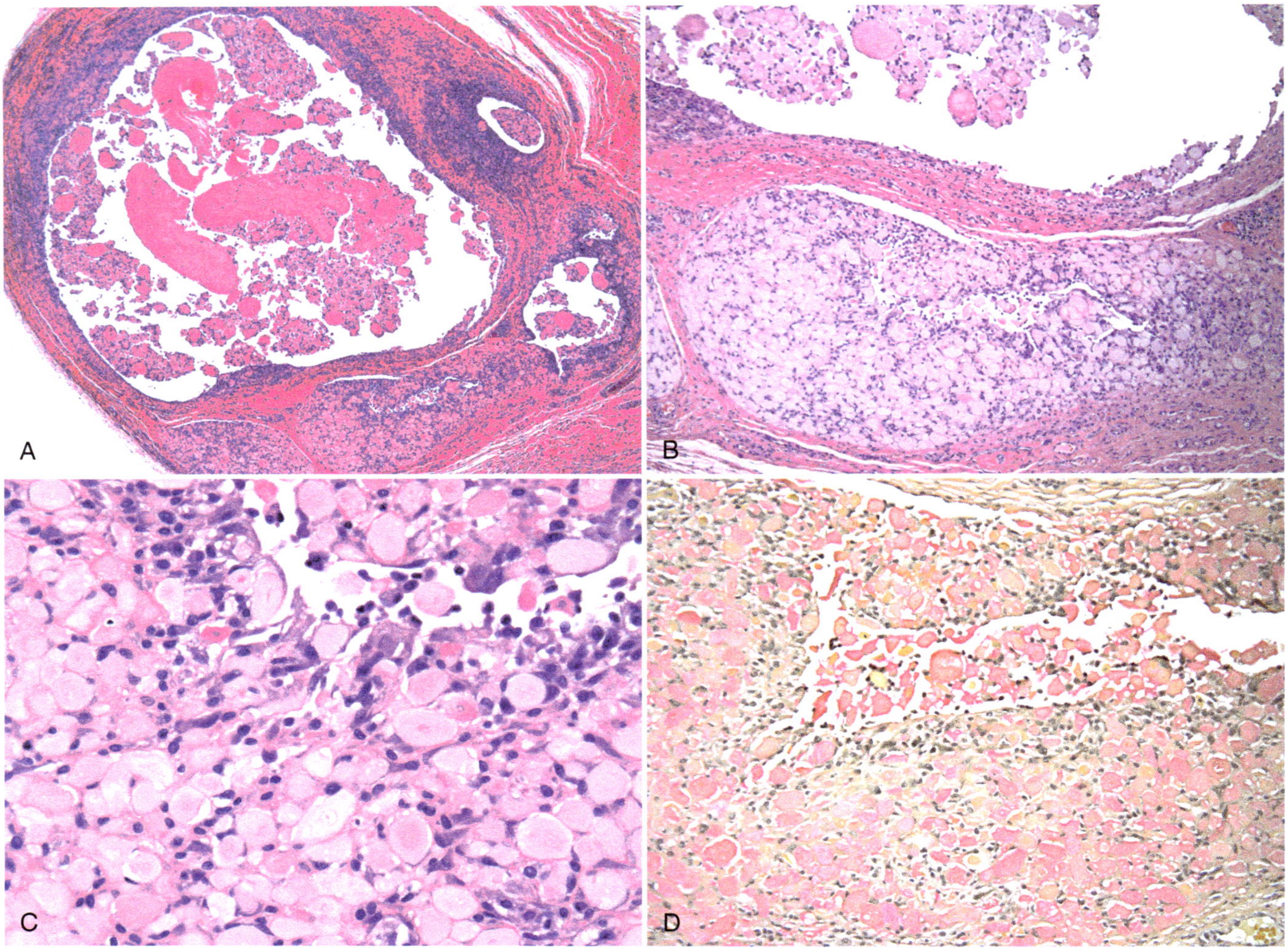

FIG 12.3 Mucocele with prominent myxoglobulosis. (A) Pool of mucin containing many eosinophilic globules. (B) Eosinophlic globules within the lumen and the wall. (C) Compact collections of mucin globules. (D) Globules are mucicarmine-positive.

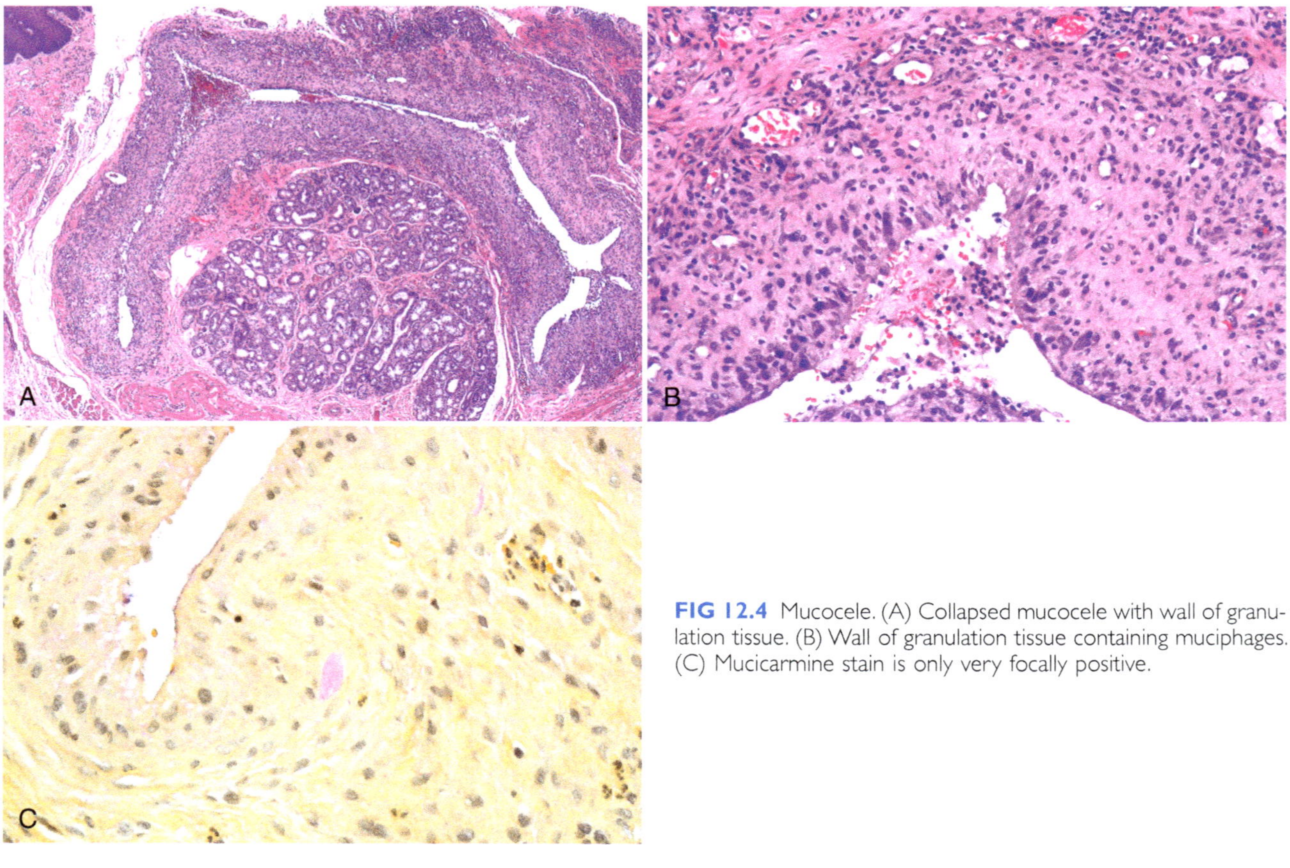

FIG 12.4 Mucocele. (A) Collapsed mucocele with wall of granulation tissue. (B) Wall of granulation tissue containing muciphages. (C) Mucicarmine stain is only very focally positive.

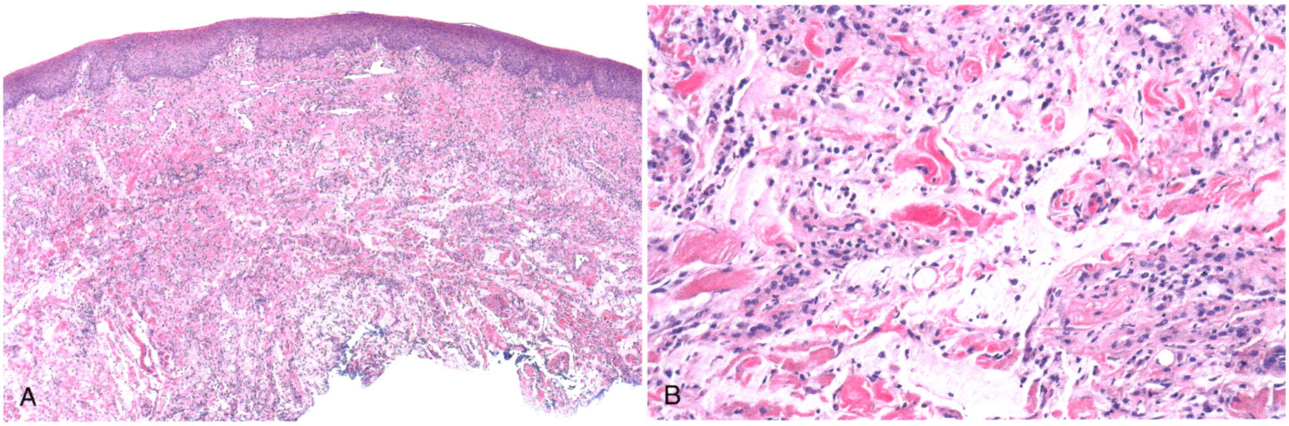

FIG 12.5 Mucocele. (A) Mucin appears diffusely in the interstitium without demarcated mucin pool. (B) Abundant interstitial mucin with muciphages.

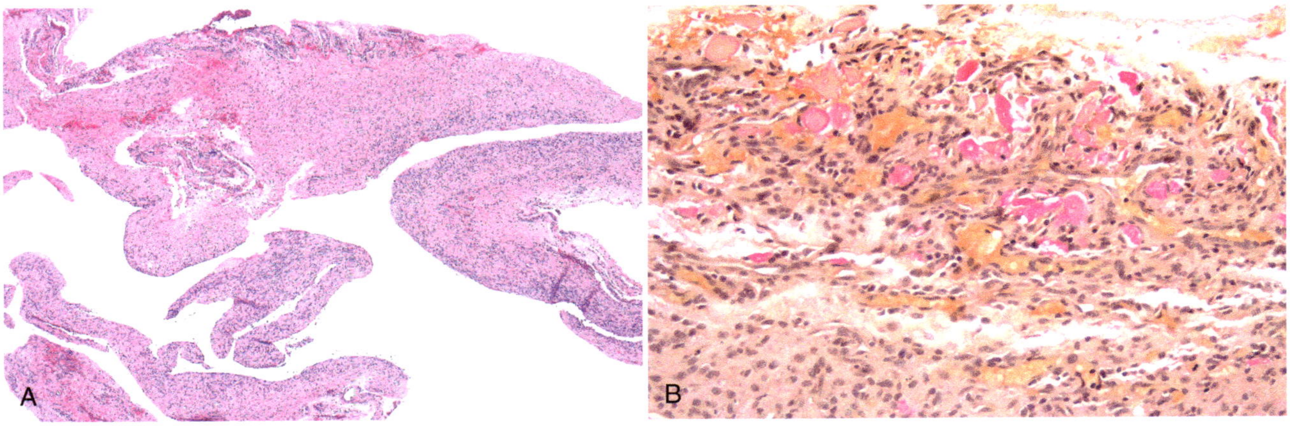

FIG 12.6 Mucocele. (A) Fragments of granulation tissue from a curetted specimen. (B) Eosinophilic mucin globules in the wall stain for mucicarmine.

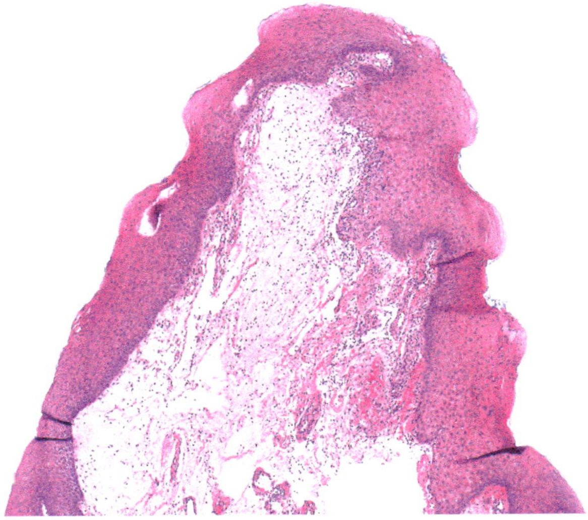

FIG 12.7 Mucocele of ventral tongue: pool of mucin and granulation tissue that is generally not as obviously walled off.

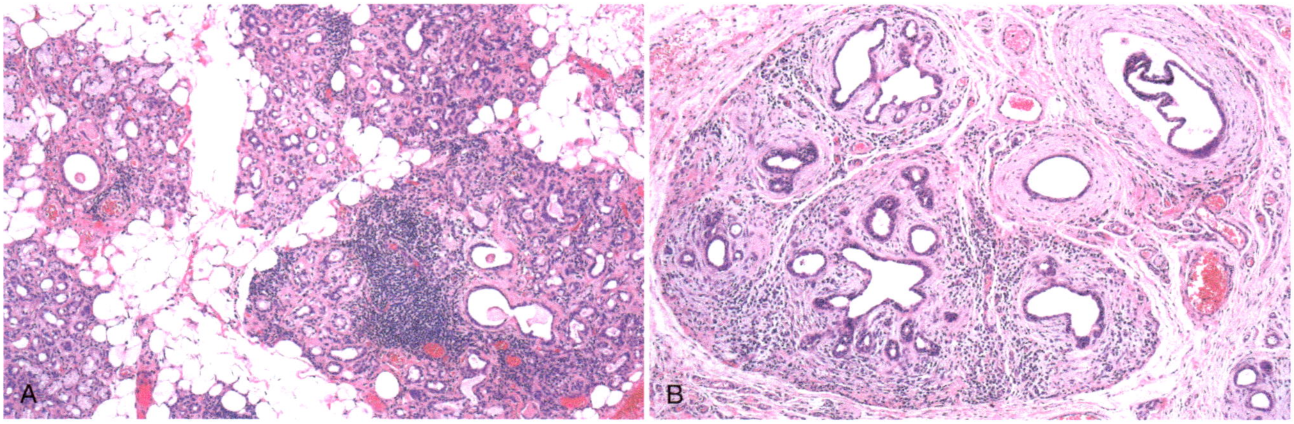

FIG 12.8 Chronic obstructive sialadenitis with maintenance of lobular architecture. (A) Diffuse involvement of glands with acinar atrophy, ductal dilatation interstitial fibrosis, and interstitial chronic inflammation. (B) Marked acinar atrophy, prominent ductal dilatation, interstitial fibrosis, and chronic inflammation.

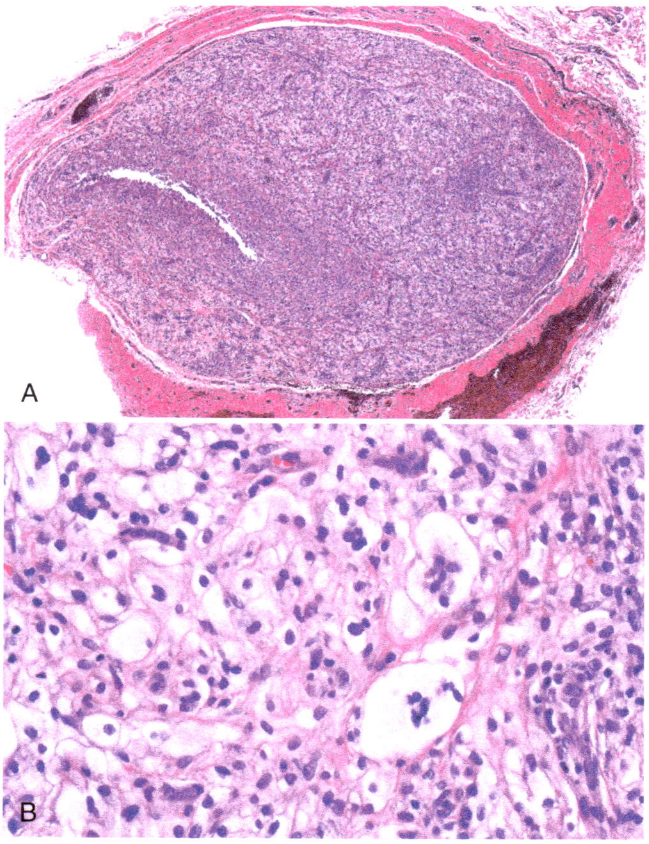

FIG 12.9 Organizing mucocele. (A) Compact mass of granulation tissue with peripheral fibrosis. (B) Compact granulation tissue with muciphages.

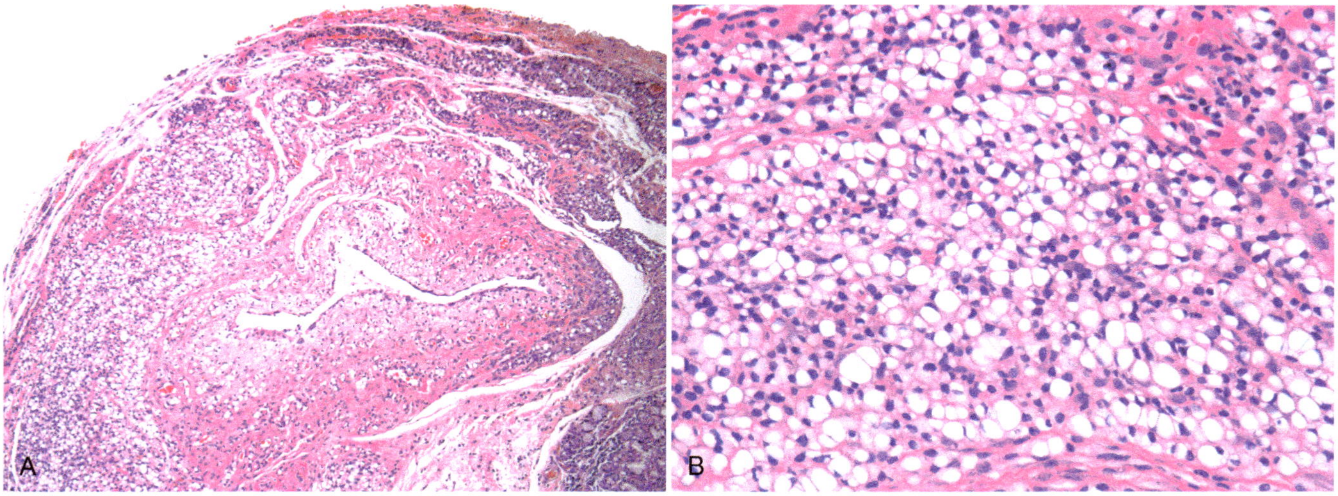

FIG 12.10 Mucocele with clear cells. (A) Granulation tissue surrounds a cystlike space. (B) Granulation tissue wall with muciphages and clear cells.

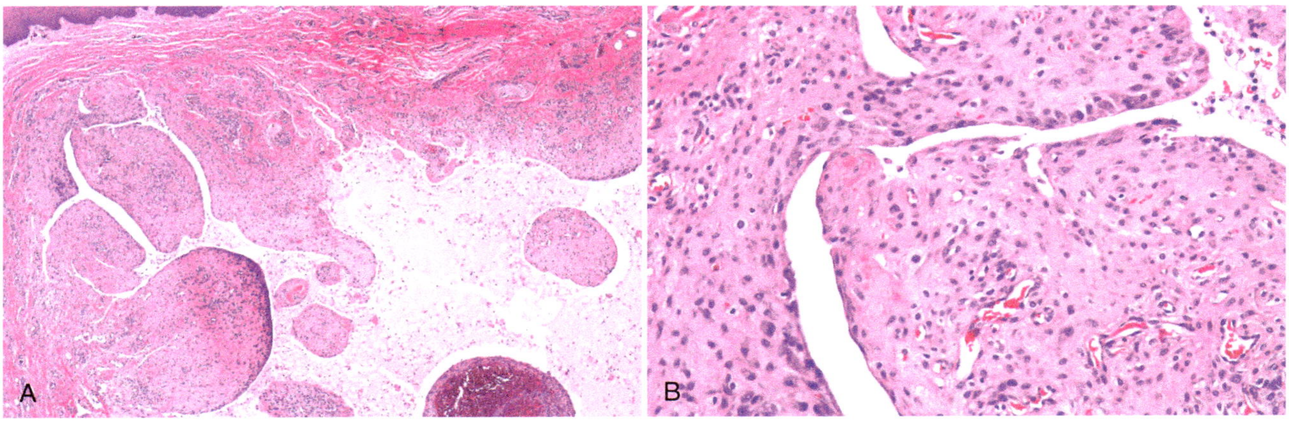

FIG 12.11 Mucocele. (A) Papillary synovium-like structures protrude into mucin pool. (B) Synovium-like areas are composed of fibroblasts, macrophages, and capillaries.

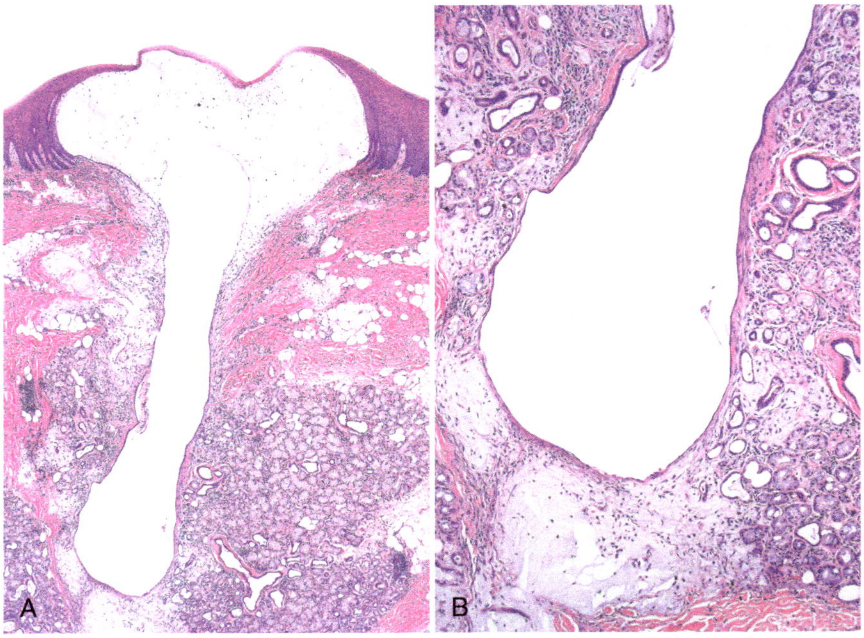

FIG 12.12 Superficial mucocele. (A) Mucin pool abuts and thins the epithelium that forms a collarette. (B) Mucin in the connective tissue with obstructive changes in salivary glands.

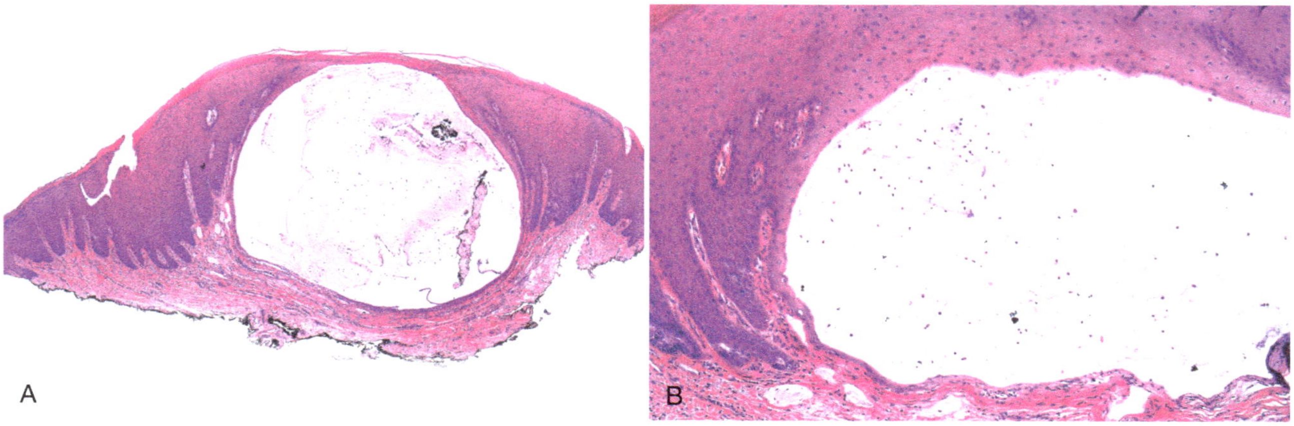

FIG 12.13 Superficial mucocele. (A) Mucin pool abuts and thins the epithelium that forms a collarette. (B) Mucin partially enclosed by surface epithelium.

SALIVARY DUCT CYST (MUCUS RETENTION CYST, SIALOCYST)

Clinical Findings

- This lesion is more common in adults and tends to occur in the maxillary and mandibular sulcus/vestibule (mucobuccal fold) and upper lip (where it is often associated with sialoliths) (Fig. 12.14); it appears as a bluish nodule that may feel hard if a sialolith is present.

Etiopathogenesis and Histopathologic Features

This cyst arises from retention of secretions within a duct from a distal obstruction, such as a sialolith or even viscid secretions, although in some cases the etiology is unclear.

- The cystically dilated excretory salivary duct may be lined by a double layer of low cuboidal-to-columnar cells or may exhibit squamous, ciliated cell, or oncocytic metaplasia (is sometimes termed *oncocytic sialocyst*); it may have slight papillary projections in the lining and a sialolith may be present (Figs. 12.15–12.17); a variable lymphoplasmacytic infiltrate is present, often just beneath the lining epithelium.
- Multiple cystically dilated ducts exhibiting oncocytic metaplasia may occur in both extralobular and intralobular locations, with the surrounding salivary gland lobules exhibiting other chronic obstructive changes such as acinar atrophy, and interstitial fibrosis and inflammation (Figs. 12.18 and 12.19).

Differential Diagnosis

- Gingival cyst of the adult that occurs on the attached gingiva often contains squamous epithelial plaques with clear cells; the occurrence of salivary gland disease on the attached gingiva is extremely rare.
- Multifocality, lack of encapsulation, or significant adenomatous hyperplasia differentiates cystic oncocytic metaplasia from cystadenoma. True oral papillary cystadenoma lymphomatosum has been reported but is rare.

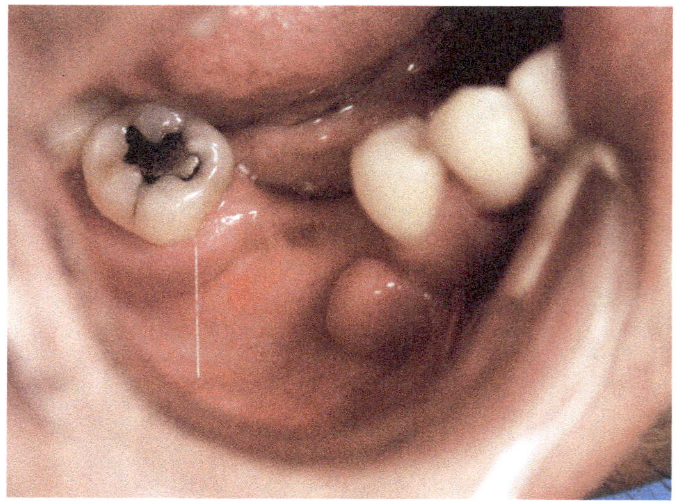

FIG 12.14 Salivary duct cyst of the mandibular vestibule.

Management

- Enucleation or excision with surrounding glands is curative.

REFERENCES

Eversole LR. Oral sialocysts. *Arch Otolaryngol.* 1987;113:51-56.

Fantasia JE, Miller AS. Papillary cystadenoma lymphomatosum arising in minor salivary glands. *Oral Surg Oral Med Oral Pathol.* 1981;52:411-416.

Takeda Y, Yamamoto H. Salivary duct cyst: its frequency in a certain Japanese population group (Tohoku districts), with special reference to adenomatous proliferation of the epithelial lining. *J Oral Sci.* 2001;43:9-13.

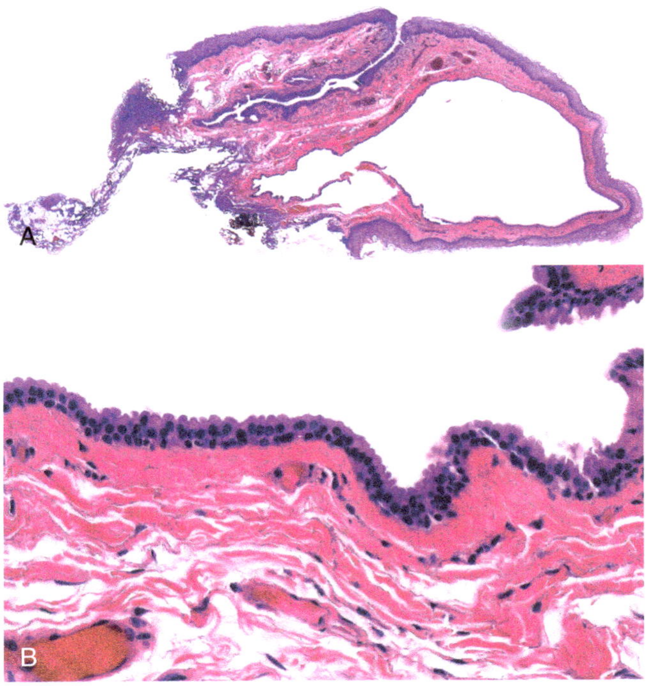

FIG 12.15 Salivary duct cyst. (A) Note the adjacent normal excretory salivary duct in continuity with the surface epithelium. (B) Lining consists of a double layer of low cuboidal-to-columnar cells.

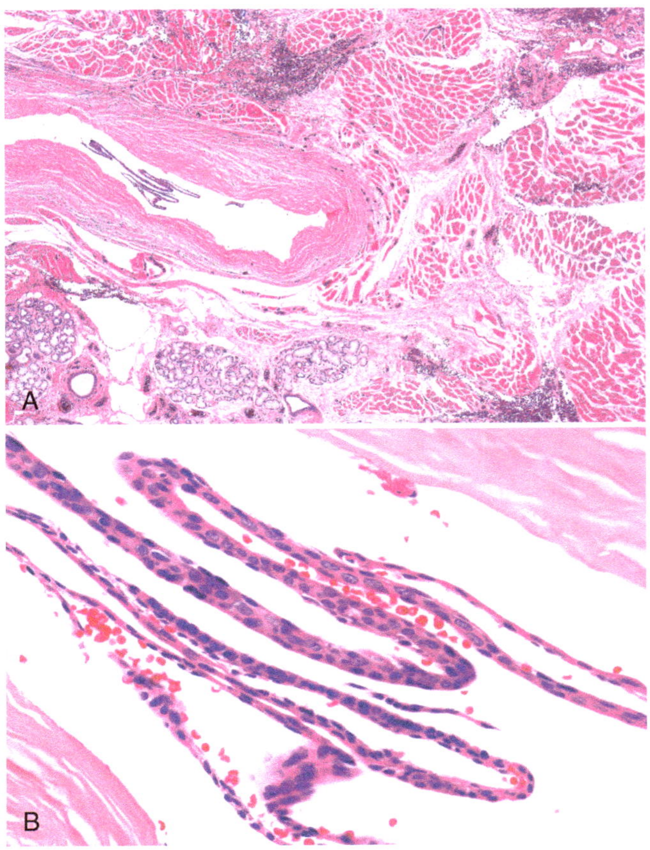

FIG 12.16 Salivary duct cyst. (A) Cyst with uniformly thin lining and thickened, hyalinized basement membrane. (B) Detached strips of epithelium composed of two to three layers of flattened cuboidal cells.

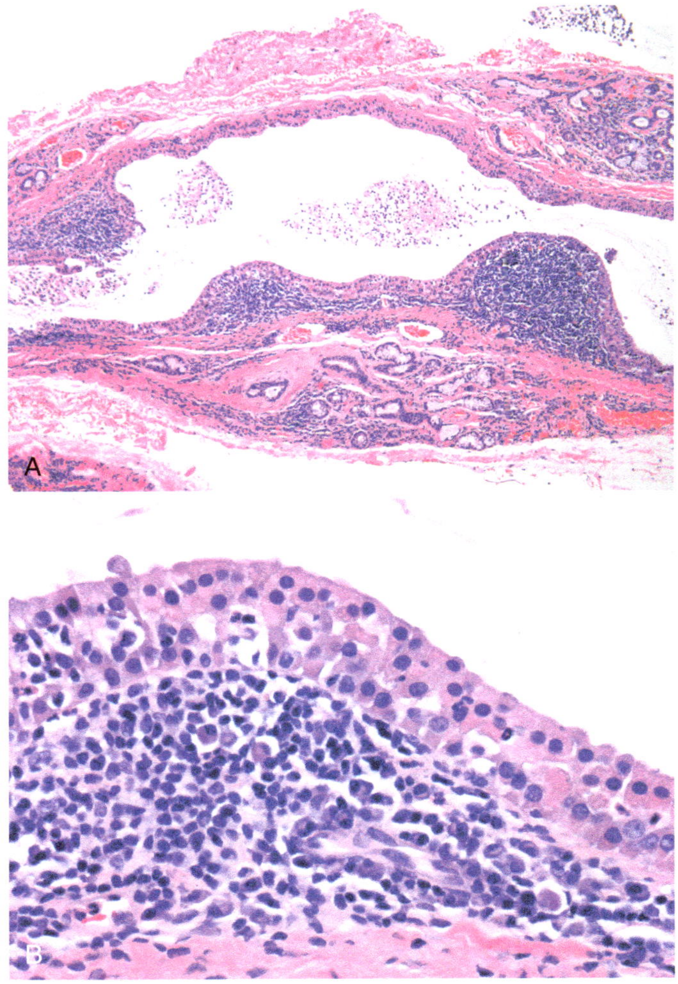

FIG 12.17 Salivary duct cyst with oncocytic metaplasia. (A) Undulating luminal surface and surrounding chronic inflammation. (B) Lining composed of oncocytes with surrounding lymphoplasmacytic infiltrate.

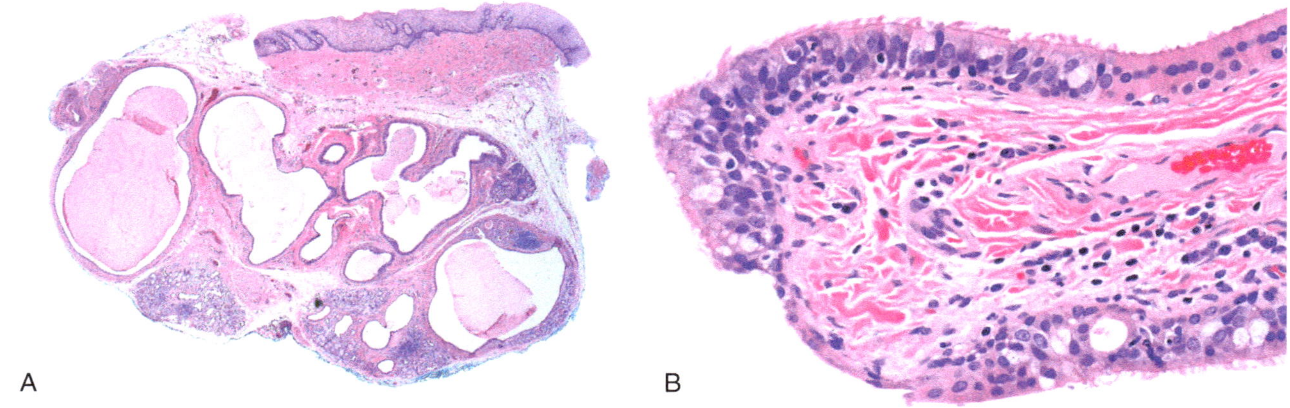

FIG 12.18 Oncocytic metaplasia in multiple ducts. (A) Dilated extralobular and intralobular ducts with marked sclerosing sialadenitis in surrounding glands. (B) Lining is composed of pseudostratifed columnar, ciliated, oncocytic *(right)*, and mucous cells.

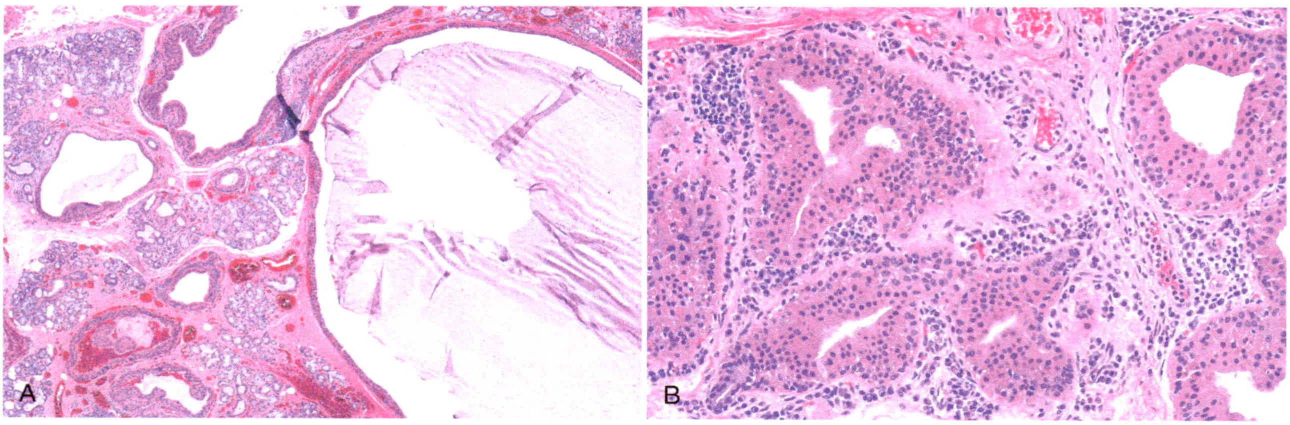

FIG 12.19 Oncocytic metaplasia in multiple ducts. (A) Dilated extralobular and intralobular ducts with obstructive changes in adjacent glands. (B) Early dilatation of ducts exhibiting oncocytic metaplasia.

SIALOLITH (SALIVARY CALCULUS)

Clinical Findings

- Sialolith of the minor salivary glands occurs most commonly in the fifth to seventh decades of life, usually in the upper lip (45% of cases) and buccal mucosa (40% of cases), and occurs as a firm-to-hard nodule, usually asymptomatic, unless ruptured and inflamed.
- Sialolith of the major glands is most common within the Wharton (submandibular) duct (80% of cases), causing pain from pressure of retained saliva just before meals (meal symptoms); it may be seen on intraoral occlusal radiographs if it is sufficiently calcified (Fig. 12.20).

Etiopathogenesis and Histopathologic Features

Sialoliths form from a central nidus of cellular debris, bacteria, or mucous plugs and are unassociated with hypercalcemic syndromes. They are more common in the Wharton duct because of the length of the duct, its tortuous course, and the relatively thick mucinous secretions.

- Basophilic concentric lamellar and globular calcifications occur within a cystically dilated duct that exhibits squamous and often mucous cell metaplasia; suppuration may be seen if there is infection (Figs. 12.21 and 12.22); the associated minor glands exhibit obstructive changes and bacteria may be identified in rare cases (Fig. 12.23).

Differential Diagnosis

- Phleboliths are usually smaller, do not have a globular component, and are present within venules.

Management

- Excision of the sialolith with surrounding minor salivary glands is curative.
- Submandibular sialoliths are removed by transoral extraction, sialoendoscopy with extraction, or extracorporeal shockwave lithotripsy.

REFERENCES

Anneroth G, Hansen LS. Minor salivary gland calculi. A clinical and histopathological study of 49 cases. *Int J Oral Surg.* 1983;12:80-89.

Brazao-Silva MT, Prosdocimi FC, Lemos-Junior CA, de Sousa SO. Clinicopathological aspects of 25 cases of sialolithiasis of minor salivary glands. *Gen Dent.* 2015;63:e22-e26.

Jensen JL, Howell FV, Rick GM, Correll RW. Minor salivary gland calculi. A clinicopathologic study of forty-seven new cases. *Oral Surg Oral Med Oral Pathol.* 1979;47:44-50.

Zenk J, Koch M, Klintworth N, et al. Sialendoscopy in the diagnosis and treatment of sialolithiasis: a study on more than 1000 patients. *Otolaryngol Head Neck Surg.* 2012;147:858-863.

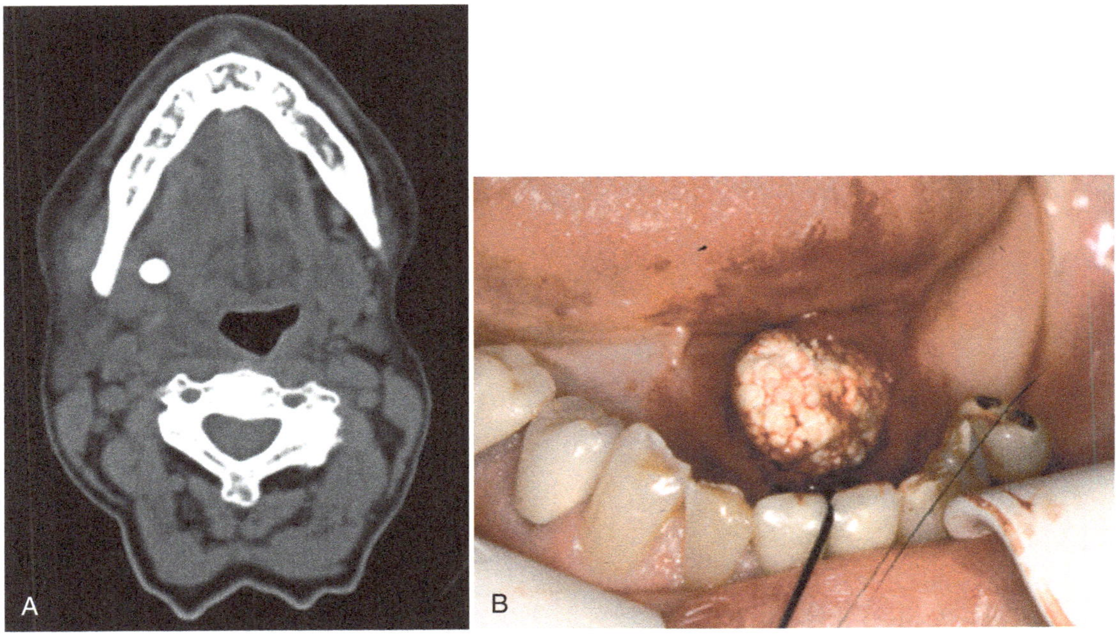

FIG 12.20 (A) Axial CT scan of a sialolith in the right submandibular duct. (B) Sialolith of submandibular duct. *(Courtesy Dr. Bonnie Padwa, Children's Hospital, Boston.)*

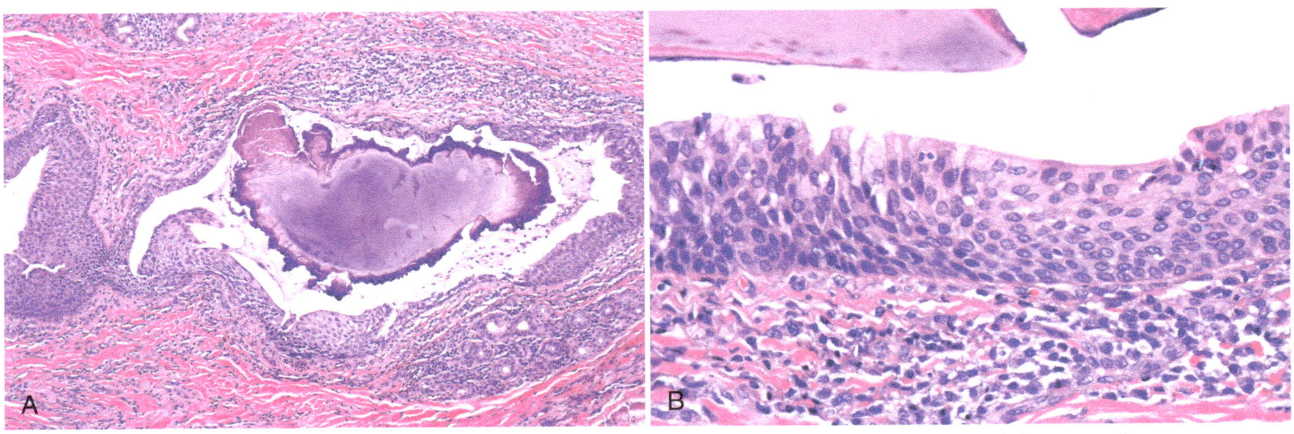

FIG 12.21 Sialolith. (A) Sialolith within an ectatic duct with squamous metaplasia, partially ruptured, with surrounding inflammation. (B) Duct epithelium exhibits squamous and mucous cell metaplasia.

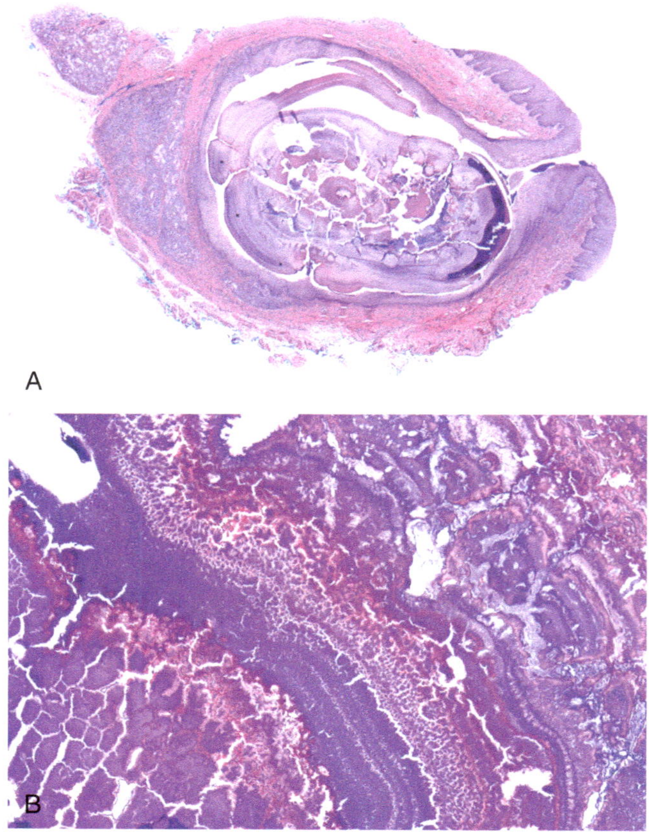

FIG 12.22 Sialolith. (A) Sialolith within ectatic duct with squamous metaplasia that opens into the oral cavity. (B) Lamellar and globular concretions.

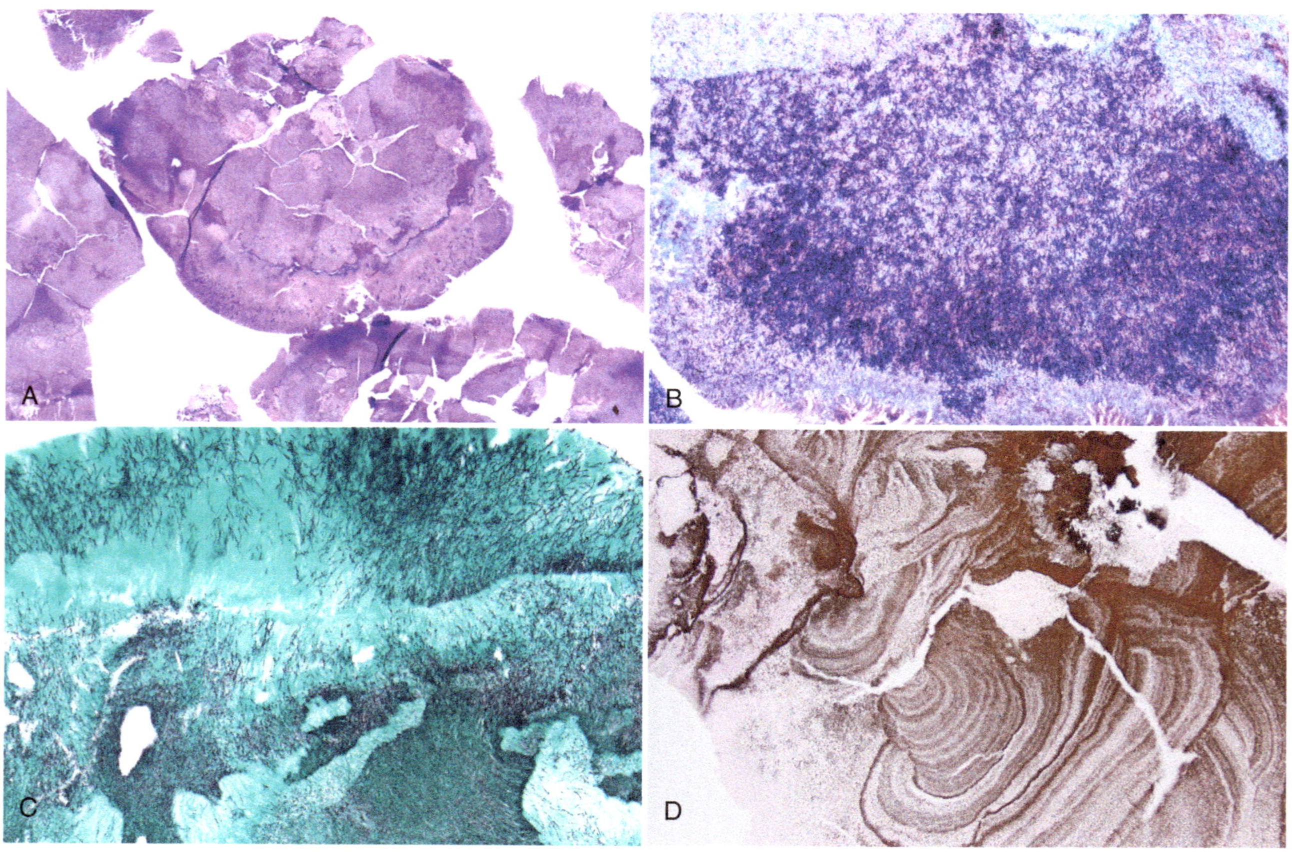

FIG 12.23 Fragments of a sialolith. (A) Fragmented, calcified structure. (B) Brown and Brenn stain showing many gram-positive cocci and rods. (C) Gomori methenamine silver stain showing many filamentous bacteria. (D) von Kossa stain showing lamellar calcifications.

CHEILITIS GLANDULARIS (STOMATITIS GLANDULARIS, CHEILITIS GLANDULARIS APOSTEMATOSA)

Clinical Findings

- This presents mostly in older adults with a 3:1 male predilection and is characterized by asymmetric, painful swelling, usually on the lower lip (95% of cases) that typically becomes everted with visible ostia from which viscous mucoid material or pus may be expelled; there may be crusting (Fig. 12.24); photodamage is usually present and simple, deep, and deep suppurative forms are recognized; cases in albinos have been reported, as has squamous cell carcinoma developing within the lesion.

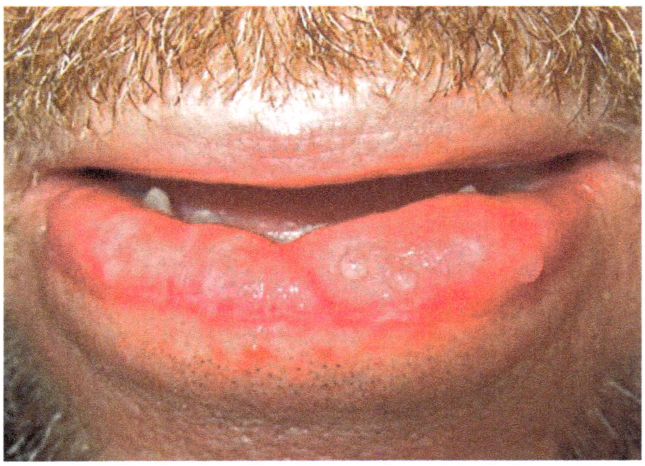

FIG 12.24 Cheilitis glancularis of lower lip with actinic cheilitis. *(Courtesy Division of Dermatology, Brigham and Women's Hospital, Boston, MA.)*

Etiopathogenesis and Histopathologic Features

This is an inflammatory condition that most likely results from actinic or other damage of the surface epithelium that extends down the ducts leading to sialadenitis, rather than resulting from primary glandular pathology.

- Cystically dilated excretory salivary ducts exhibit squamous, oncocytic, and mucous cell metaplasia with luminal secretions or suppuration, and periductal acute and chronic inflammation (Fig. 12.25).
- The overlying mucosa should be evaluated for dysplasia and/or invasive carcinoma.

Differential Diagnosis

- A ruptured and infected salivary duct cyst, with or without a sialolith, or local trauma may produce similar changes.

Management

- Antibiotics should be prescribed for infection if pain and/or suppuration is present.
- Excision of lesion is curative; dysplasia in the epithelium must be treated appropriately with excision, or topical 5-fluorouracil or imiquomod.

REFERENCES

Lourenco SV, Gori LM, Boggio P, Nico MM. Cheilitis glandularis in albinos: a report of two cases and review of histopathological findings after therapeutic vermilionectomy. *J Eur Acad Dermatol Venereol.* 2007;21:1265-1267.

Nico MM, Nakano de Melo J, Lourenco SV. Cheilitis glandularis: a clinicopathological study in 22 patients. *J Am Acad Dermatol.* 2010;62:233-238.

Reiter S, Vered M, Yarom N, et al. Cheilitis glandularis: clinico-histopathological diagnostic criteria. *Oral Dis.* 2011;17:335-339.

Swerlick RA, Cooper PH. Cheilitis glandularis: a re-evaluation. *J Am Acad Dermatol.* 1984;10:466-472.

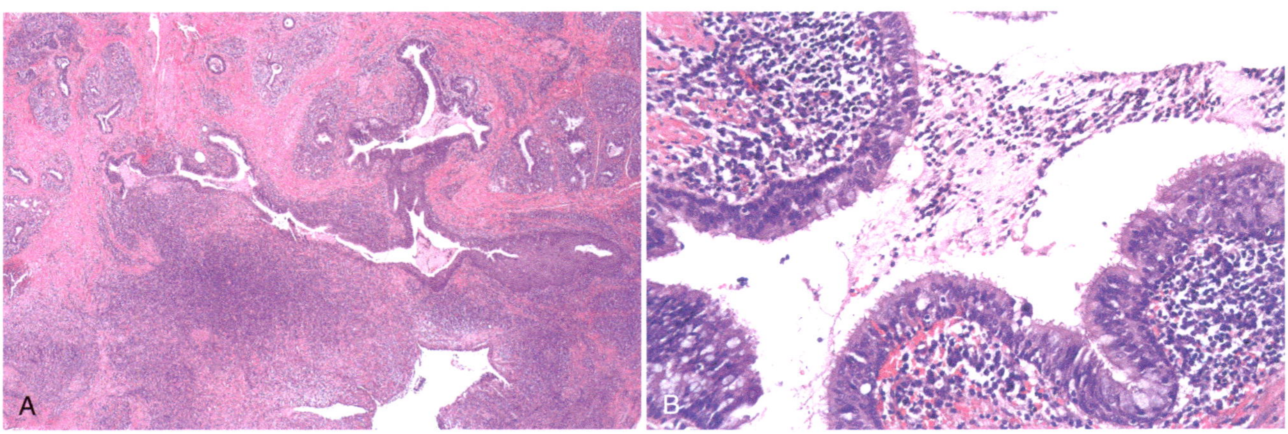

FIG 12.25 Cheilitis glandularis. (A) Tortuous and dilated ducts and surrounding glands exhibiting marked acute and chronic sialadenitis. (B) Luminal mucin and suppuration, and ciliated and mucous cell metaplasia of ducts with surrounding lymphoplasmacytic infiltrate

NECROTIZING SIALOMETAPLASIA

Clinical Findings

- This condition occurs in the fifth to sixth decades with a 4:1 female predilection with 75% of cases occurring on the posterior hard palatal mucosa.
- The lesion starts as a swelling that breaks down over a few days to weeks to form a necrotic ulcer that over the ensuing few weeks sloughs off cleanly and then heals; it may or may not be painful and some cases are bilateral (Fig. 12.26).
- Associated risk factors include having a greater palatine anesthetic block, Raynaud disease, Buerger disease, bulimia, excessive smoking and alcohol intake, local trauma, and adjacent malignancy.

Etiopathogenesis and Histopathologic Features

This condition is caused by ischemia and infarction of the salivary gland, and hypoxia-inducible factor-1-α has been identified within gland parenchyma, the endothelium, and stromal cells.

- Preservation of the lobular architecture of the glands is an important finding but is not always present.
- *Early stage:* there is spillage of mucin into the interstitial tissues of the gland parenchyma; ghostly outlines of acini with preserved basement membrane but erased acinar cell outlines are classic features (Figs. 12.27A–B and 12.28A–B).
- *Late stage:* squamous metaplasia of the ducts may be marked with some reactive atypia, but without significant pleomorphism or abnormal mitoses (see Figs. 12.27C and 12.28C–D).
- Acute and chronic inflammation is present in variable degrees, as are necrosis and secondary thrombosis.

Differential Diagnosis

- Overdiagnosing this condition as squamous cell carcinoma is an important pitfall; lack of invasion, lack of abnormal mitoses and pleomorphism, and maintenance of lobular architecture are not consistent with malignancy.
- Subacute necrotizing sialadenitis shows marked mixed inflammation with only focal necrosis.

Management

- The lesion resolves on its own without medical or surgical intervention after spontaneous exfoliation of the necrotic tissue; intralesional steroid therapy may be helpful.

REFERENCES

Abrams AM, Melrose RJ, Howell FV. Necrotizing sialometaplasia. *Cancer.* 1973;32:130-135.

Allon I, Kaplan I, Allon DM, et al. HIF-1alpha, VEGF, and EGFR: contributing factors in the pathogenesis of necrotizing sialometaplasia. *Oral Dis.* 2014;20:440-445.

Brannon RB, Fowler CB, Hartman KS. Necrotizing sialometaplasia. A clinicopathologic study of sixty-nine cases and review of the literature. *Oral Surg Oral Med Oral Pathol.* 1991;72:317-325.

Dominguez-Malagon H, Mosqueda-Taylor A, Cano-Valdez AM. Necrotizing sialometaplasia of the palatal mucosa associated with angiocentric T-cell lymphoma. *Ann Diagn Pathol.* 2009;13:60-64.

Janner SF, Suter VG, Altermatt HJ, et al. Bilateral necrotizing sialometaplasia of the hard palate in a patient with bulimia: a case report and review of the literature. *Quintessence Int.* 2014;45:431-437.

Lee DJ, Ahn HK, Koh ES, et al. Necrotizing sialometaplasia accompanied by adenoid cystic carcinoma on the soft palate. *Clin Exp Otorhinolaryngol.* 2009;2:48-51.

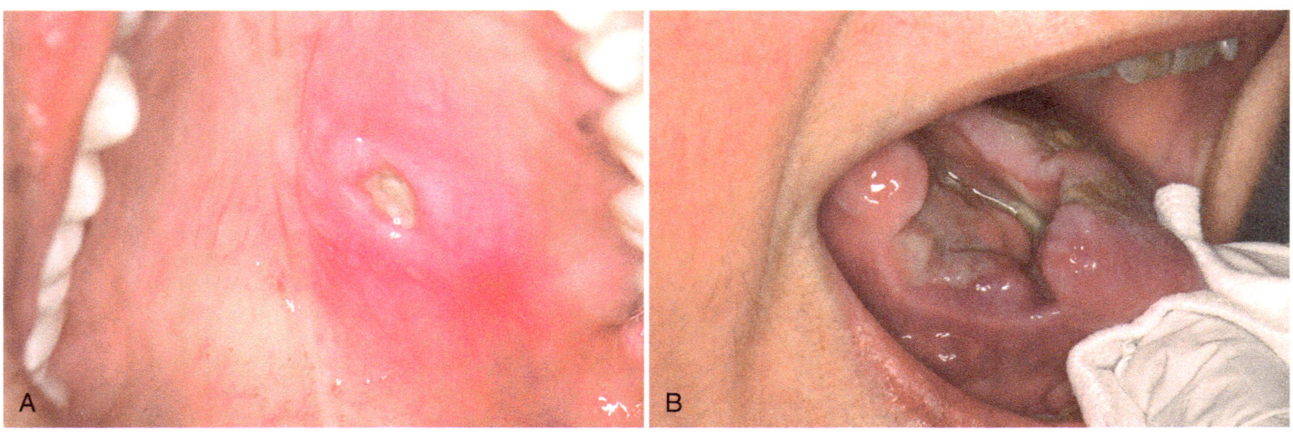

FIG 12.26 Necrotizing sialometaplasia. (A) Ulcer of the hard palatal mucosa. (B) Necrotic ulcer of the tongue after general anesthesia intubation. *(A, Courtesy Dr. Hani Mawardi, Brigham and Women's Hospital, Boston.)*

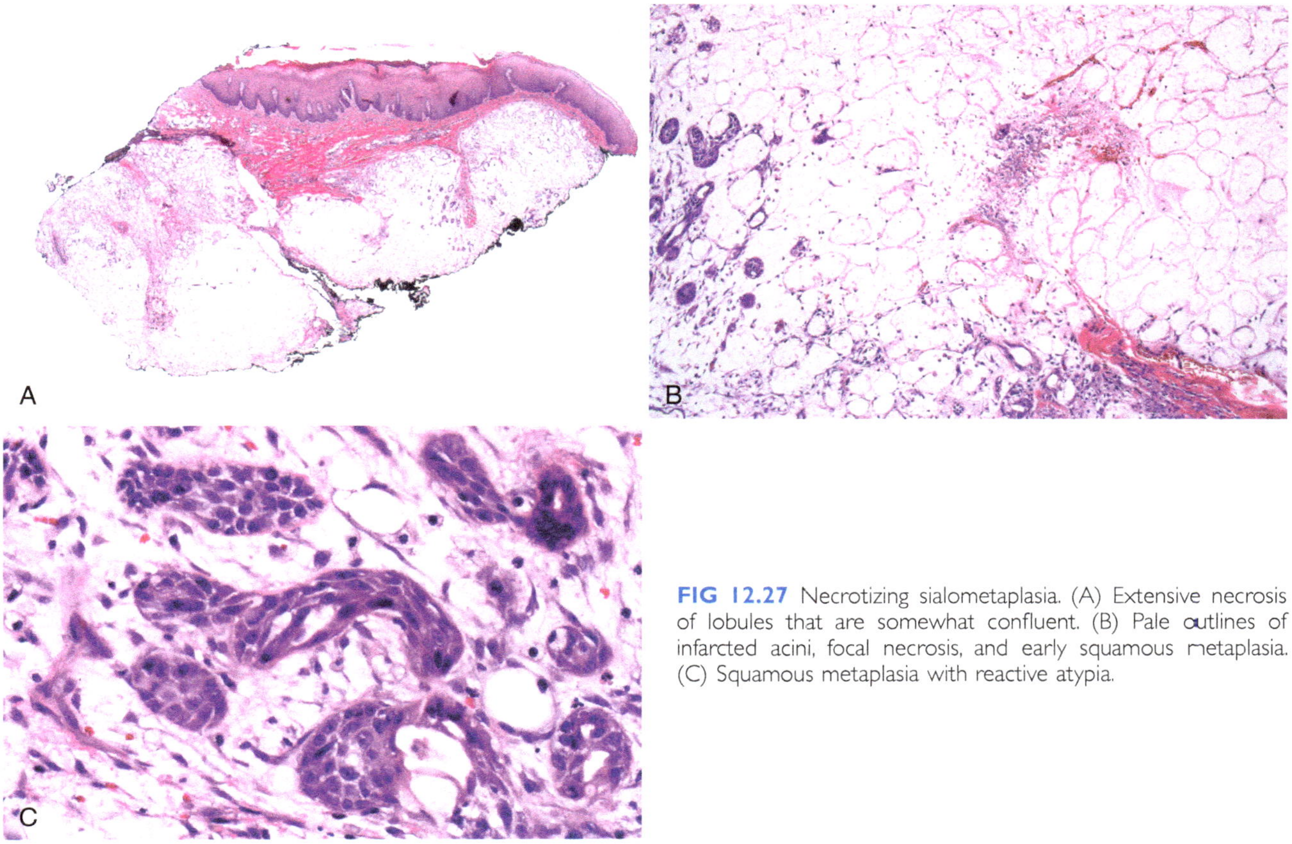

FIG 12.27 Necrotizing sialometaplasia. (A) Extensive necrosis of lobules that are somewhat confluent. (B) Pale outlines of infarcted acini, focal necrosis, and early squamous metaplasia. (C) Squamous metaplasia with reactive atypia.

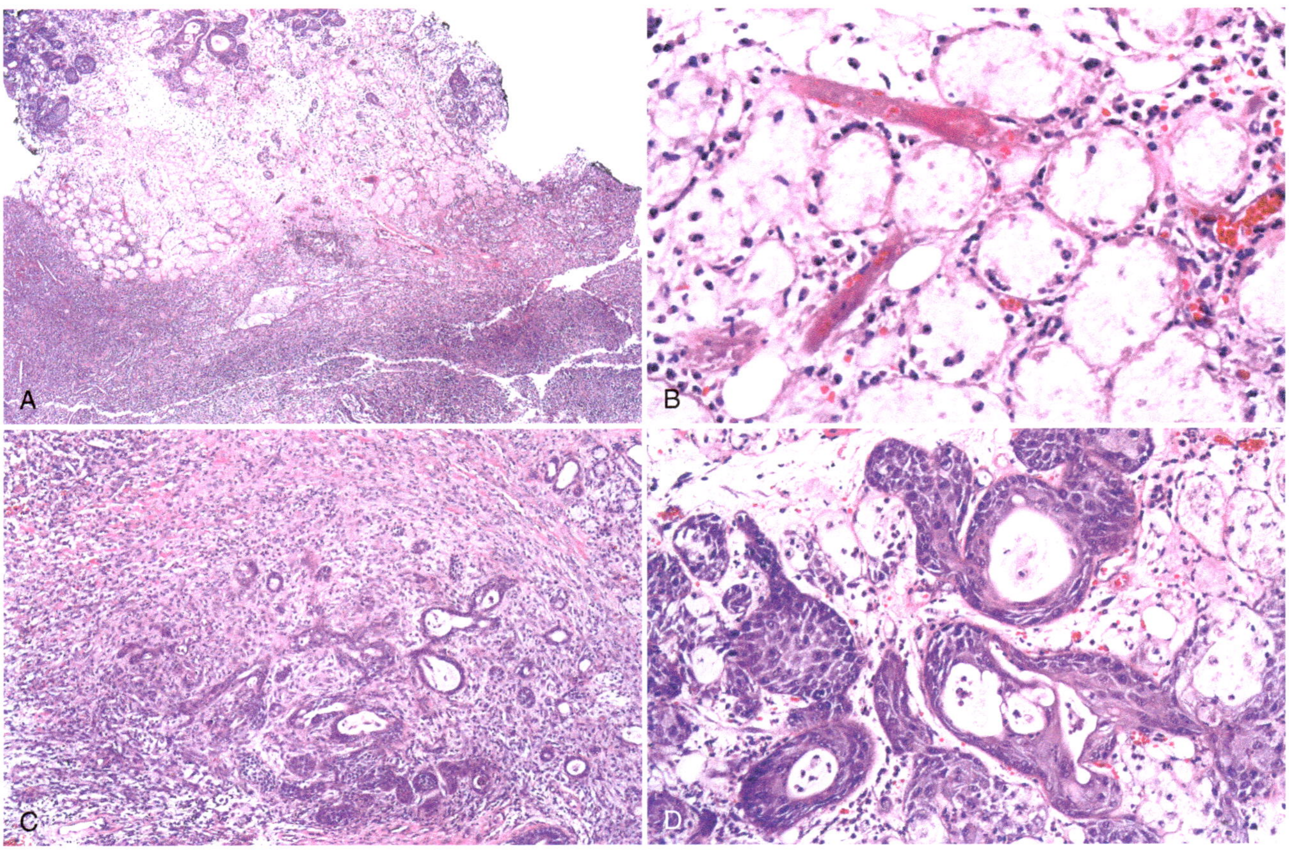

FIG 12.28 Necrotizing sialometaplasia. (A) Diffuse necrosis, inflammation, and squamous metaplasia. (B) Infarction of acini with remnant basement membrane material and acinar necrosis with many neutrophils. (C) Squamous metaplasia of ducts appearing pseudosarcomatoid with marked surrounding inflammation. (D) Squamous metaplasia of ducts with reactive atypia.

SUBACUTE NECROTIZING SIALADENITIS

Clinical Findings

This occurs in the second to third decades of life as a diffuse, nonulcerated painful swelling of the hard palatal mucosa (majority of cases), soft palate, tonsil, and, much less commonly, buccal mucosa.

Etiopathogenesis and Histopathologic Features

- The etiology is unknown, but infectious and hypersensitivity theories have been put forward. This is not a variant of necrotizing sialometaplasia.
- There is maintenance of lobular architecture with a diffuse interstitial infiltration by neutrophils, lymphocytes, plasma cells, histiocytes, and often eosinophils (Fig. 12.29A–B).
- There is multifocal acinar atrophy and necrosis, mucin spillage, and ductal dilatation with flattened ductal cells; many neutrophils are present and these may infiltrate acini and ductal epithelium (see Fig. 12.29C).

Differential Diagnosis

- Necrotizing sialometaplasia exhibits extensive ischemic necrosis characterized by ghostly outlines of the acini in early lesions and marked squamous metaplasia in later lesions.

Management

- This condition is self-limited and heals within a few weeks.

REFERENCES

Fowler CB, Brannon RB. Subacute necrotizing sialadenitis: report of 7 cases and a review of the literature. *Oral Surg Oral Med Oral Pathol Oral Radiol Endod.* 2000;89:600-609.

Geyer JT, Ferry JA, Harris NL, et al. Chronic sclerosing sialadenitis (Kuttner tumor) is an IgG4-associated disease. *Am J Surg Pathol.* 2010;34:202-210.

Kitagawa S, Zen Y, Harada K, et al. Abundant IgG4-positive plasma cell infiltration characterizes chronic sclerosing sialadenitis (Kuttner's tumor). *Am J Surg Pathol.* 2005;29:783-791.

Suresh L, Aguirre A. Subacute necrotizing sialadenitis: a clinicopathological study. *Oral Surg Oral Med Oral Pathol Oral Radiol Endod.* 2007;104:385-390.

Werning JT, Waterhouse JP, Mooney JW. Subacute necrotizing sialadenitis. *Oral Surg Oral Med Oral Pathol.* 1990;70:756-759.

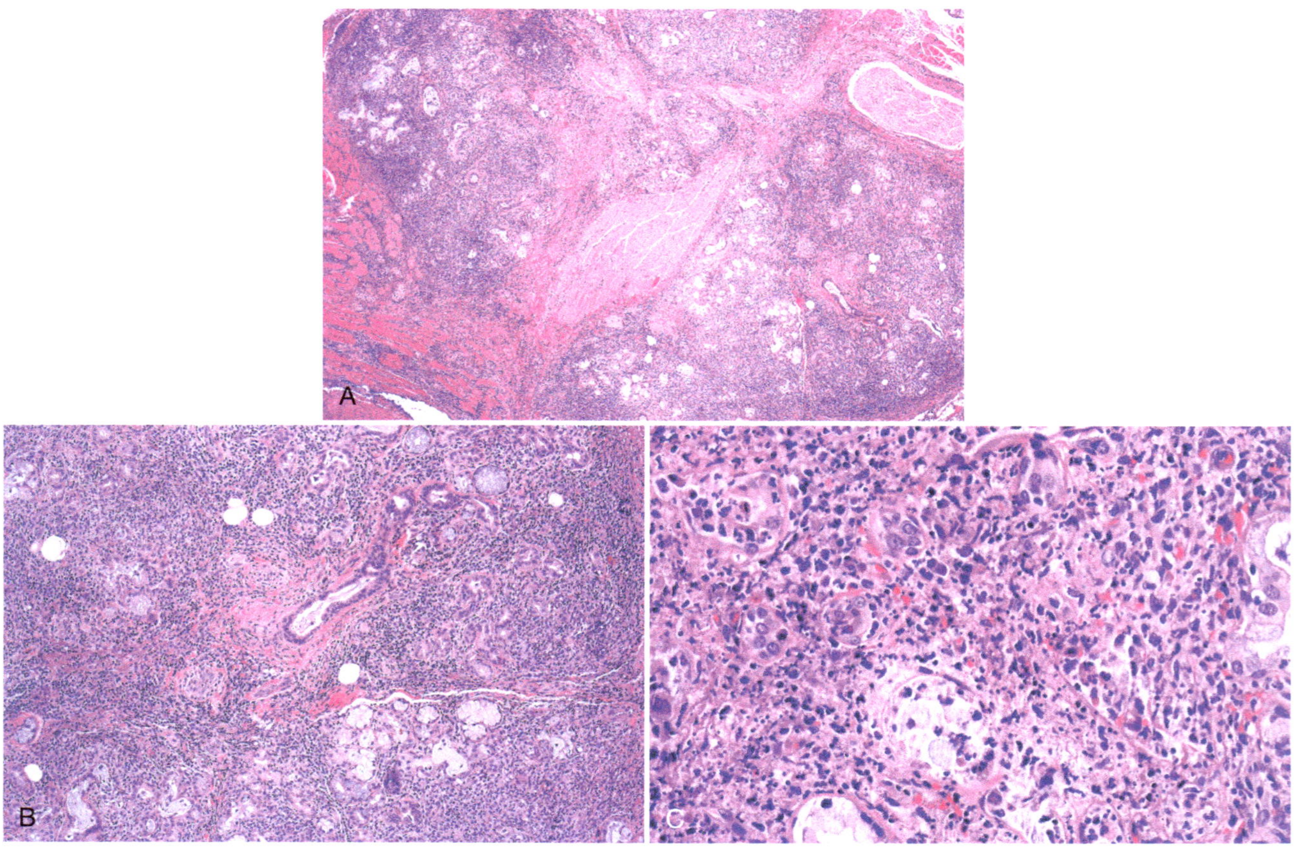

FIG 12.29 Subacute necrotizing sialadenitis. (A) Maintenance of lobular architecture with marked interstitial inflammation. (B) Acinar atrophy, interstitial fibrosis with acute and chronic inflammation. (C) Necrosis of acini with acute inflammation.

SJÖGREN SYNDROME

Sjögren syndrome is an autoimmune disease that is characterized by immune destruction of exocrine glands and, in particular, the salivary and lacrimal glands leading to dry mouth (subjective xerostomia and objective hyposalivation) and dry eyes (keratoconjunctivitis sicca). Patients have protean clinical manifestations and many serologic abnormalities. By convention, two forms are recognized: *primary* Sjögren syndrome, when there is only salivary and eye involvement, and *secondary* Sjögren syndrome, when there is another autoimmune disease present. However, the distinction between the two groups is not always that clear. There is a 16-fold increase in the probability of developing lymphoma.

Clinical Features

- This occurs in adults from the fourth decade upward, with a 9:1 female predilection; other symptoms that are frequently encountered include fatigue, arthralgia, myalgia, vasculitis and purpura, lymphadenopathy, serositis, interstitial lung disease, renal failure, peripheral and central nervous system disorders, hypothyroidism and Raynaud phenomenon; rheumatoid arthritis, systemic lupus erythematosus, and systemic sclerosis are other commonly associated autoimmune disorders.
- Patients report dry eyes and dry mouth (sicca syndrome) as well as dry nasal passages; long-standing cases exhibit bilateral parotid gland swelling, although this is likely to represent the presence of a low-grade lymphoma.
- Patients exhibit elevated titers for antinuclear antibody (ANA), rheumatoid factor (RF) and Sjögren syndrome A (SSA, Ro) and Sjögren syndrome B (SSB or La) antibodies, and there is usually hypergammaglobulinemia, hypocomplementemia, and sometimes cryoglobulinemia.
- Sialography exhibits peripheral sialectasia and ultrasonography exhibits hypoechoic areas and echogenic streaks.
- Patients must have at least two of the following three criteria for the diagnosis:
  - Positive antibodies to SSA and SSB, *or* positive ANA (at least 1:320) *and* RF
  - Labial salivary gland biopsy exhibiting focal lymphocytic sialadenitis with a focus score of at least 1 focus score/4 mm^2.
  - Keratoconjunctivitis sicca with an ocular staining score (using lissamine green and fluorescein) of at least 3.

Etiopathogenesis and Histopathologic Features

One possible mechanism suggests that a viral (or other) infection leads to dysregulation of the innate immune system and inappropriate activation of the adaptive immune system via dendritic cells, mediated by many cytokines including type 1 interferon, B cell activating factor (BAFF), and many interleukins. Increased incidence of HLA-DQA*05:01, -DQB1*02:01, -DQB1*03:01 are associated with Sjögren syndrome, and in particular, increased incidence of -DQ2 and -B8 in whites and -DR5 in Greeks and Israelis. Some patients or family members present with other autoimmune diseases. The terms benign lymphoepithelial lesion and myoepithelial sialadenitis have been replaced with lymphoepithelial sialadenitis because this form of sialadenitis has a high risk for lymphomatous transformation, and myoepithelial cells are not a prominent feature within the epithelial islands.

- *Minor salivary glands:* At least 5 glands should be present for evaluation; periductal collections of 50 or more lymphocytes within a 4 mm^2 area is called a focus (Fig. 12.30); focus score is calculated as follows: Focus score = Number of foci (maximum 12 or confluent foci) × 4/Number of mm^2 of salivary gland parenchyma; a score of at least 1 is supportive of the diagnosis of Sjögren syndrome and the higher the focus score, the more likely the diagnosis of Sjögren syndrome.
- There is minimal evidence of nonspecific obstructive changes, such as significant ductal dilatation and interstitial fibrosis.
- If lymphocytes spill out of the lobules, forming a diffuse infiltrate with effacement of lobular architecture, work-up for lymphoma is indicated (Fig. 12.31); the presence of germinal center formation should be reported because of the higher risk for development of lymphoma in these patients, likely because chronic antigenic stimulation leads to B cell activation and germinal center hypermutation resulting in B cell clones capable of inducing neoplasia; light chain restriction indicates the presence of lymphoma.
- *Major salivary glands:* Lymphoepithelial sialadenitis is characterized by islands and strands of epithelial cells in a diffuse lymphocytic infiltrate with maintenance of lobular architecture; effacement of lobular architecture and proliferation of "monocytoid" lymphoid cells around lymphoepithelial islands usually indicate the presence of evolving lymphoma (usually marginal zone and less commonly diffuse large B cell lymphoma) (Fig. 12.32).
- There is a 16 times higher risk for development of lymphoma, usually marginal zone lymphoma (see Chapter 18) with risk factors being lymphocytopenia, hypocomplementemia, skin purpura/vasculitis, cryoglobulinemia, and germinal centers within labial salivary gland biopsy with a high focus score.

Differential Diagnosis

- Lymphocytes in a periductal and interstitial location with prominent ductal ectasia and acinar atrophy are nonspecific findings often caused by obstruction (Fig. 12.33).

Management and Prognosis

- Cholinergic agents (such as bethanechol, pilocarpine, and cevimeline) help to reduce discomfort by increasing salivation only if there is residual functional gland tissue.
- Patients are at high risk for caries and should be prescribed fluorides and placed on regular dental follow-ups to restore caries and treat candidiasis.

- Rituximab shows promise in reducing fatigue, pain, and dryness; other biologics have been used with variable success but only in small studies.
- Patients must be closely followed because of the high risk for lymphoma.

REFERENCES

Daniels TE. Benign lymphoepithelial lesion and Sjögren's syndrome. In: Ellis GI, Auclair PL, Gnepp DR, eds. *Surgical Pathology of the Salivary Glands*. Philadelphia: W.B. Saunders; 1991 Chapter 6:92-98.

Daniels TE, Cox D, Shiboski CH, et al. Associations between salivary gland histopathologic diagnoses and phenotypic features of Sjögren's syndrome among 1,726 registry participants. *Arthritis Rheum.* 2011;63:2021-2030.

Ihrler S, Zietz C, Sendelhofert A, et al. Lymphoepithelial duct lesions in Sjögren-type sialadenitis. *Virchows Arch.* 1999;434:315-323.

Jonsson MV, Theander E, Jonsson R. Predictors for the development of non-Hodgkin lymphoma in primary Sjögren's syndrome. *Presse Med.* 2012;41:e511-e516.

Jordan R, Diss TC, Lench NJ, et al. Immunoglobulin gene rearrangements in lymphoplasmacytic infiltrates of labial salivary glands in Sjögren's syndrome. A possible predictor of lymphoma development. *Oral Surg Oral Med Oral Pathol Oral Radiol Endod.* 1995;79:723-729.

Papageorgiou A, Voulgarelis M, Tzioufas AG. Clinical picture, outcome and predictive factors of lymphoma in Sjögren syndrome. *Autoimmun Rev.* 2015;14:641-649.

Peri Y, Agmon-Levin N, Theodor E, Shoenfeld Y. Sjögren's syndrome, the old and the new. *Best Pract Res Clin Rheumatol.* 2012;26: 105-117.

Risselada AP, Looije MF, Kruize AA, et al. The role of ectopic germinal centers in the immunopathology of primary Sjögren's syndrome: a systematic review. *Semin Arthritis Rheum.* 2013;42:368-376.

Shiboski SC, Shiboski CH, Criswell L, et al. American College of Rheumatology classification criteria for Sjögren's syndrome: a data-driven, expert consensus approach in the Sjögren's International Collaborative Clinical Alliance cohort. *Arthritis Care Res.* 2012;64:475-487.

Theander E, Henriksson G, Ljungberg O, et al. Lymphoma and other malignancies in primary Sjögren's syndrome: a cohort study on cancer incidence and lymphoma predictors. *Ann Rheum Dis.* 2006;65:796-803.

Theander E, Vasaitis L, Baecklund E, et al. Lymphoid organisation in labial salivary gland biopsies is a possible predictor for the development of malignant lymphoma in primary Sjögren's syndrome. *Ann Rheum Dis.* 2011;70:1363-1368.

Vitali C, Bombardieri S, Jonsson R, et al. Classification criteria for Sjögren's syndrome: a revised version of the European criteria proposed by the American-European Consensus Group. *Ann Rheum Dis.* 2002;61:554-558.

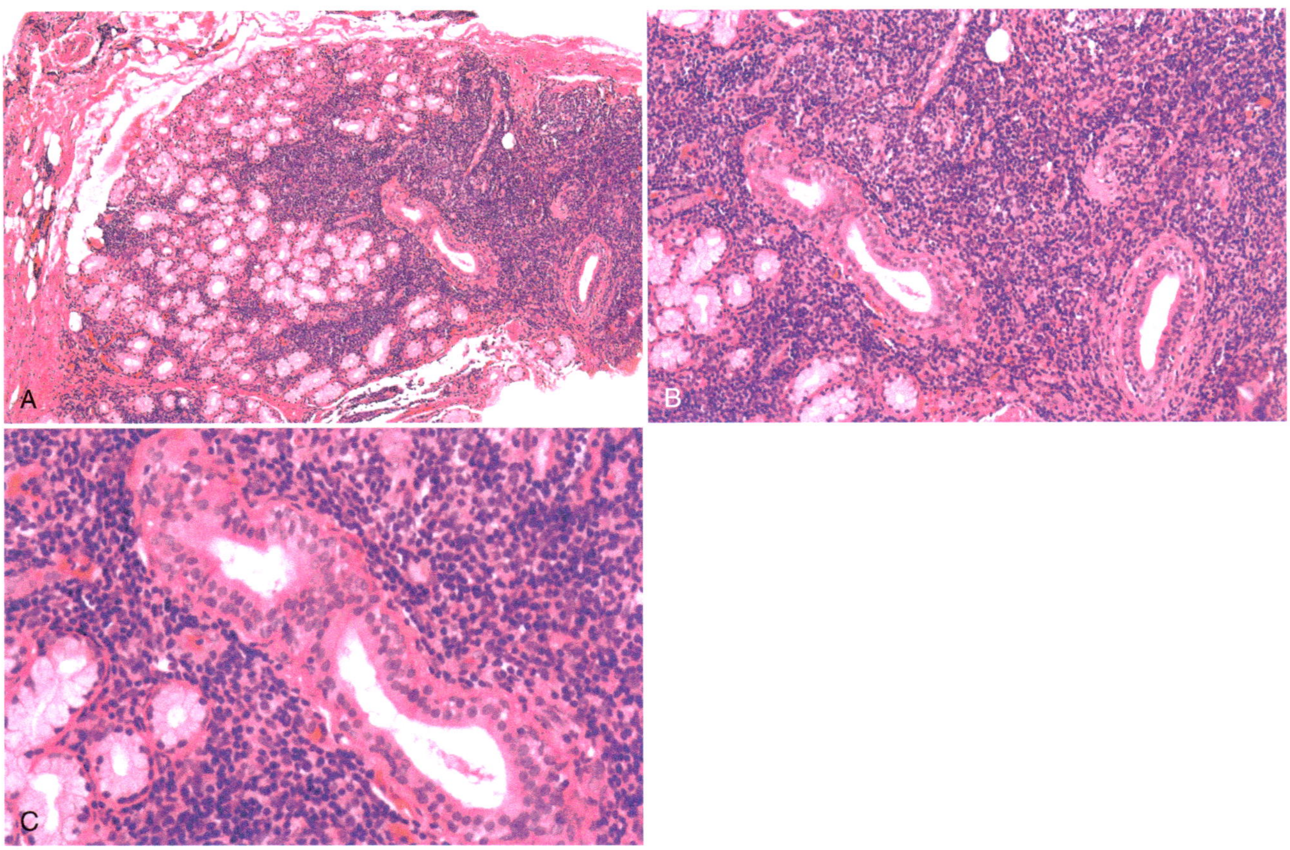

FIG 12.30 Autoimmune sialadenitis in Sjögren syndrome. (A) Maintenance of lobular architecture with marked periductal and interstitial lymphocytic infiltrate without significant obstructive changes. (B) Intense periductal lymphocytic infiltrate. (C) Lymphocytes are small and mature. *(A, Courtesy Dr. Leland Slater, Scripps Institute, San Diego, Calif.)*

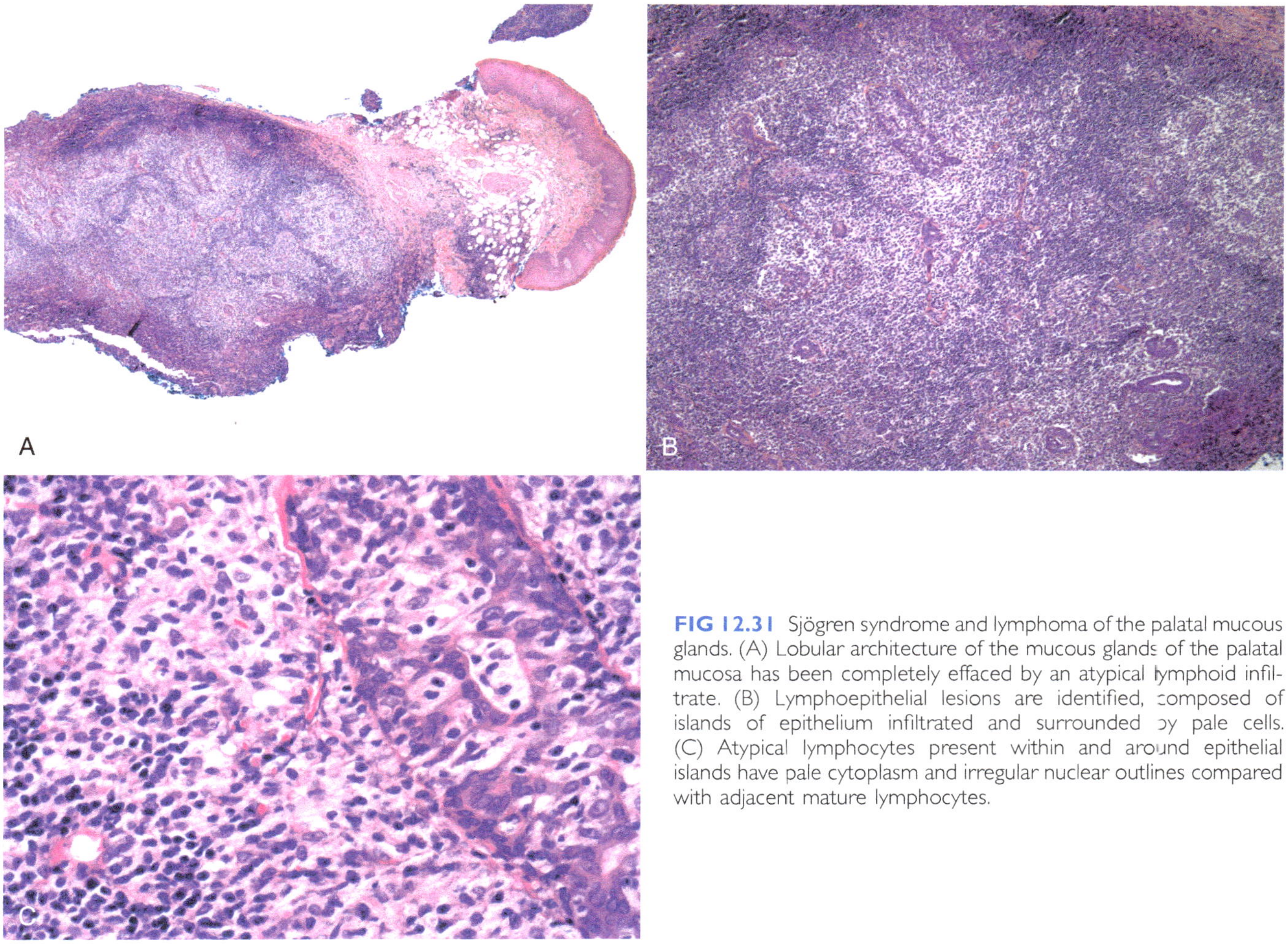

FIG 12.31 Sjögren syndrome and lymphoma of the palatal mucous glands. (A) Lobular architecture of the mucous glands of the palatal mucosa has been completely effaced by an atypical lymphoid infiltrate. (B) Lymphoepithelial lesions are identified, composed of islands of epithelium infiltrated and surrounded by pale cells. (C) Atypical lymphocytes present within and around epithelial islands have pale cytoplasm and irregular nuclear outlines compared with adjacent mature lymphocytes.

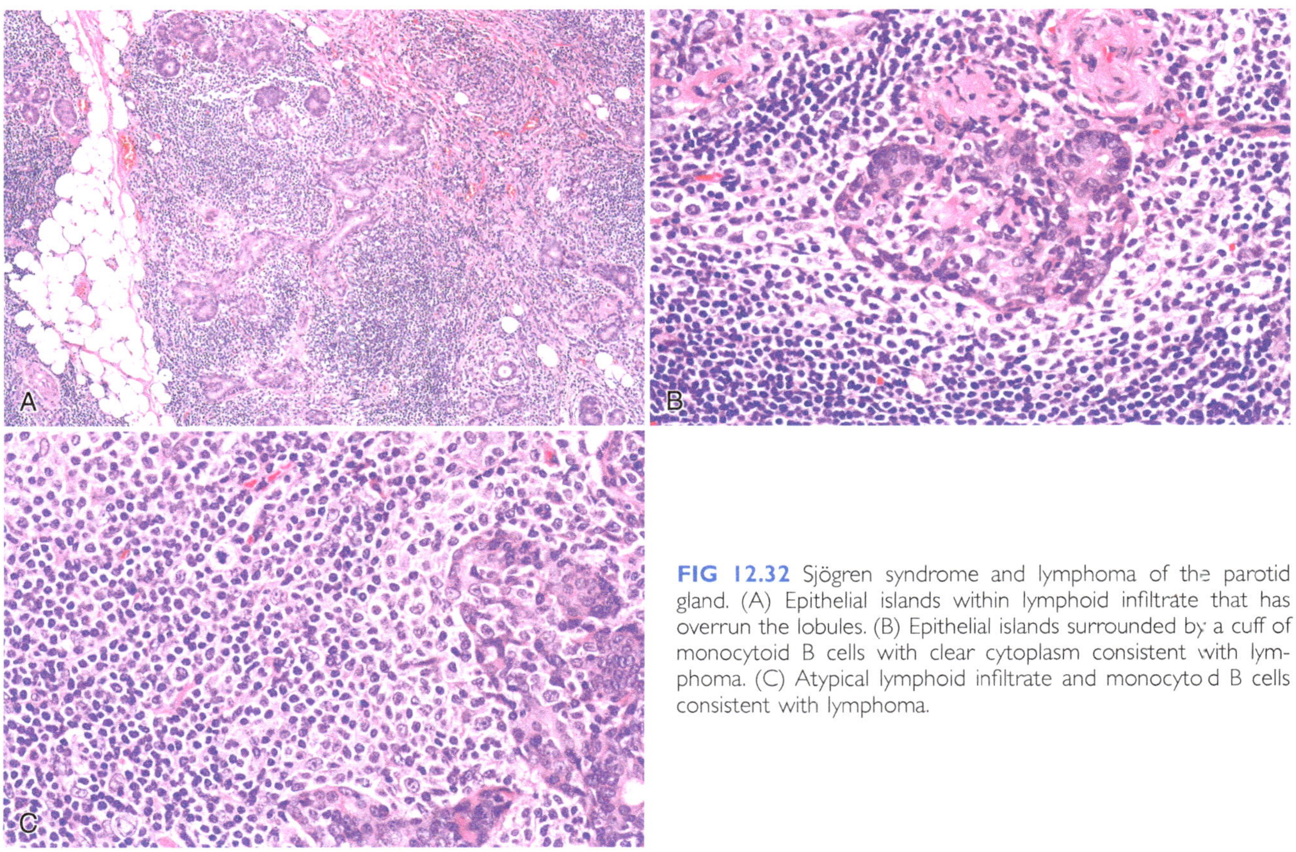

FIG 12.32 Sjögren syndrome and lymphoma of the parotid gland. (A) Epithelial islands within lymphoid infiltrate that has overrun the lobules. (B) Epithelial islands surrounded by a cuff of monocytoid B cells with clear cytoplasm consistent with lymphoma. (C) Atypical lymphoid infiltrate and monocytoid B cells consistent with lymphoma.

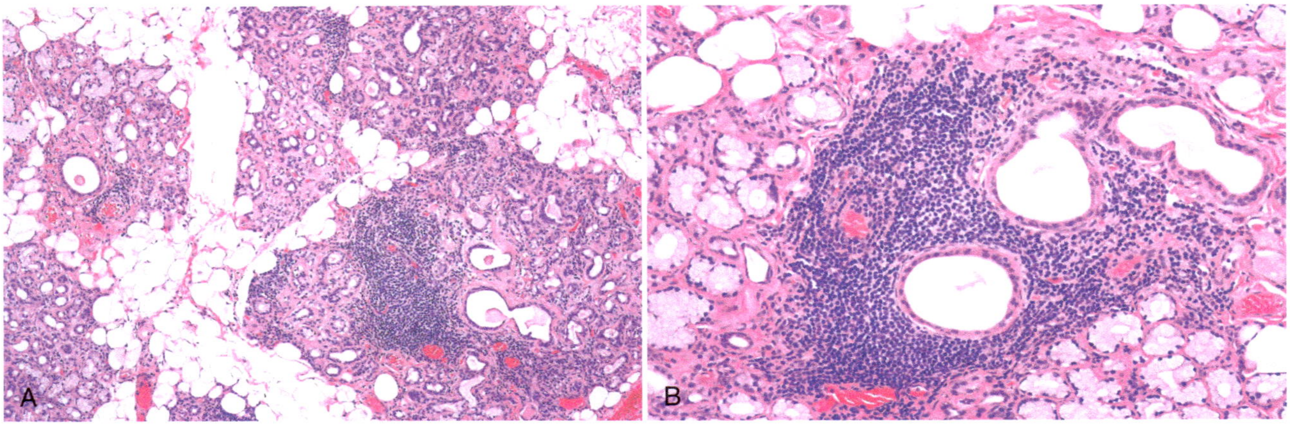

FIG 12.33 Obstructive sialadenitis. (A) Glands maintain lobular architecture but show diffuse acinar atrophy, ductal dilatation, and interstitial fibrosis and inflammation. (B) Periductal inflammation is present but ducts are dilated.

IgG4-RELATED DISEASE

IgG4-related disease is a systemic fibroinflammatory condition affecting the pancreas and hepatobiliary tract, as well as salivary glands (formerly referred to as Kuttner tumor), thyroid, lymph nodes, and retroperitoneum, resulting in tumefaction of involved glands and characterized by elevated levels of IgG4 in the serum and increased numbers of IgG4+ tissue plasma cells, although these last findings may be nonspecific. IgG4 is the least abundant of the four IgG subclasses.

Clinical Findings

- This affects patients in the sixth to eighth decade with a 4–7 : 1 male predilection and patients often have dry eyes; patients tend to be atopic and exhibit peripheral eosinophilia and increased levels of plasma IgG4, although 30% of patients have normal IgG4 levels.
- Patients present with dry mouth and bilateral swollen major salivary glands (especially submandibular glands) and infrequently, palatal perforation; rare cases are identified through labial salivary gland biopsy.
- Autoimmune pancreatitis and sclerosing cholangitis are one of the major associated conditions.
- In the Japanese population, increased susceptibility for this condition includes harboring HLA-DRB1*0401-DRB1*0405.

Etiopathogenesis and Histopathologic Features

This is a disease of immune dysregulation that leads to fibrosis and a marked lympho-plasmacytic infiltrate rich in IgG4+ plasma cells. One theory is that in the susceptible individual (usually a male), an environmental insult (possible infection) triggers tissue damage and a break in immunologic tolerance. A self-antigen-driven CD4 response leads to fibrosis and a proinflammatory cascade, including generation of IgG4-secreting plasma cells.

- Salivary glands show effacement of their architecture and exhibit florid irregular follicular lymphoid hyperplasia with germinal centers, cellular interlobular (storiform) fibrosis, pheblitis (sometimes obliterative), marked interstitial plasma cell infiltrate, periductal fibrosis, and inflammation and destruction of excretory ducts (Fig. 12.34).
- IgG4:IgG positive plasma cell ratio is at least 1 : 2, and there are 10 to greater than 50 IgG4+ plasma cells per high power field.

Differential Diagnosis

- Salivary gland biopsies in neither Sjögren syndrome nor nonspecific sialadenitis exhibit cellular interlobular fibrosis, phlebitis, or large numbers of IgG4+ plasma cells.
- Extranodal marginal zone lymphoma exhibits an atypical lymphoid infiltrate that may be plasmacytoid but would exhibit light chain restriction.

Management

- First-line therapy is with glucocorticoids but other medications that may be effective include rituximab, methotrexate, azathioprine, and mycophenolate.

REFERENCES

Baer AN, Gourin CG, Westra WH, et al. Rare diagnosis of IgG4-related systemic disease by lip biopsy in an international Sjögren syndrome registry. *Oral Surg Oral Med Oral Pathol Oral Radiol.* 2013;115:e34-e39.

Della-Torre E, Mattoo H, Mahajan VS, et al. IgG4-related midline destructive lesion. *Ann Rheum Dis.* 2014;73:1434-1436.

Deshpande V, Zen Y, Chan JK, et al. Consensus statement on the pathology of IgG4-related disease. *Mod Pathol.* 2012;25:1181-1192.

Geyer JT, Ferry JA, Harris NL, et al. Chronic sclerosing sialadenitis (Kuttner tumor) is an IgG4-associated disease. *Am J Surg Pathol.* 2010;34:202-210.

Kamisawa T, Zen Y, Pillai S, Stone JH. IgG4-related disease. *Lancet.* 2015;385:1460-1471.

Khosroshahi A, Wallace ZS, Crowe JL, et al. International Consensus Guidance Statement on the Management and Treatment of IgG4-Related Disease. *Arthritis Rheumatol.* 2015;67:1688-1699.

Kitagawa S, Zen Y, Harada K, et al. Abundant IgG4-positive plasma cell infiltration characterizes chronic sclerosing sialadenitis (Kuttner's tumor). *Am J Surg Pathol.* 2005;29:783-791.

Laco J, Ryska A, Celakovsky P, et al. Chronic sclerosing sialadenitis as one of the immunoglobulin G4-related diseases: a clinicopathological study of six cases from Central Europe. *Histopathology.* 2011;58:1157-1163.

Ota M, Katsuyama Y, Hamano H, et al. Two critical genes (HLA-DRB1 and ABCF1) in the HLA region are associated with the susceptibility to autoimmune pancreatitis. *Immunogenetics.* 2007;59:45-52.

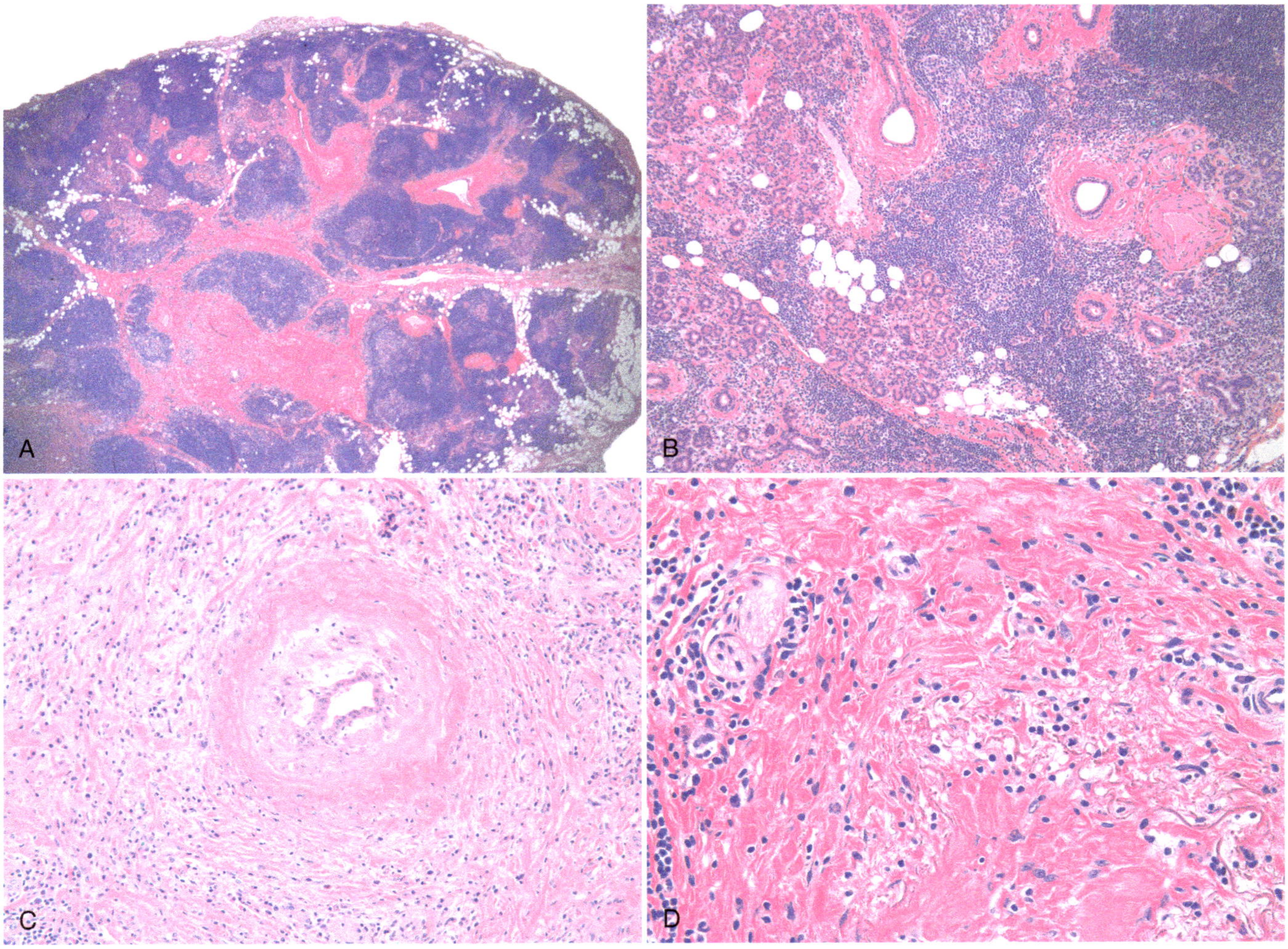

FIG 12.34 IgG-related disease of submandibular gland. (A) There is acinar atrophy and the gland is diffusely infiltrated by plasma cells and lymphocytes with germinal center formation and marked fibrosis, especially around ducts. (B) Periductal fibrosis is prominent and there is destruction of the acini and an intense lymphoplasmacytic infiltrate. (C) A duct exhibits circumferential fibrosis with infiltration by lymphocytes and destruction of the lining. (D) Remnant basement membrane–like material is present, likely of ductal origin, and there is fibrosis and chronic inflammation. *(Courtesy Dr. Jeffrey Krane, Brigham and Women's Hospital, Boston.)*

ADENOMATOID (ACINAR) HYPERPLASIA

Adenomatoid hyperplasia of the minor salivary glands involves *acinar* hyperplasia as opposed to *adenomatoid* ductal hyperplasia that occurs mostly in the parotid gland.

Clinical Findings

- This occurs in adults in the fourth to sixth decade with more than 80% occurring in the hard and soft palatal mucosa as a painless unilateral swelling usually without ulceration.

Etiopathogenesis and Histopathologic Features

This condition represents a reactive hyperplasia of acini that is often seen in smokers and denture wearers, and is found adjacent to neoplasms or necrotizing sialometaplasia. A rare case exhibited chromosomal translocation t(2,14).

- There is hyperplasia and hypertrophy of mucous acini that are back to back, often with fewer ducts than normal and with enlarged lobules (Fig. 12.35); there is usually no inflammation present although there may be focal mucus spillage and slight ductal dilatation.

Differential Diagnosis

- As with ductal adenomatoid hyperplasia of major glands, this may be an indication that a salivary gland neoplasm, benign or malignant, is in the vicinity.

Management

- Excision is curative.

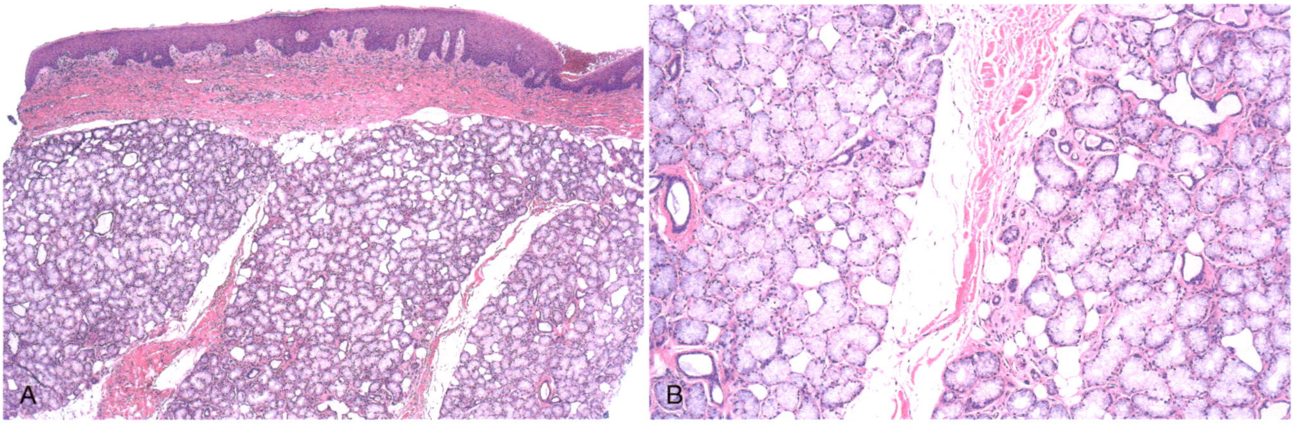

FIG 12.35 Adenomatoid hyperplasia of salivary glands. (A) Hyperplasia of salivary gland lobules filling the deep lamina propria of the hard palatal mucosa. (B) Closely packed acini are hyperplastic and hypertrophied with some ductal ectasia.

REFERENCES

Arafat A, Brannon RB, Ellis GL. Adenomatoid hyperplasia of mucous salivary glands. *Oral Surg Oral Med Oral Pathol*. 1981;52:51-55.

Barrett AW, Speight PM. Adenomatoid hyperplasia of oral minor salivary glands. *Oral Surg Oral Med Oral Pathol Oral Radiol Endod*. 1995;79:482-487.

Buchner A, Merrell PW, Carpenter WM, Leider AS. Adenomatoid hyperplasia of minor salivary glands. *Oral Surg Oral Med Oral Pathol*. 1991;71:583-587.

Manor E, Sinelnikov I, Brennan PA, Bodner L. Chromosomal aberrations in adenomatoid hyperplasia of palatal minor salivary gland. *Br J Oral Maxillofac Surg*. 2013;51:170-172.

Yu GY, Donath K. Adenomatous ductal proliferation of the salivary gland. *Oral Surg Oral Med Oral Pathol Oral Radiol Endod*. 2001;91:215-221.

13 SALIVARY GLAND NEOPLASMS

CHAPTER CONTENTS

Any salivary gland tumor in the major glands may occur in the minor glands, and only the more common benign and malignant lesions of intraoral minor glands will be discussed in this section. Intraoral minor salivary gland neoplasms account for 1% to 2% of nonhospital-based biopsy services, with 60% of these being benign. There is a female predominance with the exception of salivary duct carcinoma, which shows male predominance.

Traditionally salivary gland neoplasms have been diagnosed by histomorphology alone, although more recent advances in immunohistochemistry, molecular diagnostics, and recognition of gene fusions have greatly advanced practical diagnosis of some conditions (Table 13.1). Other gene alterations such as associated with cyclin dependent kinase, ERBB2, and in the PI3K/AKT/mTOR pathway have also been identified.

Ductal cells show cytoplasmic positivity for epithelial membrane antigen (EMA), carcinoembryonic antigen (CEA), AE1/3, K5/6, K7, K8, K19, and SOX10. Myoepithelial/basal, nonluminal cells are immunopositive for pankeratin, vimentin, calponin, smooth muscle actin (SMA), smooth muscle myosin long chain, S-100 protein, K14, glial fibrillary acidic protein (GFAP) in neoplastic cells only, p63, p40, and also SOX10. The nuclear transcription factor p40 is more specific for basal and myoepithelial cells than p63. Acinar cells are also positive for SOX10. Most tumors are thought to arise from the intercalated duct reserve cell or its precursor that differentiates into acinar, myoepithelial, and intercalated ductal cells; all such tumors are SOX10 positive. The

TABLE 13.1 Fusion Oncogenes and Other Genetic Abnormalities in Salivary Gland Tumors

Salivary Gland Tumor	Mutations, Gene Rearrangement, or Fusion Products
Pleomorphic adenoma	*PLAG1* (8q12) and *HMGA2* (12q13-15) rearrangements
Mucoepidermoid carcinoma	*CRTC1(MECT1) -MAML2* t(11;19)(q21;p13) *CRTC3(MECT3)-MAML2* t(15;19)(q21;q26)
Clear cell carcinoma	*EWSR1-ATF1* t(12;22)(q13;q12)
Mammary analog of secretory carcinoma	*ETV6-NTRK3* t(12;15)(p13;q25)
Adenoid cystic carcinoma	*MYB-NFIB* t(6:9)(q22-23;p23-24)
Polymorphous low-grade adenocarcinoma	*PRKD1* (p.Glu710Asp) mutation
Low-grade cribriform adenocarcinoma of minor salivary glands	*ARID1A-PRKD1* t(1;14)(p36;q12) *DDX3X-PRKD1* t(X;14)(p11.4;q12)

excretory duct reserve cell differentiates into excretory ductal cells and gives rise to tumors such as mucoepidermoid carcinoma and salivary duct carcinoma, and these are SOX10 negative. Striated ducts and oncocytic tumors are SOX10 negative and as such, these may arise from the excretory rather than intercalated duct reserve cell.

REFERENCES

Barnes L, Eveson J, Reichart P, Sidransky D, eds. *Pathology and Genetics of Head and Neck Tumors.* Lyon: IARC Press; 2005.

Chenevert J, Duvvuri U, Chiosea S, et al. DOG1: a novel marker of salivary acinar and intercalated duct differentiation. *Mod Pathol.* 2012;25:919-929.

Ellis GL, Auclair PL. *Tumors of the Salivary Glands.* Washington, DC: American Registry of Pathology; 2008.

Ohtomo R, Mori T, Shibata S, et al. SOX10 is a novel marker of acinus and intercalated duct differentiation in salivary gland tumors: a clue to the histogenesis for tumor diagnosis. *Mod Pathol.* 2013;26: 1041-1050.

Owosho AA, Aguilar CE, Seethala RR. Comparison of p63 and p40 (DeltaNp63) as basal, squamoid, and myoepithelial markers in salivary gland tumors. *Appl Immunohistochem Mol Morphol.* 2015; July 30;[Epub ahead of print].

Wang K, Russell JS, McDermott JD, et al. Profiling of 149 salivary duct carcinomas, carcinoma ex pleomorphic adenomas, and adenocarcinomas, not otherwise specified reveals actionable genomic alterations. *Clin Cancer Res.* 2016;[epub ahead of print].

Weinreb I. Translocation-associated salivary gland tumors: a review and update. *Adv Anat Pathol.* 2013;20:367-377.

Benign Salivary Gland Neoplasms

DUCTAL PAPILLOMAS

There are three papillary lesions, collectively referred to as ductal papillomas that involve the salivary gland excretory ducts and all are uncommon lesions: intraductal papilloma, inverted ductal papilloma, and sialadenoma papilliferum. It is still unclear whether all of these represent neoplasms or merely hyperplasias. A possible cell of origin is the excretory duct reserve cell located in the distal portions of the excretory duct.

INTRADUCTAL PAPILLOMA

Clinical Findings

- These occur in the sixth decade and present as painless nodules or masses on the lips (most common site), and buccal and palatal mucosa (Fig. 13.1).

Histopathologic Features

- This lesion arises within a cystically dilated excretory salivary duct and consists of a benign papillary proliferation of cuboidal and columnar cells (especially on the luminal aspect), squamous cells, and mucous cells with fibrovascular cores, often filling the lumen; microcysts are often present; the point of origin/attachment to the duct lumen may be evident (Fig. 13.2).

Differential Diagnosis

- Papillary cystadenoma consists of a proliferation of multiple cystic structures of varying sizes with ductal adenomatous hyperplasia that are composed of cuboidal-columnar cells forming papillary structures.
- Inverted ductal papilloma is endophytic and forms bulbous fronds of epithelium that invaginates into the connective tissue.

Management and Prognosis

- Excision is curative.

REFERENCES

Aikawa T, Kishino M, Masuda T, et al. Intraductal papilloma arising from sublingual minor salivary gland: case report and immunohistochemical study. *Oral Surg Oral Med Oral Pathol Oral Radiol Endod.* 2009;107:e34-e37.

Brannon RB, Sciubba JJ, Giulani M. Ductal papillomas of salivary gland origin: a report of 19 cases and a review of the literature. *Oral Surg Oral Med Oral Pathol Oral Radiol Endod.* 2001;92:68-77.

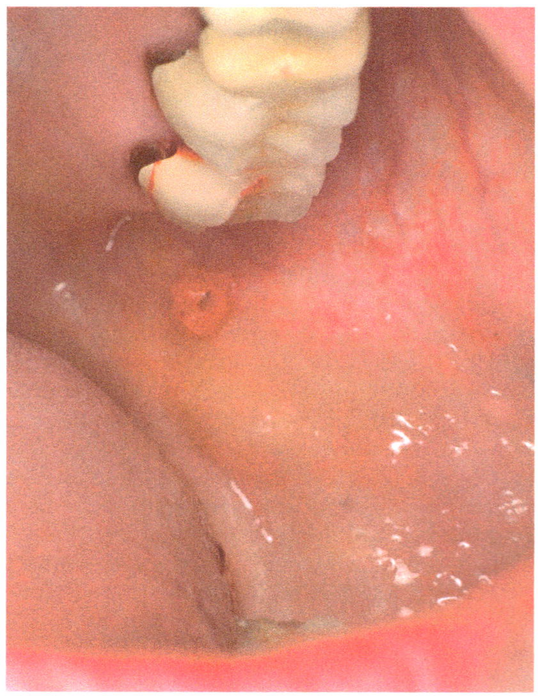

FIG 13.1 Intraductal papillomas of the left buccal mucosa. *(Courtesy Dr. Jeffrey Stone, private practice, Lowell, Mass.)*

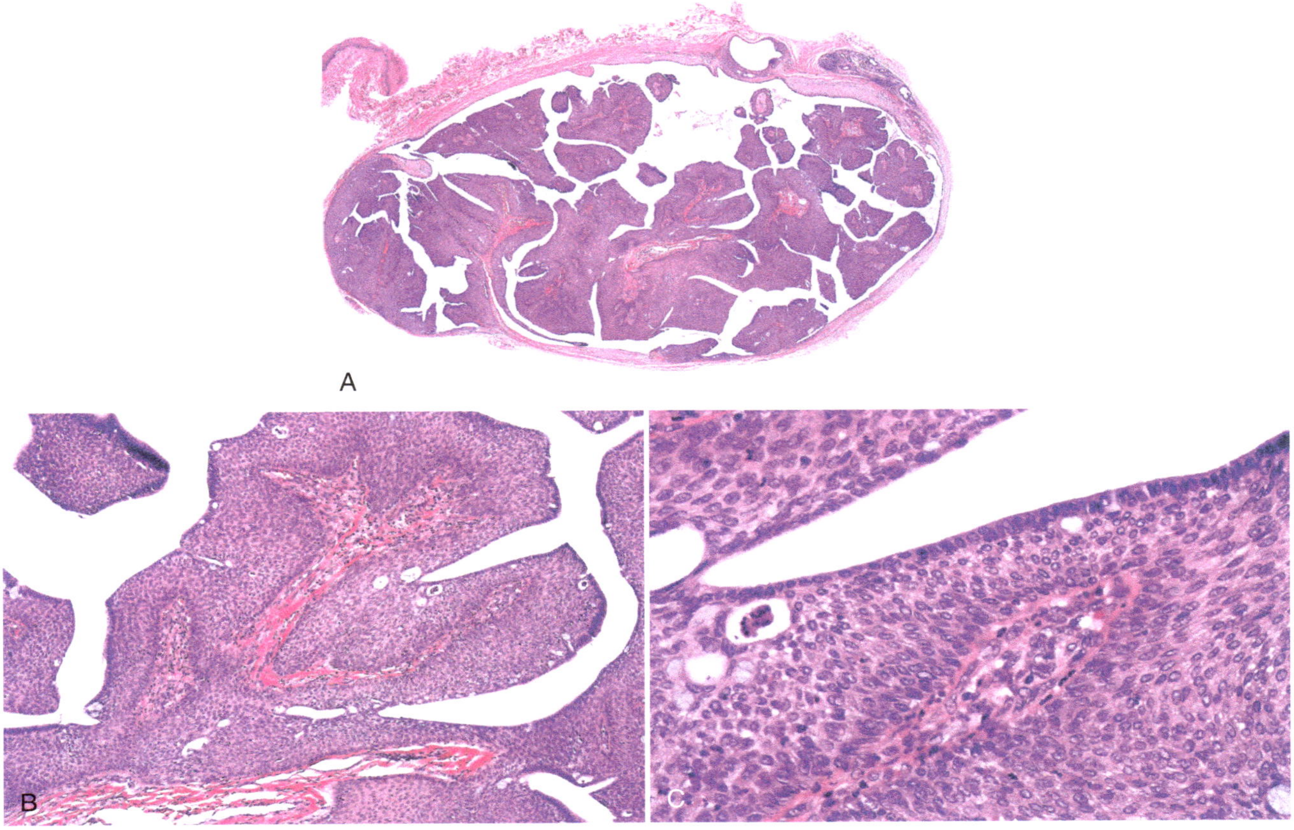

FIG 13.2 Intraductal papilloma. (A) Single, dilated excretory salivary duct with luminal papillary proliferation. (B) Well-organized papillary structures with fibrovascular cores and microcysts. (C) Surface luminal cells are cuboidal/columnar, and scattered mucous cells are present.

INVERTED DUCTAL PAPILLOMA

Clinical Findings

- This occurs most frequently in the sixth decade and half occur in the lips and one-third in the buccal mucosa as a painless nodule, sometimes with a punctum from which mucus may be expressed.

Etiopathogenesis and Histopathologic Features

This lesion is similar to a sinonasal inverted papilloma.

- There is an unencapsulated, discrete endophytic, lobular proliferation of squamous epithelium arising from an excretory salivary duct; clefts within the lobules represent extensions of the duct, and they are lined by low cuboidal-to-columnar cells; clusters of mucous cells, oncocytes, and microcysts are often seen (Fig. 13.3).
- Lesions are positive for K14 and K19; rare cases show the presence of human papillomavirus-6 and -11.

Differential Diagnosis

- Mucoepidermoid carcinoma may have a predominantly epidermoid component with only a few mucous and intermediate cells but is infiltrative and often forms small and large cysts.
- Intraductal papillomas generally have one large cystically dilated lumen with an intraluminal papilloma.

Management and Prognosis

- Excision is curative; lesion does not tend to recur.

REFERENCES

Brannon RB, Sciubba JJ, Giulani M. Ductal papillomas of salivary gland origin: a report of 19 cases and a review of the literature. *Oral Surg Oral Med Oral Pathol Oral Radiol Endod.* 2001;92:68-77.

Cabov T, Macan D, Manojlovic S, et al. Oral inverted ductal papilloma. *Br J Oral Maxillofac Surg.* 2004;42:75-77.

Haberland-Carrodeguas C, Fornatora ML, Reich RF, Freedman PD. Detection of human papillomavirus DNA in oral inverted ductal papillomas. *J Clin Pathol.* 2003;56:910-913.

Jurgens PE. Inverted ductal papilloma of the lower lip: a case report. *J Oral Maxillofac Surg.* 2004;62:1158-1161.

Kubota N, Suzuki K, Kawai Y, et al. Inverted ductal papilloma of minor salivary gland: case report with immunohistochemical study and literature review. *Pathol Int.* 2006;56:457-461.

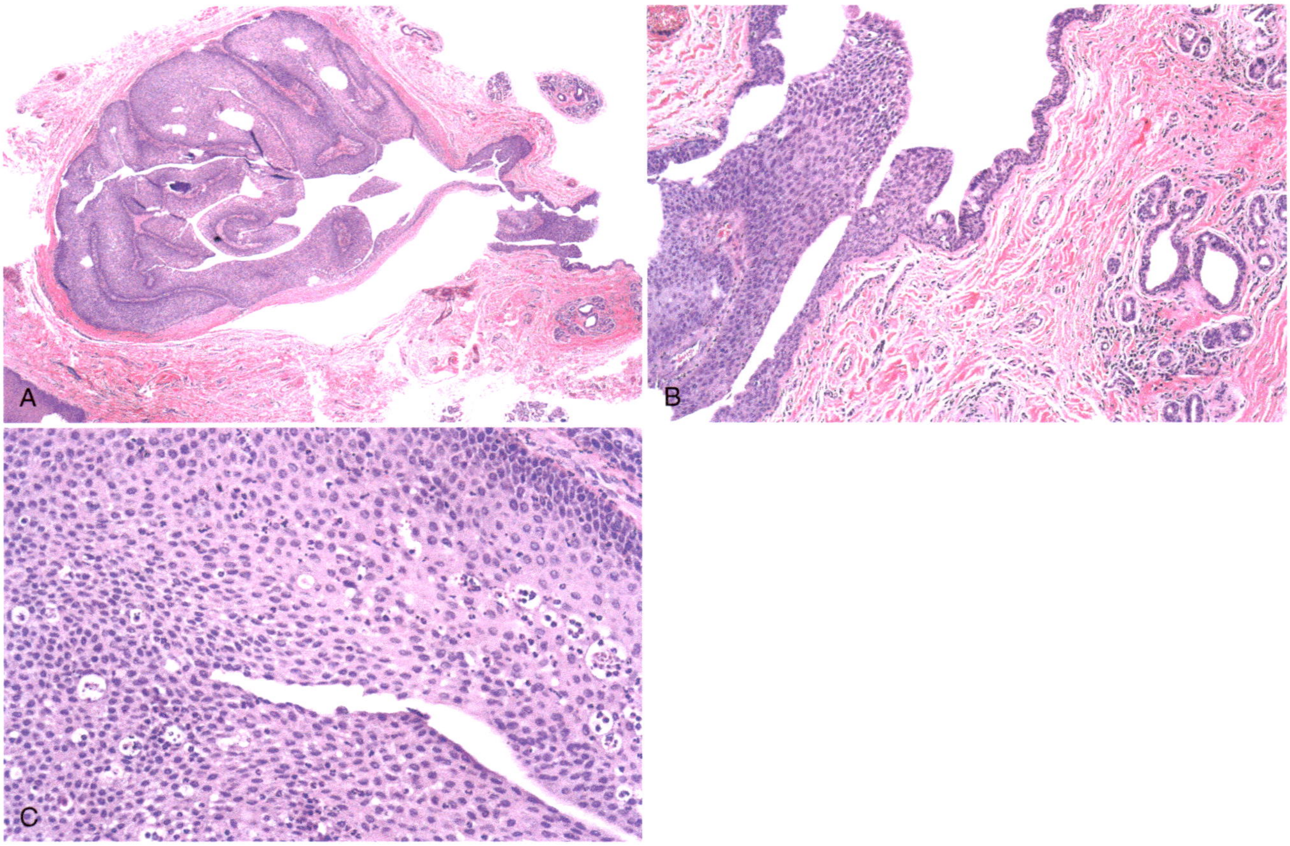

FIG 13.3 Inverted ductal papilloma. (A) Bulbous endophytic growth arising from a duct. (B) Cuboidal-to-columnar cells seen on luminal surface with scattered mucous cells. (C) Cells have bland nuclear morphology, and there is microcyst formation.

SIALADENOMA PAPILLIFERUM

Clinical Findings

- This occurs most frequently in the sixth decade with a slight male predilection and the most common location is the hard palatal mucosa (70% of cases) with the buccal mucosa affected in 10% of cases; the lesion has a rough, warty appearance similar to a squamous papilloma.

Etiopathogenesis and Histopathologic Features

This is the salivary gland equivalent of the syringocystadenoma papilliferum of the skin.

- There is a benign exophytic papillary proliferation of surface squamous epithelium similar to a papilloma, in continuity with deep adenomatous hyperplasia and dilated ducts present at the base of the lesion. There may be a subtle cribriform pattern and the ducts are irregularly shaped with papillary epithelial hyperplasia of ductal epithelium. Eosinophilic columnar luminal cells, and occasional mucous cells are present (Fig. 13.4).
- Occasional lesions have shown development of dysplasia or other salivary gland malignancies.

Differential Diagnosis

- Squamous papilloma does not show the deep adenomatous hyperplasia but this may be the rendered diagnosis if the biopsy is small and superficial.
- Papillary cystadenocarcinoma is invasive, but this may be subtle in low-grade lesions, and they do not exhibit the typical papillomatous surface change.

Management

- Excision is the treatment of choice and there is an up to 15% recurrence rate.

REFERENCES

Brannon RB, Sciubba JJ, Giulani M. Ductal papillomas of salivary gland origin: a report of 19 cases and a review of the literature. *Oral Surg Oral Med Oral Pathol Oral Radiol Endod.* 2001;92:68-77.

Ide F, Kikuchi K, Kusama K, Kanazawa H. Sialadenoma papilliferum with potentially malignant features. *J Clin Pathol.* 2010;63:362-364.

Liu W, Gnepp DR, de Vries E, et al. Mucoepidermoid carcinoma arising in a background of sialadenoma papilliferum: a case report. *Head Neck Pathol.* 2009;3:59-62.

Maiorano E, Favia G, Ricco R. Sialadenoma papilliferum: an immunohistochemical study of five cases. *J Oral Pathol Med.* 1996;25:336-342.

Ubaidat MA, Robinson RA, Belding PJ, Merryman DJ. Sialadenoma papilliferum of the hard palate: report of 2 cases and immunohistochemical evaluation. *Arch Pathol Lab Med.* 2001;125:1595-1597.

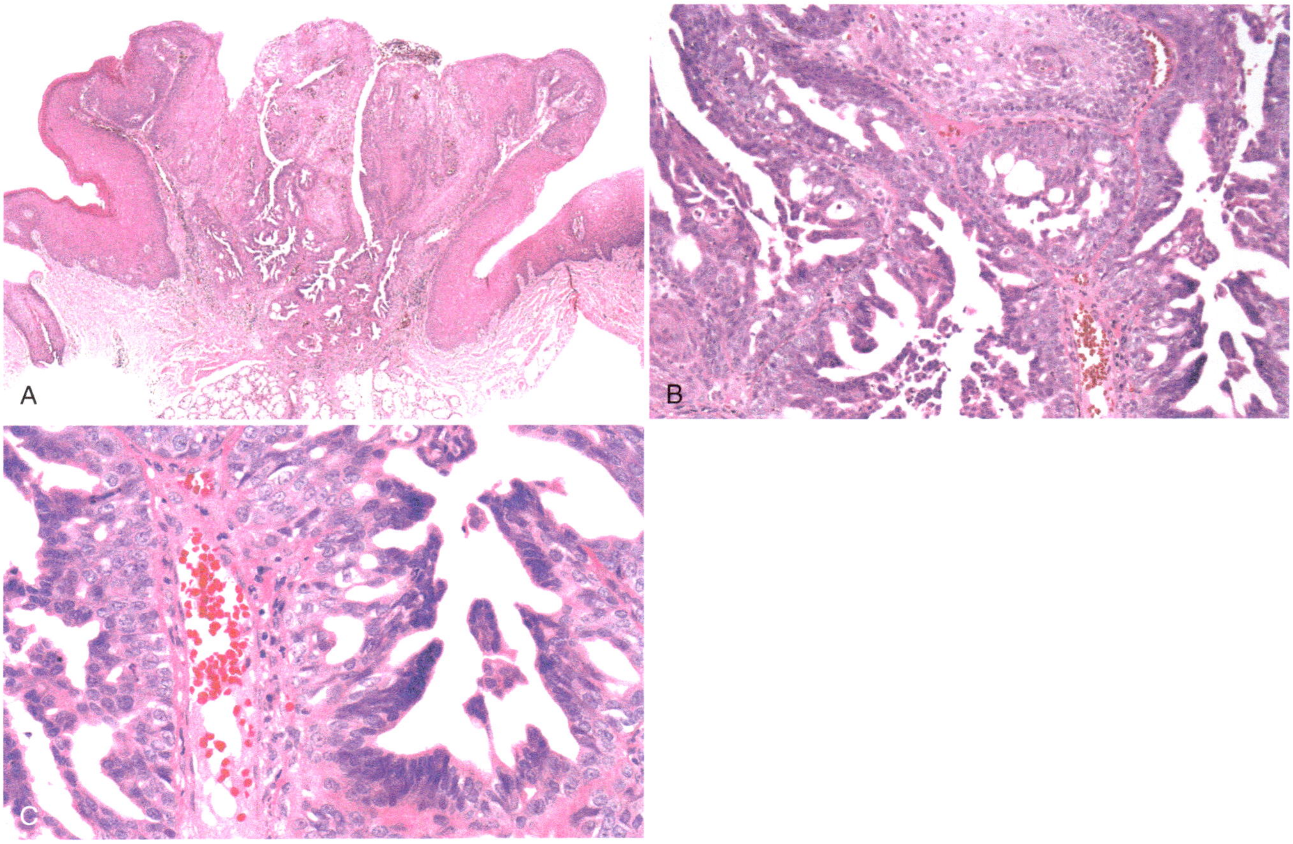

FIG 13.4 Sialadenoma papilliferum. (A) There is surface papillary squamous proliferation and adenomatous proliferation of ducts at base. (B) Adenomatous proliferation with papillary hyperplasia. (C) Luminal cells are cuboidal with spindled nuclei and there is a subtle cribriform architecture. *(A, Courtesy Dr. Paul Auclair, Portland, Me.)*

PLEOMORPHIC ADENOMA AND MYOEPITHELIOMA

Clinical Findings

Benign and malignant intraoral salivary gland tumors occur in approximately equal proportions in the oral cavity. Reports from large medical centers may show a higher proportion of malignant tumors because of referral bias. The pleomorphic adenoma (and its variant the myoepithelioma) is the most common intraoral benign neoplasm (60–80% of all cases), followed by canalicular adenoma (over 80% of which occur in the upper lip mucosa) and much less common, cystadenoma.

- Benign salivary gland neoplasms manifest similarly regardless of the final histologic diagnosis; they occur in adults in the fifth to seventh decades of life, and those on the mucosa not attached to periosteum present as mobile, firm nodules; trauma may lead to ulceration.
- The palatal mucosa is the most common site (50–60% of cases), followed by the upper lip (15–25% of cases) and buccal mucosa (Fig. 13.5).

Etiopathogenesis and Histopathologic Features

This neoplasm putatively arises from the intercalated duct reserve cell and differentiates toward ductal and myoepithelial elements. This neoplasm is pleomorphic in the variety of its architecture, as well as its variable yet distinctive stroma that is myxochondroid, and may exhibit bone, well-formed cartilage, and even adipose tissue. The term *myoepithelioma* is used by some pathologists to mean a myoepithelial cell–predominant neoplasm with few ducts, whereas others use that term only if no ducts are present, preferring the term *pleomorphic adenoma, myoepithelial predominant* for the former lesions. Over 90% of pleomorphic adenomas and myoepitheliomas are positive for *PLAG1* or *HMGA2* rearrangements.

- There is a partially encapsulated or nonencapsulated tumor exhibiting a proliferation of ducts with a cuff of epithelioid myoepithelial cells, with the myoepithelial cells streaming into the myxochondroid stroma, sometimes with infiltration of the capsule; some tumors are cellular with sheets of cells and little stroma, whereas other tumors are predominantly myxoid (Figs. 13.6–13.9).
- Squamous metaplasia, keratin pearls, keratin cysts, osteochondroid material, foci of mucous cells, oncocytes, mature fat, and tyrosine crystals are variably present (Figs. 13.10 and 13.11).
- Myoepithelial cells may be epithelioid, spindled, plasmacytoid, or clear; plasmacytoid myoepithelial cells have abundant eosinophilic cytoplasm and eccentric

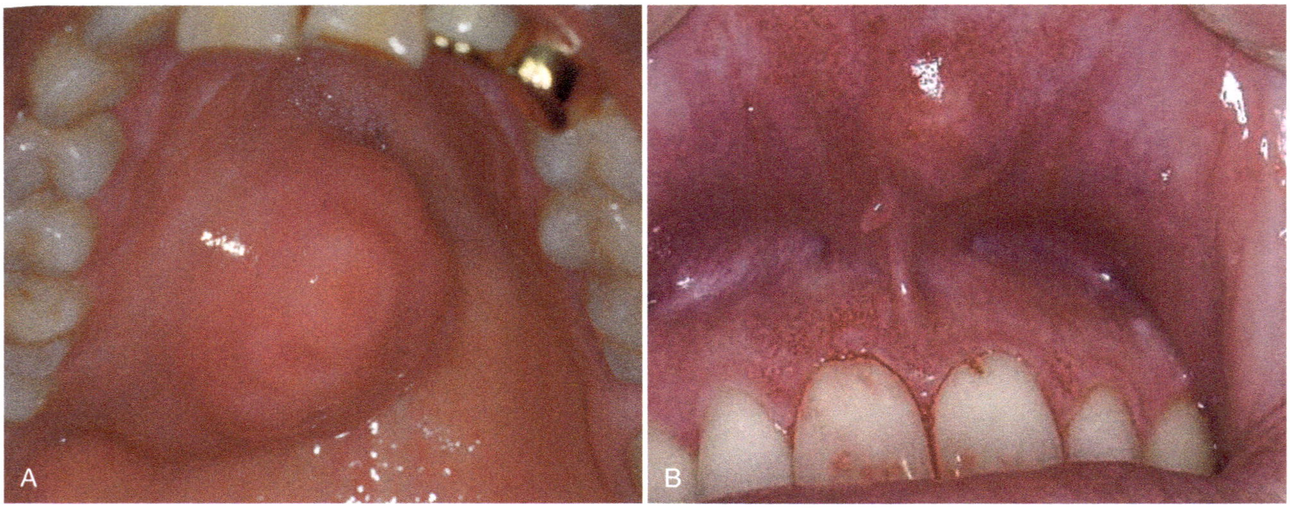

FIG 13.5 (A) Pleomorphic adenoma of the palatal mucosa. (B) Canalicular adenoma of the upper lip mucosa. *(Courtesy Dr. John Sexton, private practice, Wellesley, Mass.)*

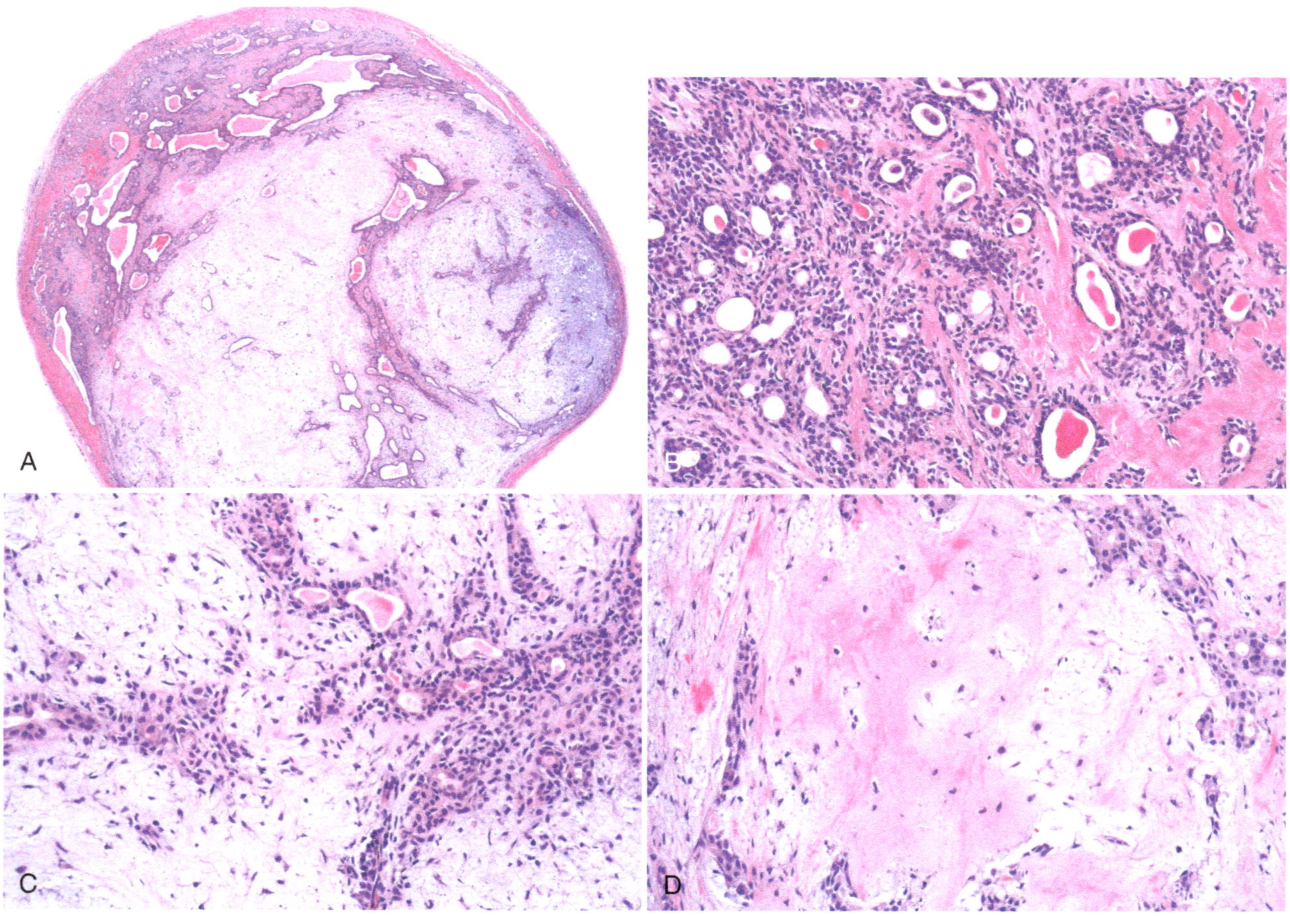

FIG 13.6 Pleomorphic adenoma. (A) Encapsulated tumor with many ducts and prominent myxochondroid areas. (B) Ducts surrounded by myoepithelial cells that merge into hyalinized stroma. (C) Ducts with surrounding epithelioid myoepithelial cells that merge into myxoid stroma that contains spindled myoepithelial cells. (D) Myxochondroid areas within the stroma.

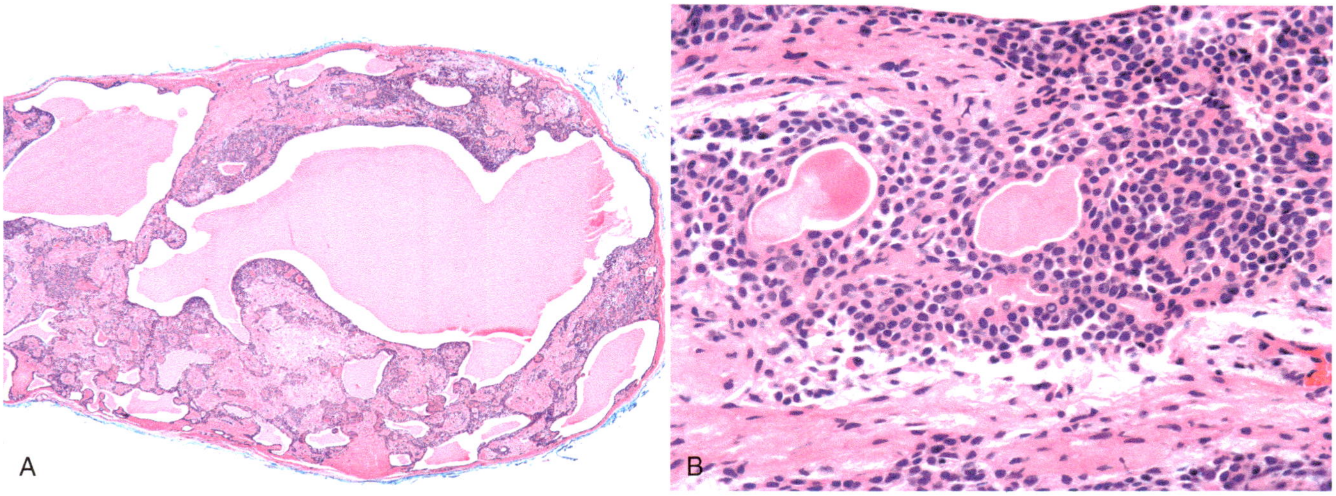

FIG 13.7 Pleomorphic adenoma. (A) Cystic tumor with myxoid and hyalinized stroma. (B) Ducts are surrounded by multiple layers of myoepithelial cells, some of which are plasmacytoid while those in the myxoid stroma are spindled.

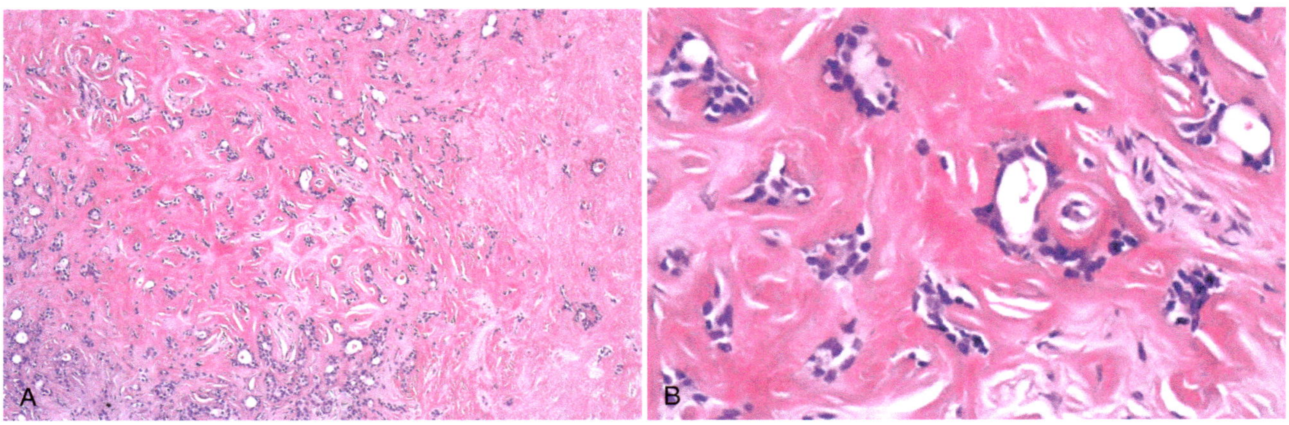

FIG 13.8 Pleomorphic adenoma. (A) Tumor with extensive hyalinization. (B) Ducts exhibit benign cytology surrounded by densely hyalinized stroma.

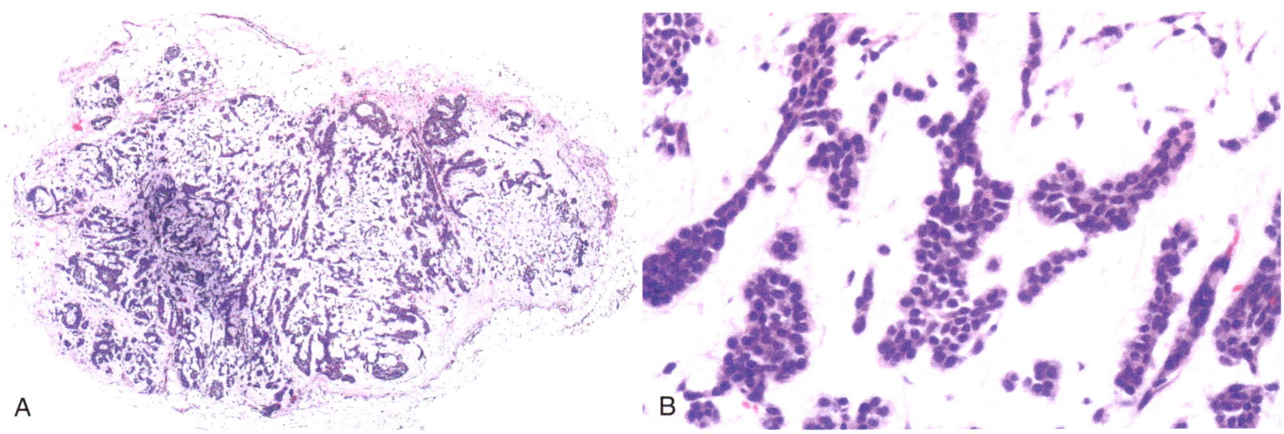

FIG 13.9 Myxoid pleomorphic adenoma. (A) Myxoid tumor containing many islands and cords of tumor cells; rare ductal structures are present. (B) Epithelioid and spindled myoepithelial cells in myxoid stroma.

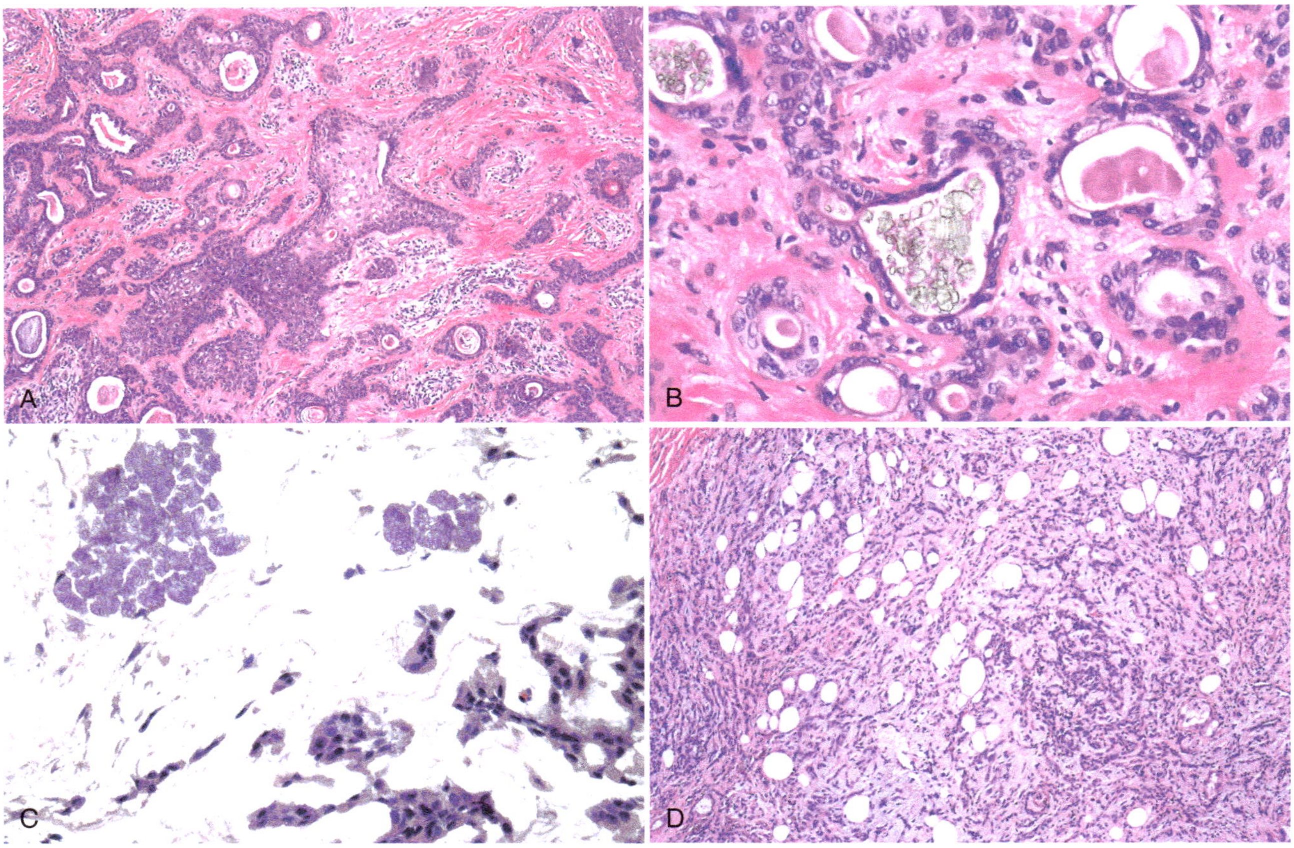

FIG 13.10 Pleomorphic adenoma. (A) Pleomorphic adenoma exhibiting squamous metaplasia and keratin formation. (B) Ducts containing mucous cells and crystalline structures. (C) Crystalline bodies within the stroma in a myxoid pleomorphic adenoma. (D) Lipometaplasia in a spindle cell myoepithelioma.

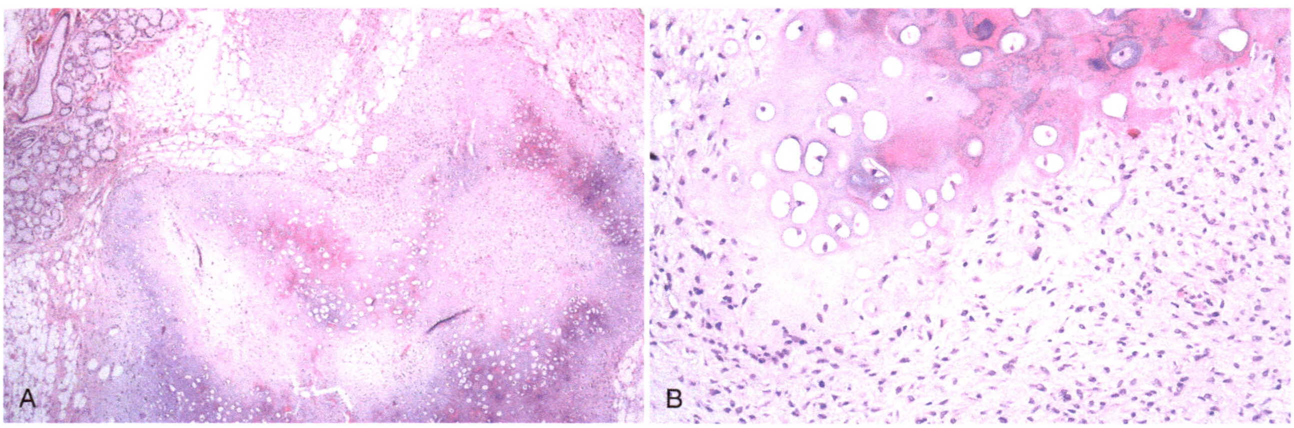

FIG 13.11 Spindle cell myoepithelioma of palate. (A) Spindle cell proliferation with formation of cartilage and fat. (B) Spindled myoepithelial cells with nuclear atypia associated with osteochondroid material.

nuclei that vary in shape and size, dispersed chromatin, and small or inconspicuous nucleoli (Figs. 13.12 and 13.13); one variant of myoepithelioma has a reticulated pattern of growth.

- Significant cytologic atypia (not just variation in nuclear shape and size) is seen in intracapsular, in situ carcinoma, or noninvasive carcinoma ex pleomorphic adenoma; these are usually strongly associated with the presence of stromal hyalinization and hyaline nodules.
- Myoepithelial cells are positive for vimentin, calponin, smooth muscle actin, maspin, smooth muscle myosin long chain, K14, S-100 protein, GFAP, p63, p40, and SOX10 (Fig. 13.14).
- Rearrangements in *PLAG1* and *HMGA2* are generally present in cases that show myxoid change or have

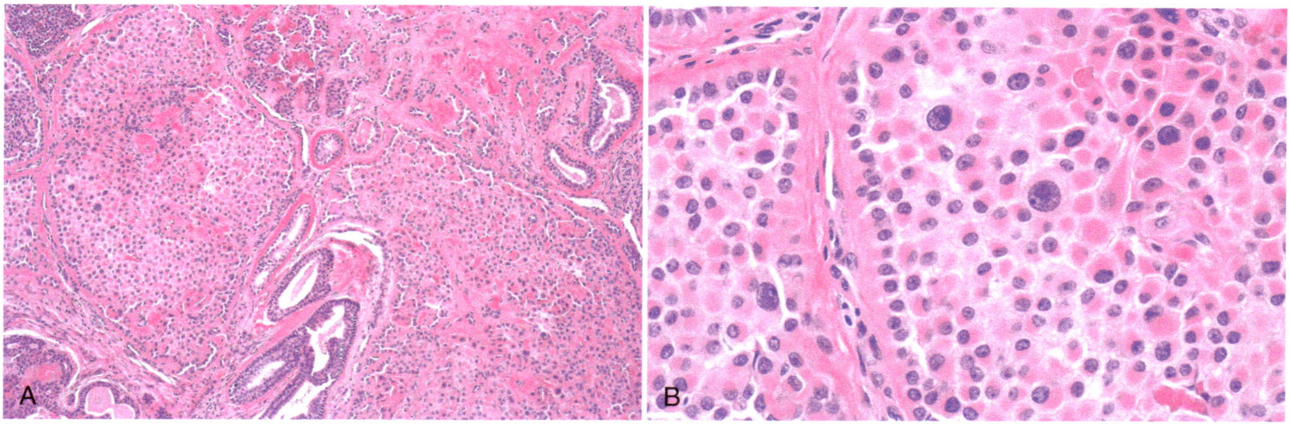

FIG 13.12 Pleomorphic adenoma. (A) Sheets of plasmacytoid myoepithelial cells with focal duct formation. (B) Cells with eccentric pleomorphic nuclei and abundant eosinophilic cytoplasm.

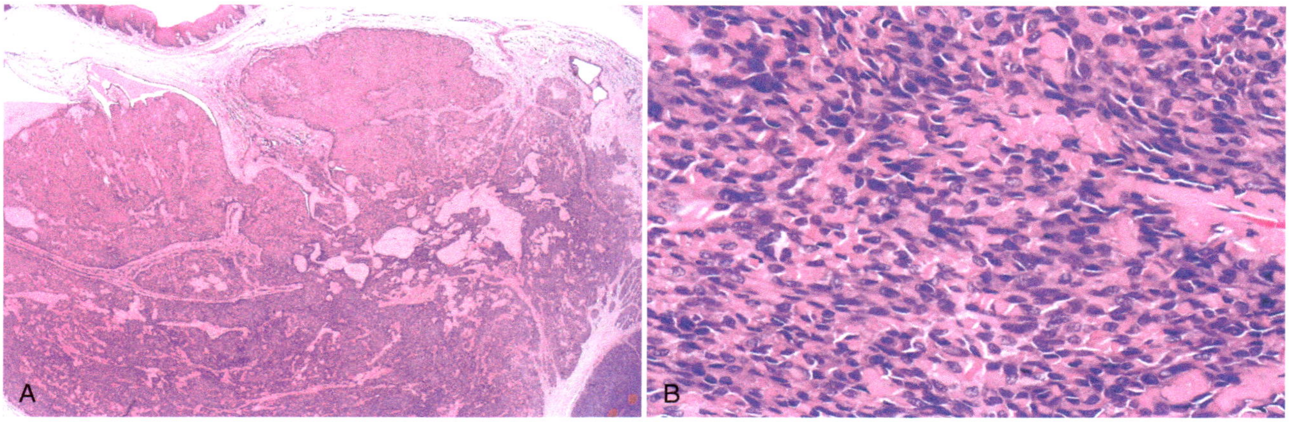

FIG 13.13 Myoepithelioma. (A) Myoepithelioma composed of sheets of myoepithelial cells without duct formation. (B) Plasmacytoid myoepithelial cells with abundant eosinophilic cytoplasm and eccentric nuclei.

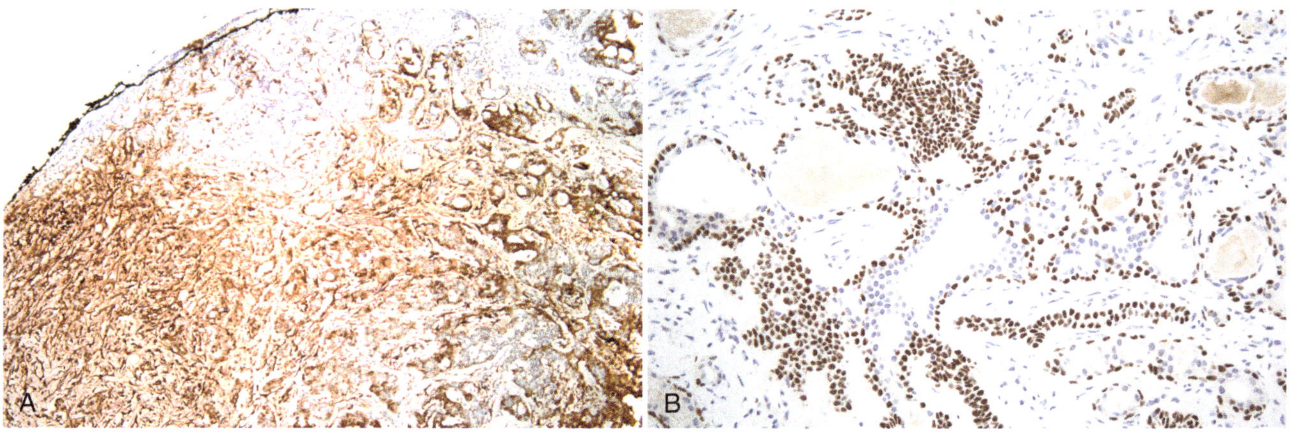

FIG 13.14 Pleomorphic adenoma: (A) Glial fibrillary acidic protein is positive within spindled myoepithelial cells and abluminal cells. (B) Abluminal cells are positive for p63.

abundant cartilage, while cellular pleomorphic adenomas are less likely to be positive.

Differential Diagnosis

- Apocrine chondroid syringoma of the skin (presenting on the lip) may appear similar, although there may be apocrine decapitation secretion within ducts and follicular and sebaceous differentiation.
- Spindle cell lipoma or other benign mesenchymal neoplasm with bone, cartilage, and fat differentiation such as osteolipoma do not show immunopositivity for keratin within the spindle cells.

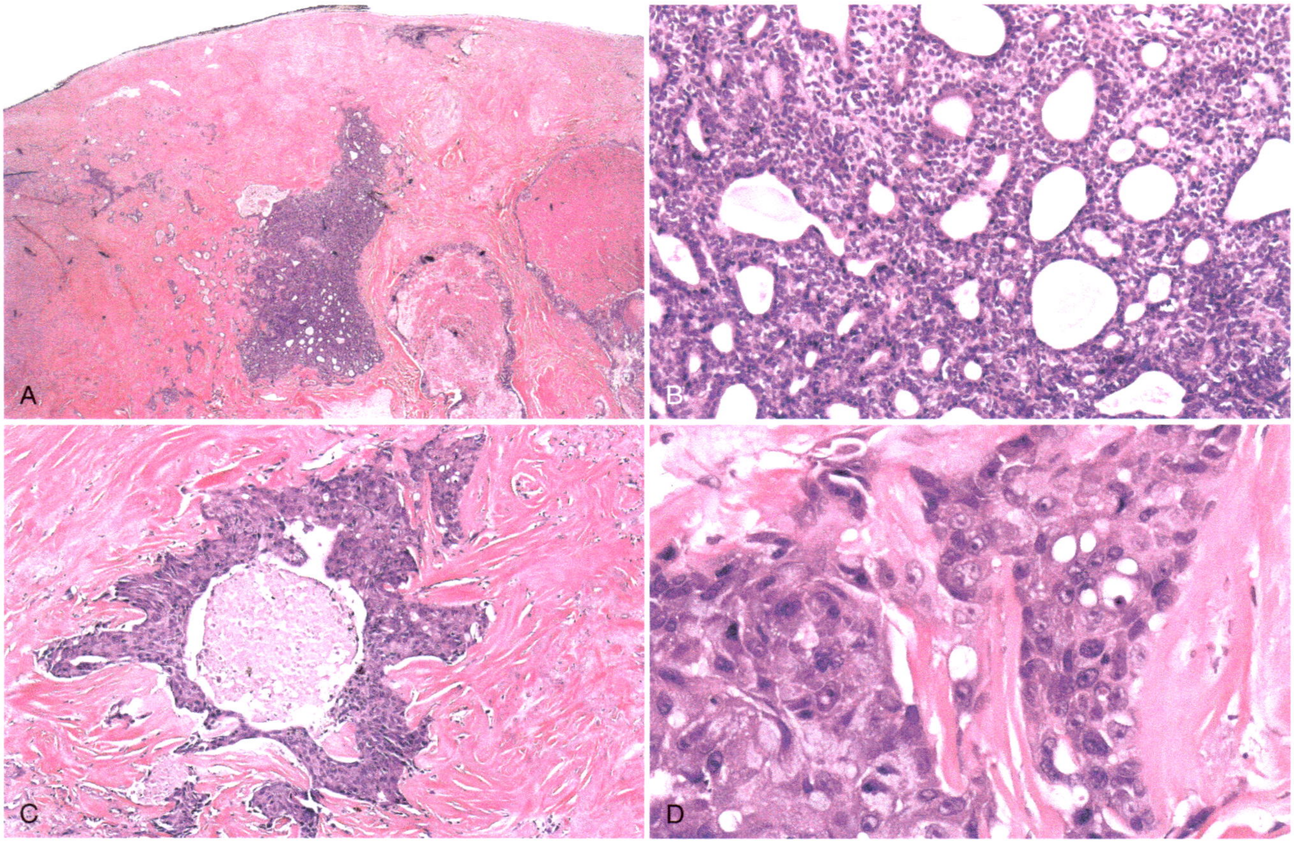

FIG 13.15 Carcinoma ex pleomorphic adenoma of the upper lip. (A) Pleomorphic adenoma with extensive hyalinization and adenocarcinoma *(right)*. (B) Remnant pleomorphic adenoma. (C) Area of adenocarcinoma with comedonecrosis. (D) Carcinoma with pleomorphic nuclei.

- Plasmacytoma has coarse "clock-face" chromatin and a clear perinuclear zone of Hopf, and tumor cells are CD138+ and negative for S-100 protein, p63, and keratin.
- The presence of significant hyalinization must prompt a search for carcinoma ex pleomorphic adenoma, the two most common of which are salivary duct carcinoma and myoepithelial carcinoma. Carcinoma ex pleomorphic adenoma is positive for *PLAG1* and *HMGA2* in approximately 85% of cases. The presence of a hyalinized nodule alone within salivary duct carcinoma or myoepithelial carcinoma is associated with *PLAG1* and *HMGA2* in 80% to 90% of cases, suggesting that these nodules represent senescent areas of pleomorphic adenoma (Fig. 13.15). The terms *noninvasive, in situ,* and *intracapsular* carcinoma ex pleomorphic adenoma are used for tumors that do not invade the capsule; the definition of *minor* invasion (*minimally invasive*) and *wide* invasion beyond the capsule is still controversial with 1.5 mm, 2.5 mm, and 5 mm as the maximal measurements defining minor invasion, with *noninvasive* and *minimally invasive* tumors having less metastases and better survival. Tumors with copy gains of both *EGFR* and *HER2* may have poor prognosis and most of these have been reported within the parotid gland and may not apply to intraoral tumors that tend not to be well encapsulated.
- Myoepithelial carcinomas rarely occur intraorally and most are of the epithelioid or clear cell type; tumor cells show significant cytologic atypia.
- Interestingly, soft tissue myoepithelioma exhibits *PLAG1* rearrangement in approximately 30% of cases as well as *EWSR1* rearrangements in approximately 45% of cases.

Management and Prognosis

- Excision with clear margins is treatment of choice for pleomorphic adenoma, and the recurrence rate is insignificant for intraoral lesions.
- Malignant transformation occurs in long-standing lesions in less than 5% of cases.

REFERENCES

Antonescu CR, Zhang L, Shao SY, et al. Frequent PLAG1 gene rearrangements in skin and soft tissue myoepithelioma with ductal differentiation. *Genes Chromosomes Cancer.* 2013;52:675-682.

Bahrami A, Perez-Ordonez B, Dalton JD, Weinreb I. An analysis of PLAG1 and HMGA2 rearrangements in salivary duct carcinoma and examination of the role of precursor lesions. *Histopathology.* 2013;63:250-262.

Buchner A, Merrell PW, Carpenter WM. Relative frequency of intra-oral minor salivary gland tumors: a study of 380 cases from northern California and comparison to reports from other parts of the world. *J Oral Pathol Med.* 2007;36:207-214.

Cheuk W, Chan JK. Advances in salivary gland pathology. *Histopathology.* 2007;51:1-20.

Gnepp DR. Mucinous myoepithelioma, a recently described new myoepithelioma variant. *Head Neck Pathol.* 2013;7(suppl 1):S85-S89.

Haskell HD, Butt KM, Woo SB. Pleomorphic adenoma with extensive lipometaplasia: report of three cases. *Am J Surg Pathol.* 2005;29:1389-1393.

Jo VY, Fletcher CD. Myoepithelial neoplasms of soft tissue: an updated review of the clinicopathologic, immunophenotypic, and genetic features. *Head Neck Pathol.* 2015;9:32-38.
Katabi N, Ghossein R, Ho A, et al. Consistent PLAG1 and HMGA2 abnormalities distinguish carcinoma ex-pleomorphic adenoma from its de novo counterparts. *Hum Pathol.* 2015;46:26-33.
Matsuyama A, Hisaoka M, Nagao Y, Hashimoto H. Aberrant PLAG1 expression in pleomorphic adenomas of the salivary gland: a molecular genetic and immunohistochemical study. *Virchows Arch.* 2011;458:583-592.
Nishijima T, Yamamoto H, Nakano T, et al. Dual gain of HER2 and EGFR gene copy numbers impacts the prognosis of carcinoma ex pleomorphic adenoma. *Hum Pathol.* 2015;46:1730-1743.
Rito M, Fonseca I. Carcinoma ex-pleomorphic adenoma of the salivary glands has a high risk of progression when the tumor invades more than 2.5 mm beyond the capsule of the residual pleomorphic adenoma. *Virchows Arch.* 2015.
Rotellini M, Palomba A, Baroni G, Franchi A. Diagnostic utility of PLAG1 immunohistochemical determination in salivary gland tumors. *Appl Immunohistochem Mol Morphol.* 2014;22:390-394.
Savera AT, Sloman A, Huvos AG, Klimstra DS. Myoepithelial carcinoma of the salivary glands: a clinicopathologic study of 25 patients. *Am J Surg Pathol.* 2000;24:761-774.
Sciubba JJ. Myoepithelioma of salivary glands: report of 23 cases. *Cancer.* 1982;47:562-572.
Wang C, Zhang Z, Ge Y, et al. Myoepithelial carcinoma of the salivary glands: a clinicopathologic study of 29 patients. *J Oral Maxillofac Surg.* 2015;73:1938-1945.
Weiler C, Zengel P, van der Wal JE, et al. Carcinoma ex pleomorphic adenoma with special reference to the prognostic significance of histological progression: a clinicopathological investigation of 41 cases. *Histopathology.* 2011;59:741-750.
Yang S, Li L, Zeng M, et al. Myoepithelial carcinoma of intraoral minor salivary glands: a clinicopathological study of 7 cases and review of the literature. *Oral Surg Oral Med Oral Pathol Oral Radiol Endod.* 2010;110:85-193.

CANALICULAR ADENOMA

Clinical Findings

- This occurs most frequently in the seventh decade with a 2 : 1 female predilection; 80% occur as a mobile, firm nodule in the upper lip mucosa with approximately 10% occurring in the buccal mucosa; rarely, synchronous tumors are noted.

Etiopathogenesis and Histopathologic Features

This tumor is likely to arise from the intercalated duct reserve cells with differentiation toward ductal cells with no myoepithelial differentiation.

- There is an encapsulated proliferation of cuboidal-to-columnar cells, usually in two layers, in interconnected trabeculae and ribbon-like strands that enclose narrow, elongated ducts and channels (canaliculi); where two strands meet, knots or beads of cells form; cells have slightly palisaded, pseudostratified, ovoid nuclei with dispersed chromatin and small nucleoli; occasional mitoses, oncocytes, and mucous cells may be seen; cystic change and hemorrhage are frequent findings (Figs. 13.16–13.18A–B).
- The stroma is collagen-poor and mucinous/myxoid with prominent ectatic capillaries; other findings include psammomatoid spherical calcifications and luminal epithelial spherules or morules.

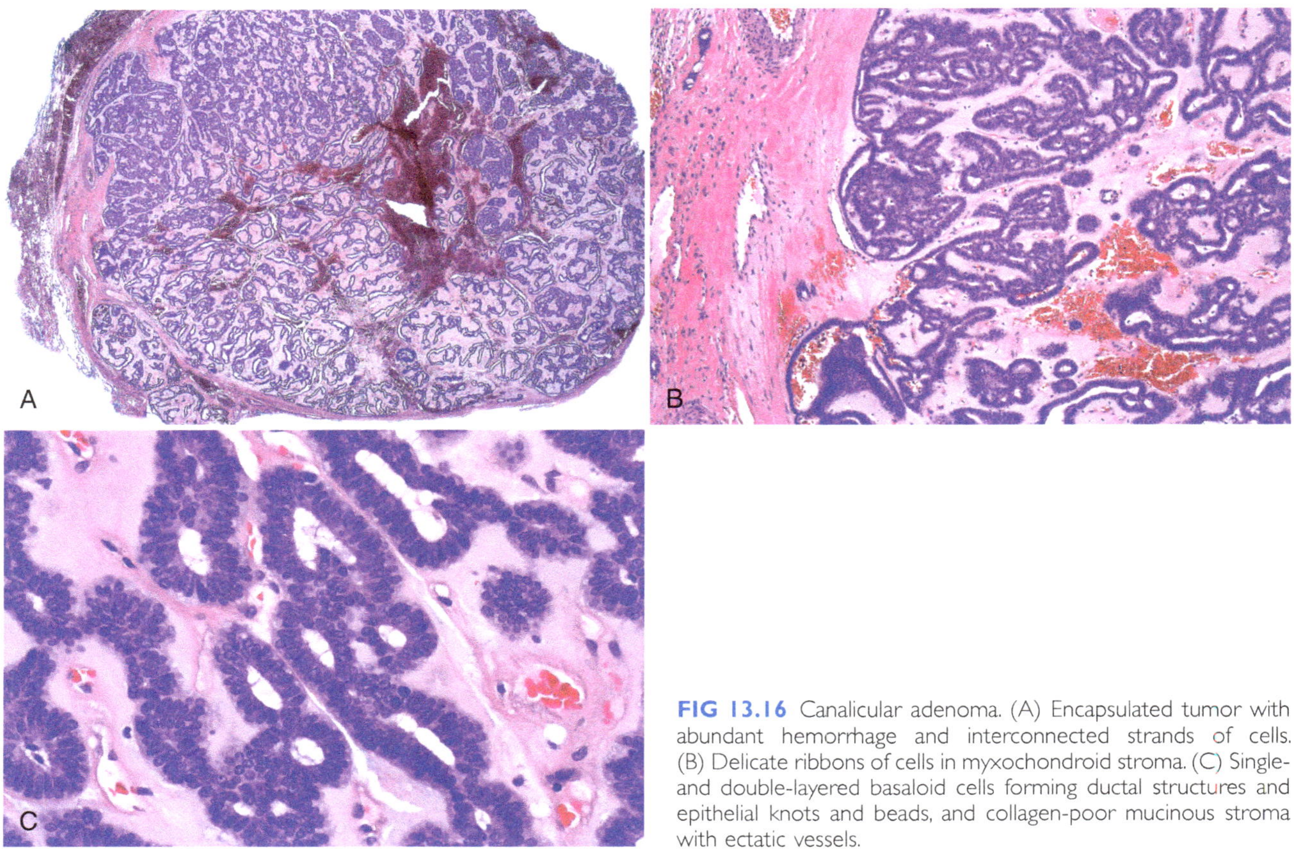

FIG 13.16 Canalicular adenoma. (A) Encapsulated tumor with abundant hemorrhage and interconnected strands of cells. (B) Delicate ribbons of cells in myxochondroid stroma. (C) Single- and double-layered basaloid cells forming ductal structures and epithelial knots and beads, and collagen-poor mucinous stroma with ectatic vessels.

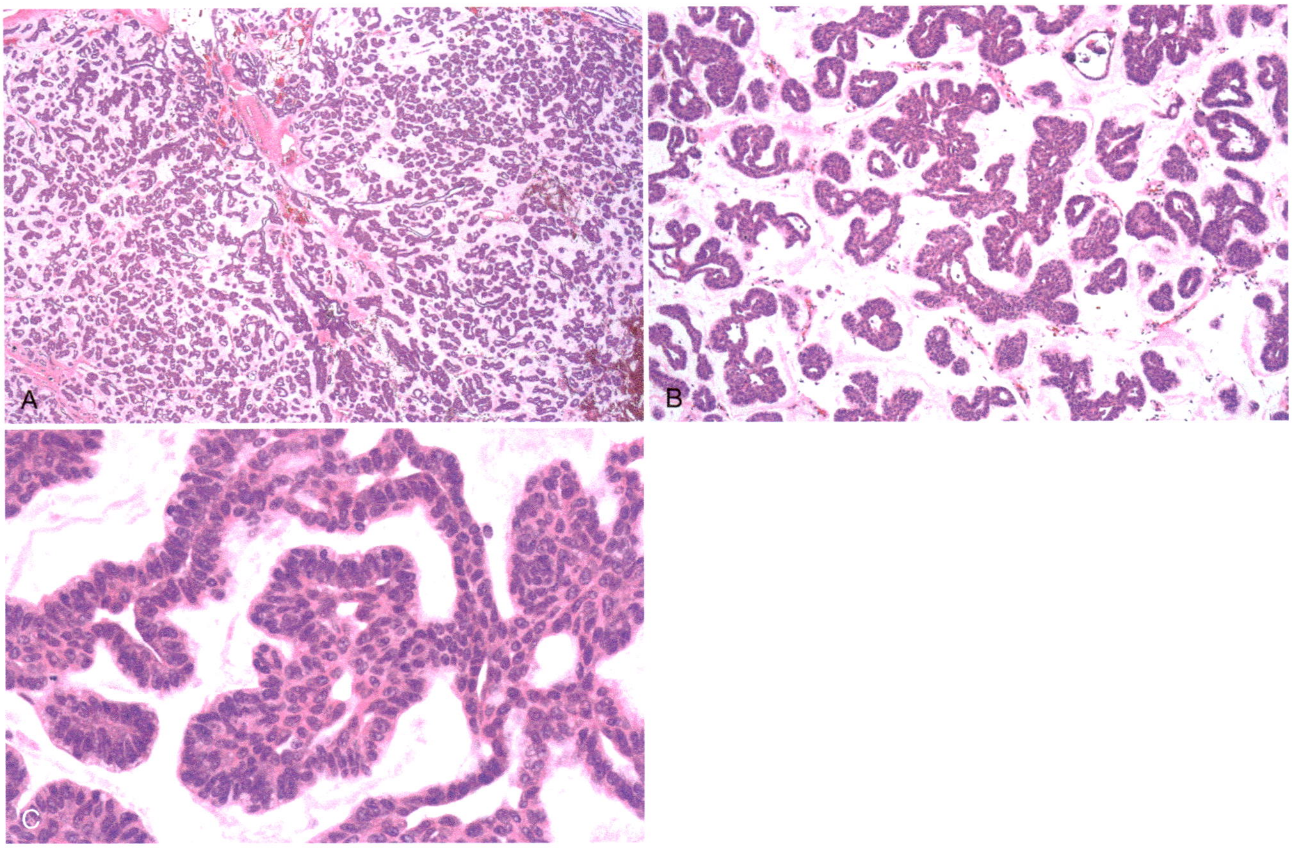

FIG 13.17 Canalicular adenoma. (A) Irregular strands and small islands of tumor cells in myxochondroid stroma. (B) Strands and islands of tumor cells, some with central lumens, delicate vessels, and collagen-poor stroma. (C) Strands are double layered or multilayered with epithelial knots or beads where tumor strands intersect.

- Cells are positive for AE1/3, CAM 5.2, K7, K19, EMA, S-100 protein, vimentin, c-kit (CD117), and SOX10, and negative for smooth muscle actin and other myoepithelial markers (Fig. 13.18C–D); the epithelial spherules are positive for p16 and p63, and GFAP is present only in tumor cells at the tumor-capsule interface.
- Foci of early canalicular adenoma within adjacent gland lobules is not unusual

Differential Diagnosis

- Trabecular basal cell adenoma is rare in the minor glands and exhibits hyalinized stroma, and contains both ductal and myoepithelial cell populations with positivity for myoepithelial markers such as p63 in the abluminal cells.
- Pleomorphic adenoma has a more variable pattern with solid sheets of cells in some areas, and the presence of myoepithelial cells and myxochondroid, and hyalinized stroma.
- Eccrine spiradenoma, a skin adnexal tumor forms lobules and broad trabeculae of tumor cells with two cell populations, and hyalinized material and lymphocytes are present.

Management

- Enucleation or excision with clear margins is curative.

REFERENCES

Edwards PC, Bhuiya T, Kelsch RD. C-kit expression in the salivary gland neoplasms adenoid cystic carcinoma, polymorphous low-grade adenocarcinoma, and monomorphic adenoma. *Oral Surg Oral Med Oral Pathol Oral Radiol Endod.* 2003;95:586-593.

Edwards PC, Bhuiya T, Kelsch RD. Assessment of p63 expression in the salivary gland neoplasms adenoid cystic carcinoma, polymorphous low-grade adenocarcinoma, and basal cell and canalicular adenomas. *Oral Surg Oral Med Oral Pathol Oral Radiol Endod.* 2004;97:613-619.

Huebner TA, Almubarak H, Drachenberg CB, Papadimitriou JC. Canalicular adenoma–search for the cell of origin: ultrastructural and immunohistochemical analysis of 7 cases and review of the literature. *Ultrastruct Pathol.* 2014;38:74-82.

Owosho AA, Aguilar CE, Seethala RR. Comparison of p63 and p40 (DeltaNp63) as basal, squamoid, and myoepithelial markers in salivary gland tumors. *Appl Immunohistochem Mol Morphol.* 2015; July 30;[Epub ahead of print].

Samar ME, Avila RE, Fonseca IB, et al. Multifocal canalicular adenoma of the minor labial salivary glands. *Int J Clin Exp Pathol.* 2014;7:8205-8210.

Siqueira CS, Fernandes KS, Vivas AP, et al. Clinical and histological features of multifocal canalicular adenomas of the upper lip. *Braz Dent J.* 2013;24:542-546.

Thompson LD, Bauer JL, Chiosea S, et al. Canalicular adenoma: a clinicopathologic and immunohistochemical analysis of 67 cases with a review of the literature. *Head Neck Pathol.* 2015;9:181-195.

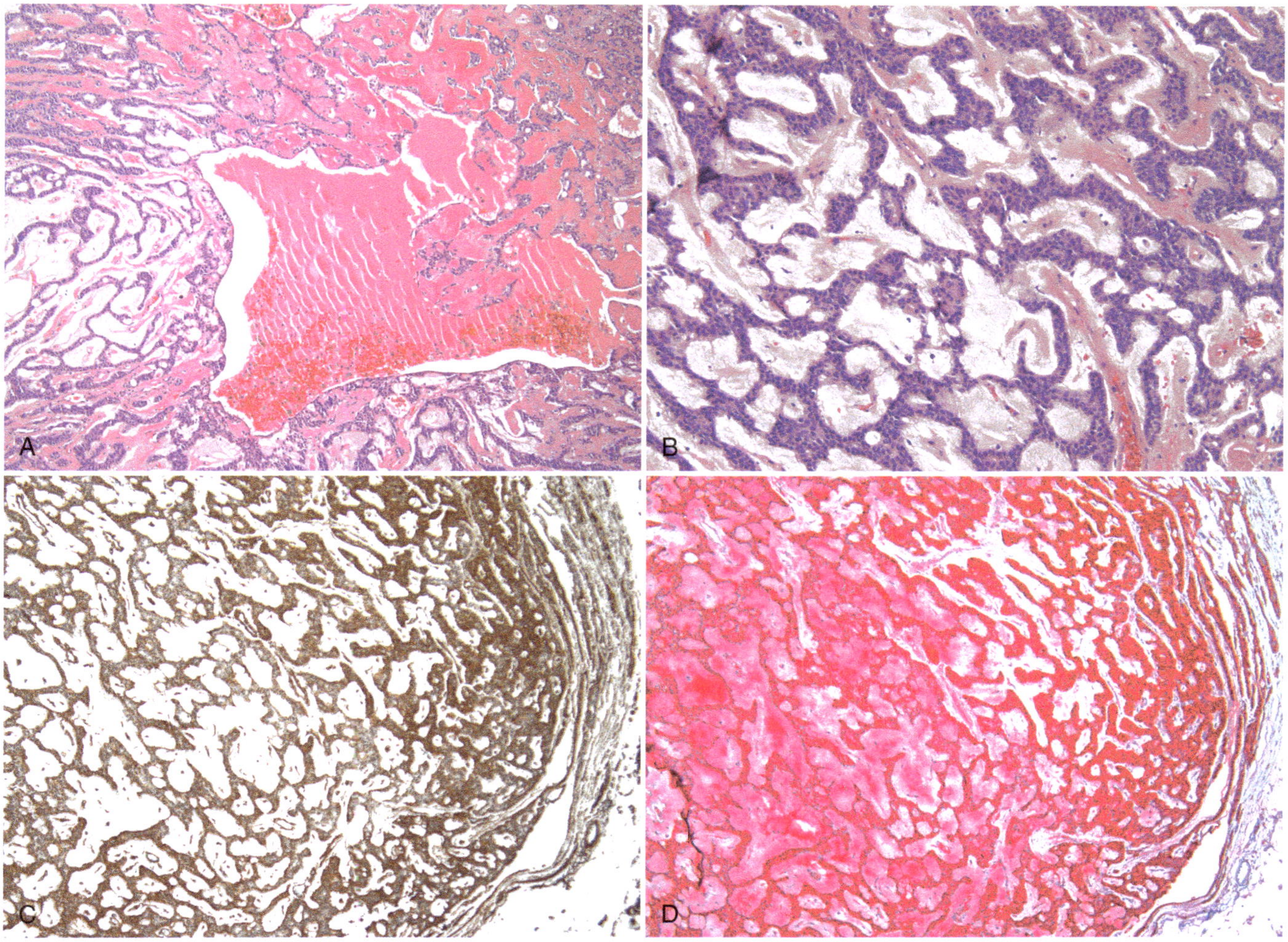

FIG 13.18 Canalicular adenoma. (A) Tumor with cystic spaces and both myxoid and hyalinized stroma. (B) Interconnected strands of basaloid cells with plexiform pattern in collagen-poor stroma and beads or knots of cells where two strands intersect. (C) Tumor cells are positive for vimentin. (D) Tumor cells are positive for S-100 protein.

CYSTADENOMA, PAPILLARY OR OTHERWISE

Etiopathogenesis and Histopathologic Features

This tumor likely arises from the intercalated duct reserve cell.

- There is an encapsulated or well-circumscribed adenomatous proliferation of low- cuboidal-to-columnar cells forming cystic structures of varying sizes; in the papillary form, papillary structures with adenomatous ductal proliferation protrude into the lumen or are constituents of the lining. Oncoytes mucous cells, apocrine cells, and epidermoid cells may be present; cells have benign morphology and there is insignificant mitotic activity (Figs. 13.19–13.21).

Differential Diagnosis

- Reactive multifocal metaplasia of ducts is nonencapsulated and shows cystically dilated ducts in multiple salivary gland lobules without adenomatous proliferation, although sometimes papillary projections may be seen (Fig. 13.22).
- Salivary duct cyst is generally a single cyst lined by cuboidal-to-columnar cells exhibiting oncocytic and mucous cell metaplasia, sometimes with subtle papillary projections and surface undulations; this is a reactive ectatic duct and other ducts in the area may show similar ectasia but should not be diagnosed as cystadenoma (see Chapter 12).
- Intraductal papilloma forms papillary structures without adenomatous ductal proliferation.
- Low-grade adenocarcinomas are nonencapsulated and infiltrative, although cytology may be bland.

Management

- Excision or enucleation with clear margins is curative.

REFERENCES

Gallego L, Junquera L, Fresno MF, de Vicente JC. Papillary cystadenoma and cystadenocarcinoma of salivary glands: two unusual entities. *Med Oral Patol Oral Cir Bucal.* 2008;13:E460-E463.

Guccion JG, Redman RS, Calhoun NR, Saini N. Papillary cystadenoma of the palate: a case report and ultrastructural study. *J Oral Maxillofac Surg.* 1997;55:759-764.

Halbritter SA, Altermatt HJ, Caversaccio M, Bornstein MM. Apocrine papillary cystadenoma of a minor salivary gland on the lower lip: case presentation. *Quintessence Int.* 2009;40:167-169.

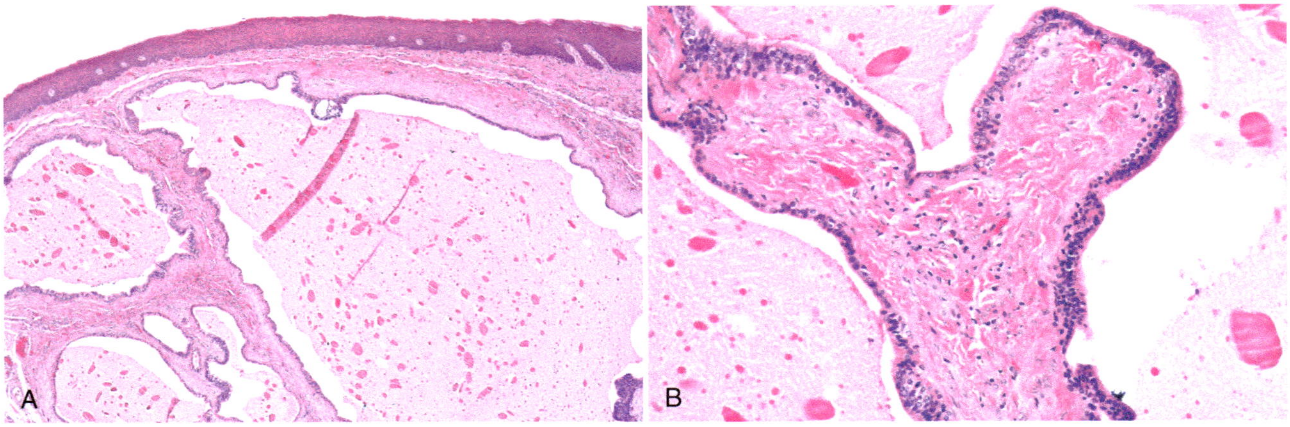

FIG 13.19 Cystadenoma. (A) Proliferation of cysts of varying sizes with focal adenomatous plaques. (B) Cysts are lined by a double layer of columnar cells with eosinophilic luminal cells.

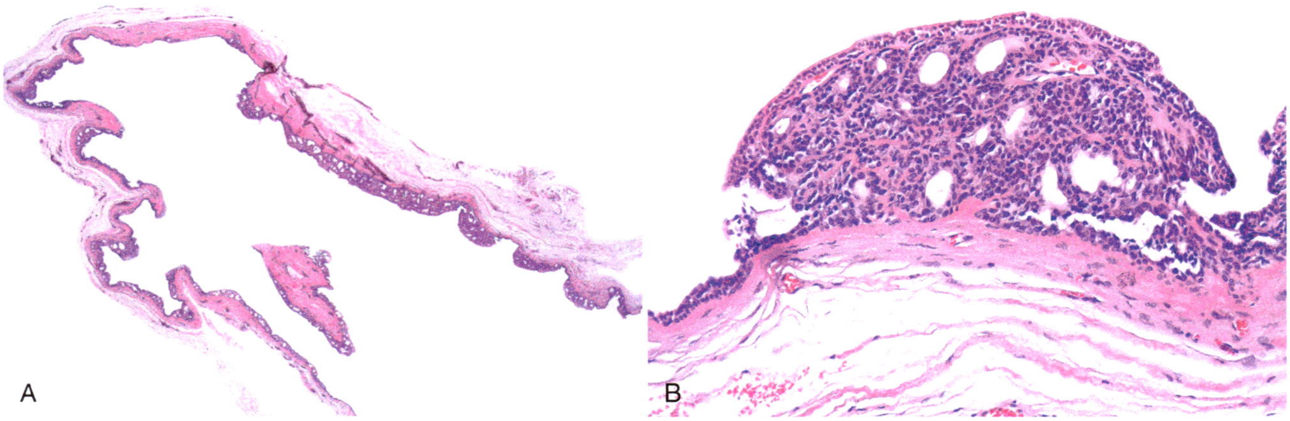

FIG 13.20 Cystadenoma. (A) Single large cyst with adenomatous proliferation of lining epithelium forming plaques. (B) Adenomatous proliferation of lining epithelium forming small ducts.

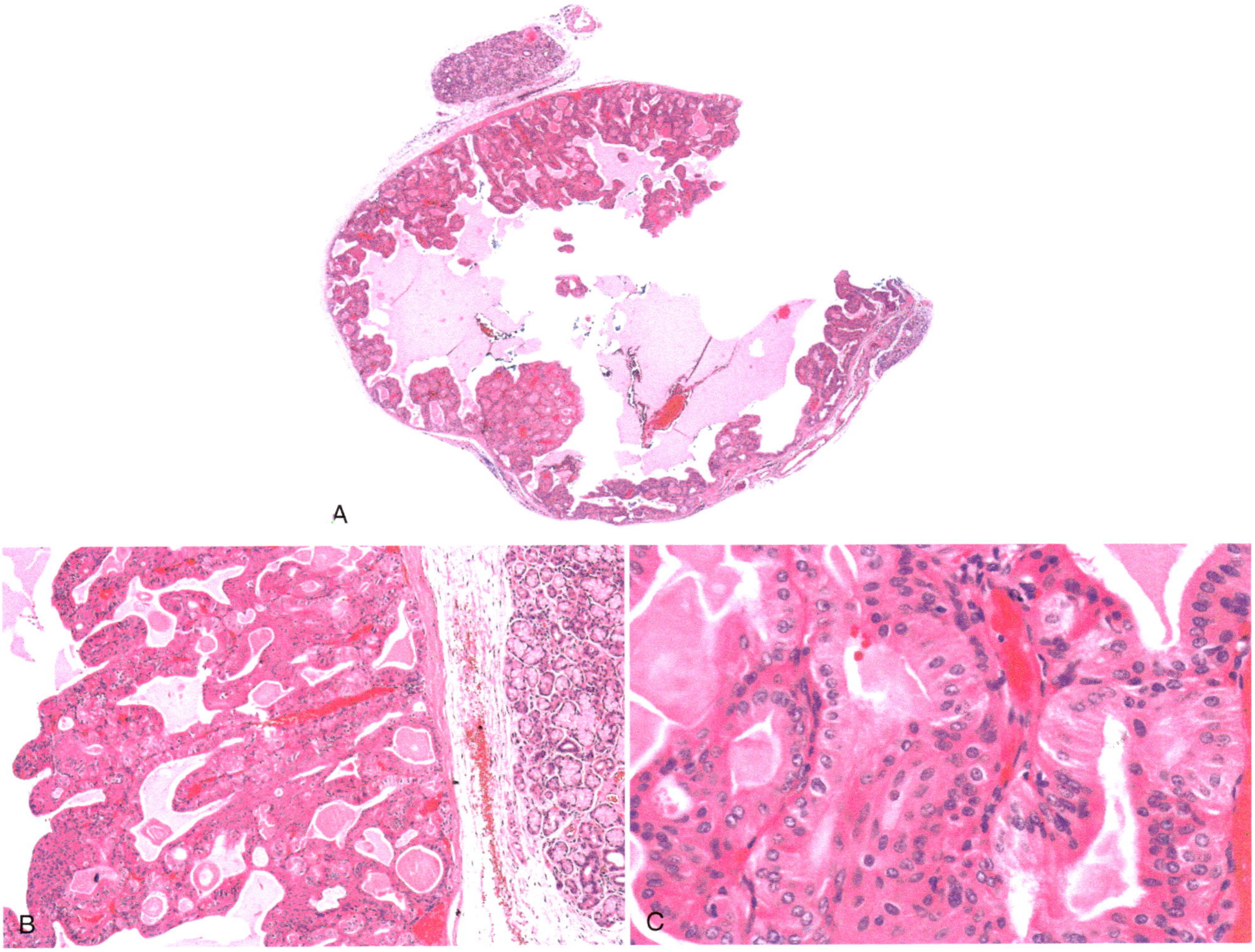

FIG 13.21 Papillary oncocytic cystadenoma. (A) Single large cyst with papillary and adenomatous proliferation of lining. (B) Papillary proliferation of oncocytes with delicate fibrovascular cores. (C) Oncocytes in adenomatous configuration with eosinophilic, granular cytoplasm.

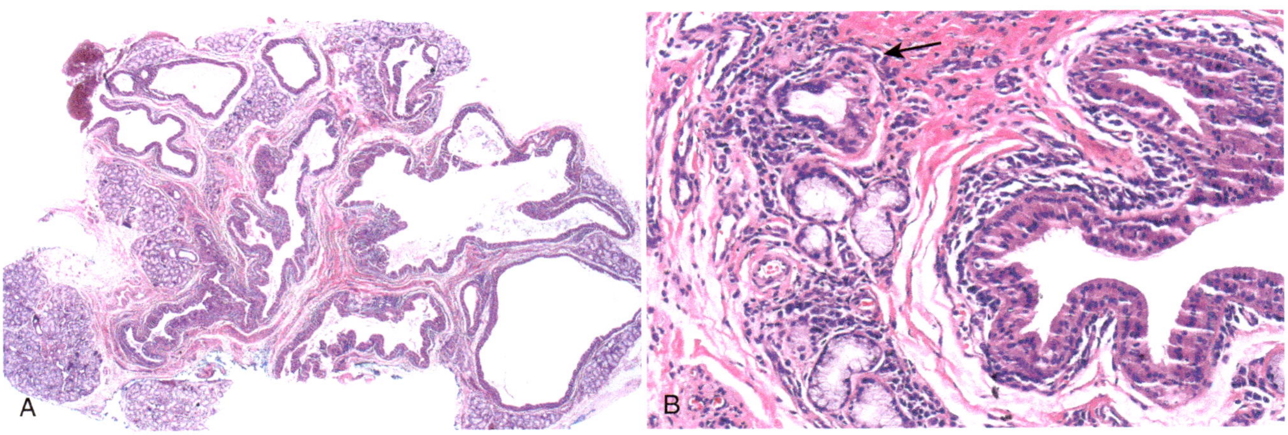

FIG 13.22 Oncocytic metaplasia from chronic obstruction of glands. (A) Salivary gland with multiple dilated ducts within multiple gland lobules. (B) Dilated ducts are lined by a double layer of oncocytes with underlying plasma cells; early changes are noted in adjacent glands *(arrow)*.

Kusafuka K, Ueno T, Kurihara K, et al. Cystadenoma of the palate: immunohistochemistry of mucins. *Pathol Int.* 2008;58:524-528.

Lim CS, Ngu I, Collins AP, McKellar GM. Papillary cystadenoma of a minor salivary gland: report of a case involving cytological analysis and review of the literature. *Oral Surg Oral Med Oral Pathol Oral Radiol Endod.* 2008;105:e28-e33.

Tjioe KC, de Lima HG, Thompson LD, et al. Papillary cystadenoma of minor salivary glands: report of 11 cases and review of the english literature. *Head Neck Pathol.* 2015;9:354-359.

Malignant Salivary Gland Neoplasms

Mucoepidermoid carcinoma is the most common intraoral salivary gland malignancy (also the most common in childhood), with the other two most common being polymorphous low-grade adenocarcinoma and adenoid cystic carcinoma.

Clinical Findings

The clinical appearance of malignant salivary gland neoplasms is similar, regardless of the final histopathologic diagnosis.

- Tumors present in middle-aged or older adults with a female predilection (except for salivary duct carcinoma which has a male predilection); they appear as firm masses, mobile or tethered, ulcerated or cystic (especially mucoepidermoid carcinoma) on the hard palatal mucosa, upper lip mucosa, floor of mouth, buccal mucosa, and tongue (Fig. 13.23).

General Histopathologic Considerations

It is believed that most tumors arise from the intercalated duct reserve cell with differentiation toward ductal, myoepithelial, and acinar cells. The mucoepidermoid carcinoma and salivary duct carcinoma arise from the excretory duct reserve cell. As noted in Table 13.1, genetic mutations are now known to drive cell proliferation for some of these tumors.

- Most malignant salivary gland tumors are diagnosed by pattern of growth and morphology of tumor cells, infiltration of the stroma and adjacent glands, and increasingly by the identification of specific gene fusions.
- Bland-appearing tumor cells and lack of mitotic activity is the norm for many low-grade salivary gland malignancies.
- Although tumors may show low recurrence and moderate to high survival rates at 5 years, recurrence and metastases often occur many years after the initial diagnosis.

MUCOEPIDERMOID CARCINOMA

This represents approximately one-quarter of all intraoral minor salivary gland tumors, and one-half of all intraoral malignant salivary gland tumors, and is the most common salivary gland malignancy in children. This neoplasm when presenting on the retromolar pad often resembles a mucocele. Differentiation of this tumor is toward mucous cells and epidermoid cells with a variable population of intermediate cells. It is associated with the fusion oncogene *MECT1/3-MAML2* in 40% to 60% of cases. Two grading systems are in use, one from the Armed Forces Institute of Pathology and one by Brandwein et al. Some believe that the former undergrades whereas others believe that the latter overgrades.

Histopathologic Features

- The tumor presents as a nonencapsulated proliferation of mucous, epidermoid, columnar, and intermediate cells that invade the stroma; cysts of varying sizes are usually present, and ductal structures are noted. Some low-grade tumors consist of a single large cyst with tumor plaques in the lining. Intermediate cells vary from small cells with scant cytoplasm and dark nuclei to larger, polygonal cells with pale nuclei and inconspicuous nucleoli; perineural invasion may be present (see Figs. 13.24 and 13.25A–B).
- Mucous cells are mucicarmine positive; most tumors are positive for p63, p40, membrane-bound mucins MUC1 and MUC4, and negative for SOX10 (Fig. 13.25C–D).

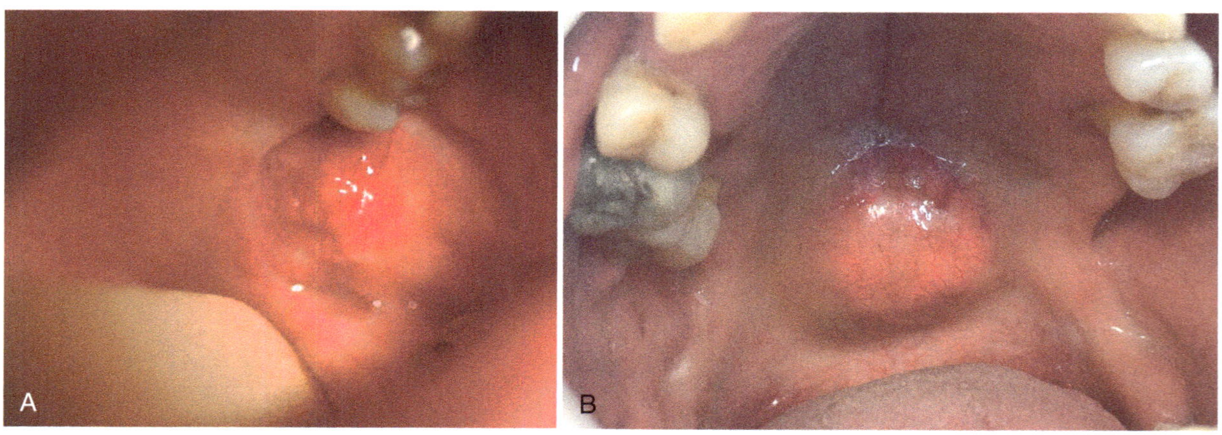

FIG 13.23 (A) Mucoepidermoid carcinoma of buccal mucosa with ulceration. (B) Adenoid cystic carcinoma of the palate. *(A, Courtesy Dr. John Sexton, private practice, Wellesley, Mass; B, Courtesy Dr. Jeffrey Reitzel, private practice, Waltham, Mass.)*

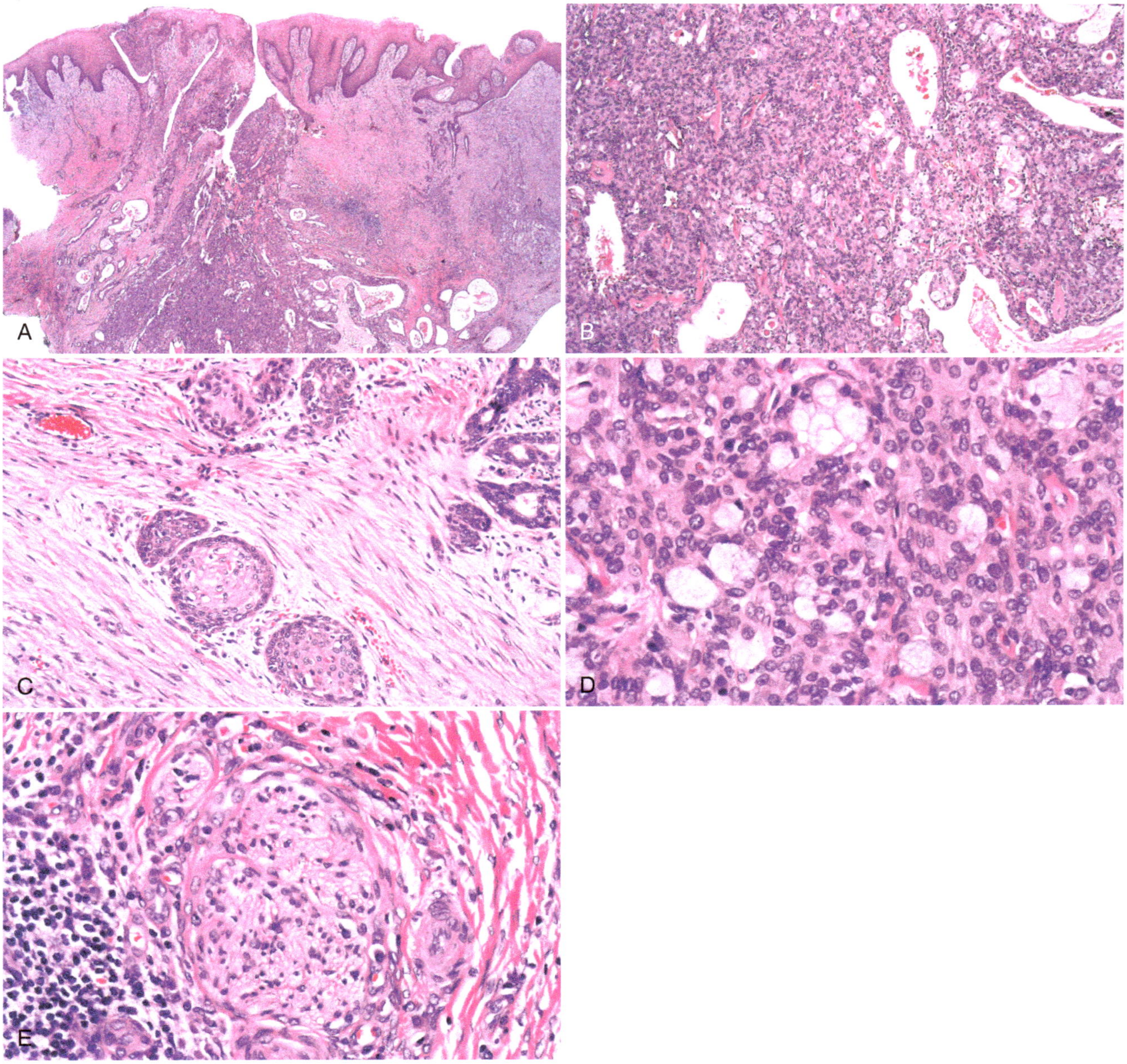

FIG 13.24 Mucoepidermoid carcinoma, intermediate to high grade. (A) Infiltrative tumor in continuity with surface epithelium, with cystic and solid components. (B) Solid areas with mucous and intermediate cells, and ductal structures. (C) Invasive islands of atypical epidermoid cells with desmoplasia. (D) Mucous and intermediate cells that have bland nuclei with small nucleoli. (E) Perineural invasion is present.

- Clear cell (glycogen or mucin positive) and oncocytic variants are noted, the latter usually in the parotid gland, but small populations of these cells may be present in conventional mucoepidermoid carcinoma (Fig 13.26).
- Sclerosing mucoepidermoid carcinoma is rare in the oral cavity and exhibits marked stromal sclerosis, many stromal eosinophils, and tumor-associated lymphocyte proliferation with lymphoid follicles, usually at the periphery of the tumor (Fig. 13.27); some cases exhibit increased numbers of IgG4+ plasma cells.
- Grading depends on the extent of cystic areas, mitotic activity, necrosis, hemorrhage, perineural invasion and invasion pattern, and correlates with the prognosis (Table 13.2); high Ki-67 index is predictive for poorer 5-year survival; the presence of MECT1/3-MAML2 fusion transcripts is associated with younger age, less necrosis, smaller lesions, more cystic lesions, and lower clinical stage (Fig. 13.28).

Differential Diagnosis

- Mucin-producing cystadenocarcinoma is often papillary and consists of a proliferation of mucous cells and columnar to cuboidal cells with infiltration of the stroma.

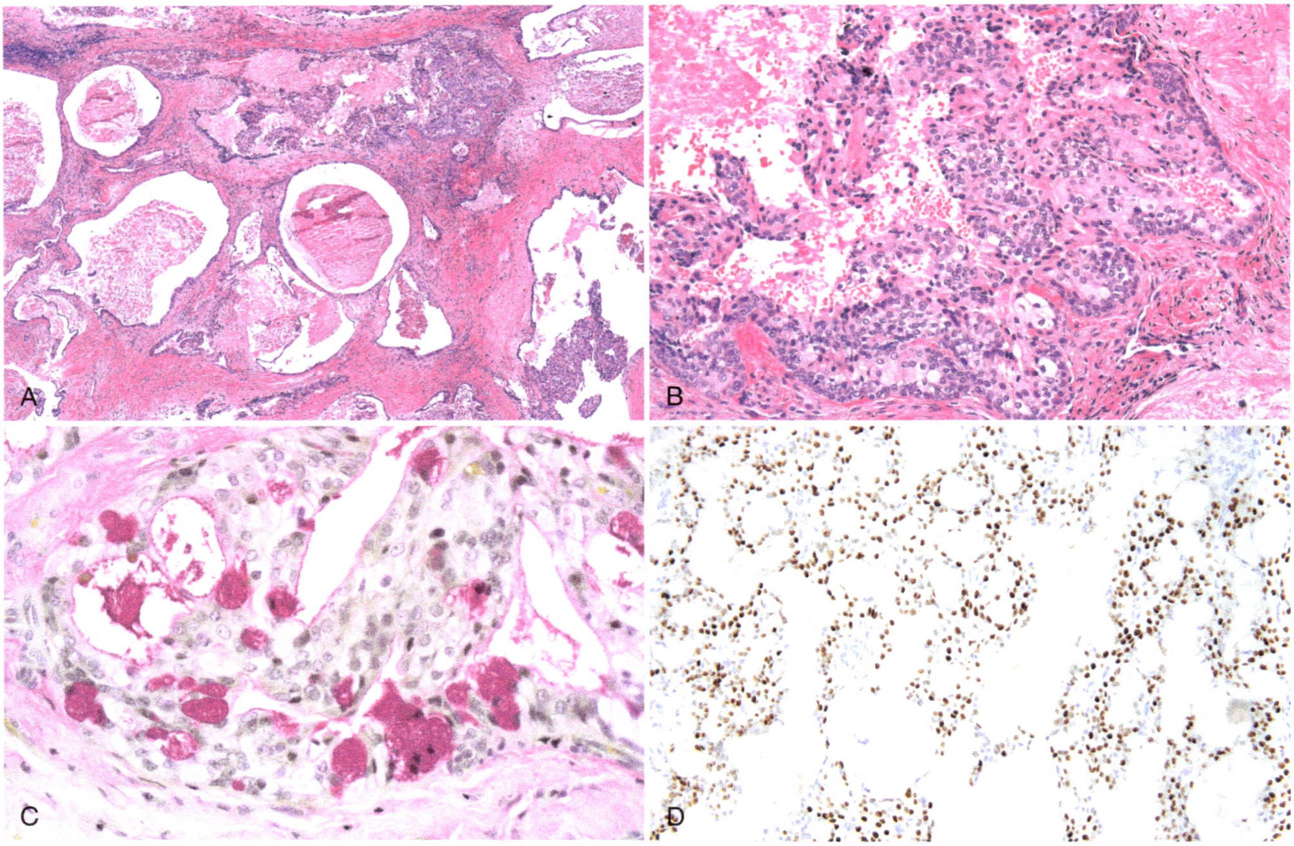

FIG 13.25 Mucoepidermoid carcinoma. (A) Tumor forms many large cysts. (B) Proliferation of mucous, epidermoid, and intermediate cells with stromal invasion. (C) Mucicarmine stain confirms many mucous cells. (D) Tumor cells are p63+.

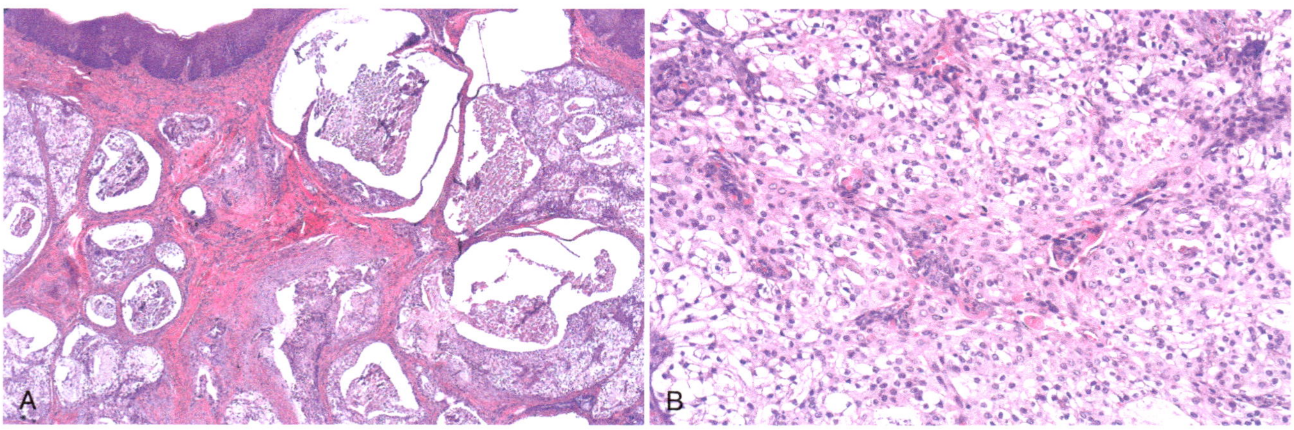

FIG 13.26 Mucoepidermoid carcinoma. (A) Tumor with solid and cystic areas. (B) Intermediate, epidermoid, and clear cells with only rare mucocytes.

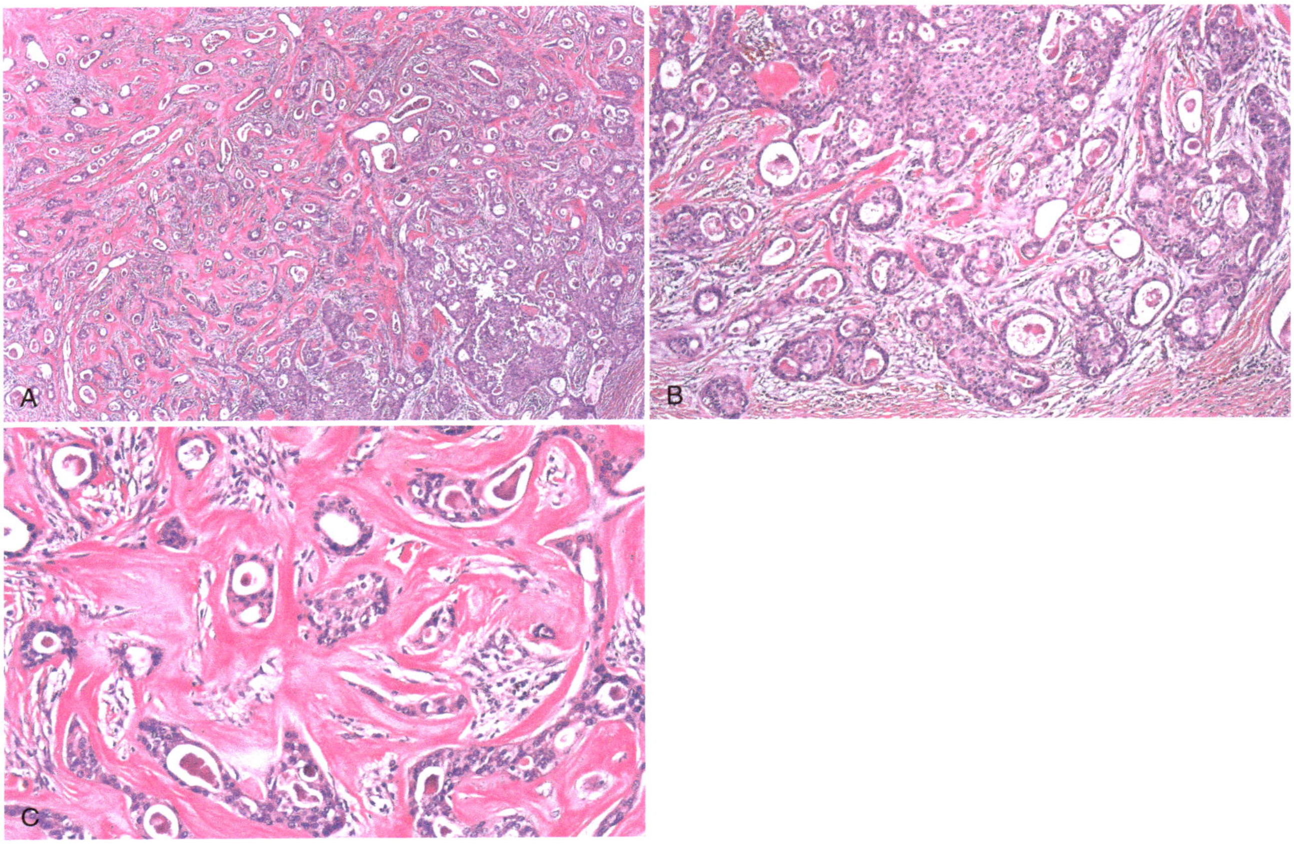

FIG 13.27 Mucoepidermoid carcinoma. (A) Tumor forms many small ductal structures with prominent sclerosis; more typical tumor at *bottom* and *right*. (B) Many ducts are present composed of epidermoid and intermediate cells with only rare mucocytes. (C) Epidermoid and intermediate cells with bland nuclear morphology forming ducts associated with stromal sclerosis.

TABLE 13.2 Parameters for Grading Mucoepidermoid Carcinoma

GOODE ET AL. (AFIP)		BRANDWEIN ET AL.	
Criteria	**Points**	**Criteria**	**Points**
Intracystic component <20%	2	Intracystic component <25%	2
Neural invasion	2	Perineural spread	3
Necrosis	3	Necrosis	3
≥4 mitoses/10 HPF	3	>4 mitoses/10 HPF	3
Anaplasia	4	Pronounced nuclear atypia	2
		Tumor invasion in small nests and islands	2
		Lymphatic and/or vascular invasion	3
		Bony invasion	3
Grade		**Grade**	
Low grade	0–4	Low grade	0
Intermediate grade	5–6	Intermediate grade	2–3
High grade	7 or more	High grade	4 or more

HPF, High-power field.

Data from Brandwein MS, Ivanov K, Wallace DI, et al. Mucoepidermoid carcinoma: a clinicopathologic study of 80 patients with special reference to histological grading. *Am J Surg Pathol.* 2001; 25:835–845; Goode RK, Auclair PL, Ellis GL. Mucoepidermoid carcinoma of the major salivary glands: clinical and histopathologic analysis of 234 cases with evaluation of grading criteria. *Cancer.* 1998; 82:1217–1224.

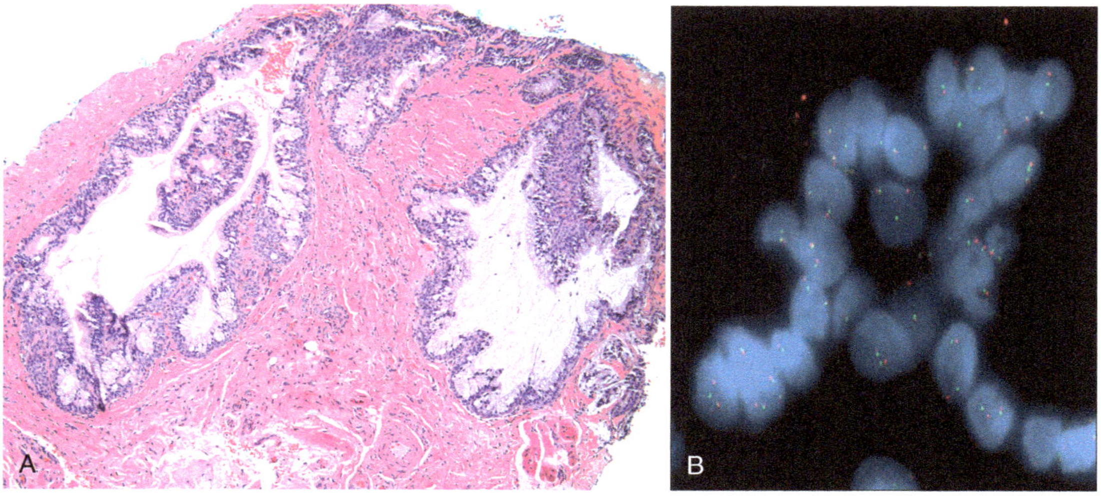

FIG 13.28 Mucoepidermoid carcinoma. (A) Low-grade mucoepidermoid carcinoma forming cystic structures with mucous and intermediate cells. (B) Fluorescent in situ hybridization study break apart rearrangement probe showing separation of 3' (green) and 5' (red) probe regions of MAML2.

- Colloid carcinoma consists of pools of mucin within which float islands of tumor cells with fewer than 50% of tumor cells in contact with collagenous stroma (Fig. 13.29).
- Mammary analog secretory carcinoma may contain clusters of mucous cells but these are a minor component and there is no epidermoid component; cells are SOX10+.
- Acinic cell carcinoma has a more uniform appearance and it contains cells with zymogen granules (periodic acid–Schiff [PAS] stain positive and diastase resistant); these tumors are positive for SOX10 and negative for p63.
- Signet ring cell, mucin-producing adenocarcinoma is a rare minor salivary gland malignancy and consists of cords, strands, and nests of tumor cells consisting mainly of signet ring cells that are filled with mucicarmine-positive material, with eccentric, crescent-shaped nuclei; these do not show papillary or cribriform structures and do not have an epidermoid component; cells are positive for CAM5.2, smooth muscle actin, HHF35, and p63, variably positive for S-100 protein, and negative for calponin.

Management and Prognosis

- Excision with clear margins is the treatment of choice; radiotherapy may help to improve local control in selected cases.
- The presence of MUC1 is associated with higher recurrence, metastases, and poorer survival while the opposite is true for the presence of MUC4.
- The presence of *MECT1/3-MAML2* is generally seen in low- and intermediate-grade tumors and is associated with improved survival. However, conventional grading is still important in prognostication of these tumors (Table 13.1); 3% and 80% of intraoral low-grade and high-grade tumors, respectively, metastasize or lead to death of the patient.

REFERENCES

Abd Elhamid IS, Elmalahy MH. Image cytometric analysis of p53 and mdm-2 expression in primary and recurrent mucoepidermoid carcinoma of parotid gland: immunohistochemical study. *Diagn Pathol.* 2010;5:72.

Aguiar MC, Bernardes VF, Cardoso SV, et al. A rare case of sclerosing mucoepidermoid carcinoma arising in minor salivary glands with immunohistochemical evaluation. *Minerva Stomatol.* 2008;57:453-457.

Auclair PL. Tumor-associated lymphoid proliferation in the parotid gland. A potential diagnostic pitfall. *Oral Surg Oral Med Oral Pathol.* 1994;77:19-26.

Bai S, Clubwala R, Adler E, et al. Salivary mucoepidermoid carcinoma: a multiinstitutional review of 76 patients. *Head Neck Pathol.* 2013;7:105-112.

Bastaki J, Summersgill K. Signet-ring cell (mucin-producing) adenocarcinoma of minor salivary glands: report of a case. *Oral Surg Oral Med Oral Pathol Oral Radiol Endod.* 2010;110:e33-e36.

Brandwein MS, Ivanov K, Wallace DI, et al. Mucoepidermoid carcinoma: a clinicopathologic study of 80 patients with special reference to histological grading. *Am J Surg Pathol.* 2001;25:835-845.

Brannon RB, Willard CC. Oncocytic mucoepidermoid carcinoma of parotid gland origin. *Oral Surg Oral Med Oral Pathol Oral Radiol Endod.* 2003;96:727-733.

Buchner A, Merrell PW, Carpenter WM. Relative frequency of intra-oral minor salivary gland tumors: a study of 380 cases from northern California and comparison to reports from other parts of the world. *J Oral Pathol Med.* 2007;36:207-214.

Cheuk W, Chan JK. Advances in salivary gland pathology. *Histopathology.* 2007;51:1-20.

Ellis GL, Auclair PL. *Tumors of the Salivary Glands.* Washington, DC: American Registry of Pathology; 2008.

Ghannoum JE, Freedman PD. Signet-ring cell (mucin-producing) adenocarcinomas of minor salivary glands. *Am J Surg Pathol.* 2004;28:89-93.

Goode RK, Auclair PL, Ellis GL. Mucoepidermoid carcinoma of the major salivary glands: clinical and histopathologic analysis of 234 cases with evaluation of grading criteria. *Cancer.* 1998;82:1217-1224.

Ide F, Mishima K, Tanaka A, et al. Mucinous adenocarcinoma of minor salivary glands: a high-grade malignancy prone to lymph node metastasis. *Virchows Arch.* 2009;454:55-60.

Kobayashi Y, Satoh K, Aizawa T, et al. Local recurrence of sclerosing mucoepidermoid carcinoma with eosinophilia in the upper lip: a case report. *J Med Case Rep.* 2015;9:41.

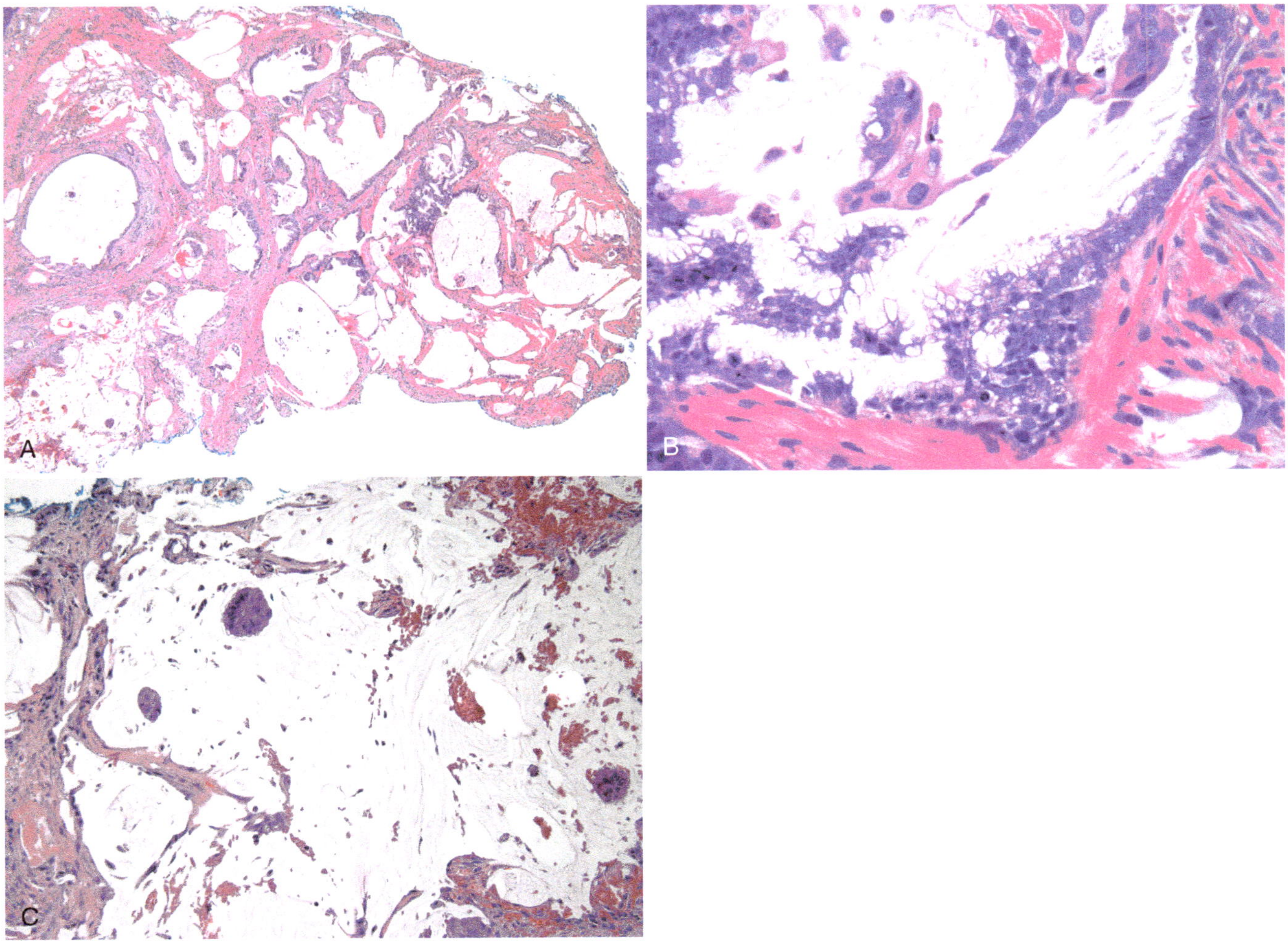

FIG 13.29 Mucin-producing cystadenocarcinoma with areas of colloid carcinoma. (A) Infiltrative tumor with cystic spaces of varying sizes, pools of stromal mucin, and focal areas of papillary tumor. (B) Tumor cells have pleomorphic nuclei and many mucous cells are present. (C) Nests of atypical tumor cells float within pools of mucin.

Luukkaa H, Klemi P, Leivo I, et al. Prognostic significance of Ki-67 and p53 as tumor markers in salivary gland malignancies in Finland: an evaluation of 212 cases. *Acta Oncol.* 2006;45:669-675.

Okumura Y, Miyabe S, Nakayama T, et al. Impact of CRTC1/3-MAML2 fusions on histological classification and prognosis of mucoepidermoid carcinoma. *Histopathology.* 2011;59:90-97.

Owosho AA, Aguilar CE, Seethala RR. Comparison of p63 and p40 (DeltaNp63) as basal, squamoid, and myoepithelial markers in salivary gland tumors. *Appl Immunohistochem Mol Morphol.* 2015; July 30;[Epub ahead of print].

Seethala RR, Dacic S, Cieply K, et al. A reappraisal of the MECT1/MAML2 translocation in salivary mucoepidermoid carcinomas. *Am J Surg Pathol.* 2010;34:1106-1121.

Tian W, Yakirevich E, Matoso A, Gnepp DR. IgG4(+) plasma cells in sclerosing variant of mucoepidermoid carcinoma. *Am J Surg Pathol.* 2012;36:973-979.

Triantafillidou K, Dimitrakopoulos J, Iordanidis F, Koufogiannis D. Mucoepidermoid carcinoma of minor salivary glands: a clinical study of 16 cases and review of the literature. *Oral Dis.* 2006;12:364-370.

Yakirevich E, Sabo E, Klorin G, et al. Primary mucin-producing tumours of the salivary glands: a clinicopathological and morphometric study. *Histopathology.* 2010;57:395-409.

ADENOID CYSTIC CARCINOMA

This represents 5% to 6% of all intraoral salivary gland tumors and 15% of all malignant intraoral salivary gland tumors, and pain is a presenting symptom in up to two-thirds of cases. This is a biphasic tumor and is associated with the fusion oncogene *MYB-NFIB* in 86% of cases using frozen tissue and approximately half of cases using formalin-fixed paraffin-embedded cases. Mutations in *PIK3CA*, *SMARCA2*, *CREBBP*, and *KDM6A* have also been noted.

Histopathologic Features

- Cribriform (classic "Swiss cheese") pattern: there are lobules and islands of tumor cells with multiple small pseudoducts or true ducts; pseudoducts contain glycosaminoglycans or basement membrane material and are surrounded by myoepithelial cells; true ducts are composed of low cuboidal cells with eosinophilic cytoplasm, round nuclei, and indistinct nucleoli and they are surrounded by myoepithelial cells. Myoepithelial cells have hyperchromatic, angulated nuclei and coarse

chromatin, small nucleoli, and clear cytoplasm (Fig. 13.30).
- Tubular pattern: this consists of true ducts surrounded by myoepithelial cells; most tumors have a combination of cribriform and tubular patterns (Fig. 13.31A–D).
- Solid pattern: cells are basaloid with less angulated and more uniform nuclei, small nucleoli, and more mitotic activity; there may be comedonecrosis (Fig. 13.32A–C); tumors with greater than 30% solid component have higher Ki-67 index, higher rate of recurrence, and poorer 5-year survival but a recent study suggests that any solid component is associated with a poorer prognosis.
- Perineural invasion is present in one third of cases.
- C-kit (CD117) is positive in the luminal cells, p63 and p40 are positive in the abluminal cells, and SOX10 is positive in both populations of cells, but more strongly in the abluminal cells (see Figs. 13.31E–F and 13.32D); CD43 is positive in 50% to 100% of cases and may be useful in diagnosis of some problematic cases; some cases are positive for p53 and BCL2; high Ki-67 index may adversely affect survival.
- Dedifferentiation leads to foci of tumor cells with high-grade, anaplastic morphology and this occurrence is more common in the major glands; it is associated with loss of biphasic morphology, high Ki67 labeling, and diffuse p53 positivity.

Differential Diagnosis

- Polymorphous low-grade adenocarcinoma has multiple patterns of growth and a single cell population with bland nuclear morphology; the cells are diffusely p63 positive rather than limited to the abluminal cells in adenoid cystic carcinoma; they are only weakly positive for c-kit (CD117) and negative for CD43 and p40.
- Adenoid cystic carcinoma-like human papillomavirus (HPV)–associated squamous carcinoma of the sinonasal tract exhibits dysplasia of the overlying epithelium, lack of *MYB* rearrangement, and positivity for p16 and HPV, usually type 33.
- Epithelial myoepithelial carcinoma is rare in the minor glands and the biphasic pattern of ductal cells with surrounding myoepithelial cells is fairly consistent throughout the tumor; this tumor lacks *MYB* rearrangement (Fig. 13.33).

Management and Prognosis

- Wide excision with clear margins is the treatment of choice and adjuvant radiotherapy helps with local control for advanced-stage tumors and for microscopic positive margins.

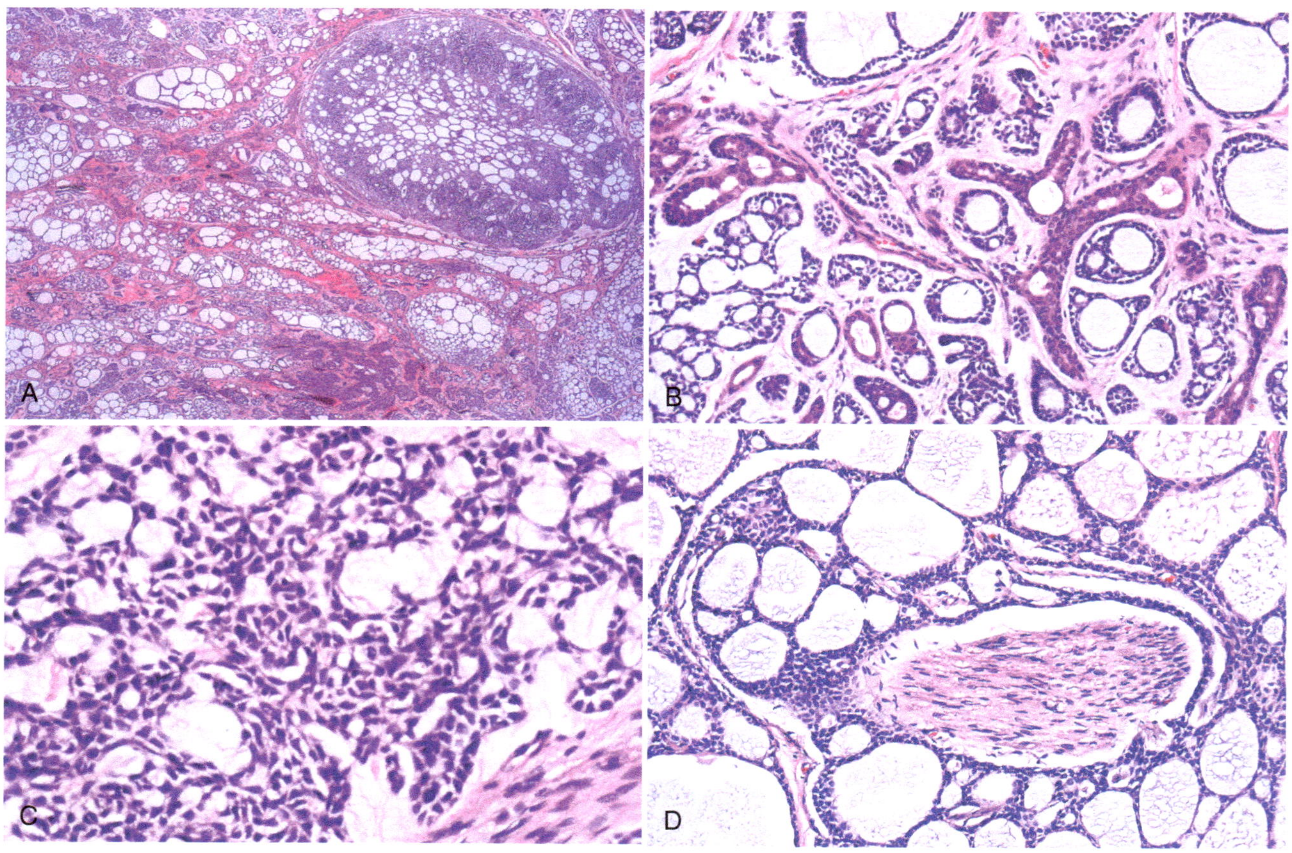

FIG 13.30 Adenoid cystic carcinoma, classic pattern. (A) Prominent cribriform pattern with focal solid component *(bottom center)*. (B) Cribriform pattern has true ducts lined by eosinophilic cuboidal cells and pseudoducts surrounded by myoepithelial cells. (C) Myoepithelial cells with angulated, hyperchromatic nuclei surround pseudoducts filled with glycosaminoglycans. (D) Perineural invasion is present within this lobule composed of pseudoducts filled with glycosaminoglycans.

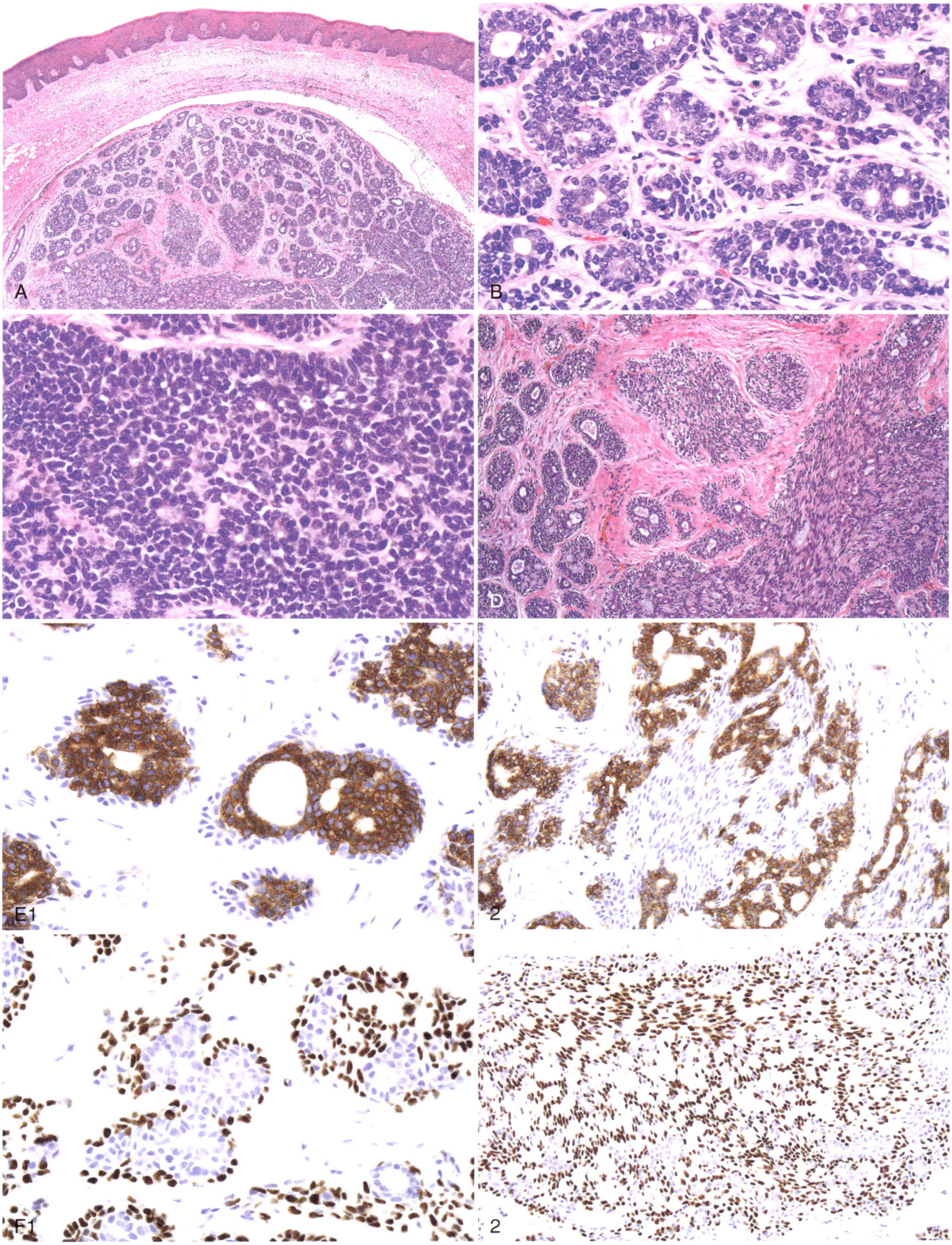

FIG 13.31 Adenoid cystic carcinoma. (A) Tumor has solid, tubular, and cribriform patterns. (B) Tubular pattern with central duct and surrounding myoepithelial cells; a mitotic figure is present (C) Solid pattern where cells are hyperchromatic, and exhibit variation in nuclear shape and size and coarse chromatin. (D) Cribriform pattern with spindled myoepithelial cells seen at *right*. (E1–2) Ductal cells are c-kit (CD117) positive. (F1–2) Myoepithelial cells (including spindle cells) are p63+.

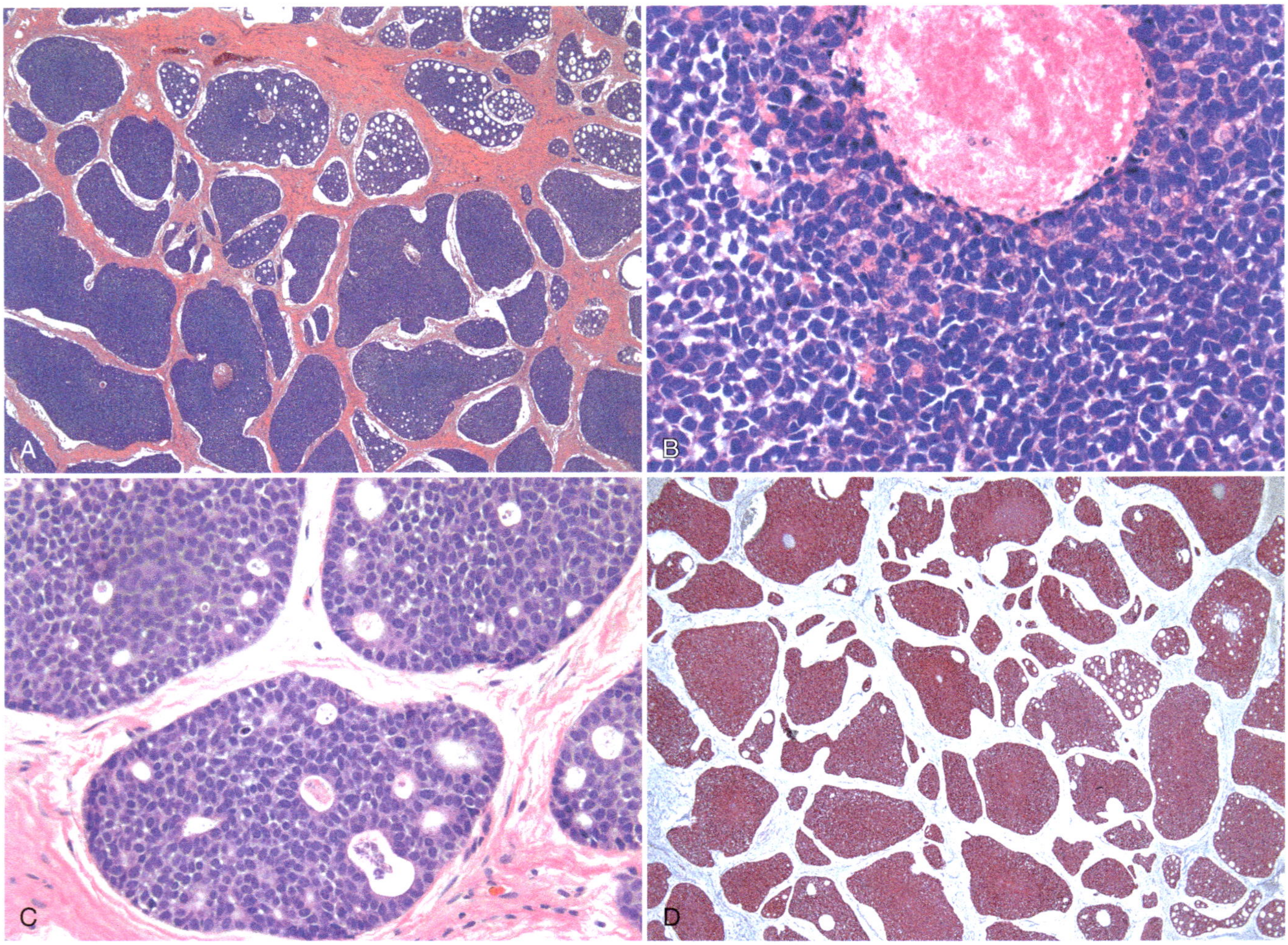

FIG 13.32 Adenoid cystic carcinoma, mostly solid variant. (A) Tumor consists of solid lobules of cells with focal cribriform (*top*) pattern and comedonecrosis. (B) Tumor cells have little cytoplasm and large, angular hyperchromatic nuclei; comedonecrosis is present. (C) Focal areas exhibit cribriform pattern with mitotic figures and true ducts composed of eosinophilic columnar cells. (D) SOX10 is diffusely positive within tumor cells.

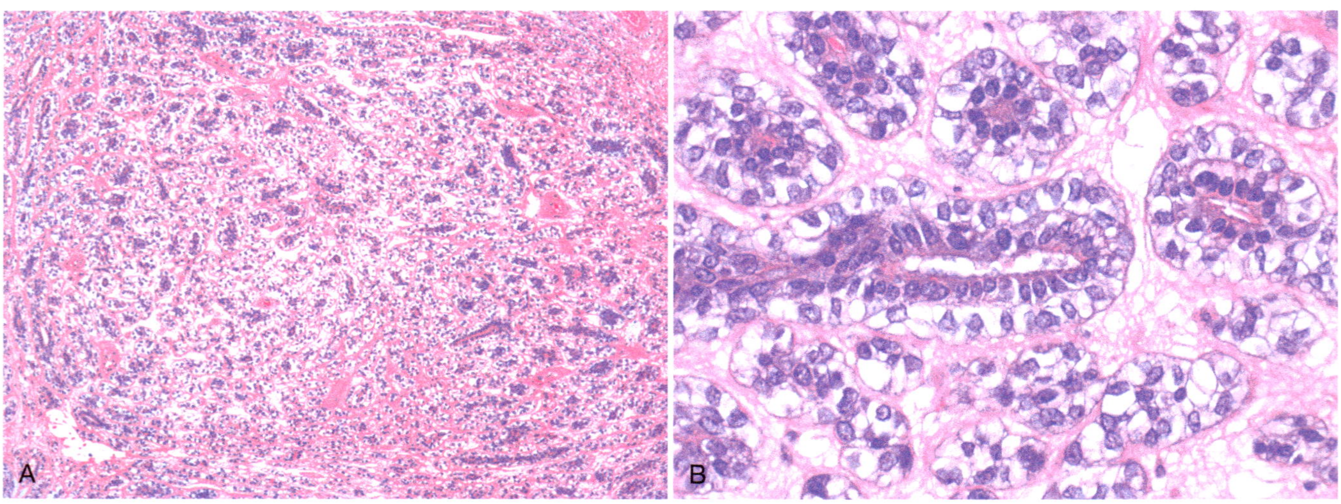

FIG 13.33 Epithelial myoepithelial carcinoma. (A) Islands of tumor cells exhibit a biphasic pattern with prominent clear cells and central eosinophilic cells. (B) Each tumor island consists of central luminal cells with eosinophilic cytoplasm forming a duct, and surrounding clear cells.

- Recurrence occurs in 40% of cases and lymph node and distant metastases are noted in 4% to 10%, and 14% to 50% of patients; 5-year and 10-year survival is 75% to 90% and 65% to 80%, respectively; tumors generally exhibit persistence and recurrence with late-onset metastases to the lungs, lymph nodes, and bones.
- Tumors with a solid component have a poorer prognosis and 5-year survival for low versus high Ki-67 index is 77% versus 50% respectively.
- Older age, solid pattern, positive margins, nodal extracapsular extension, and high tumor stage adversely affect local recurrence rate and disease-free survival; oral cavity tumors have a better prognosis than minor gland tumors at other head and neck sites and major gland lesions, and perineural invasion and histologic grade (solid pattern) may or may not affect prognosis.

REFERENCES

Agarwal JP, Jain S, Gupta T, et al. Intraoral adenoid cystic carcinoma: prognostic factors and outcome. *Oral Oncol.* 2008;44:986-993.

Argyris PP, Wetzel SL, Greipp P, et al. Clinical utility of myb rearrangement detection and p63/p40 immunophenotyping in the diagnosis of adenoid cystic carcinoma of minor salivary glands: a pilot study. *Oral Surg Oral Med Oral Pathol Oral Radiol.* 2016;121:282-289.

Bianchi B, Copelli C, Cocchi R, et al. Adenoid cystic carcinoma of intraoral minor salivary glands. *Oral Oncol.* 2008;44:1026-1031.

Bishop JA, Ogawa T, Stelow EB, et al. Human papillomavirus-related carcinoma with adenoid cystic-like features: a peculiar variant of head and neck cancer restricted to the sinonasal tract. *Am J Surg Pathol.* 2013;37:836-844.

Brill LB 2nd, Kanner WA, Fehr A, et al. Analysis of MYB expression and MYB-NFIB gene fusions in adenoid cystic carcinoma and other salivary neoplasms. *Mod Pathol.* 2011;24:1169-1176.

Carlinfante G, Lazzaretti M, Ferrari S, et al. P53, bcl-2 and Ki-67 expression in adenoid cystic carcinoma of the palate. A clinico-pathologic study of 21 cases with long-term follow-up. *Pathol Res Pract.* 2005;200:791-799.

Ciccolallo L, Licitra L, Cantu G, et al. Survival from salivary glands adenoid cystic carcinoma in European populations. *Oral Oncol.* 2009;45:669-674.

Edwards PC, Bhuiya T, Kelsch RD. C-kit expression in the salivary gland neoplasms adenoid cystic carcinoma, polymorphous low-grade adenocarcinoma, and monomorphic adenoma. *Oral Surg Oral Med Oral Pathol Oral Radiol Endod.* 2003;95:586-593.

Ellington CL, Goodman M, Kono SA, et al. Adenoid cystic carcinoma of the head and neck: Incidence and survival trends based on 1973–2007 Surveillance, Epidemiology, and End Results data. *Cancer.* 2012;118:4444-4451.

Ho AS, Kannan K, Roy DM, et al. The mutational landscape of adenoid cystic carcinoma. *Nat Genet.* 2013;45:791-798.

Luukkaa H, Klemi P, Leivo I, et al. Prognostic significance of Ki-67 and p53 as tumor markers in salivary gland malignancies in Finland: an evaluation of 212 cases. *Acta Oncol.* 2006;45:669-675.

Pires FR, Pringle GA, de Almeida OP, Chen SY. Intra-oral minor salivary gland tumors: a clinicopathological study of 546 cases. *Oral Oncol.* 2007;43:463-470.

Seethala RR, Hunt JL, Baloch ZW, et al. Adenoid cystic carcinoma with high-grade transformation: a report of 11 cases and a review of the literature. *Am J Surg Pathol.* 2007;31:1683-1694.

Seethala RR. An update on grading of salivary gland carcinomas. *Head Neck Pathol.* 2009;3:69-77.

Silverman DA, Carlson TP, Khuntia D, et al. Role for postoperative radiation therapy in adenoid cystic carcinoma of the head and neck. *Laryngoscope.* 2004;114:1194-1199.

van Weert S, Bloemena E, van der Waal I, et al. Adenoid cystic carcinoma of the head and neck: a single-center analysis of 105 consecutive cases over a 30-year period. *Oral Oncol.* 2013;49:824-829.

van Weert S, van der Waal I, Witte BI, et al. Histopathological grading of adenoid cystic carcinoma of the head and neck: analysis of currently used grading systems and proposal for a simplified grading scheme. *Oral Oncol.* 2015;51:71-76.

Woo VL, Bhuiya T, Kelsch R. Assessment of CD43 expression in adenoid cystic carcinomas, polymorphous low-grade adenocarcinomas, and monomorphic adenomas. *Oral Surg Oral Med Oral Pathol Oral Radiol Endod.* 2006;102:495-500.

POLYMORPHOUS LOW-GRADE ADENOCARCINOMA

This tumor represents 5% to 7% of all intraoral salivary gland neoplasms and 12% to 17% of malignant tumors; it rivals adenoid cystic carcinoma in frequency of occurrence and is a monophasic tumor. An activating hotspot mutation in PRDK1 has been identified in 73% of tumors.

Histopathologic Features

- This infiltrative tumor is polymorphic in architecture, forming solid sheets, ducts, tubules, trabeculae, cribriform structures, and small islands and strands of cells; linear cords of cells in single file are often seen at the periphery of the tumor and near the mucosal surface which often exhibits papillary epithelial hyperplasia; thin strands and cords of cells may have a swirling or targetoid pattern, often centered around a nerve, and the stroma is often myxochondroid or hyalinized (Figs. 13.34A–B, 13.35A–C, and 13.36A–C).
- Cells are isomorphic, round, or polygonal, with indistinct cytoplasmic outlines, pale cytoplasm, ovoid-to-round nuclei with fine, dispersed chromatin, and small nucleoli; mitotic figures are infrequent. The stroma is variably hyalinized and myxoid, and perineural invasion is seen in 50% to 75% of cases but has little prognostic significance (see Figs. 13.34C, 13.35D, and 13.36D). Invasion of bone is present in 25% of cases.
- Focal nests of oncocytes, clear cells, mucous cells, and crystalloid bodies may be seen (see Fig. 13.35B).
- A papillary configuration seen in approximately 10% of cases may be associated with up to 30% vascular invasion and a poorer prognosis.
- Cells are strongly positive for p63, S-100 protein, and vimentin, weakly reactive for GFAP and c-kit (CD117), and negative for p40 (Fig. 13.37).

Differential Diagnosis

- Pleomorphic adenoma is biphasic with ductal and myoepithelial elements and does not exhibit perineural invasion; the presence of plasmacytoid myoepithelial cells, cartilage, and fat and bone support a diagnosis of pleomorphic adenoma; GFAP is generally positive with pleomorphic adenoma but negative or focally and weakly positive in polymorphous low-grade adenocarcinoma; pleomorphic adenoma is also positive for *PLAG1* and *HMGA2* mutations.
- Adenoid cystic carcinoma cells have hyperchromatic, large angulated nuclei; the pattern is more consistently cribriform, tubular, and solid; c-kit (CD117) is strongly positive within luminal cells of true ducts, while p63 is present in the rest of the tumor cells; p40 is positive in both cell populations and negative in polymorphous low-grade adenocarcinoma; CD43 is positive in some cases.

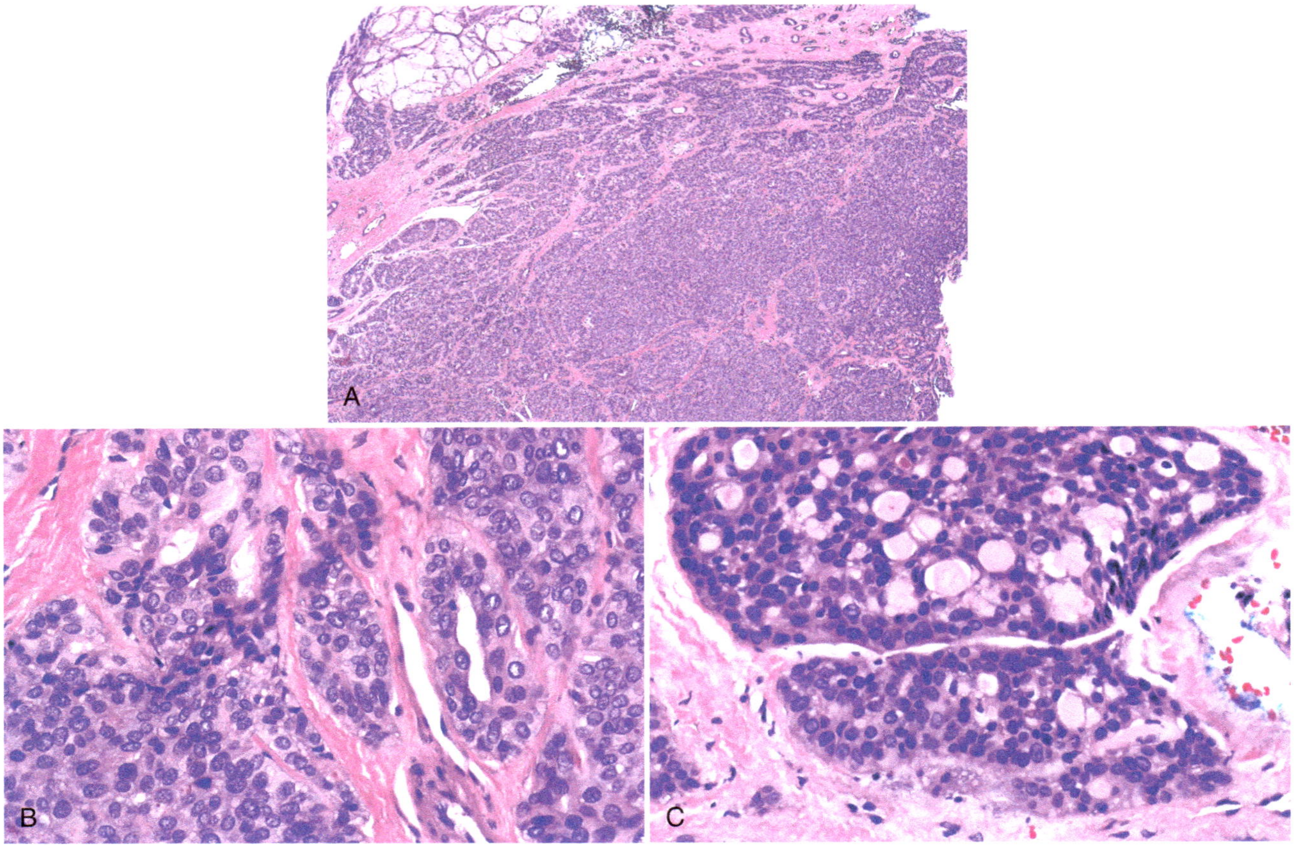

FIG 13.34 Polymorphous low-grade adenocarcinoma. (A) Sheets, ducts, and cords of cells with infiltration of adjacent glands. (B) Ductal structures are present and cells are isomorphic with bland nuclei and small, inconspicuous nucleoli. (C) A cribriform pattern is often present with pseudoducts.

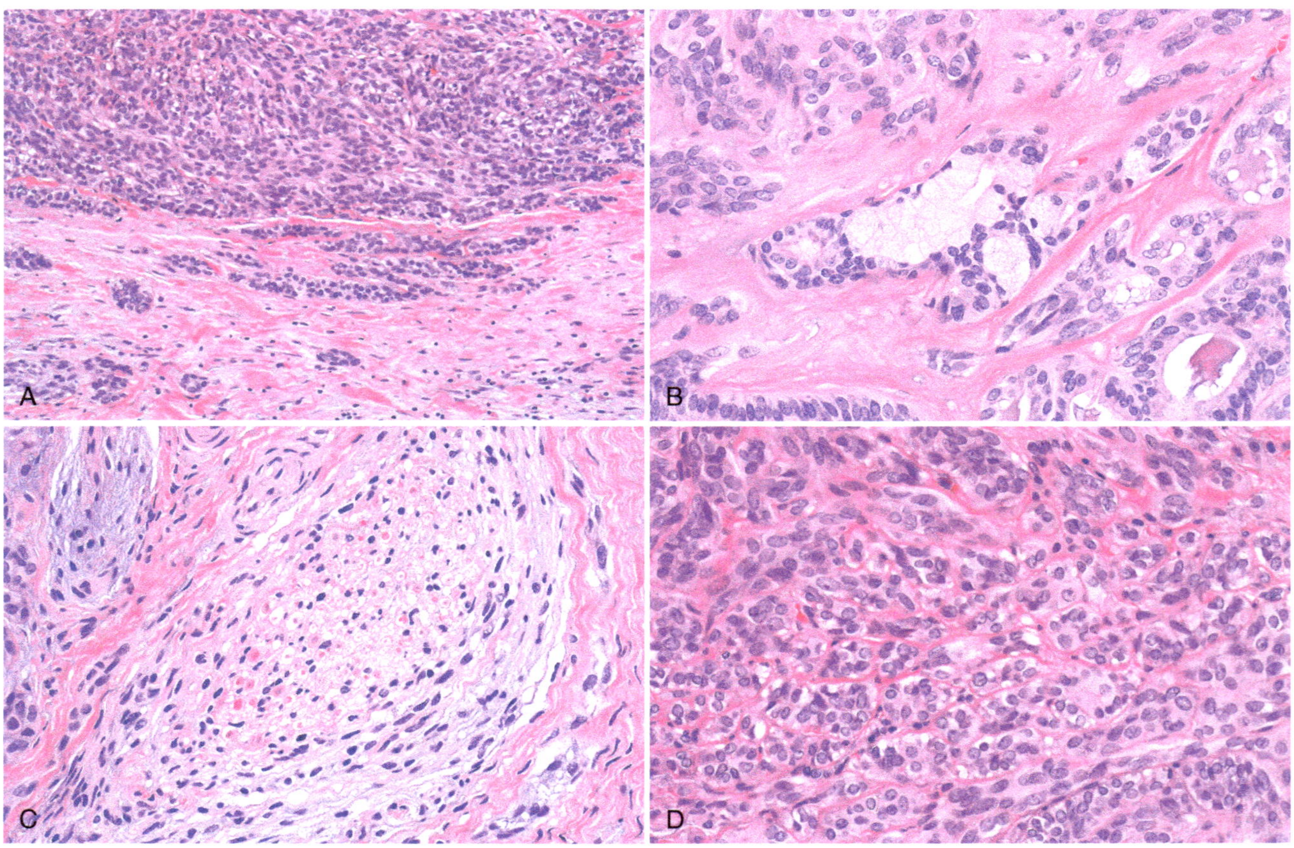

FIG 13.35 Polymorphous low-grade adenocarcinoma. (A) Solid mass of tumor cells with strands of cells at the periphery; some clear cells are present. (B) Ductal structures with clusters of mucous cells in hyalinized stroma. (C) Perineural invasion is identified. (D) Cells have pale or clear cytoplasm and nuclei have dispersed chromatin and small nucleoli.

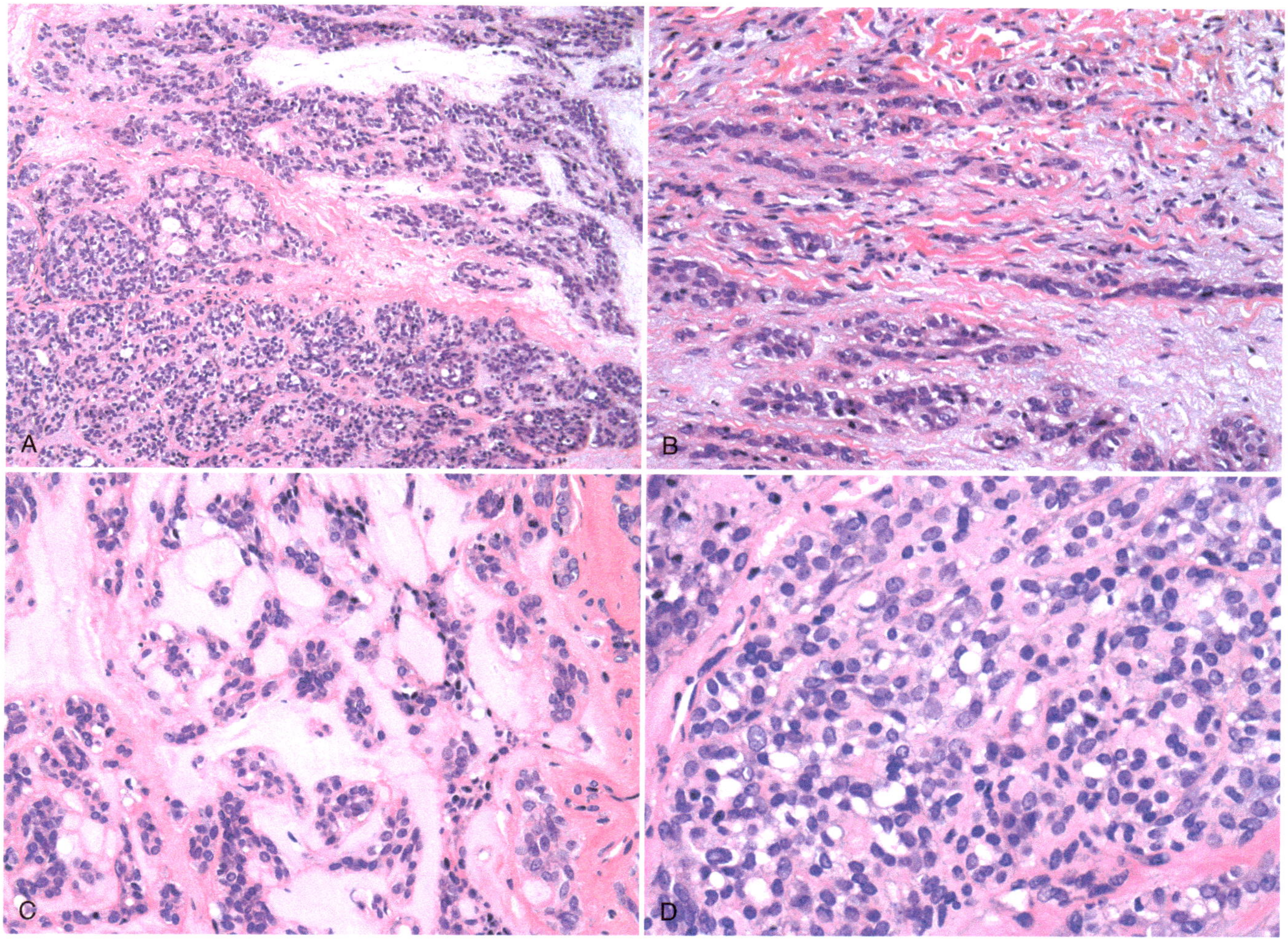

FIG 13.36 Polymorphous low-grade adenocarcinoma. (A) Nests and trabeculae of tumor cells with duct formation, focal cribriform pattern, and myxochondroid and hyalinized stroma. (B) Cords and strands of tumor cells in fibromyxoid stroma. (C) Interconnected strands and cords of tumor cells in a reticular pattern within myxochondroid stroma. (D) Isomorphic tumor cells, some with vacuolated cytoplasm and bland nuclei.

Management and Prognosis

- Complete surgical excision is the treatment of choice and adjuvant radiation therapy is used in selected cases.
- Recurrence occurs in 9% to 30% of cases, often more than 5 years from diagnosis; metastases occur in up to 9% of cases, overall survival is 97% and death from this tumor is rare.

REFERENCES

Castle JT, Thompson LD, Frommelt RA, et al. Polymorphous low grade adenocarcinoma: a clinicopathologic study of 164 cases. *Cancer.* 1999;86:207-219.

Chi AC, Neville BW. Surface papillary epithelial hyperplasia (rough mucosa) is a helpful clue for identification of polymorphous low-grade adenocarcinoma. *Head Neck Pathol.* 2015;9:244-252.

Curran AE, Allen CM, Beck FM, et al. Distinctive pattern of glial fibrillary acidic protein immunoreactivity useful in distinguishing fragmented pleomorphic adenoma, canalicular adenoma and polymorphous low grade adenocarcinoma of minor salivary glands. *Head Neck Pathol.* 2007;1:27-32.

Evans HL, Luna MA. Polymorphous low-grade adenocarcinoma: a study of 40 cases with long-term follow up and an evaluation of the importance of papillary areas. *Am J Surg Pathol.* 2000;24:1319-1328.

Hunter JB, Smith RV, Brandwein-Gensler M. Low-grade papillary adenocarcinoma of the palate: the significance of distinguishing it from polymorphous low-grade adenocarcinoma. *Head Neck Pathol.* 2008;2:316-323.

Rooper L, Sharma R, Bishop JA. Polymorphous low grade adenocarcinoma has a consistent p63+/p40- immunophenotype that helps distinguish it from adenoid cystic carcinoma and cellular pleomorphic adenoma. *Head Neck Pathol.* 2015;9:79-84.

Seethala RR, Johnson JT, Barnes EL, Myers EN. Polymorphous low-grade adenocarcinoma: the University of Pittsburgh experience. *Arch Otolaryngol Head Neck Surg.* 2010;136:385-392.

Vincent SD, Hammond HL, Finkelstein MW. Clinical and therapeutic features of polymorphous low-grade adenocarcinoma. *Oral Surg Oral Med Oral Pathol.* 1994;77:41-47.

Weinreb I, Piscuoglio S, Martelotto LG, et al. Hotspot activating PRKD1 somatic mutations in polymorphous low-grade adenocarcinomas of the salivary glands. *Nat Genet.* 2014;46:1166-1169.

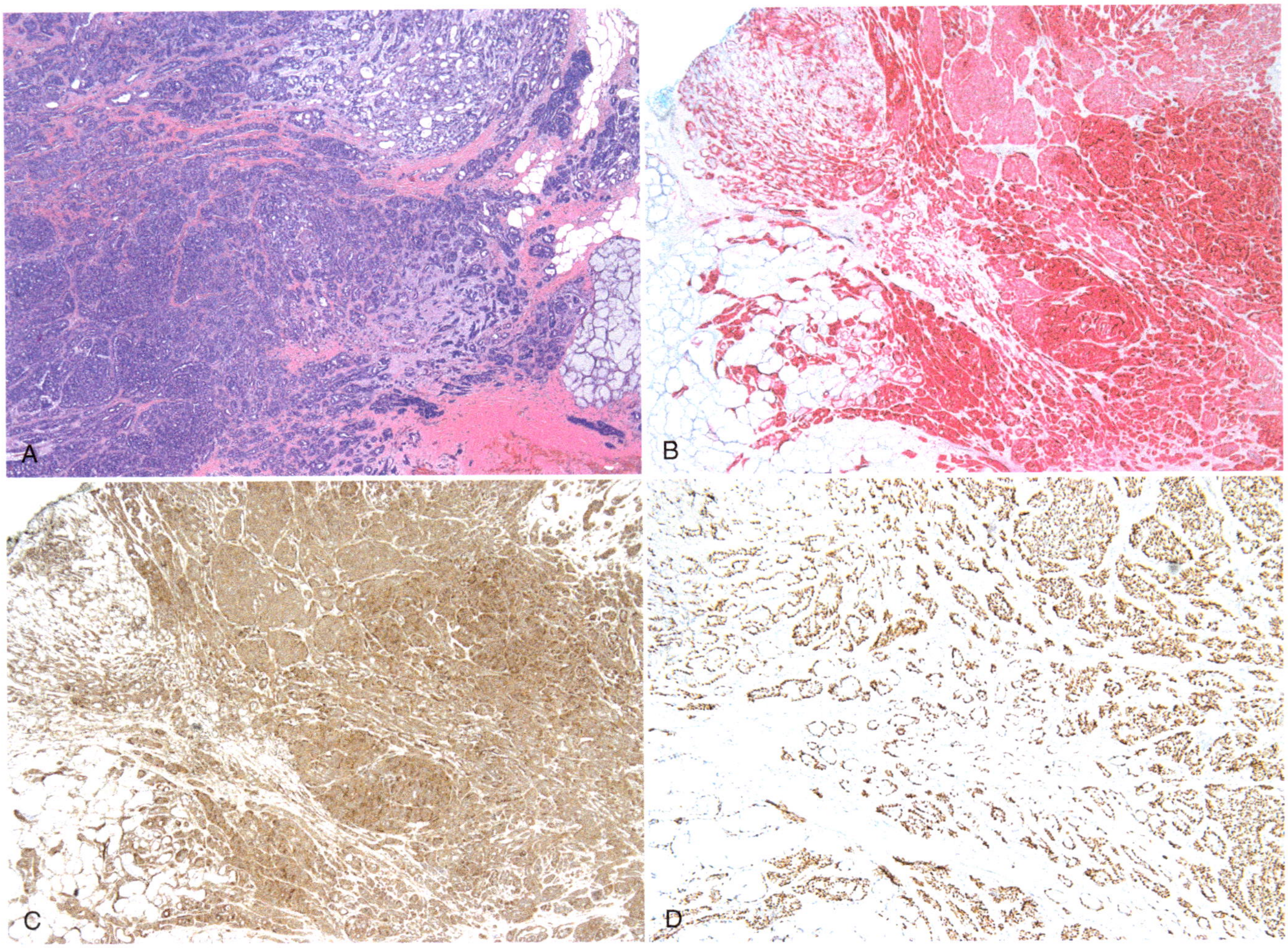

FIG 13.37 Polymorphous low-grade adenocarcinoma. (A) Infiltrative tumor with solid pattern, as well as nests and strands of tumor cells. (B) Tumor cells are positive for S-100 protein. (C) Tumor cells are positive for vimentin. (D) Tumor cells are positive for p63.

MAMMARY ANALOG SECRETORY CARCINOMA

This is the salivary gland analog of secretory carcinoma of the breast and unlike most of the other salivary gland neoplasms, this has a slight male predilection. It is most common in the parotid (75% of cases). With its recognition, many cases previously diagnosed as zymogen-poor acinic cell carcinoma have been shown to be mammary analog secretory carcinoma, harboring the fusion gene transcript *ETV6-NTRK3*. Some authorities believe that most extraparotid tumors previously diagnosed as acinic cell carcinomas are probably mammary analog secretory carcinomas. More recently it has been shown that tumors with non-*NTRK* fusions behave more aggressively.

Histopathologic Features

- The tumor is composed of a nonencapsulated, infiltrative, lobular tumor exhibiting solid areas, microcystic, macrocystic, tubular, and papillary patterns of growth; tumor cells are medium-sized, round to polygonal with moderate amounts of pale, eosinophilic and sometimes vacuolated, bubbly cytoplasm and round nuclei with dispersed chromatin and inconspicuous nucleoli; perineural invasion is not a prominent feature (Figs. 13.38 and 13.39A–C).
- Bubbly secretions (sometimes these are eosinophilic, resembling thyroid colloid) are often noted within microcystic spaces and these are positive with mucicarmine and with MUC1 and MUC4; fibrous septa are present around tumor lobules and connection to a residual duct may be present.
- Tumor cells are positive for K7, K8/18, K19, S-100 protein (may be variable), and vimentin, as well as for EMA, gross cystic disease fluid protein (GCDFP)-15, mammoglobin (100%), and STAT5a (Fig. 13.39D–F); markers for basal cell/myoepithelial cells such as K5/6, K14, calponin, smooth muscle actin, and p63 are negative, although there may be positivity in a single layer of cells surrounding tumor islands; cells are DOG1 negative.
- High grade transformation has been reported in parotid tumors.

Differential Diagnosis

- Acinic cell carcinoma is positive for PAS-positive diastase resistant zymogen granules, negative for S-100

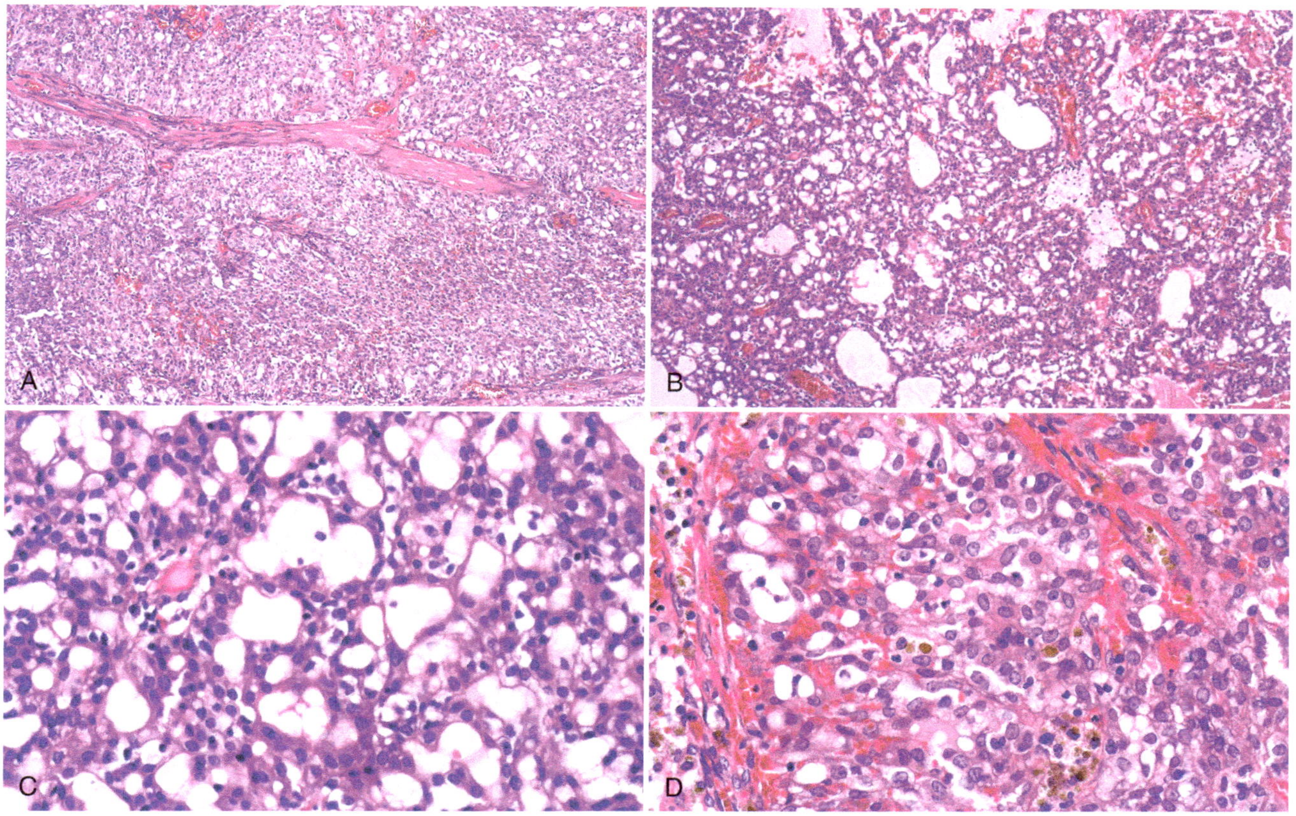

FIG 13.38 Mammary analog secretory carcinoma. (A) Tumor is present as lobules separated by hyalinized stroma. (B) A microcystic pattern is present with some clear cells. (C) Cells have pale to clear cytoplasm and bubbly secretions are present within microcystic spaces. (D) Cells have pale, vacuolated cytoplasm and bland nuclei with small nucleoli.

protein and mammoglobin, and positive for DOG1; it is negative for *ETV6-NTRK* fusion gene.

- Low-grade cribriform salivary duct carcinoma is also positive for S-100 protein and mammoglobin, but is an intraductal tumor with cribriform and papillary architecture and is negative for *ETV6-NTRK*.
- Mucoepidermoid carcinoma contains epidermoid and mucous cells and is S-100 negative, diffusely p63 positive and positive for *MECT1/3-MAML2*.

Management and Prognosis

- Wide excision is the treatment of choice with adjuvant radiation therapy as necessary.
- Local recurrence and metastases occur in 20% of cases, and 12% die of disease; mean disease-free survival is 92 months.

REFERENCES

Bishop JA, Yonescu R, Batista D, et al. Most nonparotid "acinic cell carcinomas" represent mammary analog secretory carcinomas. *Am J Surg Pathol.* 2013;37:1053-1057.

Chenevert J, Duvvuri U, Chiosea S, et al. DOG1: a novel marker of salivary acinar and intercalated duct differentiation. *Mod Pathol.* 2012;25:919-929.

Chiosea SI, Griffith C, Assaad A, Seethala RR. The profile of acinic cell carcinoma after recognition of mammary analog secretory carcinoma. *Am J Surg Pathol.* 2012;36:343-350.

Chiosea SI, Griffith C, Assaad A, Seethala RR. Clinicopathological characterization of mammary analogue secretory carcinoma of salivary glands. *Histopathology.* 2012;61:387-394.

Ito Y, Ishibashi K, Masaki A, et al. Mammary analogue secretory carcinoma of salivary glands: a clinicopathologic and molecular study including 2 cases harboring ETV6-X fusion. *Am J Surg Pathol.* 2015;39:602-610.

Kratochvil FJ 3rd, Stewart JC, Moore SR. Mammary analog secretory carcinoma of salivary glands: a report of 2 cases in the lips. *Oral Surg Oral Med Oral Pathol Oral Radiol.* 2012;114:630-635.

Majewska H, Skalova A, Stodulski D, et al. Mammary analogue secretory carcinoma of salivary glands: a new entity associated with ETV6 gene rearrangement. *Virchows Arch.* 2015;466:245-254.

Skalova A, Vanecek T, Sima R, et al. Mammary analogue secretory carcinoma of salivary glands, containing the ETV6-NTRK3 fusion gene: a hitherto undescribed salivary gland tumor entity. *Am J Surg Pathol.* 2010;34:599-608.

Skalova A, Vanecek T, Majewska H, et al. Mammary analogue secretory carcinoma of salivary glands with high-grade transformation: report of 3 cases with the ETV6-NTRK3 gene fusion and analysis of TP53, beta-catenin, EGFR, and CCND1 genes. *Am J Surg Pathol.* 2014;38:23-33.

Skalova A, Vanecek T, Simpson RH, et al. Mammary analogue secretory carcinoma of salivary glands: molecular analysis of 25 ETV6 gene rearranged tumors with lack of detection of classical ETV6-NTRK3 fusion transcript by standard RT-PCR: report of 4 cases harboring ETV6-X gene fusion. *Am J Surg Pathol.* 2016;40:3-13.

Stevens TM, Kovalovsky AO, Velosa C, et al. Mammary analog secretory carcinoma, low-grade salivary duct carcinoma, and mimickers: a comparative study. *Mod Pathol.* 2015;28:1084-1100.

Urano M, Nagao T, Miyabe S, et al. Characterization of mammary analogue secretory carcinoma of the salivary gland: discrimination from its mimics by the presence of the ETV6-NTRK3 translocation and novel surrogate markers. *Hum Pathol.* 2015;46:94-103.

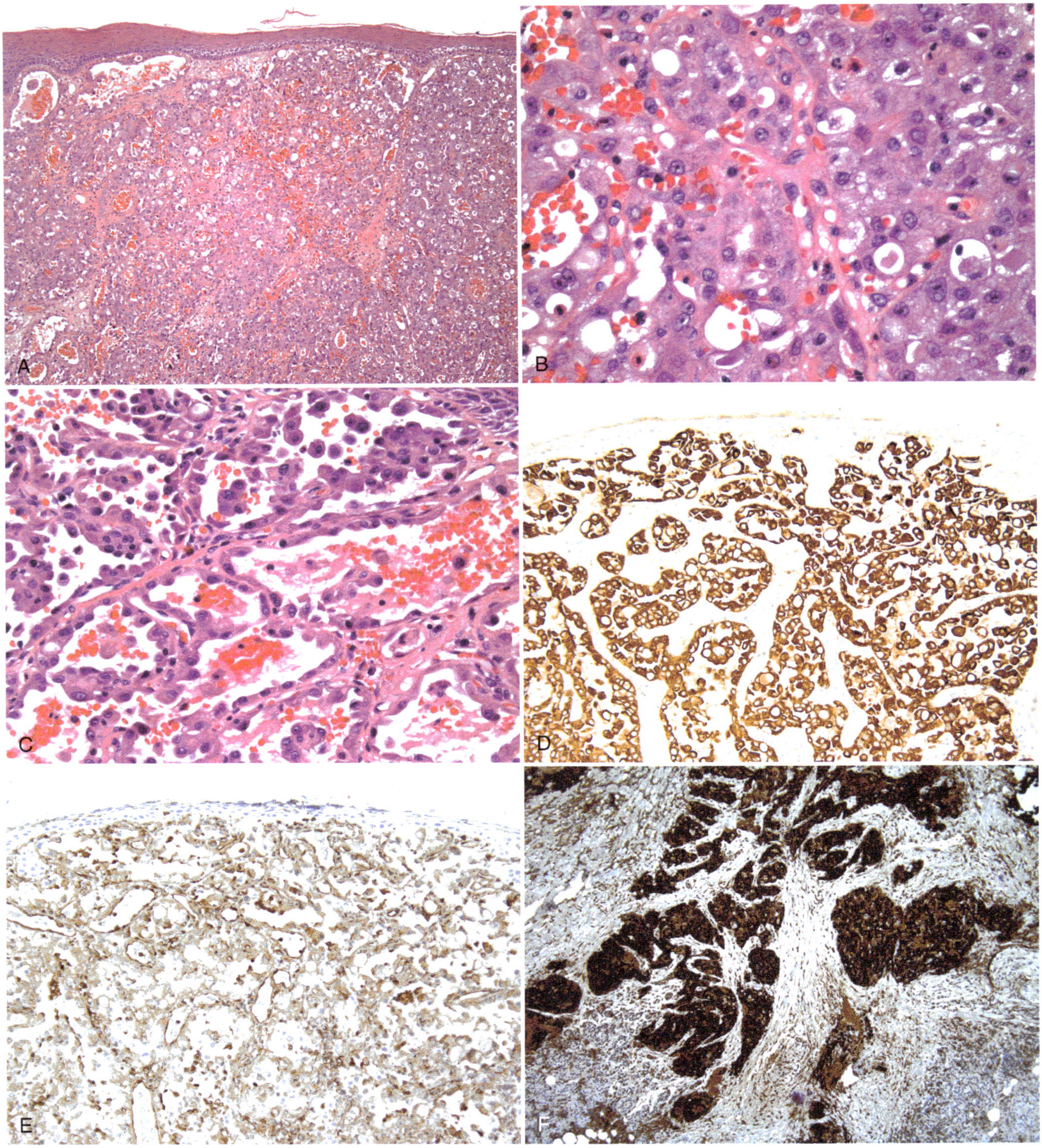

FIG 13.39 Mammary analog secretory carcinoma. (A) Microcystic pattern of growth with papillary area *(upper left)*. (B) Cells have pale, bubbly cytoplasm and bland nuclei with small nucleoli. (C) Areas with papillary growth pattern. (D) Tumor cells are positive for K7. (E) Tumor cells are positive for vimentin. (F) Tumor cells are positive for mammoglobin.

ACINIC CELL CARCINOMA

With the reclassification of many if not most acinic cell carcinomas (especially the zymogen-poor, microcystic, and papillary-cystic subtypes) as mammary analog secretory carcinoma, this category of tumors has changed considerably. Most believe that almost all acinic cell carcinomas of the minor salivary glands with a papillary-cystic pattern of grown likely to represent mammary analog secretory carcinoma.

Histopathologic Features

- The well-differentiated acinic cell carcinoma is a nonencapsulated tumor composed of solid sheets of serous acinar cells with abundant hematoxyphilic granules and small, dark, eccentric nuclei with minimal cytologic atypia (see Figs. 13.40A–C and 13.41A–C). A clear-cell variant is well recognized.
- Other tumors may have more ductal elements and exhibit a microcystic pattern, but will still exhibit significant numbers of serous cells.
- Tumor-associated lymphoid proliferation is seen in one-third of cases and these may exhibit germinal center formation (Fig. 13.40D); the stroma may show marked sclerosis.
- The PAS stain shows diastase-resistant zymogen granules and stains for amylase are positive (Fig. 13.41D). Cells that are granular with acinar differentiation are negative for K7 whereas ductal elements are positive. This tumor is SOX10+ and positive for DOG1 in more than 90% of cases. Tumor cells are negative for S100 protein, mammoglobin and ETV6 translocation. A high Ki-67 index may be associated with poorer prognosis.
- Dedifferentiated tumors occur mostly in the major glands and consist of undifferentiated and pleomorphic cells with high mitotic activity and high frequency of perineural and lymphovascular invasion.

Differential Diagnosis

- Mammary analog secretory carcinoma is positive for mammoglobin and vimentin, and negative for DOG1, as well as being positive for *ETV6-NTRK* fusion gene.
- Mucoepidermoid carcinoma contains mucous cells and epidermoid/squamous cells.
- Low grade cribriform adenocarcinoma has a delicate cribriform, sievelike pattern of growth and is negative for zymogen granules and positive for S-100 protein.

Management and Prognosis

- Surgical excision is the treatment of choice; adjuvant radiation therapy may be helpful in selected cases.
- Intraoral tumors tend to behave less aggressively compared with those in the major glands, where

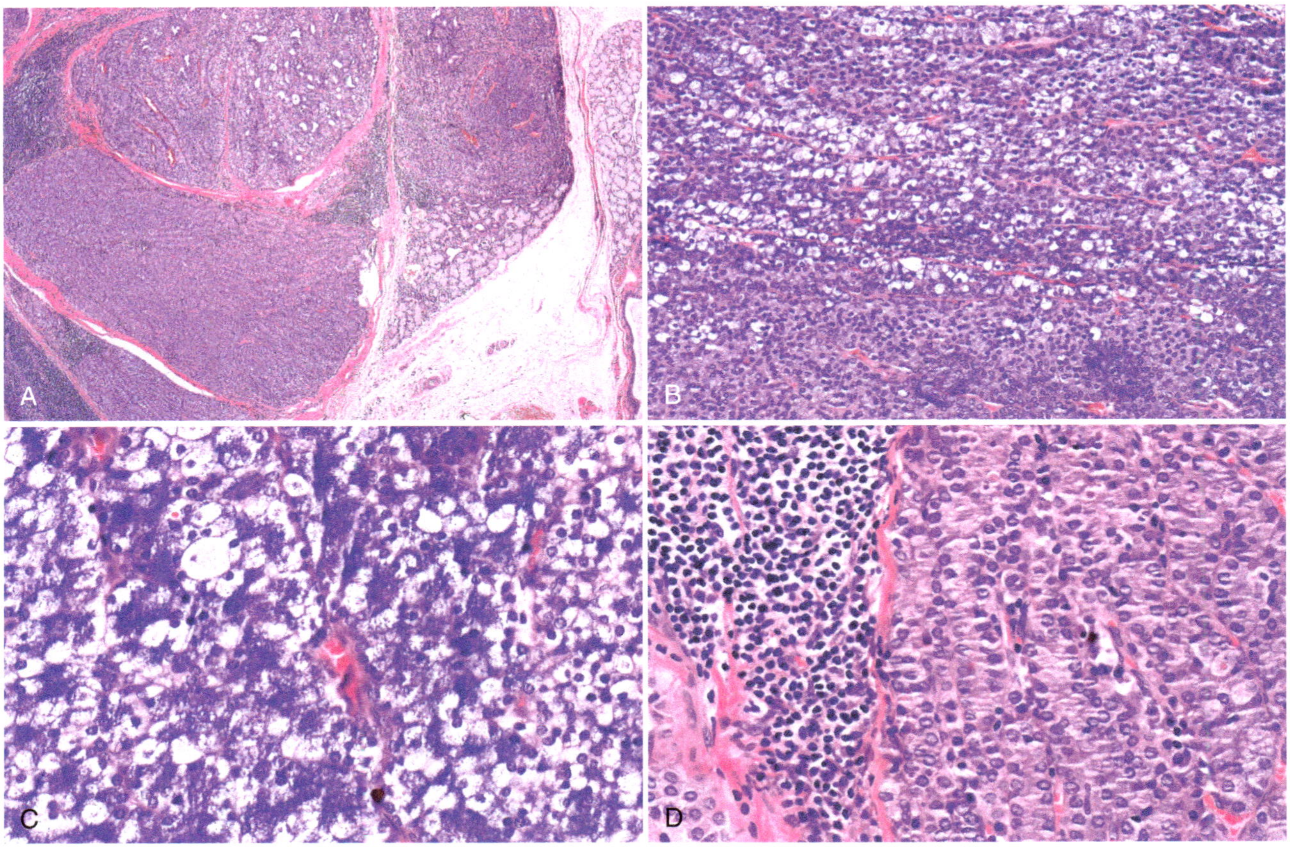

FIG 13.40 Acinic cell carcinoma. (A) Solid, lobular growth pattern with tumor-associated lymphoid stroma *(left)* and infiltration of normal glands. (B) Sheets of clear cells, and darker-staining cells. (C) Cells contain cytoplasmic zymogen granules and contain small nuclei; many clear cells are present. (D) Tumor-associated lymphoid proliferation is present adjacent to nonspecific glandular cells with pale, granular cytoplasm.

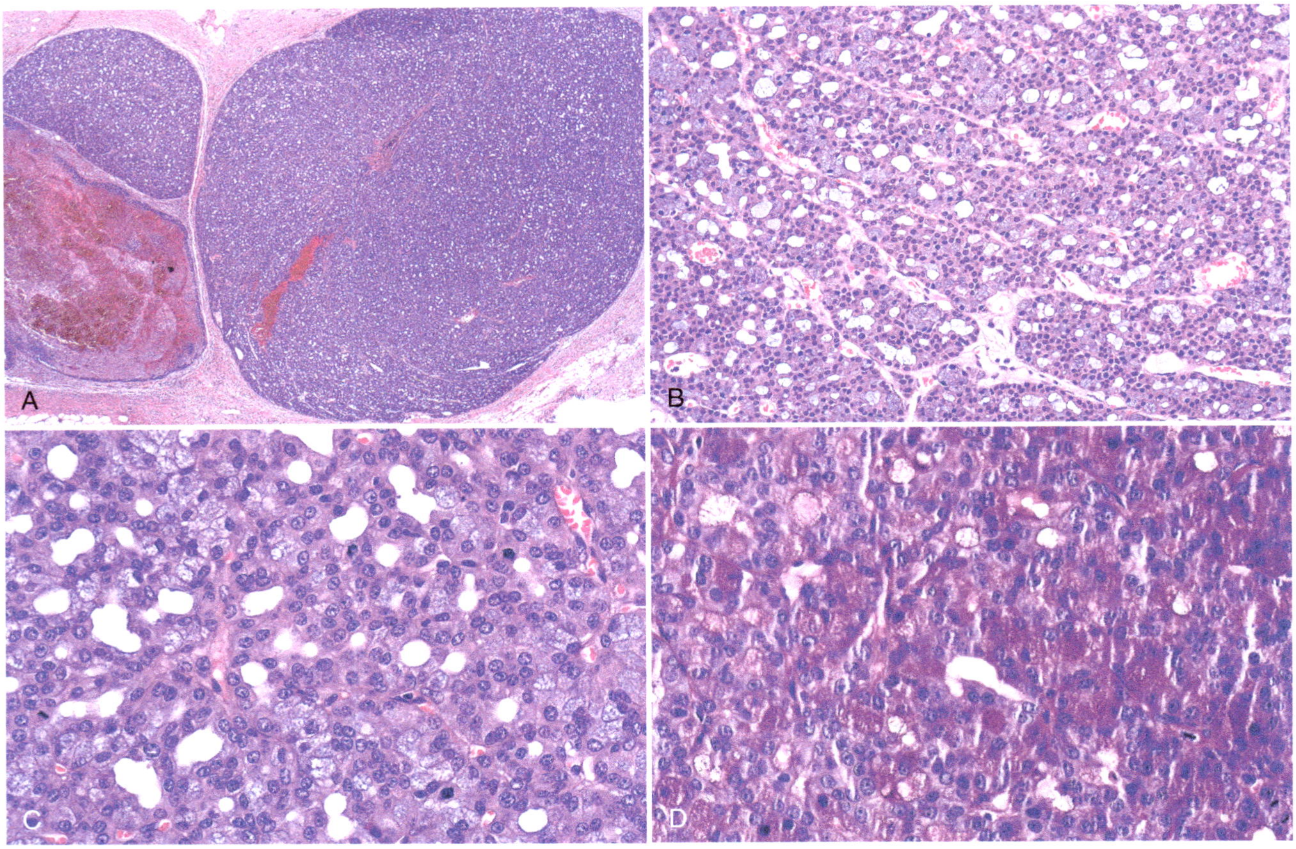

FIG 13.41 Acinic cell carcinoma. (A) Solid, lobular tumor with hemorrhage. (B) Microcystic pattern is noted with nonspecific paler cells and cells with darker, granular cytoplasm. (C) Tumor cells form small ducts with intervening cells containing hematoxyphilic granules; mitotic figures are present. (D) Zymogen granules are periodic acid–Schiff (PAS) positive and diastase resistant.

recurrence rate is 12% to 20%, 8% exhibit nodal metastases, and 6% to 10% of patients die of their disease.

- Low-grade tumors have an overall five-year survival of 100% while high-grade dedifferentiated tumors had an overall 5-year survival of 70%; atypical mitoses, pleomorphism, and necrosis are histopathologic features associated with poor prognosis.

REFERENCES

Bishop JA, Yonescu R, Batista D, et al. Most nonparotid "acinic cell carcinomas" represent mammary analog secretory carcinomas. *Am J Surg Pathol.* 2013;37:1053-1057.

Ellis GL, Corio RL. Acinic cell adenocarcinoma. A clinicopathologic analysis of 294 cases. *Cancer.* 1983;52:542-549.

Gomez DR, Katabi N, Zhung J, et al. Clinical and pathologic prognostic features in acinic cell carcinoma of the parotid gland. *Cancer.* 2009;115:2128-2137.

Hsieh MS, Chou YH, Yeh SJ, Chang YL. Papillary-cystic pattern is characteristic in mammary analogue secretory carcinomas but is rarely observed in acinic cell carcinomas of the salivary gland. *Virchows Arch.* 2015;467:145-153.

Michal M, Skalova A, Simpson RH, et al. Well-differentiated acinic cell carcinoma of salivary glands associated with lymphoid stroma. *Hum Pathol.* 1997;28:595-600.

Schwarz S, Zenk J, Muller M, et al. The many faces of acinic cell carcinomas of the salivary glands: a study of 40 cases relating histological and immunohistological subtypes to clinical parameters and prognosis. *Histopathology.* 2012;61:395-408.

Thompson LD, Aslam MN, Stall JN, et al. Clinicopathologic and immunophenotypic characterization of 25 cases of acinic cell carcinoma with high-grade transformation. *Head Neck Pathol.* 2016;10:152-160.

Triantafillidou K, Iordanidis F, Psomaderis K, Kalimeras E. Acinic cell carcinoma of minor salivary glands: a clinical and immunohistochemical study. *J Oral Maxillofac Surg.* 2010;68:2489-2496.

CRIBRIFORM ADENOCARCINOMA OF MINOR SALIVARY GLANDS

This tumor often arises in the tongue (60–75% of cases), 65% to 75% of patients present initially with lymph node metastases and it shares some features with polymorphous low-grade adenocarcinoma. Rearrangements in PRDK1-3 have been identified in 80% of cases, as well as polymorphisms in *RET* and *HRAS*.

Histopathologic Features

- There is a lobular epithelial proliferation forming solid sheets, and cribriform and microcystic patterns with ductal structures; cells are medium sized and polygonal with moderate amounts of pale cytoplasm and clear, overlapping nuclei, similar to those seen in papillary thyroid carcinoma; glomeruloid structures are typical for this tumor. The intervening stroma is densely fibrocollagenous and sometimes mucinous (Fig. 13.42).

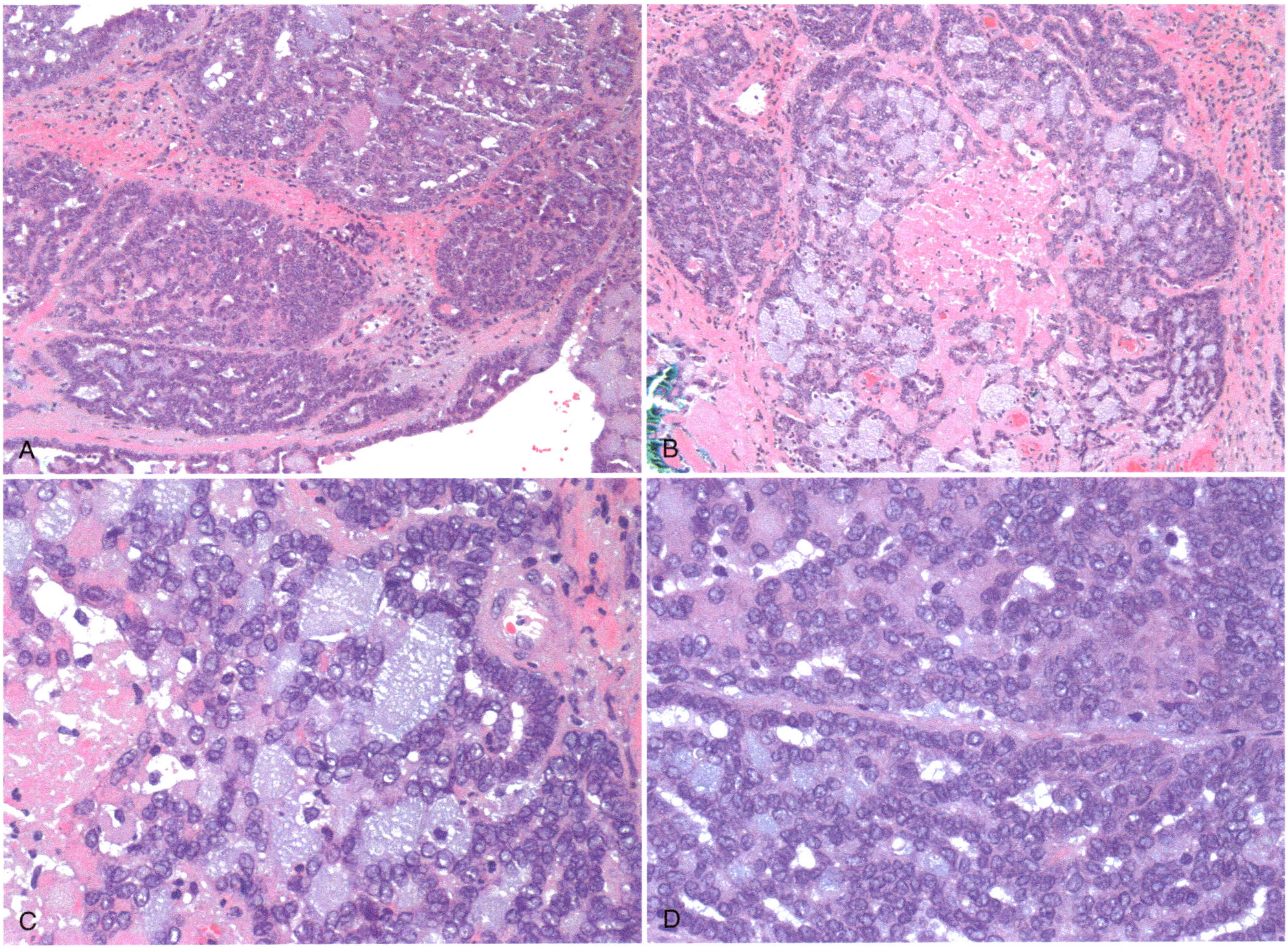

FIG 13.42 Cribriform adenocarcinoma. (A) Tumor is present in lobules with microcystic and cribriform pattern. (B) Cribriform pattern with central necrosis and myxoid stroma. (C) Tumor cells have pale-to-clear, round-to-ovoid, overlapping nuclei. (D) More cellular area with similar nuclear morphology. *(Courtesy Dr. Paul Freedman, Oral Pathology Laboratory, NY.)*

- Vascular invasion is noted in one-third of cases although perineural invasion is rare.
- Cells are positive for pankeratin, K7, vimentin, c-kit (CD117), and basal cell/myoepithelial markers such as K5/6, K14, calponin, smooth muscle actin, and p63; tumor cells are also positive for K19, galectin-3, and HBME-1, which are often positive in papillary thyroid carcinoma, but negative for TTF-1.
- Ultrastructural findings demonstrate the presence of secretory cells with microvilli and abundant rough endoplasmic reticulum that also contain myofilaments suggested of "secretory myoepithelial cells."

Differential Diagnosis

- Polymorphous low-grade adenocarcinoma has a more varied and polymorphic architecture, and strands of tumor cells are often noted just beneath the epithelium; nuclei are also not clear or overlapping.
- Metastatic papillary thyroid carcinoma to the lymph nodes is usually TTF-1+ and would normally contain psammoma bodies.

Management and Prognosis

- Treatment is wide surgical excision with lymph node dissection and, as necessary, adjuvant radiation therapy; in spite of most patients presenting with nodal metastases, patients rarely if ever die of this disease.

REFERENCES

Laco J, Kamaradova K, Vitkova P, et al. Cribriform adenocarcinoma of minor salivary glands may express galectin-3, cytokeratin 19, and HBME-1 and contains polymorphisms of RET and H-RAS proto-oncogenes. *Virchows Arch.* 2012;461:531-540.

Michal M, Skalova A, Simpson RH, et al. Cribriform adenocarcinoma of the tongue: a hitherto unrecognized type of adenocarcinoma characteristically occurring in the tongue. *Histopathology.* 1999;35:495-501.

Michal M, Kacerovska D, Kazakov DV. Cribriform adenocarcinoma of the tongue and minor salivary glands: a review. *Head Neck Pathol.* 2013;7(suppl 1):S3-S11.

Skalova A, Sima R, Kaspirkova-Nemcova J Mgr, et al. Cribriform carcinoma of minor salivary gland origin principally affecting the tongue: characterization of new entity. *Am J Surg Pathol.* 2011;35:1168-1176.

Simpson RH, Skalova A, Di Palma S, Leivo I. Recent advances in the diagnostic pathology of salivary carcinomas. *Virchows Arch.* 2014;465:371-384.

Weinreb I, Zhang L, Tirunagari LM, et al. Novel PRKD gene rearrangements and variant fusions in cribriform adenocarcinoma of salivary gland origin. *Genes Chromosomes Cancer.* 2014;53:845-856.

HYALINIZING CLEAR CELL CARCINOMA

This low-grade malignancy is primarily seen within minor salivary glands and is associated with fusion gene *EWSR1-ATF1* in 80% to 90% of cases. Clear cell odontogenic carcinoma harbors the same fusion gene in 60% of cases, suggesting that they represent central clear cell carcinoma with salivary differentiation, similar to other central salivary gland tumors arising within bone. This fusion gene transcript has also been identified in up to 40% of clear cell myoepithelial carcinomas. *EWSR1* translocations have also involved *POU5F1*, *PBX1*, and *ZNF444* in soft tissue tumors and myoepithelial tumors, as well as in ectomesenchymal chondromyxoid tumor (see Chapter 5).

Histopathologic Features

- This is a nonencapsulated infiltrative tumor composed of a proliferation of sheets, cords, islands, nests, and trabeculae of monomorphic, minimally atypical clear cells with prominent stromal hyalinization sometimes imparting a pseudocribriform appearance; the tumor cells are polygonal with mostly clear or pale, eosinophilic granular cytoplasm, and contain ovoid nuclei with dispersed chromatin and small to inconspicuous nucleoli; a basaloid cell population is often present and mitoses are rare (Fig. 13.43A–C).
- One-third of cases exhibit perineural invasion but necrosis is rare; 40% of tumors exhibit connection with surface epithelium which may exhibit pseudoepitheliomatous hyperplasia (see Fig. 13.43D).
- Cells are glycogen-rich and stain for PAS with diastase lability (see Fig. 13.43E–F); mucicarminophilic cells are present in 44% of cases; tumor cells are positive for AE1/3, K7, K14, K19, p63, and epithelial membrane antigen (EMA), and carcinoembryonic antigen (CEA) is positive in some cases; tumor cells are negative for S-100 protein, SMA, GFAP and vimentin.

Differential Diagnosis

- Clear cell mucoepidermoid carcinoma contains many mucous cells and epidermoid cells and often contains micro- or macrocystic structures; it is positive for *MECT1/3-MAML2* fusion transcript.
- Clear cell variant of acinic cell carcinoma has abundant PAS-stain positive, diastase-resistant zymogen granules within the tumor cells.
- Epithelial-myoepithelial carcinoma is rare in the oral cavity and is biphasic with ductal cells surrounded by clear myoepithelial cells. Rare cases may comprise predominantly clear cells but these are S-100 protein+.
- Clear cell myoepithelial neoplasms are diffusely immunopositive for myoepithelial markers such as S-100 protein, vimentin, smooth muscle actin, and p63.
- Metastatic renal cell carcinoma contains nests of tumor cells with numerous interspersed capillaries; tumor cells are positive for vimentin, CD10, PAX2, PAX8, and renal cell carcinoma (RCC) marker (Fig. 13.44).

Management and Prognosis

- Excision with clear margins is the treatment of choice and generally curative; radiotherapy may be indicated in some cases.
- Recurrences occur in 19% of cases and metastases develop in up to 12% of patients; most metastases are to regional nodes, and 4% of patients die of disease.

REFERENCES

Albergotti WG, Bilodeau EA, Byrd JK, et al. Hyalinizing clear cell carcinoma of the head and neck: Case series and update. *Head Neck.* 2016;38:426-433.

Antonescu CR, Katabi N, Zhang L, et al. EWSR1ATF1 fusion is a novel and consistent finding in hyalinizing clear-cell carcinoma of salivary gland. *Genes Chromosomes Cancer.* 2011;50:559-570.

Bilodeau EA, Weinreb I, Antonescu CR, et al. Clear cell odontogenic carcinomas show EWSR1 rearrangements: a novel finding and a biological link to salivary clear cell carcinomas. *Am J Surg Pathol.* 2013;37:1001-1005.

Fisher C. The diversity of soft tissue tumours with EWSR1 gene rearrangements: a review. *Histopathology.* 2014;64:134-150.

Milchgrub S, Gnepp DR, Vuitch F, et al. Hyalinizing clear cell carcinoma of salivary gland. *Am J Surg Pathol.* 1994;18:74-82.

O'Sullivan-Mejia ED, Massey HD, Faquin WC, Powers CN. Hyalinizing clear cell carcinoma: report of eight cases and a review of literature. *Head Neck Pathol.* 2009;3:179-185.

Shah AA, LeGallo RD, van Zante A, et al. EWSR1 genetic rearrangements in salivary gland tumors: a specific and very common feature of hyalinizing clear cell carcinoma. *Am J Surg Pathol.* 2013;37:571-578.

Skalova A, Weinreb I, Hyrcza M, et al. Clear cell myoepithelial carcinoma of salivary glands showing EWSR1 rearrangement: molecular analysis of 94 salivary gland carcinomas with prominent clear cell component. *Am J Surg Pathol.* 2015;39:338-348.

Solar AA, Schmidt BL, Jordan RC. Hyalinizing clear cell carcinoma: case series and comprehensive review of the literature. *Cancer.* 2009;115:75-83.

Wang B, Brandwein M, Gordon R, et al. Primary salivary clear cell tumors—a diagnostic approach: a clinicopathologic and immunohistochemical study of 20 patients with clear cell carcinoma, clear cell myoepithelial carcinoma, and epithelial-myoepithelial carcinoma. *Arch Pathol Lab Med.* 2002;126:676-685.

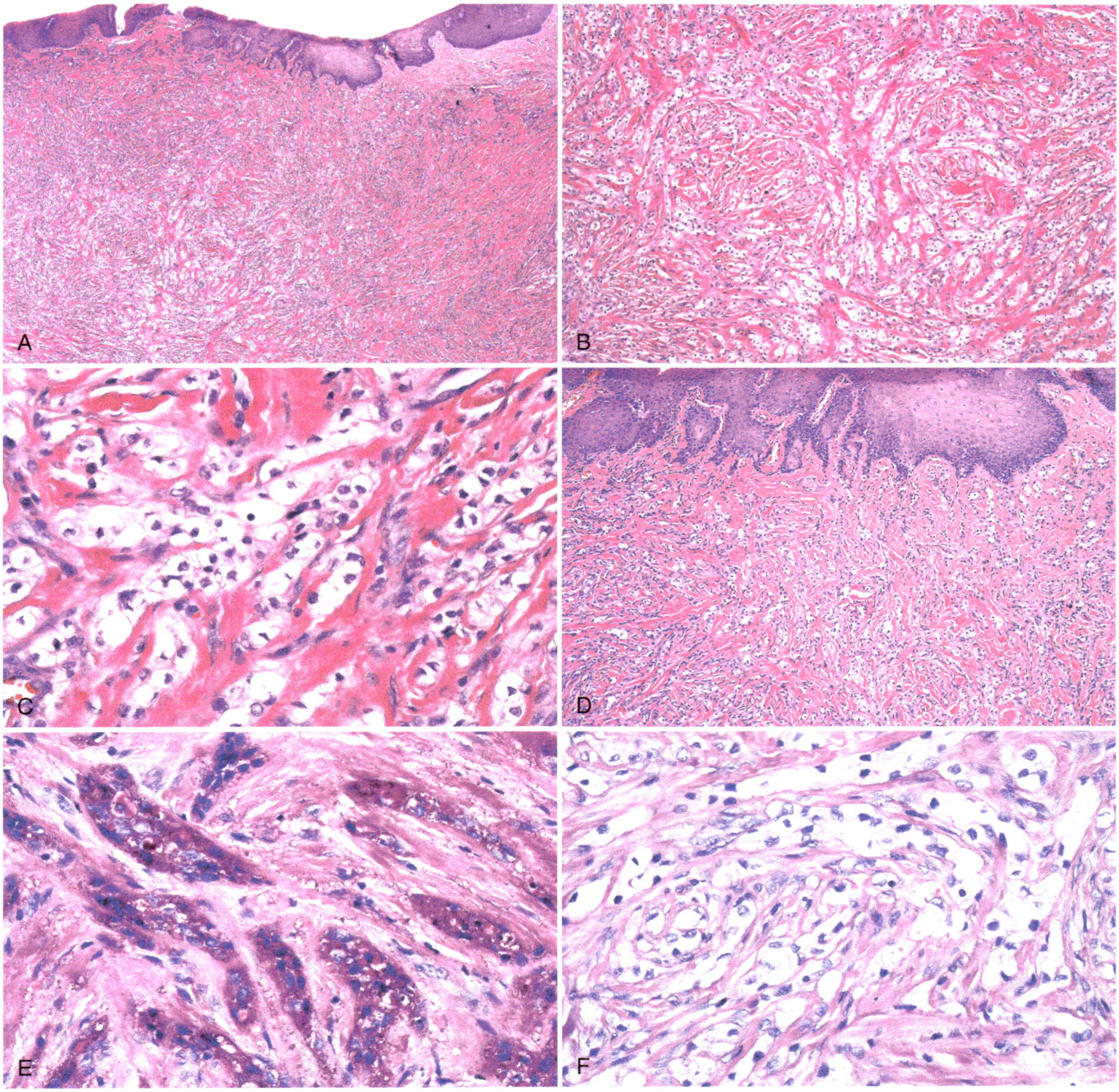

FIG 13.43 Hyalinizing clear cell carcinoma. (A) Small islands of clear cells within hyalinized stroma with infiltrative pattern. (B) Cords and nests of tumor cells with prominent stromal hyalinization. (C) Cells with clear cytoplasm and slightly irregular nuclear outlines. (D) Focal pseudoepitheliomatous hyperplasia is noted. (E) Cytoplasm contains abundant periodic acid–Schiff (PAS) positive granules. (F) Granules of glycogen digested by diastase.

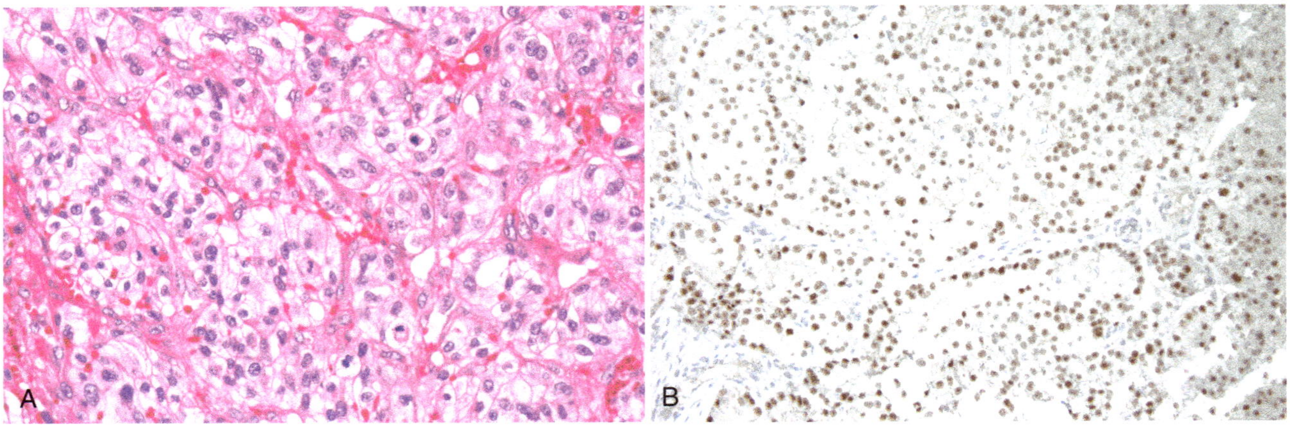

FIG 13.44 (A) Metastatic renal cell carcinoma: nests of cells with clear or granular cytoplasm are surrounded by dilated capillaries. (B) Tumor cells are positive for PAX8.

SALIVARY DUCT CARCINOMA

This is one of the most aggressive salivary gland tumors. It is uncommon in the minor salivary glands but often occurs in the setting of malignant transformation of pleomorphic adenomas, but may arise de novo. It is the equivalent of high-grade invasive ductal carcinoma of the breast and, unlike other salivary gland tumors, exhibits a male predominance (up to 4:1). Tumor cells are often positive for HER2 protein and androgen receptors. They also show genetic alterations in *TP53*, *PTEN*, *PIK3CA*, and *ERBB2*.

Histopathologic Features

- The tumor forms ductal structures exhibiting an intraluminal proliferation of ductal cells that characteristically form "Roman arches" or exhibit cribriform architecture; comedonecrosis is frequently seen. Tumor cells are large with abundant eosinophilic cytoplasm, pleomorphic nuclei with coarse chromatin and prominent nucleoli; luminal cells may exhibit apocrine features and "snouting." Many mitotic figures are present and more than 50% of cases exhibit perineural and lymphovascular invasion; mucous cells are rarely seen (Fig. 13.45).
- Papillary-cystic, micro-papillary, sarcomatoid, oncocytic, and mucin-producing variants are recognized, with micro-papillary types having a poorer prognosis.
- Tumor cells are positive for pankeratin, EMA, HER2 protein, androgen receptors (nuclear positivity), and gross cystic disease fluid protein (GCDFGP)-15; tumor cells are usually negative for S-100 protein although a layer of myoepithelial cells may be present around ducts.

Differential Diagnosis

- Low grade cribriform cystadenocarcinoma (formerly named low-grade salivary duct carcinoma) occurs mostly in the parotid gland and bears some resemblance to conventional salivary duct carcinoma except that tumor cells are small to medium sized with small bland-appearing nuclei and there is infrequent comedonecrosis or perineural invasion; the intraductal component forms delicate filigree papillary structures and sievelike spaces with a cribriform appearance; cells are positive for S-100 protein and calponin-positive myoepithelial cells form a single layer around tumor ducts except in areas of stromal invasion; most patients do not exhibit metastasis or die of this disease.
- Cystadenocarcinoma, papillary or otherwise, consists of an invasive tumor that forms micro- and macrocystic spaces lined by tumor cells that may form simple or complex papillary structures that project into the lumens; mucous cells may be present with extensive mucous production; cribriform structures and comedonecrosis are not prominent and cells are negative for HER2 protein and androgen receptors.

Management and Prognosis

- Treatment is wide excision with adjuvant radiation and chemotherapy; recurrence rate is 33% with more than 50% of cases showing distant metastases; 5-year survival is 20% to 40%.
- Targeted therapies such as anti-HER2 monoclonal antibodies and HER2 tyrosine kinase inhibitors show promise.

REFERENCES

Brandwein-Gensler M, Hille J, Wang BY, et al. Low-grade salivary duct carcinoma: description of 16 cases. *Am J Surg Pathol.* 2004;28: 1040-1044.

Chiosea SI, Williams L, Griffith CC, et al. Molecular characterization of apocrine salivary duct carcinoma. *Am J Surg Pathol.* 2015;39: 744-752.

Etit D, Ekinci N, Evcim G, et al. Papillary cystadenoma originating from a minor salivary gland with lymph node metastases. *Ear Nose Throat J.* 2011;90:e6-e7.

Foss RD, Ellis GL, Auclair PL. Salivary gland cystadenocarcinomas. A clinicopathologic study of 57 cases. *Am J Surg Pathol.* 1996;20: 1440-1447.

Nagao T, Gaffey TA, Visscher DW, et al. Invasive micropapillary salivary duct carcinoma: a distinct histologic variant with biologic significance. *Am J Surg Pathol.* 2004;28:319-326.

Simpson RH. Salivary duct carcinoma: new developments–morphological variants including pure in situ high grade lesions; proposed molecular classification. *Head Neck Pathol.* 2013;7(suppl 1):S48-S58.

van Heerden WF, Raubenheimer EJ, Swart TJ, Boy SC. Intraoral salivary duct carcinoma: a report of 5 cases. *J Oral Maxillofac Surg.* 2003;61: 126-131.

Wanjari SP, Wanjari PV, Patidar KA, Parwani RN. Papillary cystadenocarcinoma of the hard palate. *BMJ Case Rep.* 2014;2014.

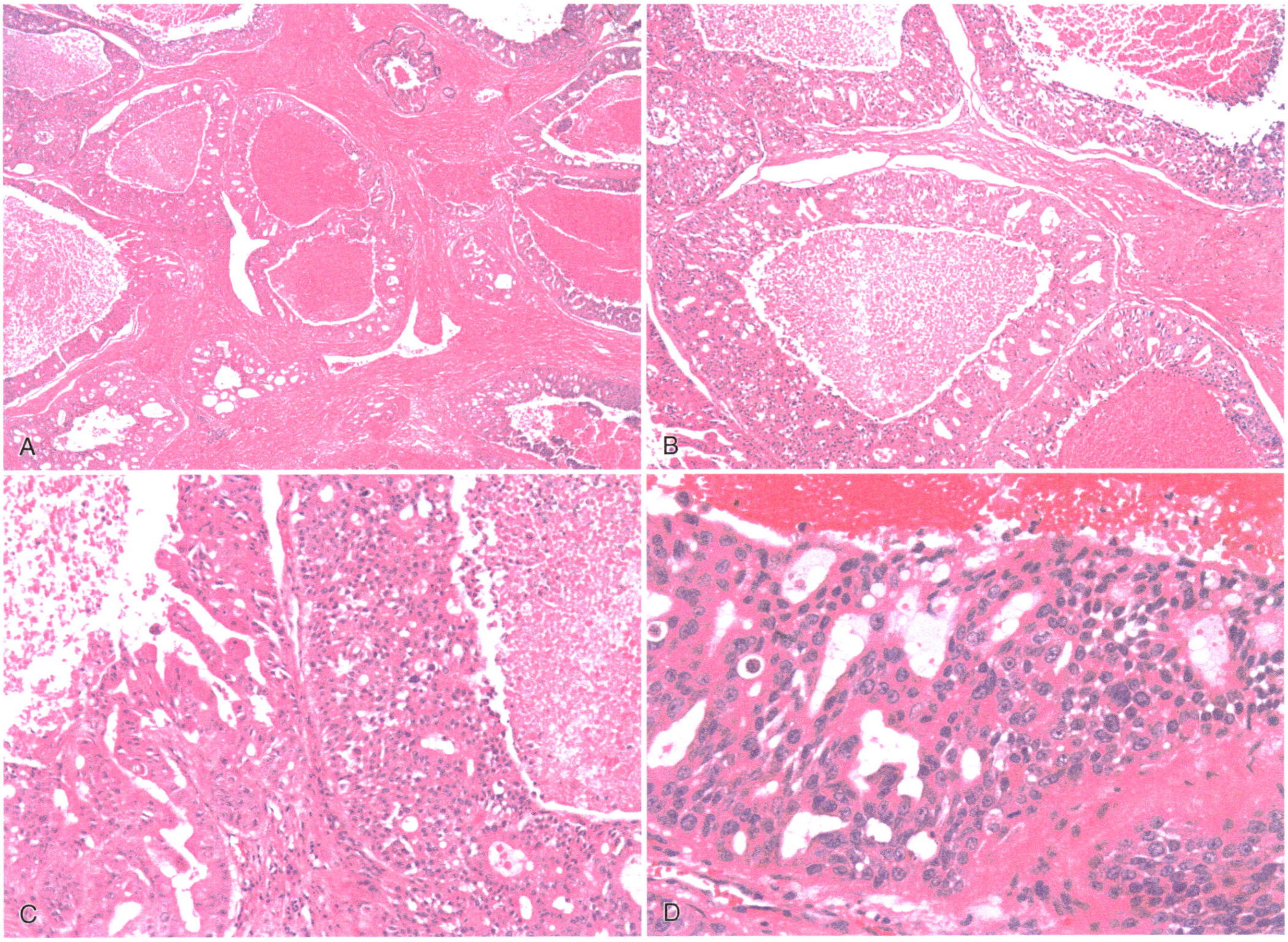

FIG 13.45 Salivary duct carcinoma. (A) Islands of tumor cells exhibit comedonecrosis. (B) There is intraluminal proliferation of tumor cells forming Roman arches and a cribriform pattern. (C) Micropapillary areas are present and there is pleomorphism. (D) Tumor cells exhibit large, pleomorphic nuclei with prominent nucleoli and mitotic activity.

ADENOCARCINOMA, NOT OTHERWISE SPECIFIED

Adenocarcinoma, not otherwise specified, involves the minor glands in 40% of cases. It constitutes less than 10% of cases of intraoral malignant salivary gland tumors, but this frequency varies greatly depending on the pathologist's interpretation and availability of special studies. The tumor forms ductal structures and it is a diagnosis that can only be made if it does not fit any of the defined salivary gland malignancies.

Histopathologic Features

- Adenocarcinoma, not otherwise specified, is an infiltrative neoplasm that forms ductal and glandular structures and may exhibit a variety of patterns including nests, tubules, cords and strands, trabeculae, or solid sheets (Fig. 13.46); because cytologic atypia is often minimal, the presence of infiltration at the tumor margin is one of the most important criteria that separates benign from malignant processes.
- Tumors can usually be graded by cytologic features into low-, intermediate-, or high-grade lesions.

Differential Diagnosis

- Metastatic adenocarcinoma must be ruled out with special studies and lack of clinical evidence of some other primary tumor.

Management and Prognosis

- Surgical excision is the treatment of choice with adjuvant radiation therapy for selected cases; 15-year survival for low-grade, intermediate-grade, and high-grade tumors are 54%, 31%, and 3% respectively.
- As expected, tumors with high-grade cytology, necrosis, perineural invasion, and infiltration of normal structures are associated with locoregional recurrence.

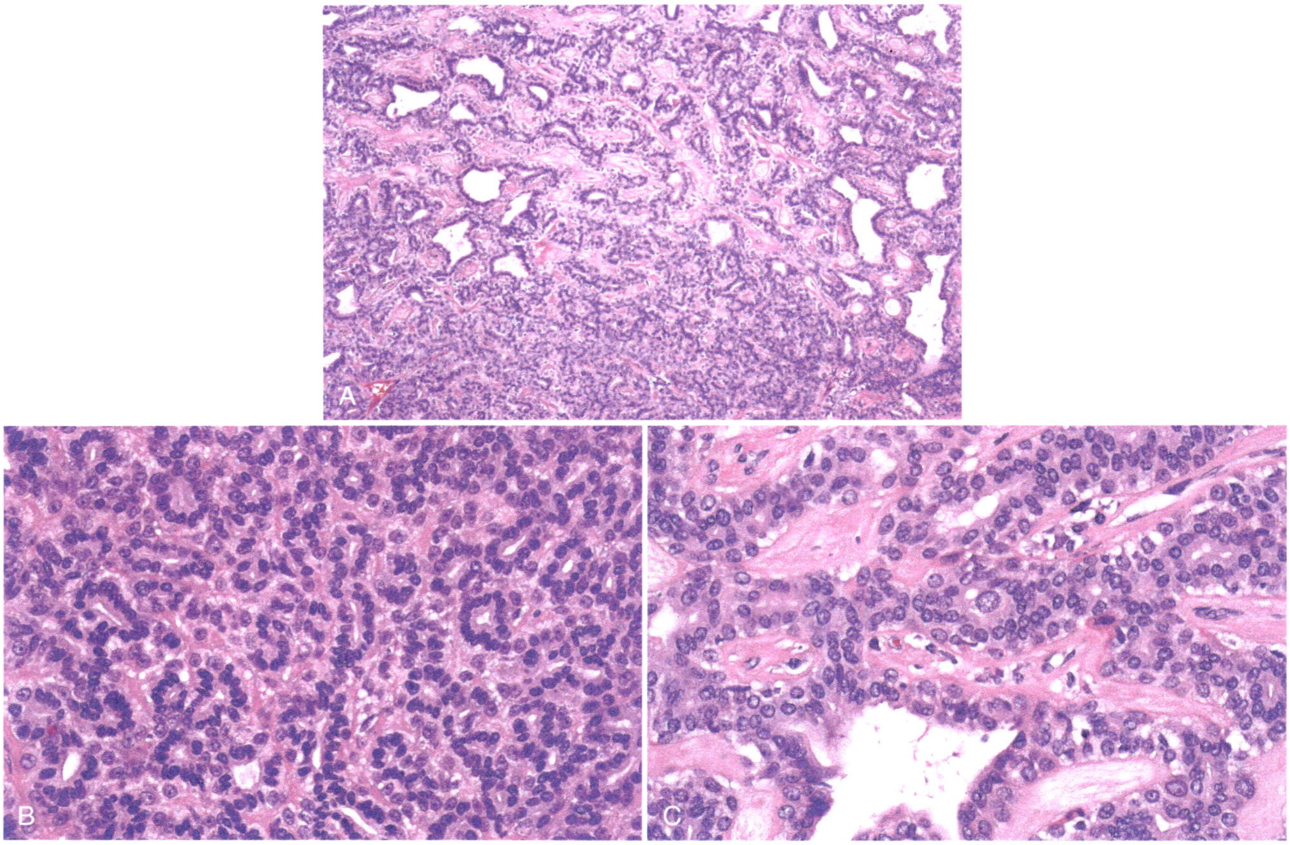

FIG 13.46 Adenocarcinoma, not otherwise specified. (A) Tumor forming ductal structures. (B) Closely packed ducts are surrounded by tumor cells with pale cytoplasm. (C) Cells show variation in nuclear shape and size and the stroma is hyalinized.

REFERENCES

Buchner A, Merrell PW, Carpenter WM. Relative frequency of intraoral minor salivary gland tumors: a study of 380 cases from northern California and comparison to reports from other parts of the world. *J Oral Pathol Med.* 2007;36:207-214.

Ellis GL, Auclair PL. *Tumors of the Salivary Glands.* Washington, DC: American Registry of Pathology; 2008.

Matsuba HM, Mauney M, Simpson JR, et al. Adenocarcinomas of major and minor salivary gland origin: a histopathologic review of treatment failure patterns. *Laryngoscope.* 1988;98:784-788.

Spiro RH, Huvos AG, Strong EW. Adenocarcinoma of salivary origin. Clinicopathologic study of 204 patients. *Am J Surg.* 1982;144: 423-431.

Salivary Gland Tumor of Uncertain Biologic Potential

SCLEROSING POLYCYSTIC ADENOSIS

This uncommon salivary gland disorder is usually seen in the parotid gland (75% of cases), and infrequently in the minor glands (15% of cases). Some clinicians consider it a pseudoneoplastic inflammatory condition, whereas others consider it a low-grade malignancy.

Clinical Findings

- This is usually seen in adults in the fourth and fifth decades and presents as a nondescript movable nodule within the mucosa.

Etiopathogenesis and Histopathologic Features

There is a mixture of metaplastic and cystic changes suggestive of fibrocystic disease and sclerosing adenosis of the breast. Changes in minor glands are not as marked, and lesions are not as sclerotic as those in the major glands. A recent study showed monoclonality for human androgen receptor (HUMARA). As such, some authorities consider this a low-grade malignancy.

- Tumors are circumscribed with tubuloacinar hyperplasia forming ducts of varying sizes usually surrounded by a layer of myoepithelial cells, with marked interstitial fibrosis, hyalinization, collagenous spherules and variable chronic inflammation; cribriform or microcystic patterns may be noted (Fig. 13.47A–B).
- Ducts have lumens of varying sizes and may be cystically dilated and exhibit oncocytic, apocrine-like, clear cell, and mucous cell metaplasia with inspissation of secretions; mucous extravasation is often associated with foamy macrophages and large eosinophilic PAS-positive inclusions are present in some acinar cells (altered zymogen granules) (see Fig. 13.47C–D); there is often

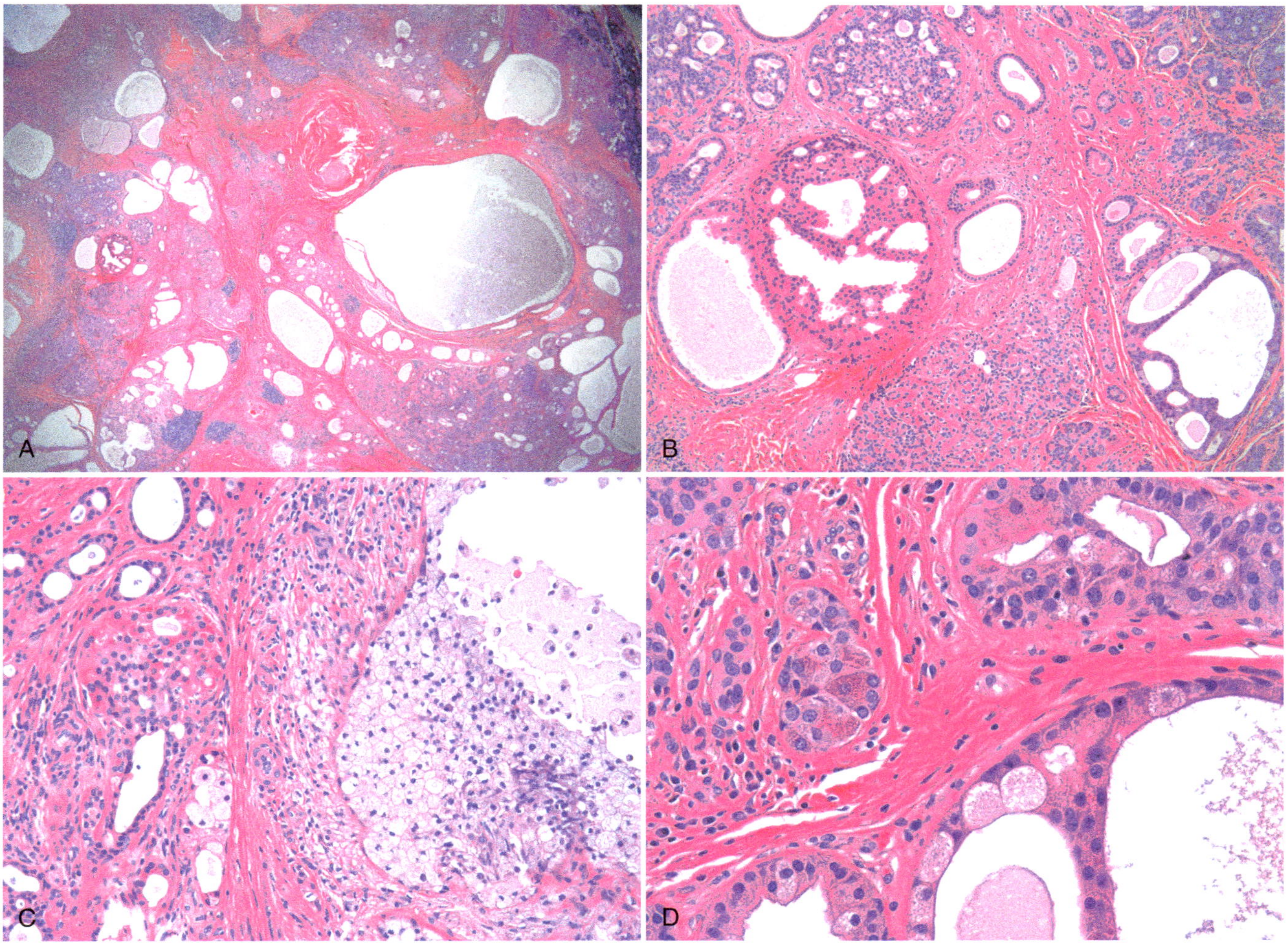

FIG 13.47 Sclerosing polycystic adenosis. (A) Dilated ducts of varying sizes, tubuloacinar hyperplasia, inflammation, and fibrosis with collagenous spherules. (B) Cribriform, microcystic, and adenomatous patterns are noted here with apocrine metaplasia. (C) Mucous extravasation associated with many foamy macrophages; note bright intracytoplasmic eosinophilic granules. (D) Brightly eosinophilic intracytoplasmic granules are noted and there is also mucous cell and squamous metaplasia.

cytologic atypia and occasionally true dysplasia (up to 50% of cases) but not stromal invasion.

- Calponin, p63, and other myoepithelial markers confirm the presence of a layer of myoepithelial cells around ducts and islands of cells.
- Epstein-Barr virus has been identified in some cases.

Differential Diagnosis

- Pleomorphic adenoma may have diverse histopathologic features but does not show such extensive oncocytic and apocrine metaplasia.
- Adenocarcinoma generally does not usually exhibit such a wide range of metaplastic changes.

Management

- Excision is treatment of choice and 10% to 20% of lesions recur, with 2% to 3% of cases developing invasive adenocarcinoma.

REFERENCES

Canas Marques R, Felix A. Invasive carcinoma arising from sclerosing polycystic adenosis of the salivary gland. *Virchows Arch.* 2014;464:621-625.

Gnepp DR. Sclerosing polycystic adenosis of the salivary gland: a lesion that may be associated with dysplasia and carcinoma in situ. *Adv Anat Pathol.* 2003;10:218-222.

Gnepp DR. Salivary gland tumor "wishes" to add to the next WHO tumor classification: sclerosing polycystic adenosis, mammary analogue of secretory carcinoma, cribriform adenocarcinoma fo the tongue and other sites, and mucinous variant of myoepithelioma. *Head Neck Pathol.* 2014;8:42-49.

Gnepp DR, Wang LJ, Brandwein-Gensler M, et al. Sclerosing polycystic adenosis of the salivary gland: a report of 16 cases. *Am J Surg Pathol.* 2006;30:154-164.

Noonan VL, Kalmar JR, Allen CM, et al. Sclerosing polycystic adenosis of minor salivary glands: report of three cases and review of the literature. *Oral Surg Oral Med Oral Pathol Oral Radiol Endod.* 2007;104:516-520.

Skalova A, Gnepp DR, Simpson RH, et al. Clonal nature of sclerosing polycystic adenosis of salivary glands demonstrated by using the polymorphism of the human androgen receptor (HUMARA) locus as a marker. *Am J Surg Pathol.* 2006;30:939-944.

Smith BC, Ellis GL, Slater LJ, Foss RD. Sclerosing polycystic adenosis of major salivary glands. A clinicopathologic analysis of nine cases. *Am J Surg Pathol.* 1996;20:161-170.

Swelam WM. The pathogenic role of Epstein-Barr virus (EBV) in sclerosing polycystic adenosis. *Pathol Res Pract.* 2010;206:565-571.

14 ODONTOGENIC CYSTS

CHAPTER CONTENTS

The tooth develops from the dental lamina, an ingrowth of the lining of the primitive stomodeum, and the dental lamina forms tooth buds for the primary and the permanent dentition (Fig. 14.1). After odontogenesis, remnant epithelium is left behind as rests. The epithelium of odontogenic cysts is thought to arise from stimulation and proliferation of such residual odontogenic rests (Fig. 14.2).

Odontogenic Cysts

Cystic lesions in the jawbones are either odontogenic or nonodontogenic; nonodontogenic cysts are discussed in Chapter 16. Odontogenic cysts are inflammatory, developmental, or less commonly, neoplastic in nature. The putative epithelium from which they derive may be rests of Malassez, dental lamina rests, reduced enamel epithelium, degenerated enamel organ, or the epithelium of the surface mucosa (Fig. 14.3). There is still controversy regarding whether the odontogenic keratocyst is a cyst with a high recurrence rate, or whether it should be reclassified as a keratocystic odontogenic tumor—a cystic neoplasm—as was done by the World Health Organization in 2005. Similarly within that classification the calcifying odontogenic cyst was renamed calcifying cystic odontogenic tumor and classified as a cystic tumor/neoplasm. In this atlas, I have classified them as cystic neoplasms; both entities are discussed in Chapter 15.

General Principles

In general, inflammatory odontogenic cysts have proliferative epithelium, and developmental odontogenic cysts have uniformly thin epithelium, although inflammation may lead to epithelial proliferation in the latter. The most common odontogenic cyst is the radicular cyst (>50% of cases) followed by the dentigerous cyst (20% of cases). Any odontogenic cyst may grow to a large size, involve multiple teeth, cause root resorption, cause clinical swelling, perforate the cortex, or involve the maxillary sinus. Because the neuroectoderm is involved in odontogenesis, melanin occasionally may be identified in odontogenic cysts and tumors.

Inflammatory Cysts

APICAL AND LATERAL RADICULAR CYST, PERIAPICAL GRANULOMA, AND PERIAPICAL SCAR

A tooth that has caries involving the pulp or that has experienced direct trauma becomes devitalized and may develop a radiolucency at the apex of the root. This may represent an apical radicular cyst, periapical granuloma, or scar.

Clinical Findings

- The radicular cyst or granuloma is usually seen in adults, may be asymptomatic or painful, and may manifest as a swelling within the maxillary or mandibular sulcus, or on the face, depending on its size. A well-circumscribed radiolucency is present at the apex (apical radicular and representing >95% of cases) or on the side (lateral radicular from a lateral accessory canal) of a nonvital tooth that may have had prior root canal/endodontic therapy (Fig. 14.4A–B).
- A residual cyst refers to any odontogenic cyst in the alveolar bone where a tooth had been extracted and is most often a residual apical radicular cyst because of statistical frequency (Fig. 14.4C).

Etiopathogenesis and Histopathologic Features

Inflammation from the pulp of necrotic teeth results in stimulation and proliferation of rests of Malassez, which are remnants of the Hertwig root sheath that helps form the roots of the teeth during odontogenesis.

- A radicular cyst is lined by nonkeratinized stratified squamous epithelium that usually proliferates in a plexiform pattern and exhibits spongiosis and neutrophilic exocytosis; the wall is composed of edematous granulation tissue and often scar tissue with many plasma cells, Russell bodies, lymphocytes, foamy macrophages, abscesses, and many cholesterol granulomas from hemorrhage (Fig. 14.5); curetted specimens may show only granulation tissue with focal lining epithelium (Fig. 14.6); curetted lesions from anterior teeth often show abundant skeletal muscle, and some lesions exhibit squamous odontogenic tumor-like proliferations (Fig. 14.7).
- Rushton bodies are hyaline lamellar or globular structures of odontogenic origin often seen within the epithelium, sometimes exhibiting dystrophic calcifications; these are composed of K17, hair keratin, and hemoglobin alpha chain (Fig. 14.8).
- Root canal filling material and cements are often present in apical biopsies: gutta-percha is yellowish or brownish green, granular, and homogenously refractile (Fig. 14.9); AH Plus is an epoxy resin that contains zirconium, iron oxides, and calcium tungstate; it is spherical and refractile in an eosinophilic background, whereas mineral trioxide aggregate (a tricalcium silicate cement) is basophilic and granular, but with refractile, crystalline particles (Fig. 14.10); amalgam tattoo may be present from a previous apicoectomy (root apex excision).
- Hyaline ring granulomas consist of hyalinized rings with central and/or surrounding giant cells; foreign material (eg, leguminous material) is sometimes identified as are dystrophic calcifications; the hyaline material is negative for Type IV collagen and does not represent vascular basement membrane as was previously believed (Fig. 14.11).
- Radicular cysts from the apices of maxillary molars may be lined by respiratory epithelium (Fig. 14.12); fragments of sinus mucosa, however, signify an oroantral communication and must be reported; fragments of sinus inflammatory polyps may be present exhibiting few to no mucous glands, eosinophilic coagulum, and eosinophils (Fig. 14.13).
- If epithelium is not present the diagnosis is periapical granuloma (not a true granuloma but an "oma" of granulation tissue); sheets of plasma cells are common in periapical granulomas, and they should not be overdiagnosed as plasmacytomas (Fig. 14.14).
- Periapical scar shows only fibrosis, sometimes with inflammation (Fig. 14.15).
- Suction artifact that appears as ovoid-to-round spaces within the soft tissues is a common finding; the spaces contain wispy amorphous material that has been identified as alcianophilic acid mucopolysaccharides (Fig. 14.15).

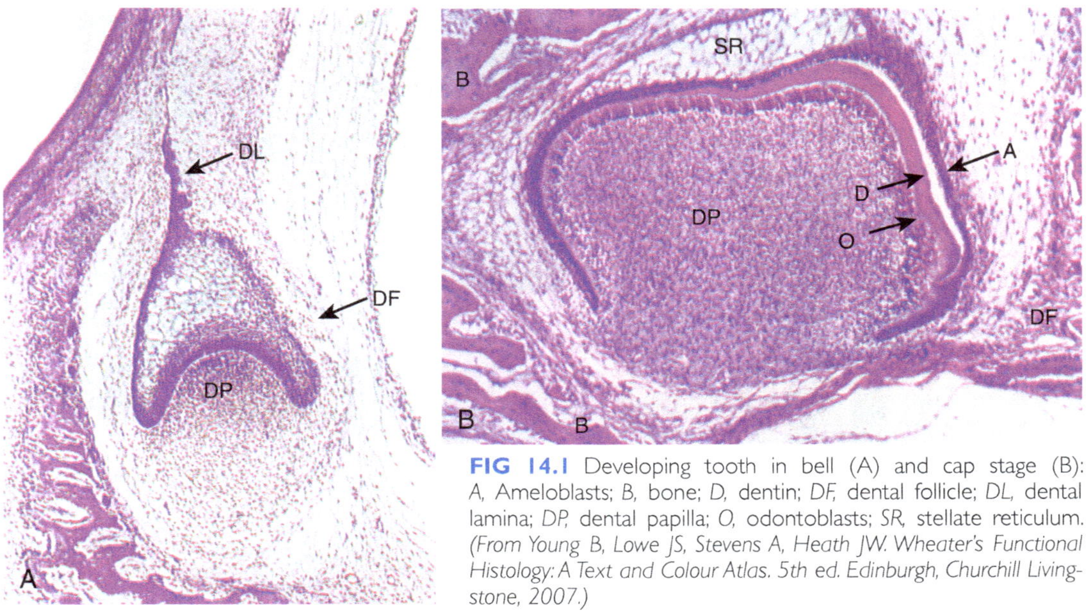

FIG 14.1 Developing tooth in bell (A) and cap stage (B): *A*, Ameloblasts; *B*, bone; *D*, dentin; *DF*, dental follicle; *DL*, dental lamina; *DP*, dental papilla; *O*, odontoblasts; *SR*, stellate reticulum. *(From Young B, Lowe JS, Stevens A, Heath JW. Wheater's Functional Histology: A Text and Colour Atlas. 5th ed. Edinburgh, Churchill Livingstone, 2007.)*

Differential Diagnosis

- An inflamed dentigerous cyst appears similar except that it surrounds an impacted tooth.
- Chronic active periodontal disease consists of granulation tissue lined by crevicular epithelium that is composed of similar nonkeratinized stratified squamous epithelium, which exhibits spongiosis and neutrophilic exocytosis often in continuity with surface keratinized epithelium, but clinically the tooth exhibits a periradicular radiolucency; disease starts either from an apical radicular cyst that grows very large and combines with an overlying periodontal bone defect, or from periodontal disease starting from the surface of the bone and extending downward to encompass the entire tooth.

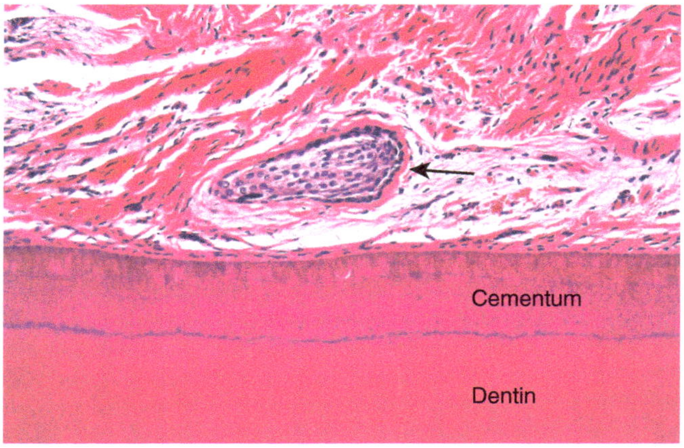

FIG 14.2 Odontogenic rest, likely rest of Malassez *(arrow)* in the periodontal ligament (fibrous tissue that attaches the tooth to bone).

Management and Prognosis

- Enucleation or curettage with apicoectomy (excision of the root tip) is curative.

REFERENCES

Gadbail AR, Chaudhary M, Patil S, Gawande M. Actual Proliferating Index and p53 protein expression as prognostic marker in odontogenic cysts. *Oral Dis.* 2009;15:490-498.

Johnson NR, Gannon OM, Savage NW, Batstone MD. Frequency of odontogenic cysts and tumors: a systematic review. *J Investig Clin Dent.* 2014;5:9-14.

Philipsen HP, Reichart PA. Pulse or hyaline ring granuloma. Review of the literature on etiopathogenesis of oral and extraoral lesions. *Clin Oral Investig.* 2010;14:121-128.

Sakamoto K, Khanom R, Hamagaki M, Yamaguchi A. Ectopic production of hair keratin constitutes Rushton's hyaline bodies in association with hematogenous deposits. *J Oral Pathol Med.* 2012;41:637-641.

Schulz M, von Arx T, Altermatt HJ, Bosshardt D. Histology of periapical lesions obtained during apical surgery. *J Endod.* 2009;35:634-642.

Wysocki GP, Gusenbauer AW, Daley TD, Sapp JP. Surgical suction damage: a common tissue artifact. *Oral Surg Oral Med Oral Pathol.* 1987;63:573-575.

Text continued on p. 360

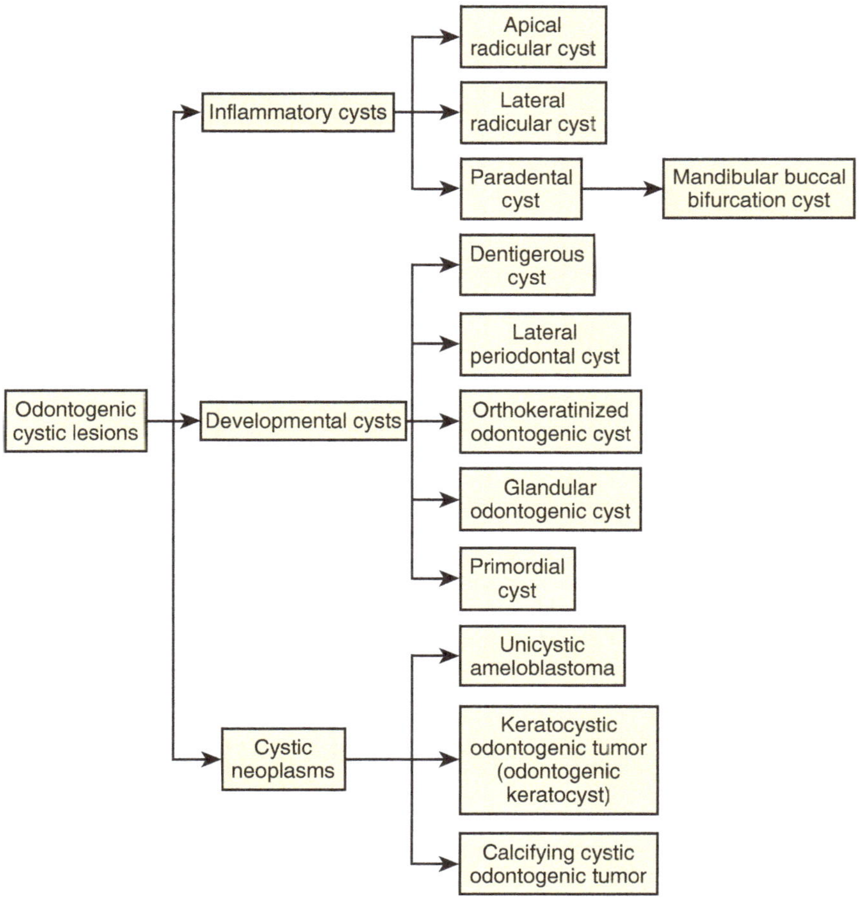

FIG 14.3 Classification of odontogenic cysts.

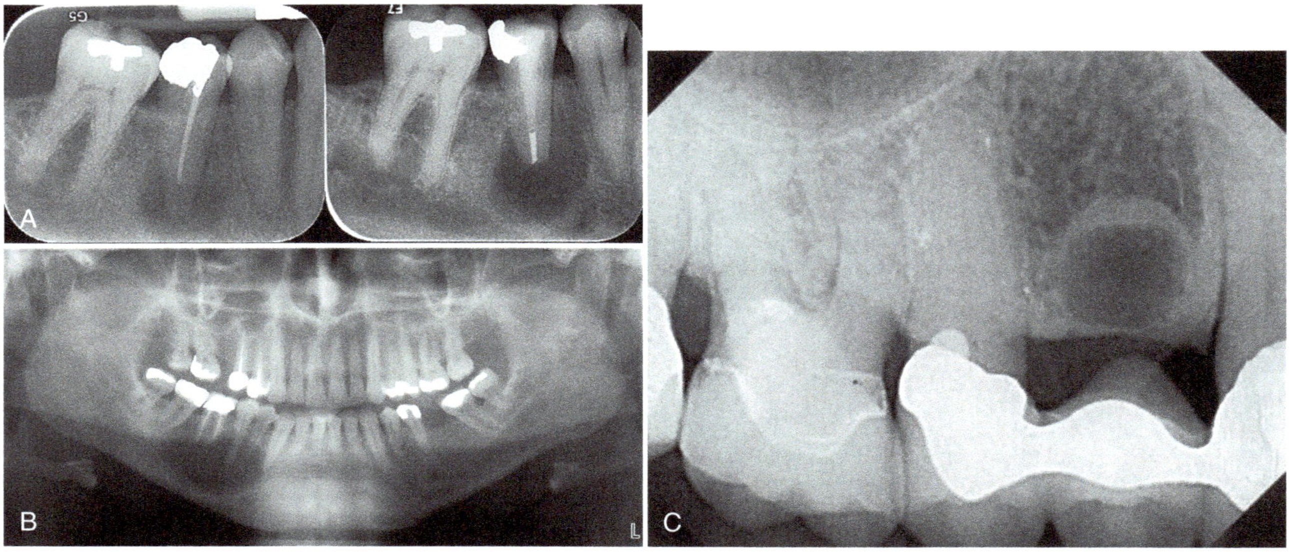

FIG 14.4 Apical radicular cyst. (A) Circumscribed radiolucency at the apex of an endodontically treated right mandibular second premolar before *(left)* and after curettage, apicoectomy, and retrofill *(right)*. (B) Large circumscribed radiolucency centered around an endodontically treated right lower first molar. (C) Residual apical radicular cyst after extraction of the right maxillary first premolar. *(B, Courtesy Dr. Manuel Diaz, private practice, Houston, Tex.)*

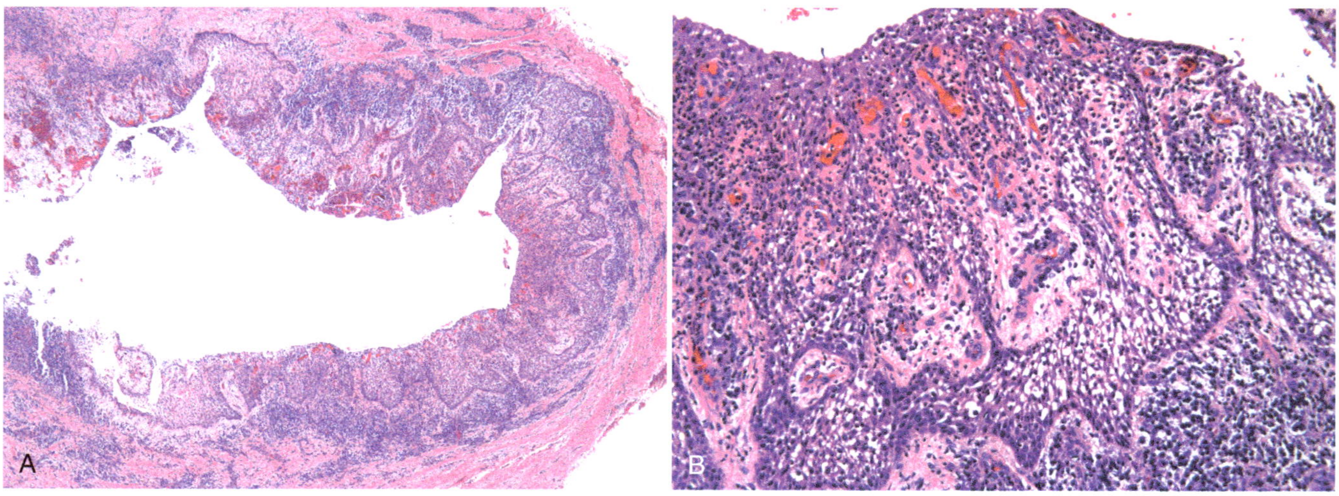

FIG 14.5 Apical radicular cyst. (A) Cyst with epithelial proliferation and inflammation. (B) Lining consists of nonkeratinized stratified squamous epithelium with plexiform proliferation, spongiosis, and neutrophilic exocytosis.

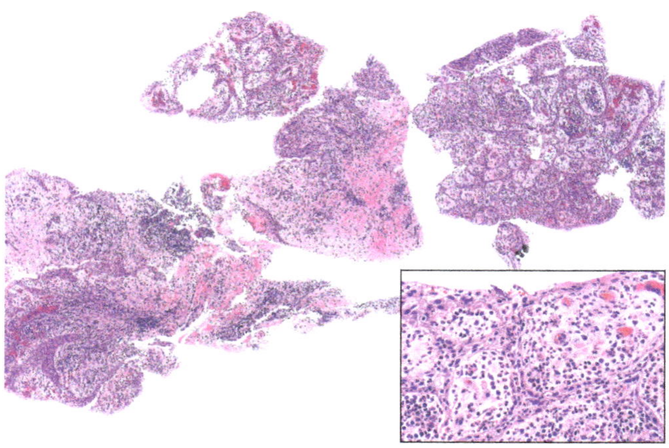

FIG 14.6 Apical radicular cyst in fragments with plexiform epithelial proliferation showing spongiosis and neutrophilic exocytosis *(inset)*.

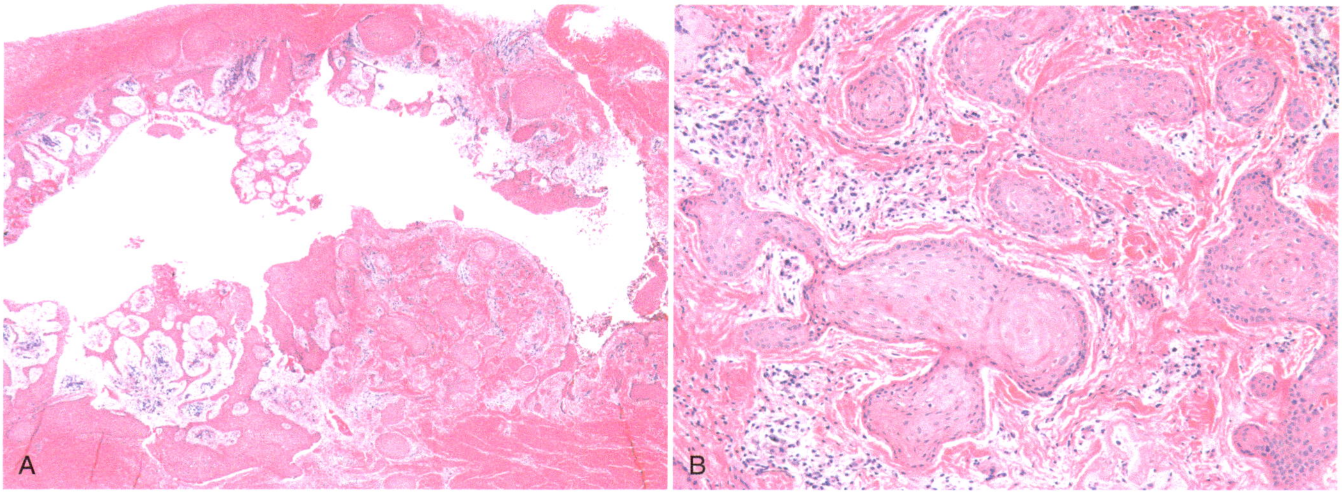

FIG 14.7 Apical radicular cyst with squamous odontogenic tumor-like proliferation. (A) Cyst with many islands of epithelium within the wall. (B) Irregular islands of epithelium with dyskeratotic cells without palisading of peripheral cells.

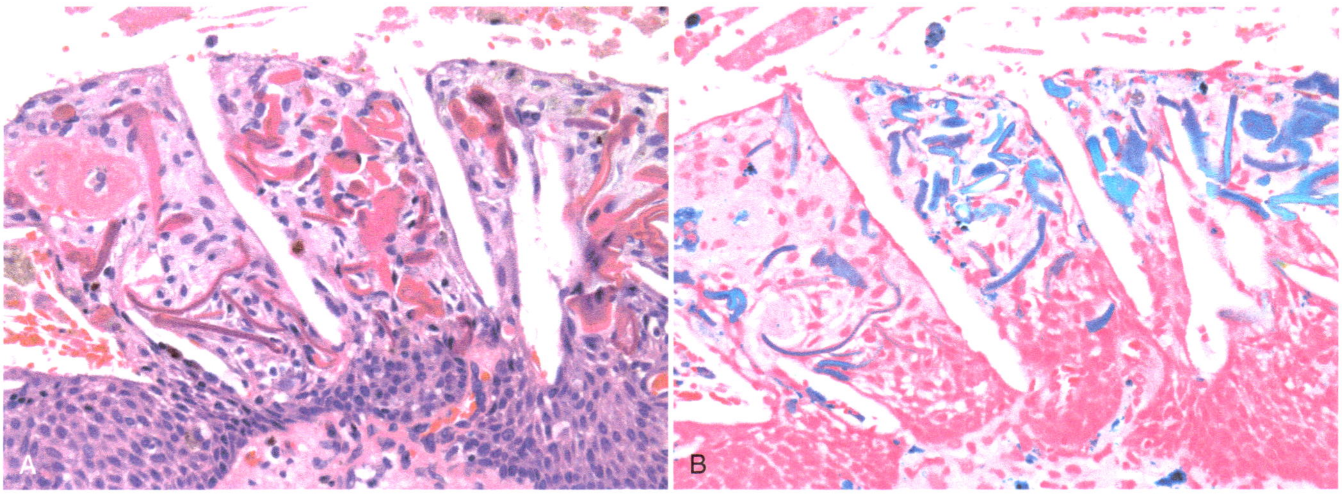

FIG 14.8 Rushton bodies within cyst epithelium. (A) Hyaline, eosinophilic globular, and laminated structures within the epithelium. (B) These stain for iron although the intensity is less strong when compared with hemosiderin (Prussian blue).

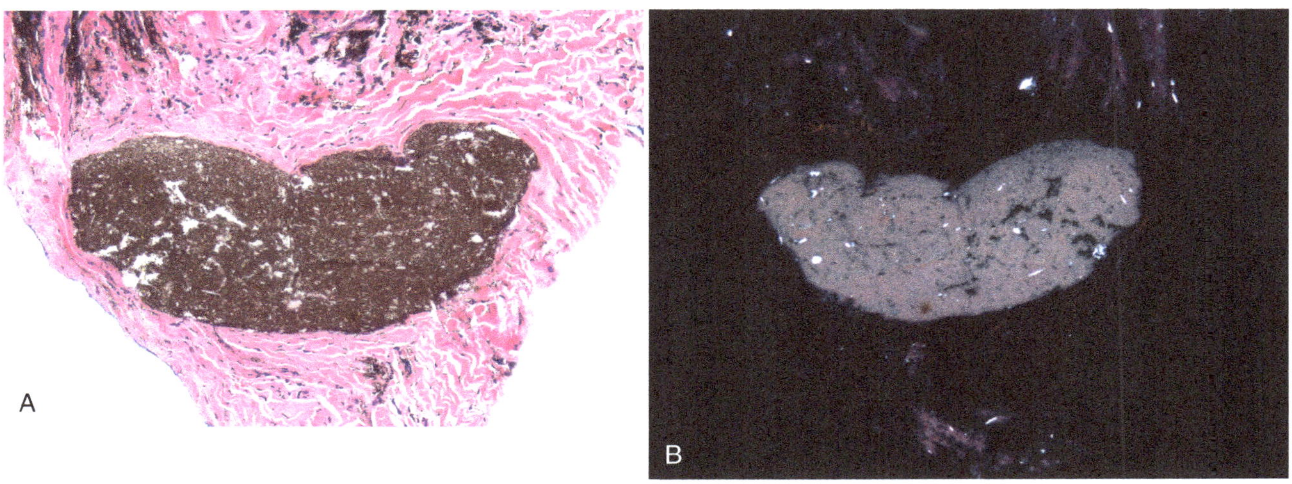

FIG 14.9 Gutta-percha (root canal filler). (A) Brown-green granular foreign body commonly seen in apical lesions. (B) Gutta-percha is homogenously refractile, and particles of root canal cement within it is more brightly refractile.

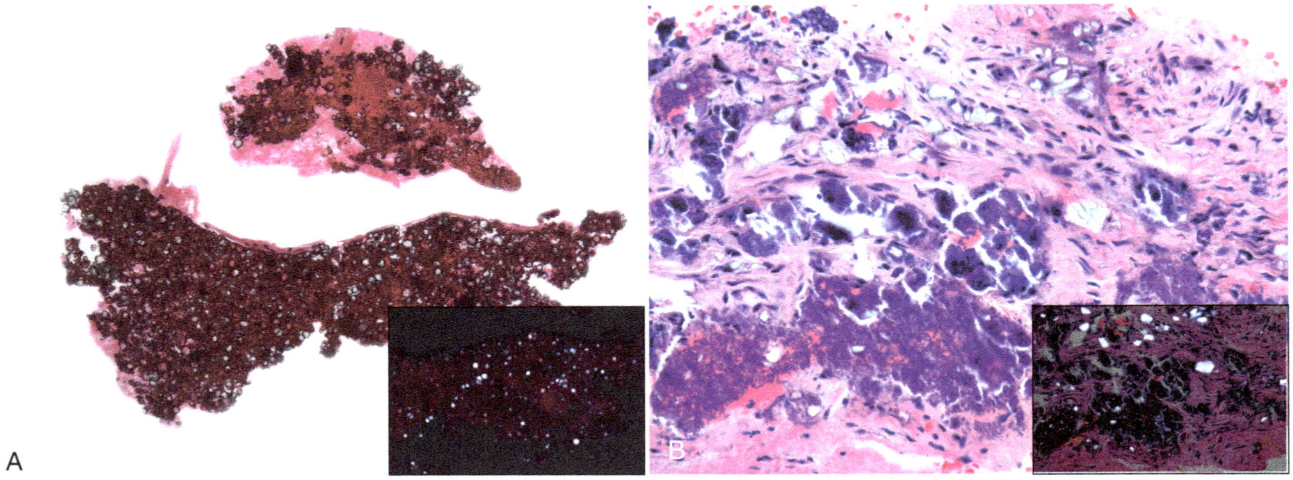

FIG 14.10 (A) Periapical granuloma with AH Plus cement composed of spherical, refractile particles in an eosinophilic background *(inset with polarized light)*. (B) Mineral trioxide aggregate consists of basophilic granular material with brightly refractile crystalline particles *(inset with polarized light)*.

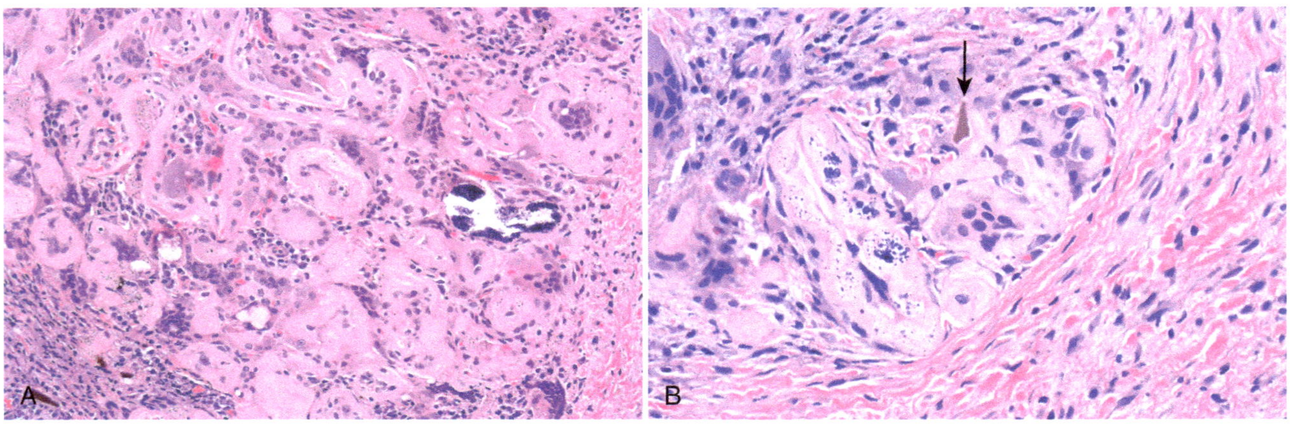

FIG 14.11 Hyaline ring granulomas. (A) Hyalinized rings often with giant cells in the center. (B) Hyaline rings with giant cells, calcifications, foreign material *(arrow)*, and dystrophic calcifications.

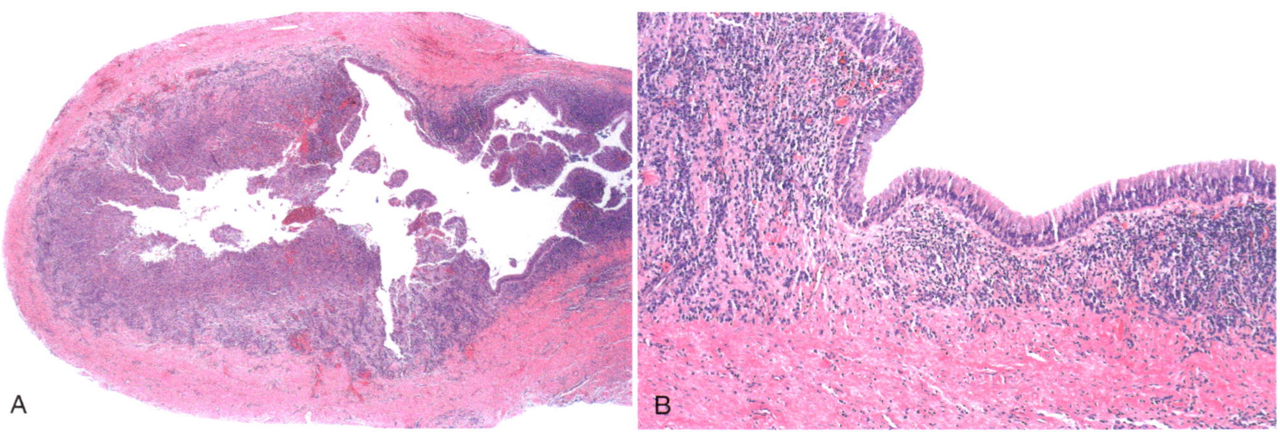

FIG 14.12 Apical radicular cyst at apex of maxillary first molar. (A) Cyst is partially lined by respiratory epithelium but without any mucous glands. (B) Typical pseudostratified columnar epithelium.

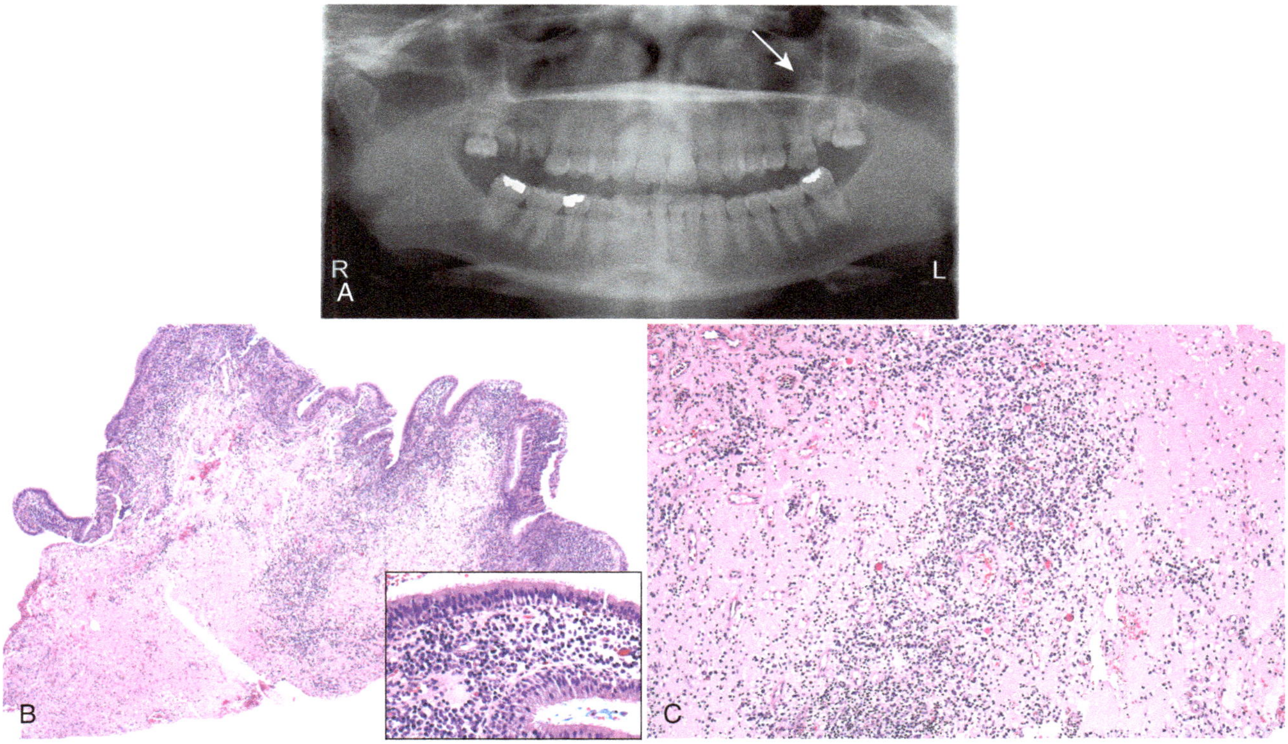

FIG 14.13 Sinus inflammatory polyp. (A) Radiograph showing dome-shaped opacity *(arrow)* in the left sinus adjacent to carious left maxillary first molar and root tips of second molar. (B) Mass of eosinophilic material and granulation tissue covered by respiratory epithelium with no mucous glands; many plasma cells and eosinophils *(inset)* (from A). (C) Abundant eosinophilic amorphous material (from A). *(A, Courtesy Dr. Jeffrey Stone, private practice, Lowell, Mass.)*

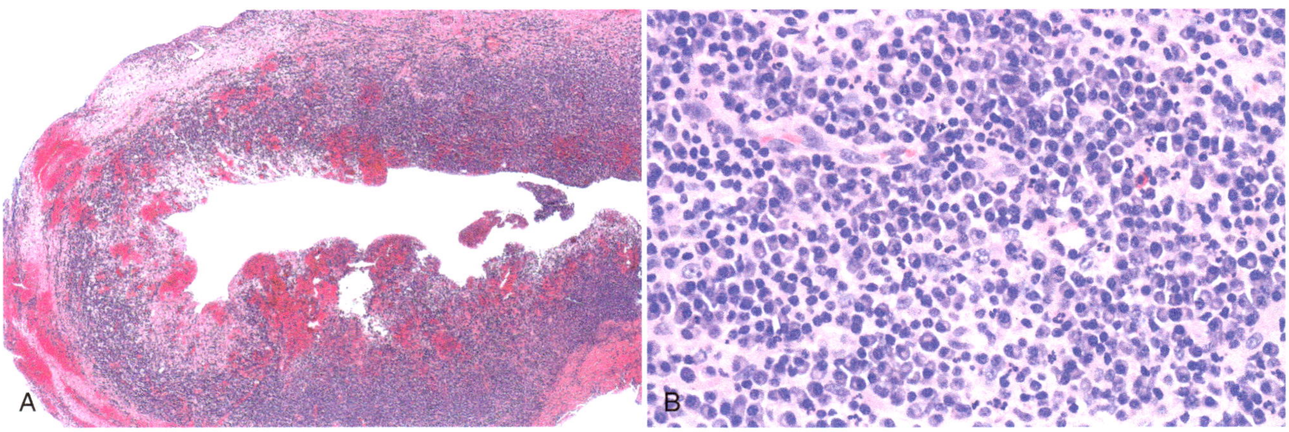

FIG 14.14 Periapical granuloma. (A) Granulation tissue arranged around a cystlike cavity with acute and chronic inflammatory cells and no lining epithelium. (B) Periapical granuloma with sheets of plasma cells.

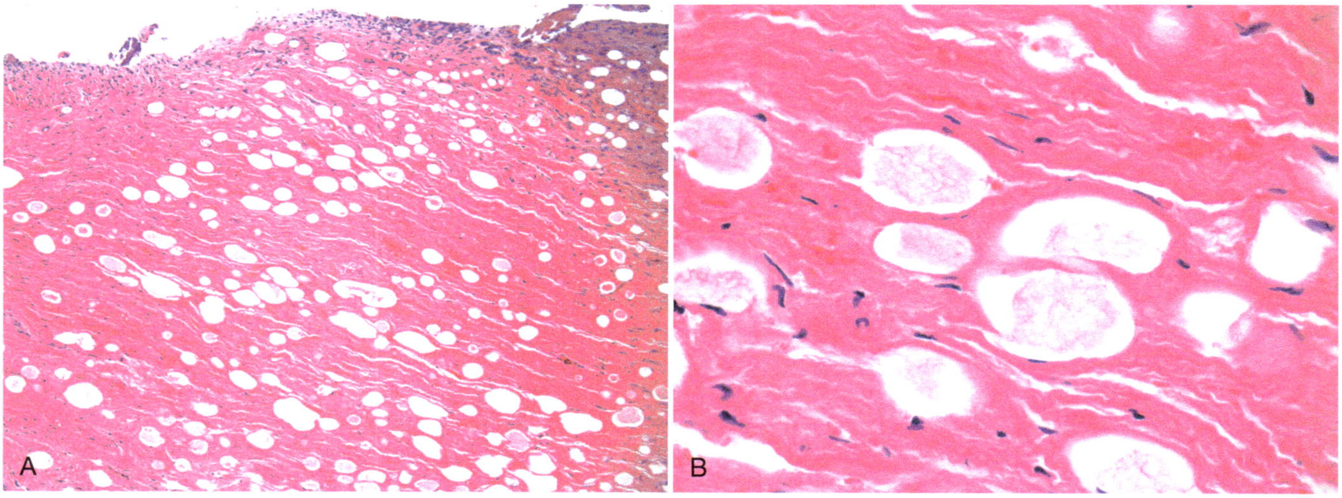

FIG 14.15 Periapical scar. (A) Dense fibrous scar tissue with suction artifact presenting as spaces in the tissue. (B) Spaces are filled with wispy amorphous material *(ground substance)*.

MANDIBULAR BUCCAL BIFURCATION CYST

Clinical Findings

- This occurs in children in the first decade with a mean age of 7 years and 38% are bilateral.
- There is swelling and pain in the area of a vital first permanent molar and a radiolucency that extends from the furcation (where roots diverge) to the apex of the tooth causing tilting of the roots lingually (best seen on occlusal radiograph); a periosteal reaction may be present (Fig. 14.16).

Etiopathogenesis and Histopathologic Features

The lining may derive from dental lamina rests or more likely crevicular epithelium. Another theory of pathogenesis is that this arises from a laterally displaced dentigerous cyst of the first molar, which could explain the high incidence of bilaterality. A third theory is that buccal enamel extensions onto the tooth root cause periodontal pocketing.

- The histopathology is similar to that of a radicular cyst with proliferative nonkeratinized stratified squamous epithelium and acute and chronic inflammation within the wall.

Differential Diagnosis

- If the tooth is nonvital and the cyst is unilateral, a lateral radicular cyst should be considered.
- Some clinicians consider the buccal bifurcation cyst a subcategory of paradental cysts, which are cysts located to the side of a tooth; however, categorizing a cyst based on anatomic site alone rather than etiopathogenesis is not useful; many so-called paradental cysts are distal to third molars and they are more likely to be dentigerous cysts (see later).

Management and Prognosis

- Enucleation of the cyst without extraction of the tooth is curative.
- Extraction of the tooth and enucleation of the paradental cyst associated with the third molar is curative.

REFERENCES

de Sousa SO, Correa L, Deboni MC, de Araujo VC. Clinicopathologic features of 54 cases of paradental cyst. *Quintessence Int.* 2001;32: 737-741.

Maruyama S, Yamazaki M, Abe T, et al. Paradental cyst is an inclusion cyst of the junctional/sulcular epithelium of the gingiva: histopathologic and immunohistochemical confirmation for its pathogenesis. *Oral Surg Oral Med Oral Pathol Oral Radiol.* 2015;120:227-237.

Parmar RM, Brannon RB, Fowler CB. Squamous odontogenic tumor-like proliferations in radicular cysts: a clinicopathologic study of forty-two cases. *J Endod.* 2011;37:623-626.

Philipsen HP, Reichart PA, Ogawa I, et al. The inflammatory paradental cyst: a critical review of 342 cases from a literature survey, including 17 new cases from the author's files. *J Oral Pathol Med.* 2004;33: 147-155.

Pompura JR, Sandor GK, Stoneman DW. The buccal bifurcation cyst: a prospective study of treatment outcomes in 44 sites. *Oral Surg Oral Med Oral Pathol Oral Radiol Endod.* 1997;83:215-221.

Zadik Y, Yitschaky O, Neuman T, Nitzan DW. On the self-resolution nature of the buccal bifurcation cyst. *J Oral Maxillofac Surg.* 2011;69: e282-e284.

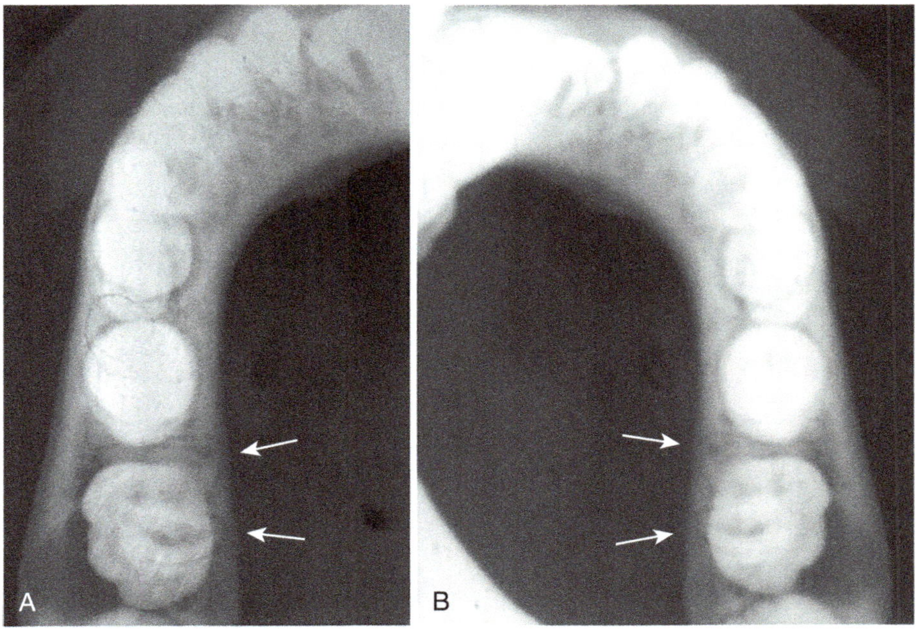

FIG 14.16 Bilateral mandibular buccal bifurcation cyst in one patient. (A) Occlusal radiograph showing lingual displacement of roots of first molar on right *(arrows)*, and buccal radiolucency. (B) Occlusal radiograph showing displacement of roots of first molar on left *(arrows)*, and buccal radiolucency. *(Courtesy Dr. Bernard Friedland, Harvard School of Dental Medicine, Boston.)*

Developmental Odontogenic Cysts

The epithelium of these cysts arises from stimulation and proliferation of dental lamina rests, squamatization and proliferation of reduced enamel epithelium, or from the epithelium of the tooth germ. These cysts are characterized by uniformly thin lining 5 to 15 cells thick, although inflammation will cause epithelial proliferation with spongiosis and neutrophilic exocytosis. The multipotentiality of the lining of dentigerous and other developmental odontogenic cysts as well as odontogenic rests are the likely origin of intraosseous salivary gland neoplasms, the most common of which is the mucoepidermoid carcinoma, with adenoid cystic carcinoma being the second most common, but with much lower frequency. Some developmental odontogenic cysts occur in a peripheral (extraosseous) location and the most frequent is the gingival cyst of the adult. The less common gingival cyst of the newborn forms from cystic dental lamina rests and resolves spontaneously (see Chapter 2, Fig. 2.30B). Erupting teeth may be associated with eruption cysts.

GINGIVAL CYST OF THE ADULT

This is considered the extraosseous counterpart of the lateral periodontal cyst.

Clinical Findings

- These usually occur in the fifth or sixth decade and appear as a bluish, slightly fluctuant, dome-shaped nodule on the attached gingiva or alveolar mucosa; these cysts are most frequent in the mandibular canine-premolar area (70–80% of cases), with the second most common site being the maxillary canine lateral incisor area; some cases are multiple or bilateral (Fig. 14.17A).

Etiopathogenesis and Histopathologic Features

Gingival cyst of the adult forms from cystic degeneration of rests of dental lamina (rests of Serres) in the gingiva (Fig. 14.17B).

- These cysts are lined by nonkeratinized, low cuboidal or squamous epithelium usually two to four cells thick; epithelial plaques containing glycogen-rich clear cells are often present sometimes with a whorled, morular architecture (Figs. 14.18–14.19); rare cases are parakeratotic, but without palisading of the basal cell nuclei. Bona fide gingival keratocystic odontogenic tumor (odontogenic keratocyst) has been reported (Fig. 14.20).

Differential Diagnosis

- Salivary duct cyst occurs on *nonkeratinized* gingiva/alveolar mucosa and is lined by stratified squamous epithelium, cuboidal cells, contains mucous cells, ciliated cells, or oncocytes, and does not show epithelial plaques with clear cells.
- A keratocystic odontogenic tumor (odontogenic keratocyst) that has eroded through bone and manifests in the soft tissues must be ruled out by a radiograph if parakeratin is present in the gingival cyst of the adult.
- A gingival cyst that occurs in the vicinity of a gingival graft lined by thin squamous epithelium that may be keratinized is more likely to represent an implantation epithelial inclusion cyst.

Management and Prognosis

- Excision is the treatment of choice for the adult form.

REFERENCES

Bell RC, Chauvin PJ, Tyler MT. Gingival cyst of the adult: a review and a report of eight cases. *J Can Dent Assoc.* 1997;63:533-535.

Buchner A, Hansen LS. The histomorphologic spectrum of the gingival cyst in the adult. *Oral Surg Oral Med Oral Pathol.* 1979;48:532-539.

Gil Escalante M, Tatakis DN. Gingival cyst of the adult as early sequela of connective tissue grafting. *Case Rep Dent.* 2015;2015:473689.

Giunta JL. Gingival cysts in the adult. *J Periodontol.* 2002;73:827-831.

Nxumalo TN, Shear M. Gingival cyst in adults. *J Oral Pathol Med.* 1992;21:309-313.

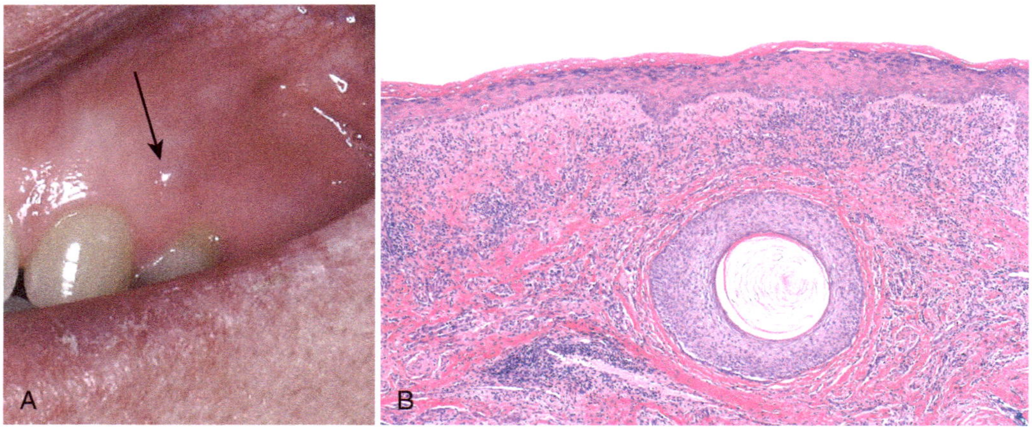

FIG 14.17 (A) Small gingival cyst of the adult appearing as a bluish dome-shaped lesion *(arrow)*. (B) A rest of Serres within the gingiva showing cystic change and keratinization.

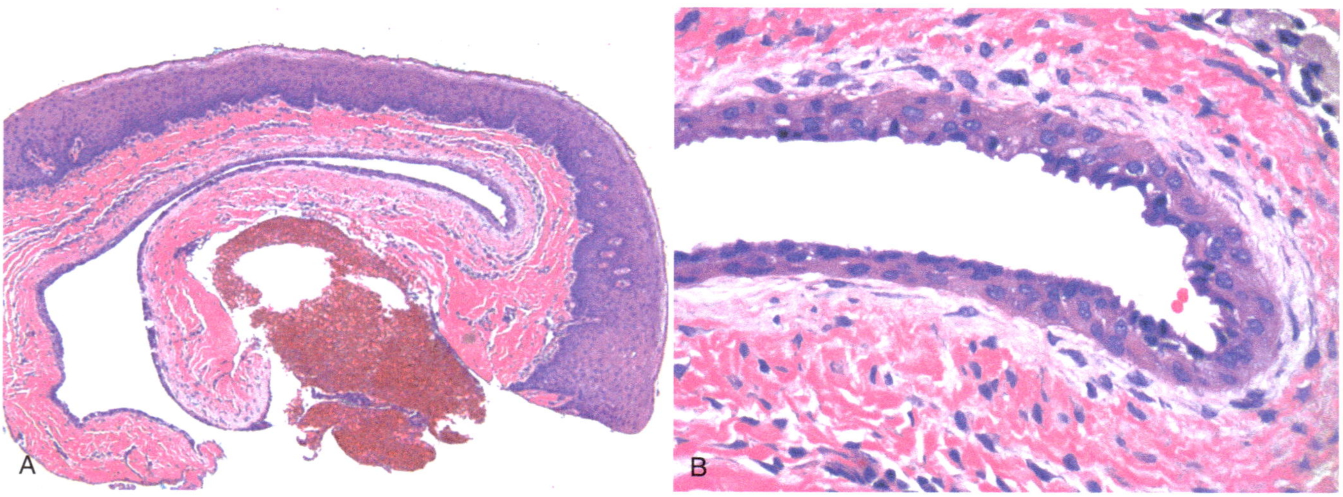

FIG 14.18 Gingival cyst of the adult. (A) The cyst is lined by uniformly thin epithelium without inflammation. (B) The cyst lining varies from 3 to 6 cells in thickness.

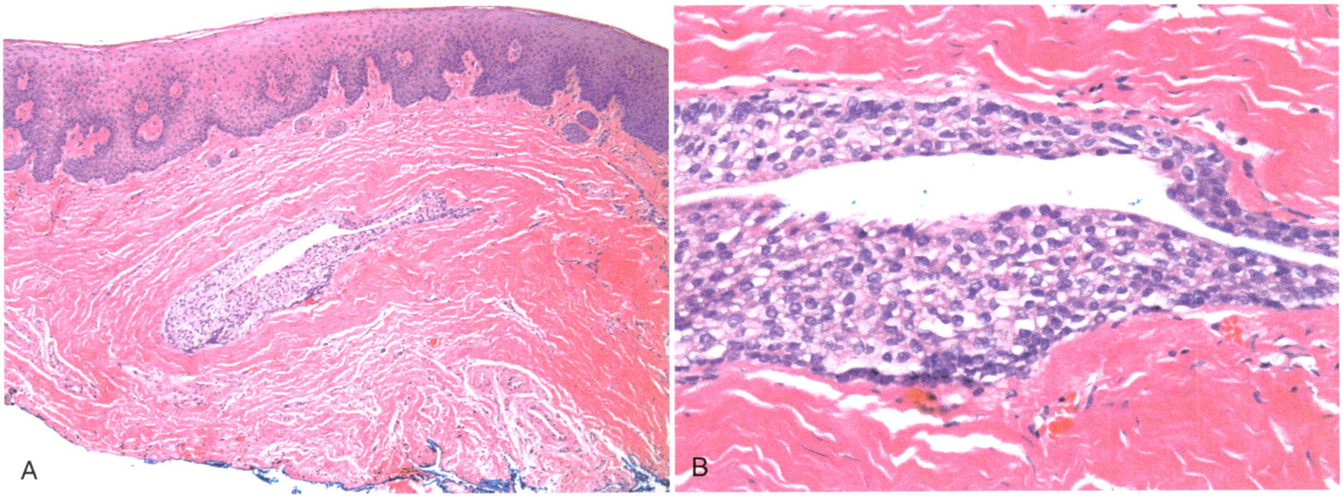

FIG 14.19 Gingival cyst of the adult. (A) The lining epithelium is uniformly 5 to 15 cells thick. (B) The epithelium contains many clear cells that are glycogen rich.

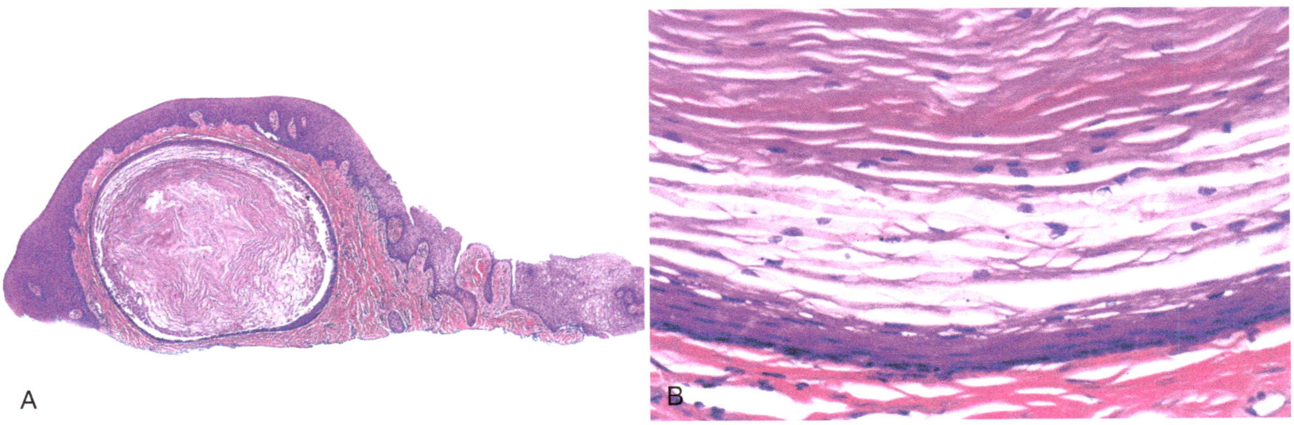

FIG 14.20 Gingival cyst of the adult. (A) Cyst in the lamina propria filled with keratin. (B) Parakeratin is present but without palisading of the basal cells.

ERUPTION CYST (ERUPTION HEMATOMA)

This is often considered the soft tissue variant of a dentigerous cyst and there is overlap between these two entities. It is more appropriately considered a separate entity because it has different clinical and demographic findings from a dentigerous cyst.

Clinical Findings

- This occurs between 4 and 8 years of age and there may be a 2:1 male predilection; it presents as a bluish bleb overlying an erupting tooth with no intervening bone (Fig. 14.21A).
- The most commonly affected teeth are the permanent first molar (50% of cases) that erupts at 6 years of age and the primary central incisor (42% of cases) that erupts at 6 months of age; natal teeth are affected in 8% of cases, and some cases are multiple.

Etiopathogenesis and Histopathologic Features

There is impedance in the eruption of a tooth that may be caused by overlying dense fibrous gingival tissue. Some cases are hemorrhagic, hence the term eruption hematoma. Some believe that this is a process of exteriorization of a dentigerous cyst.

- The cyst is lined by nonkeratinized stratified squamous epithelium, sometimes with hemorrhage or inflammation from pericoronitis (Fig. 14.21B).

Differential Diagnosis

- Gingival cyst of the adult generally does not occur in young children and infants.

Management and Prognosis

- Approximately 40% of cases will resolve on their own with tooth eruption; however, if this does not occur within a reasonable time, marsupialization or

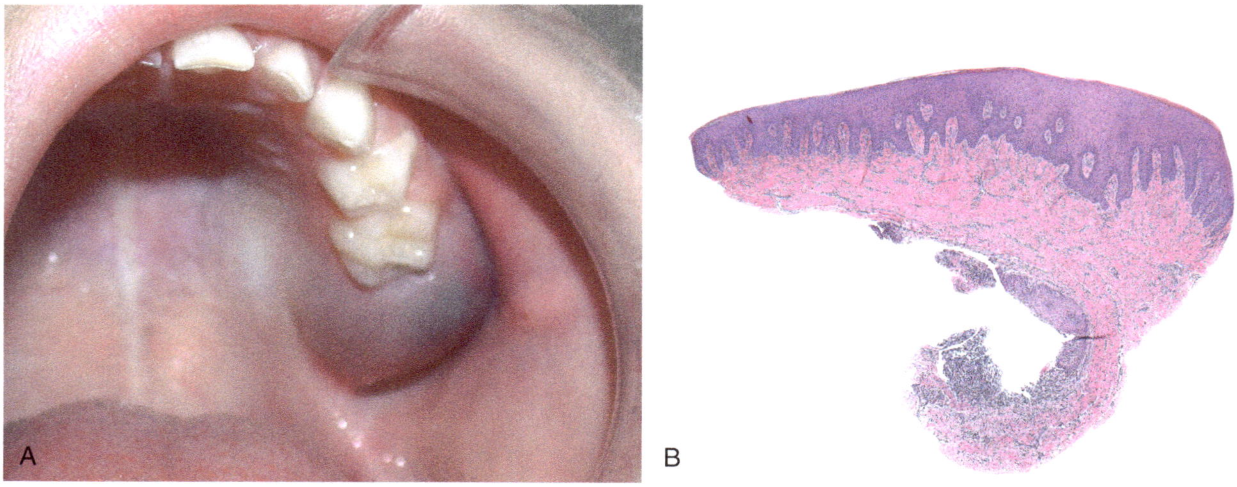

FIG 14.21 Eruption cyst. (A) Bluish, cystic lesion overlying the erupting left maxillary first permanent molar. (B) The eruption cyst presents within the deep lamina propria and there is mild chronic inflammation. *(Courtesy Dr. Bonnie Padwa, Harvard School of Dental Medicine, Boston.)*

exteriorization of the cyst allows for eruption of the underlying tooth.

- Malformed teeth such as a natal tooth associated with an eruption cyst should be extracted and the cyst excised.

REFERENCES

Aguilo L, Cibrian R, Bagan JV, Gandia JL. Eruption cysts: retrospective clinical study of 36 cases. *ASDC J Dent Child.* 1998;65:102-106.

Woldenberg Y, Goldstein J, Bodner L. Eruption cyst in the adult–a case report. *Int J Oral Maxillofac Surg.* 2004;33:804-805.

DENTIGEROUS CYST (FOLLICULAR CYST)

Clinical Findings

- This is most frequently seen in the second and third decades as a radiolucency associated with impacted teeth, usually the mandibular third molars (77% of cases), maxillary third molars (11% of cases), and maxillary canines (5% of cases), although any other teeth may be involved such as the premolars and supernumerary teeth; 3% of cases are multiple, especially around multiple impacted third molars.
- It presents as a well-demarcated unilocular radiolucency that may be around the crown of the tooth (central location, the most common), on the side of the tooth (lateral location), or completely around the tooth (circumferential location) (Fig. 14.22); some may appear multiloculated on plain radiographs because of protruding bony septa from the walls, but true multiloculation should raise suspicion for odontogenic neoplasms or nonodontogenic lesions.

Etiopathogenesis and Histopathologic Features

The epithelium is derived from reduced enamel epithelium (fused external and internal enamel epithelium after the tooth is formed) that has undergone squamous metaplasia, and fluid buildup between the crown and the reduced enamel epithelium. This epithelium is multipotent and capable of producing mucous cells, ciliated cells, and glandular structures. One study had shown that pericoronal radiolucencies of less than 4 mm followed over many years do not change, and as such do not represent cysts. Still others believe that a diagnosis of dentigerous cyst can only be made if there is clinical evidence of a cystic space between the tooth and the surrounding tissue at the time of cyst removal.

Between 1% and 2% of radiolucencies associated with impacted teeth are histologically keratocystic odontogenic tumors (odontogenic keratocysts), and another 1% to 2% represent other benign odontogenic neoplasms such as adenomatoid odontogenic tumor, ameloblastoma, or calcifying cystic odontogenic tumor; less than 1% are associated with the development of mucoepidermoid carcinoma or squamous cell carcinoma. The development of salivary gland neoplasms within the jawbones, often in the vicinity of developmental odontogenic cysts and in particular dentigerous cysts, is testament to the multipotentiality of the cyst lining as well as odontogenic epithelial rests. Other possible origins for salivary gland tumors in the jaws include entrapped retromolar salivary glands and ectopic salivary gland tissue.

- The lining consists of nonkeratinized stratified squamous epithelium 5 to 10 cells thick and generally does not exhibit spongiosis or neutrophilic exocytosis unless there is underlying inflammation; it may then be indistinguishable from an apical radicular cyst (Fig. 14.23). Cholesterol granulomas are often seen where epithelium is disrupted and there is hemorrhage, and consist of needle-shaped, clear clefts surrounded by histiocytes, and multinucleated foreign body–type giant cells (Fig. 14.24). Mucous cells and ciliated cells are present in up to 25% and 10% of cases, respectively (Fig. 14.25). The overlying oral mucosa may be inflamed

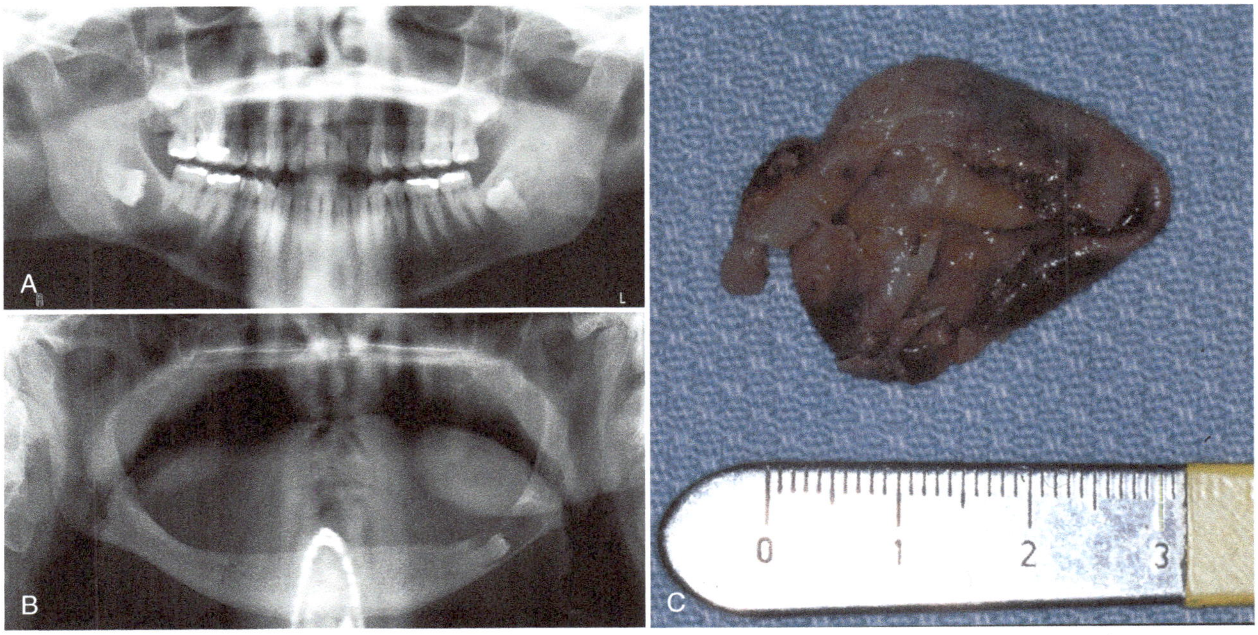

FIG 14.22 Dentigerous cyst. (A) Panoramic radiograph showing unilocular radiolucency around impacted lower right third molar with resorption of roots of the adjacent molar. (B) Panoramic radiograph showing unilocular radiolucency around retained left mandibular molar at risk for pathologic fracture. (C) Gross specimen consisting of hemorrhagic cystic sac. *(B, Courtesy Dr. Thomas Dodson, Harvard School of Dental Medicine, Boston; C, Courtesy Dr. Bonnie Padwa, Harvard School of Dental Medicine, Boston.)*

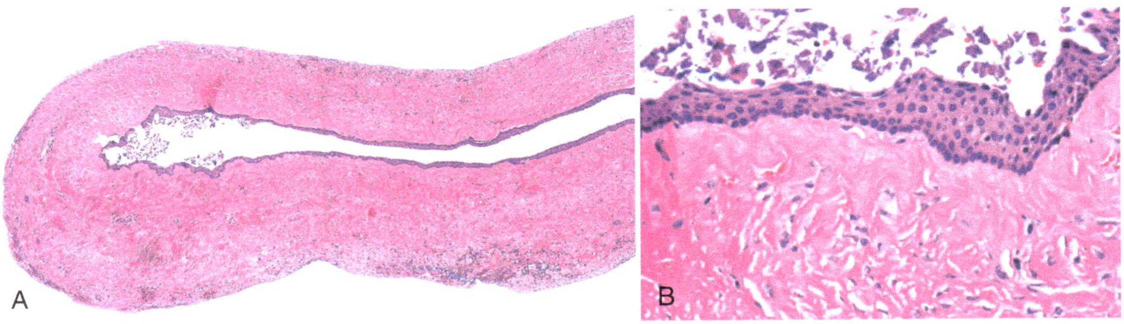

FIG 14.23 Dentigerous cyst. (A) Cyst lined by uniformly thin epithelium with little mural inflammation. (B) Lining is nonkeratinized stratified squamous epithelium 5 to 10 cells thick.

especially if the patient is symptomatic, and this should be reported as pericoronitis.

- Interestingly, *MAML2* rearrangement has been noted in 40% of dentigerous cysts (and one case of a radicular cyst) with mucous cell metaplasia.
- The dental follicle, which is the bulk of the soft tissue that envelops the tooth, is composed of delicately and sometimes more densely collagenous fibrous tissue with a distinctly myxoid/mucinous background, sometimes lined by reduced enamel epithelium composed of eosinophilic low cuboidal basal cells and columnar luminal cells (Fig. 14.26A–B); islands and strands of odontogenic epithelial rests are present to varying degrees, often with clear cells and sometimes keratin pearls; these odontogenic rests are often seen disposed parallel to or perpendicular to the lumen and identify the tissue as dental follicle; there may also be periepithelial and/or perivascular stromal hyalinization (Fig. 14.26C–H).
- Some radiolucencies described by clinicians as dentigerous cysts because of the size of the radiographic radiolucency maintain a lining of reduced enamel epithelium, and a diagnosis of dentigerous cyst is made.
- Fragments of dental papilla from an impacted tooth may be present and this is composed of delicately collagenous myxoid/mucinous tissue with spindle and stellate cells with a rounded configuration lined by odontoblasts (Fig. 14.27).
- Follicular hamartomas with psammomatoid and lamellar Liesegang-type dystrophic calcifications, "enameloid conglomerates," and epithelial rests (similar to structures seen in dental follicles around the "ghost teeth" of regional odontodysplasia) are seen in patients

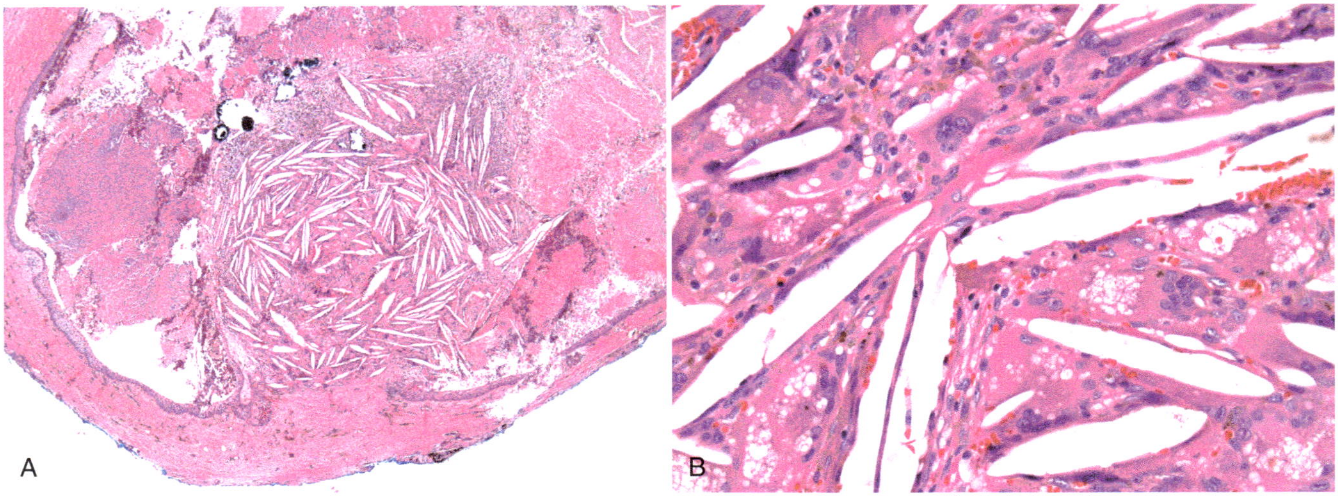

FIG 14.24 Dentigerous cyst. (A) Cholesterol granulomas are associated with disruption of the lining and hemorrhage. (B) Cholesterol granulomas consist of needle-shaped clefts associated with multinucleated giant cells and macrophages.

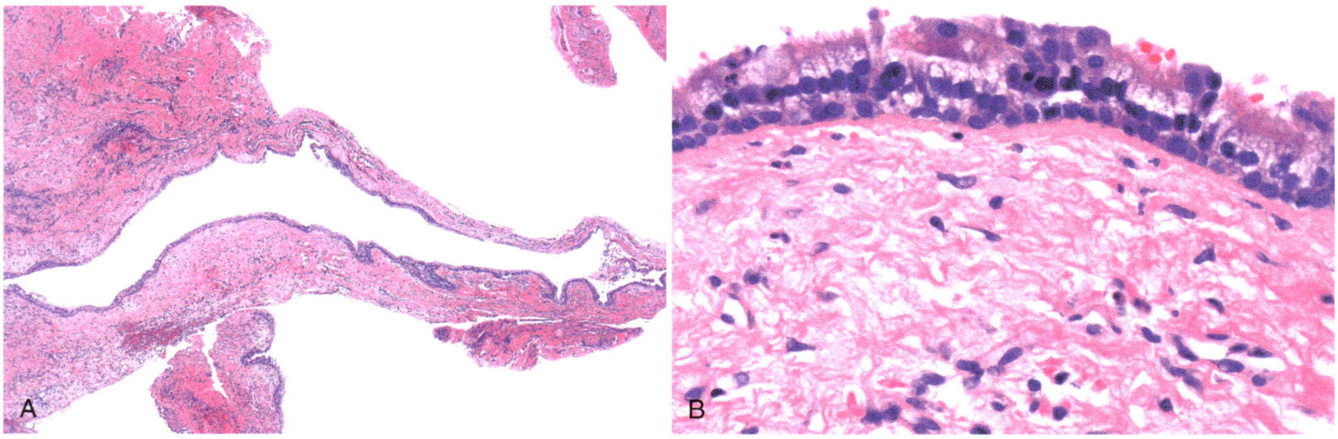

FIG 14.25 Dentigerous cyst. (A), Lining is uniformly 5 to 8 cells thick. (B) The cyst is lined by columnar, mucous, and ciliated cells.

(usually Black patients) with amelogenesis imperfecta, and gingival hyperplasia; however, they may occasionally be seen within conventional dental follicles (Fig. 14.28).

- Incipient calcifying epithelial odontogenic tumor-like areas may be seen within the follicular soft tissue composed of polyhedral cells with abundant eosinophilic cytoplasm, and slight nuclear atypia; the stroma is hyalinized resembling amyloid, although it is usually not congophilic (Fig. 14.29).
- The term "paradental cyst" has been used to describe a cyst with all the histopathologic features of a dentigerous cyst located on the buccal or distal aspect of a partially or fully erupted third molar that occurs in patients with the same demographic as a dentigerous cyst; these likely represent a buccally or distally displaced and inflamed dentigerous cyst, and most patients have a history of third molar infection/pericoronitis (Fig. 14.30); there have been recent suggestions that these arise from the crevicular epithelium because of positivity for keratins that are often seen in crevicular epithelium.

Differential Diagnosis

- Odontogenic myxomas are paucicellular tumors with scattered stellate-shaped and bipolar spindle cells with abundant mucinous/myxoid stroma resembling dental papilla, but without the latter's rounded configuration and presence of odontoblasts.
- Central odontogenic fibroma is more uniform and densely collagenous compared with the dental follicle, containing islands and strands of odontogenic epithelium and often dentinoid deposits.
- Intraosseous mucoepidermoid carcinoma is differentiated from a dentigerous cyst with mucous cell metaplasia by a proliferation of epidermoid cells, mucous cells, and intermediate cells with invasion of the stroma (Fig. 14.31); they are indistinguishable histopathologically from conventional salivary gland mucoepidermoid carcinoma and at least half (but not all) of such cases exhibit t(11:19) fusion gene transcript CRTC1-MAML2.
- Rarely, the dentigerous cyst lining may undergo malignant transformation and develop an intraosseous squamous cell carcinoma (see Chapter 15).

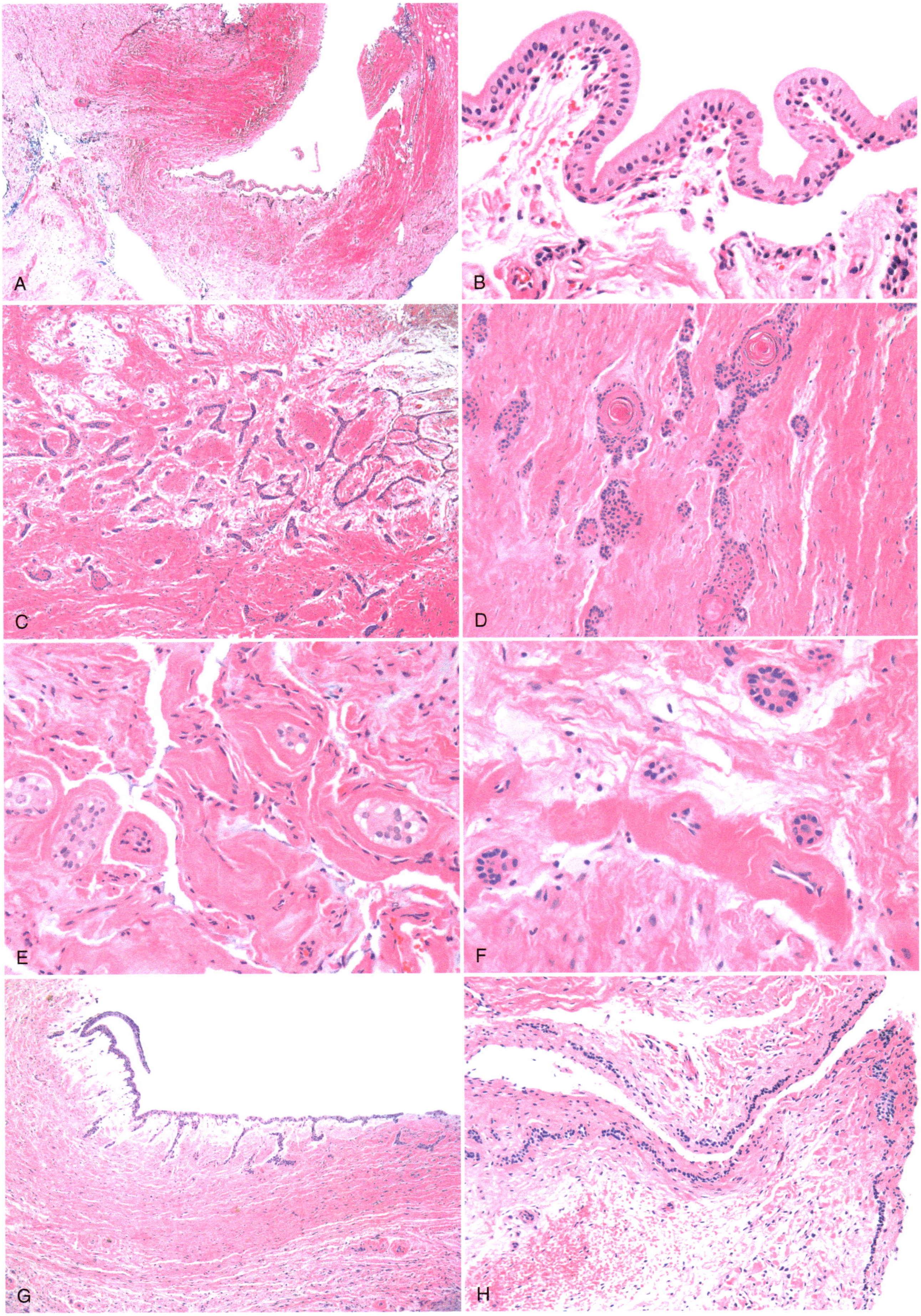

FIG 14.26 Dental follicle. (A) The follicle is lined by thin reduced enamel epithelium. (B) Reduced enamel epithelium has eosinophilic luminal columnar cells and low cuboidal basal cells. (C) Many islands of odontogenic rests may be present in the follicle. (D) Some islands may exhibit keratin pearl formation. (E) Islands may contain clear cells and exhibit periepithelial hyalinization. (F) Perivascular hyalinization is also common. (G) Epithelial islands may run perpendicular to the lumen. (H) Often islands of epithelium run parallel to the lumen.

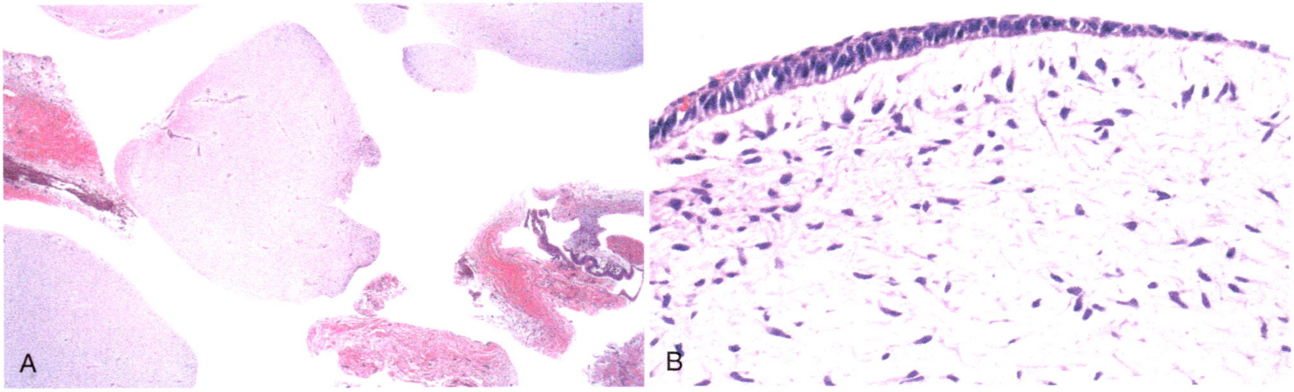

FIG 14.27 Dental papilla. (A) Several rounded fragments of delicately collagenous and mucinous/myxoid tissue; note reduced enamel epithelium and follicle on the *right*. (B) Papilla is myxoid/mucinous with plump, stellate fibroblasts, rimmed by a layer of columnar odontoblasts.

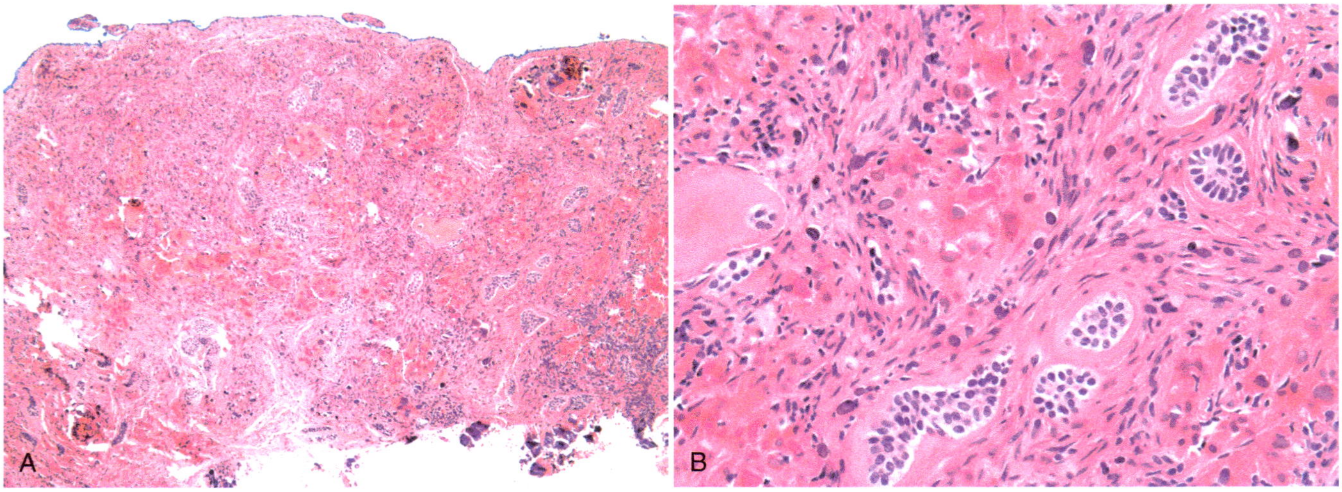

FIG 14.28 Follicle around regional odontodysplasia. (A) Fibrous tissue containing hyalinized material, psammomatoid dystrophic calcifications, and islands of odontogenic epithelium. (B) Many small islands of odontogenic epithelium, hyalinized dentinoid-like material, and basophilic psammomatoid calcifications (sometimes referred to as enameloid conglomerates).

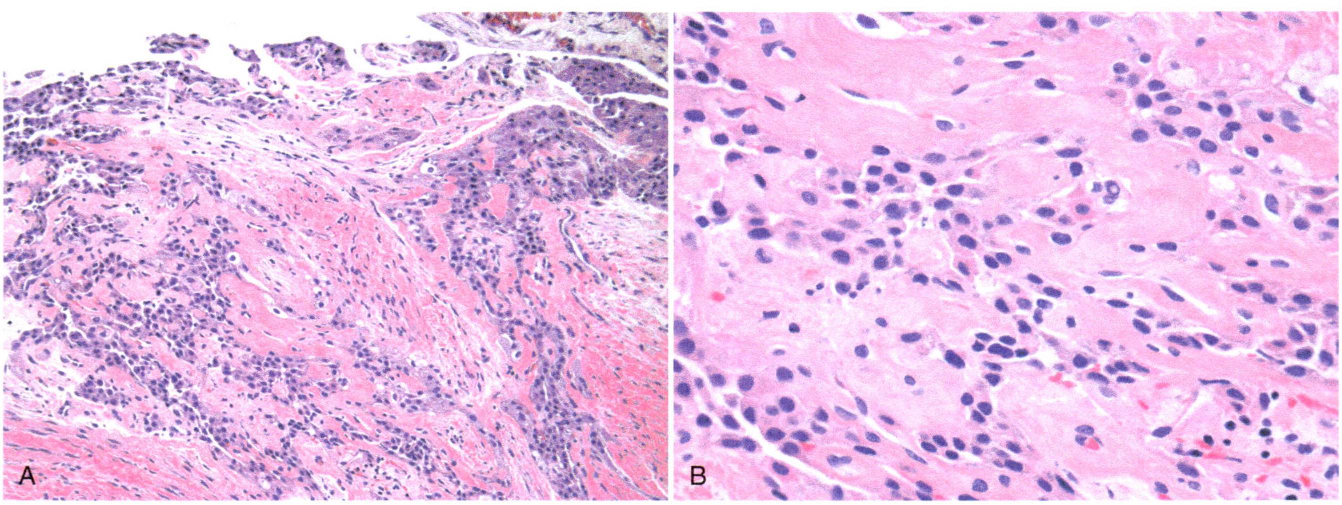

FIG 14.29 (A) Epithelial proliferation within the follicle in interconnected trabeculae resembling calcifying epithelial odontogenic tumor with hyalinization of stroma resembling amyloid. (B) Cells are polyhedral with abundant eosinophilic cytoplasm, slight nuclear atypia, and nuclear inclusions.

Management

- Enucleation or curettage with removal of the tooth is curative.

REFERENCES

Adeyemo WL. Do pathologies associated with impacted lower third molars justify prophylactic removal? A critical review of the literature. *Oral Surg Oral Med Oral Pathol Oral Radiol Endod.* 2006;102:448-452.

Argyris PP, Wehrs RN, Garcia JJ, Koutlas IG. Fluorescence in-situ hybridization identifies Mastermind-like 2 (MAML2) rearrangement in odontogenic cysts with mucous prosoplasia: a pilot study. *Histopathology.* 2015;66:791-797.

Azevedo RS, Mosqueda-Taylor A, Carlos R, et al. Calcifying epithelial odontogenic tumor (CEOT): a clinicopathologic and immunohistochemical study and comparison with dental follicles containing CEOT-like areas. *Oral Surg Oral Med Oral Pathol Oral Radiol.* 2013;116:759-768.

Bell D, Lewis C, El-Naggar AK, Weber RS. Primary intraosseous mucoepidermoid carcinoma of the jaw: Reappraisal of the MD Anderson Cancer Center experience. *Head Neck.* 2016;E312-E317.

Bodner L, Manor E, Friger MD, van der Waal I. Oral squamous cell carcinoma in patients twenty years of age or younger–review and analysis of 186 reported cases. *Oral Oncol.* 2014;50:84-89.

Buchner A, David R, Carpenter W, Leider A. Pigmented lateral periodontal cyst and other pigmented odontogenic lesions. *Oral Dis.* 1996;2:299-302.

Carlos R, Contreras-Vidaurre E, Almeida OP, et al. Regional odontodysplasia: morphological, ultrastructural, and immunohistochemical features of the affected teeth, connective tissue, and odontogenic remnants. *J Dent Child.* 2008;75:144-150.

Daley TD, Wysocki GP. The small dentigerous cyst. A diagnostic dilemma. *Oral Surg Oral Med Oral Pathol Oral Radiol Endod.* 1995;79:77-81.

Li Y, Li LJ, Huang J, et al. Central malignant salivary gland tumors of the jaw: retrospective clinical analysis of 22 cases. *J Oral Maxillofac Surg.* 2008;66:2247-2253.

Rakprasitkul S. Pathologic changes in the pericoronal tissues of unerupted third molars. *Quintessence Int.* 2001;32:633-638.

Roquebert D, Champsaur A, Gil del Real P, et al. Amelogenesis imperfecta, rough hypoplastic type, dental follicular hamartomas, and gingival hyperplasia: report of a case from Central America and review of the literature. *Oral Surg Oral Med Oral Pathol Oral Radiol Endod.* 2008;106:92-98.

Shahrabi Farahani S, Lotfalian M. A pigmented dentigerous cyst in a patient with multiple dentigerous cysts of the jaws: a case report. *J Contemp Dent Pract.* 2007;8:85-91.

Takeda Y, Oikawa Y, Furuya I, et al. Mucous and ciliated cell metaplasia in epithelial linings of odontogenic inflammatory and developmental cysts. *J Oral Sci.* 2005;47:77-81.

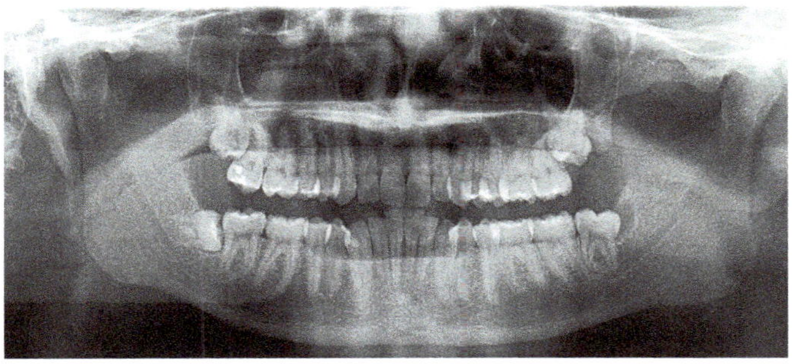

FIG 14.30 So-called paradental cyst distal to the left mandibular third molar; it is likely a distal dentigerous cyst.

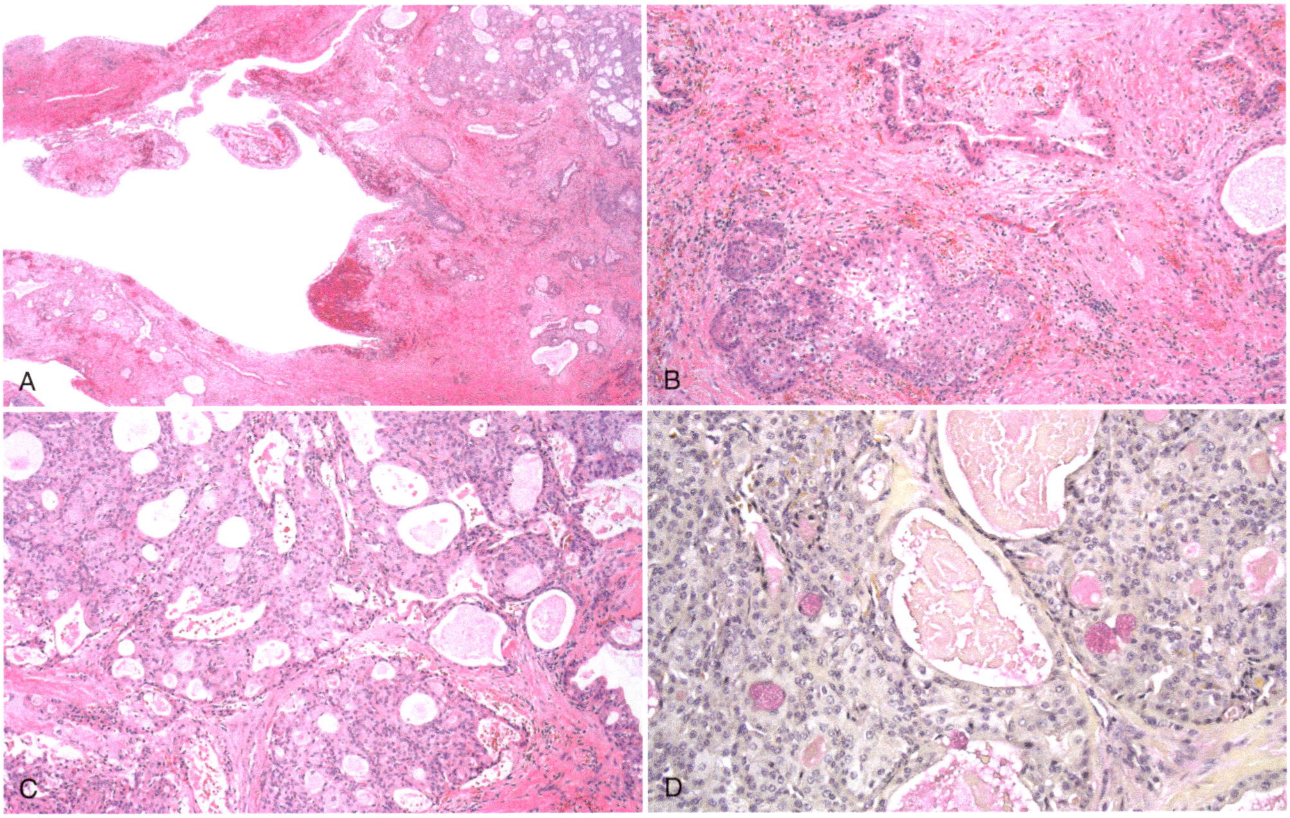

FIG 14.31 Mucoepidermoid carcinoma arising within a dentigerous cyst. (A) Infiltrative islands of tumor cells adjacent to a portion of the cyst lining. (B) Island of tumor cells adjacent to portion of a cyst lining exhibiting mucous cell metaplasia. (C) Tumor consists of epidermoid, mucous, and intermediate cells with duct formation. (D) Mucicarmine stain confirms presence of mucous cells.

Takeda Y, Yamamoto H. Case report of a pigmented dentigerous cyst and a review of the literature on pigmented odontogenic cysts. *J Oral Sci*. 2000;42:43-46.

Zhang LL, Yang R, Zhang L, et al. Dentigerous cyst: a retrospective clinicopathological analysis of 2082 dentigerous cysts in British Columbia, Canada. *Int J Oral Maxillofac Surg*. 2010;39:878-882.

LATERAL PERIODONTAL CYST AND BOTRYOID ODONTOGENIC CYST

The lateral periodontal cyst is considered the intraosseous counterpart of the gingival cyst of the adult and the botryoid odontogenic cyst is the multicystic variant.

Clinical Findings

- The lateral periodontal cyst usually affects those in the fifth to seventh decades of life and appears as an asymptomatic unilocular, round or pear-shaped radiolucency between two teeth that are vital, often resulting in splaying of the roots; 80% of cases occur in the mandible, usually in the canine-premolar area with the incisors being the next most common site (Fig. 14.32); rare cases are multifocal.
- A multiloculated radiolucency in the same location associated with vital teeth may represent a botryoid odontogenic cyst which has the same histopathology.

Etiopathogenesis and Histopathologic Features

The putative origin of the epithelium is rests of dental lamina.

- The epithelium is uniformly three to eight cells thick and composed of nonkeratinized stratified squamous or low cuboidal cells, with epithelial plaques composed of clear cells that contain glycogen and that may have a whorled, morular morphology (Figs. 14.33 and 14.34); a thickened basement membrane zone is often evident and the wall is densely collagenous and devoid of inflammation unless secondarily inflamed.
- The multicystic variant is the botryoid odontogenic cyst (Fig. 14.35).

Differential Diagnosis

- The glandular odontogenic cyst shares many features with the botryoid odontogenic cyst in that it is often complex and multicystic; in addition, there are duct-like structures and mucous cells; the luminal cells are cuboidal and eosinophilic (see later).

Management and Prognosis

- Enucleation or curettage is curative for the conventional lateral periodontal cyst.
- Botryoid odontogenic cysts have been reported to recur in as many as 18% to 30% of cases and it may be that some of these cysts represent the glandular odontogenic cyst.

REFERENCES

Buchner A, David R, Carpenter W, Leider A. Pigmented lateral periodontal cyst and other pigmented odontogenic lesions. *Oral Dis*. 1996;2:299-302.

Carter LC, Carney YL, Perez-Pudlewski D. Lateral periodontal cyst. Multifactorial analysis of a previously unreported series. *Oral Surg Oral Med Oral Pathol Oral Radiol Endod*. 1996;81:210-216.

Cohen DA, Neville BW, Damm DD, White DK. The lateral periodontal cyst. A report of 37 cases. *J Periodontol*. 1984;55:230-234.

Fantasia JE. Lateral periodontal cyst. An analysis of forty-six cases. *Oral Surg Oral Med Oral Pathol*. 1979;48:237-243.

Greer RO Jr, Johnson M. Botryoid odontogenic cyst: clinicopathologic analysis of ten cases with three recurrences. *J Oral Maxillofac Surg*. 1988;46:574-579.

Gurol M, Burkes EJ Jr, Jacoway J. Botryoid odontogenic cyst: analysis of 33 cases. *J Periodontol*. 1995;66:1069-1073.

Mendez P, Junquera L, Gallego L, Baladron J. Botryoid odontogenic cyst: clinical and pathological analysis in relation to recurrence. *Med Oral Patol Oral Cir Bucal*. 2007;12:E594-E598.

Rasmusson LG, Magnusson BC, Borrman H. The lateral periodontal cyst. A histopathological and radiographic study of 32 cases. *Br J Oral Maxillofac Surg*. 1991;29:54-57.

Santos PP, Freitas VS, Freitas Bde A, et al. Botryoid odontogenic cyst: a clinicopathologic study of 10 cases. *Ann Diagn Pathol*. 2011;15:221-224.

Siponen M, Neville BW, Damm DD, Allen CM. Multifocal lateral periodontal cysts: a report of 4 cases and review of the literature. *Oral Surg Oral Med Oral Pathol Endod*. 2011;111:225-233.

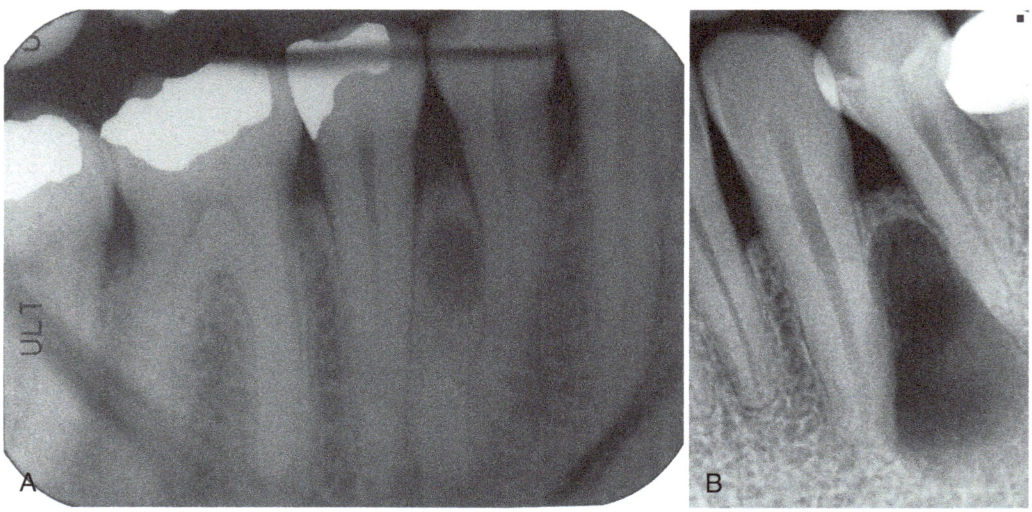

FIG 14.32 Lateral periodontal cyst. (A) Well-demarcated radiolucency between the vital right mandibular premolars. (B) Well-demarcated radiolucency between the mandibular canine and premolar with slight splaying of the roots. *(A, Courtesy Dr. Amy Field, private practice, Lowell, Mass.)*

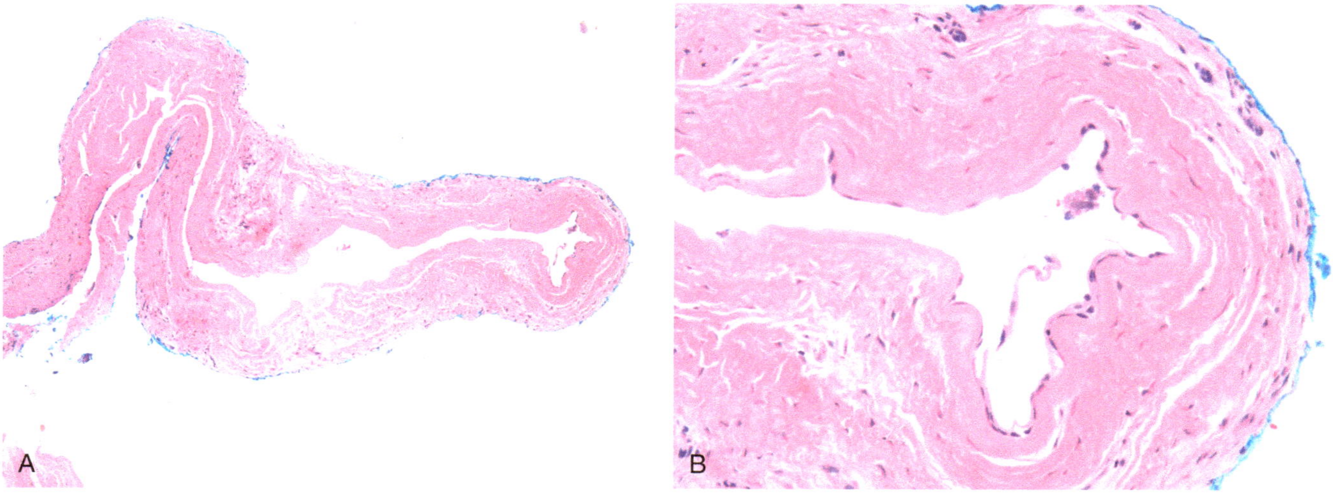

FIG 14.33 Lateral periodontal cyst. (A) The cyst has a thin lining, a thick basement membrane zone, and a fibrous wall without inflammation. (B) The lining consists of nonkeratinized stratified squamous epithelium that is only a few cells thick.

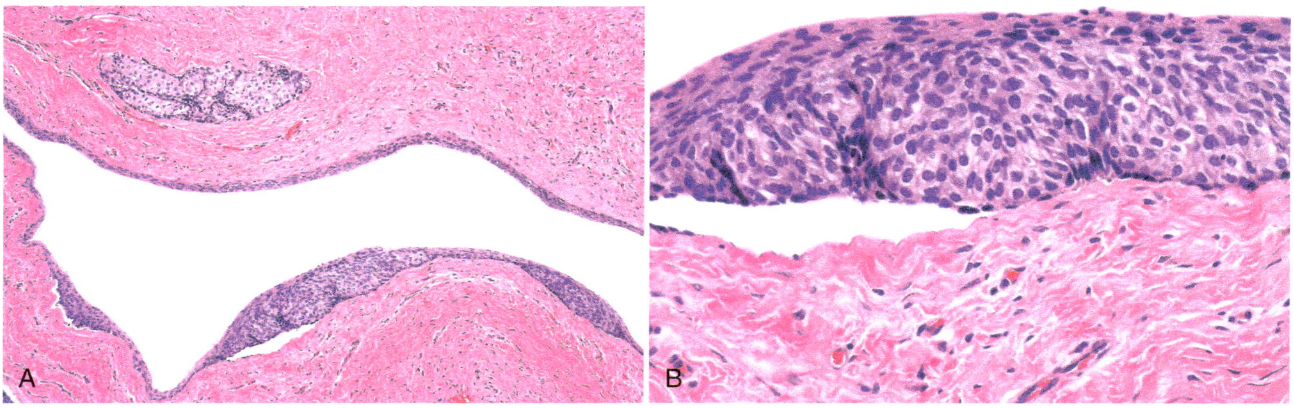

FIG 14.34 Lateral periodontal cyst. (A) The cyst lining is uniformly thin with epithelial plaques, and an odontogenic rest composed of clear cells is present in the wall that has no inflammation. (B) The epithelial plaque contains clear cells.

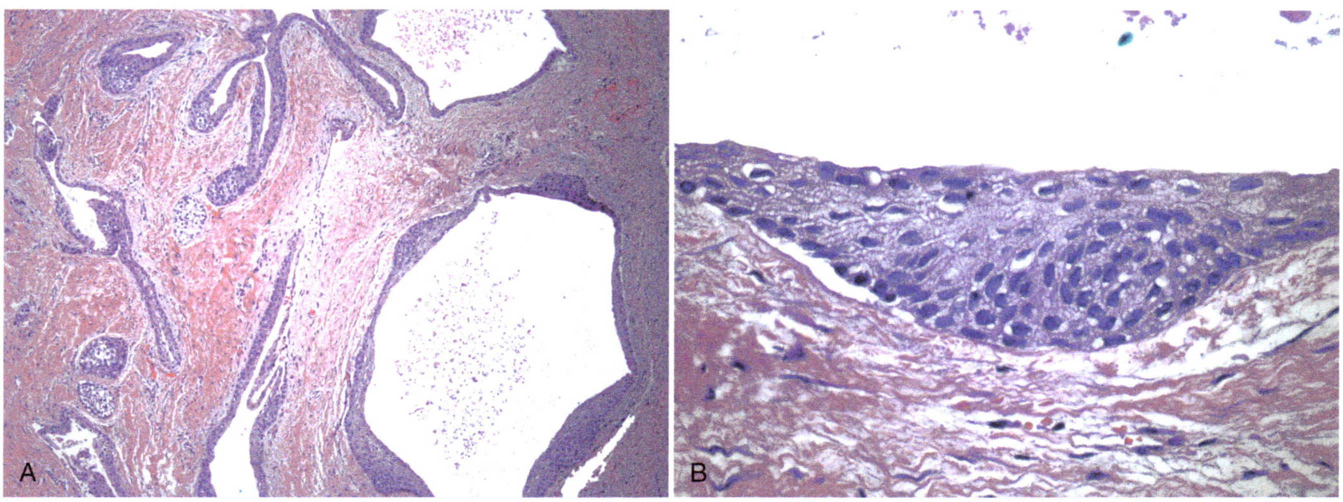

FIG 14.35 Botryoid odontogenic cyst. (A) There are multiple cystic structures lined by uniformly thin epithelium with epithelial plaques; the wall contains odontogenic rests with clear cells. (B) An epithelial plaque with slightly whorled morular morphology.

ORTHOKERATINIZED ODONTOGENIC CYST

Although this cyst is keratinizing it should not be confused with the keratocystic odontogenic tumor (odontogenic keratocyst) because of its different histopathology and behavior (see Chapter 15). This cyst constitutes 12% of keratinizing jaw cysts and cystic tumors.

Clinical Features

- The orthokeratinized odontogenic cyst is most common in the third and fourth decades with a 3:1 male predilection, and presents as a unilocular radiolucency in the mandible (90% of cases), mostly in the molar/ramus area; 5% to 10% are multilocular radiolucencies and at least 50% of cases are associated with an impacted tooth (Fig. 14.36); there is no association with nevoid basal cell carcinoma syndrome.

Etiopathogenesis and Histopathologic Features

This cyst likely arises from dental lamina rests and resembles an epithelial inclusion (epidermoid) cyst (see Chapter 2).

- The cyst epithelium is uniformly 5 to 15 cells thick and is surfaced with orthokeratin and a distinct granular layer; there is no palisading of basal cell nuclei and the interface is flat; abundant keratinaceous material fills the lumen and satellite cysts are not present (Fig. 14.37); rarely, sebaceous glands may be noted within the epithelium and cartilage within the wall.
- p63 is confined to basal and immediate parabasal cells whereas Ki-67 positivity is confined to scattered cells in the basal layer only (Fig. 14.38).

Differential Diagnosis

- If parakeratin is present, even focally, associated with basal cell palisading, a diagnosis of keratocystic odontogenic tumor (odontogenic keratocyst) must be made. Approximately 1% to 2% of keratocystic odontogenic tumors exhibit orthokeratin formation.

Management and Prognosis

- Excision or curettage is curative and the recurrence rate is insignificant.

REFERENCES

Chi AC, Neville BW, McDonald TA, et al. Jaw cysts with sebaceous differentiation: report of 5 cases and a review of the literature. *J Oral Maxillofac Surg.* 2007;65:2568-2574.

Crowley TE, Kaugars GE, Gunsolley JC. Odontogenic keratocysts: a clinical and histologic comparison of the parakeratin and orthokeratin variants. *J Oral Maxillofac Surg.* 1992;50:22-26.

Diniz MG, Galvao CF, Macedo PS, et al. Evidence of loss of heterozygosity of the PTCH gene in orthokeratinized odontogenic cyst. *J Oral Pathol Med.* 2011;40:277-280.

Dong Q, Pan S, Sun LS, Li TJ. Orthokeratinized odontogenic cyst: a clinicopathologic study of 61 cases. *Arch Pathol Lab Med.* 2010; 134:271-275.

Ide F, Saito I, Horie N, Shimoyama T. Orthokeratinized odontogenic cyst of the mandible with heterotopic cartilage. *Head Neck Pathol.* 2009;3:150-152.

Li TJ, Kitano M, Chen XM, et al. Orthokeratinized odontogenic cyst: a clinicopathological and immunocytochemical study of 15 cases. *Histopathology.* 1998;32:242-251.

Vuhahula E, Nikai H, Ijuhin N, et al. Jaw cysts with orthokeratinization: analysis of 12 cases. *J Oral Pathol Med.* 1993;22:35-40.

Wright JM. The odontogenic keratocyst: orthokeratinized variant. *Oral Surg Oral Med Oral Pathol.* 1981;51:609-618.

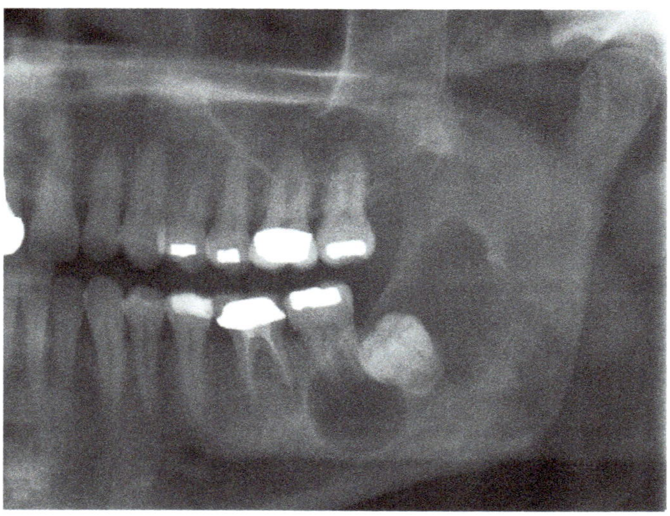

FIG 14.36 Orthokeratinized odontogenic cyst in a circumferential dentigerous relationship with the impacted left mandibular third molar. *(Courtesy Dr. David Moyer, private practice, Portland, Me.)*

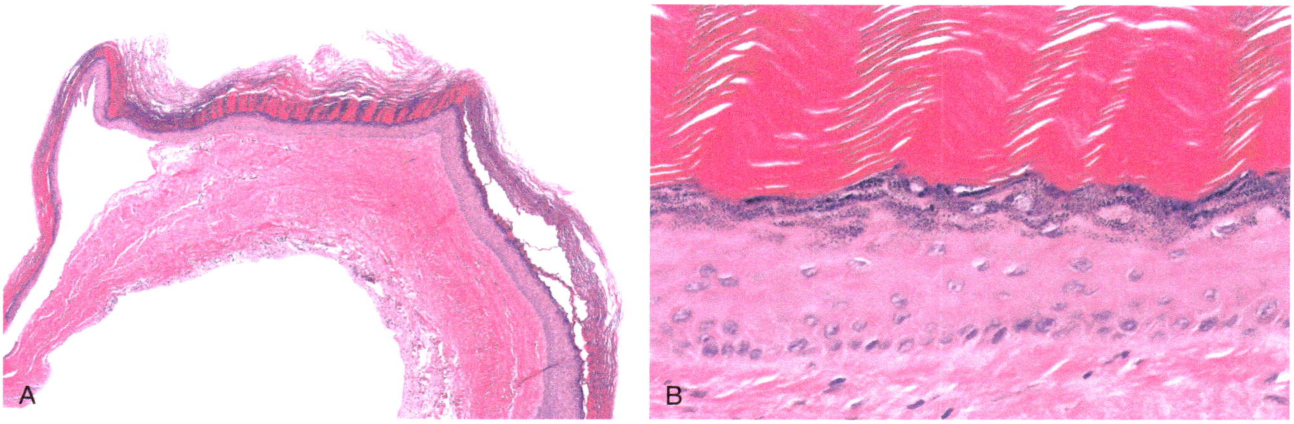

FIG 14.37 Orthokeratinized odontogenic cyst. (A) The cyst is lined by thickly orthokeratinized epithelium of variable thickness with no inflammation in the wall. (B) The epithelium is orthokeratinized with a granular layer and the basal cells do not show palisading of nuclei.

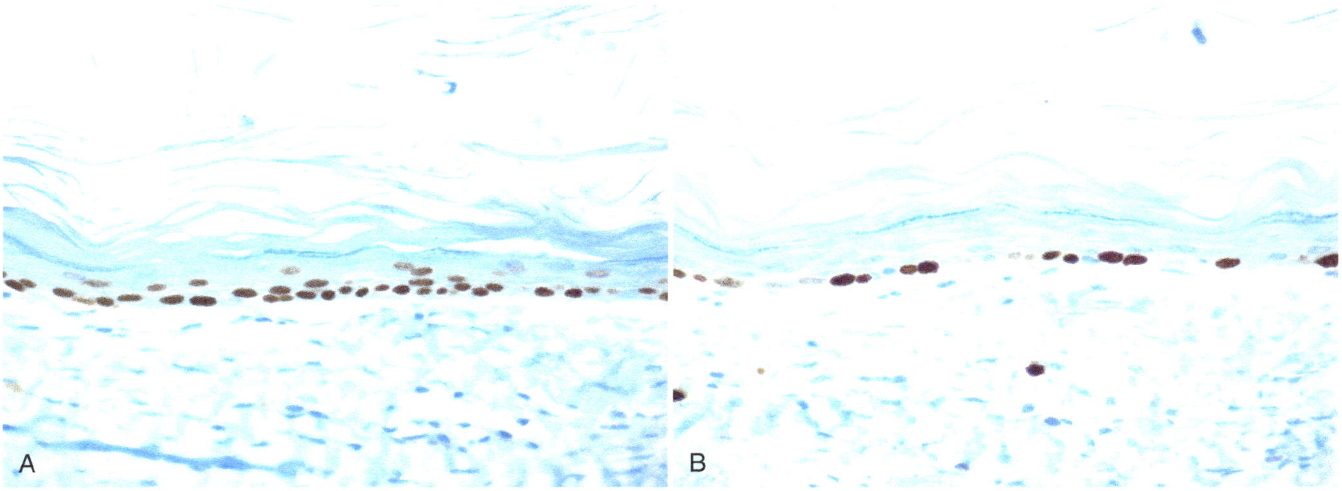

FIG 14.38 Orthokeratinized odontogenic cyst. (A) p63 is positivity noted in basal and parabasal cell nuclei. (B) Ki-67 is present in only scattered basal cell nuclei.

ODONTOGENIC CYST IN A GLOBULOMAXILLARY LOCATION

This cyst once was classified as a fissural cyst but has been reclassified as an odontogenic cyst.

Clinical Findings

- This odontogenic cyst occurs as a pear-shaped radiolucency between the maxillary canine and the lateral incisor often causing splaying of the roots of adjacent teeth (Fig. 14.39); the teeth adjacent to this cyst may be vital or nonvital.

Etiopathogenesis and Histopathologic Features

For a few decades it was believed that mesenchymal ingress rather than fusion of facial processes erased the globulomaxillary suture so that entrapment of epithelium did not occur and a fissural cyst could not develop at this site. Even though more recent evidence suggests that fusion of facial processes does exist and there is potential for entrapment of epithelium, two pieces of evidence support an odontogenic origin and refute a nonodontogenic process: (1) approximately 10% are keratocystic odontogenic tumors (odontogenic keratocysts), and (2) Rushton bodies, a product of odontogenic epithelium are sometimes noted.

- Histolopathologically they usually represent one of the following:
  - radicular cyst (if one/both of the adjacent teeth is/are nonvital) (Fig. 14.39)
  - lateral periodontal cyst
  - lateral dentigerous cyst from the maxillary canine, which tends to erupt late, is often impacted, and is often associated with a conventional dentigerous cyst (Fig. 14.40)
  - keratocystic odontogenic tumor (odontogenic keratocyst)
- The current practice is to identify the cyst specifically as one of the aforementioned entities rather than use the term *globulomaxillary cyst*.

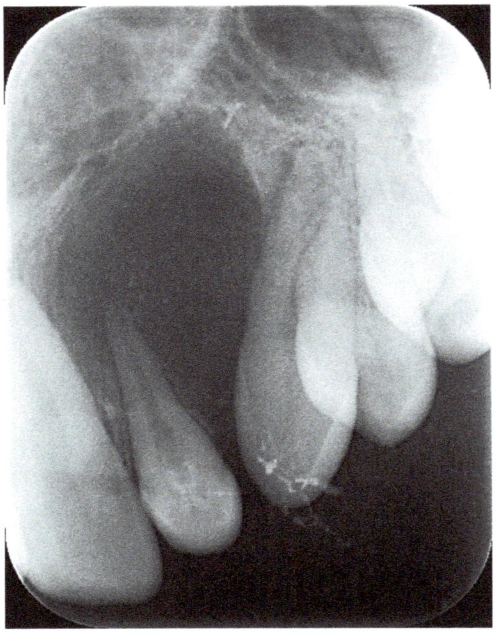

FIG 14.39 Odontogenic cyst in a globulomaxillary location causing splaying of the tooth roots. In this case, the canine was found to be nonvital and therefore this represented a radicular cyst.

Management and Prognosis

- Excision is curative.
- If a lateral radicular cyst is suspected, the adjacent teeth should be evaluated for vitality.

REFERENCES

Brannon RB. The odontogenic keratocyst. A clinicopathologic study of 312 cases. Part I. Clinical features. *Oral Surg Oral Med Oral Pathol.* 1976;42:54-72.

Dammer U, Driemel O, Mohren W, et al. Globulomaxillary cysts–do they really exist? *Clin Oral Investig.* 2014;18:239-246.

D'Silva NJ, Anderson L. Globulomaxillary cyst revisited. *Oral Surg Oral Med Oral Pathol.* 1993;76:182-184.

Wysocki GP, Goldblatt LI. The so-called "globulomaxillary cyst" is extinct. *Oral Surg Oral Med Oral Pathol.* 1993;76:185-186.

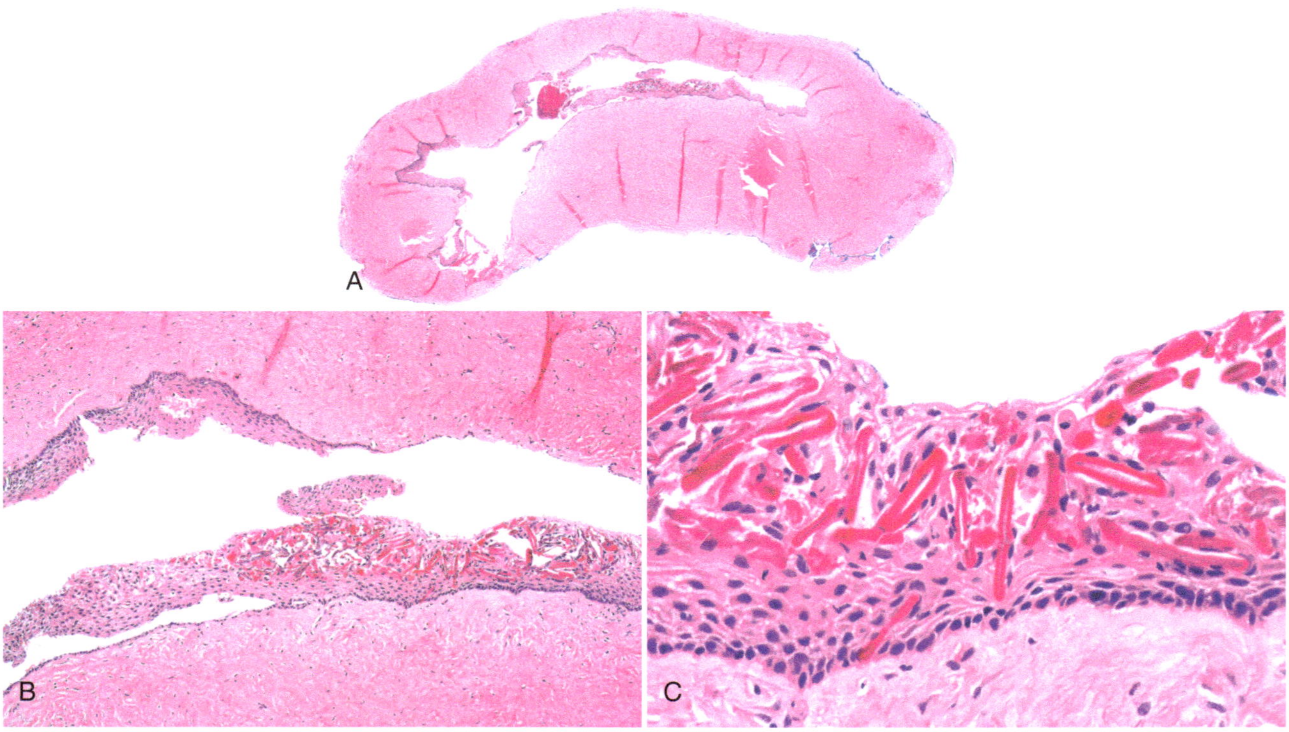

FIG 14.40 (A) Odontogenic cyst in a globulomaxillary location may sometimes represent a lateral dentigerous cyst. (B) The cyst is lined by uniformly thin epithelium with no mural inflammation. (C) Rushton bodies composed of brightly eosinophilic lamellar structures are present.

GLANDULAR ODONTOGENIC CYST (SIALOODONTOGENIC CYST)

This lesion is currently classified as a cyst but it demonstrates locally aggressive behavior and a high recurrence rate.

Clinical Findings

- The glandular odontogenic cyst occurs in adults in the fifth to seventh decade, usually in the mandible (80% of cases) and usually in the anterior (60% of cases) causing jaw expansion and facial swelling; it appears as a large unilocular or multilocular radiolucency (usually 5–6 cm), often crossing the midline with multiloculated lesions tending to be larger (Fig. 14.41).
- Lesions are associated with tooth displacement, root resorption (25–50% of cases) or impacted teeth (10–30% of cases); cortical perforation is seen in 60% of cases.

Etiopathogenesis and Histopathologic Features

The epithelium putatively arises from rests of dental lamina. It is no longer suspected to represent a precursor to central mucoepidermoid carcinoma because it lacks the *MAML2* rearrangement.

- The cyst has a complex architecture with multiple cystic compartments each lined by nonkeratinized stratified squamous epithelium with scattered mucous cells and ductlike or microcystic structures; the thickness of the epithelium is variable; luminal cells have a hobnail appearance and are often cuboidal with eosinophilic cytoplasm and exhibit “snouting”; epithelial plaques with a whorled configuration (epithelial spherules), clear cells, papillary tufts, and ciliated cells may be present (Figs. 14.42 and 14.43).
- The epithelium is positive for K19 throughout, basal cells are positive for K14, luminal cells for K8/18, and suprabasal cells for K10/13; epithelial plaques are positive for K7 and K14.

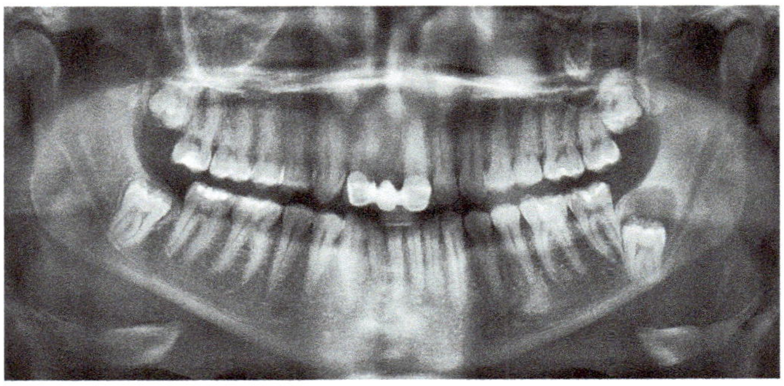

FIG 14.41 Glandular odontogenic cyst: unilocular radiolucency around impacted left mandibular third molar. *(Courtesy Dr. Steven Young, private practice, Johnston, RI.)*

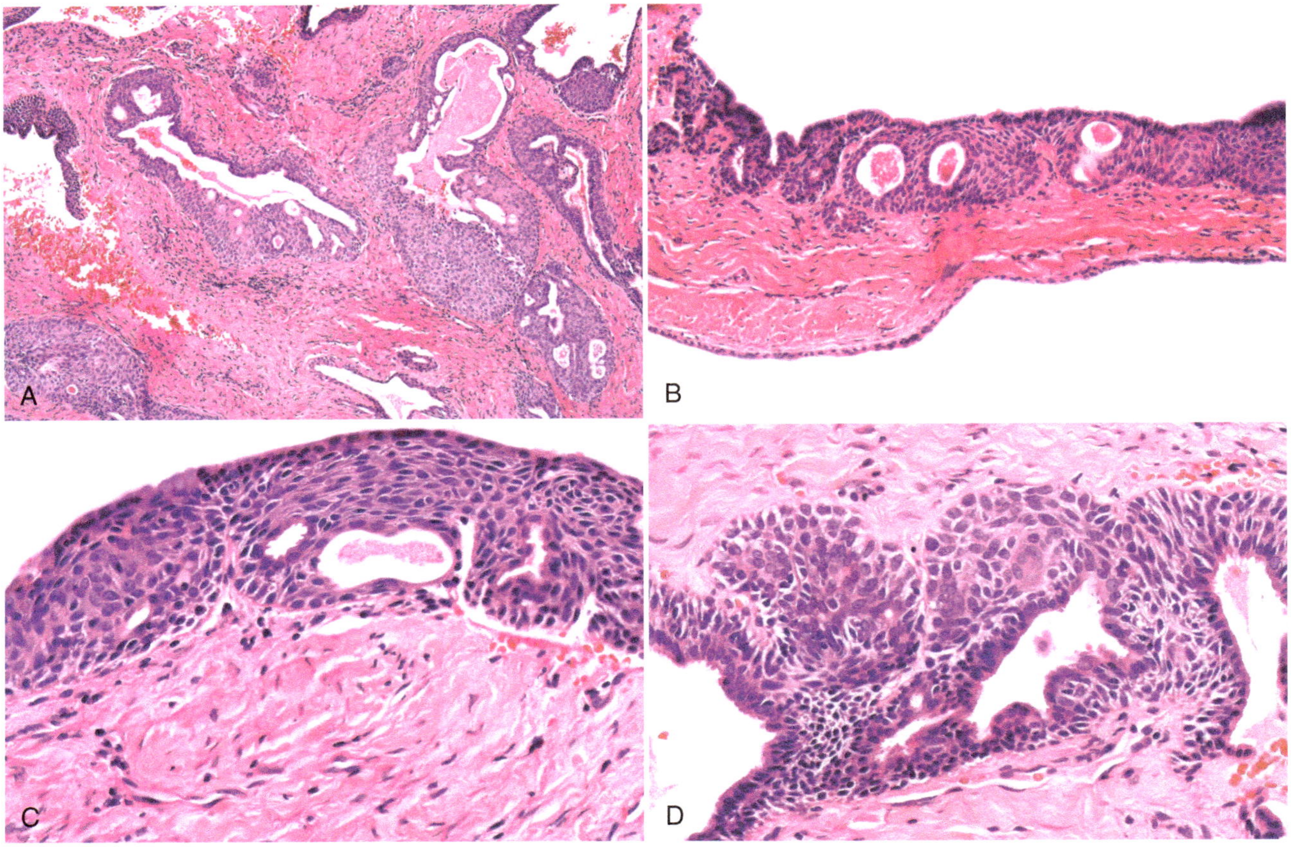

FIG 14.42 Glandular odontogenic cyst. (A) Multiple cystic structures lined by squamous cells with ductlike structures with very few mucous cells. (B) There is both simple thin cyst lining *(bottom)* and glandular cyst lining with ducts *(top)*. (C) Ducts are lined by eosinophilic cuboidal cells. (D) Luminal cells, often showing secretory activity and “snouting.”

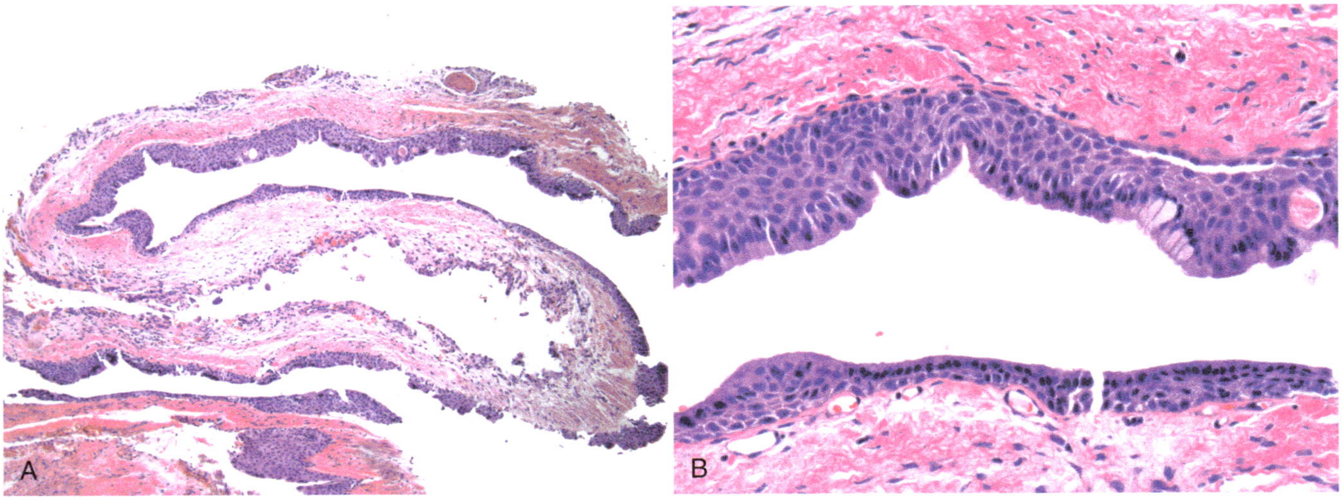

FIG 14.43 Glandular odontogenic cyst. (A) The cyst is lined by nonkeratinized stratified squamous epithelium that is uniformly thick with ductlike structures. (B) The lining contains eosinophilic, columnar luminal cells, clusters of mucous cells, a ductlike structure, and an epithelial plaque.

Differential Diagnosis

- Dentigerous cyst may show mucous cell metaplasia and ductlike structures focally but without the complexity noted in this lesion; some of these dentigerous cysts are positive for *MAML2* gene rearrangement.
- Mucoepidermoid carcinoma shows invasion of the stroma by polygonal epidermoid cells, intermediate cells, and mucous cells.
- Cystic lesions with thin epithelial lining and epithelial plaques alone are more likely botryoid odontogenic or lateral periodontal cysts.

Management and Prognosis

- Peripheral ostectomy, en bloc resection, and marginal resection are the treatments of choice; larger lesions, cortical perforation, and enucleation and curettage are associated with a higher rate of recurrence that varies from 14% to 30%.

REFERENCES

Bishop JA, Yonescu R, Batista D, et al. Glandular odontogenic cysts (GOCs) lack MAML2 rearrangements: a finding to discredit the putative nature of GOC as a precursor to central mucoepidermoid carcinoma. *Head Neck Pathol.* 2014;8:287-290.

Fowler CB, Brannon RB, Kessler HP, et al. Glandular odontogenic cyst: analysis of 46 cases with special emphasis on microscopic criteria for diagnosis. *Head Neck Pathol.* 2011;5:364-375.

Gratzinger D, Salama ME, Poh CF, Rouse RV. Ameloblastoma, calcifying epithelial odontogenic tumor, and glandular odontogenic cyst show a distinctive immunophenotype with some myoepithelial antigen expression. *J Oral Pathol Med.* 2008;37:177-184.

Kaplan I, Gal G, Anavi Y, et al. Glandular odontogenic cyst: treatment and recurrence. *J Oral Maxillofac Surg.* 2005;63:435-441.

Kaplan I, Anavi Y, Hirshberg A. Glandular odontogenic cyst: a challenge in diagnosis and treatment. *Oral Dis.* 2008;14:575-581.

Noffke C, Raubenheimer EJ. The glandular odontogenic cyst: clinical and radiological features; review of the literature and report of nine cases. *Dentomaxillofac Radiol.* 2002;31:333-338.

Shen J, Fan M, Chen X, et al. Glandular odontogenic cyst in China: report of 12 cases and immunohistochemical study. *J Oral Pathol Med.* 2006;35:175-182.

Vered M, Allon I, Buchner A, Dayan D. Is maspin immunolocalization a tool to differentiate central low-grade mucoepidermoid carcinoma from glandular odontogenic cyst? *Acta Histochem.* 2010;112:161-168.

PRIMORDIAL CYST

Clinical Features

- The primordial cyst is a unilocular radiolucency that develops in place of a tooth, although the tooth may be a supernumerary such as a mesiodens that occurs in the midline of the maxilla.

Etiopathogenesis and Histopathologic Features

Theoretically, the epithelium is derived from degeneration of the enamel organ without formation of a tooth, although others suggest that it may arise from dental lamina rests. This is an uncommon cyst and 40% to 50% of cases represent a keratocystic odontogenic tumor (odontogenic keratocyst) histopathologically. A diagnosis of primordial cyst can only be rendered if there is a clear history of a tooth being absent at the site of the cyst without a history of previous extraction.

- If not a keratocystic odontogenic tumor (see Chapter 15), the epithelium is that of a developmental odontogenic cyst, that is, nonkeratinized stratified squamous and generally 5 to 10 layers thick without inflammation within the lining or wall.

Differential Diagnosis

- A residual dentigerous cyst should be considered if an impacted tooth had been extracted from the same area.

Management and Prognosis

- Enucleation or complete curettage is curative unless the histopathology is that of a keratocystic odontogenic tumor (see Chapter 15).

REFERENCES

Brannon RB. The odontogenic keratocyst. A clinicopathologic study of 312 cases. Part I. Clinical features. *Oral Surg Oral Med Oral Pathol.* 1976;42:54-72.

Neville BW, Damm DD, Brock T. Odontogenic keratocysts of the midline maxillary region. *J Oral Maxillofac Surg.* 1997;55:340-344.

Woo SB, Eisenbud L, Kleiman M, Assael N. Odontogenic keratocysts in the anterior maxilla: report of two cases, one simulating a nasopalatine cyst. *Oral Surg Oral Med Oral Pathol.* 1987;64:463-465.

15 ODONTOGENIC TUMORS

CHAPTER CONTENTS

Odontogenic tumors are classified as follows: (1) epithelial tumors with mature fibrous stroma without ectomesenchyme, (2) epithelial tumors with production of ectomesenchyme, and (3) ectomesenchymal tumors with or without epithelium (usually rests) (Fig. 15.1). Epithelial tumors are likely to derive from rests of dental lamina, and mesenchymal tumors from precursor mesenchymal cells that recapitulate formation of the dental papilla, follicle, periodontal tissues, and osteocementum. Those that produce significant amounts of calcified tissues will exhibit radiopacities on imaging studies. Some odontogenic neoplasms exhibit histopathologic patterns of several tumors, and these are called *combined* or *hybrid odontogenic tumors.* Attention has been focused on molecular findings in odontogenic tumors, particularly on changes in the Wnt signaling pathway that may be involved in odontogenesis, cell proliferation and migration, and cell fate specification, as well as mutations in *BRAF* (specifically $BRAF^{V600E}$) that lead to production of mutant protein kinases leading to dysregulation of the mitogen-activated protein kinase (MAPK) signaling pathway.

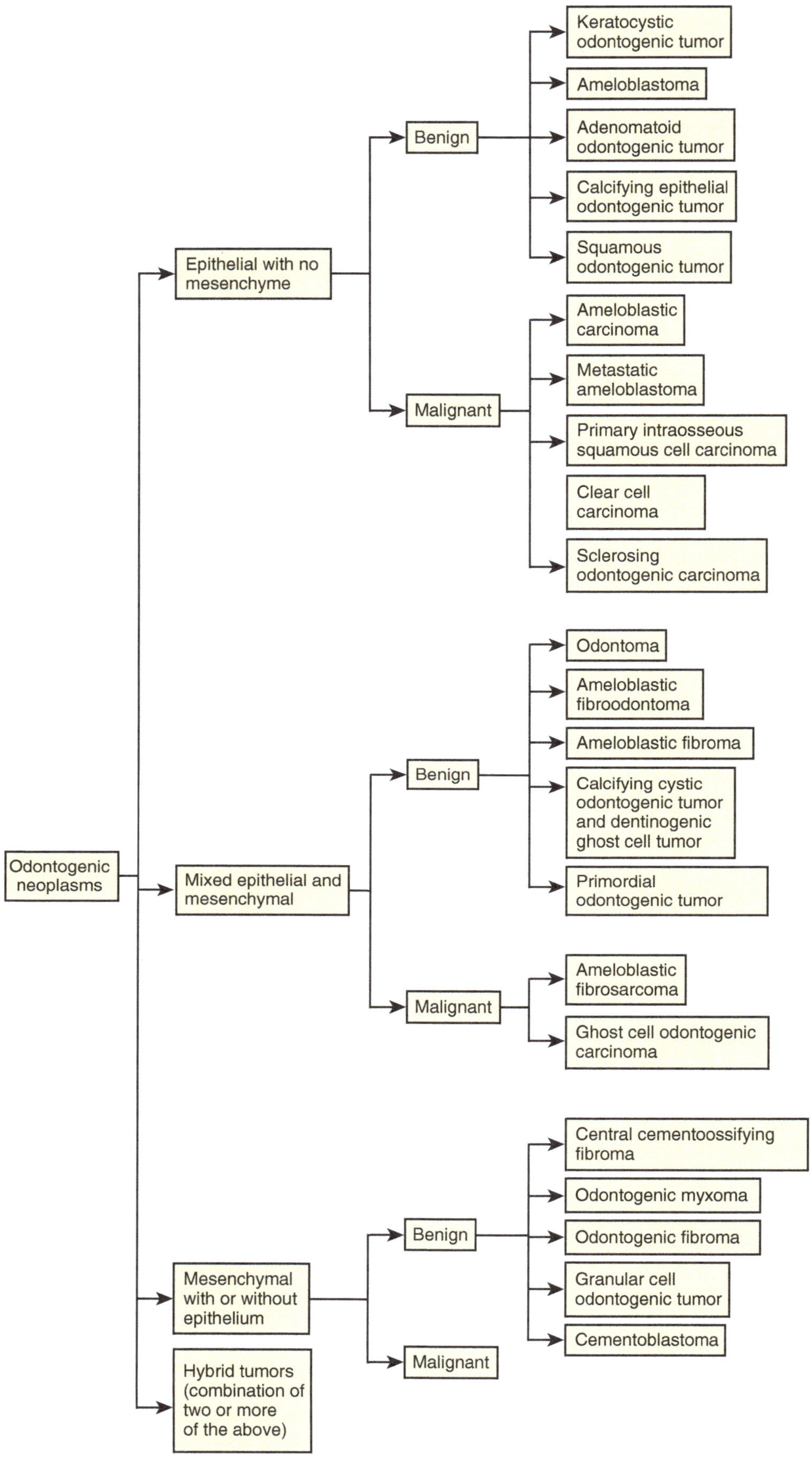

FIG 15.1 Classification of odontogenic tumors.

Extraosseous Odontogenic Neoplasms

Any odontogenic tumor may occur within the soft tissue of the gingiva (peripheral or extraosseous). The most common odontogenic tumors are the peripheral odontogenic fibroma (approximately 50% of all cases of peripheral odontogenic tumors), peripheral ameloblastoma, and peripheral calcifying cystic odontogenic tumor (CCOT). Even odontomas may occur in an extraosseous site, and all behave in a benign fashion. Theoretically, any of the tumors may have malignant counterparts and only the well-characterized ones are discussed in this chapter.

Epithelial Tumors Without Ectomesenchyme

KERATOCYSTIC ODONTOGENIC TUMOR (ODONTOGENIC KERATOCYST)

This is one of the conditions that occurs almost always in the nevoid basal cell carcinoma syndrome (Gorlin-Goltz or Gorlin syndrome). In 2005, this lesion was reclassified by the World Health Organization as a cystic neoplasm because of its locally aggressive behavior, high proliferation indices, mutation of *PTCH1* in most syndromic cases and some nonsyndromic cases, and high recurrence rate. Those arguing against such a reclassification cite a lack of clonality, loss of heterozygosity of *PTCH1* in other developmental odontogenic cysts, and alteration of the cystic lining or even resolution of the lesion with decompression.

Clinical Findings

- Forty percent of sporadic cases occur in the third and fourth decades of life, with a 2:1 male predilection. Cysts in syndromic cases are generally diagnosed in the first and second decades of life, and patients tend to develop multiple lesions. Swelling tends to occur in larger, long-standing lesions.
- Approximately 80% of cases present as unilocular and the rest as multilocular radiolucencies, usually in the posterior mandible and/or ramus area (70% of cases). The radiolucency expands along the long axis of the jaw bones anteroposteriorly rather than buccal-lingually or superoinferiorly. Twenty-five to thirty-three percent of cases are associated with an impacted tooth (Fig. 15.2A–C).
- Those arising in the midline of the maxilla in the vicinity of the incisive (nasopalatine) canal occur in patients in the seventh decade of life or older, with a 3:1 male predilection. This may represent a primordial cyst from a mesiodens.
- Patients with the nevoid basal cell carcinoma syndrome, an autosomal dominant condition associated with mutation of *PTCH1*, have not only multiple cystic lesions in the jaw in early childhood (Fig. 15.2D) but also many basal cell carcinomas starting within the first three decades of life, as well as hypertelorism, rib abnormalities (such as bifid, missing, or fused ribs), calcification of the falx cerebri, palmar-plantar pits, cutaneous epidermal cysts, ovarian fibromas, medulloblastomas, and other malformations. This cystic tumor has been reported in peripheral or extraosseous sites, such as the gingiva, as well as in the buccal mucosa.

Etiopathogenesis and Histopathologic Features

This tumor is believed to arise from proliferation of dental lamina rests. Mutations in *PTCH1*, a tumor suppressor gene mapped to chromosome 9q22.3-q31, are seen in keratocystic odontogenic tumor (odontogenic keratocyst) in the nevoid basal cell carcinoma syndrome, an autosomal dominant condition, in over 80% of cases and in approximately 30% of sporadic cases of this cystic tumor. Allelic losses have also been identified for other tumor suppressor genes (namely, *MTS1*, *TP53*, and *MCC*).

- The epithelium is uniformly 5 to 10 cells thick, with parakeratosis, often with a corrugated surface, palisading of the basal cell nuclei, and a flat interface. Basal cell hyperplasia and dysmaturation with occasional mitotic figures are not uncommon, as are epithelial buds. However, if inflammation is present, these typical features are lost or may be subtle or focal, and may lead to a misdiagnosis. Focal areas may be covered by orthokeratin, and the lining may show mucous and ciliated cell metaplasia (Figs. 15.3–15.5).
- Satellite cysts are often present within the wall and sometimes within the deep lamina propria of the oral mucosa if the cortical plate is perforated. The latter may be associated with a higher recurrence rate and should be reported (Fig. 15.6). Syndromic cases have a higher frequency of satellite cysts.
- Marsupialization or exteriorization of the cyst and flushing with a caustic agent results in loss of the parakeratin layer. Cartilage and melanin pigment may be seen. A solid variant has been reported and is composed of back-to-back cysts filled with keratin. The relationship of this cyst with keratoameloblastoma is unclear (see later). Keratin 4 (K4), K13, K17, and K19, as well as BCL2, have been identified in the cyst epithelium.
- Compared with other odontogenic cysts, there are high proliferating cell nuclear antigen and Ki-67 indices, and positivity for p53 and p63 involving basal and suprabasal cells (see Fig. 15.3C–D). Recurrence may be associated with cases exhibiting higher labeling indices for Ki-67.

Differential Diagnosis

Orthokeratinized odontogenic cyst is lined entirely by orthokeratin with a granular layer, does not exhibit palisaded basal cells or satellite cysts, and has a low Ki-67 index and a low recurrence rate (see Chapter 14).

- Some basal cell hyperplasia and dysmaturation is acceptable and, unless other features of atypia are present, should not be diagnosed as dysplasia.
- Cystic ameloblastoma has no parakeratosis, although the luminal cells are large, with abundant eosinophilic cytoplasm, and exhibit stellate reticulum–like areas

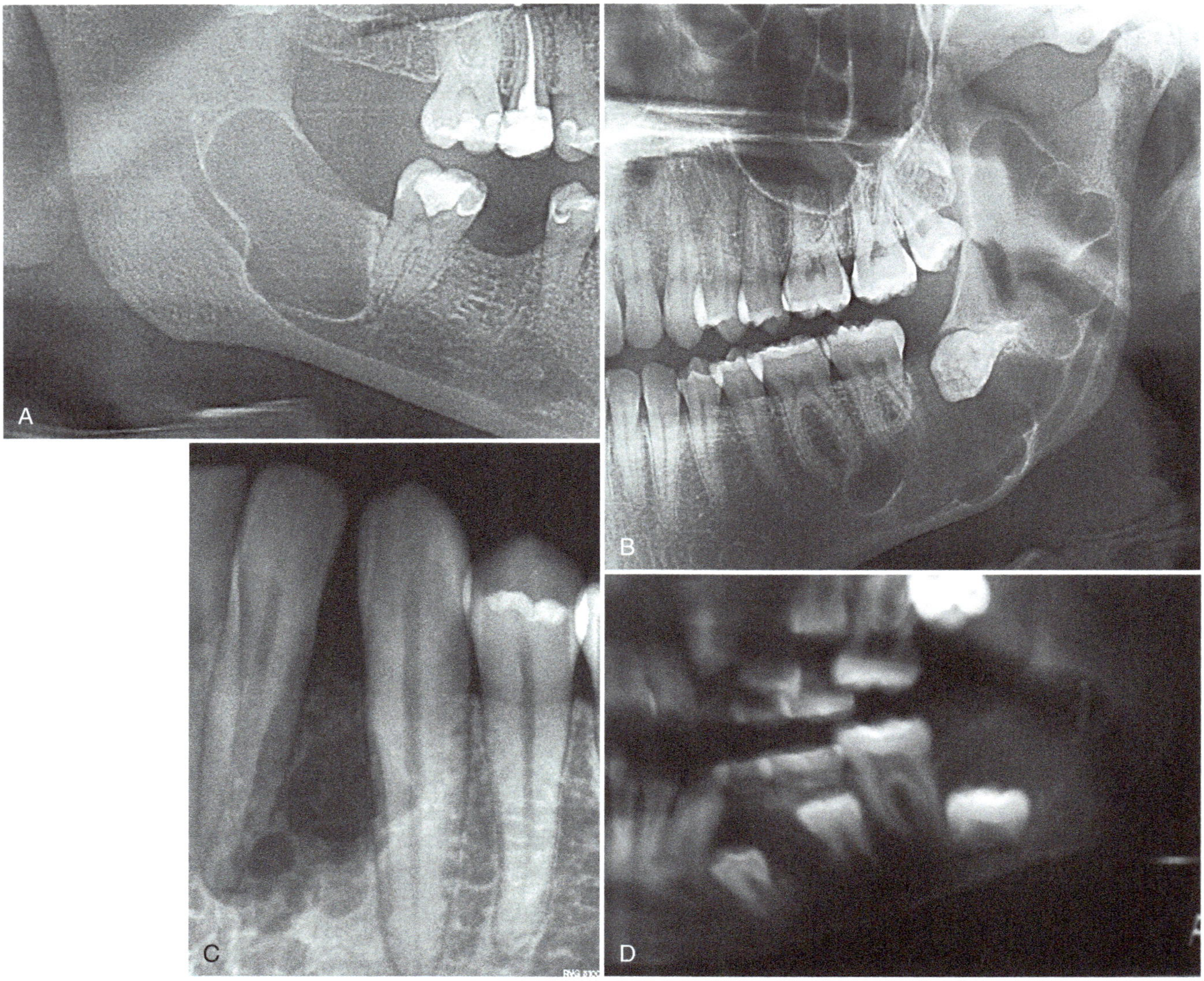

FIG 15.2 Keratocystic odontogenic tumor. (A) Unilocular radiolucency of the right posterior mandible. (B) Multilocular radiolucency of the left mandible. (C) Multiloculated radiolucency between two vital teeth noted on periapical film. (D) Anterior and left mandibular cystic tumors overlying impacted teeth in a child with nevoid basal cell carcinoma syndrome. *(A, Courtesy Dr. David Moyer, private practice, South Portland, Me; B, Courtesy Dr. John Biernacki, private practice, Cumberland, RI; C, Courtesy Dr. Melissa Hamilton, private practice, Taunton, Mass; D, Courtesy Dr. Dr. Leonard Kaban, Massachusetts General Hospital, Boston.)*

and palisaded basal cell nuclei with reverse nuclear polarization.

Management and Prognosis

- Recurrence rate varies from 10% to 40%, depending on how the tumor is managed and the experience of the surgeon, with curettage associated with the highest recurrence rate.
- Enucleation with adjunctive measures such as application of Carnoy solution, peripheral ostectomy, cryosurgery, and electrocautery is associated with a low recurrence rate and is tissue-sparing.
- Marsupialization and daily irrigation followed by cystectomy is also associated with a low recurrence rate and is organ-sparing.
- En bloc excision may be necessary for recurrent lesions that have failed other therapies and is not usually first-line therapy.
- Vismodegib, a hedgehog pathway inhibitor, has been shown to shrink these cystic tumors in syndromic patients.

REFERENCES

Agaram NP, Collins BM, Barnes L, et al. Molecular analysis to demonstrate that odontogenic keratocysts are neoplastic. *Arch Pathol Lab Med.* 2004;128:313-317.

Ally MS, Tang JY, Joseph T, et al. The use of vismodegib to shrink keratocystic odontogenic tumors in patients with basal cell nevus syndrome. *JAMA Dermatol.* 2014;150:542-545.

Aragaki T, Michi Y, Katsube K, et al. Comprehensive keratin profiling reveals different histopathogenesis of keratocystic odontogenic

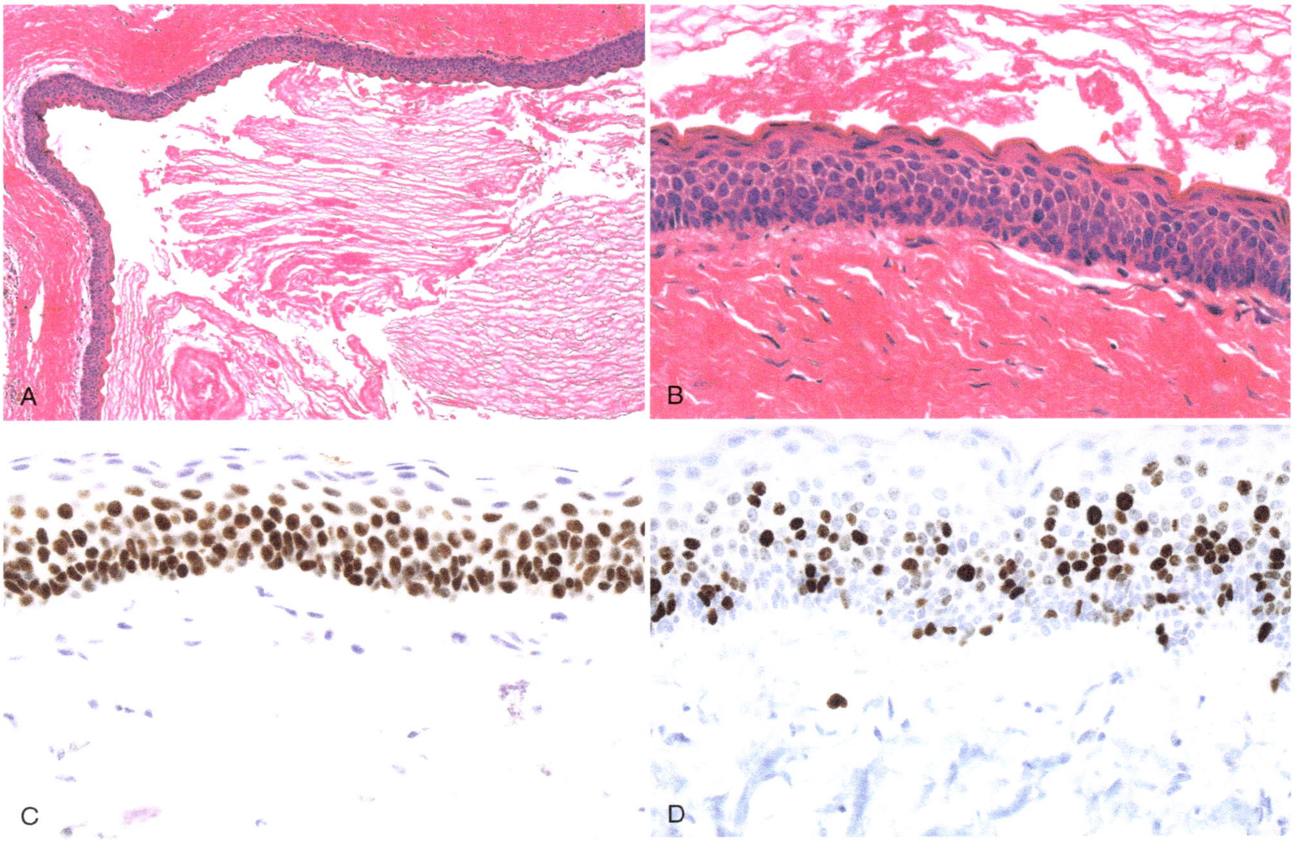

FIG 15.3 Odontogenic keratocyst. (A) Cyst lined by uniformly thin epithelium with abundant keratin in the lumen. (B) Lining is 5–15 cells thick with parakeratosis, surface corrugations, and palisading of basal cell nuclei. (C) Strong nuclear staining of most cells for p63, excluding parakeratin. (D) Strong nuclear staining for Ki-67 in at least 30% of nuclei scattered throughout the epithelium.

tumor and orthokeratinized odontogenic cyst. *Hum Pathol.* 2010;41: 1718-1725.

August M, Faquin WC, Troulis MJ, Kaban LB. Dedifferentiation of odontogenic keratocyst epithelium after cyst decompression. *J Oral Maxillofac Surg.* 2003;61:678-683, discussion 683–684.

Boffano P, Ruga E, Gallesio C. Keratocystic odontogenic tumor (odontogenic keratocyst): preliminary retrospective review of epidemiologic, clinical, and radiologic features of 261 lesions from University of Turin. *J Oral Maxillofac Surg.* 2010;68:2994-2999.

Brannon RB. The odontogenic keratocyst: a clinicopathologic study of 312 cases. Part II. Histologic features. *Oral Surg Oral Med Oral Pathol.* 1977;43:233-255.

Buchner A, Merrell PW, Carpenter WM. Relative frequency of central odontogenic tumors: a study of 1,088 cases from Northern California and comparison to studies from other parts of the world. *J Oral Maxillofac Surg.* 2006;64:1343-1352.

Chi AC, Owings JR Jr, Muller S. Peripheral odontogenic keratocyst: report of two cases and review of the literature. *Oral Surg Oral Med Oral Pathol Oral Radiol Endod.* 2005;99 71-78.

Dominguez FV, Keszler A. Comparative study of keratocysts, associated and non-associated with nevoid basal cell carcinoma syndrome. *J Oral Pathol.* 1988;17:39-42.

Fornatora ML, Reich RF, Chotkowski G, Freedman PD. Odontogenic keratocyst with mural cartilaginous metaplasia: a case report and a review of the literature. *Oral Surg Oral Med Oral Pathol Oral Radiol Endod.* 2001;92:430-434.

Geng N, Lv D, Chen QM, et al. Solid variant of keratocystic odontogenic tumor with ameloblastomatous transformation: a case report and review of the literature. *Oral Surg Oral Med Oral Pathol Oral Radiol.* 2012;114:223-229.

Gurgel CA, Ramos EA, Azevedo RA, et al. Expression of Ki-67, p53 and p63 proteins in keratocyst odontogenic tumours: an immunohistochemical study. *J Mol Histol.* 2008;39:311-316.

Henley J, Summerlin DJ, Tomich C, et al. Molecular evidence supporting the neoplastic nature of odontogenic keratocyst: a laser capture microdissection study of 15 cases. *Histopathology.* 2005;47: 582-586.

John AM, Schwartz RA. Basal cell nevus syndrome: an update on genetics and treatment. *Br J Dermatol.* 2016;174:68-76.

Kaminagakura E, Almeida JD, Carvalho YR, et al. Keratocyst of the buccal mucosa: case report and immunohistochemical comparative study with sporadic intraosseous keratocystic odontogenic tumor. *Oral Surg Oral Med Oral Pathol Oral Radiol.* 2013;116: e387-e392.

Kolar Z, Geierova M, Bouchal J, et al. Immunohistochemical analysis of the biological potential of odontogenic keratocysts. *J Oral Pathol Med.* 2006;35:75-80.

Kuroyanagi N, Sakuma H, Miyabe S, et al. Prognostic factors for keratocystic odontogenic tumor (odontogenic keratocyst): analysis of clinico-pathologic and immunohistochemical findings in cysts treated by enucleation. *J Oral Pathol Med.* 2009;38:386-392.

Myoung H, Hong SP, Hong SD, et al. Odontogenic keratocyst: review of 256 cases for recurrence and clinicopathologic parameters. *Oral Surg Oral Med Oral Pathol Oral Radiol Endod.* 2001;91:328-333.

Wright JM, Odell EW, Speight PM, Takata T. Odontogenic tumors, WHO 2005: where do we go from here? *Head Neck Pathol.* 2014;8: 373-382.

Wushou A, Zhao YJ, Shao ZM. Marsupialization is the optimal treatment approach for keratocystic odontogenic tumour. *J Craniomaxillofac Surg.* 2014;42:1540-1544.

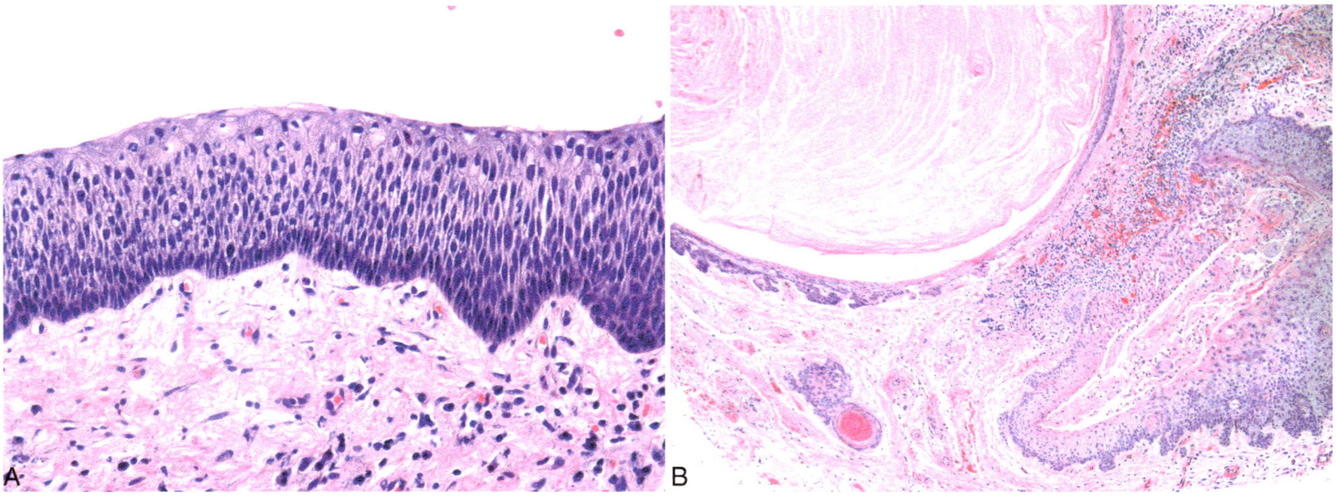

FIG 15.4 Odontogenic keratocyst. (A) Lining shows dysmaturation in the form of basal cell hyperplasia. (B) Lining shows budding of the basal cells, and there are satellite cysts and keratin pearls within satellites.

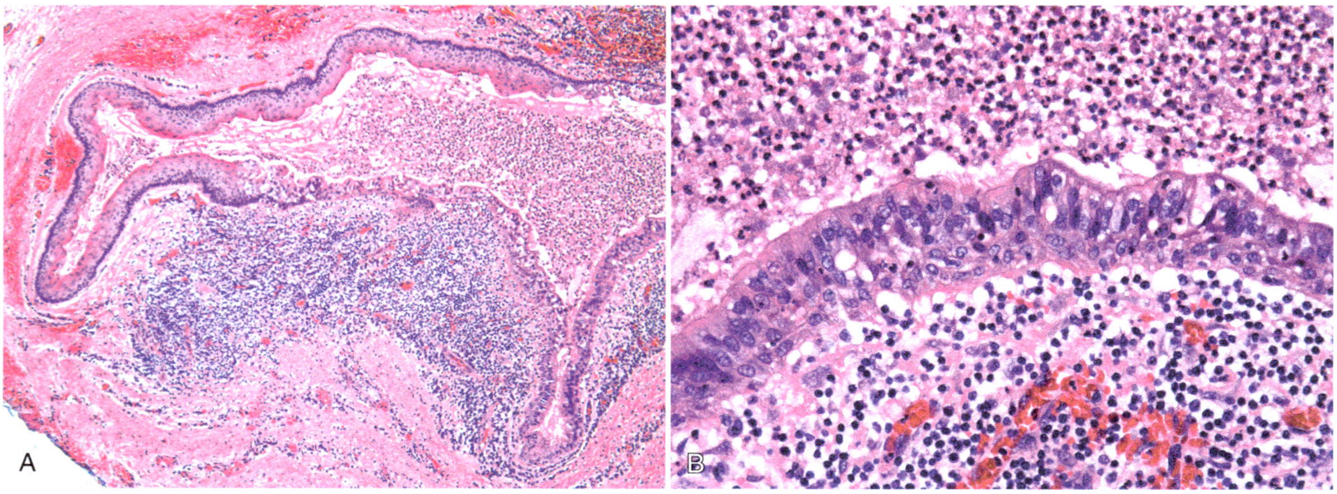

FIG 15.5 Odontogenic keratocyst. (A) The typical cyst lining is lost where there is inflammation. (B) This image shows ciliated and mucous cell metaplasia.

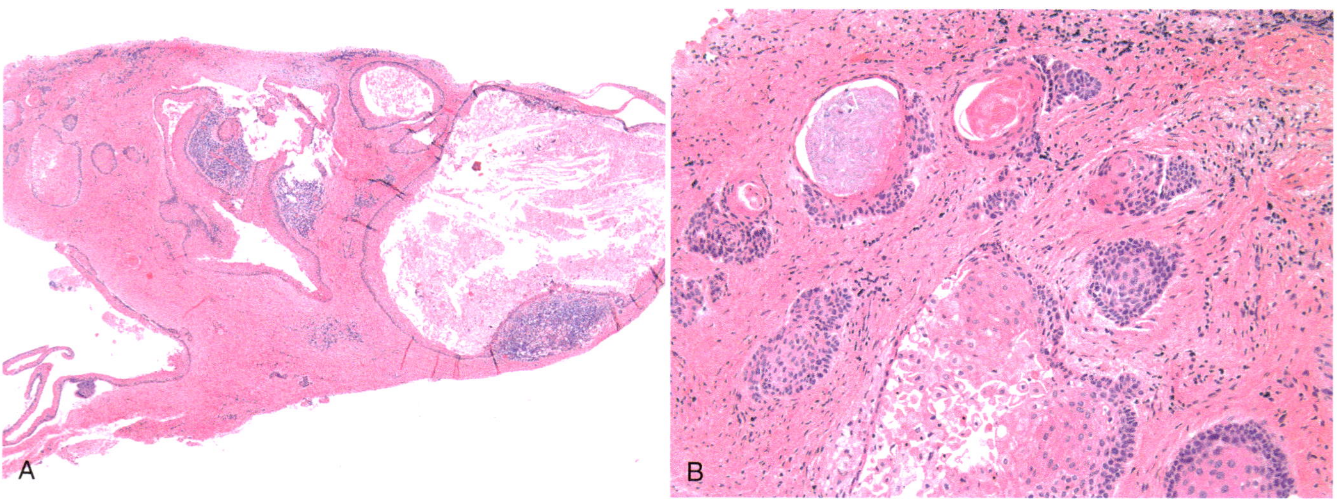

FIG 15.6 Odontogenic keratocyst with satellite cysts. (A) Many satellite cysts of varying sizes are present in the wall. (B) Satellite cysts may form keratin pearls and should not be mistaken for development of a squamous cell carcinoma.

AMELOBLASTOMA

Central (intraosseous) ameloblastoma, the third most common odontogenic tumor after keratocystic odontogenic tumor (odontogenic keratocyst) and odontoma, is a locally aggressive neoplasm, whereas peripheral (extraosseous) ameloblastoma behaves in an indolent fashion.

Clinical Findings

- *Solid ameloblastoma:* This is generally seen in the fourth to fifth decades of life and may cause swelling of the face if large. It is usually described as a solid tumor at surgery, although microcystic spaces may be present. It presents as a unilocular or multilocular radiolucency, most often in the mandible (80% of cases) and usually in the posterior mandible and/or ramus area, although in Black patients it may have a predilection for lesions in the anterior mandible. Some ameloblastomas are associated with impacted teeth (Fig. 15.7A–B).
- *Desmoplastic (scirrhous) ameloblastoma:* This variant has equal mandibular and maxillary frequency and presents as a mixed radiolucent-radiopaque mass in 50% of cases (suggesting a fibroosseous lesion), often affecting the anterior maxilla (see Fig. 15.7C). Keratoameloblastoma, which produces abundant keratin, may also have a mixed radiolucent-radiopaque appearance
- *Unicystic or unicystic plexiform ameloblastoma:* This represents 5% to 8% of ameloblastomas and presents in the second and third decades of life, often with jaw and facial swelling. It occurs as a unilocular radiolucency in the posterior mandible and is often associated with an impacted tooth (see Fig. 15.7D). It is described as a cystic lesion at surgery.
- *Peripheral (extraosseous) ameloblastoma:* This represents less than 5% of ameloblastomas and occurs in the fifth to sixth decades of life, usually as a nodule on the mandibular gingiva in the premolar-molar area. Radiographs must be taken to rule out an intraosseous ameloblastoma with perforation of the cortical bone. Rare cases occur at extragingival sites such as the buccal mucosa, although some authorities believe that these represent an unusual form of salivary gland tumor.

Etiopathogenesis and Histopathologic Features

Ameloblastomas putatively arise from rests of dental lamina and differentiate toward ameloblast-like enamel epithelium and stellate reticulum of the developing tooth germ, without deposition of dental hard tissues or their matrix. Activating mutations within the MAPK pathway have been noted, with 60% to 70% representing *BRAF*^{V600E} mutations. This, together with *RAS* and *FGFR2* mutations, constitutes 80% to 90% of mutations in intraosseous ameloblastomas, and these mutations are generally mutually exclusive. Most of the *BRAF* mutations tend to occur in mandibular lesions. Mutations in *SMO* (20–40% of cases), *CTNNB1*, *PIK3CA*, and *SMARCB1* have also been reported. Most *SMO* mutations occur in the plexiform pattern of ameloblastoma in the maxilla. Peripheral ameloblastoma arises from rests of Serres in the gingiva, although others have suggested that this lesion arises from the basal cell layer of the surface epithelium.

Ameloblastoma is classified histopathologically by gross pattern and constituent cells.

- Solid ameloblastoma patterns:
  - *Follicular ameloblastoma* exhibits islands or follicles of epithelial cells, typically with peripheral basal cells showing nuclear palisading and reverse polarization of the nuclei. Areas of microcystic and macrocystic change within the epithelial islands are common (Fig. 15.8).
  - *Plexiform ameloblastoma* shows interlacing trabeculae and cords of epithelial cells with basal cell nuclear palisading and reverse nuclear polarization, although these changes may be subtle in this pattern (Fig. 15.9).
- Constituent cells:
  - *Classic lesions* exhibit loose, stellate reticulum–like areas (see Fig. 15.8).
  - *Acanthomatous lesions* exhibit large, polygonal squamous cells with abundant eosinophilic cytoplasm or keratinization (see Figs. 15.8B, 15.10B).
  - *Granular cell lesions* contain large, pale cells with granular cytoplasm rich in lysosomes (Fig. 15.11).
  - *Basal cell lesions* contain mostly basaloid cells; this is a rare variant.
  - *Classic* and *acanthomatous variants* are the most common and often coexist.
  - *Keratoameloblastoma* is a follicular ameloblastoma producing cystic spaces filled with compact parakeratin and orthokeratin, some with intraluminal papilliferous projections. Its relationship with solid keratocystic odontogenic tumor (odontogenic keratocyst) is unclear (Fig. 15.12).
- *Desmoplastic* or *scirrhous ameloblastoma* is a variant of the follicular ameloblastoma in which islands of epithelium appear compressed by markedly desmoplastic stroma; the epithelium is present as slender cords and stellate-shaped islands of hyperchromatic cells. *Classic* and *acanthomatous* cytology are seen in some of the larger tumor islands (Fig. 15.13).
- *Unicystic ameloblastoma:* The cyst lining is generally 5 to 15 cells thick and exhibits eosinophilic (acanthomatous) luminal cells, underlying stellate reticulum–like cells, and palisaded basal cell nuclei with reverse polarization, giving the lining a "red-white-blue' appearance (Fig. 15.14). These changes are referred to as the *Vickers-Gorlin criteria* and are identical to those seen in cystic changes within epithelial islands in solid ameloblastoma (see Fig. 15.10C). This simple pattern is also sometimes called *luminal unicystic ameloblastoma.*
  - In plexiform unicystic ameloblastoma, there is, in addition to changes within the cyst lining, a plexiform proliferation of ameloblastomatous epithelium in an intraluminal pattern (Fig. 15.15A–C). Inflammation results in loss of the diagnostic features of this lesion and may lead to misdiagnosis of this cystic tumor as a radicular cyst or an inflamed odontogenic cyst, not otherwise specified (see Fig. 15.15D).
  - If there is mural proliferation within the wall of a unicystic ameloblastoma, this must be reported because it will behave in a fashion similar to a solid ameloblastoma.

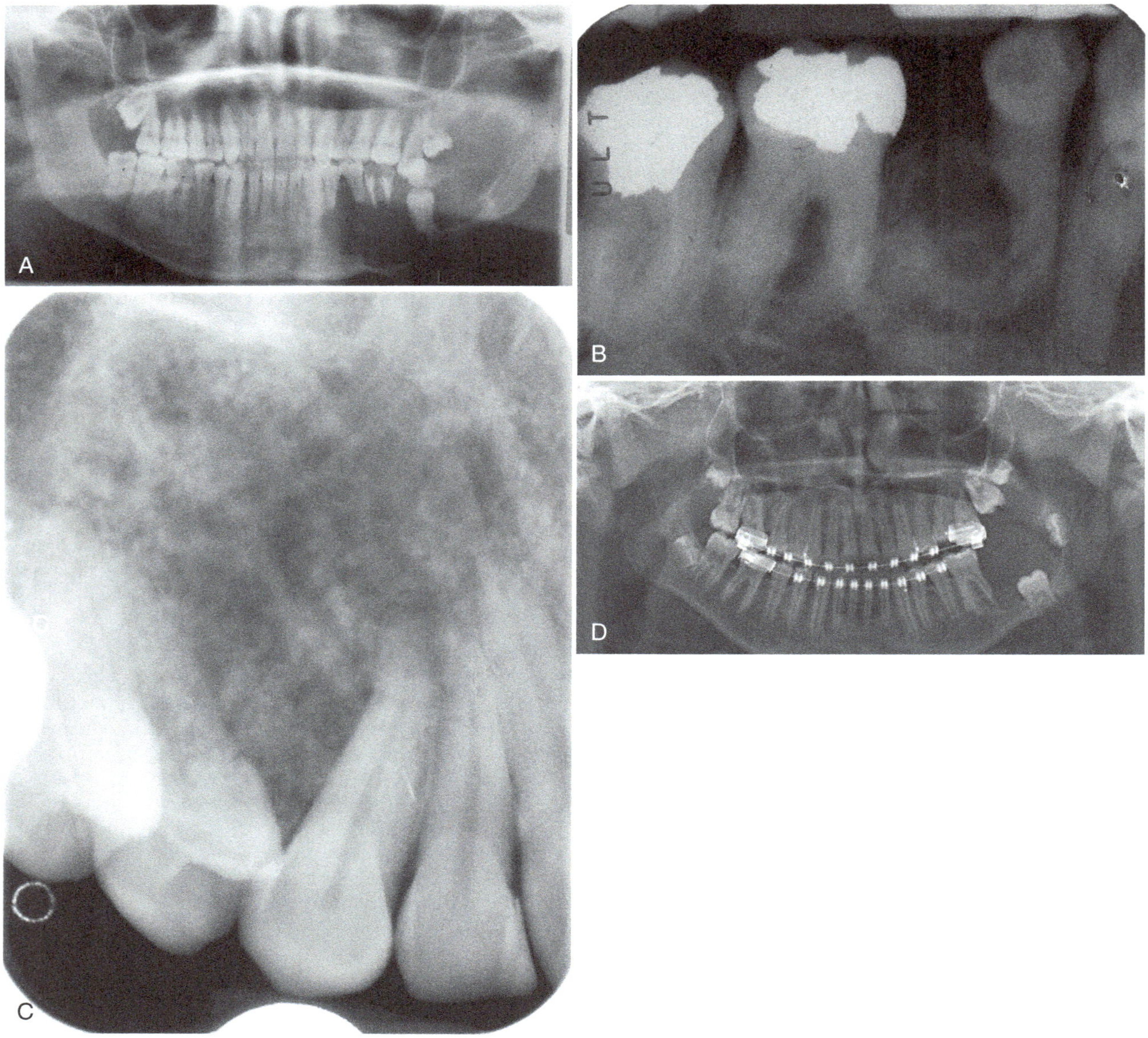

FIG 15.7 Ameloblastoma. (A) Multiloculated radiolucency in a dentigerous relationship with the left mandibular molar. (B) Ameloblastoma presenting as a unilocular radiolucency in the edentulous alveolar ridge. (C) Desmoplastic ameloblastoma presenting as a poorly demarcated, mixed radiolucent-radiopaque lesion resembling a fibroosseous lesion. (D) Plexiform unicystic ameloblastoma: unilocular radiolucency displacing mandibular second molar. *(A, Courtesy Dr. Thomas Dodson, Harvard School of Dental Medicine, Boston; B, Courtesy Dr. Pushkar Mehra, Boston University, Boston; D, Courtesy Dr. Euger Lin, private practice, Marlboro, Mass.)*

- Calretinin is positive within the stellate reticulum cells of solid ameloblastoma and the luminal cells of unicystic ameloblastoma (Fig. 15.16A). High Ki-67 labeling and large numbers of $CD10^{+}$ stromal cells may correlate with recurrence. Two-thirds of tumors are positive for BRAF (Fig. 15.16B). Tumor cells exhibit cytoplasmic positivity for K14 and K19 and are negative for K7 and K18.
- Tumors with areas of hypercellularity, pleomorphism, and mitotic activity should be diagnosed as ameloblastoma with atypia and must be carefully evaluated for malignant transformation.
- Ameloblastomas may develop in association with an odontoma, possibly from the dentigerous cyst around it. The term *odontoameloblastoma* has sometimes been used, but it is more appropriate to diagnose these as ameloblastoma with associated odontoma.
- *Adenoid ameloblastoma* (also referred to as *dentinoameloblastoma*) is an entity with a pattern of plexiform ameloblastoma, but forming ductlike structures (degenerated stroma) with a pseudocribriform architecture, basophilic stroma, whorled epithelium, and presence of dentinoid ghost cells and hyaline droplets, resembling adenomatoid odontogenic tumor. It tends to occur in

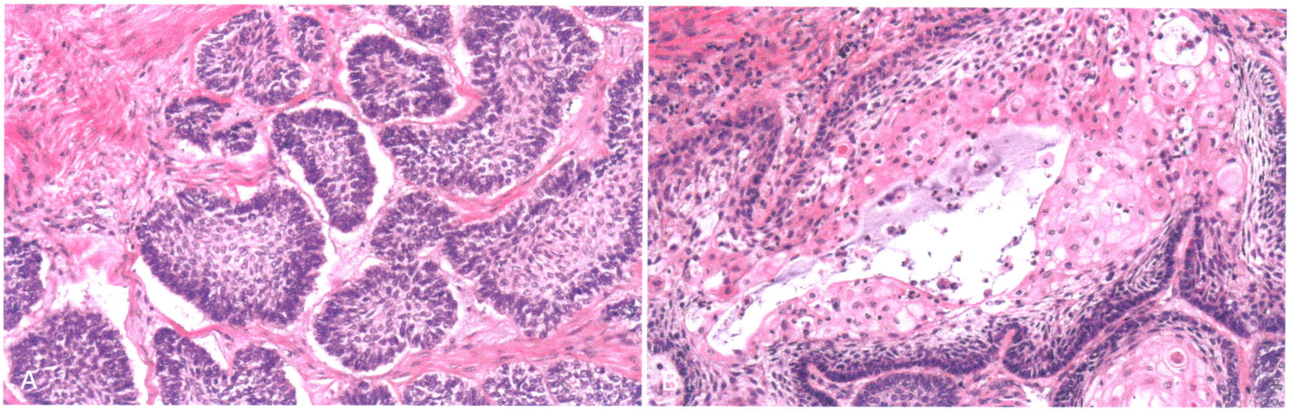

FIG 15.8 Ameloblastoma, follicular pattern. (A) Follicular pattern, classic type, composed of islands of epithelium surrounded by mature fibrous stroma. Palisading of basal cells and reverse nuclear polarization are present. (B) Follicular pattern, classic and acanthomatous type, with cystic change.

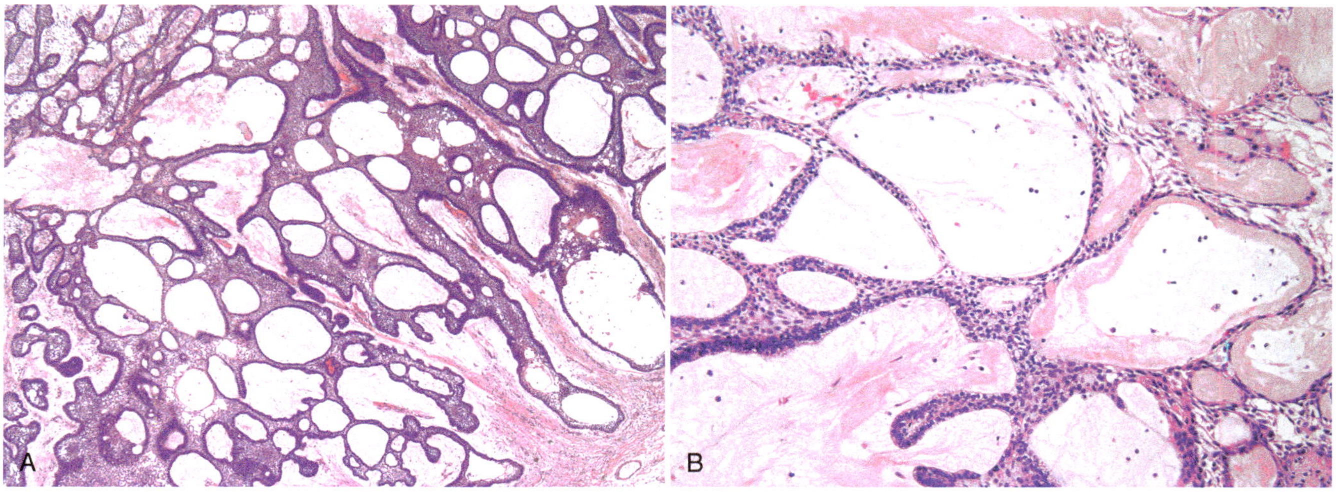

FIG 15.9 Ameloblastoma, plexiform pattern, classic and acanthomatous cell type. (A) Interlacing trabeculae and strands of epithelial cells enclose islands of fibrovascular tissue. (B) Strands of tumor cells show nuclear palisading and reverse polarization. Stroma is delicately collagenous and myxoid.

the maxilla (80% of cases) and has a high recurrence rate (Fig. 15.17).

- A rare osteoplastic type that induces bone formation within fibrous stroma has been reported.
- *Peripheral ameloblastoma:* This usually represents a *follicular* ameloblastoma, *classic* and/or *acanthomatous* type. Fifty percent of cases are in continuity with the overlying epithelium (Figs. 15.18 and 15.19).

Differential Diagnosis

- Dentigerous cyst or other odontogenic cyst does not exhibit the Vickers-Gorlin criteria, as noted in unicystic ameloblastoma; however, if the unicystic ameloblastoma is inflamed, these criteria may be lost. Squamous odontogenic tumor consists of islands of squamous cells but does not show palisading of the peripheral basal cells. Ameloblastic carcinoma shows obvious features of malignancy with hypercellularity, pleomorphic cells, many mitotic figures, and sometimes necrosis. Basaloid squamous cell carcinoma of the mucosa shows significant epithelial atypia and synchronous conventional squamous cell carcinoma. Basal cell carcinoma has been reported to occur on gingiva that is BerEP4+, similar to cutaneous basal cell carcinoma.

Management and Prognosis

- Recurrence varies greatly, depending on the surgical modality, surgical technique, and experience of the surgeon.
- *Solid ameloblastoma:* The recurrence rate is 5% to 17% if treated with marginal or segmental resection, and 30% to 35% if the tumor is curetted and/or enucleated.
- *Unicystic ameloblastoma:* The recurrence rates for those without and with mural proliferation are 6% and 37%, respectively, and most authorities recommend treating a unicystic ameloblastoma with mural proliferation as a solid ameloblastoma.
- *Peripheral (extraosseous) ameloblastoma:* This is treated with simple excision and does not recur. Malignant transformation occurs in less than 1% of cases. One patient with a metastatic ameloblastoma with the *BRAF*^{V600E} mutation showed shrinkage of the metastasis with vemurafenib, a BRAF inhibitor.

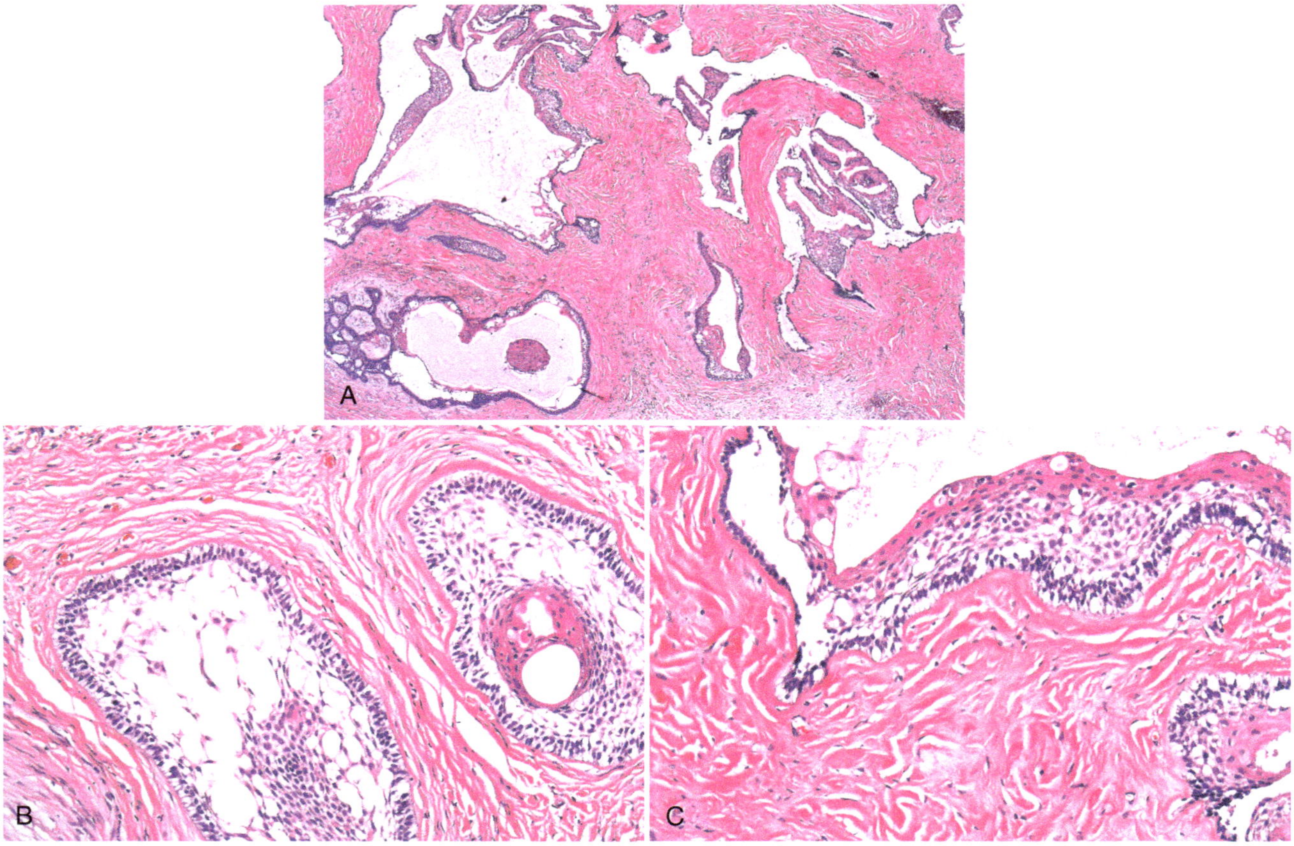

FIG 15.10 Ameloblastoma, follicular pattern, classic and acanthomatous. (A) Islands of tumor cells are present within mature fibrous stroma. (B) Classic stellate reticulum–like areas are present, and there are acanthomatous areas with early cystic change. (C) Eosinophilic luminal cells overlie stellate reticulum–like areas, and basal cells exhibit reverse nuclear polarization for a "red-white-blue" appearance.

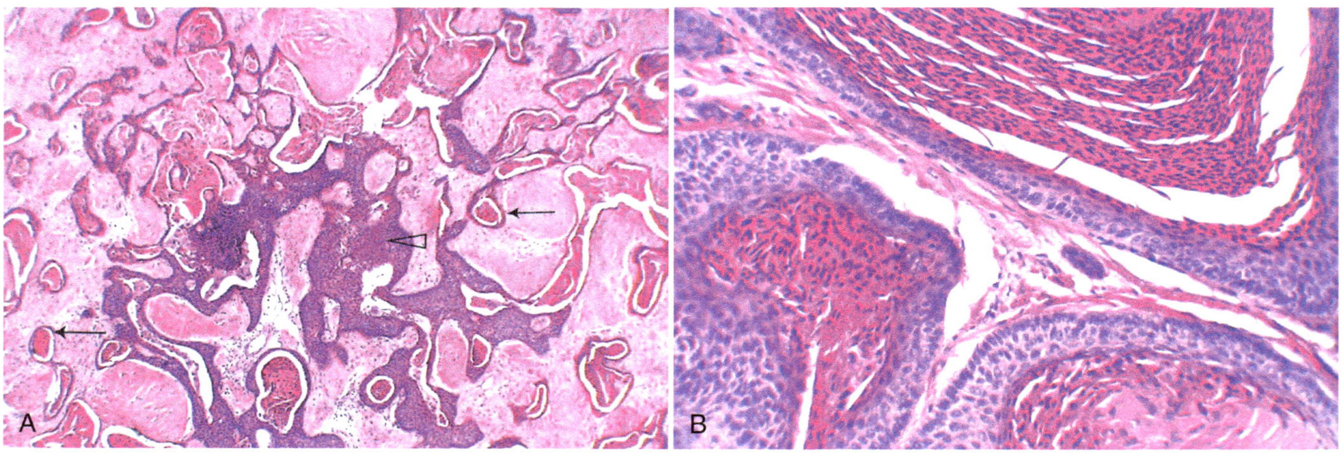

FIG 15.11 Keratoameloblastoma. (A) Photomicrograph exhibiting a plexiform pattern of odontogenic epithelial proliferation *(arrowhead)* within a collagenous, hyalinized connective tissue stroma. There are scattered microcysts packed with parakeratin *(arrows)* (hematoxylin and eosin; original magnification, ×25). (B) Photomicrograph exhibiting multiple follicles of odontogenic epithelium. The central areas are packed with layers of parakeratin. The basilar epithelial cells exhibit hyperchromatism and palisading (hematoxylin and eosin; original magnification, ×100). *(From Whitt JC, Dunlap CL, Sheets JL, Thompson ML. Keratoameloblastoma: a tumor sui generis or a chimera? Oral Surg Oral Med Oral Pathol Oral Radiol 2007;104:368–376.)*

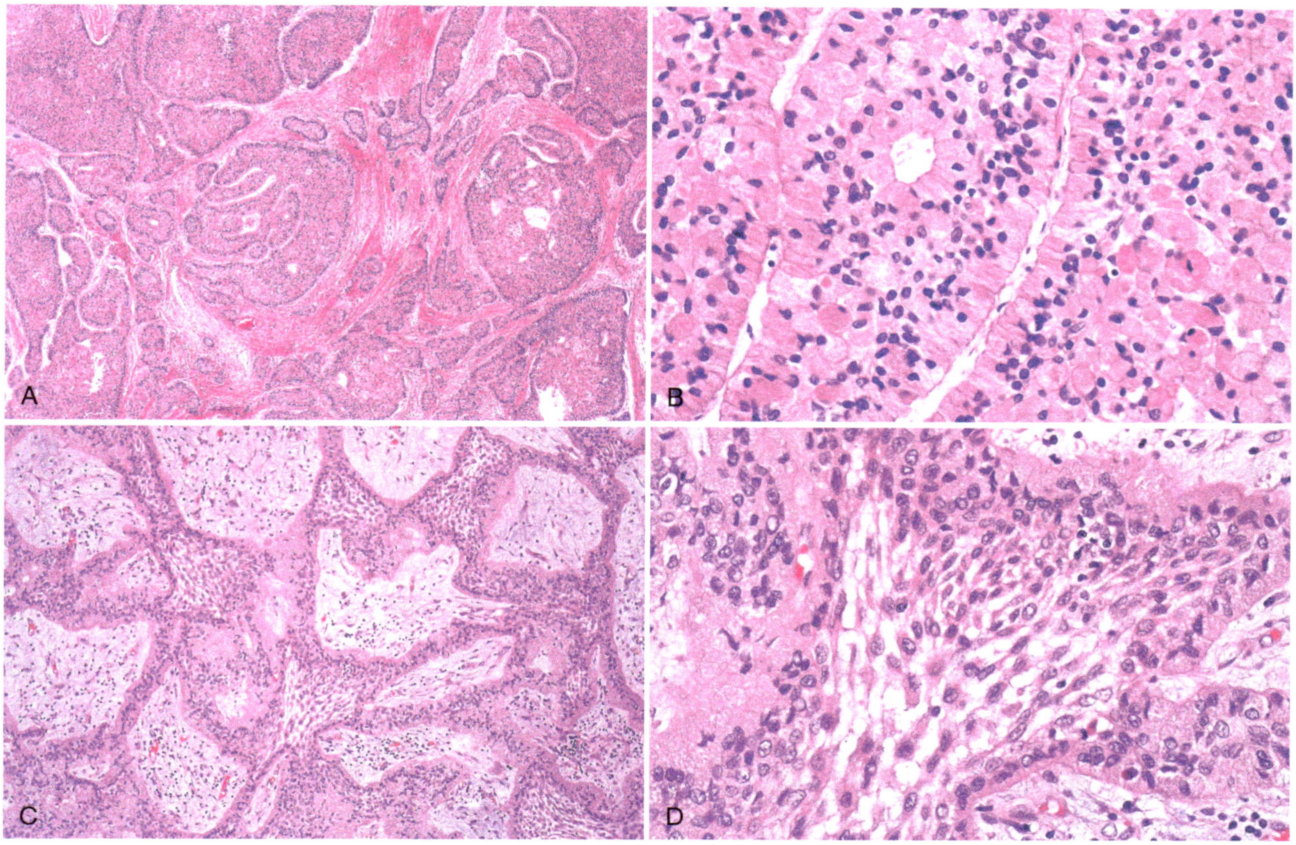

FIG 15.12 Ameloblastoma with granular cells. (A) Follicular pattern: islands of tumor containing pale, eosinophilic granular cells with palisaded basal cells. (B) Both basal cells (with reverse nuclear polarization) and cells in center of islands have granular cytoplasm. (C) Plexiform pattern: interlacing trabeculae of epithelium with palisaded basal nuclei, pale granular cells, and stellate reticulum–like areas. (D) This image displays both classic and granular cell histology.

REFERENCES

Abdel-Aziz A, Amin MM. EGFR, CD10 and proliferation marker Ki67 expression in ameloblastoma: possible role in local recurrence. *Diagn Pathol.* 2012;7:14.

Ahlem B, Wided A, Amani L, et al. Study of Ki67 and CD10 expression as predictive factors of recurrence of ameloblastoma. *Eur Ann Otorhinolaryngol Head Neck Dis.* 2015;132:275-279.

Brown NA, Betz BL. Ameloblastoma: a review of recent molecular pathogenetic discoveries. *Biomarker Cancer.* 2015;7(suppl 2):19-24.

Carlson ER, Marx RE. The ameloblastoma: primary, curative surgical management. *J Oral Maxillofac Surg.* 2006;64:484-494.

DeVilliers P, Liu H, Suggs C, et al. Calretinin expression in the differential diagnosis of human ameloblastoma and keratocystic odontogenic tumor. *Am J Surg Pathol.* 2008;32:256-260.

Hong J, Yun PY, Chung IH, et al. Long-term follow up on recurrence of 305 ameloblastoma cases. *Int J Oral Maxillofac Surg.* 2007;36: 283-288.

Ide F, Mishima K, Miyazaki Y, et al. Peripheral ameloblastoma in-situ: an evidential fact of surface epithelium origin. *Oral Surg Oral Med Oral Pathol Oral Radiol Endod.* 2009;108:763-767.

Isomura ET, Okura M, Ishimoto S, et al. Case report of extragingival peripheral ameloblastoma in buccal mucosa. *Oral Surg Oral Med Oral Pathol Oral Radiol Endod.* 2009;108:577-579.

Itoh Y, Nakahara H, Itoh R, et al. Osteoplastic ameloblastoma: a case report and literature review. *Oral Surg Oral Med Oral Pathol Oral Radiol.* 2012;113:e23-e28.

Kaye FJ, Ivey AM, Drane WE, et al. Clinical and radiographic response with combined BRAF-targeted therapy in stage 4 ameloblastoma. *J Natl Cancer Inst.* 2014;107:378.

Kishino M, Murakami S, Fukuda Y, Ishida T. Pathology of the desmoplastic ameloblastoma. *J Oral Pathol Med.* 2001;30:35-40.

Kishino M, Murakami S, Yuki M, et al. A immunohistochemical study of the peripheral ameloblastoma. *Oral Dis.* 2007;13:575-580.

Lau SL, Samman N. Recurrence related to treatment modalities of unicystic ameloblastoma: a systematic review. *Int J Oral Maxillofac Surg.* 2006;35:681-690.

Lee C, Park BJ, Yi WJ, et al. Keratoameloblastoma: a case report and a review of the literature on its radiologic features. *Oral Surg Oral Med Oral Pathol Oral Radiol.* 2015;120:e219-e225.

Li TJ, Wu YT, Yu SF, Yu GY. Unicystic ameloblastoma: a clinicopathologic study of 33 Chinese patients. *Am J Surg Pathol.* 2000;24:1385-1392.

Loyola AM, Cardoso SV, de Faria PR, et al. Adenoid ameloblastoma: clinicopathologic description of five cases and systematic review of the current knowledge. *Oral Surg Oral Med Oral Pathol Oral Radiol.* 2015;120:368-377.

Mosqueda-Taylor A, Carlos-Bregni R, Ramírez-Amador V, et al. Odontoameloblastoma: clinico-pathologic study of three cases and critical review of the literature. *Oral Oncol.* 2002;38:800-805.

Philipsen HP, Reichart PA, Nikai H, et al. Peripheral ameloblastoma: biological profile based on 160 cases from the literature. *Oral Oncol.* 2001;37:17-27.

Philipsen HP, Reichart PA. Unicystic ameloblastoma: a review of 193 cases from the literature. *Oral Oncol.* 1998;34:317-325.

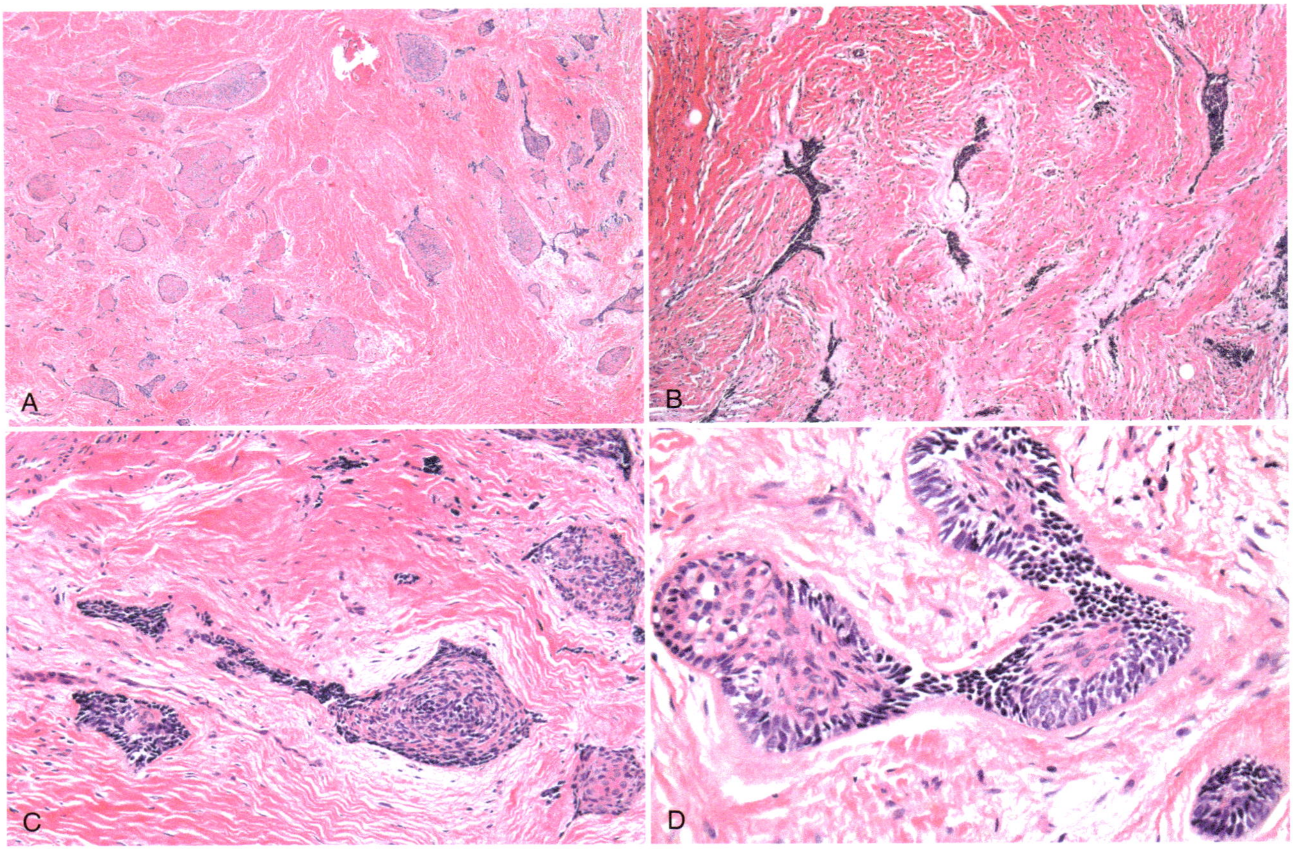

FIG 15.13 Desmoplastic ameloblastoma. (A) Irregularly shaped large islands and slender strands of squamoid tumor cells and scirrhous stroma. (B) The compressed islands consist of basaloid cells. Note the densely collagenous stroma. (C) The less compressed islands exhibit squamous cells and peripheral hyperchromatic basaloid cells. (D) Some islands are typical for follicular ameloblastoma, acanthomatous type.

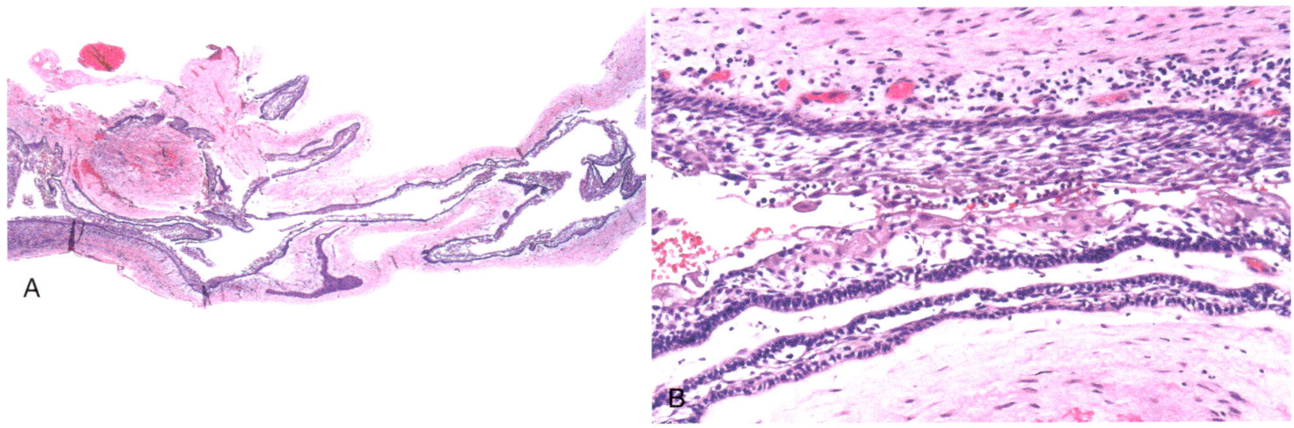

FIG 15.14 Unicystic ameloblastoma. (A) Single, large cystic space with prominent basal cells in the lining and little inflammation. (B) Eosinophilic luminal cells overlie stellate reticulum–like areas, and basal cells exhibit palisaded nuclei in a "red-white-blue" pattern.

Reichart PA, Philipsen HP, Sonner S. Ameloblastoma: biological profile of 3677 cases. *Eur J Cancer B Oral Oncol.* 1995;31B:86-99.

Sun ZJ, Wu YR, Cheng N, Zwahlen RA, Zhao YF. Desmoplastic ameloblastoma – a review. *Oral Oncol.* 2009;45:752-759.

Sweeney RT, McClary AC, Myers BR, et al. Identification of recurrent *SMO* and *BRAF* mutations in ameloblastomas. *Nat Genet.* 2014;46: 722-725. [A published corrigendum appears in *Nat Genet.* 2015 Jan;47:97.].

Waldron CA, el-Mofty SK. A histopathologic study of 116 ameloblastomas with special reference to the desmoplastic variant. *Oral Surg Oral Med Oral Pathol.* 1987;63:441-451.

Woods TR, Cohen DM, Islam MN, et al. Intraoral basal cell carcinoma, a rare neoplasm: report of three new cases with literature review. *Head Neck Pathol.* 2014;8:339-348.

Zhang J, Gu Z, Jiang L, et al. Ameloblastoma in children and adolescents. *Br J Oral Maxillofac Surg.* 2010;48:549-554.

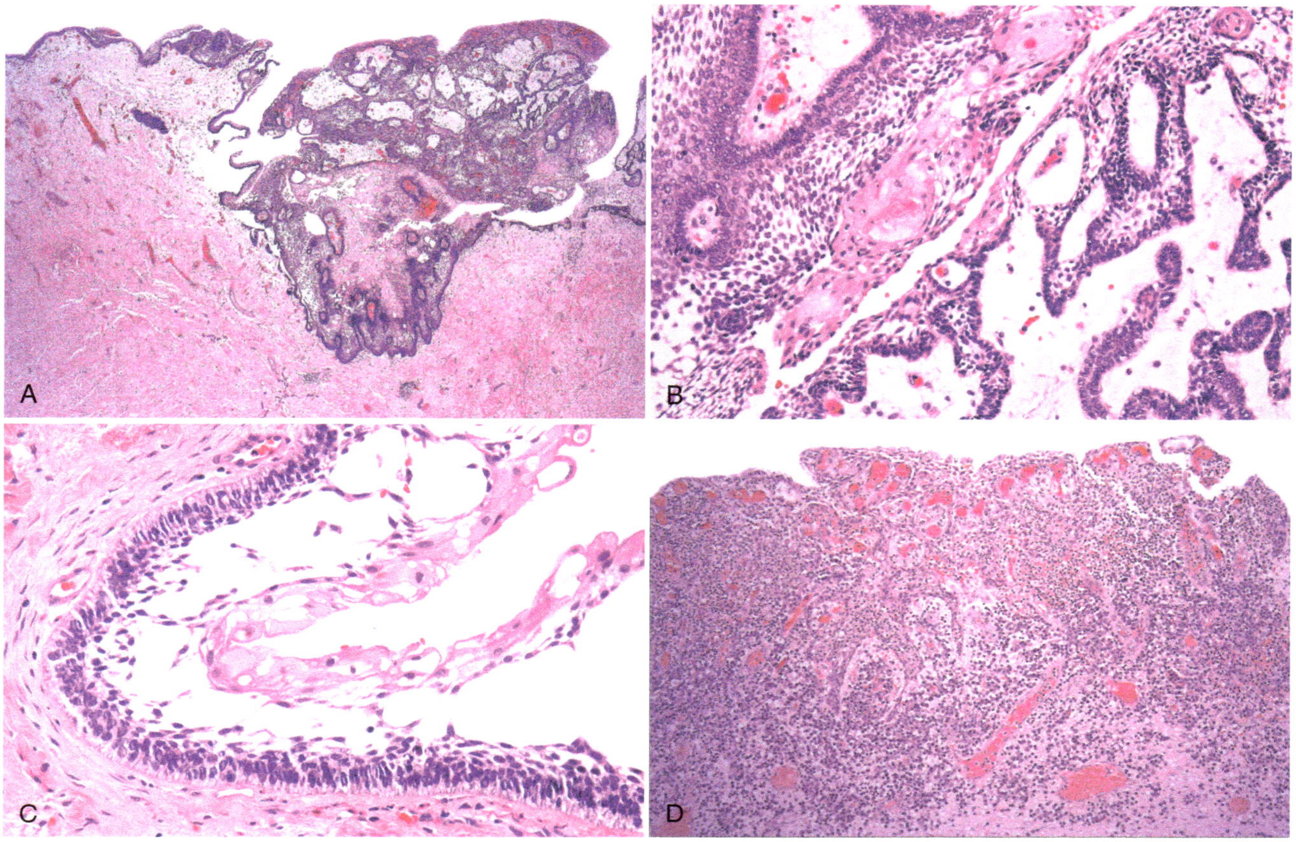

FIG 15.15 Plexiform unicystic ameloblastoma. (A) Single cystic structure with plexiform luminal and slight endophytic epithelial proliferation. (B) Plexiform epithelial proliferation exhibits classic and acanthomatous histology. (C) Thin lining exhibits luminal eosinophilic cells, stellate reticulum–like changes, and palisaded hyperchromatic basal cells in a "red-white-blue" pattern. (D) Inflammation leads to spongiosis and leukocyte exocytosis, which may easily lead to a misdiagnosis.

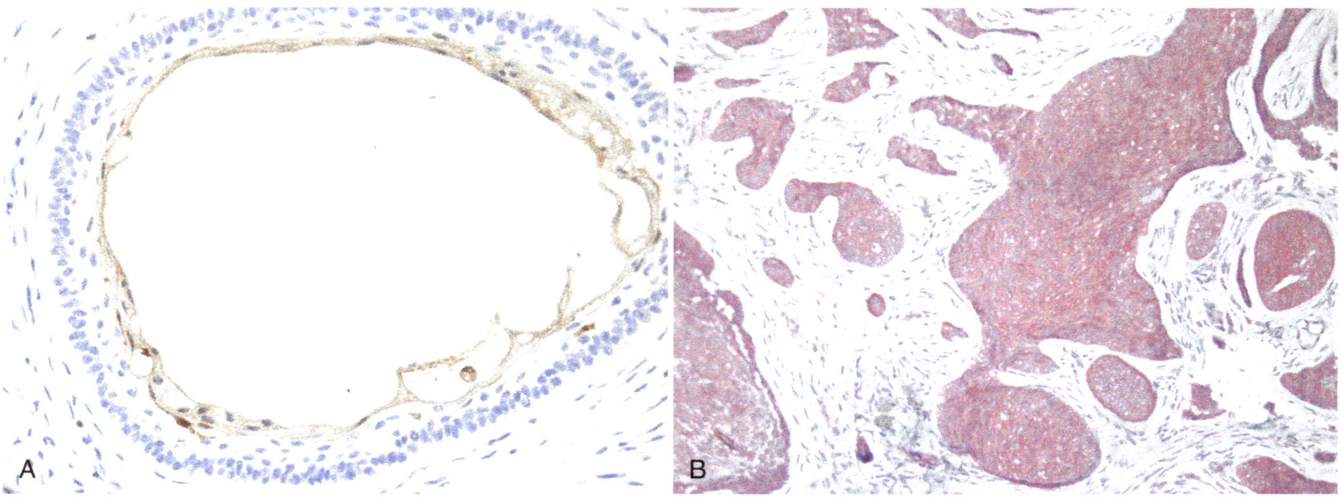

FIG 15.16 (A) Calretinin-positive cells primarily within the luminal cells. (B) BRAF positivity of follicular ameloblastoma.

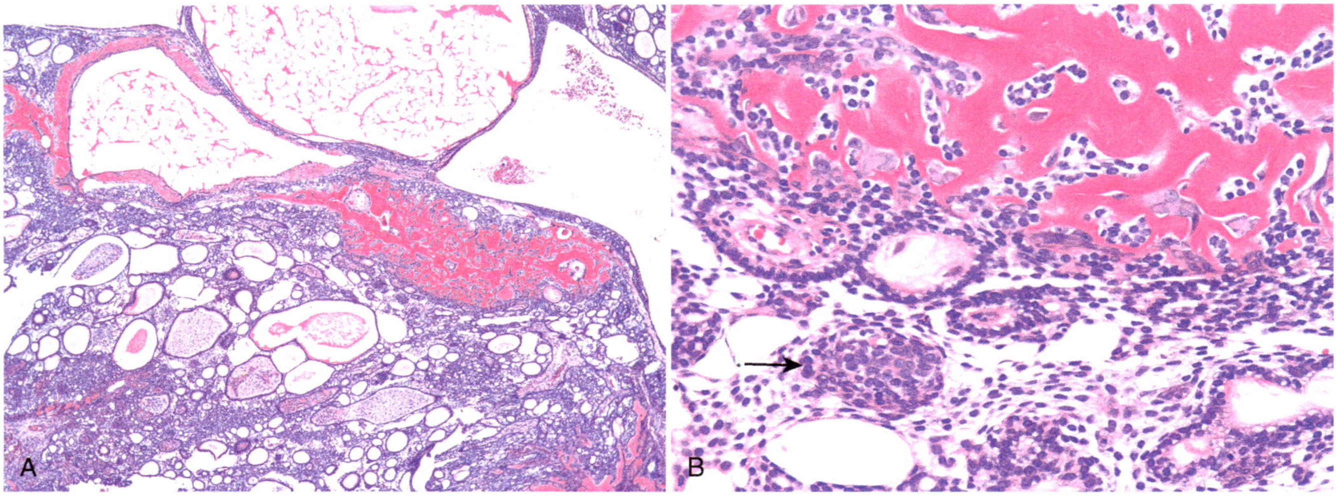

FIG 15.17 Ameloblastoma with adenoid features and dentinoid. (A) Plexiform ameloblastoma with dentinoid formation. (B) Dentinoid deposition with characteristic epithelial whorl *(arrow)*. Note that the "adenoid spaces" represent degenerated stroma.

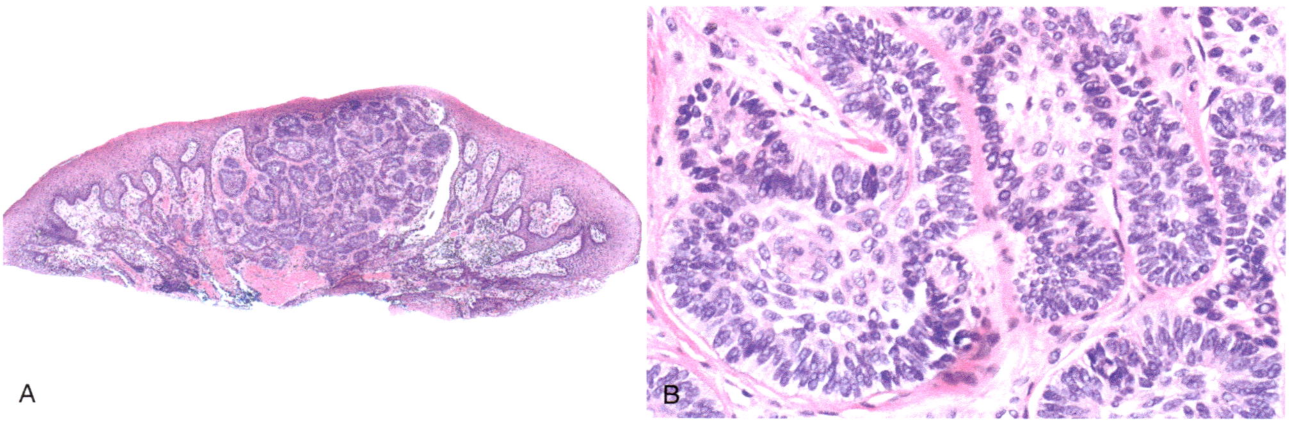

FIG 15.18 Peripheral ameloblastoma, follicular pattern, classic type. (A) There is a follicular pattern of epithelial proliferation that is in continuity with surface epithelium. (B) Palisading and reverse nuclear polarization of basal cells are shown.

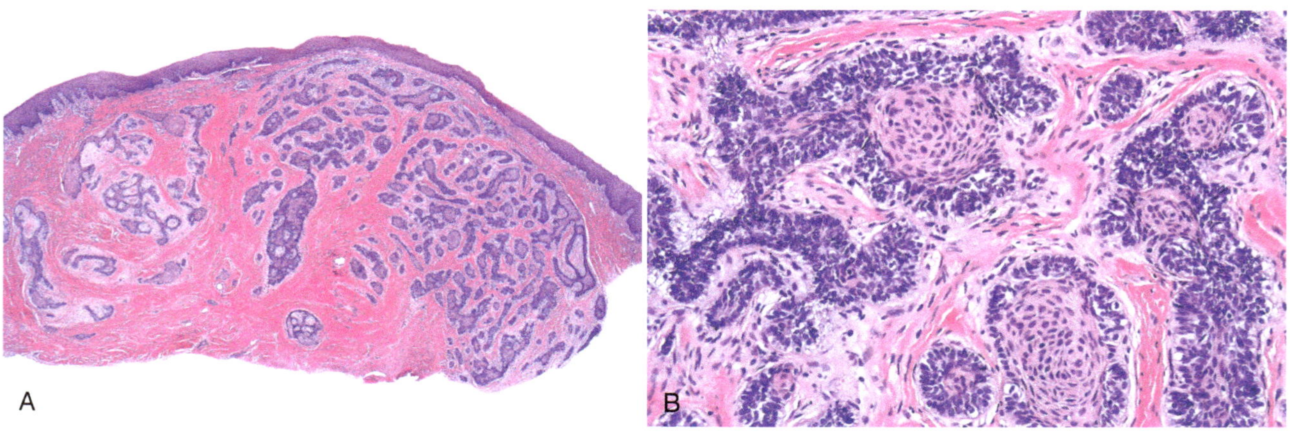

FIG 15.19 Peripheral ameloblastoma, follicular pattern, acanthomatous type. (A) Follicular ameloblastoma without obvious connection to the surface epithelium. (B) There is subtle palisading of basal cells with central acanthomatous histology.

ADENOMATOID ODONTOGENIC TUMOR

Clinical Findings

- This occurs most frequently in the second decade of life, with a 2 : 1 female predilection. At least two-thirds of cases occur in the maxilla, and two-thirds are associated with the maxillary canine. There may be slight swelling, but the most common complaint is failure of eruption of a tooth.
- It presents as a unilocular radiolucency and variable radiopaque flecks ("snowflake" opacities) around the crown of an impacted tooth (*follicular* type) (Fig. 15.20). Those unassociated with a tooth are referred to as *extrafollicular tumors*. Extraosseous lesions are rare.

Etiopathogenesis and Histopathologic Features

The tumor likely arises from rests of dental lamina.

- The tumor has a thick capsule and consists of sheets, nodules, whorls, and strands of spindled, cuboidal, and polygonal epithelial cells forming ductlike and rosette-like structures. The cells have pale or clear cytoplasm and pale nuclei with dispersed chromatin and small nucleoli. Reticular strands of epithelium surrounding the nodules contain darker nuclei with more eosinophilic cytoplasm; the stroma is delicate and often myxoid/mucinous (Figs. 15.21 and 15.22).
- Eosinophilic, deep pink, or basophilic droplets of amorphous material termed *enameloid* are characteristic, and this likely represents a matrix protein, amelotin (Figs. 15.21D and 15.22D).
- Dentinoid and calcifications may be present. Areas resembling calcifying epithelial odontogenic tumor are common, are considered to be within the normal histopathologic spectrum of this tumor, and are seen in 25% of cases.

Differential Diagnosis

- Adenoid ameloblastoma does not have a thick capsule, reticular strands of epithelium, or formation of enameloid but rather exhibits dentinoid deposition and sometimes, ghost cells.
- Adenomatoid dentinoma and adenomatoid odontogenic hamartomas have ductlike structures but also abundant dentinoid. These may represent developing odontomas with an unusual adenomatoid epithelial proliferation.

Management and Prognosis

- Excision is curative, and the recurrence rate is insignificant.

REFERENCES

Allen CM, Neville BW, Hammond HL. Adenomatoid dentinoma: report of four cases of an unusual odontogenic lesion. *Oral Surg Oral Med Oral Pathol Oral Radiol Endod.* 1998;86:313-317.

Carlos-Bregni R, Vargas PA, Santos Silva AR, et al. Adenomatoid odontogenic hamartoma: concerns about correct nomenclature and 2 additional case reports. *J Oral Maxillofac Surg.* 2009;67:1779-1780, author reply 1780.

Crivelini MM, Felipini RC, Miyahara GI, de Sousa SC. Expression of odontogenic ameloblast-associated protein, amelotin, ameloblastin, and amelogenin in odontogenic tumors: immunohistochemical analysis and pathogenetic considerations. *J Oral Pathol Med.* 2012;41:272-280.

de Matos FR, Nonaka CF, Pinto LP, de Souza LB, de Almeida Freitas R. Adenomatoid odontogenic tumor: retrospective study of 15 cases with emphasis on histopathologic features. *Head Neck Pathol.* 2012;6:430-437.

Ide F, Mishima K, Saito I, Kusama K. Rare peripheral odontogenic tumors: report of 5 cases and comprehensive review of the literature. *Oral Surg Oral Med Oral Pathol Oral Radiol Endod.* 2008;106:e22-e28.

Leon JE, Mata GM, Fregnani ER, et al. Clinicopathological and immunohistochemical study of 39 cases of adenomatoid odontogenic tumour: a multicentric study. *Oral Oncol.* 2005;41:835-842.

Mosqueda-Taylor A, Carlos-Bregni R, Ledesma-Montes C, et al. Calcifying epithelial odontogenic tumor-like areas are common findings in adenomatoid odontogenic tumors and not a specific entity. *Oral Oncol.* 2005;41:214-215.

Philipsen HP, Reichart PA, Siar CH, et al. An updated clinical and epidemiological profile of the adenomatoid odontogenic tumour: a collaborative retrospective study. *J Oral Pathol Med.* 2007;36:383-393.

Philipsen HP, Reichart PA. Adenomatoid odontogenic tumour: facts and figures. *Oral Oncol.* 1999;35:125-131.

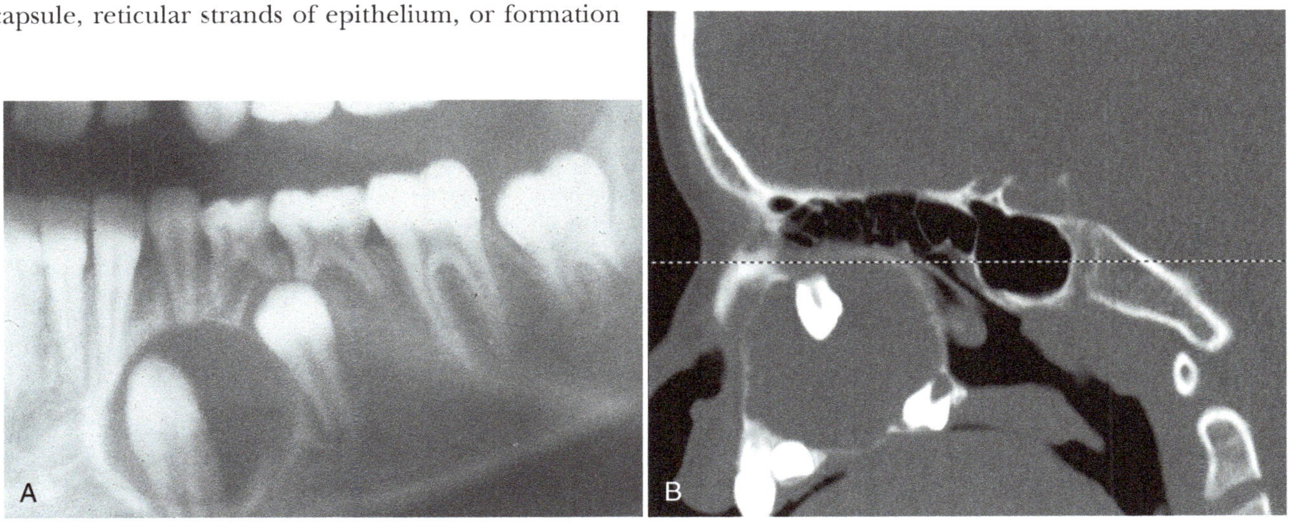

FIG 15.20 Adenomatoid odontogenic tumor. (A) Well-circumscribed radiolucency around impacted mandibular permanent canine. (B) Well-circumscribed radiolucency around impacted maxillary permanent canine. *(A, Courtesy Dr. Sadru Kabani, private practice, Cambridge, Mass.)*

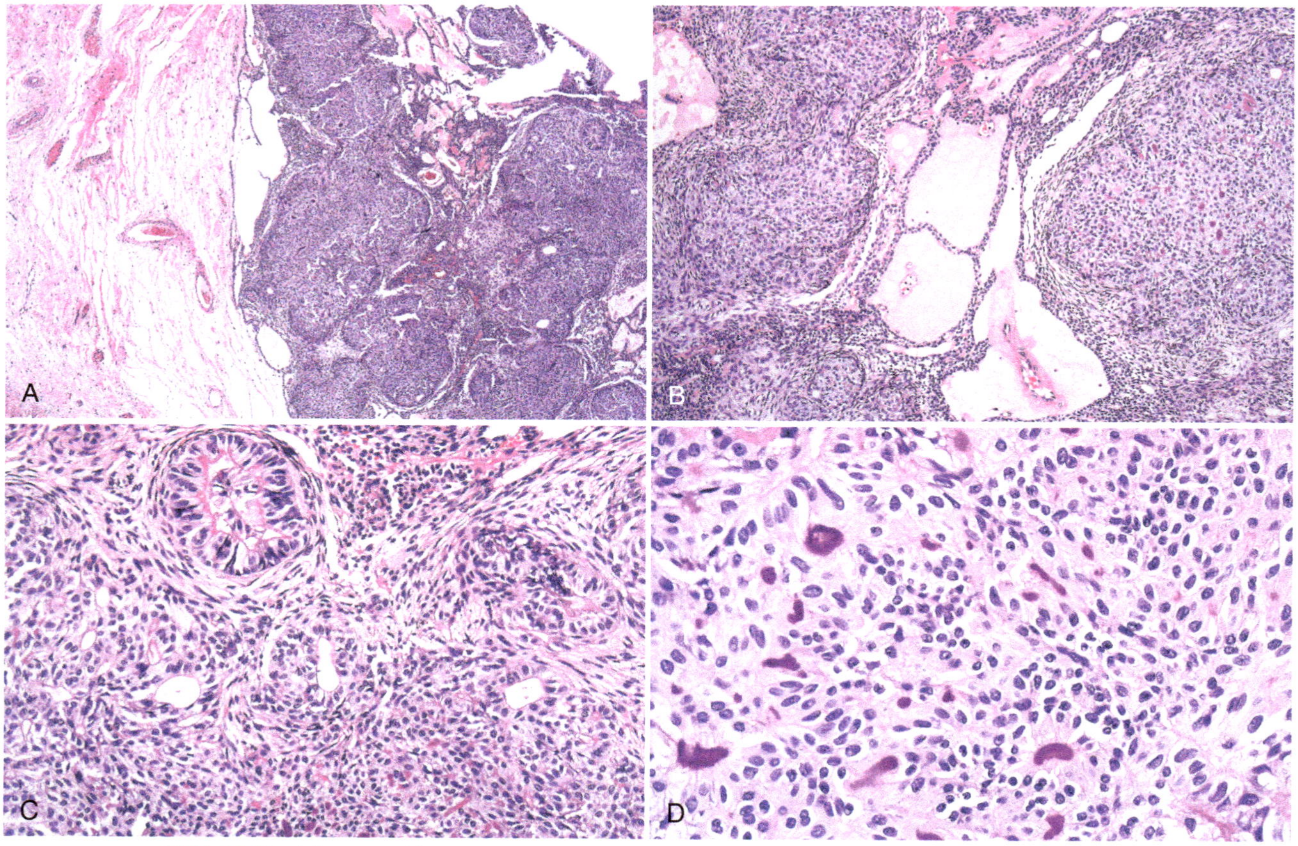

FIG 15.21 Adenomatoid odontogenic tumor. (A) Thick capsule surrounds tumor that has solid, nodular, and reticular areas. (B) Solid and reticular pattern is present with ductlike structures and delicate, mucinous stroma. (C) Spindle cells, columnar cells around ductlike structures, and polygonal cells with clear pale or clear cytoplasm are present. (D) Cells with pale cytoplasm forming rosette-like structures and darkly eosinophilic material termed *enameloid* are present.

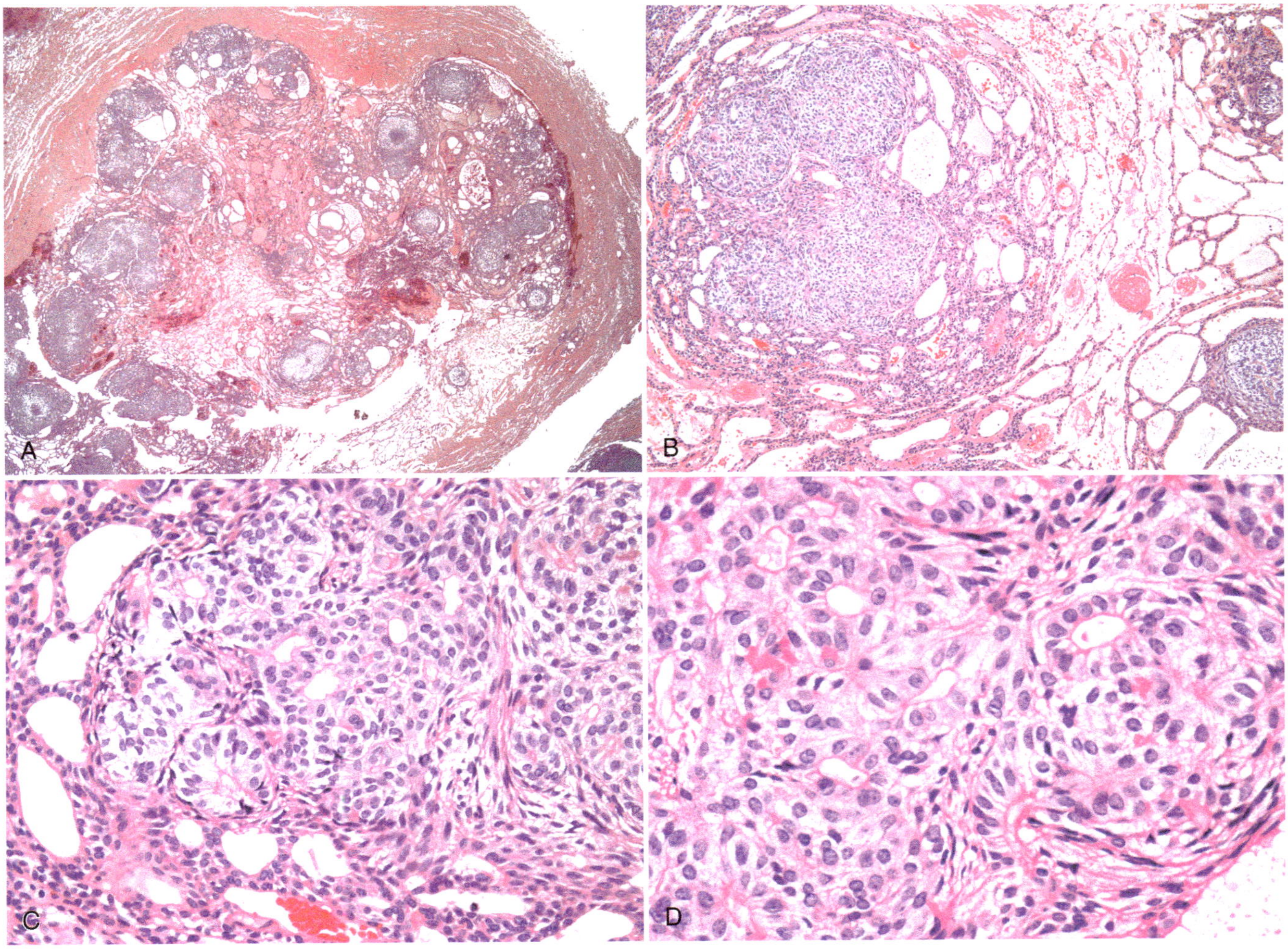

FIG 15.22 Adenomatoid odontogenic tumor. (A) A thick capsule surrounds the tumor, which has nodular, whorled, and reticular areas. (B) Nodules of pale polygonal cells and interconnected reticulated strands of epithelium with delicate, mucinous stroma. (C) Ductlike structures and small eosinophilic deposits of enameloid are shown. (D) Cuboidal cells with pale to clear cytoplasm form ductlike structures and deposit bright eosinophilic enameloid.

CALCIFYING EPITHELIAL ODONTOGENIC TUMOR (PINDBORG TUMOR)

Clinical Findings

- This is most frequent in the third to fifth decades of life, and the mandible is involved in 60% to 70% of cases, mostly in the posterior aspect; a swelling may be present. It presents usually as a unilocular (and much less often multilocular) radiolucency with variable calcifications (70% of cases), and 50% are associated with an impacted tooth (Fig. 15.23). Five to six percent are extraosseous.

Etiopathogenesis and Histopathologic Features

This tumor likely arises from dental lamina rests and is postulated to recapitulate the stratum intermedium of the enamel organ. Mutation of *PTCH1* has been reported. The tumor consists of cords, islands, and sometimes sheets of large, often polygonal cells with abundant eosinophilic cytoplasm and sometimes intercellular bridges. Variation in nuclear shape and size and pseudoinclusions are common, but mitotic activity is not seen unless the tumor is malignant (an extremely rare occurrence). Some islands may have a cribriform architecture because of the deposition of congophilic amyloid (identified as odontogenic ameloblast-associated protein) between tumor cells (Fig. 15.24).

- Variable amount of calcification occurs, and this sometimes takes the form of concentric lamellar rings (Liesegang rings). In spite of its name, calcifications are sometimes completely absent.
- Clear cells appear in 8% of tumors, and a clear cell variant has been described (Fig. 15.25). Langerhans cells have also been reported within tumor islands, and rarely lesions are cystic.
- Foci of calcifying epithelial odontogenic tumor are often seen within an adenomatoid odontogenic tumor, as are incipient lesions within the follicle of dentigerous cysts. Malignant forms are extremely rare. Peripheral lesions are less likely to exhibit calcifications.

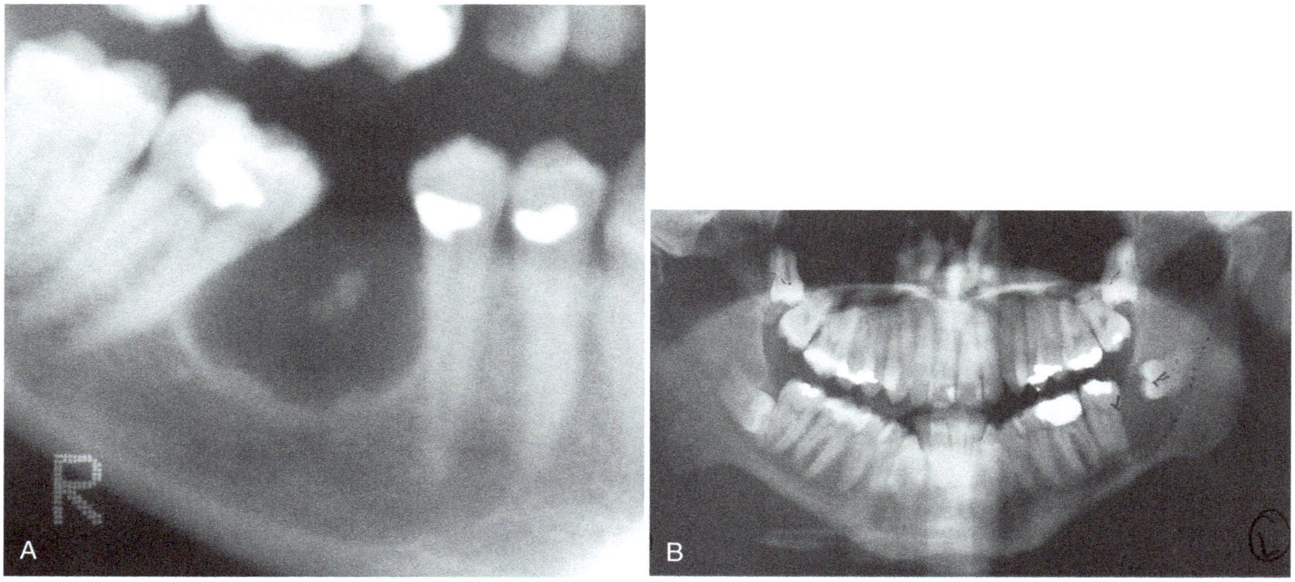

FIG 15.23 Calcifying epithelial odontogenic tumor. (A) Circumscribed radiolucency with small central radiopacity in the area of a previously extracted right mandibular first molar. (B) Circumscribed radiolucency around the crown of an impacted left mandibular third molar. *(B, Courtesy Dr. Leonard Waldman, private practice, Nashua, NH.)*

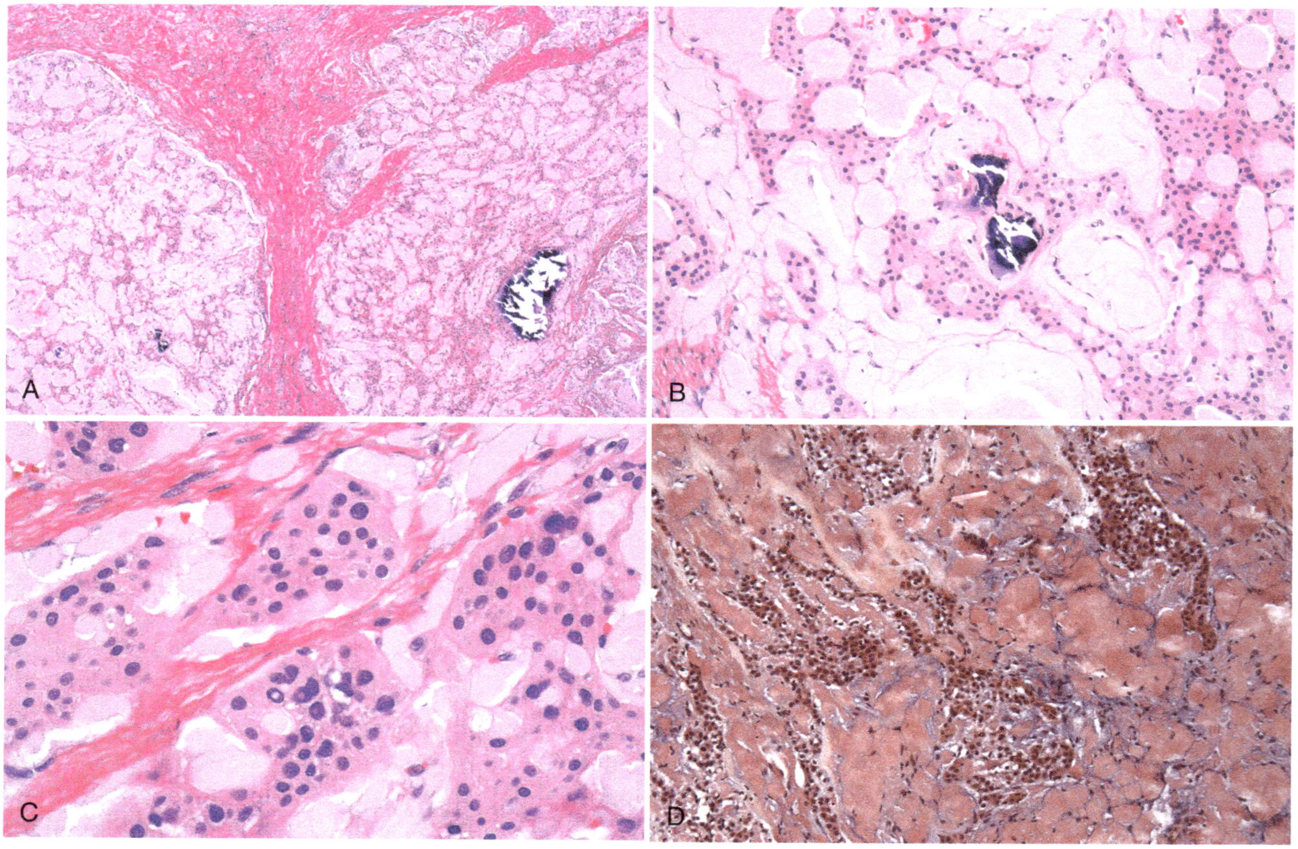

FIG 15.24 Calcifying epithelial odontogenic tumor. (A) Strands and interlacing cords of tumor cells with abundant amyloid and focal calcifications. (B) Tumor cells have an interlacing pattern of growth that may appear cribriform. (C) Cells are large and polygonal with abundant eosinophilic cytoplasm and typically with nuclear pleomorphism and nuclear pseudoinclusions. (D) Amyloid is congophilic (Congo Red stain).

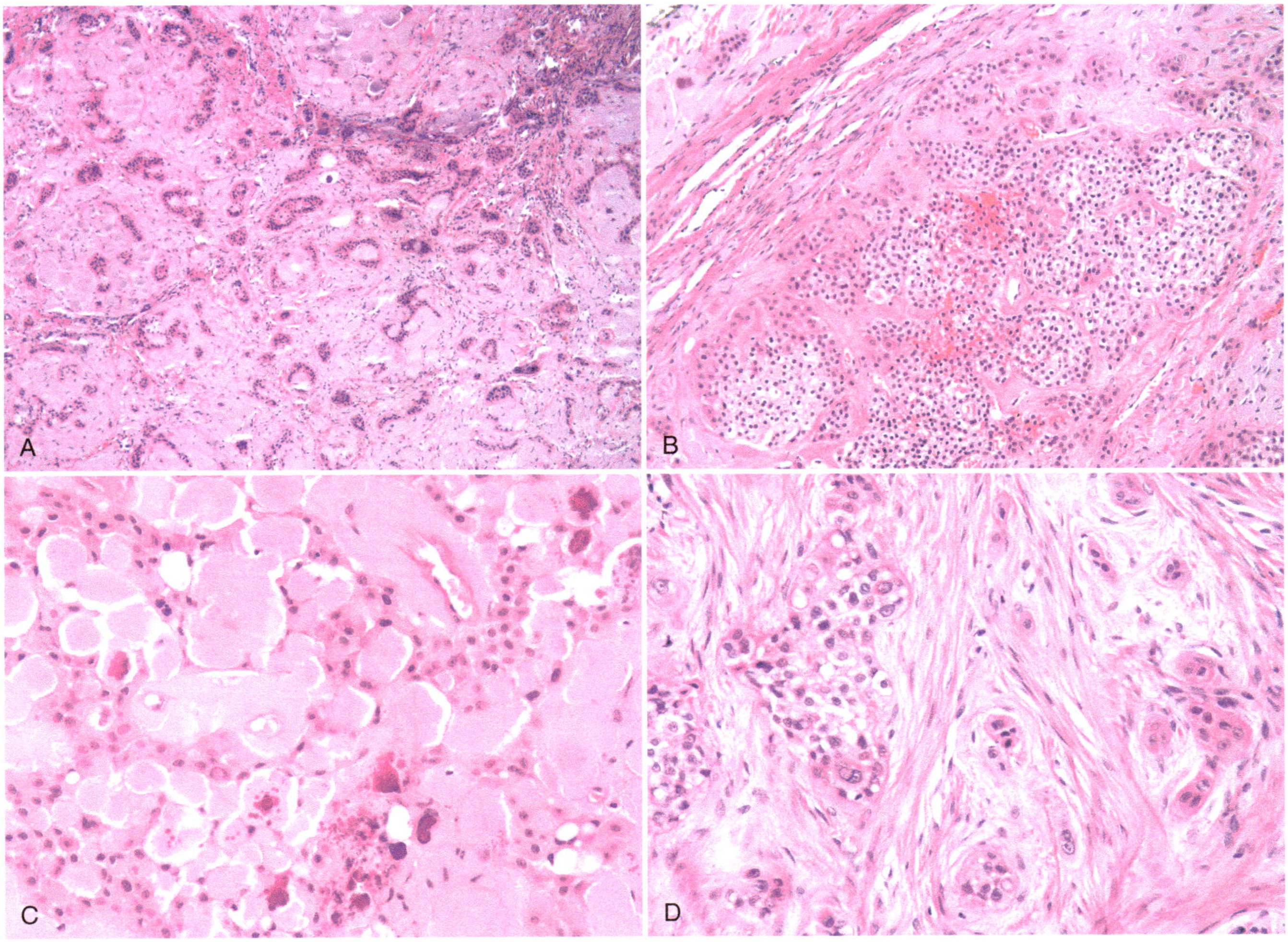

FIG 15.25 Calcifying epithelial odontogenic tumor. (A) Islands of epithelial cells surrounded by amyloid. (B) Islands of clear cells are present. (C) Tumor cells exhibit moderate nuclear pleomorphism with nuclear pseudoinclusions. Amyloid and calcifications are present. (D) Clear cells and cells with abundant eosinophilic cytoplasm within a fibrous stroma are present.

Differential Diagnosis

- Malignant calcifying epithelial odontogenic tumor exhibits hypercellularity, hyperchromatic nuclei with coarse chromatin, mitotic figures, and other features of malignancy.
- Metastatic carcinomas have significantly more atypia, mitotic activity, and desmoplasia and generally lack amyloid.
- Primary clear cell odontogenic carcinoma does not produce amyloid and exhibits features of malignancy.

Management and Prognosis

- Complete excision or enucleation is the treatment of choice, and the recurrence rate is up to 15%, especially if the tumor is curetted.

REFERENCES

Abrahao AC, Camisasca DR, Bonelli BR, et al. Recurrent bilateral gingival peripheral calcifying epithelial odontogenic tumor (Pindborg tumor): a case report. *Oral Surg Oral Med Oral Pathol Oral Radiol Endod.* 2009;108:e66-e71.

Afrogheh A, Schneider J, Mohamed N, Hille J. Calcifying epithelial odontogenic tumour with clear Langerhans cells: a novel variant, report of a case and review of the literature. *Head Neck Pathol.* 2014;8:214-219.

Anavi Y, Kaplan I, Citir M, Calderon S. Clear-cell variant of calcifying epithelial odontogenic tumor: clinical and radiographic characteristics. *Oral Surg Oral Med Oral Pathol Oral Radiol Endod.* 2003;95:332-339.

de Oliveira MG, Chaves AC, Visioli F, et al. Peripheral clear cell variant of calcifying epithelial odontogenic tumor affecting 2 sites: report of a case. *Oral Surg Oral Med Oral Pathol Oral Radiol Endod.* 2009;107:407-411.

Demian N, Harris RJ, Abramovitch K, et al. Malignant transformation of calcifying epithelial odontogenic tumor is associated with the loss of p53 transcriptional activity: report of a case with review of the literature. *J Oral Maxillofac Surg.* 2010;68:1964-1973.

Gopalakrishnan R, Simonton S, Rohrer MD, Koutlas IG. Cystic variant of calcifying epithelial odontogenic tumor. *Oral Surg Oral Med Oral Pathol Oral Radiol Endod.* 2006;102:773-777.

Kestler DP, Foster JS, Macy SD, et al. Expression of odontogenic ameloblast-associated protein (ODAM) in dental and other epithelial neoplasms. *Mol Med.* 2008;14:318-326.

Mosqueda-Taylor A, Carlos-Bregni R, Ledesma-Montes C, et al. Calcifying epithelial odontogenic tumor-like areas are common findings in adenomatoid odontogenic tumors and not a specific entity. *Oral Oncol.* 2005;41:214-215.

Peacock ZS, Cox D, Schmidt BL. Involvement of *PTCH1* mutations in the calcifying epithelial odontogenic tumor. *Oral Oncol.* 2010;46: 387-392.

Philipsen HP, Reichart PA. Calcifying epithelial odontogenic tumour: biological profile based on 181 cases from the literature. *Oral Oncol.* 2000;36:17-26.

Sedghizadeh PP, Wong D, Shuler CF, et al. Multifocal calcifying epithelial odontogenic tumor. *Oral Surg Oral Med Oral Pathol Oral Radiol Endod.* 2007;104:e30-e34.

Wang YP, Lee JJ, Wang JT, et al. Non-calcifying variant of calcifying epithelial odontogenic tumor with Langerhans cells. *J Oral Pathol Med.* 2007;36:436-439.

SQUAMOUS ODONTOGENIC TUMOR

Clinical Findings

- This rare odontogenic tumor occurs most frequently in the fourth decade of life, equally affecting the posterior mandible and anterior maxilla, and presents as a well-demarcated radiolucency around the roots of teeth. One-third are multicentric (Fig. 15.26).

Etiopathogenesis and Histopathologic Features

- The tumor consists of irregularly shaped islands of mature squamous cells containing scattered dyskeratotic cells without a peripheral layer of basaloid cells. Some islands may exhibit cystic change or may contain globular, eosinophilic, amorphous secretions or calcifications (Figs. 15.27 and 15.28).

Differential Diagnosis

- Follicular ameloblastoma, acanthomatous type, shows palisading of basal cell nuclei.

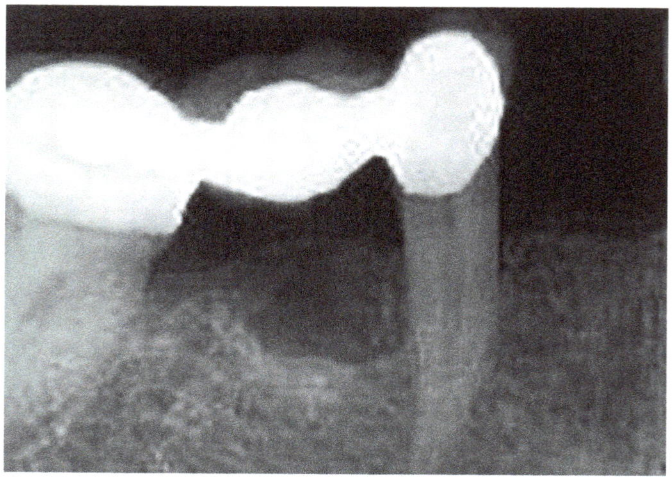

FIG 15.26 Squamous odontogenic tumor presenting as a demarcated radiolucency in the alveolus close to the roots of teeth.

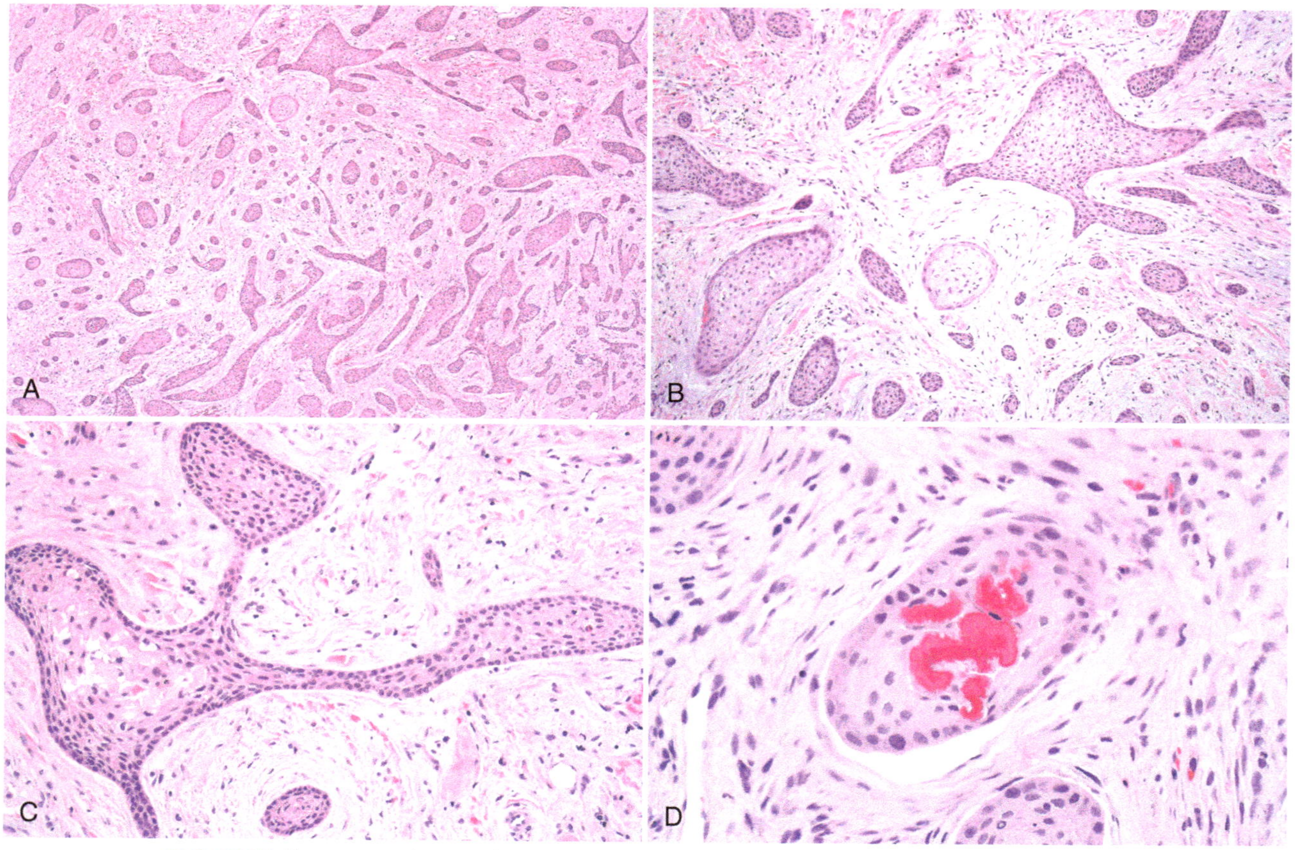

FIG 15.27 Squamous odontogenic tumor. (A) Islands of squamous epithelium within fibrous stroma. (B) Irregularly shaped islands of squamous cells within delicately fibrous stroma; one resembles a fish. (C) Peripheral cells are low cuboidal or squamous without palisading or reverse polarization of nuclei. Dyskeratotic cells are noted, and there is dyscohesion. (D) Epithelial islands may contain brightly eosinophilic hyaline material resembling Rushton bodies or other odontogenic product.

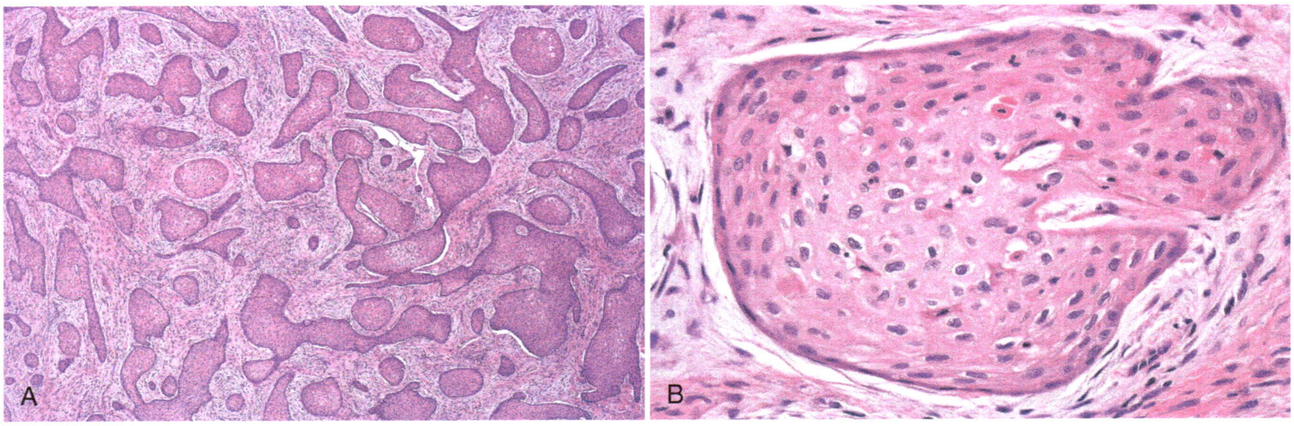

FIG 15.28 Squamous odontogenic tumor. (A) Irregularly shaped islands of squamous cells within fibrous stroma. (B) Epithelial islands contain dyskeratotic cells, and peripheral cells are squamous and flattened.

- Primary intraosseous and metastatic carcinomas show significant cytologic atypia.
- Squamous odontogenic-like proliferations composed of similar irregular islands of benign epithelium are sometimes seen in the walls of radicular cysts (see Chapter 14).

Management and Prognosis

- Enucleation, curettage, or excision is curative. Recurrence is rare.

REFERENCES

Goldblatt LI, Brannon RB, Ellis GL. Squamous odontogenic tumor: report of five cases and review of the literature. *Oral Surg Oral Med Oral Pathol.* 1982;54:187-196.

Jones BE, Sarathy AP, Ramos MB, Foss RD. Squamous odontogenic tumor. *Head Neck Pathol.* 2011;5:17-19.

Kim K, Mintz SM, Stevens J. Squamous odontogenic tumor causing erosion of the lingual cortical plate in the mandible: a report of 2 cases. *J Oral Maxillofac Surg.* 2007;65:1227-1231.

Lin YL, White DK. Squamous odontogenic tumor. *Oral Maxillofac Surg Clin North Am.* 2004;16:355-357.

Parmar RM, Brannon RB, Fowler CB. Squamous odontogenic tumor-like proliferations in radicular cysts: a clinicopathologic study of forty-two cases. *J Endod.* 2011;37:623-626.

Philipsen HP, Reichart PA. Squamous odontogenic tumor (SOT): a benign neoplasm of the periodontium. A review of 36 reported cases. *J Clin Periodontol.* 1996;23:922-926.

ODONTOGENIC CARCINOMA

Odontogenic carcinomas are rare and putatively arise from proliferation of odontogenic rests, likely dental lamina rests within the bone. Some tumors show overt differentiation toward odontogenic tissues, such as the ameloblastic carcinoma, or even toward salivary gland tissue. It is likely that the multipotent nature of the lining of the embryonic stomodeum that gives rise to salivary glands and teeth may also give rise to intraosseous salivary gland tumors both benign and malignant that are morphologically identical to conventional salivary gland tumors. A list of odontogenic carcinomas is presented in Table 15.1.

TABLE 15.1 Modified World Health Organization Classification of Odontogenic Carcinoma

Odontogenic Carcinomas
1. Tumors with odontogenic differentiation
Ameloblastic carcinoma
Metastatic ameloblastoma
Odontogenic carcinoma with dentinoid production
Ghost cell odontogenic carcinoma
2. Primary intraosseous squamous cell carcinoma
3. Sclerosing odontogenic carcinoma
4. Tumors with salivary gland differentiation
Central mucoepidermoid carcinoma
Clear cell odontogenic carcinoma
Other adenocarcinomas
5. Odontogenic carcinosarcoma

AMELOBLASTIC CARCINOMA AND METASTATIC (MALIGNANT) AMELOBLASTOMA

Ameloblastic carcinoma, the more common of the two, displays all the features of ameloblastoma, except that it has malignant cytology, behaves in an aggressive manner, may metastasize, and has a poor prognosis. Metastatic (malignant) ameloblastoma, a very rare condition, shows minimal cytologic atypia, although it has metastasized and is a retrospective diagnosis. It exhibits locally invasive growth at the metastatic site but otherwise has a more indolent course.

Clinical Findings

- *Ameloblastic carcinoma:* The average age of occurrence is in the fifth decade of life, with a 2:1 male predilection, and more than two-thirds occur in the mandible, mostly posteriorly. Pain, mucosal ulceration, and paresthesia are often noted. Lesions appear as poorly demarcated, destructive radiolucencies.
- *Metastatic ameloblastoma:* These occur an average of 18 years after the initial diagnosis of ameloblastoma in the jaws and after an average of four recurrences, with

approximately 80% of lesions presenting as lung nodules, often bilaterally. Sixty percent of the original tumors are treated by enucleation or curettage. Hypercalcemia has been reported in some cases with pulmonary metastases.

Etiopathogenesis and Histopathologic Features

The majority of ameloblastic carcinomas arise de novo, with less than 5% arising from preexisting ameloblastomas, sometimes referred to as *dedifferentiated lesions.* Metastatic ameloblastoma occurs by hematogenous spread (lymph nodes are infrequently affected). A hypothesis is that this may occur as a result of multiple surgical manipulations of multiple recurrences of the primary tumor.

- *Ameloblastic carcinoma:*
  - These tumors have features of conventional ameloblastoma and in addition exhibit necrosis, hypercellularity, hyperchromasia, pleomorphism, mitotic activity (average of 4 per high-power field), and atypical mitotic figures. Sometimes peripheral palisading is subtle or lost (Fig. 15.29).
  - Clear cells, keratinization, ghost cells, and focal dentinoid production may be present. A spindle cell variant has been reported.
  - There is a high Ki-67 proliferation index as expected; K18 may be present; and SOX2 expression has been shown to be a sensitive (77%) and specific (86%) marker for ameloblastic carcinoma. PITX2, a transcription factor in the Wnt signaling pathway, is also highly expressed in these tumors.
- *Metastatic ameloblastoma:*
  - The cytology is that of a conventional ameloblastoma without or with minimal evidence of cytologic atypia.

Differential Diagnosis

- Primary intraosseous squamous cell carcinoma and de novo ameloblastic carcinoma are likely related lesions, with the former showing less ameloblastic differentiation, in that basal cell palisading or formation of stellate reticulum–like areas is minimal or insignificant. Metastatic carcinoma must be ruled out.
- Odontogenic carcinoma with dentinoid (also reported as clear cell odontogenic carcinoma with dentinoid) is a rare, low-grade odontogenic carcinoma that consists of cords, trabeculae, and sheets of epithelial cells with pale, eosinophilic, or clear cytoplasm with dentinoid deposition. These tumors have low proliferative indices but are locally destructive and may exhibit perineural invasion. They occur with a mean age in the fourth decade of life, with the mandible twice as likely to be affected as the maxilla (Fig. 15.30).

Management and Prognosis

- *Ameloblastic carcinoma:* En bloc resection with radiation and/or chemotherapy as appropriate results in a 30% recurrence rate. Twenty-two percent develop metastases, and half of those exhibit distant metastases to lungs, bone, and brain. Five-year survival overall and with metastasis are approximately 70% and 20%, respectively.
- *Metastatic ameloblastoma:* This behaves similarly to conventional ameloblastoma, being locally aggressive at the metastatic site but otherwise running an indolent course. Patients are treated with adjunctive chemotherapy or radiation, and 50% exhibit longer than 10-year survival, while death as a result of the tumor occurs within 3 years.

REFERENCES

Barnes L, Eveson J, Reichart P, Sidransky D, eds. *Pathology and Genetics of Head and Neck Tumours.* Lyon, France: IARC Press; 2005.

Chou YH, Jhuang JY, Chang MH, et al. Metastasizing ameloblastoma with localized interstitial spread in the lung: report of two cases. *Int J Surg Pathol.* 2014;22:343-346.

Dissanayake RK, Jayasooriya PR, Siriwardena DJ, Tilakaratne WM. Review of metastasizing (malignant) ameloblastoma (METAM): pattern of metastasis and treatment. *Oral Surg Oral Med Oral Pathol Oral Radiol Endod.* 2011;111:734-741.

García-Muñoz A, Rodríguez MA, Licéaga-Escalera C, et al. Expression of the transcription factor *PITX2* in ameloblastic carcinoma. *Arch Oral Biol.* 2015;60:799-803.

Ghiam A, Al Zahrani A, Feld R. A case of recurrent metastatic ameloblastoma and hypercalcaemia successfully treated with carboplatin and paclitaxel: long survival and prolonged stable disease. *Ecancermedicalscience.* 2013;7:323.

Hall JM, Weathers DR, Unni KK. Ameloblastic carcinoma: an analysis of 14 cases. *Oral Surg Oral Med Oral Pathol Oral Radiol Endod.* 2007;103:799-807.

Lei Y, Jaradat JM, Owosho A, et al. Evaluation of SOX2 as a potential marker for ameloblastic carcinoma. *Oral Surg Oral Med Oral Pathol Oral Radiol.* 2014;117:608-616.e1.

Matsushita Y, Fujita S, Yanamoto S, et al. Spindle cell variant of ameloblastic carcinoma: a case report and literature review. *Oral Surg Oral Med Oral Pathol Oral Radiol.* 2016;121:e54-e61.

Mosqueda-Taylor A, Neville BW, Tatemoto Y, et al. Odontogenic carcinoma with dentinoid: a new odontogenic carcinoma. *Head Neck Pathol.* 2014;8:421-431.

Richardson MS, Muller S. Malignant odontogenic tumors: an update on selected tumors. *Head Neck Pathol.* 2014;8:411-420.

Van Dam SD, Unni KK, Keller EE. Metastasizing (malignant) ameloblastoma: review of a unique histopathologic entity and report of Mayo Clinic experience. *J Oral Maxillofac Surg.* 2010;68:2962-2974.

Yoon HJ, Hong SP, Lee JI, et al. Ameloblastic carcinoma: an analysis of 6 cases with review of the literature. *Oral Surg Oral Med Oral Pathol Oral Radiol Endod.* 2009;108:904-913.

Yoon HJ, Jo BC, Shin WJ, et al. Comparative immunohistochemical study of ameloblastoma and ameloblastic carcinoma. *Oral Surg Oral Med Oral Pathol Oral Radiol Endod.* 2011;112:767-776.

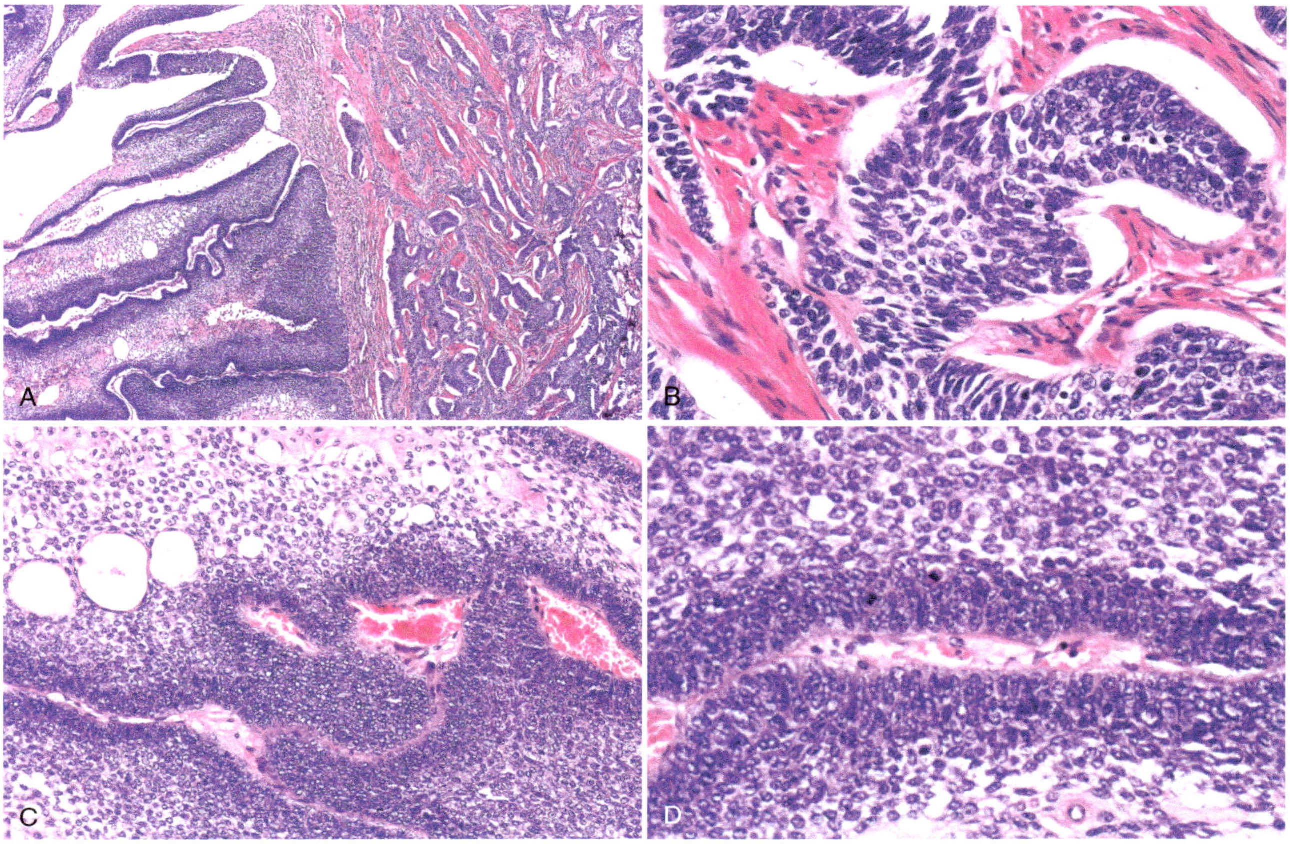

FIG 15.29 Ameloblastic carcinoma. (A) Recognizable follicular ameloblastoma, acanthomatous type, shown on *left* exhibits hypercellularity; dedifferentiated infiltrative tumor is shown on *right*. (B) Infiltrative, less well-differentiated hypercellular area of tumor composed of atypical basaloid cells. (C) Area of recognizable ameloblastoma with stellate reticulum–like and acanthomatous areas with palisaded basal cells. (D) Tumor exhibits hypercellularity, hyperchromatic nuclei, and mitoses.

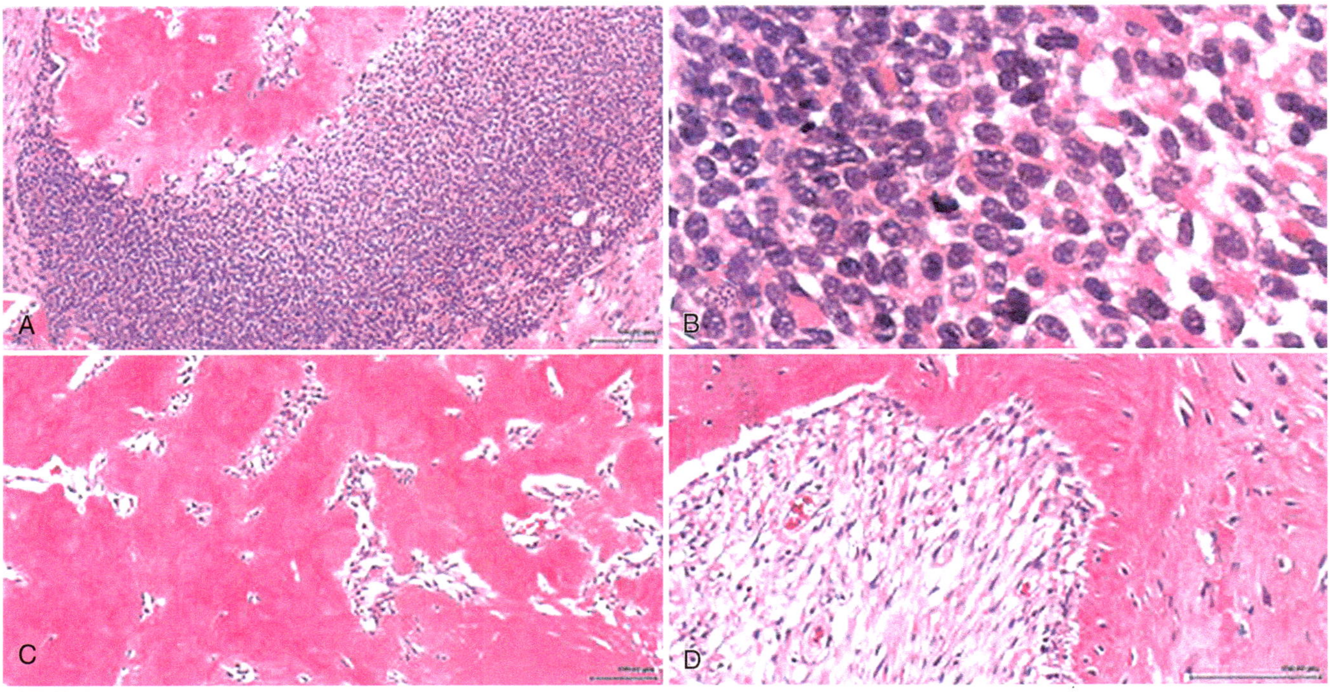

FIG 15.30 Odontogenic carcinoma with dentinoid deposition. (A) Dentinoid associated with sheets of ovoid and polygonal tumor cells. (B) Higher-power view of the tumor cells shown in A, which exhibit pleomorphism and some mitotic figures *(center)*. (C) The eosinophilic masses of dentinoid have occasional nests of tumor cells included. (D) Irregular tubules can be identified in some areas at the periphery of the dentinoid material. *(From Mosqueda-Taylor A, Neville BW, Tatemoto Y, et al. Odontogenic carcinoma with dentinoid: a new odontogenic carcinoma. Head Neck Pathol. 2014;8:421–431.)*

PRIMARY INTRAOSSEOUS SQUAMOUS CELL CARCINOMA AND OTHER ODONTOGENIC CARCINOMAS

Clinical Features

- This occurs in the sixth and seventh decades of life, with a 2:1 male predilection, and pain, mobility of teeth, and paresthesia are common. Eighty to ninety percent occur in the mandible, and it presents as a poorly demarcated radiolucency of the mandible, often with cortical perforation (Fig. 15.31).

Etiopathogenesis and Histopathologic Features

Tumors arise either from preexisting odontogenic cysts and tumors (more common) or de novo from odontogenic rests. Approximately 60% are associated with a residual or radicular cyst, 16% with a dentigerous cyst, and 14% from a keratocystic odontogenic tumor (odontogenic keratocyst). There is likely overlap between this entity and the ameloblastic carcinoma because both putatively arise from odontogenic rests within the jaw bones, except that one has a squamous cell carcinoma phenotype and the other a clearly ameloblastomatous phenotype.

- Primary intraosseous squamous cell carcinomas are infiltrating squamous cell carcinomas (>90% of cases), with approximately half being well-differentiated and keratinizing. Most arise from odontogenic cysts, the lining of which exhibits varying degrees of dysplasia or carcinoma in situ (Fig. 15.32).
- Features suggesting odontogenic differentiation may be seen in approximately half the cases and include a follicular pattern, palisading of the peripheral basal cells, and the presence of clear cells (Fig. 15.33). Tumors may manifest as verrucous or papillary squamous carcinoma or sarcomatoid carcinoma.

Differential Diagnosis

- Ameloblastic carcinoma shows obvious palisading of the peripheral cells. Differentiation between this and primary intraosseous carcinoma may be moot because both are primary carcinomas in bone and likely arise from odontogenic rests.
- Primary squamous cell carcinoma of the overlying mucosa or the maxillary sinus, as well as metastatic squamous cell carcinoma, must be ruled out.
- Mucoepidermoid carcinoma contains mucous cells and is not generally keratinizing. Ductal structures may be present.
- Desmoplastic (scirrhous) ameloblastoma contains irregularly shaped islands of basaloid cells, but some islands show typical ameloblastoma, and the stroma is desmoplastic.
- Odontogenic carcinosarcomas have been reported, but they are extremely rare and would be difficult to distinguish from a primary intraosseous sarcomatoid squamous cell carcinoma.

Management and Prognosis

- Resection is the treatment of choice with or without lymph node dissection, with adjuvant radiation therapy and/or chemotherapy as appropriate. The recurrence rate is 60%. Ten percent develop distant metastases to lungs, bones, and brain, and 2-year and 5-year survival are 60% to 70% and 30% to 40%, respectively.

REFERENCES

Bodner L, Manor E, Shear M, van der Waal I. Primary intraosseous squamous cell carcinoma arising in an odontogenic cyst: a clinicopathologic analysis of 116 reported cases. *J Oral Pathol Med.* 2011;40:733-738.

Chaisuparat R, Coletti D, Kolokythas A, et al. Primary intraosseous odontogenic carcinoma arising in an odontogenic cyst or de novo: a clinicopathologic study of six new cases. *Oral Surg Oral Med Oral Pathol Oral Radiol Endod.* 2006;101:194-200.

Chikosi R, Segall N, Augusto P, Freedman P. Odontogenic carcinosarcoma: case report and literature review. *J Oral Maxillofac Surg.* 2011;69:1501-1507.

Huang JW, Luo HY, Li Q, Li TJ. Primary intraosseous squamous cell carcinoma of the jaws: clinicopathologic presentation and prognostic factors. *Arch Pathol Lab Med.* 2009;133:1834-1840.

Mosqueda-Taylor A, Neville BW, Tatemoto Y, et al. Odontogenic carcinoma with dentinoid: a new odontogenic carcinoma. *Head Neck Pathol.* 2014;8:421-431.

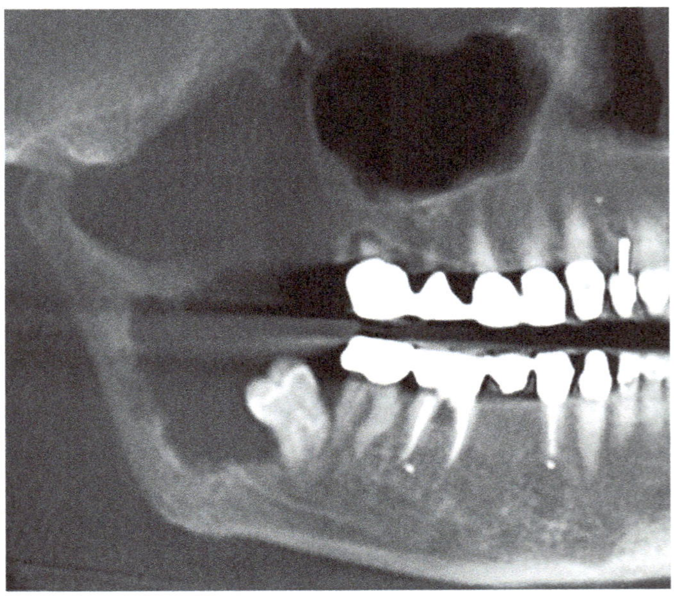

FIG 15.31 Primary intraosseous squamous cell carcinoma presenting as a poorly demarcated radiolucency arising from a dentigerous cyst associated with the right mandibular third molar. *(Courtesy Dr. Robert Schaedel, Boynton Beach, Fla.)*

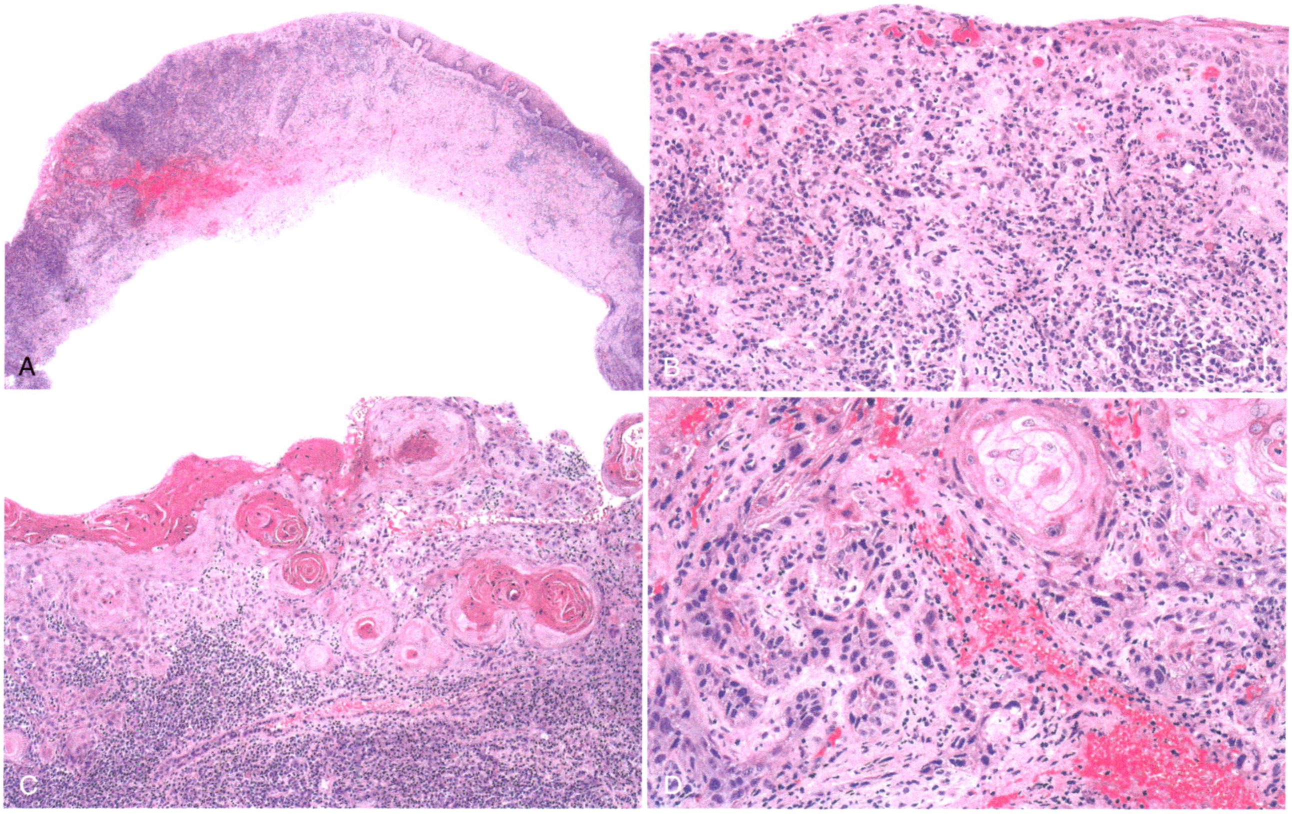

FIG 15.32 Primary intraosseous squamous cell carcinoma. (A) Cystic lining showing malignant transformation on the *left*. (B) Poorly differentiated infiltrating carcinoma arising from the cyst lining. (C) Other areas show keratinizing and infiltrating carcinoma arising from cyst lining that is dysplastic. (D) Tumor exhibits keratin pearl formation and contains pleomorphic cells.

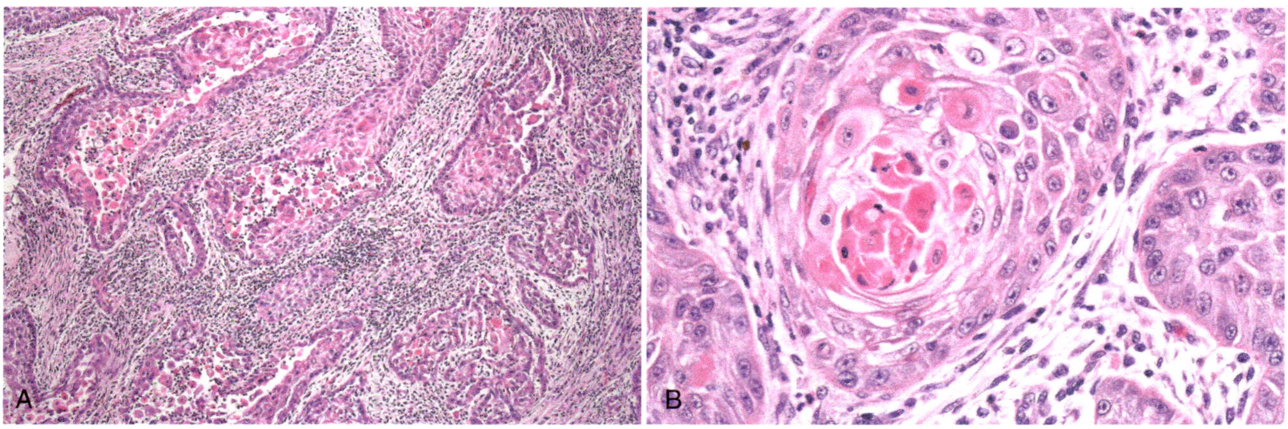

FIG 15.33 Primary intraosseous squamous cell carcinoma. (A) Infiltrating tumor islands have a vaguely follicular ameloblastomatous appearance, but without palisading of basal cells. (B) Keratin pearl formation, dyskeratosis, and nuclear atypia without peripheral palisaded cells are present.

CLEAR CELL ODONTOGENIC CARCINOMA

Clinical Findings

- The median age of occurrence of this tumor is in the sixth decade of life, with a 2:1 female predisposition. Pain, loosening of teeth, and paresthesia are often present. Seventy-five to eighty-five percent of cases occur in the mandible and it presents as a poorly demarcated radiolucency.

Etiopathogenesis and Histopathologic Features

This tumor shares many histopathologic features with salivary gland clear cell carcinoma. Salivary gland clear cell carcinomas and clear cell odontogenic carcinomas exhibit translocation of *EWSR1* in 92% and 63% of cases, respectively.

- This is an infiltrative tumor that is composed of islands and lobules of round or polyhedral cells with well-delineated borders and pale eosinophilic or clear cytoplasm that is glycogen rich. Tumor cells contain small, round-to-ovoid, hyperchromatic nuclei with small nucleoli. Atypia may be minimal, and mitoses may be present. The stroma is densely collagenous and/or hyalinized (Fig. 15.34).
- The *monophasic* variant is composed of only clear cells.
- The *biphasic* variant consists of clear cells as well as interspersed polygonal cells with denser, eosinophilic cytoplasm.
- The *ameloblastomatous* variant exhibits subtle palisading of the basal cell nuclei with reverse nuclear polarization.
- Cells are positive for keratin (AE1/AE3, K5/6, K19), p63, and epithelial membrane antigen and negative for K7, S100 protein, smooth muscle actin (SMA), and calponin.
- Fluorescence in situ hybridization studies have identified *EWSR1* rearrangements in 63% of cases.

Differential Diagnosis

- Clear cell calcifying epithelial odontogenic tumor has amyloid in the stroma and usually has calcifications.
- Clear cell mucoepidermoid carcinoma has mucous and epidermoid components, even if present focally.
- Metastatic renal cell carcinoma has nests of atypical clear cells that are positive for CD10, renal cell carcinoma antigen, PAX2, and PAX8, with dilated vessels surrounding tumor islands. Other metastatic tumors can be ruled out with appropriate immunohistochemical stains and identification of the primary site.

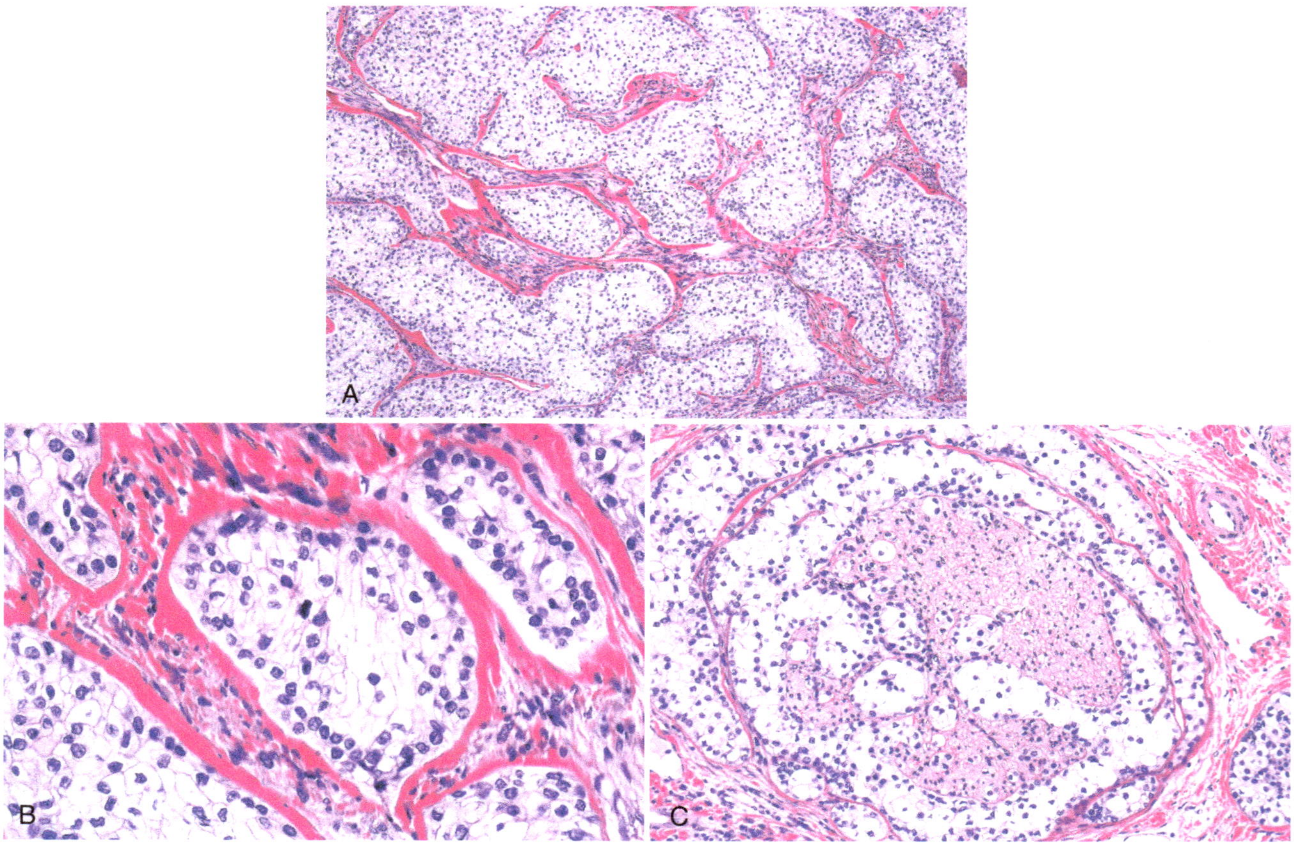

FIG 15.34 Clear cell odontogenic carcinoma. (A) Lobules of clear cells separated by hyalinized fibrous septa. (B) Cells have clear cytoplasm, mild nuclear atypia, and subtle palisading of nuclei at the periphery of lobules. A mitotic figure is present. (C) Perineural and intraneural invasion are present in this tumor.

Management and Prognosis

- En bloc resection is the treatment of choice, and adjuvant radiotherapy is employed in selected cases. Recurrence rates are 30% for resected tumors and 87% for curetted and/or enucleated lesions. Metastases are to lymph nodes, lung, and bones, and 13% of patients die as a result of the disease.

REFERENCES

August M, Faquin W, Troulis M, Kaban L. Clear cell odontogenic carcinoma: evaluation of reported cases. *J Oral Maxillofac Surg.* 2003;61:580-586.

Bilodeau EA, Hoschar AP, Barnes EL, et al. Clear cell carcinoma and clear cell odontogenic carcinoma: a comparative clinicopathologic and immunohistochemical study. *Head Neck Pathol.* 2011;5:101-107.

Bilodeau EA, Weinreb I, Antonescu CR, et al. Clear cell odontogenic carcinomas show EWSR1 rearrangements: a novel finding and a biological link to salivary clear cell carcinomas. *Am J Surg Pathol.* 2013;37:1001-1005.

Iezzi G, Rubini C, Fioroni M, Piattelli A. Clear cell odontogenic carcinoma. *Oral Oncol.* 2002;38:209-213.

Li TJ, Yu SF, Gao Y, Wang EB. Clear cell odontogenic carcinoma: a clinicopathologic and immunocytochemical study of 5 cases. *Arch Pathol Lab Med.* 2001;125:1566-1571.

Loyola AM, Cardoso SV, de Faria PR, et al. Clear cell odontogenic carcinoma: report of 7 new cases and systematic review of the current knowledge. *Oral Surg Oral Med Oral Pathol Oral Radiol.* 2015;120:483-496.

Zhang J, Liu L, Pan J, et al. Clear cell odontogenic carcinoma: report of 6 cases and review of the literature. *Med Oncol.* 2011;28(suppl 1):S626-S633.

SCLEROSING ODONTOGENIC CARCINOMA

The term *sclerosing odontogenic tumor* has also been proposed for this rare condition. No metastases have been recorded, but the number of reported cases is small.

Clinical Features

- This rare tumor occurs in the fifth to eighth decades of life and presents as a radiolucency in the mandible (60–70% of cases) with cortical perforation.

Etiopathogenesis and Histopathologic Features

As with other such tumors, this one likely arises from dental lamina rests in the bone.

- There are small islands and thin cords of epithelium that exhibit cytologic atypia in a densely hyalinized and sclerotic stroma. The cells are polygonal with distinct cell borders and nuclei that contain prominent nucleoli but usually no mitotic activity. Clear cells may be seen, and there may be squamous differentiation and cementum-like calcifications (Fig. 15.35).
- There is usually prominent perineural, intraneural, and intramuscular invasion. A case has been reported associated with a benign fibroosseous lesion.
- Tumor islands are positive for AE1/3, K5/6, K19, p63, and e-cadherin and variably for K7. They are negative for K20, carcinoembryonic antigen, CAM 5.2, vimentin, S100 protein, and amelogenin.

Differential Diagnosis

- Metastatic carcinoma must be ruled out in all cases with a clinical workup and immunohistochemical studies.
- Central odontogenic fibroma contains abundant mature fibrous tissue and many small islands and strands of odontogenic epithelium without cytologic evidence of malignancy and no perineural invasion.
- Calcifying epithelial odontogenic tumor contains islands of epithelium that often show significant nuclear pleomorphism but not perineural invasion, and it also contains amyloid and calcifications.
- Desmoplastic ameloblastoma contains irregularly shaped and stellate islands of epithelium with hyperchromatic nuclei, and some islands show palisading of the basal cell nuclei and stellate reticulum–like areas.

Management and Prognosis

- Treatment is resection with clear margins, and tumors do not tend to metastasize.

REFERENCES

Hussain O, Rendon AT, Orr RL, Speight PM. Sclerosing odontogenic carcinoma in the maxilla: a rare primary intraosseous carcinoma. *Oral Surg Oral Med Oral Pathol Oral Radiol.* 2013;116:e283-e286.

Irie T, Ogawa I, Takata T, et al. Sclerosing odontogenic carcinoma with benign fibro-osseous lesion of the mandible: an extremely rare case report. *Pathol Int.* 2010;60:694-700.

Koutlas IG, Allen CM, Warnock GR, Manivel JC. Sclerosing odontogenic carcinoma: a previously unreported variant of a locally aggressive odontogenic neoplasm without apparent metastatic potential. *Am J Surg Pathol.* 2008;32:1613-1619.

Tan SH, Yeo JF, Kheem Pang BN, Petersson F. An intraosseous sclerosing odontogenic tumor predominantly composed of epithelial cells: relation to (so-called) sclerosing odontogenic carcinoma and epithelial-rich central odontogenic fibroma. *Oral Surg Oral Med Oral Pathol Oral Radiol.* 2014;118:e119-e125.

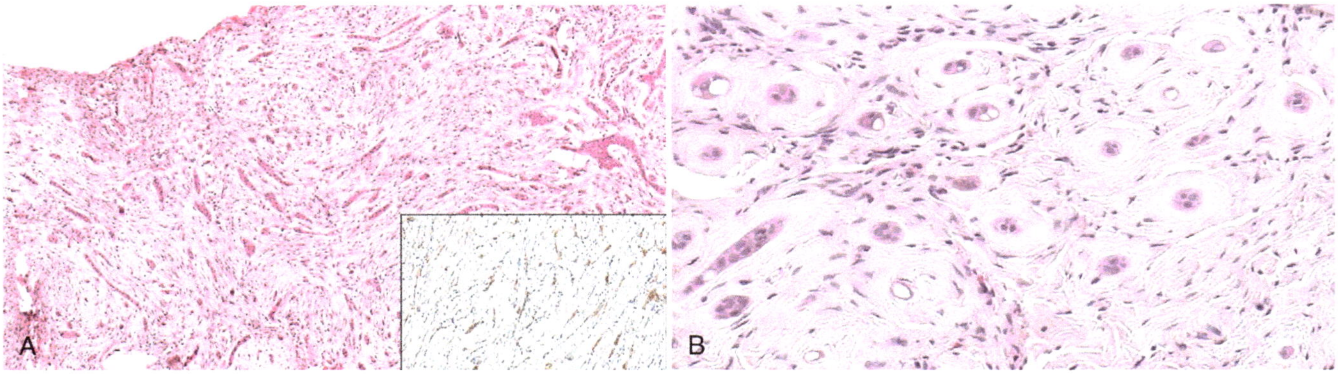

FIG 15.35 Sclerosing odontogenic carcinoma. (A) Thin cords and small nests proliferate in a densely collagenized stroma. The *inset* depicts immunoreactivity for CK19, revealing very thin cords of neoplastic cells compressed by the sclerosis (patient 2; *inset*: patient 1). *CK*, cytokeratin. (B) Occasional cytoplasmic clearing can be appreciated in all cases. Focally, a signet, ringlike pattern can be seen. *(From Koutlas IG, Allen CM, Warnock GR, Manivel JC. Sclerosing odontogenic carcinoma: a previously unreported variant of a locally aggressive odontogenic neoplasm without apparent metastatic potential. Am J Surg Pathol. 2008;32:1613–1619.)*

Mixed Epithelial and Ectomesenchymal Tumors

ODONTOMA

This is the second most common odontogenic tumor after keratocystic odontogenic tumor (odontogenic keratocyst).

Clinical Features

- Odontomas usually occur in the second and third decades of life, with complex odontomas more common in the posterior mandible and compound odontomas most common in the anterior maxilla. The mesiodens is a supernumerary or anomalous tooth located between maxillary central incisors.
- These present as a single radiopacity or multiple radiopacities with a surrounding radiolucent rim. Recognizable tooth structures or denticles are present in compound odontomas, while complex odontomas manifest as globular, calcified masses that may be very large (Fig. 15.36). Often they overlie teeth, and delayed eruption of a tooth is a presenting sign. Peripheral odontoma has been reported.

Etiopathogenesis and Histopathologic Features

Odontomas are considered by some authorities to be hamartomas, and they recapitulate the development of a tooth in either an organized (compound odontoma) or disorganized (complex odontoma) fashion.

- *Compound odontoma:* This consists of enamel matrix with a basophilic fish-scale appearance, tubular dentin, cementum, and dental papilla (myxoid and/or mucinous material with stellate fibroblasts) present in the configuration of a tooth with varying amounts of odontogenic epithelium. The term *anomalous tooth* is sometimes used for a single toothlike structure, and if this is in the midline of the maxilla, the term *mesiodens* is applied (Fig. 15.37). A dental follicle surrounds the lesion.
- *Complex odontoma:* This is composed of a mass of enamel matrix, tubular dentin, eosinophilic dentinoid, and cementoosseous material that is haphazardly arranged. Strands and islands of odontogenic epithelium, primitive dental papilla, ghost cells, lamellar calcifications, amorphous dystrophic calcifications, dentinoid, enameloid, amyloid-like material, and even melanin may be present (Figs. 15.38 and 15.39). Odontomas may be associated with other odontogenic lesions, in particular CCOT and many are associated with a dentigerous cyst.

Differential Diagnosis

- Ameloblastic fibroodontoma has components of odontoma and ameloblastic fibroma. However, some authorities consider the ameloblastic fibroodontoma to be an immature form of odontoma. Adenomatoid dentinoma and adenomatoid odontogenic hamartoma may represent developing odontomas with unusual adenomatoid epithelial proliferation, although enamel matrix is not reported in adenomatoid dentinoma. The so-called ameloblastic odontoma or odontoameloblastoma consists of an odontoma and a typical ameloblastoma and will behave as an ameloblastoma.

Management and Prognosis

- Excision or enucleation is curative.

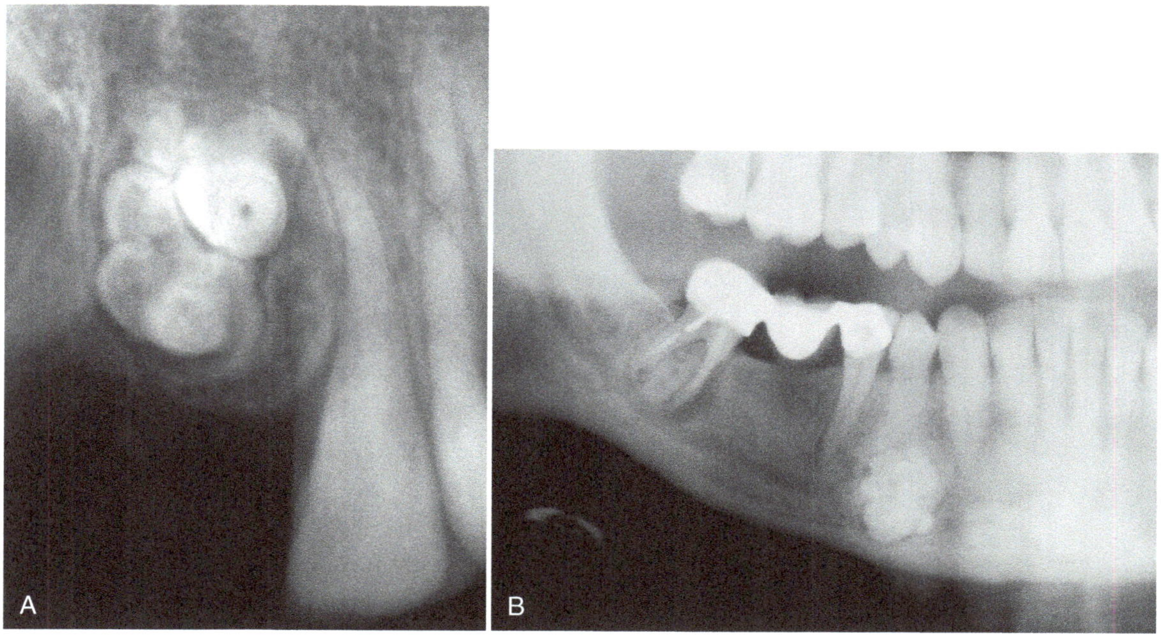

FIG 15.36 (A) Compound odontoma: recognizable toothlike structures surrounded by a thin, radiolucent rim. (B) Complex odontoma: globular masses of calcified material near the apex of the left mandibular first premolar. *(A, Courtesy Dr. John Sexton, private practice, Wellesley, Mass; B, Courtesy Dr. Bruce Sullivan, private practice, Norwood, Mass.)*

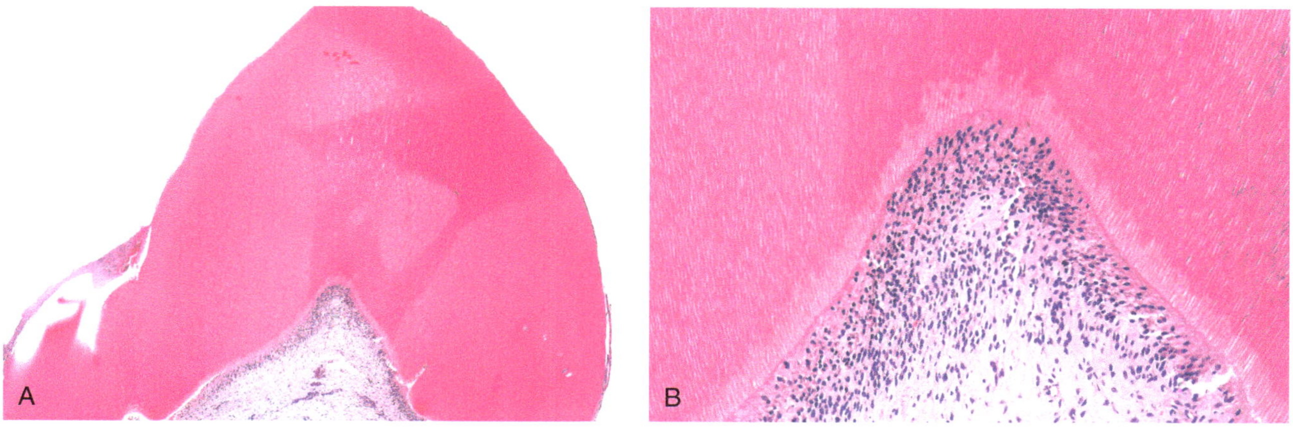

FIG 15.37 Compound odontoma or anomalous tooth if solitary. (A) Toothlike structure with dentinal tubules, enamel matrix (*left*), and dental papilla. (B) Tubular dentin formed by odontoblasts within myxoid and primitive dental papilla.

REFERENCES

Allen CM, Neville BW, Hammond HL. Adenomatoid dentinoma: report of four cases of an unusual odontogenic lesion. *Oral Surg Oral Med Oral Pathol Oral Radiol Endod.* 1998;86:313-317.

Carlos-Bregni R, Vargas PA, Santos Silva AR, et al. Adenomatoid odontogenic hamartoma: concerns about correct nomenclature and 2 additional case reports. *J Oral Maxillofac Surg.* 2009;67:1779-1780, author reply 1780.

Cohen DM, Bhattacharyya I. Ameloblastic fibroma, ameloblastic fibro-odontoma, and odontoma. *Oral Maxillofac Surg Clin North Am.* 2004;16:375-384.

Ide F, Mishima K, Saito I, Kusama K. Rare peripheral odontogenic tumors: report of 5 cases and comprehensive review of the literature. *Oral Surg Oral Med Oral Pathol Oral Radiol Endod.* 2008;106:e22-e28.

Owens BM, Schuman NJ, Mincer HH, et al. Dental odontomas: a retrospective study of 104 cases. *J Clin Pediatr Dent.* 1997;21:261-264.

Philipsen HP, Reichart PA, Praetorius F. Mixed odontogenic tumours and odontomas: considerations on interrelationship. Review of the literature and presentation of 134 new cases of odontomas. *Oral Oncol.* 1997;33:86-99.

Soluk Tekkesin M, Pehlivan S, Olgac V, et al. Clinical and histopathological investigation of odontomas: review of the literature and presentation of 160 cases. *J Oral Maxillofac Surg.* 2012;70:1358-1361.

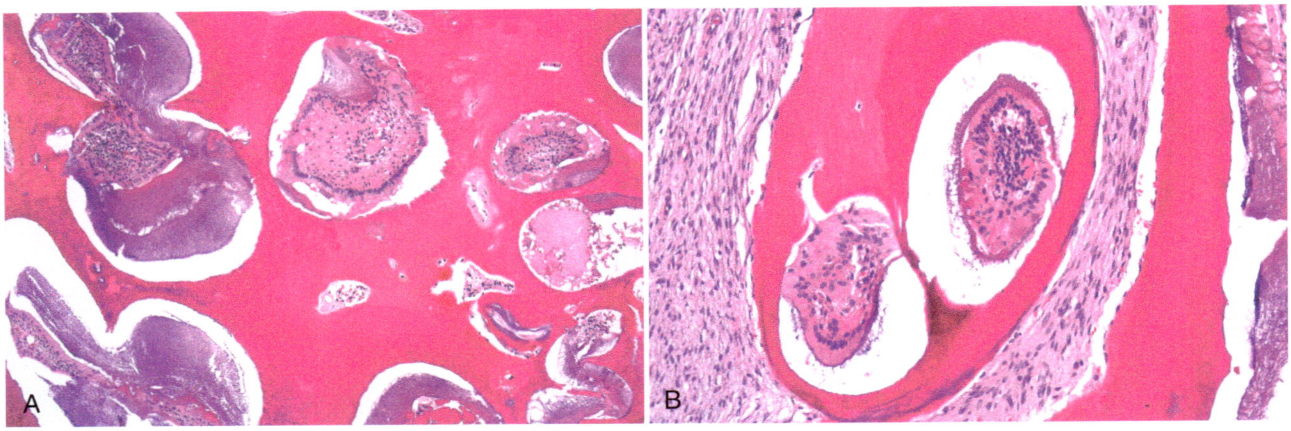

FIG 15.38 Complex odontoma. (A) Haphazard arrangement of basophilic enamel matrix, tubular dentin, and dentinoid. (B) Enamel matrix *(right)*; tubular dentin; dentinoid; and columnar, pale eosinophilic odontogenic epithelium.

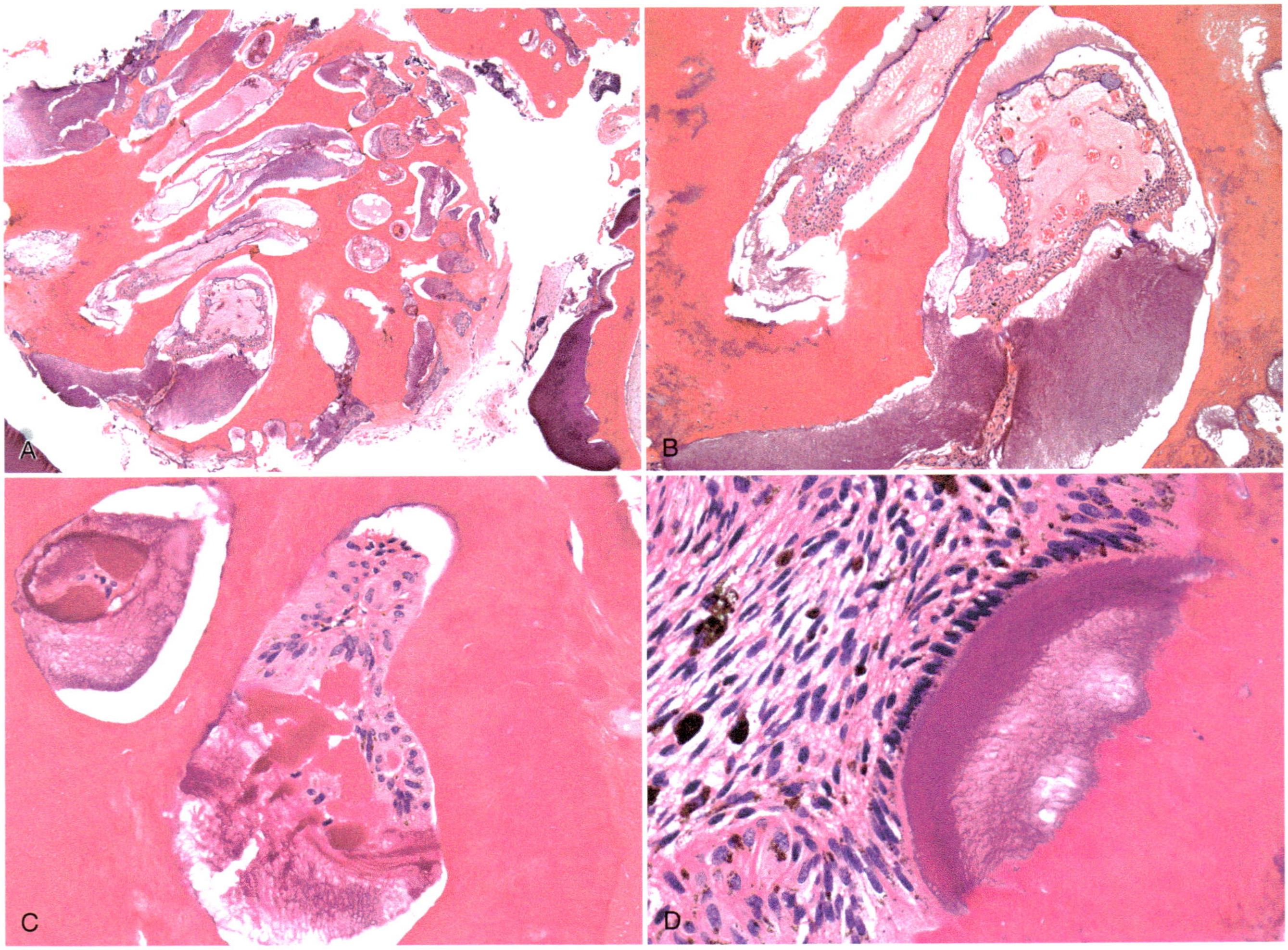

FIG 15.39 Complex odontoma. (A) Haphazard arrangement of enamel matrix, eosinophilic dentin and dentinoid, and odontogenic epithelium. (B) Enamel matrix *(bottom)*, dentinoid and columnar odontogenic epithelium. (C) Tubular dentin *(right)*, dentinoid, basophilic enamel matrix, and dark pink enameloid. (D) Enamel epithelium abutting enamel matrix and spindled odontogenic epithelium contain melanin.

AMELOBLASTIC FIBROODONTOMA

Some pathologists believe that ameloblastic fibroodontoma and odontoma are a spectrum of the same condition, with odontoma being the more mature lesion and as such, occurring in older patients; other pathologists consider them separate entities.

Clinical Features

- Most cases (98%) occur in the first and second decades of life, with a mean age of 9 years. Fifty percent occur in the posterior mandible, and 25% occur in the posterior maxilla. The most common presentation is a mixed radiolucent-radiopaque mass overlying a tooth (often a permanent mandibular first molar), causing failure of eruption (Fig. 15.40).

Etiopathogenesis and Histopathologic Features

This tumor recapitulates the developing tooth with both ectomesenchymal and epithelial components.

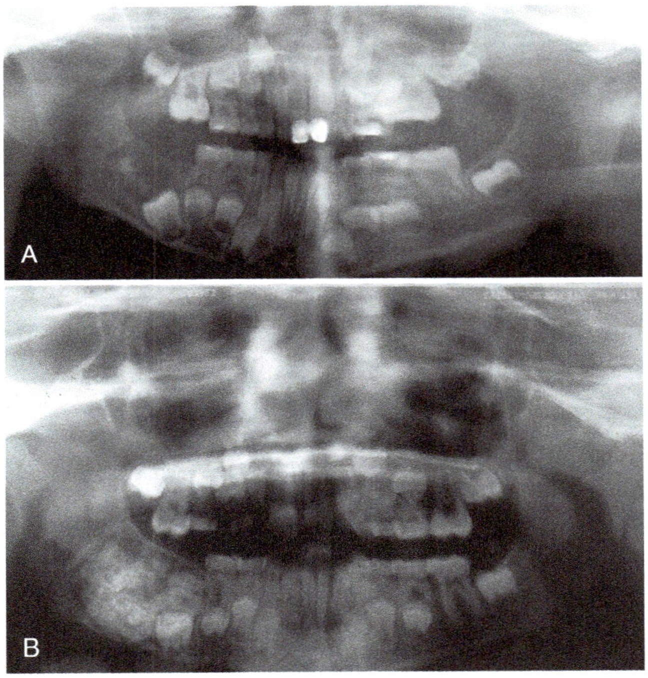

FIG 15.40 Ameloblastic fibroodontoma. (A) Well-circumscribed radiolucency with radiopacities above crown of inferiorly displaced right permanent first molar. (B) Well-circumscribed radiolucency with dense radiopaque mass above crown of inferiorly displaced right permanent mandibular first molar. *(A, Courtesy Dr. Lawrence M. Juvet, private practice, Brockton, Mass.)*

- Typical ameloblastic fibroma (see later) is present, composed of often vaguely nodular proliferation of myxoid and/or mucinous stroma containing spindle and stellate cells, within which are embedded islands and strands of ameloblastomatous epithelium with the usual central stellate reticulum and peripheral basal cells with reverse nuclear polarization; an odontoma is present, usually of the complex type. The odontoma is composed of a haphazard deposition of tubular dentin, enamel matrix ("fish scale" appearance), cementum, dentinoid, ringlike calcifications, and often ghost cells and odontogenic epithelium (Figs. 15.41 and 15.42). Melanin-containing stromal cells may be present.

Differential Diagnosis

- Ameloblastic fibroma does not produce enamel, dentin, or cementum, but a small number of cases of ameloblastic fibroma may represent very early ameloblastic fibroodontomas or odontomas.
- Complex odontoma has no ameloblastic fibroma-like component.
- Cases of ameloblastic fibrodentinoma that show an ameloblastic fibroma with dentinoid should be leveled deeper to look for enamel matrix.
- Archegonous cystic odontoma is likely an immature odontoma and is cystic, with a subepithelial hypercellular cambium zone, lobular ameloblastic fibroma-like area, and deposition of dentinoid.

Management and Prognosis

- Enucleation or excision is curative.

REFERENCES

Argyris PP, Wetzel SL, Pambuccian SE, et al. Primordial odontogenic cyst with induction phenomenon (zonal fibroblastic hypercellularity) and dentinoid material versus archegonous cystic odontoma: you choose! *Head Neck Pathol.* 2016;10:237-244.

Boxberger NR, Brannon RB, Fowler CB. Ameloblastic fibro-odontoma: a clinicopathologic study of 12 cases. *J Clin Pediatr Dent.* 2011;35:397-403.

Philipsen HP, Reichart PA, Praetorius F. Mixed odontogenic tumours and odontomas: considerations on interrelationship. Review of the literature and presentation of 134 new cases of odontomas. *Oral Oncol.* 1997;33:86-99.

Phillips MD, Closmann JJ, Baus MR, et al. Hybrid odontogenic tumor with features of ameloblastic fibro-odontoma, calcifying odontogenic cyst, and adenomatoid odontogenic tumor: a case report and review of the literature. *J Oral Maxillofac Surg.* 2010;68:470-474.

Slootweg PJ. An analysis of the interrelationship of the mixed odontogenic tumors—ameloblastic fibroma, ameloblastic fibro-odontoma, and the odontomas. *Oral Surg Oral Med Oral Pathol.* 1981;51:266-276.

Takeda Y, Sato H, Satoh M, et al. Immunohistochemical expression of neural tissue markers (neuron-specific enolase, glial fibrillary acidic protein, S100 protein) in ameloblastic fibrodentinoma: a comparative study with ameloblastic fibroma. *Pathol Int.* 2000;50:610-615.

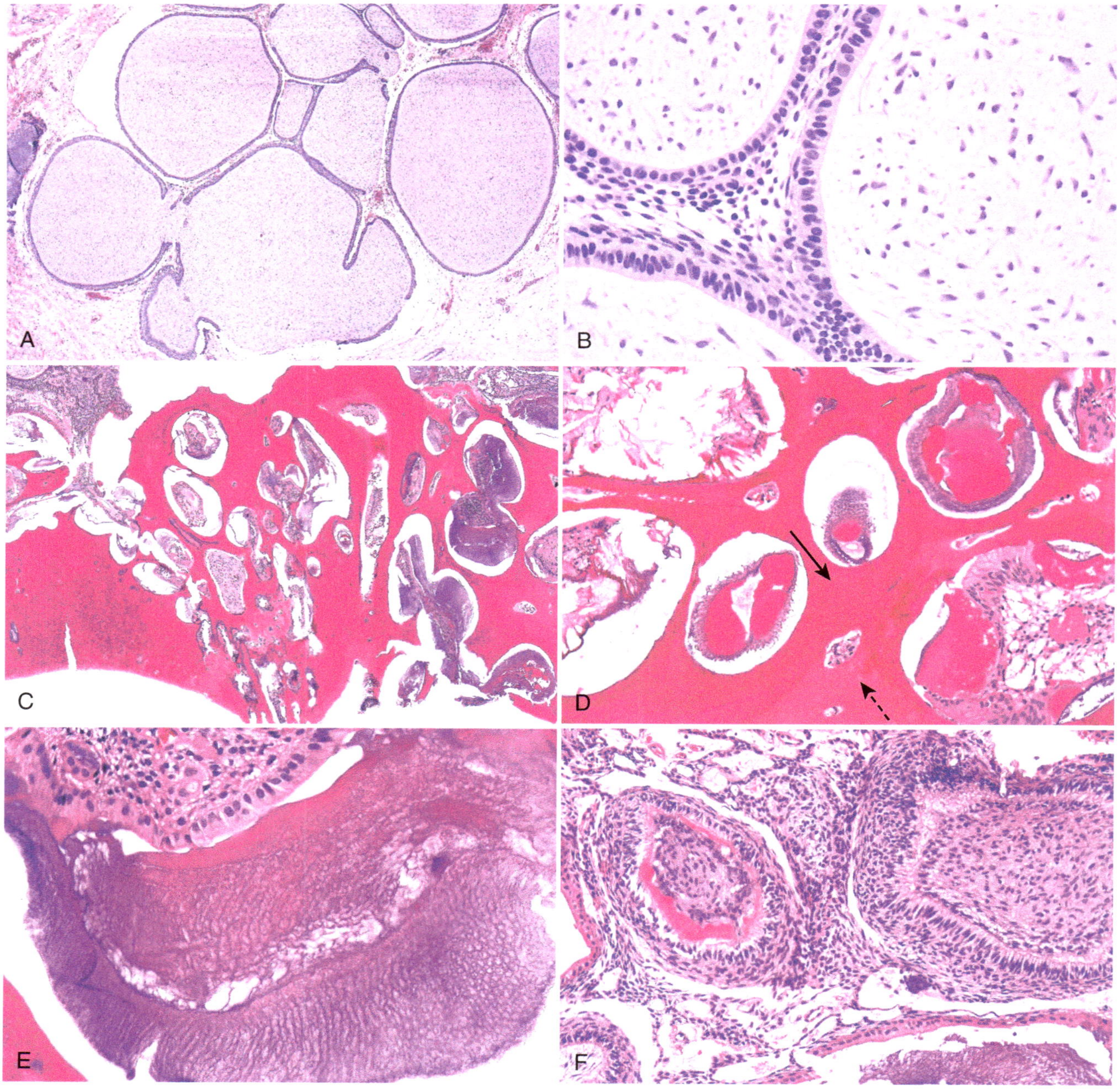

FIG 15.41 Ameloblastic fibroodontoma. (A) Ameloblastic fibroma with proliferation of epithelium and spindle cells in myxoid stroma. (B) Ameloblastoma-like epithelium with subtle palisading of basal cells and stellate reticulum–like areas. Many stellate fibroblast–like cells in myxoid stroma are present. (C) Complex odontoma composed of masses of tubular dentin and dentinoid. (D) Tubular dentin *(solid arrow)*, dentinoid *(dashed arrow)*, hematoxyphilic enamel matrix, and odontogenic epithelium. (E) Enamel matrix with fish-scale appearance and odontogenic epithelium. (F) Organoid structures with odontogenic epithelium and eosinophilic dentinoid is suggestive of abortive odontogenesis.

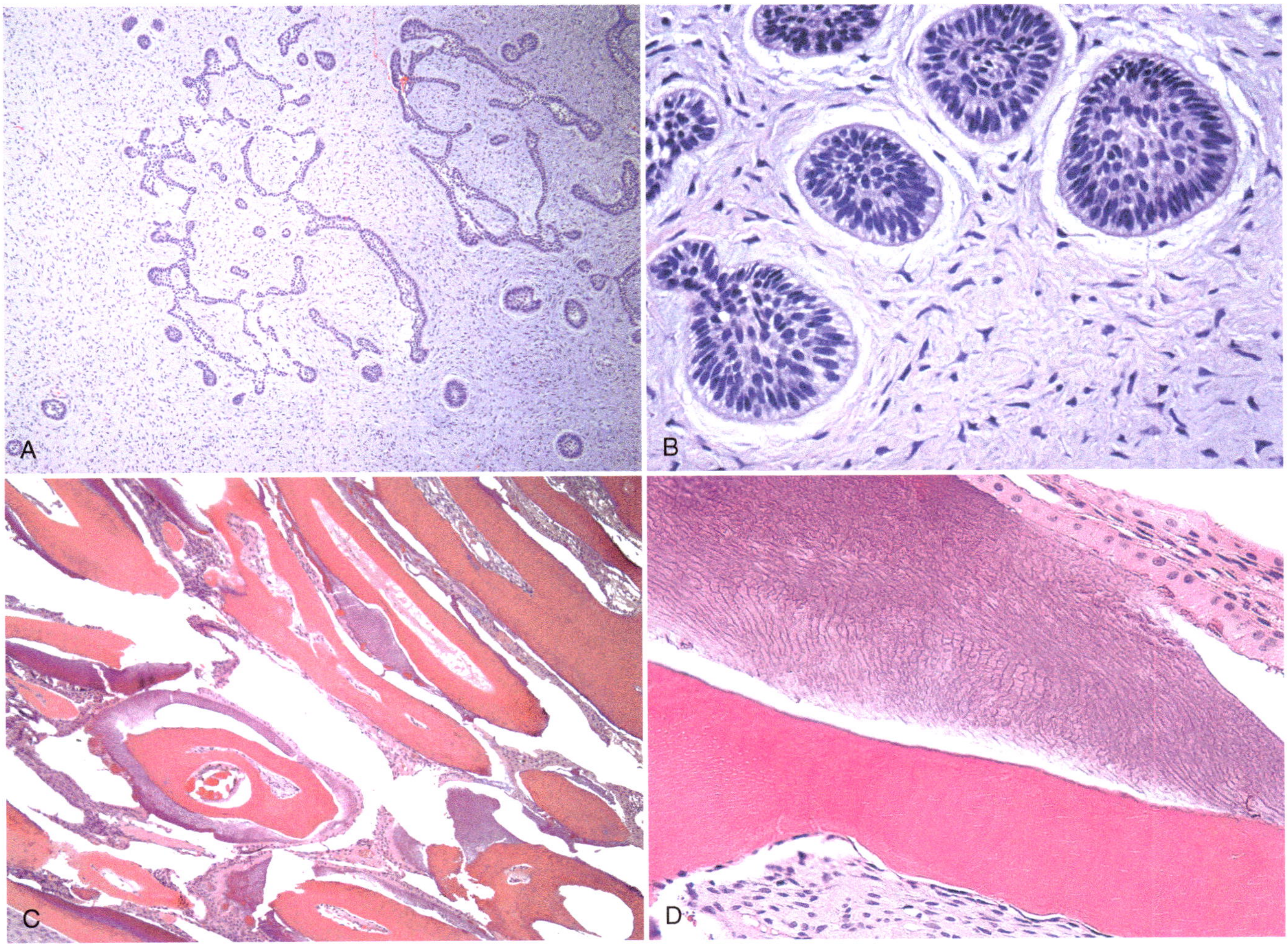

FIG 15.42. Ameloblastic fibroodontoma. (A) Ameloblastic fibroma with proliferation of strands and islands of odontogenic epithelium and spindle cells in myxoid stroma. (B) Ameloblastoma-like epithelium with palisading of basal cells and reverse nuclear polarization. Many spindle and stellate fibroblast-like cells in myxoid stroma are present. (C) Compound odontoma composed of masses of eosinophilic tubular dentin and basophilic enamel matrix in a haphazard arrangement. (D) Tubular dentin, enamel matrix with a fish-scale appearance, and odontogenic epithelium.

AMELOBLASTIC FIBROMA

Clinical Findings

- This uncommon tumor is most frequently encountered in the first to third decades of life, with 75% of cases presenting before age 20 years. Lesions may be very large and cause facial swelling. Seventy to ninety percent of cases occur in the mandible, and 90% of cases are located in the posterior aspects of the jaws. It presents as a unilocular and sometimes multilocular radiolucency (in larger tumors) (Fig. 15.43).

Etiopathogenesis and Histopathologic Features

Differentiation of this tumor is toward ameloblastomatous epithelium and dental papilla before the deposition of dental hard tissues. There is ongoing controversy regarding the relationship of this tumor to ameloblastic fibroodontoma, ameloblastic fibrodentinoma, and odontoma. Current understanding suggests that some lesions (smaller ones in children in the first decade of life) may represent developing odontomas. The evidence for this is as follows: in some tumors that were incompletely removed, lesions progressed and the subsequent removal demonstrated ameloblastic fibrodentinoma, ameloblastic fibroodontoma, or odontoma. However, the histopathologic features of these lesions that mature and those of true neoplasms with the potential for malignant transformation, are indistinguishable. One theory suggests that ameloblastic fibromas that arise after completion of odontogenesis (if that can be clearly established), are more likely to be neoplastic.

- This is a biphasic tumor with an epithelial component that is typical for follicular ameloblastoma, with the basal cells exhibiting reverse nuclear polarization and stellate reticulum–like areas in the center of the follicles. In addition, there is a cellular proliferation of spindled and stellate fibroblast-like cells with dispersed nuclear chromatin and small or inconspicuous nuclei in an extremely myxoid and/or mucinous background with delicate collagen (Fig. 15.44).

Differential Diagnosis

- If dentinoid is present, the diagnosis is ameloblastic fibrodentinoma. In such cases, deeper levels should be performed because these may reveal the presence of enamel matrix, in which case the diagnosis is ameloblastic fibroodontoma.
- Ameloblastic fibroodontoma has identical soft tissue histopathology, but an odontoma is also present.
- Ameloblastic fibrosarcoma may arise de novo, but 40% to 50% arise from a preexisting ameloblastic fibroma, usually in the fourth decade of life, one decade later than de novo lesions. The tumor contains islands of benign epithelium typical for ameloblastoma, and there is a hypercellular proliferation of spindle cells that show malignant morphology with hyperchromatic atypical nuclei, mitoses, and sometimes necrosis (Fig. 15.45). Twenty-five percent recur, and 5% develop metastases.

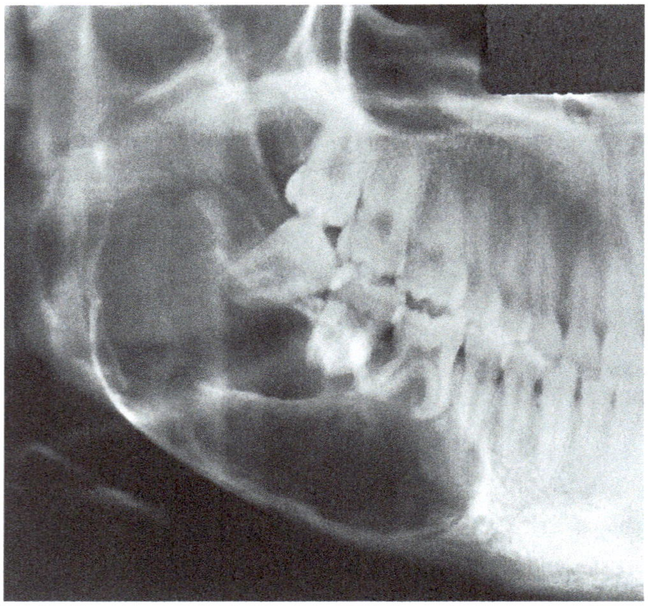

FIG 15.43 Ameloblastic fibroma: multiloculated radiolucency of the right posterior mandible body and ramus. *(From White SC, Pharoah MJ. Oral Radiology: Principles and Interpretation. 6th ed. St Louis, Mosby, 2009:381.)*

Management and Prognosis

- Excision or resection is the treatment of choice, and curettage is associated with a higher recurrence rate (likely progression of disease from incomplete removal). The recurrence is 15% to 30%, depending on the primary treatment modality, and 10% to 20% undergo malignant transformation to ameloblastic fibrosarcoma, with younger presentation associated with increased risk. Tumors do not tend to metastasize.

REFERENCES

Abughazaleh K, Andrus KM, Katsnelson A, et al. Peripheral ameloblastic fibroma of the maxilla. *Oral Surg Oral Med Oral Pathol Oral Radiol Endod.* 2008;105:e36-e48.

Buchner A, Vered M. Ameloblastic fibroma: a stage in the development of a hamartomatous odontoma or a true neoplasm? Critical analysis of 162 previously reported cases plus 10 new cases. *Oral Surg Oral Med Oral Pathol Oral Radiol.* 2013;116:598-606.

Chau E, Daley T, Darling MR, Hamilton D. The expression and immunohistochemical localization of periostin in odontogenic tumors of mixed epithelial/mesenchymal origin. *Oral Surg Oral Med Oral Pathol Oral Radiol.* 2013;116:214-220.

Chen Y, Wang JM, Li TJ. Ameloblastic fibroma: a review of published studies with special reference to its nature and biological behavior. *Oral Oncol.* 2007;43:960-969.

Lai J, Blanas N, Higgins K, Klieb H. Ameloblastic fibrosarcoma: report of a case, study of immunophenotype, and comprehensive review of the literature. *J Oral Maxillofac Surg.* 2012;70:2007-2012.

Muller S, Parker DC, Kapadia SB, et al. Ameloblastic fibrosarcoma of the jaws: a clinicopathologic and DNA analysis of five cases and review of the literature with discussion of its relationship to ameloblastic fibroma. *Oral Surg Oral Med Oral Pathol Oral Radiol Endod.* 1995;79:469-477.

Philipsen HP, Reichart PA, Praetorius F. Mixed odontogenic tumours and odontomas: considerations on interrelationship. Review of the literature and presentation of 134 new cases of odontomas. *Oral Oncol.* 1997;33:86-99.

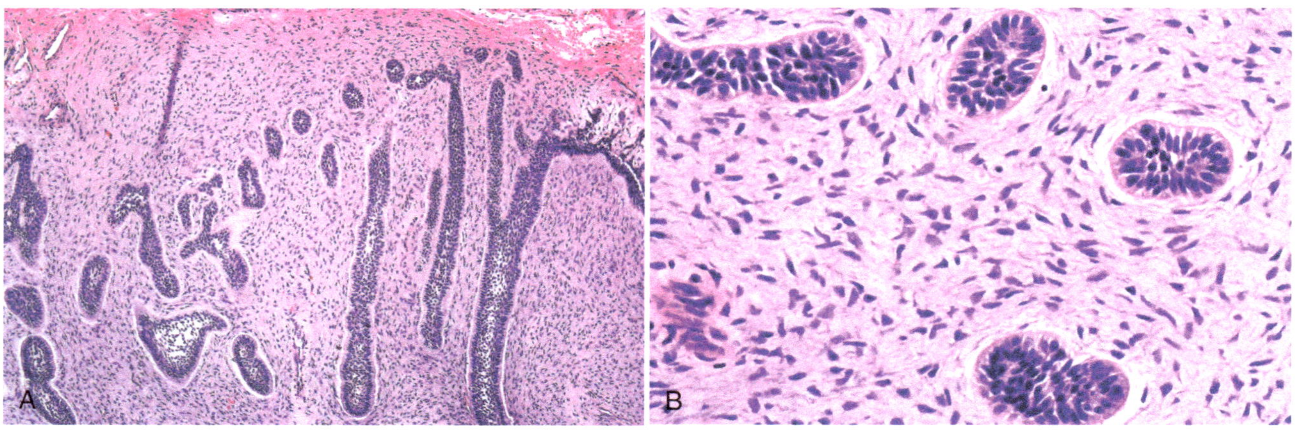

FIG 15.44 Ameloblastic fibroma. (A) Proliferation of ameloblastoma-like epithelium in a follicular pattern with a cellular spindle cell proliferation within myxoid stroma. (B) Plump, stellate, and spindled fibroblast-like cells without atypia are present in a myxoid-mucinous stroma; odontogenic islands exhibit palisading of basal cell nuclei..

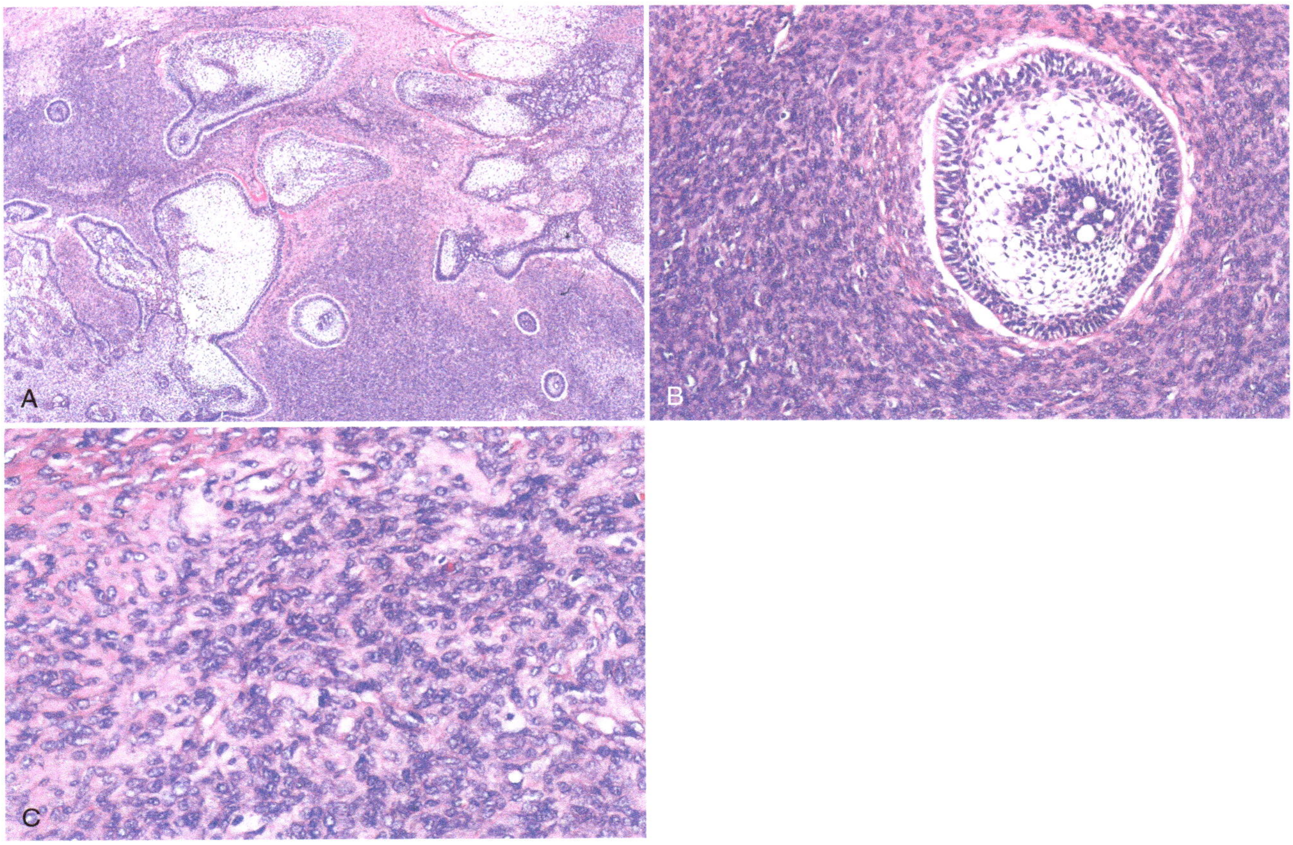

FIG 15.45 Ameloblastic fibrosarcoma. (A) Ameloblastoma and hypercellular spindle cell proliferation. (B) Typical ameloblastoma with stellate reticulum–like areas, and highly cellular proliferation of atypical spindle cells. (C) Atypical spindle cells with pleomorphic overlapping nuclei.

Slater LJ. Odontogenic sarcoma and carcinosarcoma. *Semin Diagn Pathol.* 1999;16:325-332.

Takeda Y, Sato H, Satoh M, et al. Immunohistochemical expression of neural tissue markers (neuron-specific enolase, glial fibrillary acidic protein, S100 protein) in ameloblastic fibrodentinoma: a comparative study with ameloblastic fibroma. *Pathol Int.* 2000;50:610-615.

CALCIFYING CYSTIC ODONTOGENIC TUMOR (CALCIFYING ODONTOGENIC CYST, GORLIN CYST), DENTINOGENIC GHOST CELL TUMOR, AND GHOST CELL ODONTOGENIC CARCINOMA

These lesions have in common the abundance of ghost cells and deposition of *dentinoid*, a term that refers to a hyalinized, eosinophilic substance that is closely apposed to odontogenic epithelium. It is likely a form of aberrant dentinal matrix.

Clinical Features

- *Calcifying cystic odontogenic tumor (CCOT):* The average age of patients is in the fourth decade of life, with equal involvement of the maxilla and mandible, although in the maxilla 75% occur in the anterior region. This cystic lesion manifests as a unilocular radiolucency or mixed radiolucency-radiopacity especially if associated with odontoma. Forty to fifty percent are associated with an unerupted tooth (Fig. 15.46A–B).
- *Dentinogenic ghost cell tumor (DGCT):* This solid variant represents less than 5% of ghost cell lesions. The mean age is in the fourth decade of life, with a 2:1 male predilection. Seventy-eight percent of cases are unilocular, and 67% are mixed radiolucent and/or radiopaque, with a mean size of 4 cm.
- *Peripheral (extraosseous) CCOT* and *DGCT*: Both present as a swelling of the gingiva, and the peripheral *CCOT* constitutes 13% of all peripheral odontogenic tumors, occurring in the fourth decade of life usually in the anterior jaws (see Fig. 15.46C). The peripheral *DGCT* is much less common.
- *Ghost cell odontogenic carcinoma (GCOC):* The mean age at occurrence is in the fifth decade of life, with a 3:1 to 4:1 male predilection. The maxilla is involved in 65% to 75% of cases, and 78% present as mixed radiolucency and/or radiopacity with poorly demarcated borders.

Etiopathogenesis and Histopathologic Features

The equivalent skin lesion is the pilomatrixoma or calcifying epithelioma of Malherbe. Somatic β-catenin mutations have been found in *CCOT*s, and this suggests that dysregulation of the Wnt signaling pathway, which helps to regulate odontogenesis, plays a role in the development of this cystic tumor. Approximately 50% of adamantinomatous craniopharyngiomas that develop from neoplastic transformation of remnants of Rathke pouch

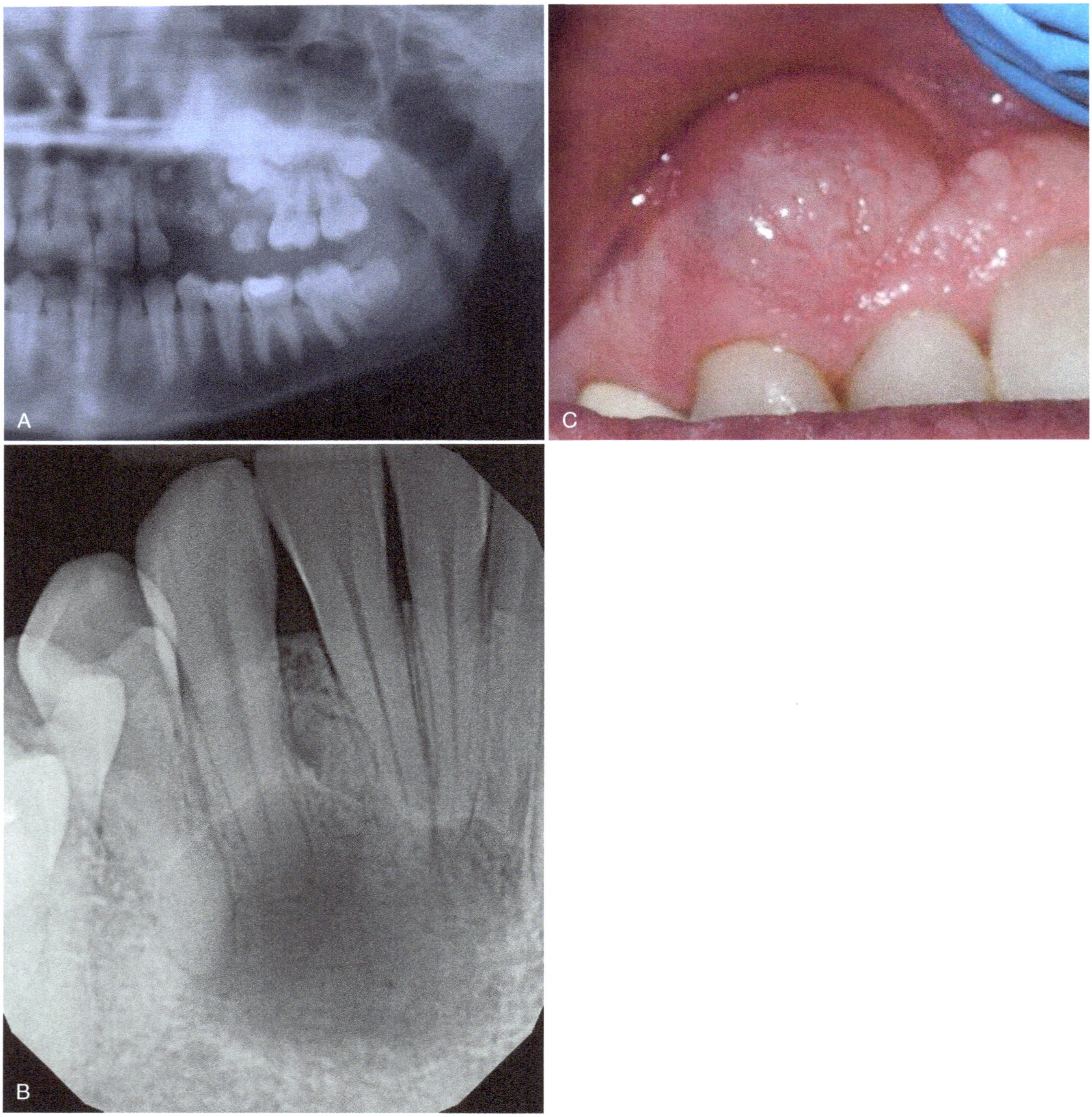

FIG 15.46 Calcifying cystic odontogenic tumor. (A) Radiolucency with multiple opacities (odontomas), associated with the impacted left maxillary canine. (B) Radiolucency at the apices of mandibular teeth. (C) Peripheral tumor presenting as a mass on the gingiva. (*C, Courtesy Dr. James Wu, private practice, Tewksbury, Mass.*)

have histopathologic features that are very similar to *CCOT*, and they also show mutations in *CTNNB1*, leading to activation of the Wnt signaling pathway, as well as the presence of enamel proteins such as amelogenin. GCOCs arise de novo in 40% of cases, from preexisting CCOTs in 37% of cases, from ameloblastomas in 13% of cases, and from DGCTs in 3% of cases, and the rest arise from other odontogenic tumors and cysts.

- *CCOT:* The following histopathologic subtypes are recognized:
  - *Simple cystic:* This represents 65% of all cases. There is a cyst lined by squamous or stellate reticulum–like cells with slight palisading of basal cells. Ghost cells are present, and these consist of large cells with eosinophilic cytoplasm, an empty space in place of the nucleus, and sometimes dystrophic

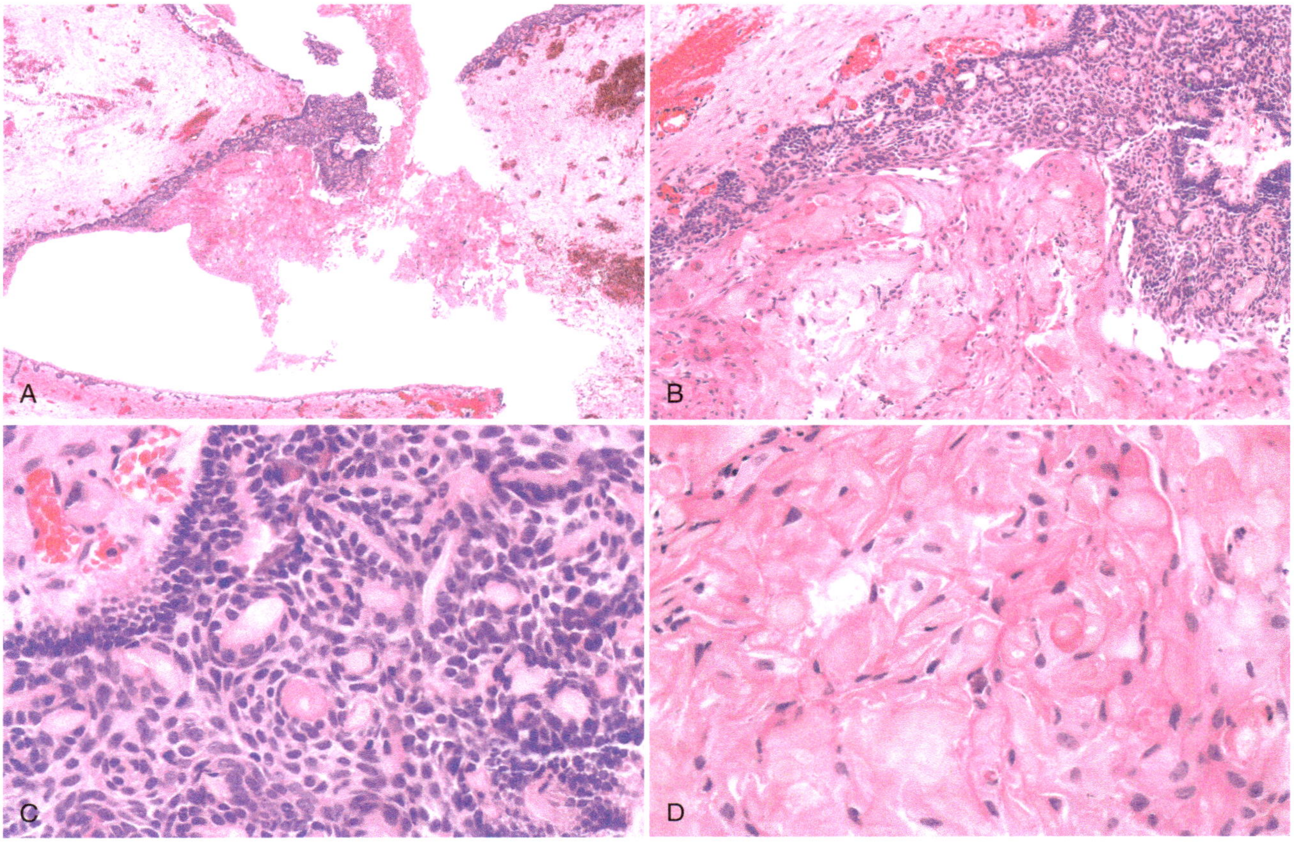

FIG 15.47 Calcifying cystic odontogenic tumor. (A) The cyst is lined by basaloid epithelium with many ghost cells. (B) Epithelial proliferation and many ghost cells are present. (C) The lining epithelium contains a few ghost cells, and basal cells are slightly palisaded. (D) Typical ghost cells with abundant eosinophilic cytoplasm and a space where the nucleus should be.

calcifications appearing as droplets within the cytoplasm. Dentinoid is variably present and often juxtaepithelial (Fig. 15.47). Melanin pigment is seen infrequently.

- *Odontoma-associated:* This represents 22% of all cases where a simple cystic *CCOT* is associated with an odontoma.
- *Ameloblastomatous:* These show ameloblastomatous proliferation with stellate reticulum–like areas and basal cells exhibiting reverse nuclear polarization (Fig. 15.48).

CCOTs exhibit nuclear and cytoplasmic positivity for β-catenin.

- *DGCT:* Components similar to those of *CCOT* are present, but DGCTs are present as solid masses and sheets of slightly basaloid cells. Ghost cells are abundant, and there may be extensive dentinoid deposition and extensive dystrophic calcifications. Cells that deposit dentinoid often show eccentric nuclei resembling osteoblasts, and some tumors may have areas resembling ameloblastoma. Melanin may be present, and β-catenin is usually present in both the nucleus and cytoplasm (Fig. 15.49).
- *GCOC:* The tumor may be cystic or solid, and tumor cells exhibit moderate atypia and pleomorphism, with variable numbers of ghost cells (Fig. 15.50). Dentinoid is usually but not invariably present. Palisading of cells at the periphery of tumor islands is often noted; mitotic activity and necrosis may be present; and Ki-67 indices are usually high.
- Peripheral lesions have the same histopathology as central lesions (Fig. 15.51).

Differential Diagnosis

- Adenoid ameloblastoma has similar histopathology to the ameloblastomatous variant of CCOT and will also contain ghost cells and dentinoid but with a pseudocribriform morphology.
- Odontogenic carcinoma with dentinoid formation usually shows minimal ghost cell formation and exhibits infiltration of the stroma and adjacent structures.

Management and Prognosis

- *CCOT:* Enucleation and/or excision is the treatment of choice. The cystic variant has a recurrence rate of 5%.
- *DGCT:* Recurrence varies, depending on the primary treatment modality. Enucleation and resection are associated with recurrence rates of 73% and 33%, respectively. GCOC is treated with resection.

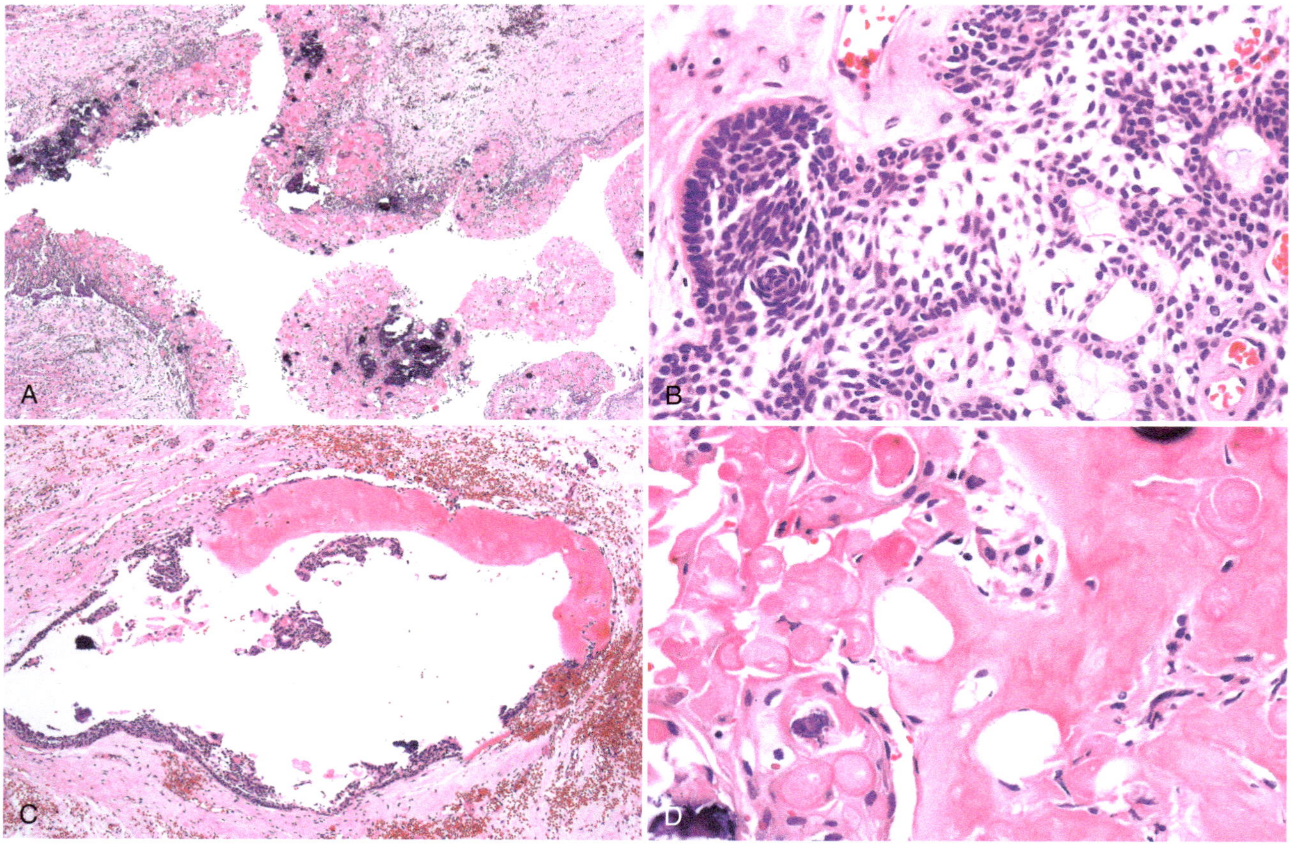

FIG 15.48 Calcifying cystic odontogenic tumor. (A) Cystic lesion with many ghost cells and dystrophic calcifications within the lining. (B) Ameloblastomatous areas with basal cell nuclear palisading and stellate reticulum–like areas. (C) Juxtaepithelial dentinoid deposition. (D) Dentinoid encircling ghost cells that exhibit early dystrophic calcifications.

REFERENCES

Arashiyama T, Kodama Y, Kobayashi T, et al. Ghost cell odontogenic carcinoma arising in the background of a benign calcifying cystic odontogenic tumor of the mandible. *Oral Surg Oral Med Oral Pathol Oral Radiol.* 2012;114:e35-e40.

Buchner A, Akrish SJ, Vered M. Central dentinogenic ghost cell tumor: an update on a rare aggressive odontogenic tumor. *J Oral Maxillofac Surg.* 2016;74:307-314.

Buchner A, Merrell PW, Hansen LS, Leider AS. Peripheral (extraosseous) calcifying odontogenic cyst: a review of forty-five cases. *Oral Surg Oral Med Oral Pathol.* 1991;72:65-70.

Buchner A. The central (intraosseous) calcifying odontogenic cyst: an analysis of 215 cases. *J Oral Maxillofac Surg.* 1991;49:330-339.

Candido GA, Viana KA, Watanabe S, Vencio EF. Peripheral dentinogenic ghost cell tumor: a case report and review of the literature. *Oral Surg Oral Med Oral Pathol Oral Radiol Endod.* 2009;108:e86-e90.

Gomes da Silva W, Ribeiro Bartholomeu dos Santos TC, Cabral MG, et al. Clinicopathologic analysis and syndecan-1 and Ki-67 expression in calcifying cystic odontogenic tumors, dentinogenic ghost cell tumor, and ghost cell odontogenic carcinoma. *Oral Surg Oral Med Oral Pathol Oral Radiol.* 2014;117:626-633.

Gong Y, Wang L, Wang H, et al. The expression of NF-κB, Ki-67 and MMP-9 in CCOT, DGCT and GCOC. *Oral Oncol.* 2009;45:515-520.

Hong SP, Ellis GL, Hartman KS. Calcifying odontogenic cyst: a review of ninety-two cases with reevaluation of their nature as cysts or neoplasms, the nature of ghost cells, and subclassification. *Oral Surg Oral Med Oral Pathol.* 1991;72:56-64.

Ledesma-Montes C, Gorlin RJ, Shear M, et al. International collaborative study on ghost cell odontogenic tumours: calcifying cystic odontogenic tumour, dentinogenic ghost cell tumour and ghost cell odontogenic carcinoma. *J Oral Pathol Med.* 2008;37:302-308.

Li BH, Cho YA, Kim SM, et al. Recurrent odontogenic ghost cell carcinoma (OGCC) at a reconstructed fibular flap: a case report with immunohistochemical findings. *Med Oral Patol Oral Cir Bucal.* 2011;16:e651-e656.

Li TJ, Yu SF. Clinicopathologic spectrum of the so-called calcifying odontogenic cysts: a study of 21 intraosseous cases with reconsideration of the terminology and classification. *Am J Surg Pathol.* 2003;27:372-384.

Paulus W, Stockel C, Krauss J, et al. Odontogenic classification of craniopharyngiomas: a clinicopathological study of 54 cases. *Histopathology.* 1997;30:172-176.

Resende RG, Brito JA, Souza LN, et al. Peripheral calcifying odontogenic cyst: a case report and review of the literature. *Head Neck Pathol.* 2011;5:76-80.

Sekine S, Sato S, Takata T, et al. β-catenin mutations are frequent in calcifying odontogenic cysts, but rare in ameloblastomas. *Am J Pathol.* 2003;163:1707-1712.

Sekine S, Takata T, Shibata T, et al. Expression of enamel proteins and LEF1 in adamantinomatous craniopharyngioma: evidence for its odontogenic epithelial differentiation. *Histopathology.* 2004;45:573-579.

Sun G, Huang X, Hu Q, et al. The diagnosis and treatment of dentinogenic ghost cell tumor. *Int J Oral Maxillofac Surg.* 2009;38:1179-1183.

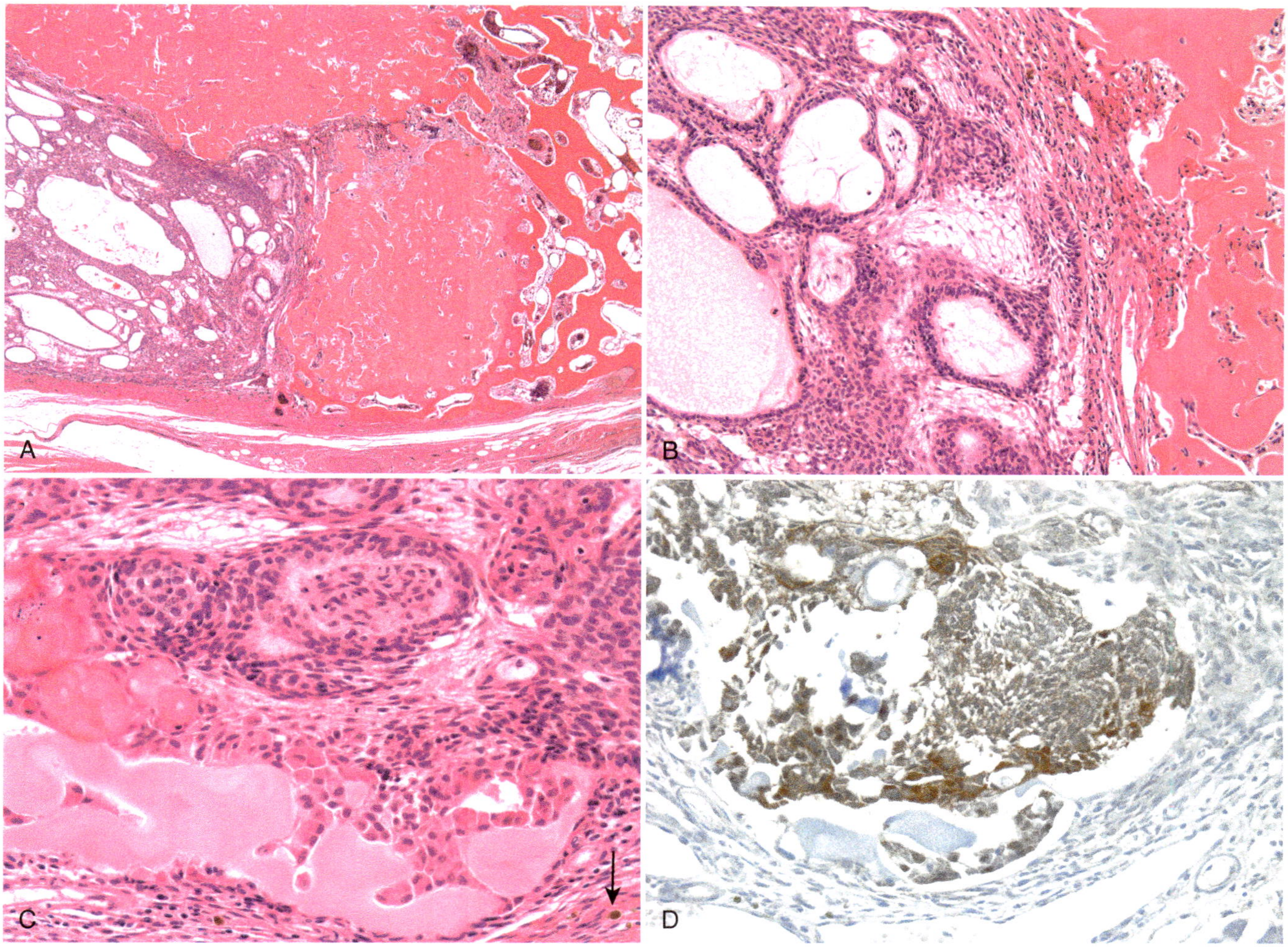

FIG 15.49 Dentinogenic ghost cell tumor. (A) The tumor produces abundant dentinoid and abuts and infiltrates the adjacent bone *(right)*. (B) Tumor epithelium has a slightly ameloblastomatous appearance with palisading of basal cells and stellate reticulum–like areas. The ductlike structures represent degenerated stroma. (C) Polygonal tumor cells transition into cells with eccentric nuclei that deposit dentinoid. Melanin is present *(arrow)*. (D) β-Catenin is positive within the cytoplasm and some nuclei of tumor cells.

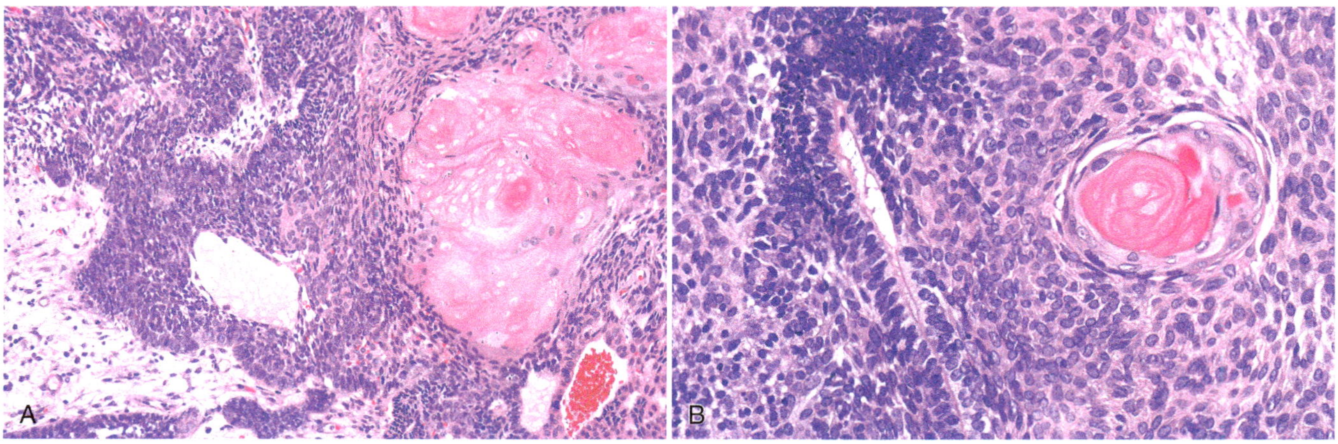

FIG 15.50 Ghost cell odontogenic carcinoma. (A) There is an infiltrative cellular proliferation of basaloid cells with many ghost cells. (B) Hypercellular and atypical odontogenic epithelium is present with palisaded basal cell nuclei.

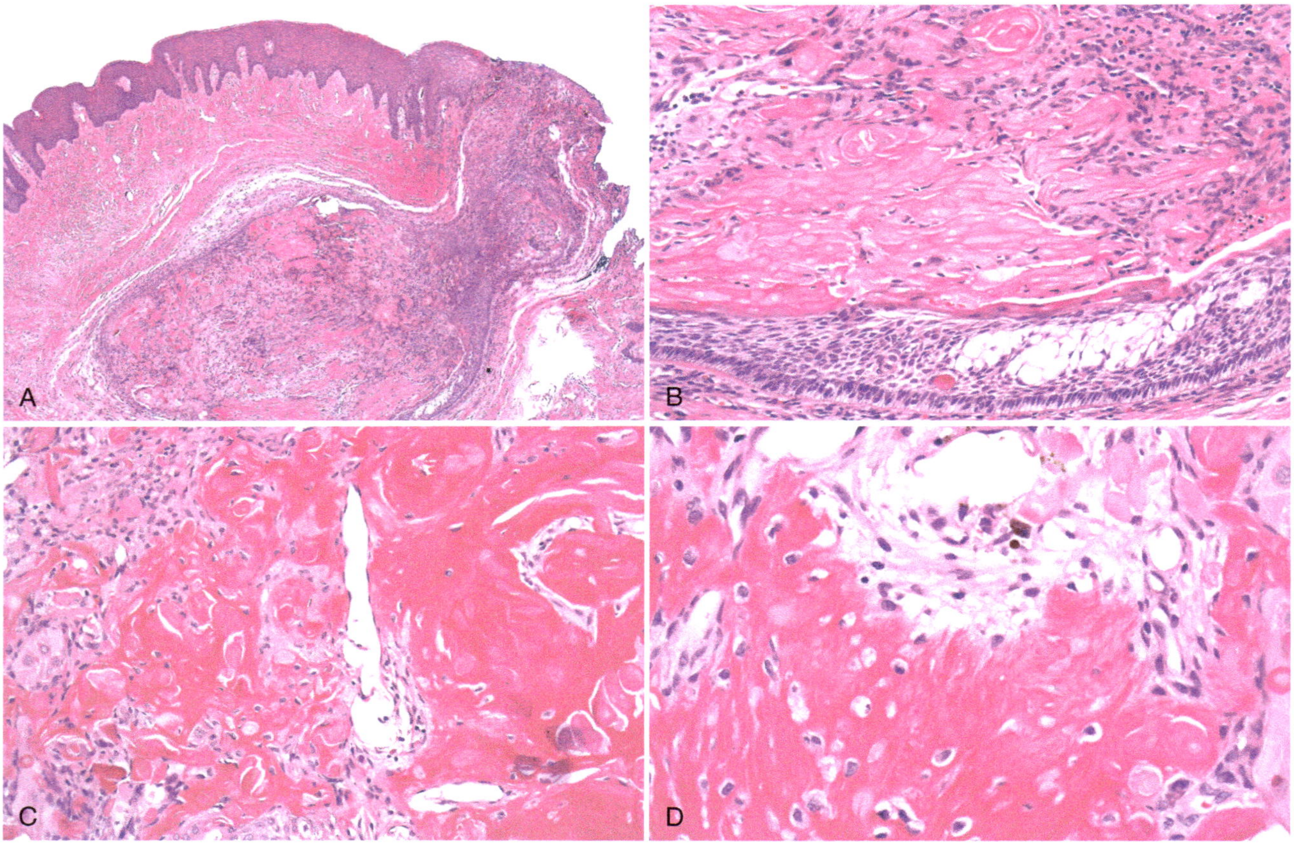

FIG 15.51 Peripheral dentinogenic ghost cell tumor. (A) Tumor is in continuity with the surface epithelium. (B) The epithelium resembles ameloblastoma with reverse polarization of nuclei, stellate reticulum–like areas, and many ghost cells. (C) Ghost cells and dentinoid. (D) Dentinoid encircling ghost cells *(lower right)* and melanin are present *(middle to upper area)*.

PRIMORDIAL ODONTOGENIC TUMOR

Clinical Findings

- This rare tumor occurs before the age of 20 years and presents as a well-demarcated, unilocular radiolucency, sometimes with scalloped margins associated with the crown of an impacted tooth (usually mandibular third molar), with displacement of adjacent teeth and root resorption. The median size is between 5 and 6 cm, and there is significant buccal swelling (Fig. 15.52).

Etiopathogenesis and Histopathologic Features

This is a primitive neoplasm that shows rudimentary differentiation toward a tooth germ, but without significant deposition of dental hard tissues.

- There is proliferation of spindle and stellate mesenchymal cells in myxoid and/or mucinous stroma that is covered on the surface by columnar epithelium similar to ameloblasts with reverse nuclear polarization, sometimes with adjacent stellate reticulum–like areas. A more densely cellular "cambium" layer of mesenchymal cells is noted just beneath the epithelium, whereas the center of the tumor is more densely collagenous. Invaginations into the stroma have the appearance of a rudimentary tooth germ, and clear cells are often present, sometimes with dentinoid and enameloid deposition (Fig. 15.53).

Differential Diagnosis

- Archegonous cystic odontoma is likely an immature odontoma and is cystic, with a subepithelial hypercellular cambium zone, a lobular ameloblastic fibroma-like area, and deposition of dentinoid.

Management and Prognosis

- Enucleation is the treatment of choice and is curative.

REFERENCES

Argyris PP, Wetzel SL, Pambuccian SE, et al. Primordial odontogenic cyst with induction phenomenon (zonal fibroblastic hypercellularity) and dentinoid material versus archegonous cystic odontoma: you choose! *Head Neck Pathol.* 2016;10:237-244.

Mosqueda-Taylor A, Pires FR, Aguirre-Urizar JM, et al. Primordial odontogenic tumour: clinicopathological analysis of six cases of a previously undescribed entity. *Histopathology.* 2014;65:606-612.

Slater LJ, Eftimie LF, Herford AS. Primordial odontogenic tumor: report of a case. *J Oral Maxillofac Surg.* 2016;74:547-551.

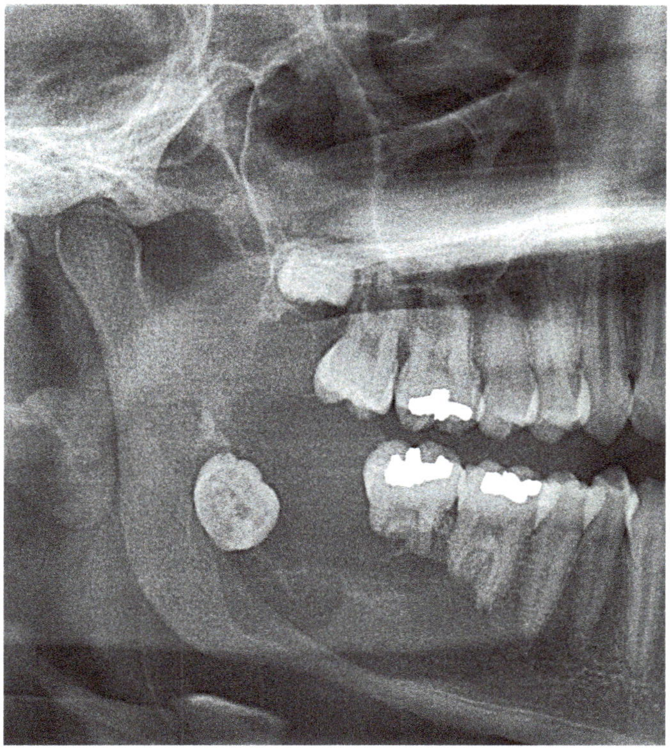

FIG 15.52 Primordial odontogenic tumor presenting as a large radiolucency of the right posterior mandible with root resorption of molars. *(Courtesy Dr. David Collette, private practice, Albuquerque, NM.)*

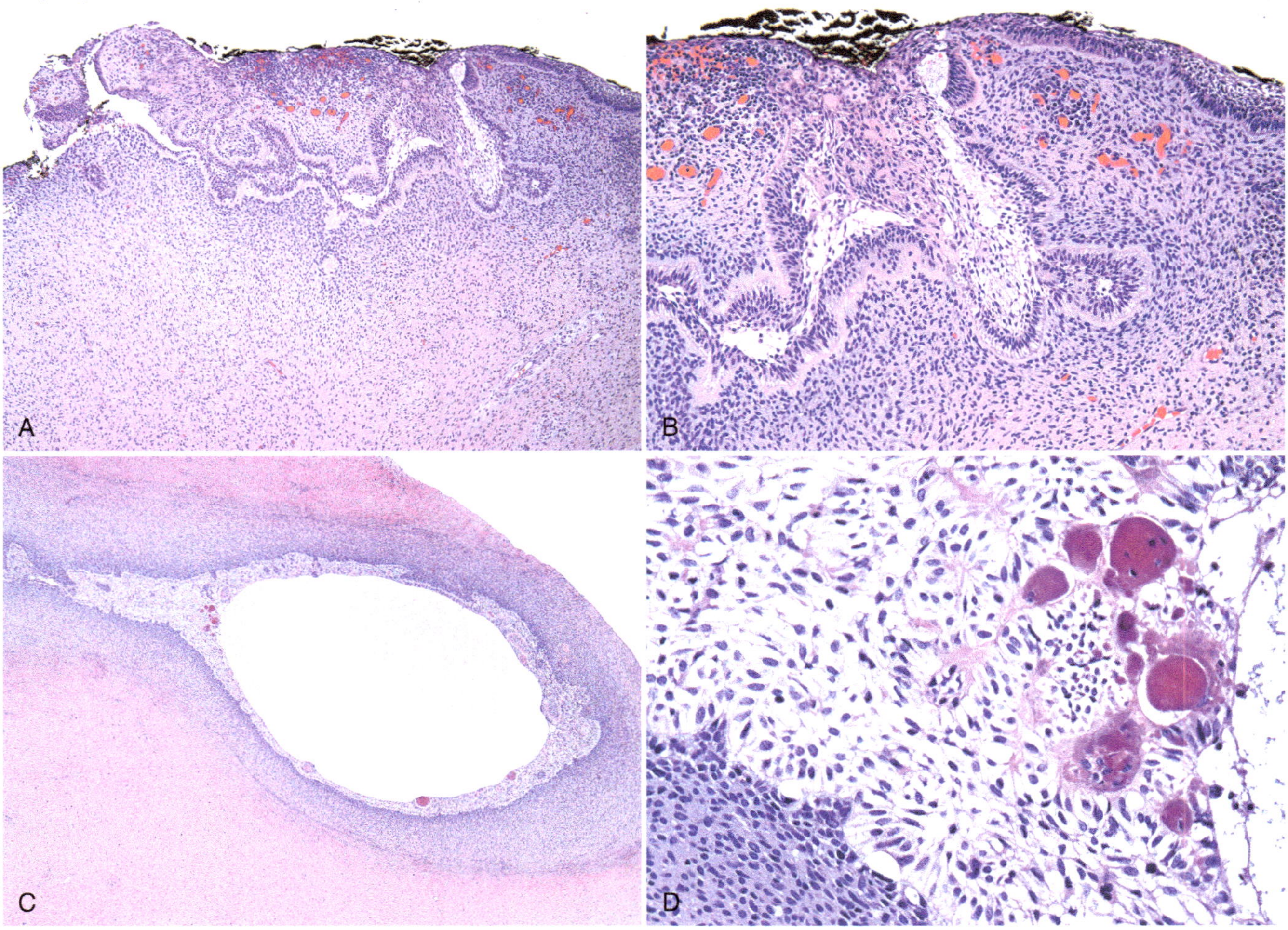

FIG 15.53 Primordial odontogenic tumor. (A) There is a proliferation of spindle and stellate cells with a mucinous stroma surfaced by columnar epithelial cells. (B) The epithelial component resembles ameloblastoma with stellate reticulum–like areas and basal cells with reverse nuclear polarization, and an underlying cellular cambium layer of stellate and spindle cells. (C) Rudimentary organization into a tooth germ is noted. (D) There are nests of epithelial cells with clear cytoplasm and deposition of enameloid-like material.

HYBRID ODONTOGENIC TUMOR

Some odontogenic tumors exhibit features of two or more distinct odontogenic tumors. CCOT is the most common tumor to be associated with another odontogenic tumor, such as ameloblastic fibroma, adenomatoid odontogenic tumor, and odontoma. Ameloblastomas are also often seen with adenomatoid odontogenic tumor and calcifying epithelial odontogenic tumor.

REFERENCES

Phillips MD, Closmann JJ, Baus MR, et al. Hybrid odontogenic tumor with features of ameloblastic fibro-odontoma, calcifying odontogenic cyst, and adenomatoid odontogenic tumor: a case report and review of the literature. *J Oral Maxillofac Surg.* 2010;68:470-474.

Yamazaki M, Maruyama S, Abe T, et al. Hybrid ameloblastoma and adenomatoid odontogenic tumor: report of a case and review of hybrid variations in the literature. *Oral Surg Oral Med Oral Pathol Oral Radiol.* 2014;118:e12-e18.

Mesenchymal Tumors

CENTRAL CEMENTOOSSIFYING FIBROMA

This is discussed in detail in Chapter 16 under the entity *fibroosseous lesions,* which has been the convention for decades. However, these neoplasms are likely to be odontogenic neoplasms arising from mesenchymal stem cells within the periodontal membrane, related to cementoosseous dysplasia, and distinct from true osseous neoplasms such as the psammomatoid and trabecular ossifying fibromas.

REFERENCES

Woo SB. Central cemento-ossifying fibroma: primary odontogenic or osseous neoplasm? *J Oral Maxillofac Surg.* 2015;73(suppl 12): S87-S93.

Wright JM, Odell EW, Speight PM, Takata T. Odontogenic tumors, WHO 2005: where do we go from here? *Head Neck Pathol.* 2014;8:373-382.

ODONTOGENIC MYXOMA

This is the most common mesenchymal odontogenic neoplasm and constitutes 5% to 10% of all odontogenic neoplasms.

Clinical Findings

- This occurs in the second to fourth decades of life, with a 2:1 female predilection, and it is often associated with displacement of teeth, perforation of the cortex, and jaw expansion. It presents as a well-demarcated or poorly demarcated multilocular (60% of cases), honeycombed or "tennis racket" radiolucency usually in the posterior maxilla or mandible (Fig. 15.54). Multilocular lesions tend to be larger, and mandibular lesions may involve the ramus extensively, while maxillary lesions often involve the sinus.

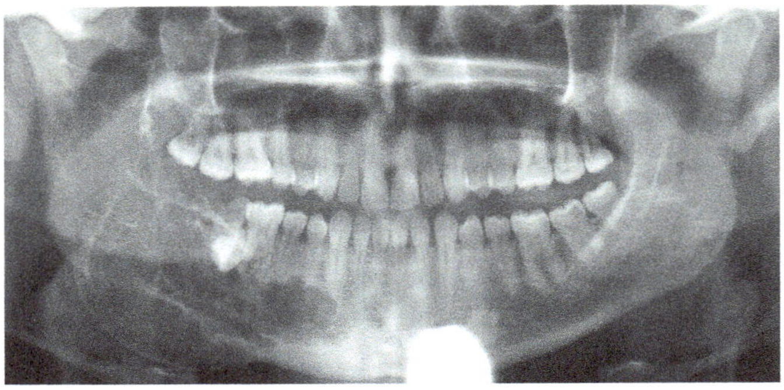

FIG 15.54 Odontogenic myxoma presenting as a multilocular radiolucency of the right mandible and ramus. *(Courtesy Dr. Jennifer Smith-Williams, private practice, Boston.)*

Etiopathogenesis and Histopathologic Features

This tumor recapitulates the dental papilla. Downregulation of *PRKAR1A*, a gene often mutated in Carney complex, which is associated with cardiac and other myxomas, may be involved because some cases of odontogenic myxomas exhibit mutation of this gene with loss of protein expression.

- There is an unencapsulated and infiltrative proliferation of spindle, bipolar, and stellate cells exhibiting bland nuclei with inconspicuous nucleoli, within a mucinous and/or myxoid stroma that contains abundant hyaluronic acid. Islands of odontogenic epithelium are noted in 10% to 25% of cases, and dystrophic calcifications may be present (Figs. 15.55 and 15.56).
- Spindle cells are S100 protein–. Approximately 45% are SMA+, and up to 25% are HHF45+, suggesting the presence of myofibroblasts. Mast cells are present in more than 70% of cases. Epithelial islands are positive for AE1/3 and K14 and usually negative for K19.

Differential Diagnosis

- Hyperplastic dental follicle is much smaller, not as homogenously myxoid, and presents around impacted teeth.
- Dental papilla (immature dental pulp from a developing tooth or odontoma) is ovoid in shape and exhibits a rim of odontoblasts at the periphery (see Fig. 14.26B).
- Some odontogenic myxomas exhibit osteocementum formation and more densely collagenous tissue, and these may represent central odontogenic myxofibromas.
- Intraosseous nerve sheath tumors are positive for S100 protein.
- Chondromyxoid fibromas contain chondroid areas, are less homogeneous with areas of cellularity, and are often multilobular.

Management and Prognosis

- The recurrence rate is up to 33%, with the highest recurrence noted for curetted or enucleated lesions. Marginal resection is recommended for smaller tumors, and segmental resection is recommended for larger tumors.

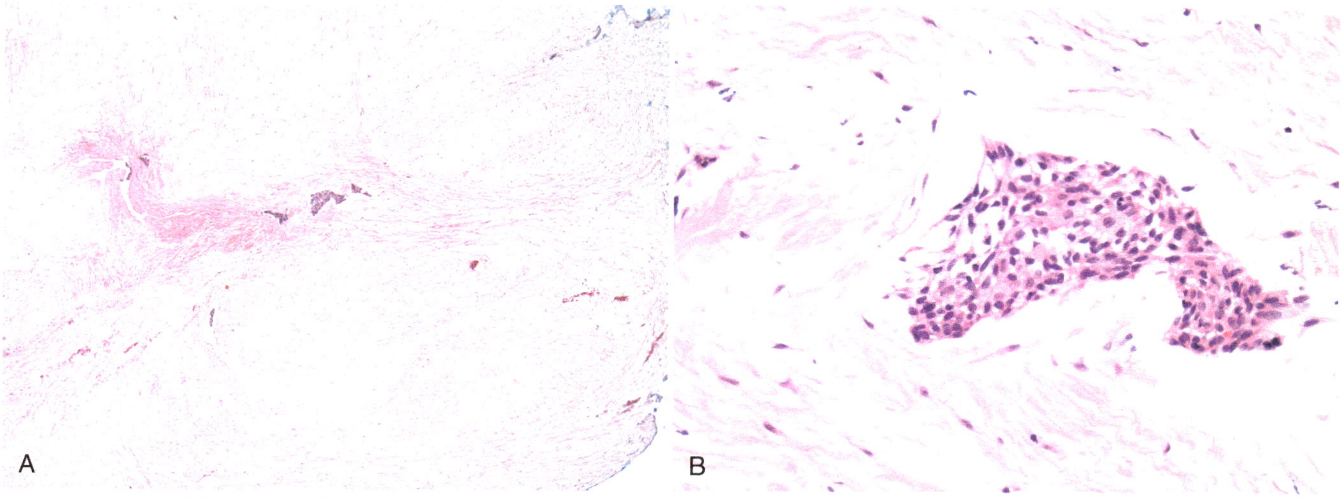

FIG 15.55 Odontogenic myxoma. (A) There is a proliferation of spindle cells in markedly myxoid-mucinous stroma with islands of odontogenic epithelium. (B) Island of odontogenic epithelium without palisading of basal cells. Spindle tumor cells have trailing cytoplasmic processes and benign nuclei.

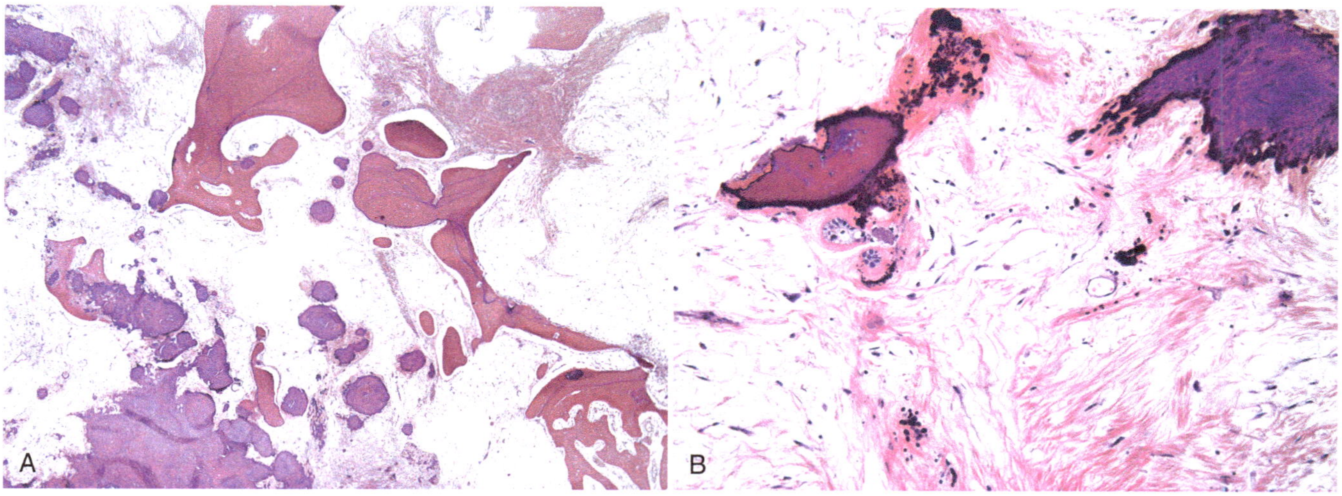

FIG 15.56 Odontogenic myxoma. (A) The tumor infiltrates bone and exhibits dystrophic calcifications. (B) Spindle cells are dispersed within a delicately and densely collagenous, and mucinous stroma with dystrophic calcifications.

REFERENCES

Lahey E, Woo SB, Park HK. Odontogenic myxoma with diffuse calcifications: a case report and review of the literature. *Head Neck Pathol.* 2013;7:97-102.

Li TJ, Sun LS, Luo HY. Odontogenic myxoma: a clinicopathologic study of 25 cases. *Arch Pathol Lab Med.* 2006;130:1799-1806.

Lo Muzio L, Nocini P, Favia G, et al. Odontogenic myxoma of the jaws: a clinical, radiologic, immunohistochemical, and ultrastructural study. *Oral Surg Oral Med Oral Pathol Oral Radiol Endod.* 1996;82:426-433.

Martinez-Mata G, Mosqueda-Taylor A, Carlos-Bregni R, et al. Odontogenic myxoma: clinico-pathological, immunohistochemical and ultrastructural findings of a multicentric series. *Oral Oncol.* 2008;44:601-607.

Noffke CE, Raubenheimer EJ, Chabikuli NJ, Bouckaert MM. Odontogenic myxoma: review of the literature and report of 30 cases from South Africa. *Oral Surg Oral Med Oral Pathol Oral Radiol Endod.* 2007;104:101-109.

Perdigão PF, Stergiopoulos SG, De Marco L, et al. Molecular and immunohistochemical investigation of protein kinase a regulatory subunit type 1A (*PRKAR1A*) in odontogenic myxomas. *Genes Chromosomes Cancer.* 2005;44:204-211.

Simon EN, Merkx MA, Vuhahula E, et al. Odontogenic myxoma: a clinicopathological study of 33 cases. *Int J Oral Maxillofac Surg.* 2004;33:333-337.

ODONTOGENIC FIBROMA

These lesions have been classified as (1) simple or epithelium-poor type, composed mostly of fibrous tissue with little to no epithelial rests or dentinoid, and (2) the epithelium-rich type, where epithelium is invariably present, sometimes with dentinoid. The epithelium-poor variant either is very rare, if it exists at all, or may represent dental follicle. In such cases, the clinical findings (swelling and radiographic appearance of a space-occupying lesion) help with the diagnosis.

Clinical Features

- The median age of occurrence is in the fourth decade of life, and there may be a female predilection. Unlike most odontogenic neoplasms, 65% of cases occur in the maxilla and most cases occur anterior to the first molars. It presents as a unilocular (70% of cases) or multilocular radiolucency and often is intimately around the roots of teeth (Fig. 15.57).

- Dimpling or clefting of the palatal mucosa overlying the lesion is characteristic although uncommon.
- Central odontogenic fibroma-like lesions have been reported in patients with enamel dysplasia or amelogenesis imperfecta.
- The peripheral variant found on the gingiva is the most common peripheral odontogenic neoplasm, constituting up to 50% of cases, and presents as a gingival nodule, usually in the area of incisors and canines with an equal maxillary and mandibular distribution.

Etiopathogenesis and Histopathologic Features

Differentiation of this neoplasm is toward the dental follicle and periodontal membrane.

- There is a proliferation of spindle cells in a densely collagenous stroma. Some tumors have a focally myxoid stroma and more delicate collagen. Islands of odontogenic epithelium may be sparse or abundant and often contain clear cells. Dentinoid, hyaline globules, basement membrane–like material, or ductlike structures may be present (Figs. 15.58 and 15.59). Periepithelial hyalinization is often present.
- Perineural and intraneural "invasion" (neurotropism) has been reported.

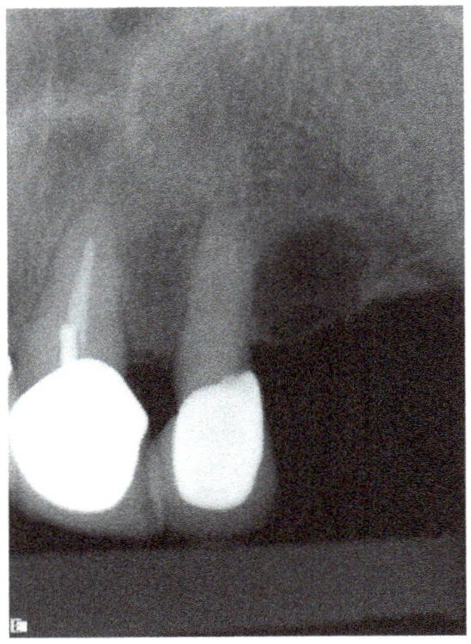

FIG 15.57 Central odontogenic fibroma. Radiolucency at site of previously extracted left maxillary canine. *(Courtesy Dr. Evetta Shwartzman, private practice, Canton, Mass.)*

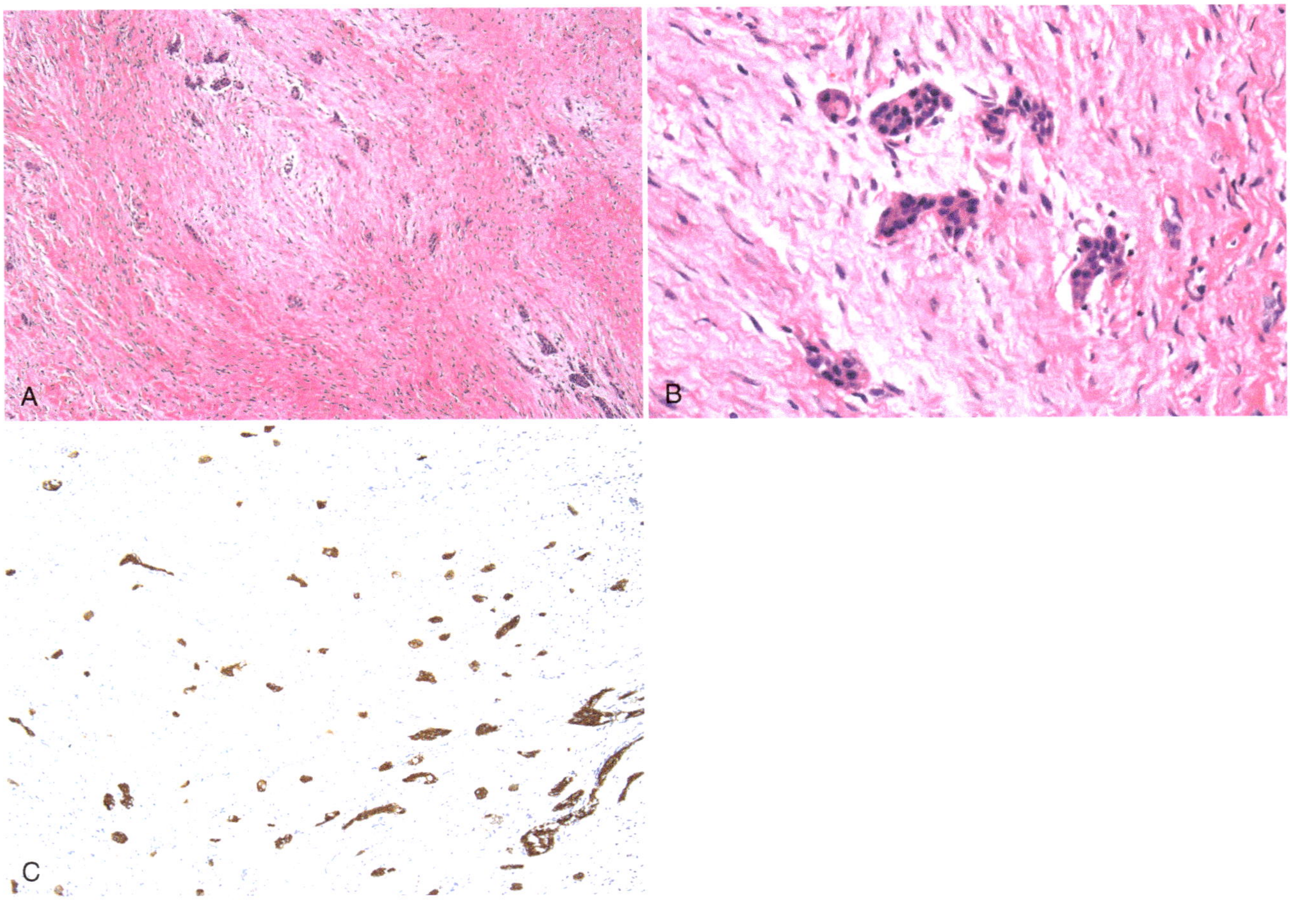

FIG 15.58 Central odontogenic fibroma. (A) There is a proliferation of densely collagenous fibrous tissue with odontogenic rests. (B) Epithelial rests with eosinophilic cytoplasm and a few hyaline globules. (C) Epithelial rests are positive for K19.

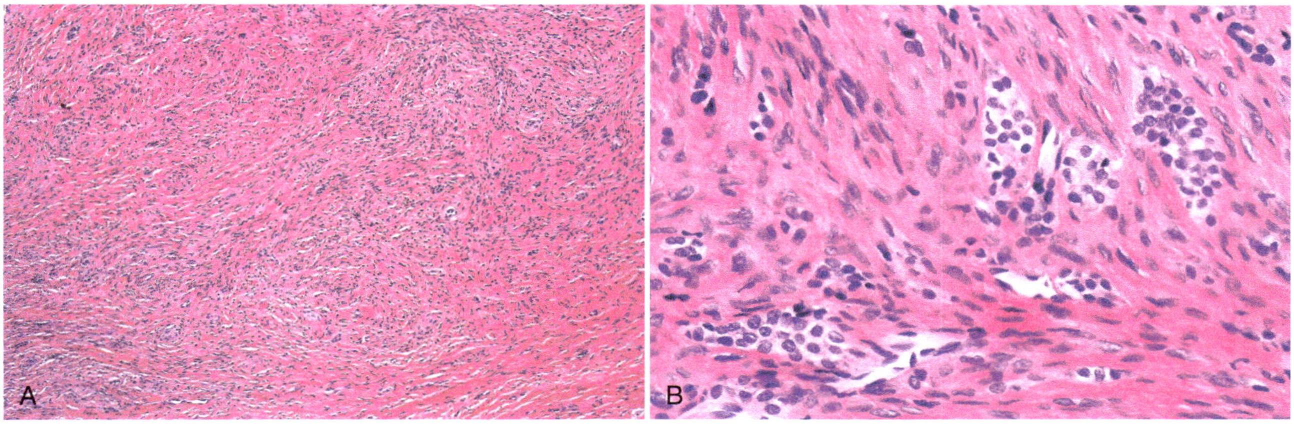

FIG 15.59 Central odontogenic fibroma. (A) There is a cellular proliferation of spindle cells and dense fibrous tissue. (B) Odontogenic rests are composed of cells with pale or clear cytoplasm.

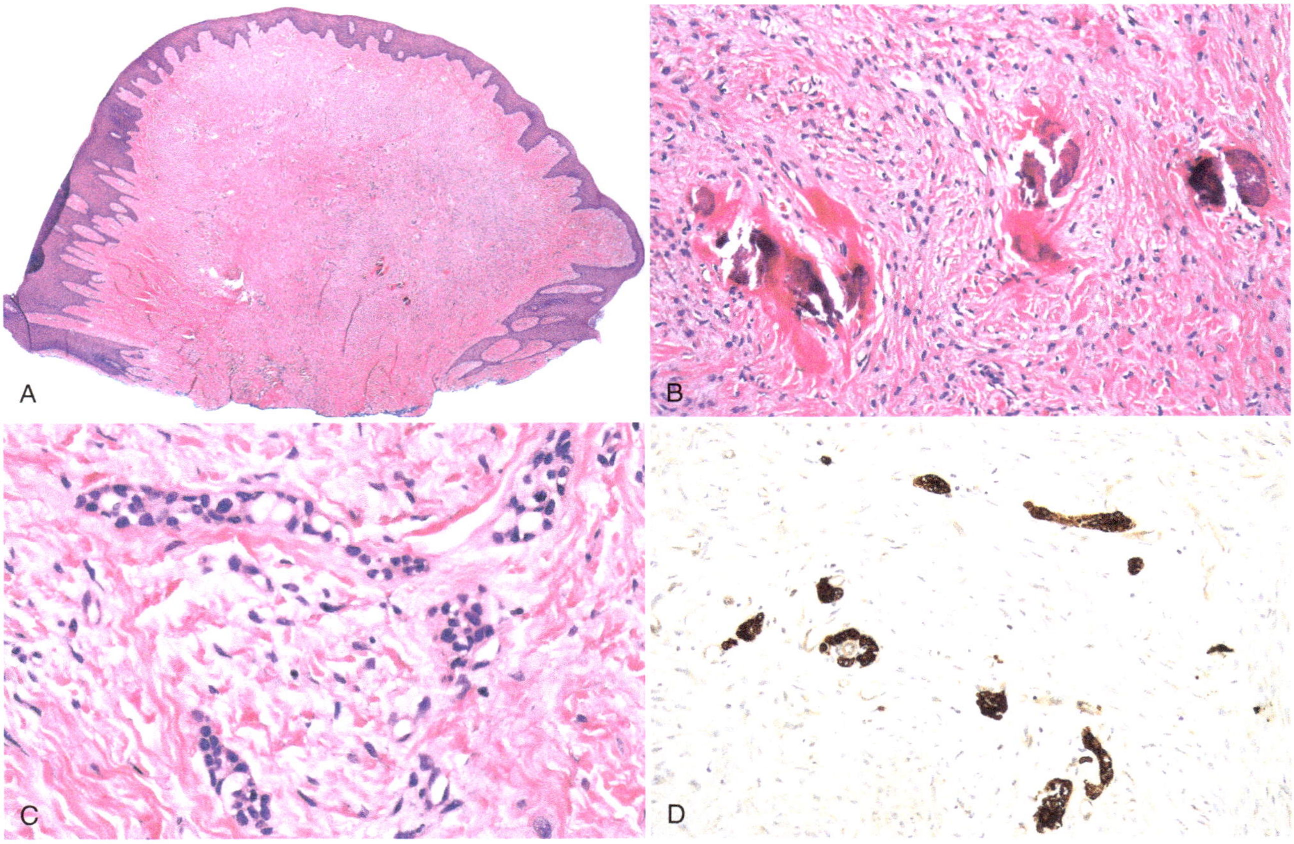

FIG 15.60 Peripheral odontogenic fibroma. (A) There is a nonencapsulated proliferation of spindle cells with calcifications. (B) Proliferation of spindle cells in collagenous stroma with calcifications. (C) Odontogenic epithelium containing clear cells. (D) Odontogenic islands are positive for pankeratin.

- The epithelium is positive for AE1/3, K8/18, K14, and K19 and often contains CD1a+ Langerhans cells.
- Clusters of multinucleated giant cells and mononuclear cells in a hemorrhagic stroma similar to central giant cell granuloma are present in up to 10% of cases (see Chapter 16).
- Peripheral odontogenic fibromas have a similar histopathology and are unencapsulated, occurring within the lamina propria. Calcifications are present in 50% of cases (Fig. 15.60).

Differential Diagnosis

- Similar-appearing tissue that occurs around the crowns of impacted teeth are almost always hyperplastic dental follicles.
- Odontogenic fibromyxoma, which tends to be epithelium-poor and very mucinous and/or myxoid, does not usually produce significant calcified tissues.
- Desmoplastic fibroma is more densely collagenous and does not contain epithelium or dentinoid. It is often

β-catenin-positive and behaves in a locally aggressive fashion.
- Sclerosing odontogenic carcinoma shows significant cytologic atypia and behaves in an aggressive fashion.
- Metastatic carcinoma exhibits cytologic atypia and desmoplasia around epithelial islands.

Management and Prognosis

- Enucleation or curettage is the treatment of choice. The recurrence rate is 4%, and lesions associated with giant cell granuloma are particularly prone to recur (up to 13% of cases).

REFERENCES

Brannon RB. Central odontogenic fibroma, myxoma (odontogenic myxoma, fibromyxoma), and central odontogenic granular cell tumor. *Oral Maxillofac Surg Clin North Am.* 2004;16:359-374.

Buchner A, Merrell PW, Carpenter WM. Relative frequency of peripheral odontogenic tumors: a study of 45 new cases and comparison with studies from the literature. *J Oral Pathol Med.* 2006;35:385-391.

Eversole LR. Odontogenic fibroma, including amyloid and ossifying variants. *Head Neck Pathol.* 2011;5:335-343.

Ficarra G, Sapp JP, Eversole LR. Multiple peripheral odontogenic fibroma, World Health Organization type, and central giant cell granuloma: a case report of an unusual association. *J Oral Maxillofac Surg.* 1993;51:325-328.

Handlers JP, Abrams AM, Melrose RJ, Danforth R. Central odontogenic fibroma: clinicopathologic features of 19 cases and review of the literature. *J Oral Maxillofac Surg.* 1991;49:46-54.

Ide F, Kikuchi K, Sakashita H, et al. Neurovascular involvement in central odontogenic fibroma: a potential source of confusion with invasive carcinoma. *Histopathology.* 2015;66:1044-1046.

Ide F, Sakashita H, Kusama K. Ameloblastomatoid, central odontogenic fibroma: an epithelium-rich variant. *J Oral Pathol Med.* 2002;31:612-614.

Mosqueda-Taylor A, Martinez-Mata G, Carlos-Bregni R, et al. Central odontogenic fibroma: new findings and report of a multicentric collaborative study. *Oral Surg Oral Med Oral Pathol Oral Radiol Endod.* 2011;112:349-358.

Odell EW, Lombardi T, Barrett AW, et al. Hybrid central giant cell granuloma and central odontogenic fibroma-like lesions of the jaws. *Histopathology.* 1997;30:165-171.

Ritwik P, Brannon RB. Peripheral odontogenic fibroma: a clinicopathologic study of 151 cases and review of the literature with special emphasis on recurrence. *Oral Surg Oral Med Oral Pathol Oral Radiol Endod.* 2010;110:357-363.

Roquebert D, Champsaur A, Gil del Real P, et al. Amelogenesis imperfecta, rough hypoplastic type, dental follicular hamartomas and gingival hyperplasia: report of a case from Central America and review of the literature. *Oral Surg Oral Med Oral Pathol Oral Radiol Endod.* 2008;106:92-98.

Siar CH, Ng KH. Clinicopathological study of peripheral odontogenic fibromas (WHO-type) in Malaysians (1967–95). *Br J Oral Maxillofac Surg.* 2000;38:19-22.

GRANULAR CELL ODONTOGENIC TUMOR

The former name for this condition was *granular cell odontogenic fibroma.*

Clinical Findings

- This occurs most frequently in the fifth to sixth decades of life, with a 3:1 female predilection, and presents usually as a unilocular radiolucency, with 75% occurring in the mandible, usually posteriorly.
- Peripheral lesions are rare.

Etiopathogenesis and Histopathologic Features

- There are clusters and sometimes sheets of large, polygonal cells with abundant eosinophilic, granular cytoplasm and eccentric, round or ovoid, slightly pleomorphic nuclei, and inconspicuous nucleoli.
- Islands of odontogenic epithelium are present that do not exhibit palisading of basal cells, and clear cells may be present. Periepithelial hyalinization and dentinoid or dystrophic calcifications may be present (Figs. 15.61 and 15.62A–C).
- Granular cells are CD68+, S100 protein– and, keratin–, and ultrastructural studies confirm the presence of lysosomes (see Fig. 15.62D). Some cases are SMA+. The epithelium is positive for K5, K7, K8, K14, and K19.

Differential Diagnosis

- Ameloblastoma, granular cell type, exhibits palisading and reverse nuclear polarization of basal cells, and the granular cells are keratin+.

Management and Prognosis

- Enucleation or curettage is the treatment of choice, and recurrence is rare.

REFERENCES

Brannon RB, Goode RK, Eversole LR, Carr RF. The central granular cell odontogenic tumor: report of 5 new cases. *Oral Surg Oral Med Oral Pathol Oral Radiol Endod.* 2002;94:614-621.

Brannon RB. Central odontogenic fibroma, myxoma (odontogenic myxoma, fibromyxoma), and central odontogenic granular cell tumor. *Oral Maxillofac Surg Clin North Am.* 2004;16:359-374.

Lotay HS, Kalmar J, DeLeeuw K. Central odontogenic fibroma with features of central granular cell odontogenic tumor. *Oral Surg Oral Med Oral Pathol Oral Radiol Endod.* 2010;109:e63-e66.

Mesquita AT, Santos CR, Gomez RS, et al. Central granular cell odontogenic tumor: a histopathologic and immunohistochemical study. *Ann Diagn Pathol.* 2009;13:405-412.

Rinaggio J, Cleveland D, Koshy R, et al. Peripheral granular odontogenic fibroma. *Oral Surg Oral Med Oral Pathol Oral Radiol Endod.* 2007;104:676-679.

Sarode SC, Sarode GS, Vaidya K. Central granular cell odontogenic tumor: a systematic review. *J Oral Pathol Med.* 2014;43:167-176.

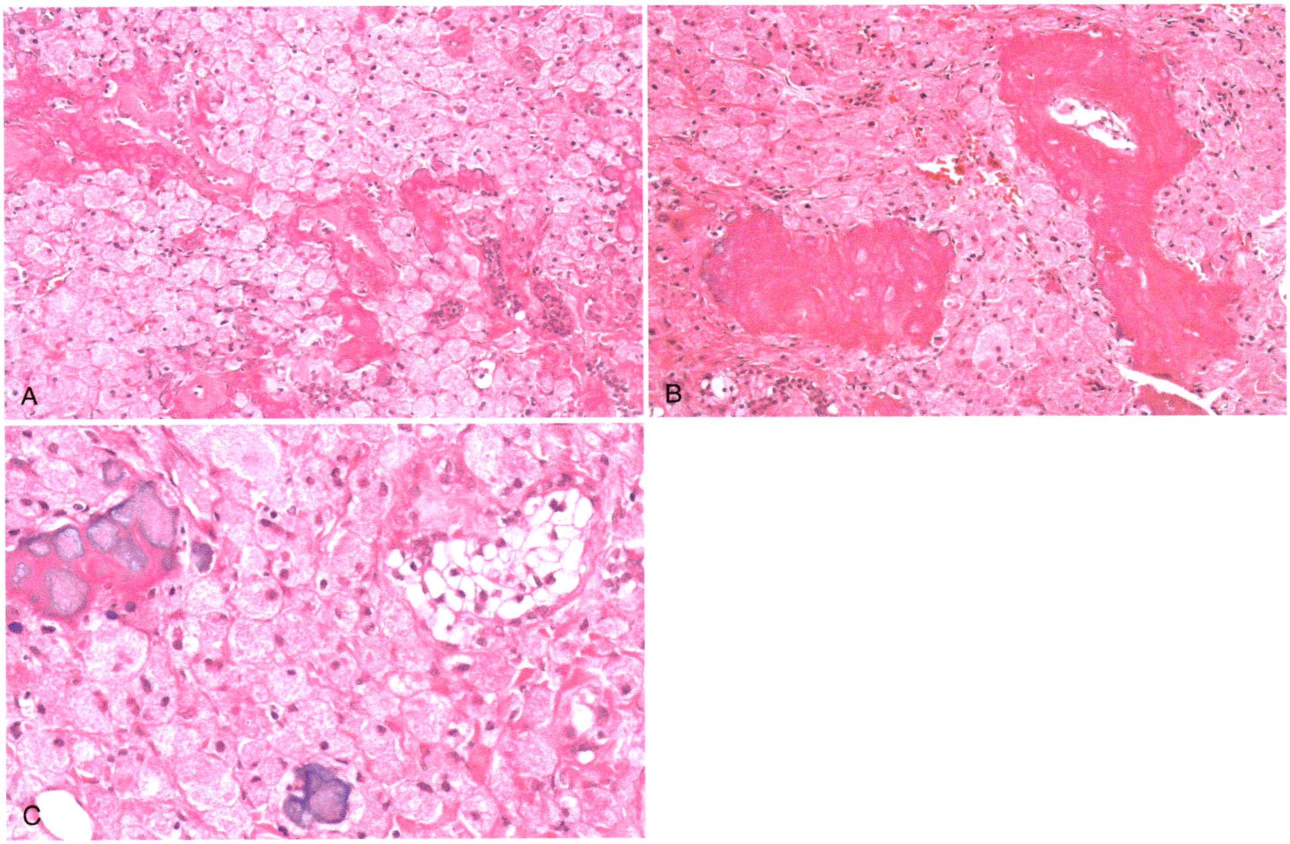

FIG 15.61 Granular cell odontogenic tumor. (A) There are sheets of granular cells, periepithelial dentinoid, and epithelial islands. (B) Granular cells surround dentinoid that in this field, is not periepithelial. (C) Granular cells have benign nuclei. An epithelial rest is composed of clear cells, and there are dystrophic globular calcifications.

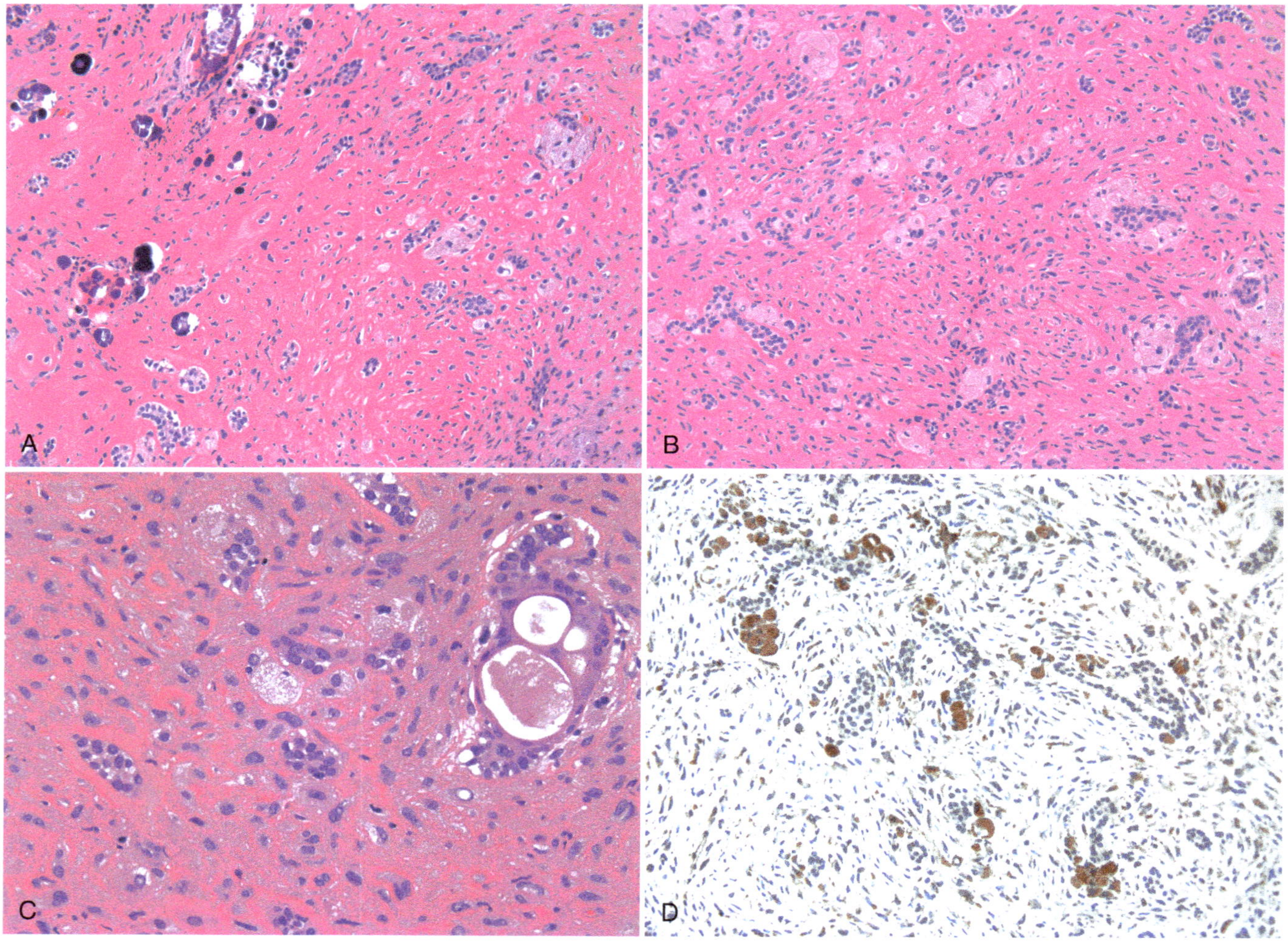

FIG 15.62 Granular cell odontogenic tumor. (A) Clusters of granular cells with epithelial islands and globular calcifications within densely collagenous stroma. (B) Benign odontogenic epithelium without palisading of basal cells, and clusters of granular cells within collagenous stroma. (C) Some epithelial islands exhibit microcystic change forming duct-like structures, and many granular cells are present. (D) Granular cells show cytoplasmic positivity for CD68.

CEMENTOBLASTOMA

Clinical Findings

- This occurs most frequently in the second and third decades of life, and the mandible is two to three times more often affected than the maxilla. Up to 60% of patients report pain and/or swelling. There is a radiopaque mass (often with a surrounding radiolucent rim) fused to the apex of a tooth, usually the mandibular first molar (50%) or a premolar. The lamina dura is usually continuous around the tooth and lesion, and root resorption is often present (Fig. 15.63). Early lesions are radiolucent only, but this is a rare finding.
- The teeth are generally vital. The tooth may have been extracted and the root fractured, leaving behind a radiopaque mass in an edentulous area. Rarely, this is associated with a primary tooth.

Etiopathogenesis and Histopathologic Features

Differentiation of this neoplasm is toward cementoblasts derived from stem cells in the periodontal soft tissues, which deposit cementum. Its bone-forming counterpart is osteoblastoma.

- There is a proliferation of cementoblasts (that appear similar to osteoblasts), which deposit cementum, as well as osteoid-like and woven bone-like material in masses and radiating columns, the latter best seen at the periphery. Resting and reversal lines are often present, and the attached root may be resorbed.
- Cementoblasts are large, with eccentric nuclei that may be slightly atypical but contain dispersed chromatin and small nucleoli. Osteoclast-like cells and dilated vessels may be seen (Figs. 15.64 and 15.65).

Differential Diagnosis

- Osteoblastoma does not have the same relationship with a tooth and, in particular, the peripheral radiating cementum seams.
- Cementoosseous dysplasia exhibits a cellular proliferation of spindle cells and deposition of globular cementum droplets, osteoid, and short trabeculae of woven bone. It is sclerotic and dense in the later stage but does not exhibit the parallel cementum seams.
- Hypercementosis manifests as thickened cellular and acellular cementum attached to the tooth, without proliferation of cementoblasts.
- Osteosarcoma may resorb the tooth but is not usually attached to it; there are no radiating or organized osteoid seams, and cells exhibit significant atypia.

Management and Prognosis

- Excision or en bloc resection of the tumor with the tooth is the treatment of choice, and the recurrence rate is 10% to 20%, depending on the treatment modality.

REFERENCES

Brannon RB, Fowler CB, Carpenter WM, Corio RL. Cementoblastoma: an innocuous neoplasm? A clinicopathologic study of 44 cases and review of the literature with special emphasis on recurrence. *Oral Surg Oral Med Oral Pathol Oral Radiol Endod.* 2002;93:311-320.

Hirai E, Yamamoto K, Kounoe T, et al. Benign cementoblastoma of the anterior maxilla. *J Oral Maxillofac Surg.* 2010;68:671-674.

Slootweg PJ. Cementoblastoma and osteoblastoma: a comparison of histologic features. *J Oral Pathol Med.* 1992;21:385-389.

Ulmansky M, Hjørting-Hansen E, Praetorius F, et al. Benign cementoblastoma: a review and five new cases. *Oral Surg Oral Med Oral Pathol.* 1994;77:48-55.

Vieira AP, Meneses JM Jr, Maia RL. Cementoblastoma related to a primary tooth: a case report. *J Oral Pathol Med.* 2007;36:117-119.

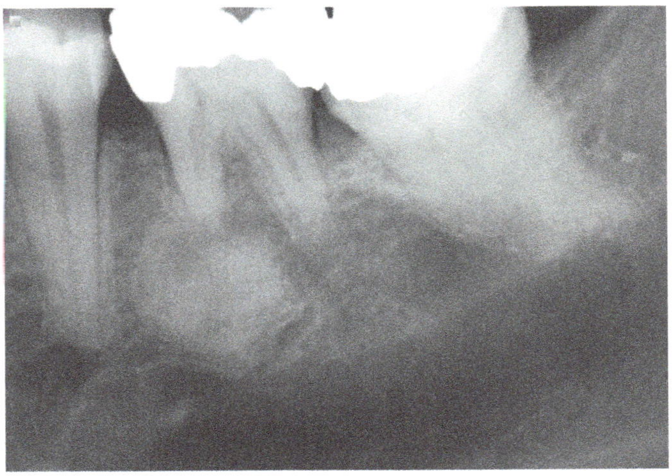

FIG 15.63 Cementoblastoma. Radiopaque mass at the apex of the left mandibular first molar mesial root with root resorption.

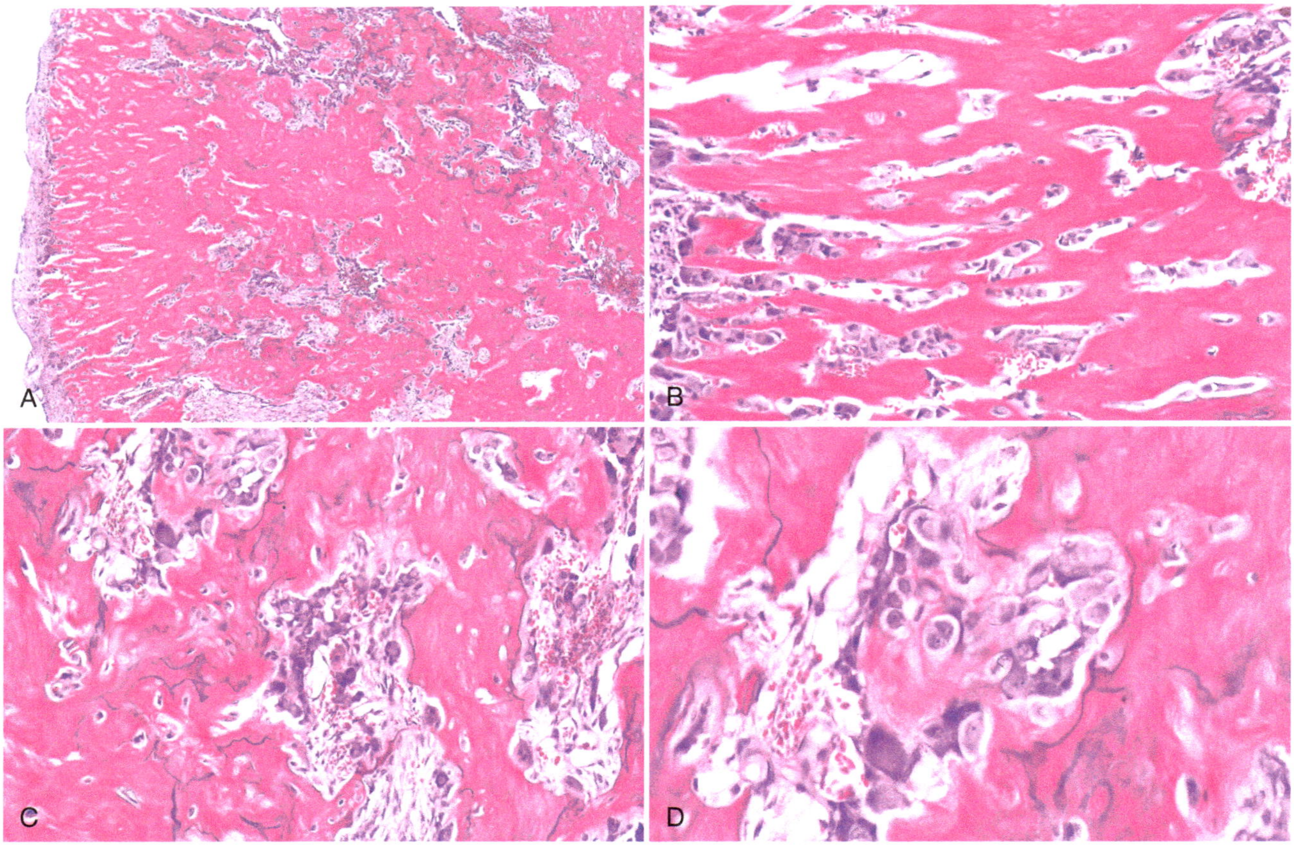

FIG 15.64 Cementoblastoma. (A) Periphery of encapsulated tumor shows parallel trabeculae of cementum. (B) Proliferation of large cementoblasts between parallel cementum seams. (C) Multiple layers of cementoblasts and osteoclast-like cells. (D) Plump, atypical-appearing cementoblasts with large benign nuclei and dispersed chromatin.

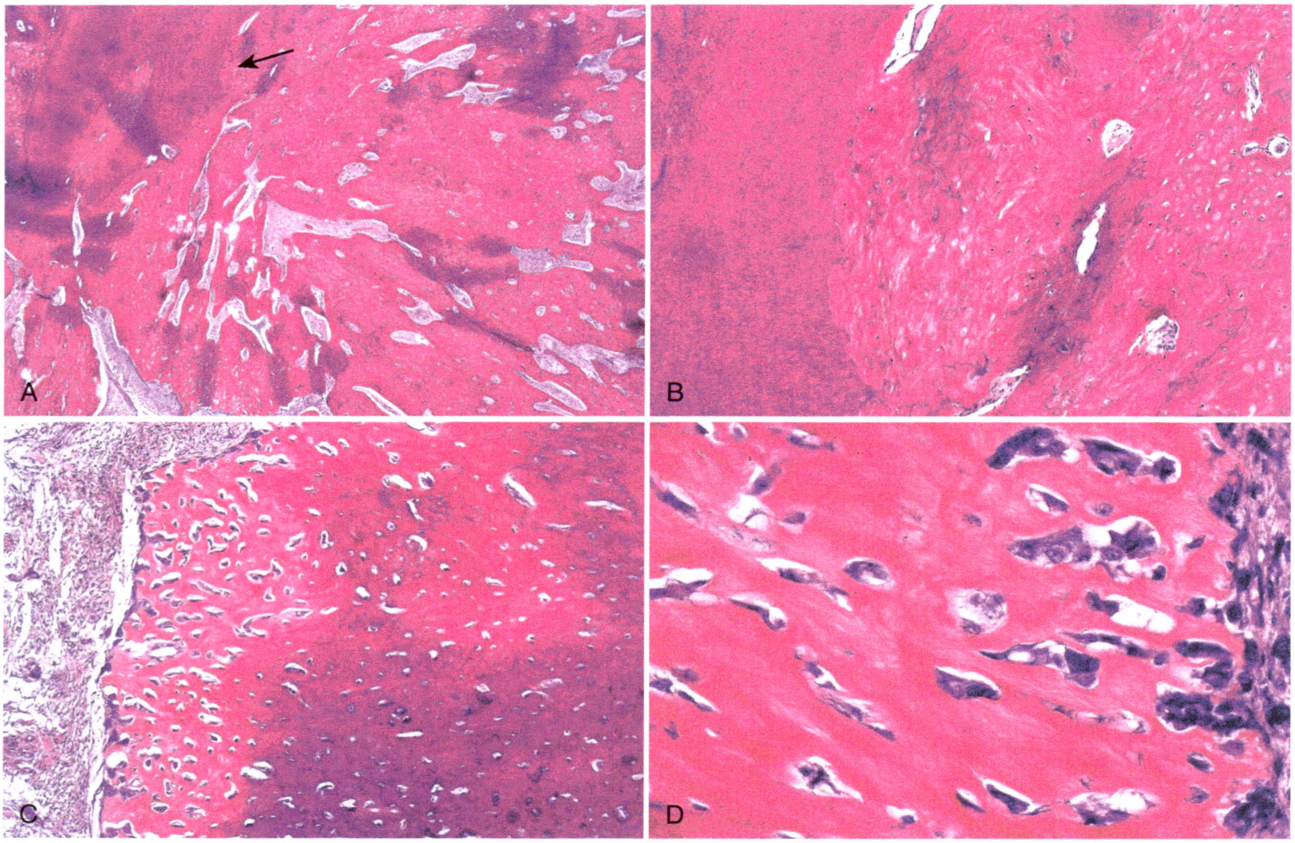

FIG 15.65 Cementoblastoma. (A) The tumor is attached to the root of the tooth, which shows resorption *(arrow)*. (B) The tumor has eroded and fused with the dentin of tooth *(left)*. (C) Encapsulated mass of cementum with cementoblasts in an organized orderly array at the periphery. (D) Cementoblasts with large, eccentric, atypical nuclei.

16 INTRABONY NONODONTOGENIC CYSTS, CYSTLIKE LESIONS, AND MISCELLANEOUS ENTITIES

CHAPTER CONTENTS

True Cysts

NASOPALATINE DUCT (INCISIVE CANAL) CYST

Clinical Findings

- This is most frequently encountered in the fourth and fifth decades of life with a slight male predilection, and it presents as a painless swelling of the anterior palate posterior to the central incisors; teeth are vital but may have been endodontically treated.
- The cyst presents as a well-demarcated, unilocular, round, ovoid, or symmetrically heart-shaped radiolucency (because of the superimposed nasal spine seen in intraoral radiographs) between the maxillary central incisors, causing root divergence (Fig. 16.1).

Etiopathogenesis and Histologic Features

The epithelium derives from remnants of the nasopalatine duct that runs from the floor of the posterior nasal cavity anteriorly to the midline of the palate.

- The cyst is lined by one of the following: nonkeratinized, stratified squamous epithelium (most common); pseudostratified, columnar, and ciliated epithelium with scattered mucous cells (30% of cases); low cuboidal epithelium; and often a combination. The basement membrane may be densely hyalinized. The nasopalatine neurovascular bundle is present in approximately half the cases (Figs. 16.2 and 16.3).

Differential Diagnosis

- A cyst with the same histopathology removed in the same area but not within bone is the cyst of the incisive papilla (see Chapter 2).

Management and Prognosis

- Curettage or enucleation is curative, and the recurrence rate is insignificant.

REFERENCES

Escoda Francolí J, Almendros Marqués N, Berini Aytés L, Gay Escoda C. Nasopalatine duct cyst: report of 22 cases and review of the literature. *Med Oral Patol Oral Cir Bucal.* 2008;13:E438-E443.

Perumal CJ. An unusually large destructive nasopalatine duct cyst: a case report. *J Maxillofac Oral Surg.* 2013;12:100-104.

Suter VG, Sendi P, Reichart PA, Bornstein MM. The nasopalatine duct cyst: an analysis of the relation between clinical symptoms, cyst dimensions, and involvement of neighboring anatomical structures using cone beam computed tomography. *J Oral Maxillofac Surg.* 2011;69:2595-2603.

Swanson KS, Kaugars GE, Gunsolley JC. Nasopalatine duct cyst: an analysis of 334 cases. *J Oral Maxillofac Surg.* 1991;49:268-271.

Vasconcelos R, de Aguiar MF, Castro W, et al. Retrospective analysis of 31 cases of nasopalatine duct cyst. *Oral Dis.* 1999;5:325-328.

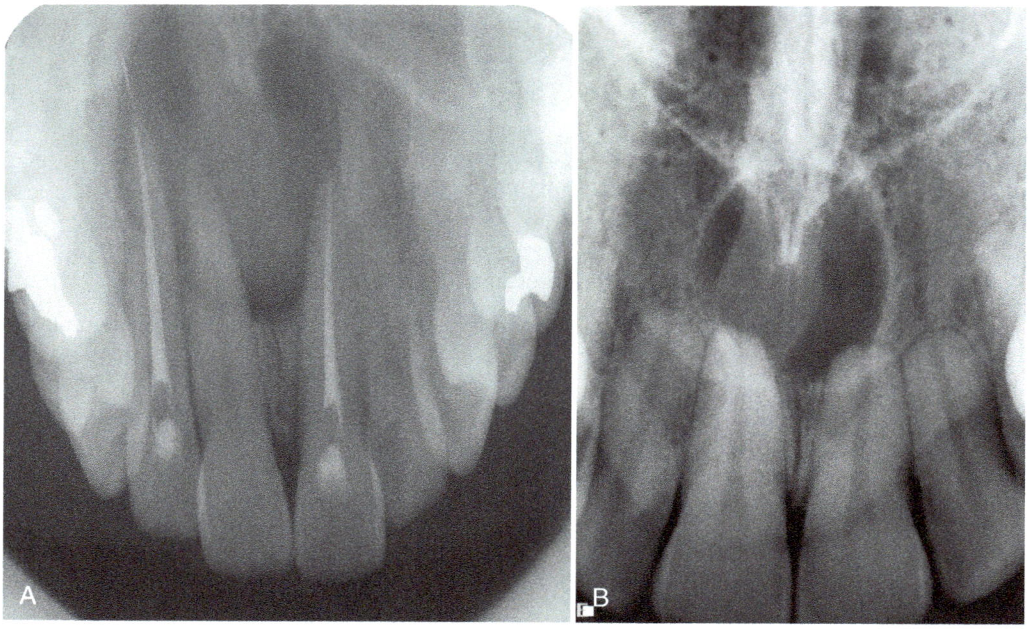

FIG. 16.1 Nasopalatine duct cyst. (A) Symmetric, heart-shaped radiolucency in occlusal radiograph between the upper central incisors. (B) Round radiolucency in the midline between the central incisors that are vital. *(A, Courtesy Dr. Martin Elson, Cranston, RI.)*

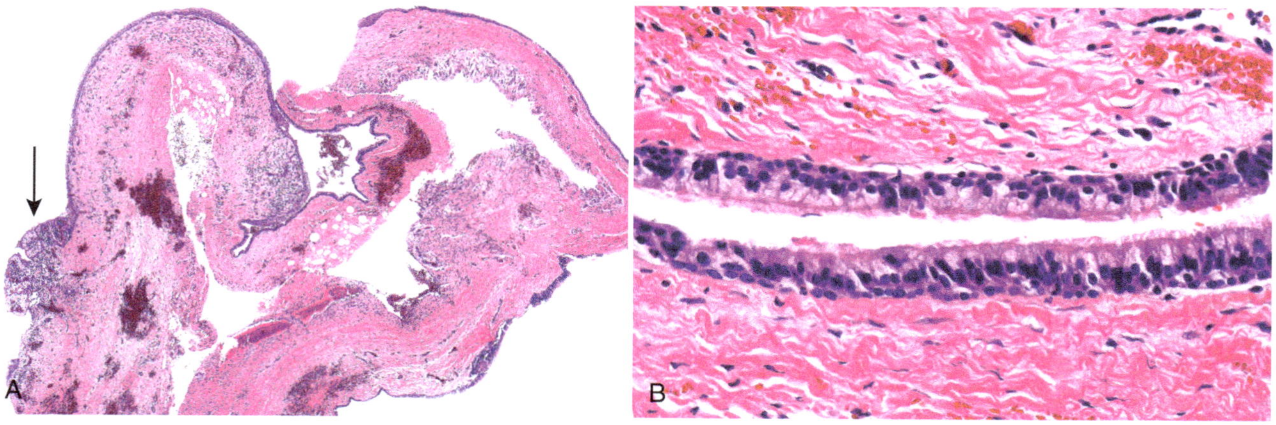

FIG. 16.2 Nasopalatine duct cyst. (A) Cyst lined by uniformly thin epithelium. The epithelium becomes proliferative if inflamed *(arrow)*. (B) Lining composed of ciliated, pseudostratified columnar epithelium.

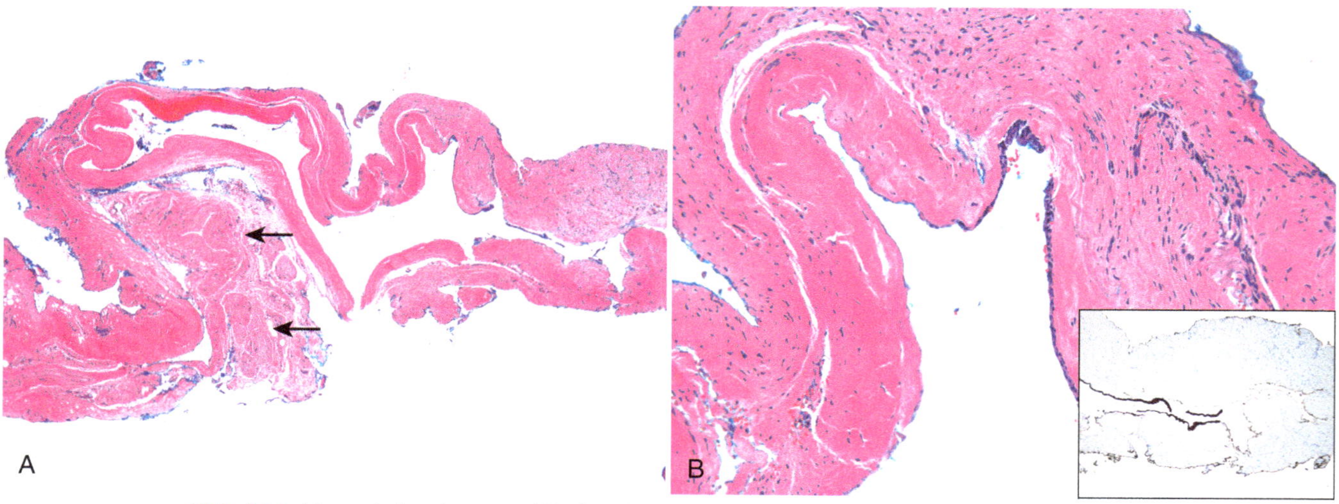

FIG. 16.3 Nasopalatine duct cyst. (A) Cyst is only focally lined by epithelium, but has a very thick basement membrane zone. Neurovascular bundles are noted within the wall *(arrows)*. (B) The cyst lining is composed of nonkeratinized, flattened squamous epithelium that is CK19+ *(inset)*.

SURGICAL CILIATED CYST (POSTOPERATIVE MAXILLARY CYST, SURGICAL IMPLANTATION CYST)

Clinical Findings

- This cyst occurs in the third to sixth decades of life, and it manifests as a swelling of the maxilla. There is a unilocular radiolucency of the posterior maxilla with a history of surgery involving the sinuses and radiographic evidence of surgical hardware (Fig. 16.4). On the rare occasion when it presents in the mandible, it is always associated with a history of concurrent sinus surgery.
- Up to 20% of Japanese patients develop this cyst after sinus surgery.

Etiopathogenesis and Histopathologic Features

The cyst epithelium is derived from surgical (traumatic) implantation of sinus respiratory epithelium during procedures such as a Le Fort I or Caldwell-Luc procedure involving the maxilla. Mandibular cysts occur if mandibular surgery is performed immediately after sinomaxillary surgery using the same instruments.

- The cyst is lined by ciliated, pseudostratified, columnar, and cuboidal epithelium two to five cells thick with mucous cells in most cases. Squamous epithelium may be present; the basement membrane zone may be thickened and there is variable inflammation (Fig. 16.5).

Differential Diagnosis

- An apical radicular cyst in the posterior maxilla may be lined by respiratory epithelium, but it is always associated with a nonvital tooth without a history of sinus surgery.

Management and Prognosis

- Excision is curative.

REFERENCES

Cai M, Shen G, Lu X, Wang X. Two mandibular surgical ciliated cysts after Le Fort I osteotomy and genioplasty. *Br J Oral Maxillofac Surg.* 2015;53:1040-1042.

Kaneshiro S, Nakajima T, Yoshikawa Y, et al. The postoperative maxillary cyst: report of 71 cases. *J Oral Surg.* 1981;39:191-198.

Koutlas IG, Gillum RB, Harris MW, Brown BA. Surgical (implantation) cyst of the mandible with ciliated respiratory epithelial lining: a case report. *J Oral Maxillofac Surg.* 2002;60:324-325.

Li CC, Feinerman DM, MacCarthy KD, Woo SB. Rare mandibular surgical ciliated cysts: report of two new cases. *J Oral Maxillofac Surg.* 2014;72:1736-1743.

Maruyama M, Onodera K, Ooya K. A histopathological and lectin-histochemical study of the lining epithelium in postoperative maxillary cysts. *Oral Dis.* 2002;8:241-248.

Yamamoto H, Takagi M. Clinicopathologic study of the postoperative maxillary cyst. *Oral Surg Oral Med Oral Pathol.* 1986;62:544-548.

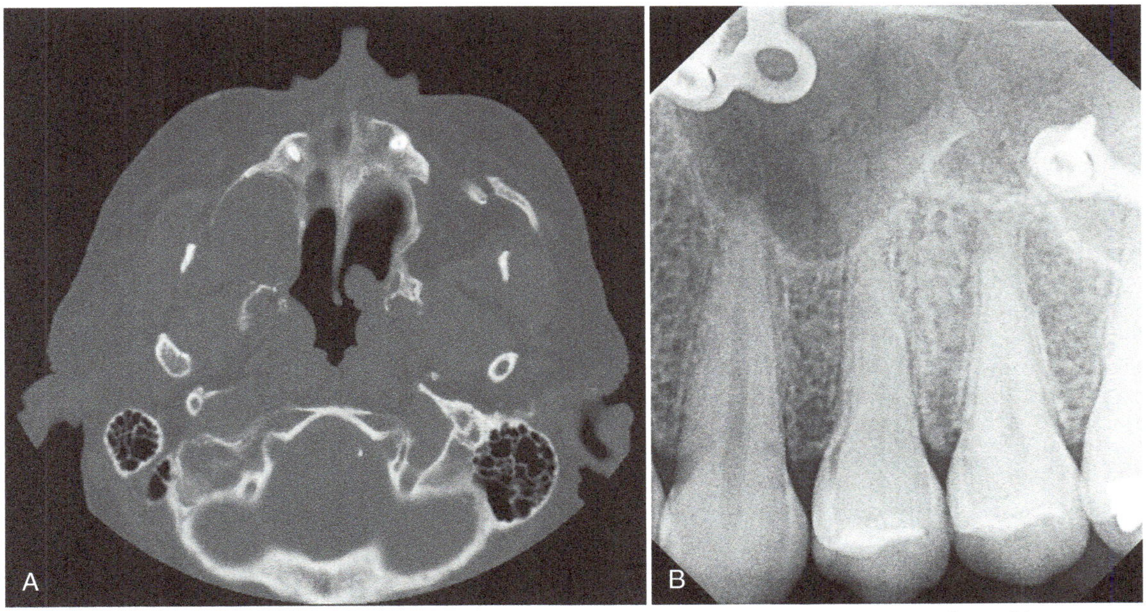

FIG. 16.4 Surgical ciliated cyst. (A) Unilocular radiolucency of the right maxilla in a patient with a history of surgery at that site. (B) Well-demarcated radiolucency at the apices of the left maxillary canine and first premolar; note surgical hardware. *(A, Courtesy Dr. Jeffrey Stone, private practice, Lowell, Mass.)*

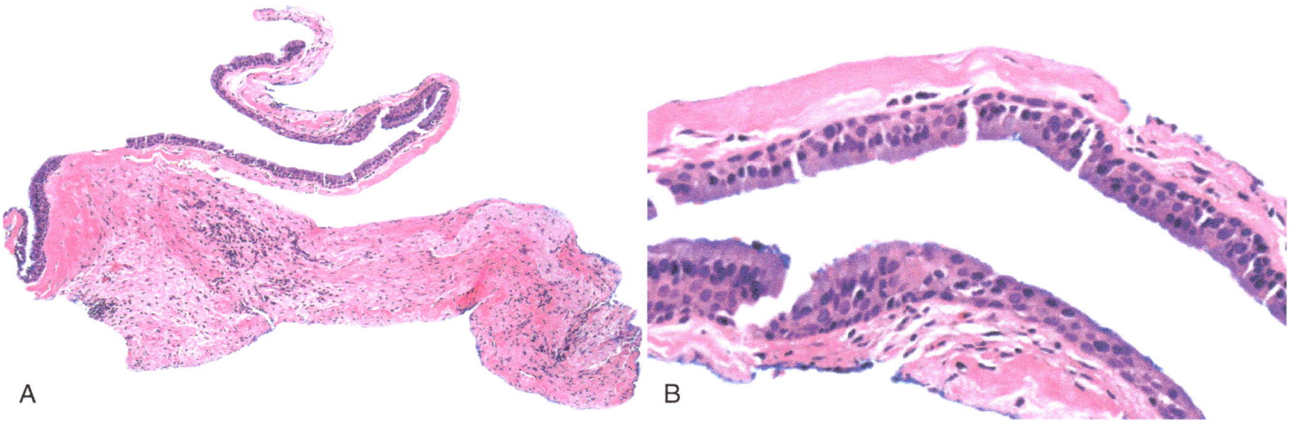

FIG. 16.5 Surgical ciliated cyst. (A) The cyst is lined by uniformly thin epithelium with mild chronic inflammation in the wall. (B) The cyst is lined by ciliated, pseudostratified columnar epithelium with many mucous cells.

MEDIAN PALATAL/PALATINE CYST

This is an extremely rare cyst, and its existence has been questioned.

Clinical Findings

- This cyst occurs in the fourth decade of life, has a 4:1 male predilection, and presents as a swelling in the midline of the palate posterior to, and not in communication with, the nasopalatine foramen.
- It presents as a well-demarcated, round or ovoid, unilocular radiolucency in the midline of the hard palate (Fig. 16.6).

Etiopathogenesis and Histopathologic Features

The lining putatively arises from entrapped epithelium during fusion of the lateral palatal shelves. Some question whether a cyst in this location could represent a nasopalatine duct cyst that developed from remnants of the nasopalatine duct in the posterior palate.

- The cyst is lined by ciliated, pseudostratified columnar or uniformly thin, nonkeratinized, stratified squamous epithelium.

Differential Diagnosis

- Posterior extension of the nasopalatine duct cyst should be considered if it communicates with the nasopalatine foramen.
- If it is parakeratinized and fulfills the histopathologic criteria for a keratocystic odontogenic tumor (odontogenic keratocyst), then it is likely a posterior extension of a primordial cyst of a mesiodens.

Management and Prognosis

- Enucleation or curettage is curative.

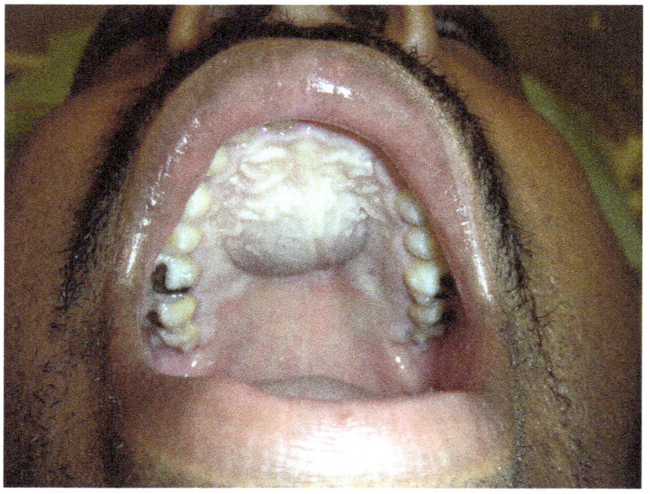

FIG. 16.6 Median palatal cyst. Swelling of the midline of the palate posterior to the nasopalatine foramen. *(From Manzon S, Graffeo M, Philbert R. Median palatal cyst: case report and review of literature. J Oral Maxillofac Surg. 2009;67:926-930.)*

REFERENCES

Gingell JC, Levy BA, DePaola LG. Median palatine cyst. *J Oral Maxillofac Surg.* 1985;43:47-51.

Kim SW, Seo BF, Baek SO, Jung SN. Large median palatine cyst. *J Craniofac Surg.* 2012;23:e288-e290.

Manzon S, Graffeo M, Philbert R. Median palatal cyst: case report and review of literature. *J Oral Maxillofac Surg.* 2009;67:926-930.

Pseudocysts

ANEURYSMAL BONE CYST

This condition is most common in the metaphases of long bones and the vertebrae, and up to 2% occur in the jaw bones.

Clinical Findings

- The majority occur before the age of 20 years, and there is a slight female predilection. Patients develop swelling of the face (sometimes rapid) that may be painful, and the mandible is affected in 75% to 90% of cases. The lesion manifests as a uniloculated or, more often, multiloculated (60% of cases) expansile radiolucency with a sclerotic rim of reactive bone and delicate intralesional trabeculae (Fig. 16.7); fluid level from hemorrhage is noted on imaging studies, and aspiration yields blood. Ten percent of lesions perforate the cortex.
- The lesion may occur secondary to another condition, such as fibrous dysplasia, ossifying fibroma, central giant cell lesion, or other intraosseous neoplasms.

Etiopathogenesis and Histopathologic Features

Primary extracranial aneurysmal bone cysts show translocation t(16;17)(q22;p13), leading to a fusion gene transcript *CDH11/USP6* in approximately 70% of cases; however, this translocation was not identified in secondary lesions, which may have a different etiology.

- Variably sized blood-filled spaces are surrounded by spindle mononuclear cells and multinucleated osteoclast-type giant cells. Fresh hemorrhage and siderophages are noted (Fig. 16.8). Reactive or residual bone is a frequent finding and should not be overdiagnosed as a synchronous fibroosseous lesion.
- An aneurysmal bone cyst may be seen in association with other lesions, especially cementoossifying fibromas, central giant cell granulomas, and fibrous dysplasias, in approximately 15% of cases (Fig. 16.9).

Differential Diagnosis

- Central giant cell granuloma and giant cell lesions of Noonan complex do not contain large, blood-filled spaces, although it may be difficult to see these in a curetted specimen. It is unclear what the relationship of a central giant cell granuloma is to the solid variant of the aneurysmal bone cyst in the jawbones. Giant cell tumors of the long bones are associated with mutation in *H3F3A*.
- Cherubism also contains giant cells but has specific clinical and radiographic features and is positive for the *SH3BP2* mutation.

Management and Prognosis

- Curettage, excision, resection (especially for recurrent and persistent lesions), cryotherapy, sclerotherapy, and low-dose radiotherapy are variably successful treatment modalities. Incomplete removal, especially via curettage, results in recurrence in 10% to 15% of cases; rarely, cases regress spontaneously.

REFERENCES

Arora SS, Paul S, Arora S, Kapoor V. Secondary jaw aneurysmal bone cyst (JABC)—a possible misnomer? A review of literature on secondary JABCs, their pathogenesis and oncogenesis. *J Oral Pathol Med.* 2014;43:647-651.

Cottalorda J, Bourelle S. Current treatments of primary aneurysmal bone cysts. *J Pediatr Orthop B.* 2006;15:155-167.

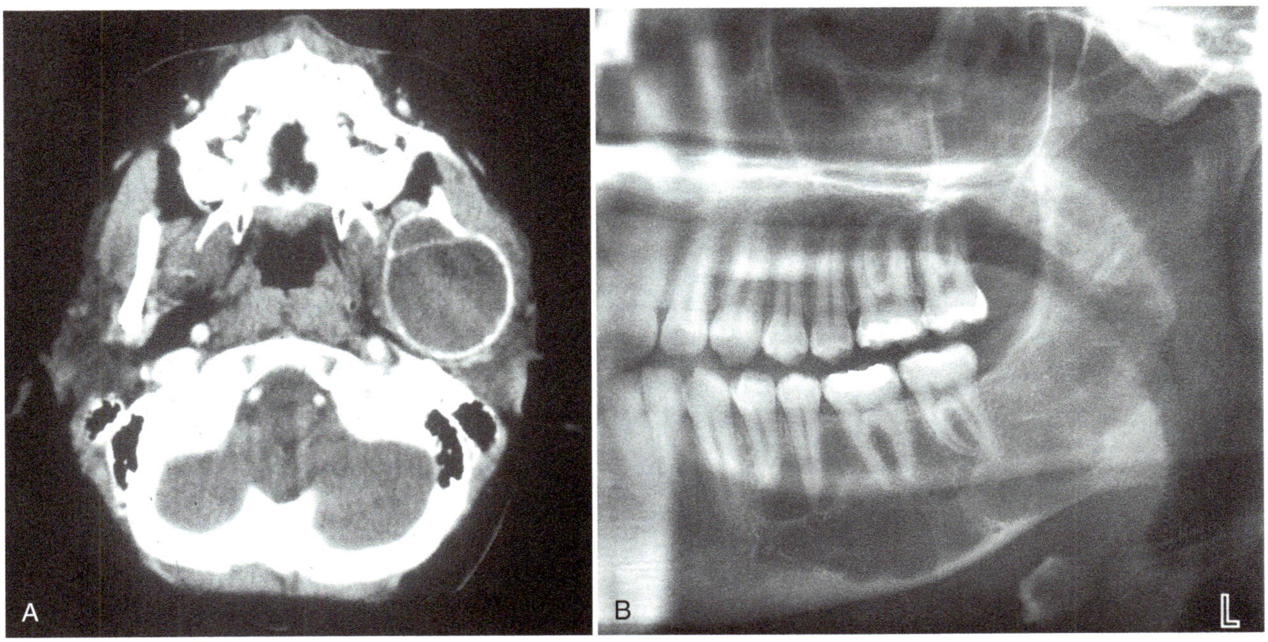

FIG. 16.7 Aneurysmal bone cyst. (A) Biloculated, expansile radiolucency of left mandibular ramus. (B) Multiloculated radiolucency of the left body and ramus of the mandible. *(A, Courtesy Dr. Charles E. Tomich, Indiana University School of Dentistry, Indianapolis, Ind; B, Courtesy Dr. Jeffrey Stone, private practice, Lowell, Mass.)*

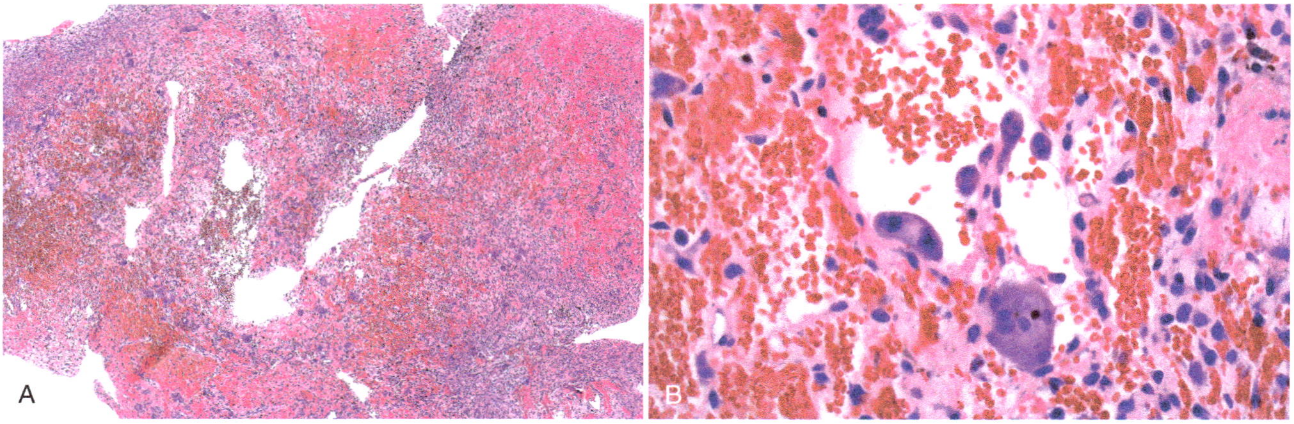

FIG. 16.8 Aneurysmal bone cyst. (A) Cystlike spaces surrounded by fibrous and granulation tissue containing many spindle and multinucleated giant cells. Extensive hemorrhage is present. (B) Giant cells rimming cystlike spaces. *(A, Courtesy Dr. Harry Kozakewich, Harvard Medical School, Boston.)*

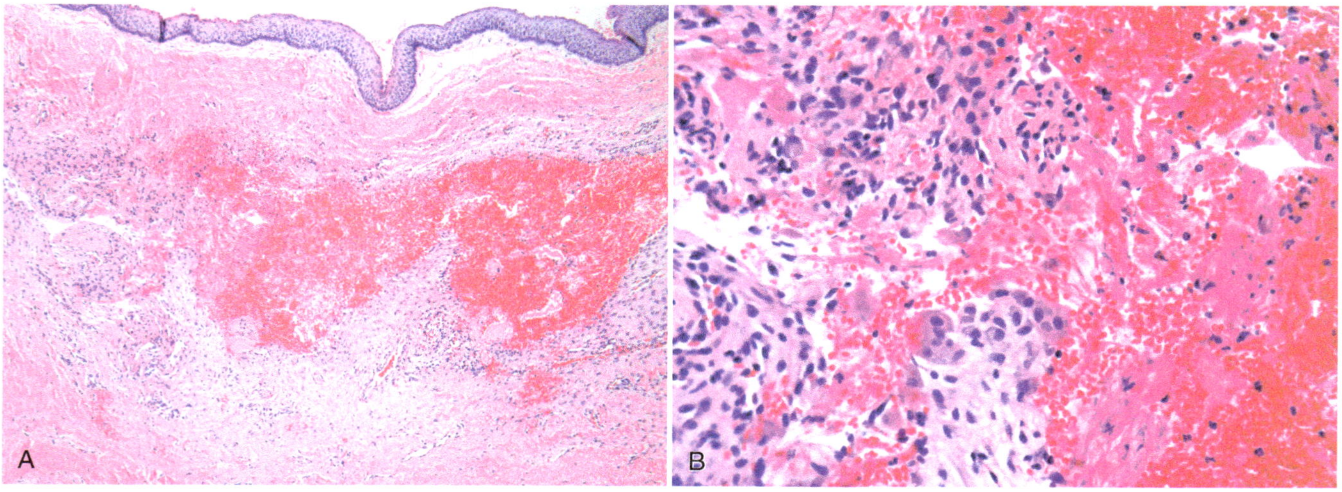

FIG. 16.9 Aneurysmal bone cyst. (A) Keratocystic odontogenic tumor (odontogenic keratocyst) with aneurysmal bone cyst within the wall, composed of a cystlike space filled with hemorrhage. (B) Space is lined by multinucleated giant cells and spindle cells.

Mankin HJ, Hornicek FJ, Ortiz-Cruz E, et al. Aneurysmal bone cyst: a review of 150 patients. *J Clin Oncol.* 2005;23:6756-6762.

Mendenhall WM, Zlotecki RA, Gibbs CP, et al. Aneurysmal bone cyst. *Am J Clin Oncol.* 2006;29:311-315.

Motamedi MH, Navi F, Eshkevari PS, et al. Variable presentations of aneurysmal bone cysts of the jaws: 51 cases treated during a 30-year period. *J Oral Maxillofac Surg.* 2008;66:2098-2103.

Oliveira AM, Perez-Atayde AR, Inwards CY, et al. *USP6* and *CDH11* oncogenes identify the neoplastic cell in primary aneurysmal bone cysts and are absent in so-called secondary aneurysmal bone cysts. *Am J Pathol.* 2004;165:1773-1780.

Sun ZJ, Zhao YF, Yang RL, Zwahlen RA. Aneurysmal bone cysts of the jaws: analysis of 17 cases. *J Oral Maxillofac Surg.* 2010;68:2122-2128.

SIMPLE BONE CYST (TRAUMATIC BONE CYST, SOLITARY BONE CYST, IDIOPATHIC BONE CAVITY, UNICAMERAL BONE CYST)

Clinical Findings

- Seventy-five percent of uncomplicated simple bone cysts are seen in the first two decades of life, with a slight male predilection. Lesions are asymptomatic, rarely cause swelling, and are usually noted on routine radiographic examination. Seventy-five to ninety percent are in the mandible, mostly in the molar-premolar area, with 13% crossing the midline. Some cases involve just the condyle. It rarely occurs in the maxilla.

- A simple bone cyst presents as a unilocular radiolucency, ovoid or round, often with a cone-shaped appearance at the periphery (tapering and angled), measuring up to several centimeters, and often scalloping between the roots of teeth (Fig. 16.10A–C). Hairline fractures may be seen in 28% of cases, and up to 13% may be multifocal
- A concomitant fibroosseous lesion may be noted with radiopacities within the radiolucency, which occurs mostly in females in the fifth decade of life and may cause facial swelling.
- Clinicians report the presence of either serosanguineous fluid or an empty cavity with only small wisps of tissue clinging to the walls (see Fig. 16.10D). Patients rarely recall an associated history of trauma.

Etiopathogenesis and Histopathologic Features

The etiology of this disorder is unknown. One theory is that trauma causes a hematoma, venous stasis, and bone ischemia. Most patients do not report a history of trauma, although the mouth is a trauma-intense environment. In support of this theory is the finding that approximately one-fourth of cases exhibit microfractures radiographically. The fact that focal cementoosseous dysplasia is frequently associated with this condition suggests an etiology related to aberrant bone homeostasis in some cases.

- There are small fragments of fibrovascular tissue, hemorrhage, and viable bone or calcified debris, disproportionate to the size of the clinical lesion (Fig. 16.11).

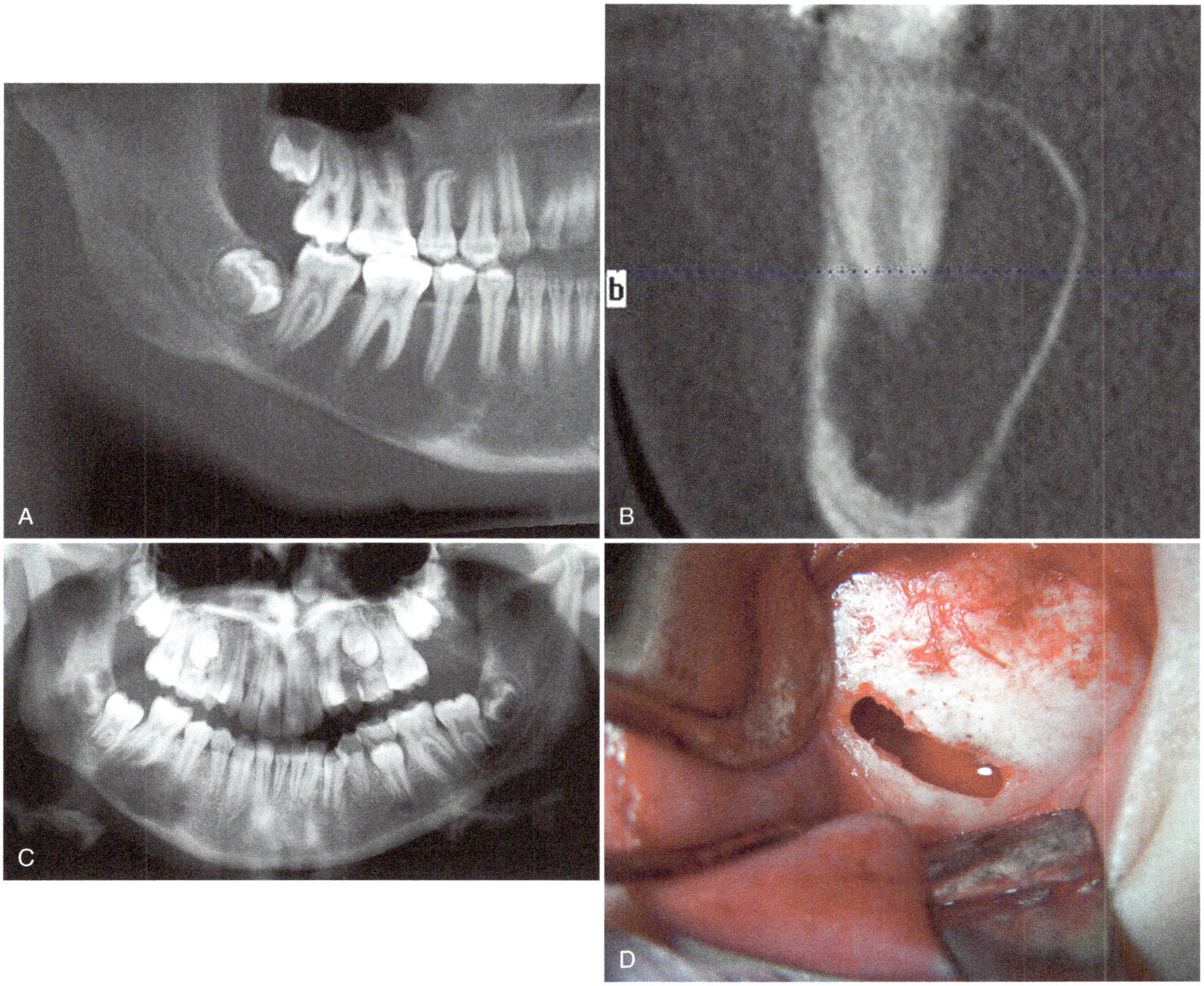

FIG. 16.10 Simple bone cyst. (A) Radiolucency with fine intralesional trabeculae, extending between the teeth roots. (B) Cone beam computerized tomogram shows lingual extent of lesion from Fig. 16.9A. (C) Multilocular radiolucency of the right posterior mandible. Note the slight cone-shaped extension between the roots of the premolar and molar. (D) At surgery, the lesion may be filled with serosanguineous fluid but is otherwise without tissue.

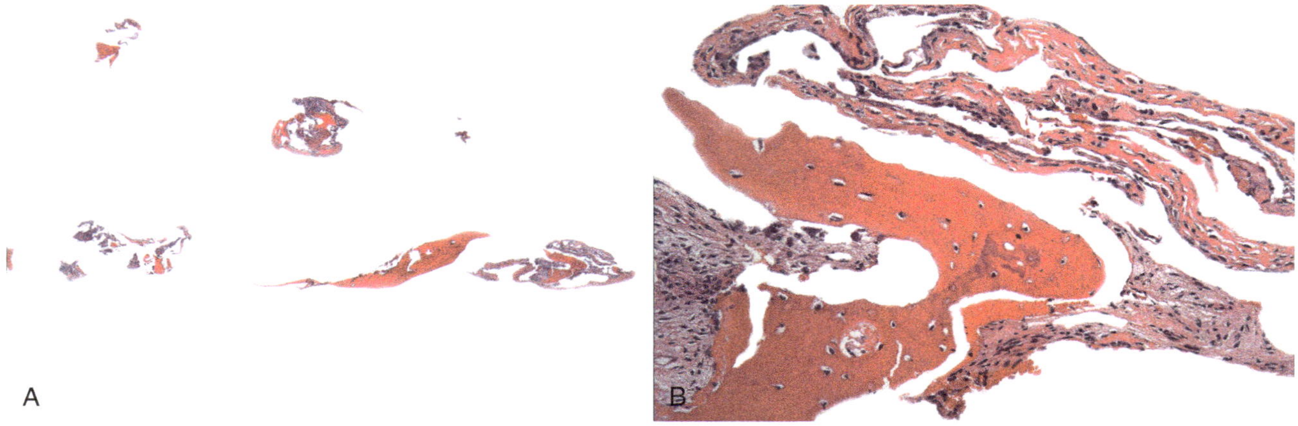

FIG. 16.11 Simple bone cyst. (A) Small fragments of fibrovascular tissue and bone curetted from the walls of an empty cavity at surgery. (B) Fibrovascular tissue and viable bone.

- Cementum droplets and osteoid within a cellular fibrous stroma are indications of the presence of a fibroosseous lesion, which is present in 9% to 23% of cases.

Management and Prognosis

- Curettage to induce a clot and granulation tissue formation with subsequent reorganization to form bone leads to resolution in 75% of cases.
- Up to 20% of cases recur, usually within the first 3 years of treatment. Risk factors for recurrence include the presence of jaw expansion, multifocality, and the presence of a benign fibroosseous lesion.

REFERENCES

Chadwick JW, Alsufyani NA, Lam EW. Clinical and radiographic features of solitary and cemento-osseous dysplasia-associated simple bone cysts. *Dentomaxillofac Radiol.* 2011;40:230-235.

Copete MA, Kawamata A, Langlais RP. Solitary bone cyst of the jaws: radiographic review of 44 cases. *Oral Surg Oral Med Oral Pathol Oral Radiol Endod.* 1998;85:221-225.

Harnet JC, Lombardi T, Klewansky P, et al. Solitary bone cyst of the jaws: a review of the etiopathogenic hypotheses. *J Oral Maxillofac Surg.* 2008;66:2345-2348.

Kuhmichel A, Bouloux GF. Multifocal traumatic bone cysts: case report and current thoughts on etiology. *J Oral Maxillofac Surg.* 2010;68: 208-212.

Magliocca KR, Edwards SP, Helman JI. Traumatic bone cyst of the condylar region: report of 2 cases. *J Oral Maxillofac Surg.* 2007;65: 1247-1250.

Mahomed F, Altini M, Meer S, Coleman H. Cemento-osseous dysplasia with associated simple bone cysts. *J Oral Maxillofac Surg.* 2005;63: 1549-1554.

Martins-Filho PR, de Santana Santos T, Cavalcanti de Araújo VL, et al. Traumatic bone cyst of the mandible: a review of 26 cases. *Braz J Otorhinolaryngol.* 2012;78:16-21.

Matsumura S, Murakami S, Kakimoto N, et al. Histopathologic and radiographic findings of the simple bone cyst. *Oral Surg Oral Med Oral Pathol Oral Radiol Endod.* 1998;85:619-625.

Suei Y, Taguchi A, Tanimoto K. Simple bone cyst of the jaws: evaluation of treatment outcome by review of 132 cases. *J Oral Maxillofac Surg.* 2007;65:918-923.

Tariq MU, Din NU, Ahmad Z, et al. Cementum-like matrix in solitary bone cysts: a unique and characteristic but yet underrecognized feature of promising diagnostic utility. *Ann Diagn Pathol.* 2014;18:1-4.

HEMATOPOIETIC BONE MARROW DEFECT (OSTEOPOROTIC BONE MARROW DEFECT)

Clinical Findings

- This is most frequently diagnosed in the fourth to sixth decades of life, and it has a 3 : 1 female predilection. It is generally asymptomatic and may occur in an area of a previously extracted tooth (23% of cases). It presents as a poorly demarcated radiolucency containing faint bone trabeculations, usually in the mandible (>90% of cases) and often in the molar area, discovered on routine radiographs. It may also appear as enlarged marrow spaces, especially at the periphery of the lesion (Fig. 16.12).

Etiopathogenesis and Histopathologic Features

Increased amounts of hematopoietic marrow in the mandible may represent reactive marrow hyperplasia because of increased demand or residual fetal marrow.

- Normal hematopoietic marrow is present with all three lineages—megakaryocytes, erythrocyte precursors, and myelocytes—in various stages of maturation. Fatty marrow may be present (Fig. 16.13).

Differential Diagnosis

- Extensive extramedullary hematopoiesis leads to diffuse, symmetric enlargement of the maxilla and mandible that appears osteoporotic on radiographs. This is seen particularly in thalassemia and sickle cell anemia (Fig. 16.14).

Management and Prognosis

- No treatment is required once the diagnosis is established.

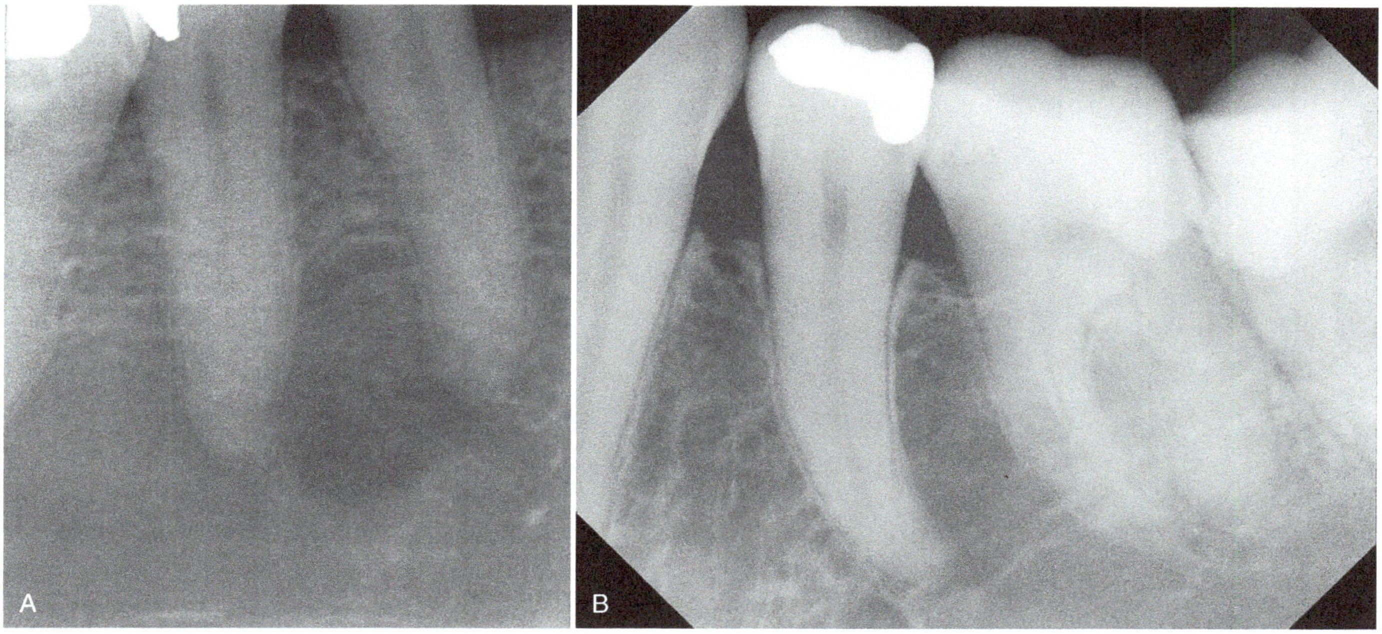

FIG. 16.12 Hematopoietic bone marrow defect. (A) Poorly circumscribed, subtle radiolucency around the roots of premolars. (B) Enlarged marrow spaces forming a poorly demarcated radiolucency with many trabeculations.

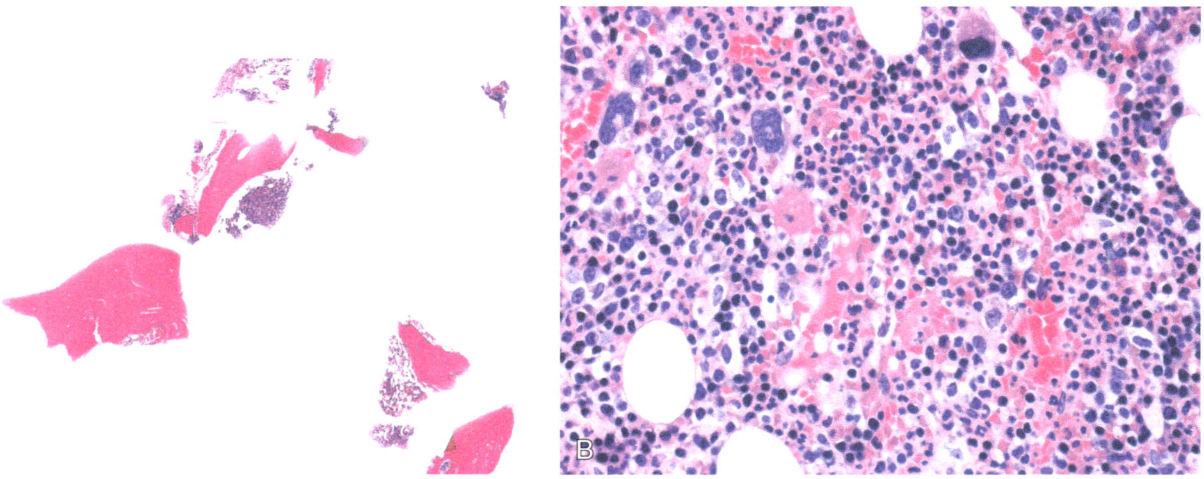

FIG. 16.13 Hematopoietic bone marrow defect. (A) Fragments of viable bone and hematopoietic marrow. (B) Megakaryocytes, erythrocyte precursors, and myelocytes are present.

REFERENCES

Almeida LY, Kato RB, Ribeiro MC, Leon JE. Focal osteoporotic bone marrow defect mimicking a mandibular cystic lesion. *J Craniofac Surg.* 2014;25:e324-e326.

Barker BF, Jensen JL, Howell FV. Focal osteoporotic bone marrow defects of the jaws: an analysis of 197 new cases. *Oral Surg Oral Med Oral Pathol.* 1974;38:404-413.

Lipani CS, Natiella JR, Greene GW Jr. The hematopoietic defect of the jaws: a report of sixteen cases. *J Oral Pathol.* 1982;11:411-416.

Makek M, Lello GE. Focal osteoporotic bone marrow defects of the jaws. *J Oral Maxillofac Surg.* 1986;44:268-273.

Schneider LC, Mesa ML, Fraenkel D. Osteoporotic bone marrow defect: radiographic features and pathogenic factors. *Oral Surg Oral Med Oral Pathol.* 1988;65:127-129.

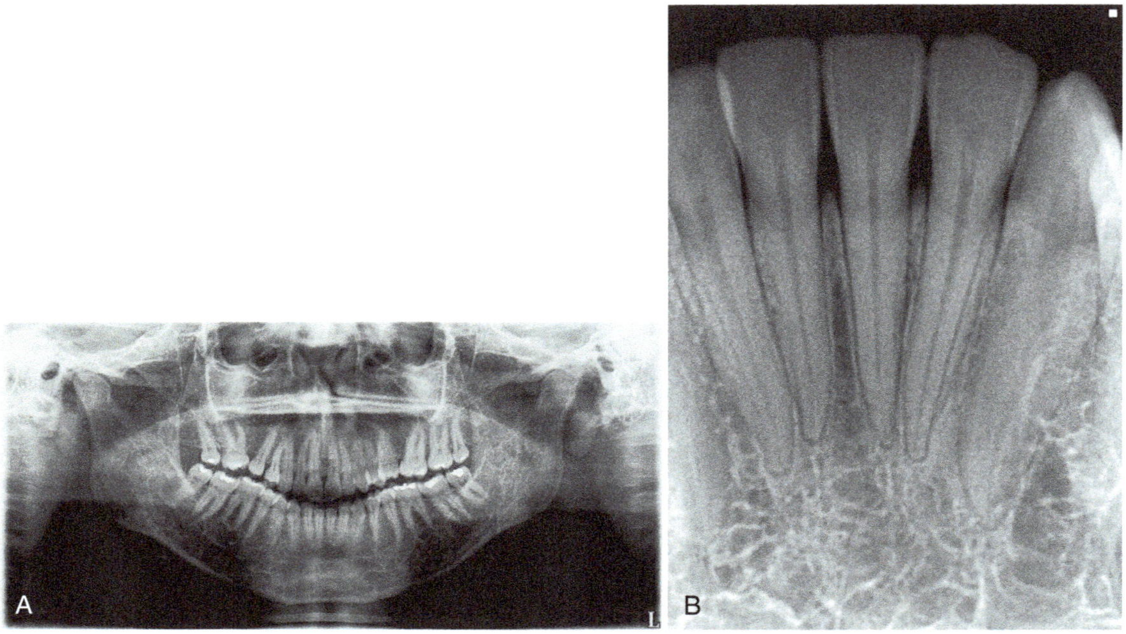

FIG. 16.14 (A) Panoramic radiograph of a patient with thalassemia exhibiting extensive extramedullary hematopoiesis and leading to osteoporotic appearance of bone and obliteration of the maxillary sinus. (B) Periapical film of anterior mandibular teeth shows markedly dilated marrow spaces with delicate bone trabeculae.

STAFNE BONE CAVITY (STAFNE BONE CYST, LINGUAL MANDIBULAR SALIVARY GLAND DEPRESSION)

Clinical Findings

- This occurs in the fifth to seventh decades of life and has a 3:1 to 6:1 male predilection. The lesions are asymptomatic and discovered incidentally. They consist of a well-demarcated radiolucency 0.5 to 2 cm in diameter, almost always unilateral in the lingual posterior mandible beneath the inferior alveolar canal (85% of cases), in the anterior mandible (12% of cases), or within the lingual ramus (2% of cases) (Fig. 16.15). In some cases, the defect extends to the buccal cortex.

Etiopathogenesis and Histopathologic Features

An entrapped lobe of the sublingual or submandibular (rarely parotid) salivary gland is present in an indentation within the lingual cortex of the mandible.

- Lobules of normal seromucinous glands are present (Fig. 16.16). Some cases consist of fibro fatty tissue only, but this may be due to the gland being displaced during surgery or to a sampling error.

Management and Prognosis

- The lesion is well visualized and diagnostic in three-dimensional imaging studies, and a biopsy is not indicated in most cases.

REFERENCES

Bornstein MM, Wiest R, Balsiger R, Reichart PA. Anterior Stafne's bone cavity mimicking a periapical lesion of endodontic origin: report of two cases. *J Endod.* 2009;35:1598-1602.

Buchner A, Carpenter WM, Merrell PW, Leider AS. Anterior lingual mandibular salivary gland defect: evaluation of twenty-four cases. *Oral Surg Oral Med Oral Pathol.* 1991;71:131-136.

Mourão CF, Miranda ÁM, Santos EJ, Pires FR. Lingual cortical mandibular bone depression: frequency and clinical-radiological features in a Brazilian population. *Braz Dent J.* 2013;24:157-162.

Philipsen HP, Takata T, Reichart PA, et al. Lingual and buccal mandibular bone depressions: a review based on 583 cases from a world-wide literature survey, including 69 new cases from Japan. *Dentomaxillofac Radiol.* 2002;31:281-290.

Shimizu M, Osa N, Okamura K, Yoshiura K. CT analysis of the Stafne's bone defects of the mandible. *Dentomaxillofac Radiol.* 2006;35:95-102.

Sisman Y, Miloglu O, Sekerci AE, et al. Radiographic evaluation on prevalence of Stafne bone defect: a study from two centres in Turkey. *Dentomaxillofac Radiol.* 2012;41:152-158.

Turkoglu K, Orhan K. Stafne bone cavity in the anterior mandible. *J Craniofac Surg.* 2010;21:1769-1775.

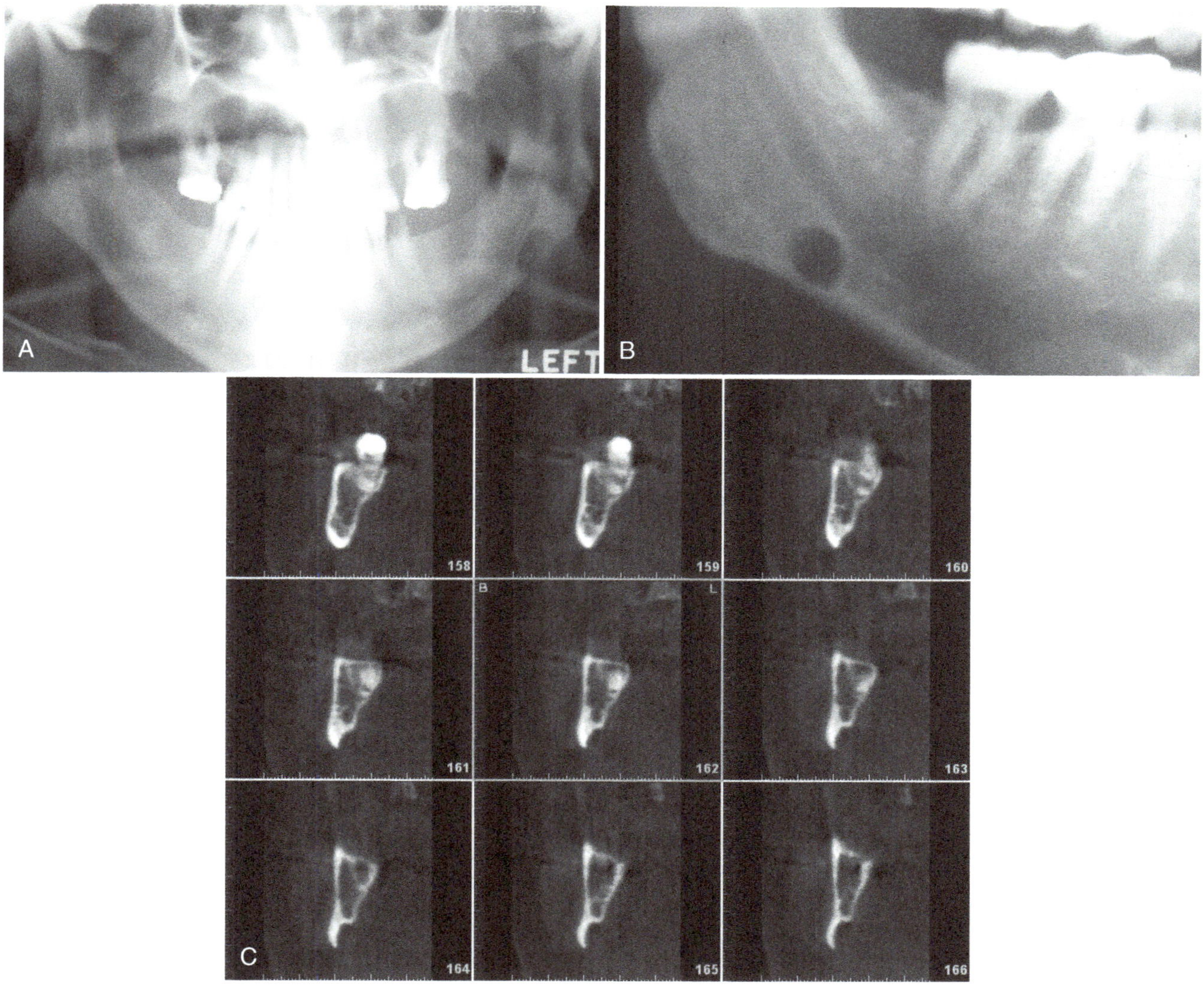

FIG. 16.15 Stafne bone cavity. (A) Circumscribed radiolucency at the left inferior border of the mandible, beneath the inferior alveolar canal. (B) Circumscribed radiolucency beneath the right inferior alveolar canal. (C) Computed tomographic scans show lingual depression just beneath inferior alveolar canal. *(A and C, Courtesy Dr. Bernard Friedland, Harvard School of Dental Medicine, Boston; B, Courtesy Dr. George Wysocki, London, ON, Canada.)*

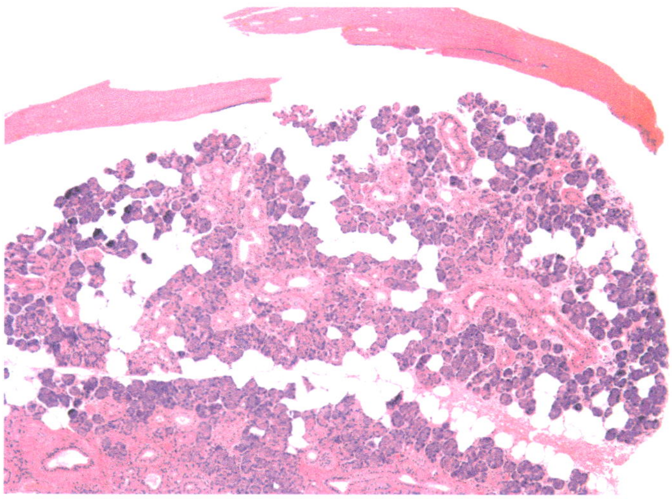

FIG. 16.16 Contents of the Stafne bone cavity consist of salivary gland tissue abutting cortical bone.

Miscellaneous Entities

MYOSPHERULOSIS (SPHERULOCYTOSIS, SPHERULOCYSTIC DISEASE OF SKIN, PARAFFINOMA)

Clinical Findings

- A persistent radiolucency is visible at the site of a previous tooth extraction, and there is a history of the site being packed or treated for dry socket, usually with a petrolatum-based material. The lesion may be present for years. Typically, the tissue specimen appears tarry, oily, and black.
- This has also been reported in sinuses that have been packed with an antibiotic ointment, and after chronic intralesional injections of the skin.

Etiopathogenesis and Histopathologic Features

Myospherulosis is caused by petrolatum- or lanolin-based packing products (usually used in conjunction with antibiotics) that undergo an emulsification process with red blood cells.

- Altered erythrocytes appear as yellowish-brown, spherical or crescent-shaped bodies within clear, cystlike spaces from leached-out lipid material. There is surrounding fibrosis and foreign body reaction. Some have "parent bodies" with endobodies within (Fig. 16.17).

Differential Diagnosis

- Fungal organisms stain with methenamine silver or periodic acid–Schiff.

Management and Prognosis

- Curettage is curative.

REFERENCES

Coulier B, Desgain O, Gielen I. Sinonasal myospherulosis and paraffin retention cysts suggested by CT: report of a case. *Head Neck Pathol.* 2012;6:270-274.

Culviner WT, Leonard DW, Wilhelmsen CL, Bolger WE. Experimental myospherulosis of the paranasal sinuses: a histologic rabbit study. *Am J Rhinol.* 2000;14:131-137.

Dunlap CL, Barker BF. Myospherulosis of the jaws. *Oral Surg Oral Med Oral Pathol.* 1980;50:238-243.

Flagothier C, Piérard GE, Quatresooz P. Cutaneous myospherulosis and membranous lipodystrophy: extensive presentation in a patient with severe steroid-induced dermal atrophy. *J Eur Acad Dermatol Venereol.* 2006;20:457-460.

Kakizaki H, Shimada K. Experimental study of the cause of myospherulosis. *Am J Clin Pathol.* 1993;99:249-256.

Lynch DP, Newland JR, McClendon JL. Myospherulosis of the oral hard and soft tissues. *J Oral Maxillofac Surg.* 1984;42:349-355.

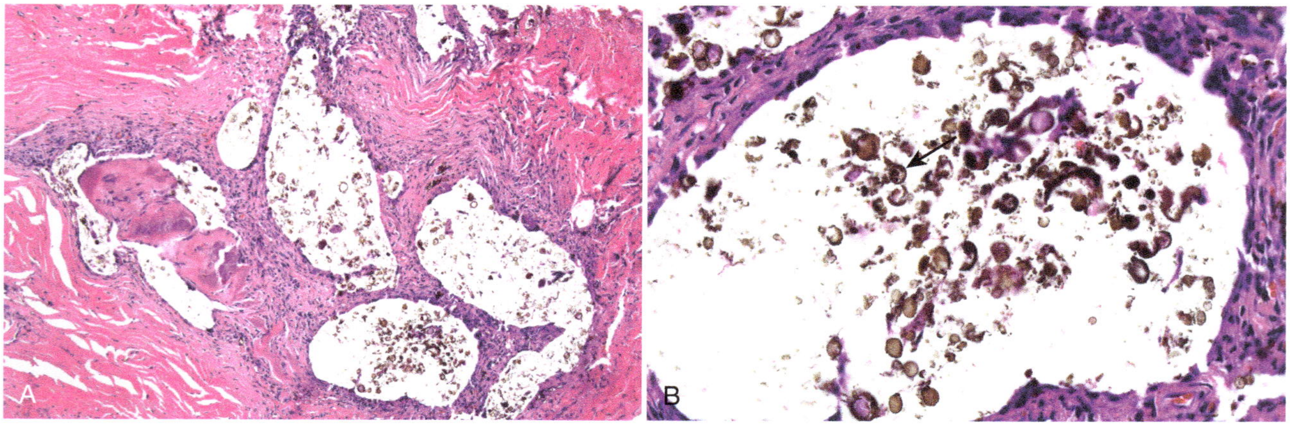

FIG. 16.17 Myospherulosis. (A) Clear spaces containing yellowish-brown particulate material surrounded by a histiocytic and giant cell reaction with fibrous and hyalinized stroma. (B) Spherical and crescent-shaped bodies and smaller fragments of similarly pigmented debris. The parent body has smaller endobodies inside *(arrow)*.

CENTRAL VASCULAR LESIONS

The most common location for central vascular lesions is the vertebral bodies, followed by the craniofacial skeleton (including the jaw bones) and the metaphyses of long bones. Many cases represent vascular malformations rather than hemangiomas, and these may be low-flow or high-flow lesions.

Clinical Findings

- Most cases are diagnosed within the first two decades of life and present as a diffuse, poorly demarcated radiolucency, often multiloculated (66%), and usually of the mandible (77% of cases) (Fig. 16.18). Rare cases have involved the condyle.
- There may be tooth mobility, bluish discoloration of the gingiva, gingival bleeding, and swelling of the face or overlying skin discoloration. In some cases, there is sudden progression in the second decade of life.
- Failure to suspect this condition may lead to life-threatening bleeding after extraction.

Etiopathogenesis and Histopathologic Features

As with other vascular lesions in young patients, these are likely caused by dysembryogenesis of vessels.

- Hemangioma is characterized by the formation of numerous capillary channels that may be dilated and tortuous or have poorly formed lumens. These are usually not associated with the presence of nerve fibers.
- Arteriovenous, arterial, or venous malformation (far more common than hemangioma) is characterized by the presence of venules with a muscle wall of varying thickness and/or arterioles with elastic lamina (Fig. 16.19). These are almost always associated with the presence of nerve fibers identified by the presence of S100 protein.

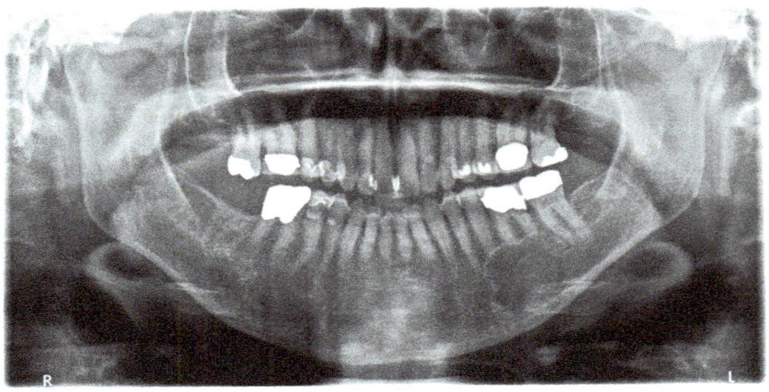

FIG. 16.18 Central venous malformation. There is a unilocular, well-demarcated radiolucency in the left bocy of the mandible. *(Courtesy Dr. Blaise Eckert, private practice, Belmont, Mass.)*

Differential Diagnosis

- Gorham disease is characterized by angiomatosis, but the clinical findings are those of progressive and diffuse destruction of the bone. The cell mediating bone destruction is of monocyte lineage, and progression of disease is propelled by cytokines that lead to osteoclastogenesis and angiogenesis.

Management and Prognosis

- If this is suspected, angiography of the external carotid artery is very useful to identify the feeder vessel, which may be ligated during surgery.
- Embolization with sclerosing agents (such as foam, sodium tetradecyl sulfate, or morrhuate sodium) followed by surgery is the treatment of choice, followed by reconstruction. Recurrence (or progression of residual disease) occurs in up to 33% of cases.

REFERENCES

Adegboyega PA, Qiu S. Hemangioma versus vascular malformation: presence of nerve bundle is a diagnostic clue for vascular malformation. *Arch Pathol Lab Med.* 2005;129:772-775.

Alves S, Junqueira JL, de Oliveira EM, et al. Condylar hemangioma: report of a case and review of the literature. *Oral Surg Oral Med Oral Pathol Oral Radiol Endod.* 2006;102:e23-e27.

Colucci S, Taraboletti G, Primo L, et al. Gorham-Stout syndrome: a monocyte-mediated cytokine propelled disease. *J Bone Miner Res.* 2006;21:207-218.

Drage NA, Whaites EJ, Hussain K. Haemangioma of the body of the mandible: a case report. *Br J Oral Maxillofac Surg.* 2003;41:112-114.

el-Sheikh MM, Zeitdoun IM, el-Massry M, Medra AM. Vascular malformations of the jaw bones: report on nine patients. *J Craniomaxillofac Surg.* 1993;21:9-14.

Giaoui L, Princ G, Chiras J, et al. Treatment of vascular malformations of the mandible: a description of 12 cases. *Int J Oral Maxillofac Surg.* 2003;32:132-136.

Persky MS, Yoo HJ, Berenstein A. Management of vascular malformations of the mandible and maxilla. *Laryngoscope.* 2003;113:1885-1892.

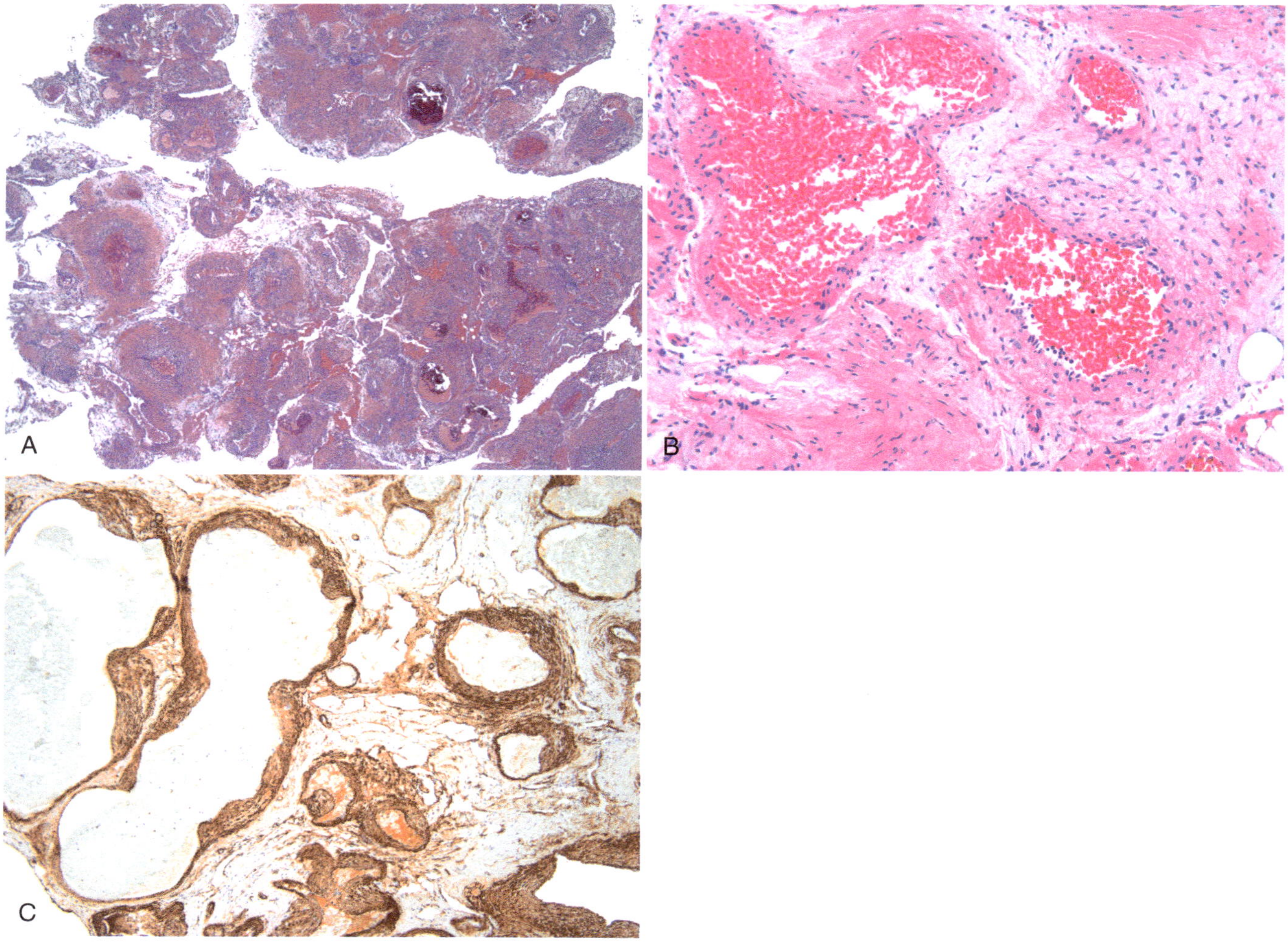

FIG. 16.19 Central venous malformation (from case in Fig. 16.18). (A) Many vessels with walls of varying thickness are visible. (B) Vessels consist of endothelium-lined spaces with muscle coats of variable thickness. (C) Study for smooth muscle actin highlights muscle walls of variable thickness.

17 NONODONTOGENIC INTRAOSSEOUS TUMORS

CHAPTER CONTENTS

As with odontogenic cysts and tumors, any nonodontogenic tumor may cause jaw and facial swelling, pain, mobility of teeth, resorption of teeth roots, teeth displacement, and paresthesia, depending on the size of lesions, how long the lesions have been present, how rapidly they are growing, whether they are benign or malignant, and the proximity of nerves.

TORI, EXOSTOSES, AND SUBPONTIC OSSEOUS HYPERPLASIA

Clinical Findings

- Tori: These occur in up to 30% of adults and present as exophytic, hard, uninodular or multinodular bony masses covered by mucosa. Torus palatinus and torus mandibularis are located on the midline of palate and lingual mandible (usually bilateral and symmetric) respectively, and may grow to a large size (Fig. 17.1A–B). They are readily traumatized and ulcerated because of their protuberant nature or may exhibit frictional keratosis; 2% of cases have both palatal and mandibular tori.
- Exostosis: This occurs in up to 27% of adults with a 5:1 male predilection and presents as an outgrowth of bone, polypoid or sessile, frequently on buccal aspects of the mandible, maxilla, or ascending arch of the palate, with more than 90% of cases having concurrent tori (Fig. 17.1C–D); exostoses may show rapid growth in some patients.
- Subpontic osseous hyperplasia (subpontic exostosis): This is an outgrowth of bone beneath a pontic (artificial tooth on a bridge that replaces a missing tooth), and radiographically is indistinguishable from normal bone, although there may be some sclerosis (Fig. 17.1E).

Etiopathogenesis and Histopathologic Features

Tori are inherited in an autosomal dominant fashion and may exhibit ethnic differences. Exostoses may develop as a result of genetic and environmental factors. Subpontic osseous hyperplasia results from irritation of bone beneath the pontic, leading to bone deposition.

- There is dense lamellar bone with well-spaced small osteocytes within lacunae, fibrovascular tissue in haversian canals, and variable osteoblastic rimming, especially if inflamed (Fig. 17.2A); fatty marrow is often present.
- Long, sweeping collagen bundles (lamellae) are noted using polarized light (Fig. 17.2B).

Differential Diagnosis

- Osteomas have identical histopathology but are usually central; pedicled "peripheral" osteomas may represent exostoses.

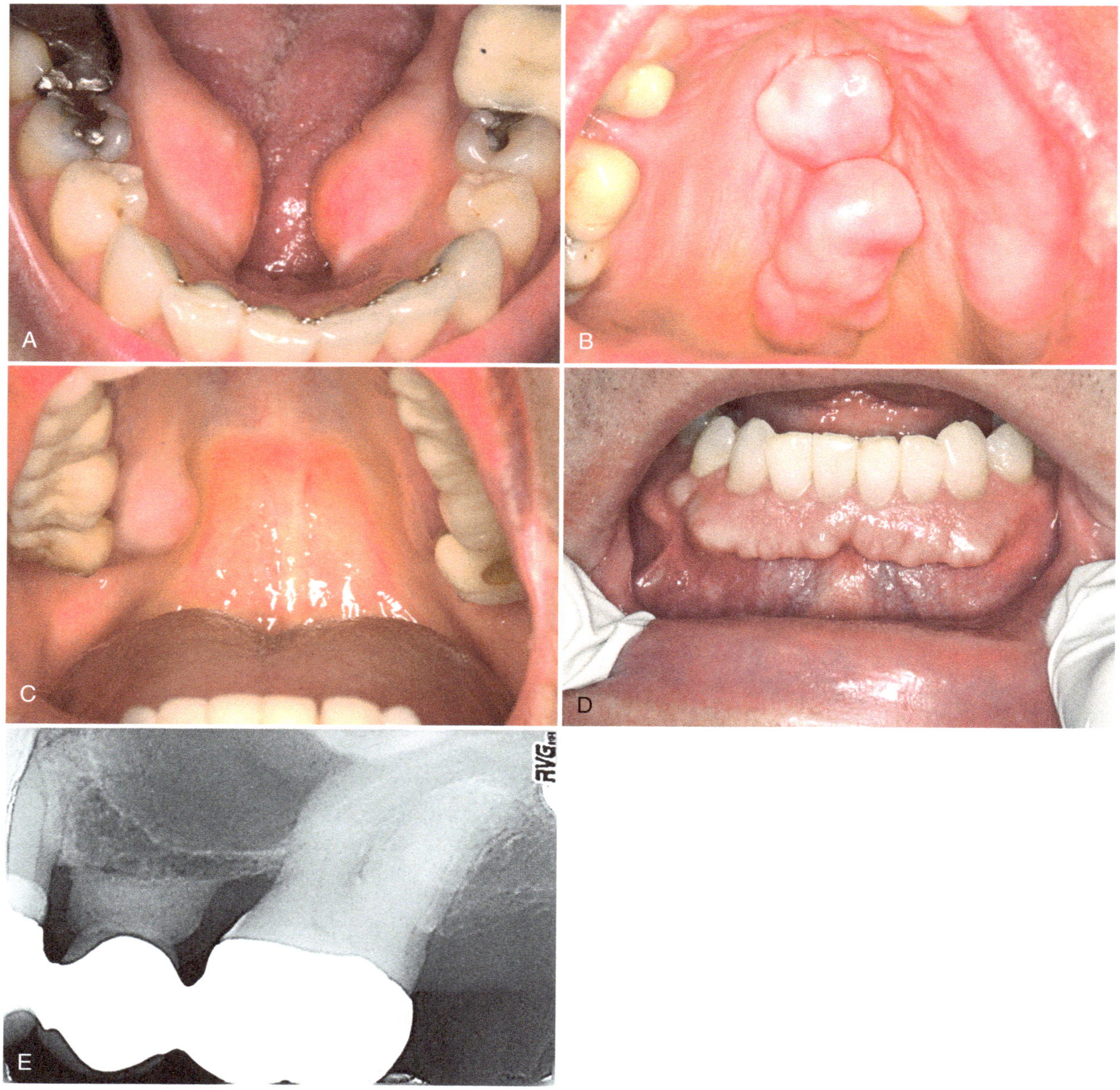

FIG 17.1 (A) Torus mandibularis: bilaterally symmetric, sessile bony masses on the lingual aspect of the mandible. (B) Torus palatinus: multinodular bony masses on the midline of the palate. (C) Palatal exostosis: bony mass on the ascending arch of the right palate. (D) Facial exostosis: a shelf of bone on the facial aspect of the anterior mandible. (E) Subpontic osseous hyperplasia: exophytic mass of sclerotic bone beneath the pontic.

- Osteochondromas occur mostly on the coronoid and condylar processes and appear as a nodule of bone with a benign cartilaginous cap.

Management and Prognosis

- Excision is performed usually in preparation for denture fabrication, or if the lesion is constantly ulcerated from trauma.

REFERENCES

Auskalnis A, Bernhardt O, Putniene E, et al. Oral bony outgrowths: Prevalence and genetic factor influence. Study of twins. *Medicina.* 2015;51:228-232.

Aydin U, Yildirim D, Bozdemir E. Subpontic osseous hyperplasia: Three case reports and literature review. *Eur J Dent.* 2013;7:363-367.

Chohayeb AA, Volpe AR. Occurrence of torus palatinus and mandibularis among women of different ethnic groups. *Am J Dent.* 2001;14:278-280.

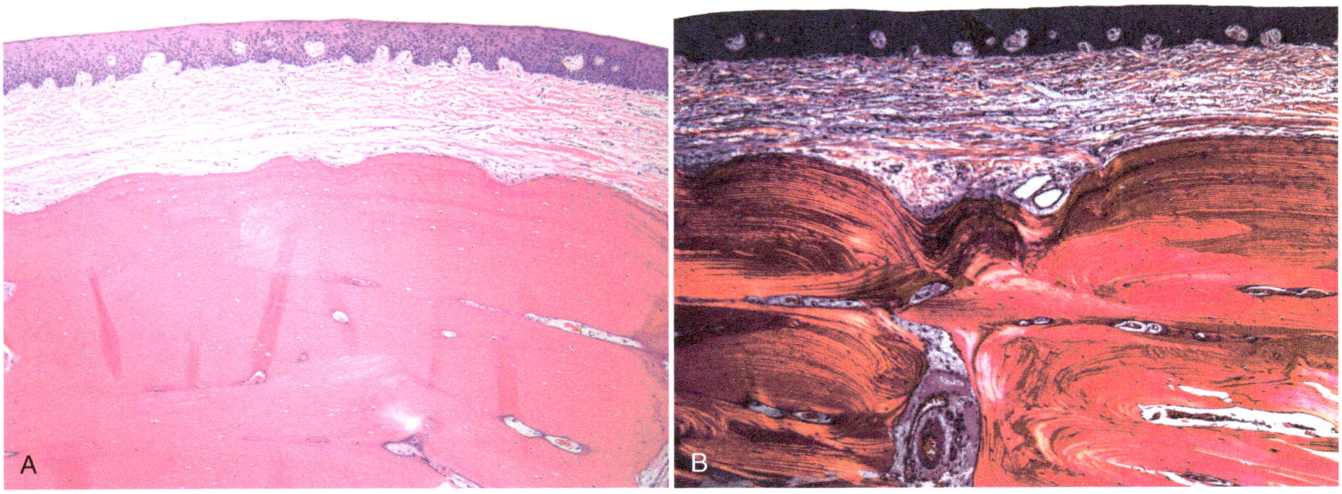

FIG 17.2 Torus. (A) Dense viable lamellar bone with small osteocytes within lacunae. (B) Polarized light reveals long sweeping fascicles of collagen typical for lamellar bone.

Gorsky M, Bukai A, Shohat M. Genetic influence on the prevalence of torus palatinus. *Am J Med Genet.* 1998;75:138-140.

Islam MN, Cohen DM, Waite MT, Bhattacharyya I. Three cases of subpontic osseous hyperplasia of the mandible: a report. *Quintessence Int.* 2010;41:299-302.

Jainkittivong A, Langlais RP. Buccal and palatal exostoses: prevalence and concurrence with tori. *Oral Surg Oral Med Oral Pathol Oral Radiol Endod.* 2000;90:48-53.

Karacayli U, Gocmen-Mas N, Kaya A, Koymen R. Clinical and stereologic evaluation of osteochondroma. *Oral Surg Oral Med Oral Pathol Oral Radiol Endod.* 2009;108:e52-e56.

Larrea-Oyarbide N, Valmaseda-Castellon E, Berini-Aytes L, Gay-Escoda C. Osteomas of the craniofacial region. Review of 106 cases. *J Oral Pathol Med.* 2008;37:38-42.

Ortakoglu K, Akcam T, Sencimen M, et al. Osteochondroma of the mandible causing severe facial asymmetry: a case report. *Oral Surg Oral Med Oral Pathol Oral Radiol Endod.* 2007;103:e21-e28.

REACTIVE AND INFLAMMATORY BONE CONDITIONS

CONDENSING OSTEITIS AND IDIOPATHIC OSTEOSCLEROSIS (DENSE BONE ISLAND, BONE SCAR, ENOSTOSIS)

These are likely related conditions that result in sclerosis of bone.

Clinical Findings

- Condensing osteitis: This occurs in 1% to 6% of the population and there is an asymptomatic poorly demarcated but discrete homogeneous radiopacity seen around the apices and roots of teeth. These are usually mandibular premolars and molars that are nonvital and/or have been endodontically treated. The periodontal ligament space may be widened (Fig. 17.3A).
- Idiopathic osteosclerosis (dense bone island, bone scar, enostosis): This occurs in approximately 1% to 5% of the population presenting as an asymptomatic poorly demarcated but discrete radiopacity that is usually not located at the apices of teeth. It occurs in the mandible in greater than 80% of cases, is discovered on routine radiography, and is unassociated with pain or swelling. If associated with apices of teeth, vitality testing of teeth should be performed (Fig. 17.3B); it may be more prevalent in the Far East.

Etiopathogenesis and Histopathologic Features

Condensing osteitis is caused by inflammation of odontogenic origin (usually from a nonvital tooth) leading to reactive bone formation and sclerosis. Idiopathic osteosclerosis is of unknown etiology.

- Both have similar histopathology and exhibits densely sclerotic bone with few or small Haversian canals; fibrosis, fatty marrow, and mild chronic inflammation may be present.

Differential Diagnosis

- True osteomas are usually present within the bone as round or ovoid homogeneous radiopacities without a surrounding radiolucent rim, and are associated with Gardner syndrome, one form of the familial adenomatous polyposis syndrome, which is an autosomal dominant condition associated with mutation in the APC gene located on 5p21. Gardner syndrome is associated with the development of osteomas of the jaws and other bones, supernumerary teeth, colonic polyps that are highly associated with the development of carcinoma, desmoid tumors, fibromas, thyroid carcinomas, and epidermoid cysts.

Management and Prognosis

- Biopsy is not necessary if the lesion is recognized for what it is on the radiograph. In some cases of idiopathic osteosclerosis at the apices of teeth the teeth should be evaluated for vitality.

REFERENCES

Galiatsatos P, Foulkes WD. Familial adenomatous polyposis. *Am J Gastroenterol.* 2006;101:385-398.

Green TL, Walton RE, Clark JM, Maixner D. Histologic examination of condensing osteitis in cadaver specimens. *J Endod.* 2013;39:977-979.

MacDonald-Jankowski DS. Idiopathic osteosclerosis in the jaws of Britons and of the Hong Kong Chinese: radiology and systematic review. *Dentomaxillofac Radiol.* 1999;28:357-363.

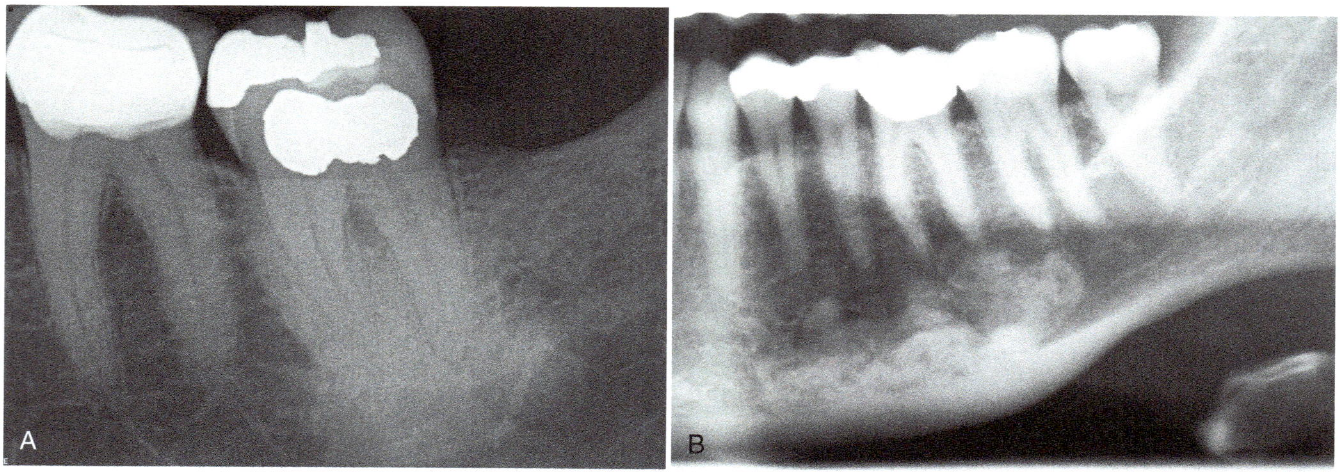

FIG 17.3 (A) Condensing osteitis: poorly demarcated uniform radiopacity around the roots of a nonvital left mandibular first molar. (B) Idiopathic osteosclerosis: radiopacities in the left mandible not related to apices of teeth. *(B, Courtesy Dr. Thomas Mone, private practice, Braintree, Mass.)*

Miloglu O, Yalcin E, Buyukkurt MC, Acemoglu H. The frequency and characteristics of idiopathic osteosclerosis and condensing osteitis lesions in a Turkish patient population. *Med Oral Patol Oral Cir Bucal.* 2009;14:e640-e645.

Verzak Z, Celap B, Modric VE, et al. The prevalence of idiopathic osteosclerosis and condensing osteitis in Zagreb population. *Acta Clin Croat.* 2012;51:573-577.

Wijn MA, Keller JJ, Giardiello FM, Brand HS. Oral and maxillofacial manifestations of familial adenomatous polyposis. *Oral Dis.* 2007;13:360-365.

Yonetsu K, Yuasa K, Kanda S. Idiopathic osteosclerosis of the jaws: panoramic radiographic and computed tomographic findings. *Oral Surg Oral Med Oral Pathol Oral Radiol Endod.* 1997;83:517-521.

OSTEOMYELITIS AND OSTEONECROSIS

Unlike other bones, infection and inflammation of the jaw bones (osteitis) is a common occurrence because teeth frequently become infected, either from caries or periodontal disease, with spread of such infection into the bone. Periapical lesions, such as periapical granuloma and apical radicular cysts, when large result in intramedullary inflammation, usually without sequestrum formation. Even large periapical abscesses heal after curettage, often without the necessity for prolonged antibiotic use.

Acute and *chronic suppurative bacterial osteomyelitis* of the jaws is usually the result of chronic odontogenic and/or jaw bone infection and is associated with sequestrum formation. A second form of osteomyelitis is not associated with bacterial infection, and the terms *primary chronic osteomyelitis, primary diffuse sclerosing osteomyelitis,* and more recently *nonbacterial chronic osteomyelitis* are used to describe this condition. It is likely related to *chronic recurrent multifocal osteomyelitis* (CRMO), which includes the syndrome consisting of synovitis, acne, pustulosis, hyperostosis, and osteomyelitis (SAPHO), and which also manifests in the oral cavity.

Osteonecrosis of the jaw is defined as the presence of sequestrum often exposed to the oral cavity and has a number of causative factors (Table 17.1). Unlike the long bones, the presence of sequestrum does not necessarily connote osteomyelitis. The best example of this is *benign spontaneous sequestration of the lingual plate* in addition to stage 1 medication-related osteonecrosis of the jaws, both of which are painless and often resolve spontaneously. As such, osteonecrosis may, but not invariably, result in osteomyelitis.

Clinical Findings

- *Suppurative osteomyelitis, acute* and *chronic:* This usually occurs in adults and is associated with a chronic tooth infection, postextraction of infected teeth, or a poorly healed jaw fracture with the presenting symptom of a mottled, poorly demarcated radiolucency with radiopaque sequestrum.
  - There is pain, swelling, and suppuration. Sinus tracts and acute exacerbations of chronic osteomyelitis are also common.
  - Patients with focal or multifocal cementoosseous dysplasia with sclerotic avascular bone are at risk for developing such osteomyelitis (Fig. 17.4A).
- *Primary diffuse osteomyelitis, primary diffuse sclerosing osteomyelitis, nonbacterial chronic (sclerosing) osteomyelitis:* The majority (>95% of cases) occur before age 20 with a 2:1 female predilection, and almost all cases involve the mandible; there is intermittent pain, swelling, trismus, and intermittent fever with little response to antibiotics. Radiographs show a diffuse expansion of the mandible with osteosclerosis and small osteolytic foci (Fig. 17.4B).
  - Patients may have osteomyelitis of other bones in addition to skin lesions such as pustulosis, acne, psoriasis, neutrophilic dermatosis, and inflammatory bowel disease; elevated erythrocyte sedimentation rate (ESR) and C-reactive protein (CRP), and elevated HLA-B27, and antinuclear antibodies are noted in less than 10% of cases.
- *Osteonecrosis:* This presents as bony sequestrum, usually exposed, with or without pain (Fig. 17.5A–D); in the case of medication-related osteonecrosis, chronic sinus tracts and nonhealing extraction sockets are common manifestations. Radiographs reveal thickened lamina dura and osteosclerosis; advanced cases exhibit mottled

TABLE 17.1 Etiologies for Osteonecrosis of the Jaws

Etiology	Clinical Findings	Management and Prognosis
Medication-induced: antiresorptive agents such as bisphosphonates and denosumab, and anti-angiogenic agents such as bevacizumab, sunitinib, and ziv-ablifercept; occurs in 1–3% of cancer patients on bisphosphonates and 1 in 2000–5000 patients on bisphosphonates for nononcologic indications.	Staging (for bisphosphonates group): 0sa or 0ss: no bone exposure, may have sinus tracts, periodontal pocketing, and/or radiolucency/opacity that cannot be attributed to odontogenic infection; may or may not be painful Stage 1: bone exposure, no symptoms Stage 2: bone exposure, symptomatic Stage 3: extensive necrosis and/or pathologic fracture, and involvement of the maxillary sinus Maxilla/mandible = 1:2; often at sites of extraction, odontogenic infection, or tori	Stages 0sa and 1: chlorhexidine rinse and follow-up; nonsurgical sequestrectomy (dislodgement of bone) Stages 0ss, 2, and 3: chlorhexidine rinse, antibiotic therapy (amoxicillin, clindamycin, or metronidazole), nonsurgical or surgical sequestrectomy/excision; pain control Prognosis: metachronous or recurrent lesions often occur
Radiation injury (damage to osteoclast precursors and sclerosis of vessels; hypovascularity); up to 5% frequency after irradiation with >6000 cGys.	Exposed bone Maxilla/mandible = 1:9 (mandible has less collateral circulation compared with maxilla)	Surgical excision, antibiotics, chlorhexidine rinse, hyperbaric oxygen, pain control Prognosis: often difficult to control with progression or recurrence, a common finding
Mechanical Trauma		
Intubation-associated or spontaneous benign sequestration of lingual plate	Both on mylohyoid ridge	Nonsurgical sequestrectomy or allow bone to exfoliate; chlorhexidine rinse; topical analgesia Prognosis: does not recur
Chemical Trauma		
Cocaine Caustic dental materials (eg, root canal)	Cocaine necrosis often seen on palate Site where dental materials placed	Cocaine necrosis: plastic surgery Prognosis: recurrence if cocaine habit maintained Dental materials: topical steroid therapy and gentle salt water rinses Prognosis: good
Infection		
Odontogenic infection or fracture site	Site of infected tooth, extraction of infected tooth or fracture site	Antibiotics, curettage, debridement, surgery, pain control
Varicella-zoster	Unilateral exposed bone, with preceding gingival/palatal ulceration	May need to excise if necrotic bone does not exfoliate; antibiotics, chlorhexidine rinse, pain control Prognosis: no recurrence
Noma, necrotizing ulcerative stomatitis (NUS)	Noma/NUS: around teeth and soft tissues; immunocompromised or HIV/AIDS-related	Improve nutrition, antibiotics, plastic surgery to correct soft tissue defects Prognosis: may recur if underlying medical issues not adequately addressed
Sclerotic bone disease such as mature cementoosseous dysplasia (especially multifocal type), Paget disease, and osteopetrosis (hypovascular bone) in presence of odontogenic infection	Where bone disease and odontogenic infection coexist with/without history of extraction and oral surgery	Antibiotics, curettage, debridement, surgery, pain control Prognosis: may recur

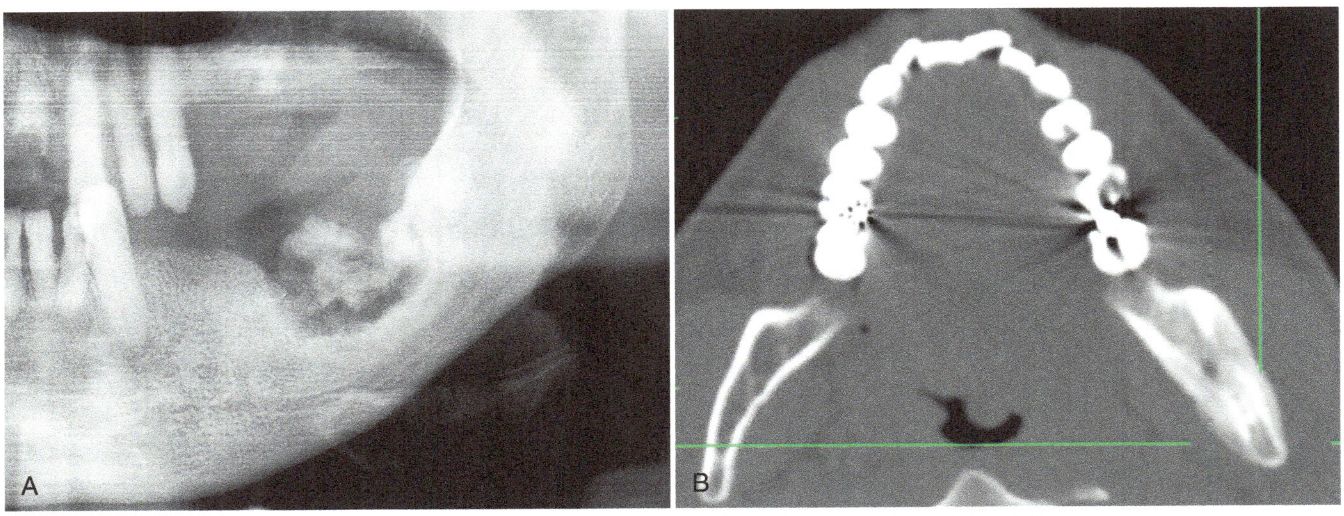

FIG 17.4 (A) Chronic osteomyelitis with sequestrum formation in a patient with multifocal cementoosseous dysplasia. (B) Primary nonbacterial chronic sclerosing osteomyelitis of the left mandible exhibiting typical diffuse sclerosis with periosteal reaction. *(B, Courtesy Dr. Andrew Salama, Boston University Medical Center, Boston.)*

radiolucency and radiopacities consistent with sequestra (Table 17.1; Fig. 17.5E–F).

- *Benign spontaneous sequestration of the lingual plate* occurs in healthy individuals, usually with a male predilection, and consists of small, 1 mm to 4 mm sequestra only (Fig. 17.5G). These heal spontaneously after the sequestrum exfoliates or is removed.

Etiopathogenesis and Histopathologic Features

Suppurative osteomyelitis is caused by a bacterial infection from a tooth. Most cases (66%) are polymicrobial although streptococcus viridians is the most commonly isolated organism. *Primary nonbacterial sclerosing osteomyelitis* of the mandible in children and adolescents is an autoinflammatory rheumatologic condition and is likely the monostotic form of CRMO that usually affects the lower limbs, pelvis, and clavicle with skin lesions as noted earlier. SAPHO syndrome is the adult equivalent. Causes of *osteonecrosis* include suppression of bone turnover, vascular compromise, and trauma (see Table 17.1).

- *Suppurative osteomyelitis:* There are nonviable bony sequestra and granulation tissue with acute and chronic inflammation and abscesses; a sclerotic mass of nonvital globular sclerotic cementum may be present if there is a preexisting cementoosseous dysplasia (Fig. 17.6).
- *Primary nonbacterial sclerosing osteomyelitis:* The reactive and reparative osteoid forms parallel bone trabeculae or exhibit an interlacing pattern; there is prominent stromal fibrosis, mild to insignificant chronic inflammation, dilated sinusoidal vessels, and rarely sequestrum; other features include a fibrous dysplasia–like pattern and atypical osteoid formation (Fig. 17.7).
- *Medication-related osteonecrosis and osteoradionecrosis:* There are nonviable bony sequestra with empty lacunae and ragged borders, usually with extensive bacterial colonization especially with *Actinomycetes* species as a biofilm (Fig. 17.8); a diagnosis of actinomycosis (actinomycotic osteomyelitis) should be made only if sulfur granules are present, surrounded by suppuration with Splendore-Hoeppli effect; *Eikenella corrodens* is often present. Osteoclasts may be seen and osteomyelitis may develop with acute and chronic inflammation, and granulation tissue (Fig. 17.9). Cases of osteoradionecrosis often exhibit thickening and fibrosis of vessel walls.

Differential Diagnosis

- Atypical osteoid and fibrous dysplasia–like areas in primary nonbacterial sclerosing osteomyelitis must always be correlated with the clinical findings; an incorrect diagnosis may be rendered when these features are taken out of context and especially if the biopsy is small.

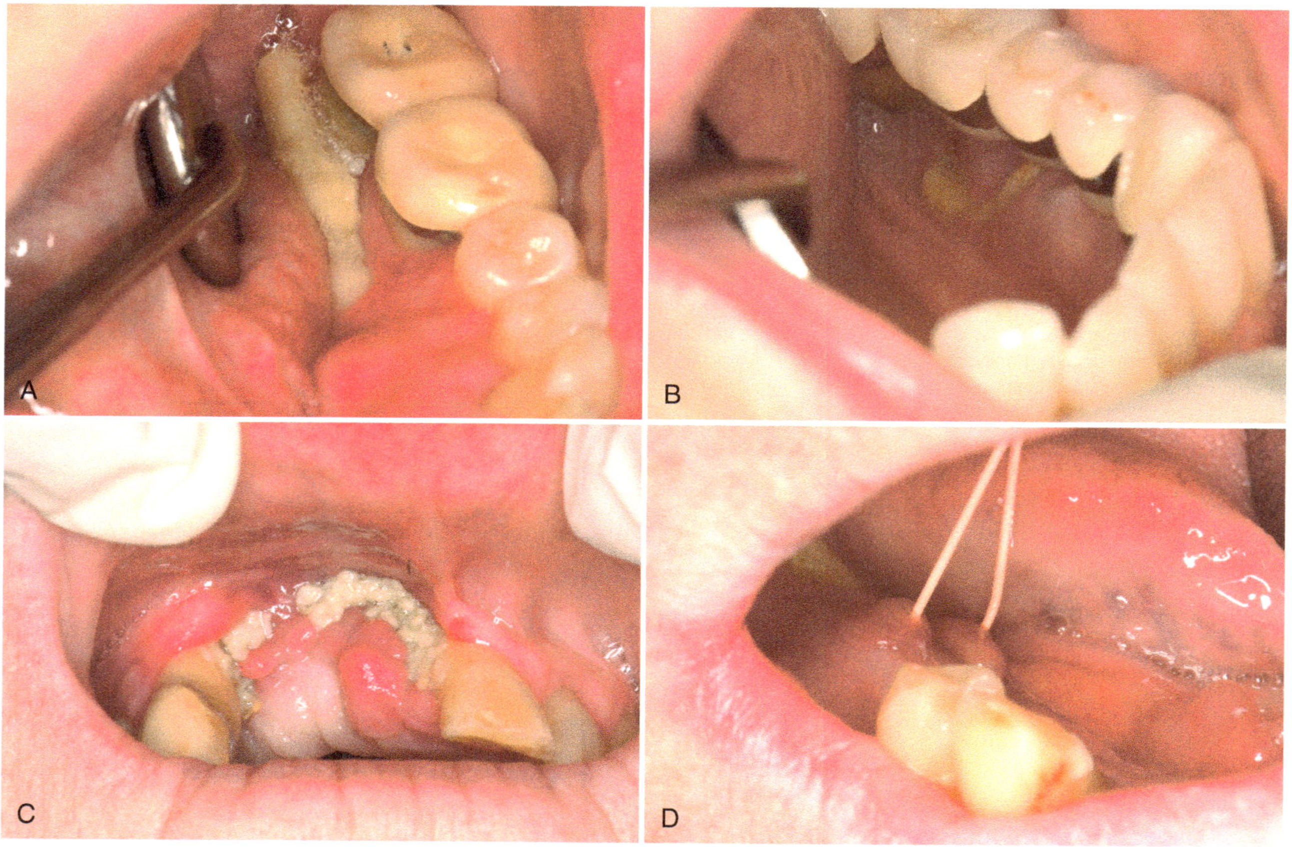

FIG 17.5 Medication (bisphosphonate)-related osteonecrosis (A–D). (A) Typical exposed sequestrum located on the mylohyoid ridge. (B) Sequestrum located beneath a subpontic exostosis. (C) Necrotic bone on the anterior maxillary ridge. (D) Sinus tracts are a common finding and may be the only finding in early lesions; note sequestrum posterior to the sinus tracts.

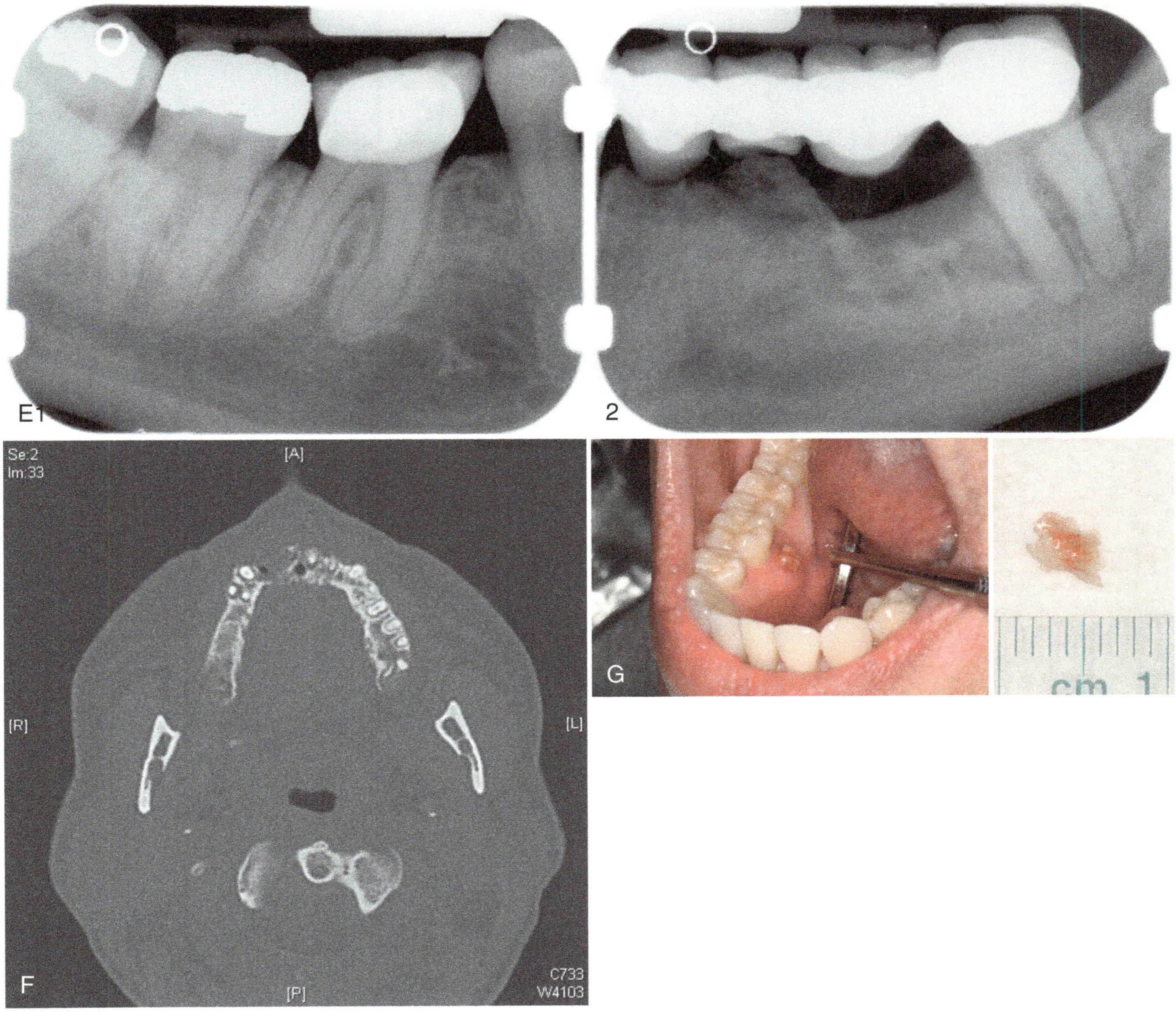

FIG 17.5, cont'd (E) Radiograph (from patient in B) showing necrotic subpontic osseous hyperplasia *(right panel)* and teeth with thickened lamina dura on the opposite side *(left panel)*. (F) CT scan of patient in C showing mottled radiolucency of the right anterior maxilla. (G) Benign sequestration of the lingual plate *(left panel)*; tiny fragment of bone removed from lesion *(right panel)*.

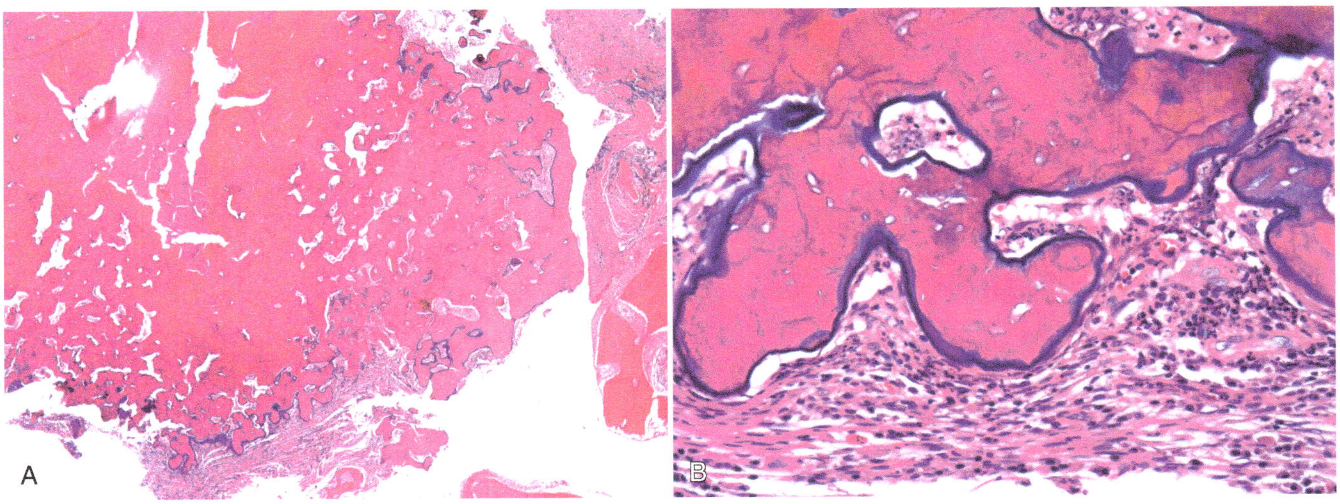

FIG 17.6 Osteomyelitis secondary to cementoosseous dysplasia. (A) Masses of nonvital sclerotic, globular cementum-like material. (B) Nonvital globular cementum-like material with empty lacunae surrounded by granulation tissue with many neutrophils.

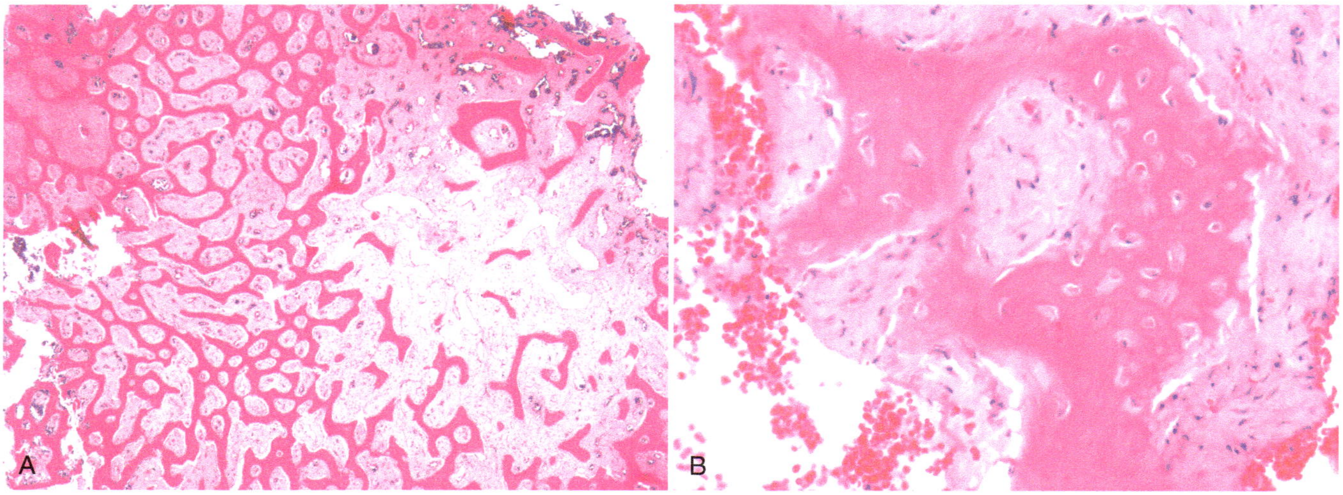

FIG 17.7 Primary nonbacterial sclerosing osteomyelitis. (A) Interlacing trabeculae of bone *(left)* with delicate fibrous dysplasia-like trabeculae *(right)*, fibrosis, and sinusoidal vessels. (B) Plump osteocytes within lacunae of woven bone.

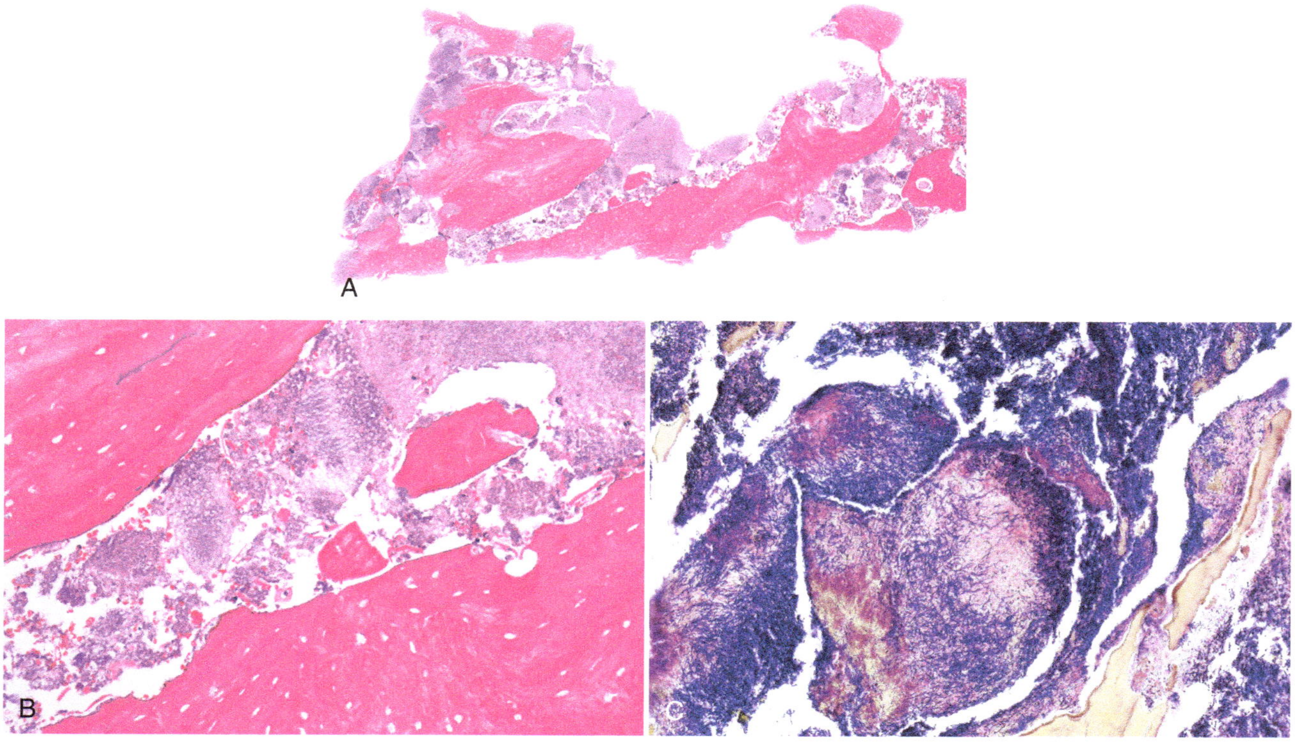

FIG 17.8 Medication-related osteonecrosis. (A) Nonviable bony sequestrum (removed by nonsurgical sequestrectomy) with ragged margins surrounded by bacterial biofilm. (B) Dense colonies of filamentous bacteria. (C) Brown and Brenn stain reveals filamentous bacteria consistent with colonization by actinomycetes, but does not constitute actinomycosis because there are no sulfur granules and there is no suppuration.

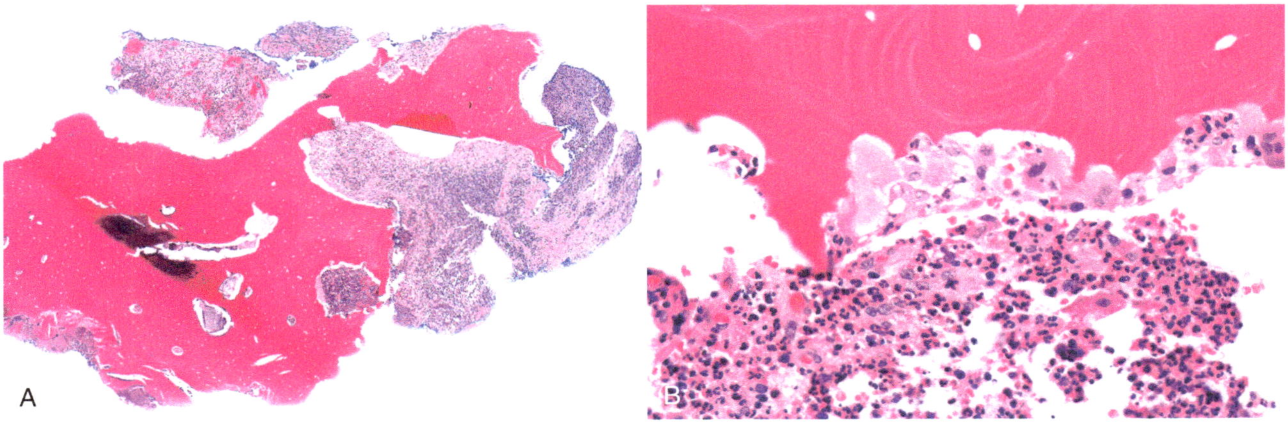

FIG 17.9 Medication-related osteonecrosis and osteomyelitis. (A) Nonviable bony sequestrum surrounded by granulation tissue with abscesses. (B) Nonviable bone is rimmed by osteoclasts within Howship lacunae; abscesses are present.

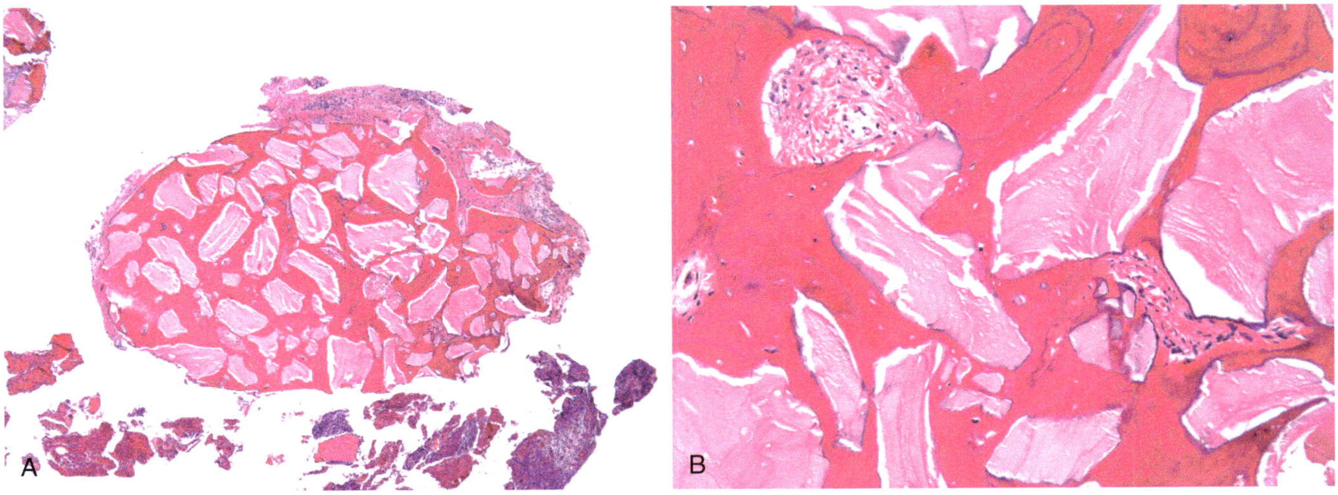

FIG 17.10 Bone graft material. (A) Fragments of bone with pale, amorphous graft material between trabeculae. (B) Pale graft material surrounded by viable woven bone.

- A search should be made for primary bone malignancy (such as myeloma) or metastatic disease for patients with cancer who develop medication-related osteonecrosis; recurrent squamous cell carcinoma is a consideration for those with radiation-induced osteonecrosis.
- Bone graft material (sometimes freeze-dried bone) is identified by the regularity in shape and size and even distribution of the osseous particles; it also shows appositional host bone on the surface in some cases (Fig. 17.10).

Management and Prognosis

- *Suppurative osteomyelitis:* Sequestrectomy and debridement, long-term antibiotics (β-lactams and clindamycin), and hyperbaric oxygen are recommended treatments.
- Primary nonbacterial sclerosing osteomyelitis is treated primarily with nonsteroidal antiinflammatory medications and corticosteroids; other effective measures include methotrexate, azathioprine, anti–tumor necrosis factor alpha (TNFα) inhibitors, and bisphosphonates.
- *Medication-related osteonecrosis:* Nonviable bone is often readily removed by nonsurgical sequestrectomy or dislodgement, surgical sequestrectomy and debridement, or resection and antibiotics depending on the stage (Table 17.1; Fig. 17.11); hyperbaric oxygen may be useful in severe cases.

REFERENCES

Almazrooa SA, Woo SB. Bisphosphonate and nonbisphosphonate-associated osteonecrosis of the jaw: a review. *J Am Dent Assoc.* 2009;140:864-875.

Almazrooa SA, Chen K, Nascimben L, et al. Case report osteonecrosis of the mandible after laryngoscopy and endotracheal tube placement. *Anesth Analg.* 2010;111:437-441.

Eyrich GK, Baltensperger MM, Bruder E, Graetz KW. Primary chronic osteomyelitis in childhood and adolescence: a retrospective analysis of 11 cases and review of the literature. *J Oral Maxillofac Surg.* 2003;61:561-573.

Girschick HJ, Huppertz HI, Harmsen D, et al. Chronic recurrent multifocal osteomyelitis in children: diagnostic value of histopathology and microbial testing. *Hum Pathol.* 1999;30:59-65.

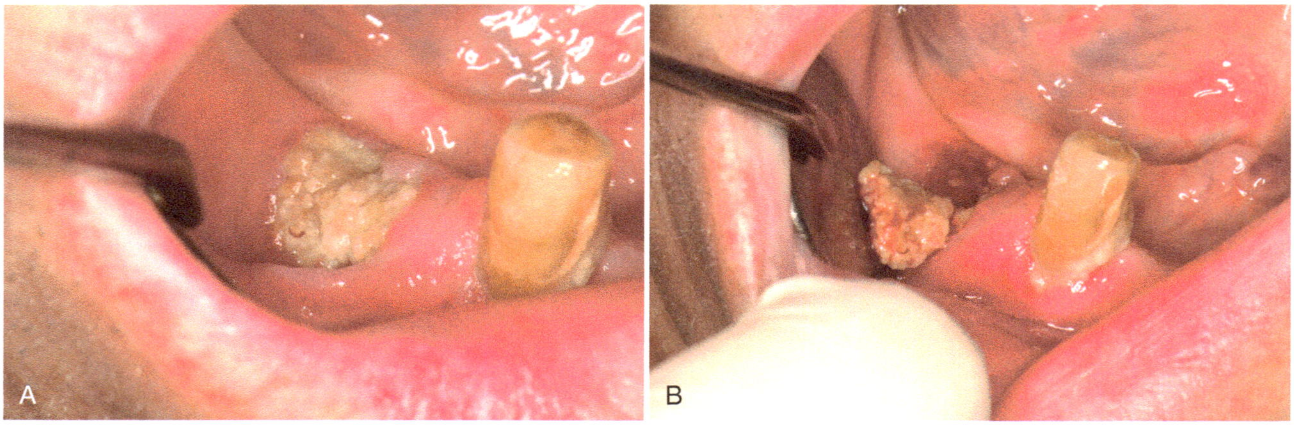

FIG 17.11 Medication-related osteonecrosis. (A) Nonviable sequestrum on mandibular ridge. (B) Bone fragment is readily dislodged (nonsurgical sequestrectomy) leaving behind a bed of hemorrhagic granulation tissue.

Hansen T, Kunkel M, Weber A, Kirkpatrick CJ. Osteonecrosis of the jaws in patients treated with bisphosphonates—histomorphologic analysis in comparison with infected osteoradionecrosis. *J Oral Pathol Med.* 2006;35:155-160.

Krakowiak PA. Alveolar osteitis and osteomyelitis of the jaws. *Oral Maxillofac Surg Clin North Am.* 2011;23:401-413.

Kumar SK, Gorur A, Schaudinn C, et al. The role of microbial biofilms in osteonecrosis of the jaw associated with bisphosphonate therapy. *Curr Osteoporos Rep.* 2010;8:40-48.

Mawardi H, Enzinger P, McCleary N, et al. Osteonecrosis of the jaw associated with ziv-ablifercept. *J Gastrointest Oncol.* 2016;[Epub ahead of print].

Nguyen MT, Borchers A, Selmi C, et al. The SAPHO syndrome. *Semin Arthritis Rheum.* 2012;42:254-265.

Obel G, Krogdahl A, Thygesen T, Godballe C. Juvenile mandibular chronic osteomyelitis: 3 cases and a literature review. *J Oral Maxillofac Surg.* 2013;71:305-309.

Padwa BL, Dentino K, Robson CD, et al. Pediatric chronic nonbacterial osteomyelitis of the jaw: clinical, radiographic and histopathologic features. *J Oral Maxillofac Surg.* 2016;[Epub ahead of print].

Peters E, Lovas GL, Wysocki GP. Lingual mandibular sequestration and ulceration. *Oral Surg Oral Med Oral Pathol.* 1993;75:739-743.

Pigrau C, Almirante B, Rodriguez D, et al. Osteomyelitis of the jaw: resistance to clindamycin in patients with prior antibiotics exposure. *Eur J Clin Microbiol Infect Dis.* 2009;28:317-323.

Ruggiero SL, Dodson TB, Fantasia J, et al. American Association of Oral and Maxillofacial Surgeons position paper on medication-related osteonecrosis of the jaw–2014 update. *J Oral Maxillofac Surg.* 2014;72:1938-1956.

Tlougan BE, Podjasek JO, O'Haver J, et al. Chronic recurrent multifocal osteomyelitis (CRMO) and synovitis, acne, pustulosis, hyperostosis, and osteitis (SAPHO) syndrome with associated neutrophilic dermatoses: a report of seven cases and review of the literature. *Pediatr Dermatol.* 2009;26:497-505.

Wipff J, Adamsbaum C, Kahan A, Job-Deslandre C. Chronic recurrent multifocal osteomyelitis. *Joint Bone Spine.* 2011;78:555-560.

FIBROOSSEOUS LESIONS

Fibroosseous lesions are a heterogeneous group of lesions composed of inflammatory/reactive conditions, developmental/metabolic bone disorders, and neoplasms. They are characterized by a proliferation of fibroblast-like cells and deposition of osseous or spherular, hypocellular, basophilic calcifications that have been traditionally referred to as cementum-like material, and are differentiated from woven bone by morphology alone. The histopathologic features of these entities overlap depending on the stage in which the biopsies are obtained, and an accurate diagnosis can be rendered only after correlation of clinical and radiographic data. Differentiation between lesions is essential so that appropriate therapy can be instituted, or just as important, no therapy, and even avoidance of a biopsy.

The terminology for these conditions continues to evolve. The term *florid cementoosseous dysplasia* is used to connote multifocal disease that may not always be florid, and here the term *multifocal cementoosseous dysplasia* is used. The terms *juvenile ossifying fibroma* and *juvenile active ossifying fibroma* refer to the same entity although the WHO prefers the term *juvenile aggressive ossifying fibroma* even though adults beyond the age of 30 are occasionally affected. Over the last two decades thinking has shifted from classifying *central cementoossifying fibroma* as a primary osseous neoplasm to placing it in the category of a mesenchymal odontogenic neoplasm arising from multipotent cells within the periodontium. In support of this are the following: a) cementoossifying fibroma does not occur outside the jaw bones; it almost always occurs in the tooth-bearing areas of the jaw bones; b) a similar condition occurs on the gingival soft tissues referred to as peripheral ossifying fibroma that is believed to arise from multipotent cells within the periodontium as a response to local inflammation. However, because of its histopathologic similarity to fibrous dysplasia and aggressive ossifying fibroma (a true primary osseous neoplasm), these will all be considered together in this section.

Clinical Findings

- Please see Table 17.2 and Figs. 17.12–17.17.

Etiopathogenesis and Histopathologic Features

Fibrous Dysplasia

This condition is associated with a mutation in *GNAS1* that results in alterations in proliferation and differentiation of preosteoblasts, and potentiation of the WNT pathway; there are monostotic (85–90% of cases) and polyostotic types; the latter is seen in McCune-Albright syndrome and also the variant Mazabraud syndrome associated with soft tissue myxomas.

TABLE 17.2 Clinical Findings in Benign Fibroosseous Lesions

Condition	Demographics	Site	Radiographic Appearance
Fibrous dysplasia	Occurs most frequently in the second and third decades with painless or painful swelling of the upper jaw and midface; polyostotic type seen in McCune-Albright syndrome with café-au-lait pigmentation with irregular borders (coast of Maine) and endocrine abnormalities (such as precocious puberty, diabetes mellitus, and thyroid disease), and its variant Mazabraud syndrome (includes soft tissue myxomas) Lesions persist throughout life and pregnancy may cause exacerbation	70–90% of cases are monostotic and generally involve craniofacial bones; lesions are unilateral affecting the maxilla and often maxillary sinus and contiguous facial bones (craniofacial fibrous dysplasia), sometimes with displacement of the orbital floor; involvement of skull base foramina results in nerve-specific neural symptoms	Diffuse ground-glass appearance of bone that merges with normal bone (see Fig. 17.12); there is loss of lamina dura; in the mandible, the inferior alveolar canal may be displaced if long-standing
Focal cementoosseous dysplasia	Usually occurs in the fourth to fifth decade, 80–90% of patients are female and 30–60% are black; 20–30% experience pain and/or swelling but most are diagnosed incidentally	Mandible is affected in 70–80% of cases and usually involves the apex/apices of vital teeth, usually mandibular first or second molar	Well-demarcated periapical radiolucency with a sclerotic rim in continuity with the lamina dura; increasing opacities develop over time and long-standing lesions may be densely sclerotic (see Fig. 17.13A)
Periapical cementoosseous dysplasia	Usually occurs in the fourth to fifth decade with predilection for black females, and usually an incidental finding	Apices of vital anterior mandibular incisors or canines and usually more than one tooth is involved	Same as focal cementoosseous dysplasia (see Fig. 17.13B)
Mutlifocal (florid) cementoosseous dysplasia	Usually occurs in the fourth and fifth decade in black females; patients may develop facial swelling if simple bone cysts occur	Apices of vital teeth in multiple quadrants	Same as focal cementoosseous dysplasia involving multiple teeth (see Fig. 17.14); simple bone cysts occur in long-standing lesions
Cementoossifying fibroma	Occurs usually in the third to fifth decade with increasing swelling of the face; there is a 2:1 female predilection and 20–40% of patients are black	70–80% occur in the mandible; synchronous or multifocal lesions may be evident	Well-demarcated radiolucency with a sclerotic rim in the tooth-bearing areas of the jaws, with variable radiopacities; there may be bowing of the inferior border of the mandible (see Fig. 17.15)
Juvenile (aggressive) ossifying fibroma	Psammomatoid type (4 times more common than the trabecular type): usually occurs in second and third decades Trabecular type: usually occurs in the first and second decades Both have slight male predilection and present with rapid growth and facial swelling	Psammomatoid type: 60–70% affect the paranasal sinuses and orbital bones, 20% the maxilla and 10% the mandible Trabecular type: affects the maxilla and mandible equally and rarely the sinonasal tract	Each presents as a fairly large radiolucency, generally well-demarcated with variable radiopacities; sometimes with destruction of cortical plates and root resorption (see Fig. 17.16)
Familial gigantiform cementoma	Arises in childhood causing severe facial deformity by teenage; some patients experience pathologic fractures of the long bones	Involves the mandible bilaterally and often also the maxilla bilaterally	Expansile radiolucency with radiopacities present bilaterally (see Fig. 17.17)

- There is a proliferation of spindle cells and delicate fibrocollagenous tissue and either small, delicate, or curvilinear trabeculae (taking the form of the letters "Y", "U", or "C") of woven bone in early lesions, or thicker and denser trabeculae of woven or lamellar bone in older lesions; the more complex "Chinese characters" are more often seen in limb and axial bones. Osteoblastic rimming and occasional osteoclasts may be seen focally, especially in early and inflamed lesions and there is variable vascularity (Figs. 17.18 and 17.19). Peritrabecular clefting, aneurysmal bone cystlike areas and cystic change may be seen, but globular deposits of basophilic cementum-like material are not seen.

Cementoosseous Dysplasia

The cause is unknown but it tends to affect black females.

- Early lesions consist of a cellular proliferation of spindle fibroblast-like cells and deposition of osteoid, woven bone and/or globular, basophilic cementum-like droplets, with abundant hemorrhage; bony trabeculae are thicker than in fibrous dysplasia ("ginger root" appearance), and cells that rim bone and cementum-like droplets are often osteoblast-like with eccentric nuclei (Figs. 17.20 and 17.21). Long-standing lesions often contain masses of coalesced cementum-like material that has a rounded, globular appearance with a few cementocytes; these are sometimes referred to as sclerotic cemental

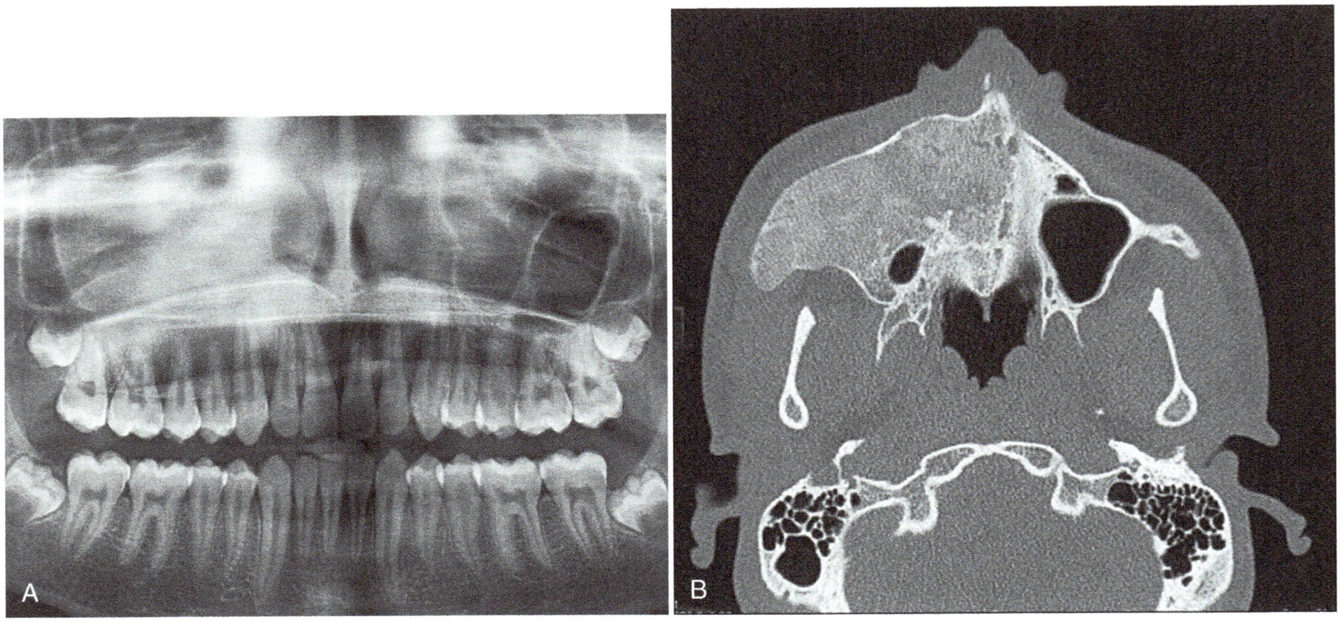

FIG 17.12 Fibrous dysplasia. (A) Panoramic radiograph showing ground-glass appearance of the right maxilla. (B) CT of the same patient showing a similar ground-glass appearance of the bone and expansion into the right sinus.

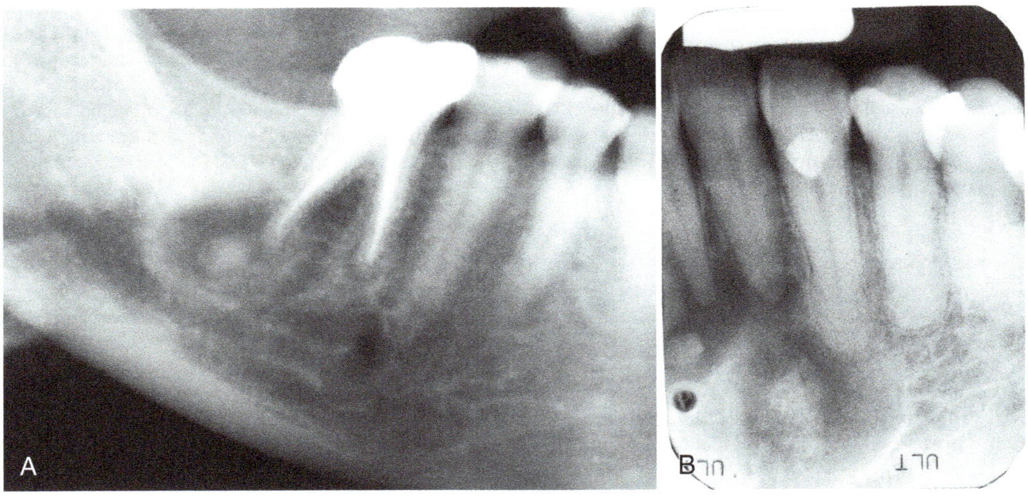

FIG 17.13 Focal cementoosseous dysplasia. (A) Circumscribed radiolucency with sclerotic rim and central calcification around the distal root of the right mandibular first molar. (B) Variant: periapical cementoosseous dysplasia. Radiolucency at the apices of vital mandibular anterior teeth with faint opacities. *(A, Courtesy Dr. Rafik Abdelsayed, Medical College of Georgia, School of Dentistry, Augusta, Ga; B, Courtesy Dr. Bernard Friedland, Harvard School of Dental Medicine, Boston.)*

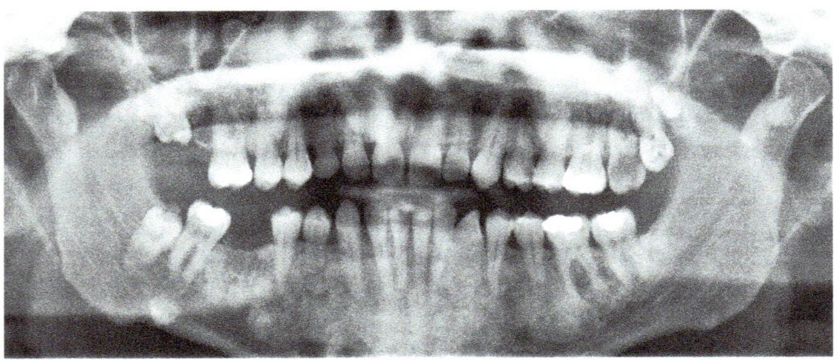

FIG 17.14 Multifocal/florid cementoosseous dysplasia: multiple radiolucencies with variable opacities around the apices of multiple teeth in the mandible and maxilla.

masses (Fig. 17.22). A simple bone cyst may be present in mature cases composed of an empty cavity surrounded by bone exhibiting the features of cementoosseous dysplasia; some lesions develop osteomyelitis especially after extraction (see Fig. 17.6).

Cementoossifying Fibroma

This is an odontogenic neoplasm likely from mesenchymal stem cells with differentiation towards periodontal structures and in particular bone and cementum-like material. Although loss of heterozygosity of hyperparathyroidism-jaw tumor syndrome 2 (*HRPT2*) encoding parafibromin has been identified, this is not associated with a somatic mutation of the gene.

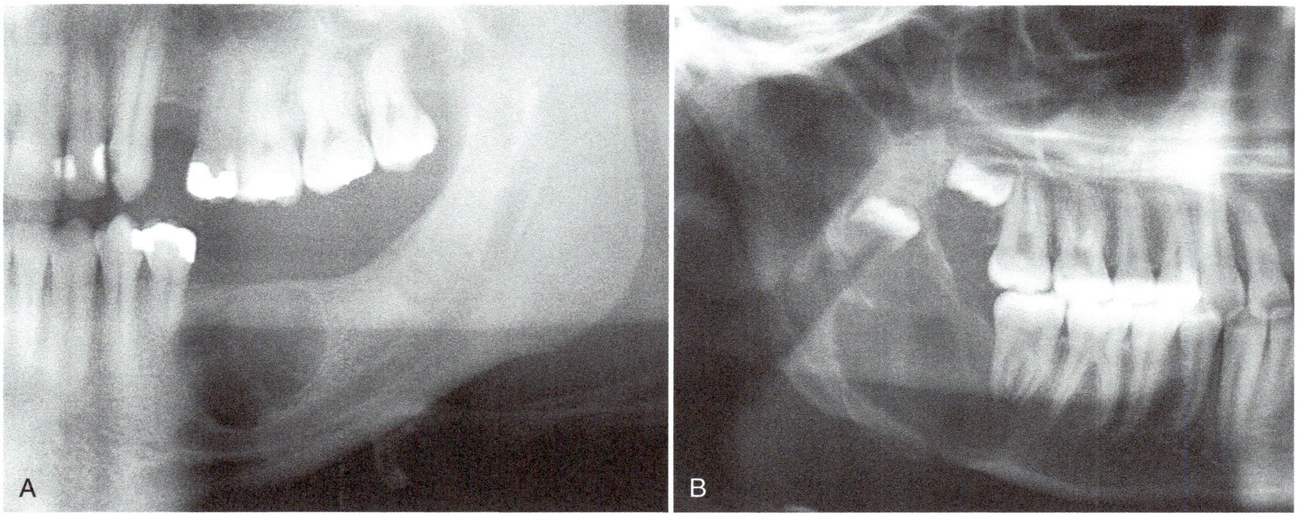

FIG 17.15 Central cementoossifying fibroma: (A) Well-demarcated radiolucency in the body of the left mandible with central faint opacities. (B) Large, slightly loculated radiolucency of the right mandible that has displaced the third molar; it exhibits minimal calcifications and has bowed the inferior border of the mandible *(Courtesy Dr. Leonard Kaban, Massachusetts General Hospital, Boston.)*

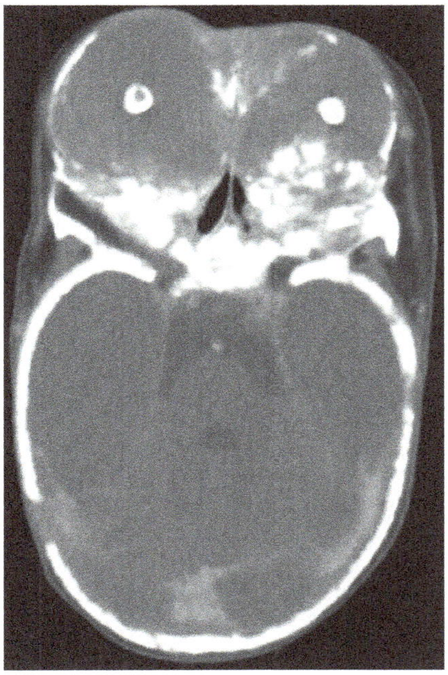

FIG 17.16 Aggressive ossifying fibroma: huge radiolucent and radiopaque lesion of the maxilla. *(Courtesy Dr. Bonnie Padwa, Harvard School of Dental Medicine, Boston.)*

- This consists of cellular proliferation of spindled fibroblast-like cells that deposit osteoid, trabeculae of woven bone, and cementum-like droplets in varying proportions; osteoblastic rimming is common and some lesions are extremely collagenous with minimal calcification (Fig. 17.23–17.24). Aneurysmal bone cystlike areas, or central giant cell granuloma may be present (Fig. 17.25).

Juvenile (Aggressive) Ossifying Fibroma

These tumors have shown fusion of breakpoints on Xq26 and 2q33, and 69% showed amplification of *MDM2* and *RASAL1* on chromosome 12, but without overexpression of MDM2.

- Both variants consist of a cellular proliferation of plump and stellate fibroblast-like cells with large, slightly atypical nuclei; the spindle cells may be cellular with a fasciculated or storiform appearance and there may be infiltration of native bone.
  - *Psammomatoid type:* There are basophilic, globular, or irregularly shaped ossicles, most of which are of uniform size with a few osteocytes within lacunae (Fig. 17.26); hematoxyphilic acellular spherical bodies resembling psammoma bodies are also present and aneurysmal bone cystlike areas are seen in 10% to 30% of cases.
  - *Trabecular type:* There is abundant osteoid and woven bone in single or interlacing trabeculae containing plump slightly atypical osteocytes with large ovoid nuclei and dispersed chromatin; recapitulation of Sharpey fibers renders a trailing "paintbrush" appearance to the osteoid that surround bone trabeculae; hematoxyphilic acellular osteoid may be present and there are often clusters of multinucleated giant cells and fresh hemorrhage (Figs. 17.27–17.29).

Familial Gigantiform Cementoma

This is an inherited disorder.

- The histopathology is similar to ossifying fibroma, especially the psammomatoid type with globular cementum-like bodies that are hypocellular with scattered osteocytes.

Differential Diagnosis

- Renal osteodystrophy from end-stage renal disease and secondary hyperparathyroidism has similar histopathology to fibrous dysplasia; clinical features of renal failure with hypercalcemia differentiate between the two.

Text continued on p. 460

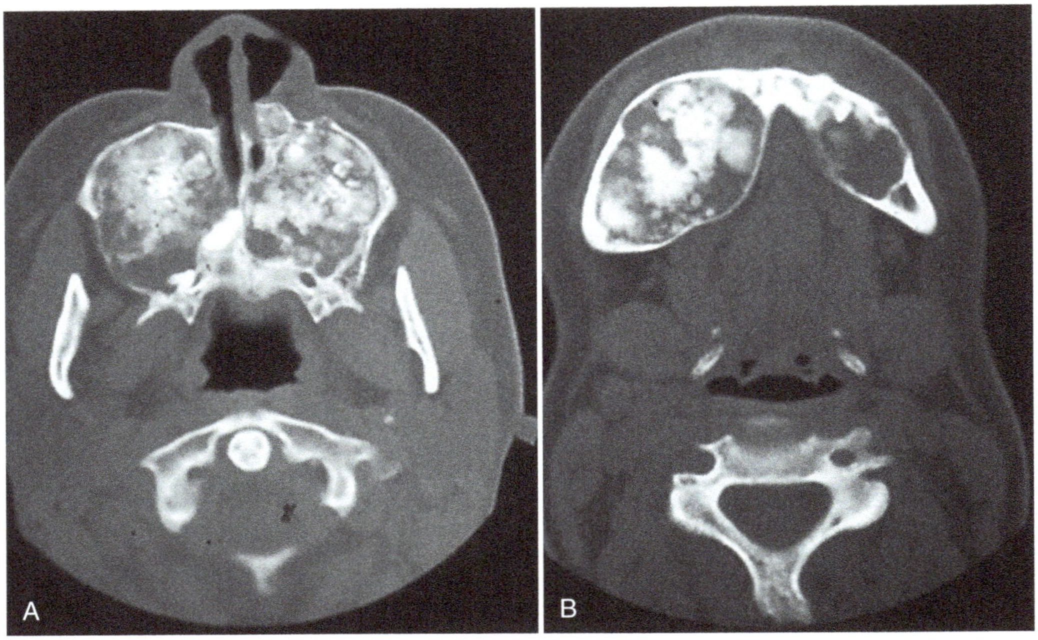

FIG 17.17 Familial gigantiform cementomas: marked expansion of maxilla (A) and mandible (B) by radiolucent-radiopaque process. *(From Abdelsayed RA, Eversole LR, Singh BS, Scarbrough FE. Gigantiform cementoma: clinicopathologic presentation of 3 cases. Oral Surg Oral Med Oral Pathol Oral Radiol Endod. 2001;91:438–444.)*

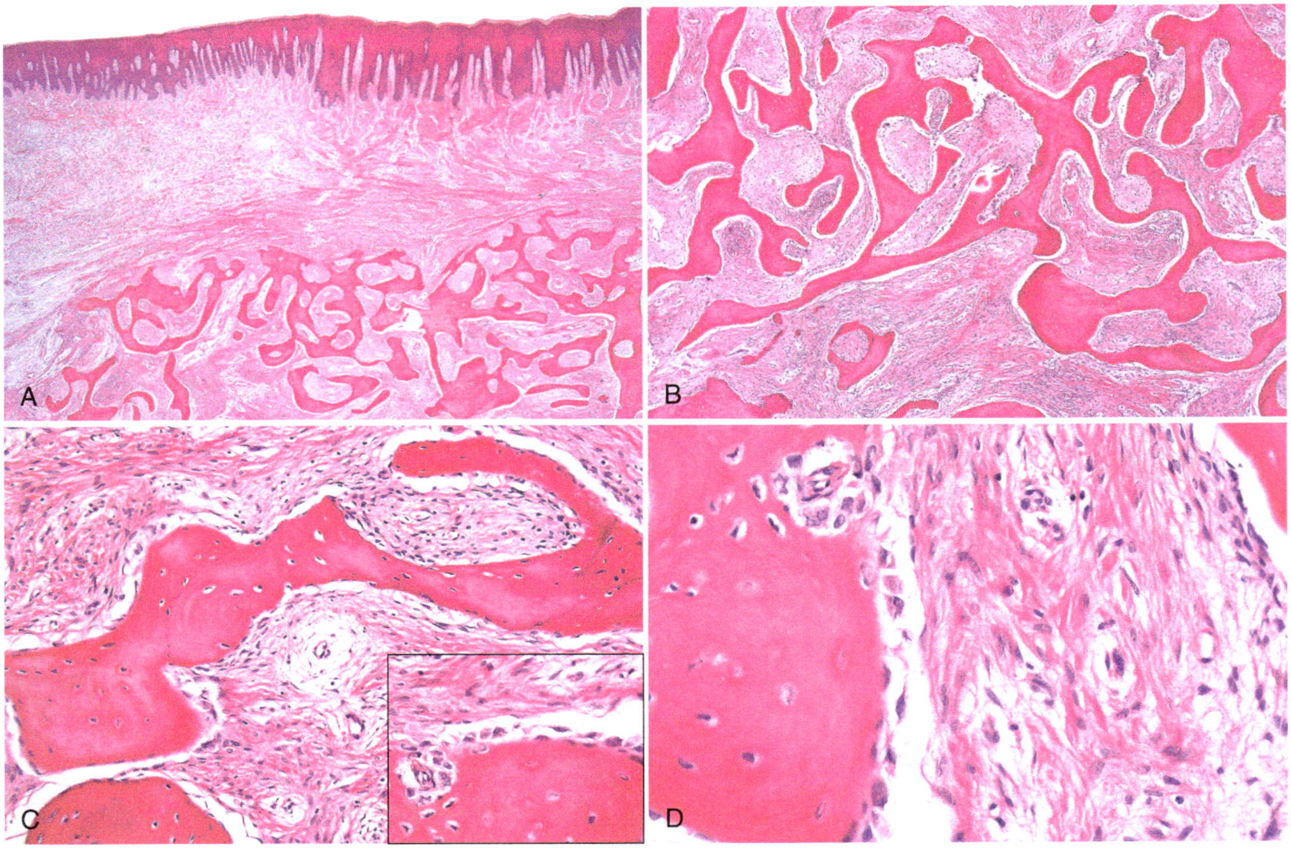

FIG 17.18 Fibrous dysplasia. (A) Delicate trabeculae of bone in fibrous stroma abut the mucosa with no intervening cortical lamellar bone. (B) Delicate interlacing trabeculae of woven bone in fibrous stroma with peritrabecular clefting. (C) Woven bone with surrounding fibrocollagenous tissue. (D) Focal osteoblastic rimming is present.

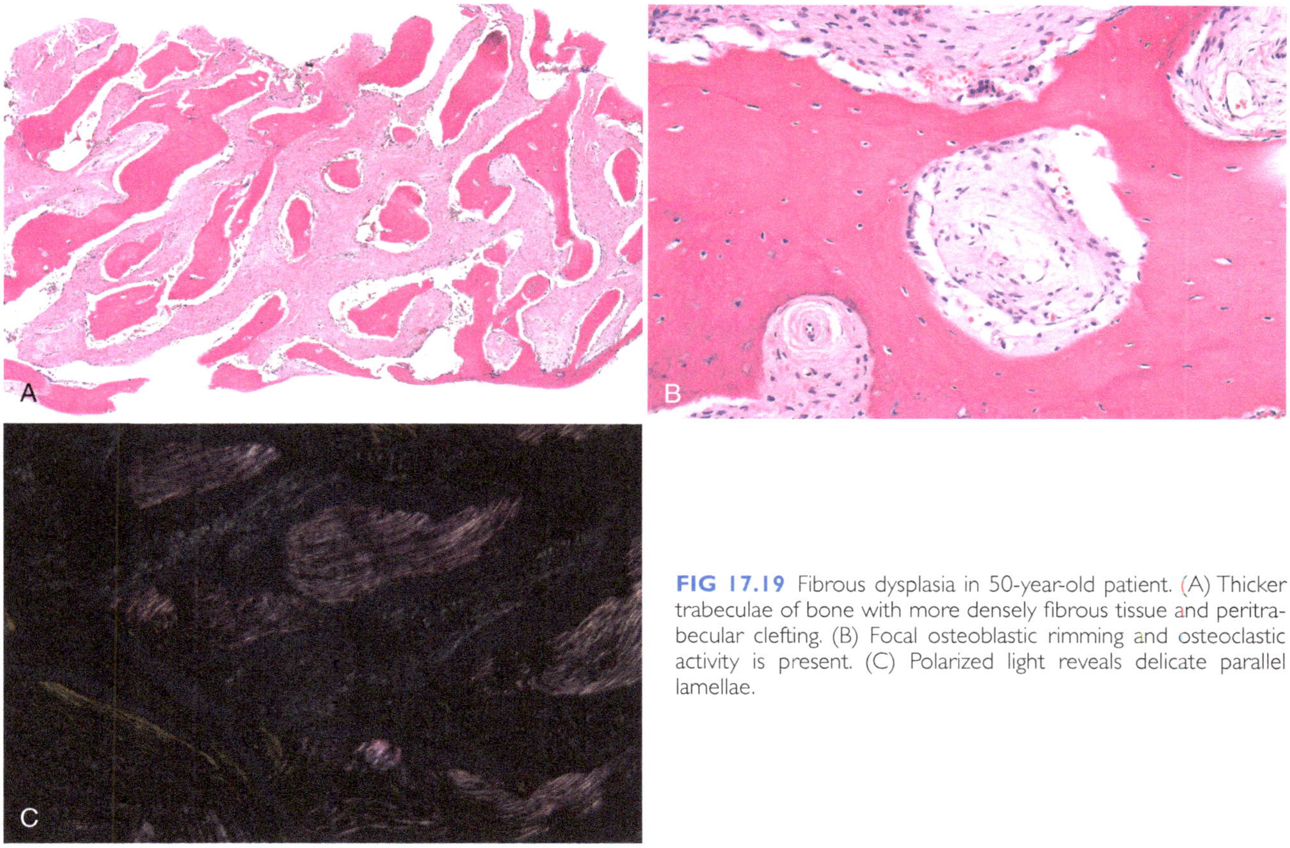

FIG 17.19 Fibrous dysplasia in 50-year-old patient. (A) Thicker trabeculae of bone with more densely fibrous tissue and peritrabecular clefting. (B) Focal osteoblastic rimming and osteoclastic activity is present. (C) Polarized light reveals delicate parallel lamellae.

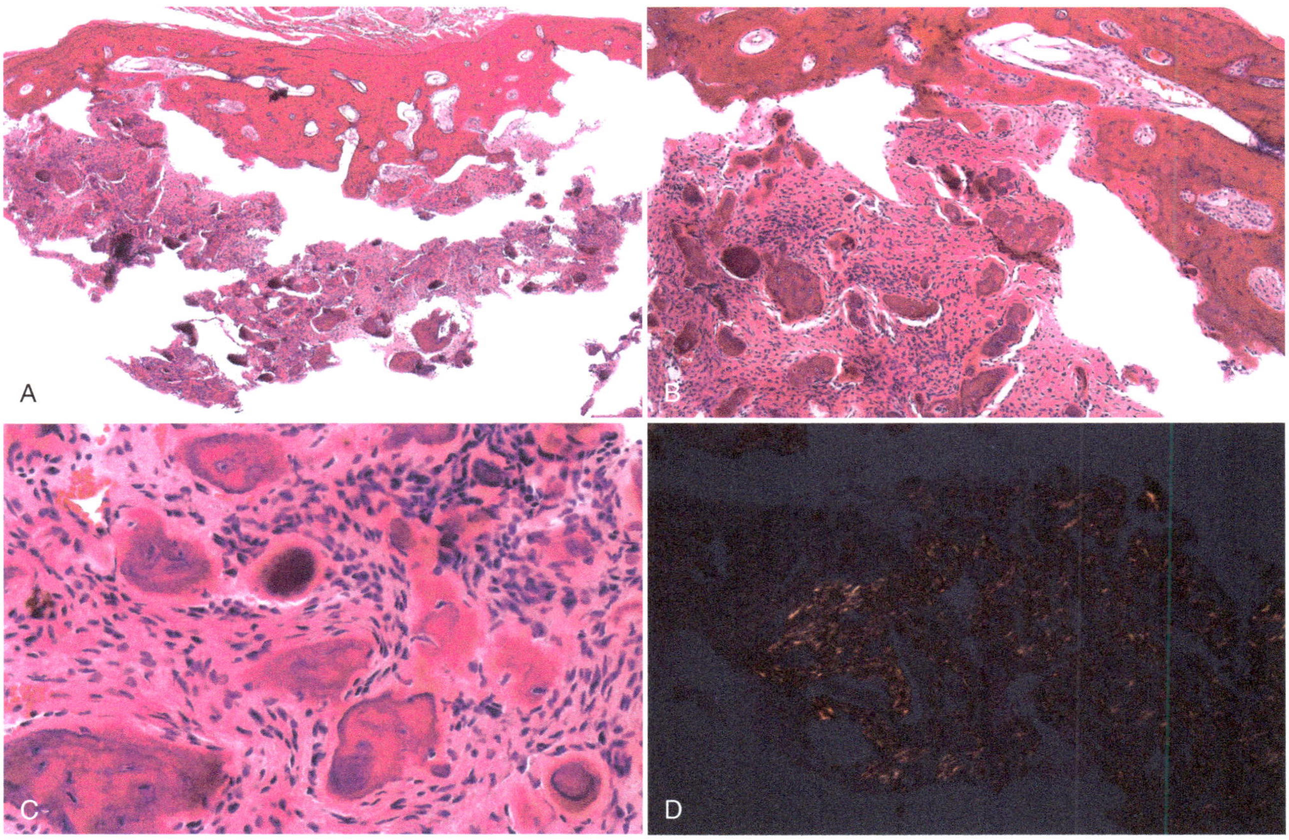

FIG 17.20 Focal cementoosseous dysplasia. (A) Nonencapsulated lesion abutting normal lamellar bone *(top)*. (B) Proliferation of spindle cells with cementum droplets and woven bone. (C) Plump spindle cells with acellular cementum droplets and woven bone containing osteocytes. (D) Polarized light reveals short collagen bundles.

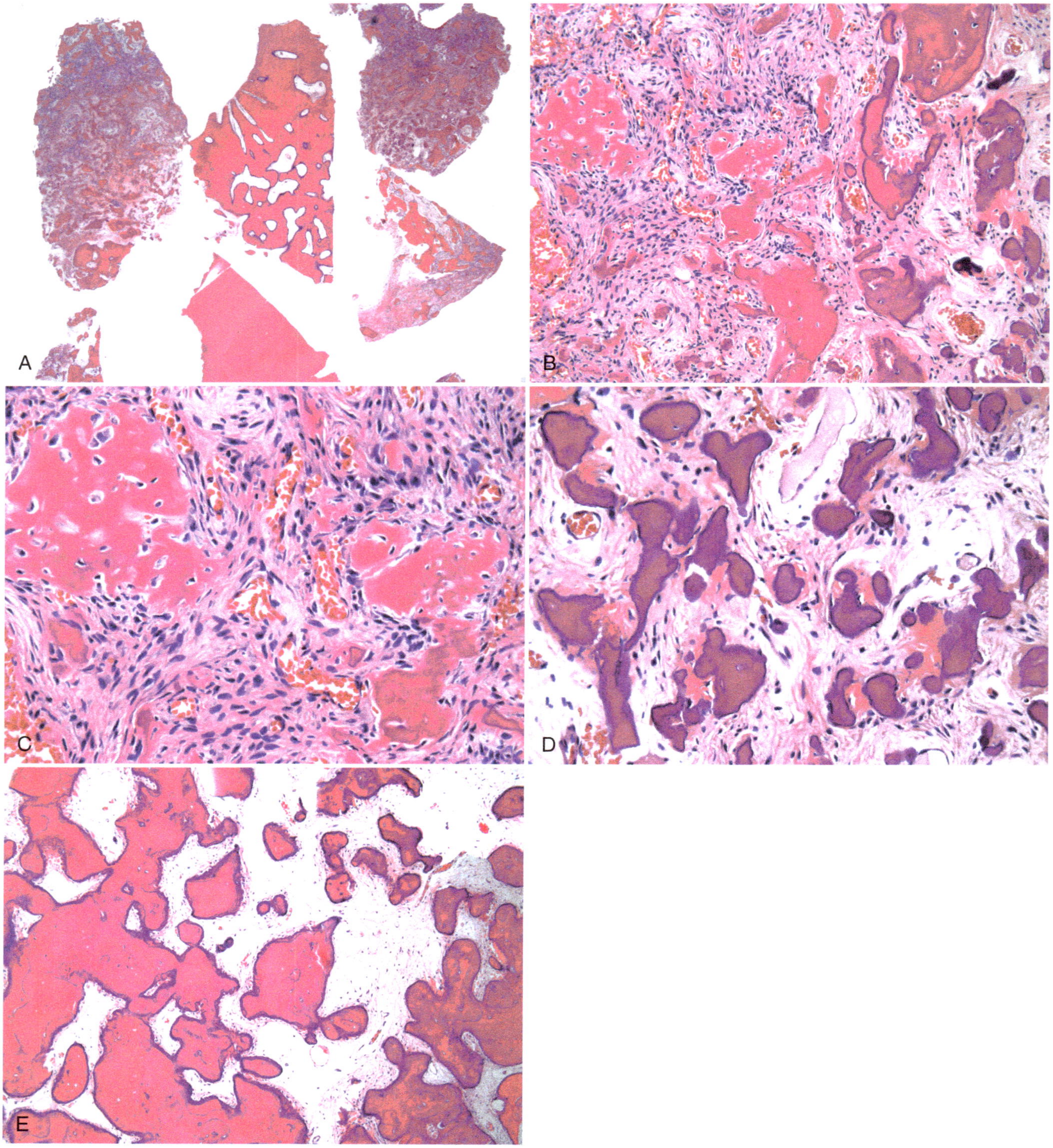

FIG 17.21 Focal cementoosseous dysplasia. (A) Many small fragments of bone and cellular fibrous tissue and cemental mass *(center)*. (B) Spindle cells depositing trabeculae of woven bone *(left)* and hematoxyphilic cementum-like material *(right)*. (C) Osteoid with many plump osteocytes focally rimmed by osteoblasts with many surrounding plump spindle cells. (D) Hematoxyphilic globular cementum-like material. (E) Coalescent hypocellular, globular cementum-like material with less cellular matrix.

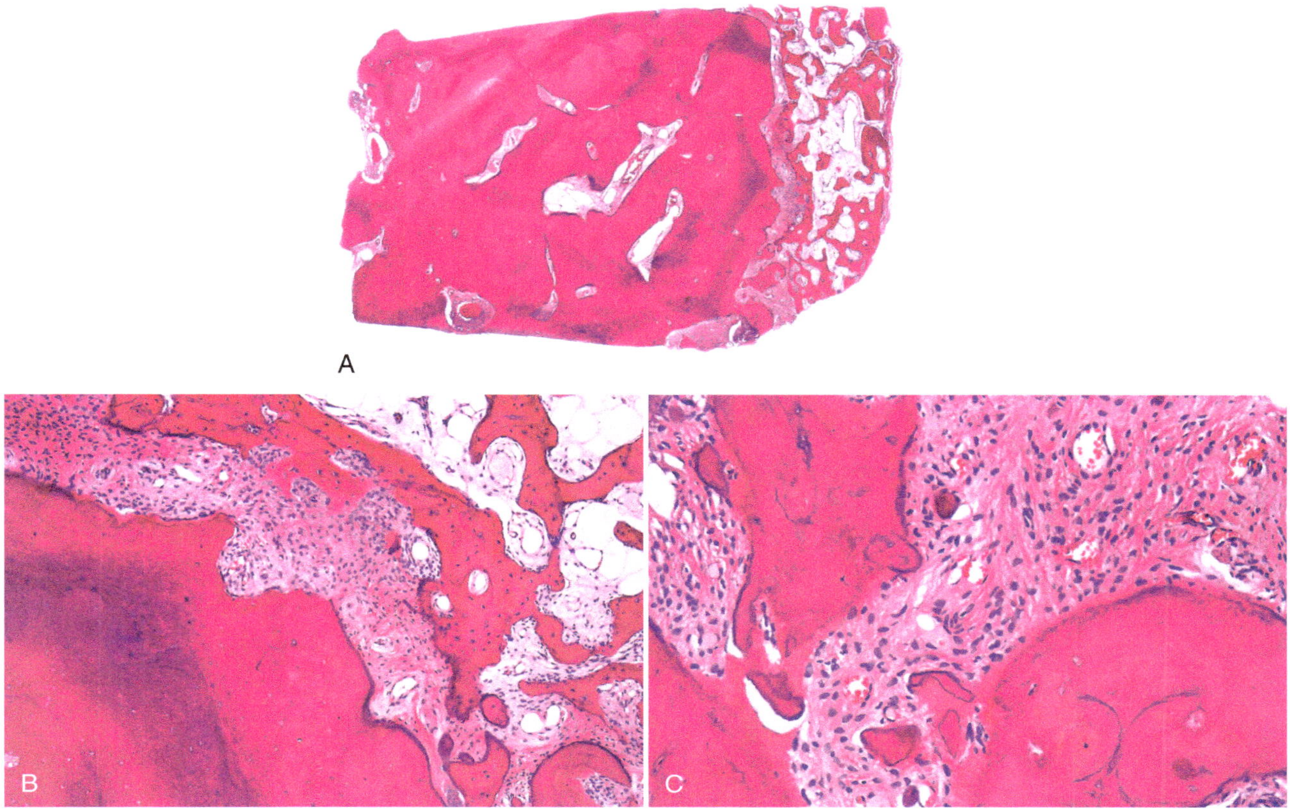

FIG 17.22 Focal cementoosseous dysplasia. (A) Long-standing lesion with large sclerotic cemental mass adjacent to lamellar cortical bone. (B) Focal area of cellular spindle cell proliferation adjacent to dense, hypocellular globular cementum-like material. (C) Spindle cells and globular cementum.

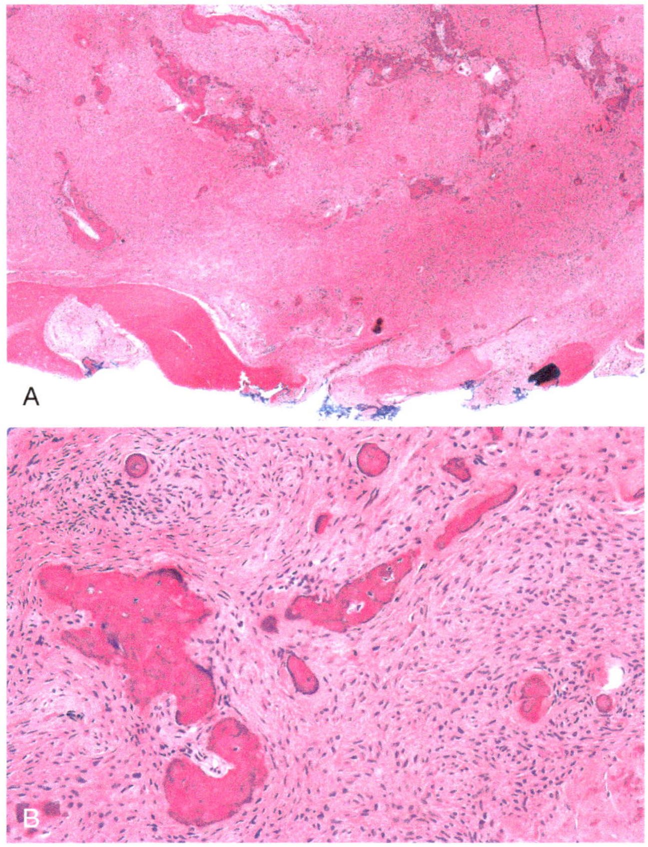

FIG 17.23 Central cementoossifying fibroma. (A) Proliferation of spindle cells with deposition of woven bone and cementum. (B) Trabeculae of woven bone with plump osteocytes and acellular globular cementum droplets and woven bone.

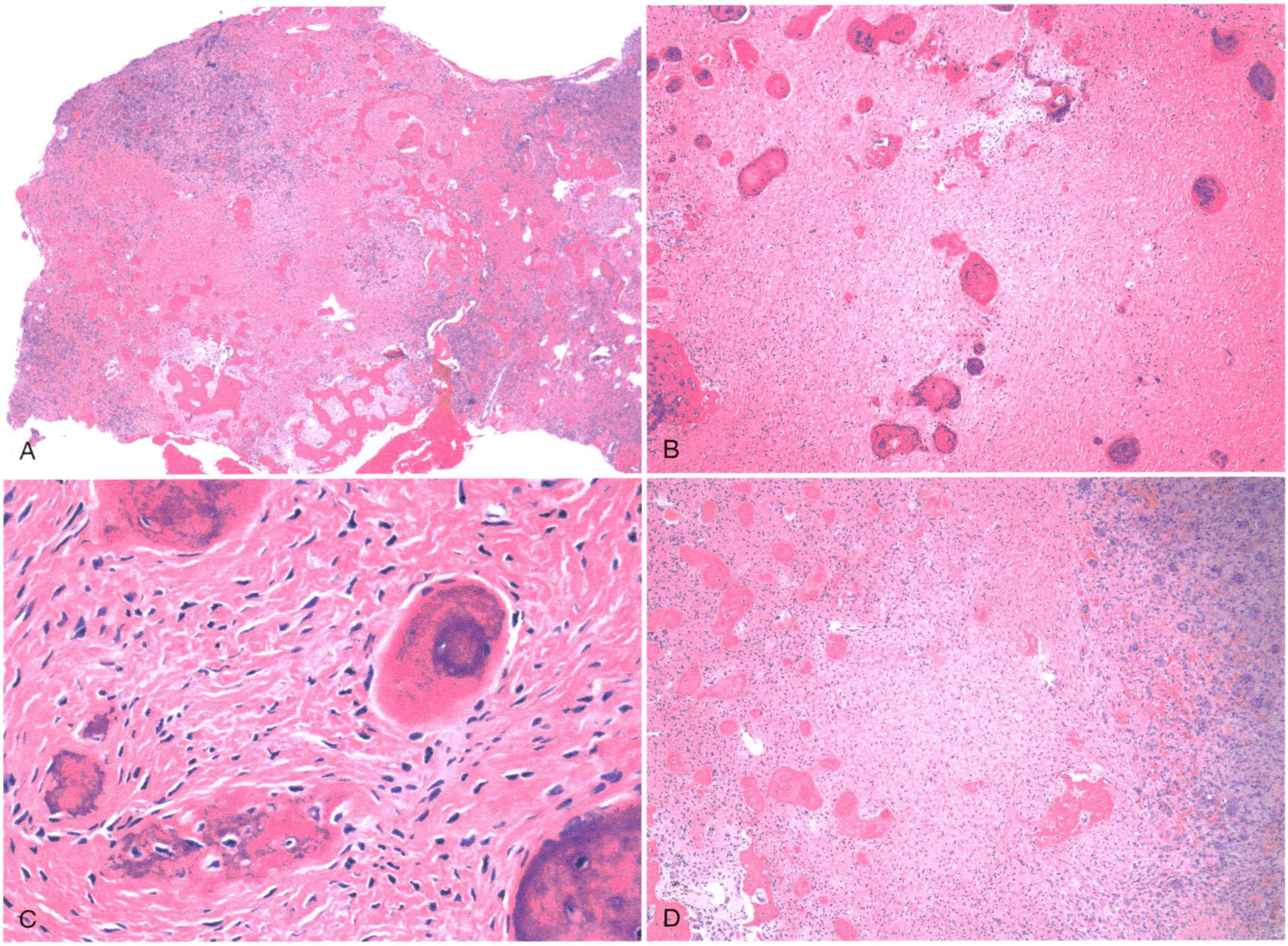

FIG 17.24 Central cementoossifying fibroma and central giant cell granuloma. (A) Proliferation of spindle cells with deposition of osteoid and clusters of giant cells *(top, left)*. (B) Spindle cells with deposition of globular cementum-like spherules and woven bone; parts of the stroma are hyalinized. (C) Spindle and stellate cells deposit globular hematoxyphilic acellular cementum droplets and osteoid. (D) Presence of central giant cell granuloma *(right)*.

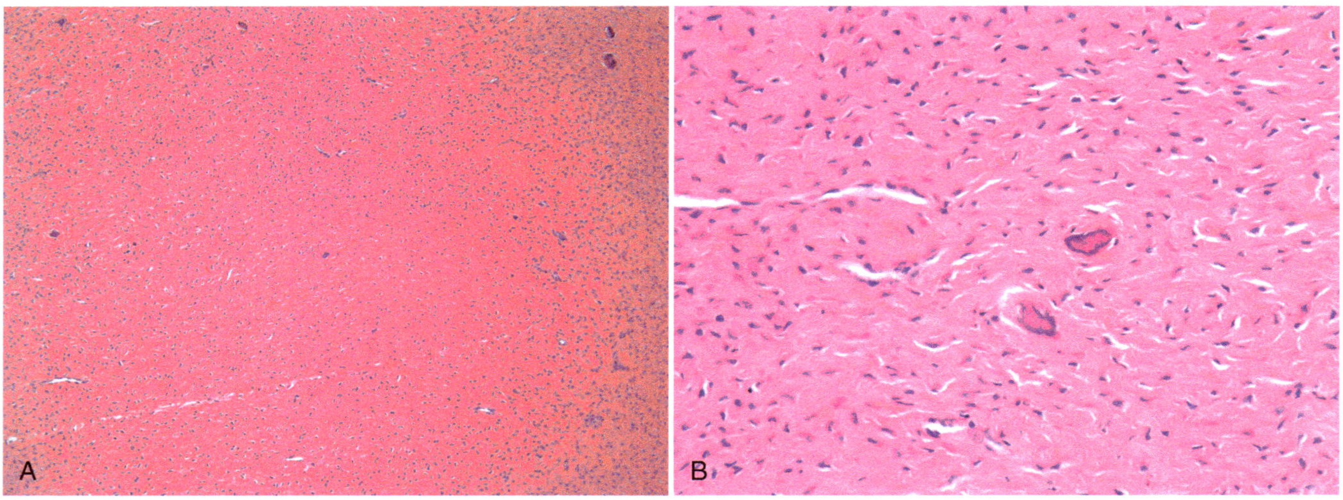

FIG 17.25 Cementoossifying fibroma. (A) Proliferation of spindle and stellate cells in hyalinized collagenous stroma with only a few cementum spherules. (B) Benign spindle and stellate cells with deposition of cementicles.

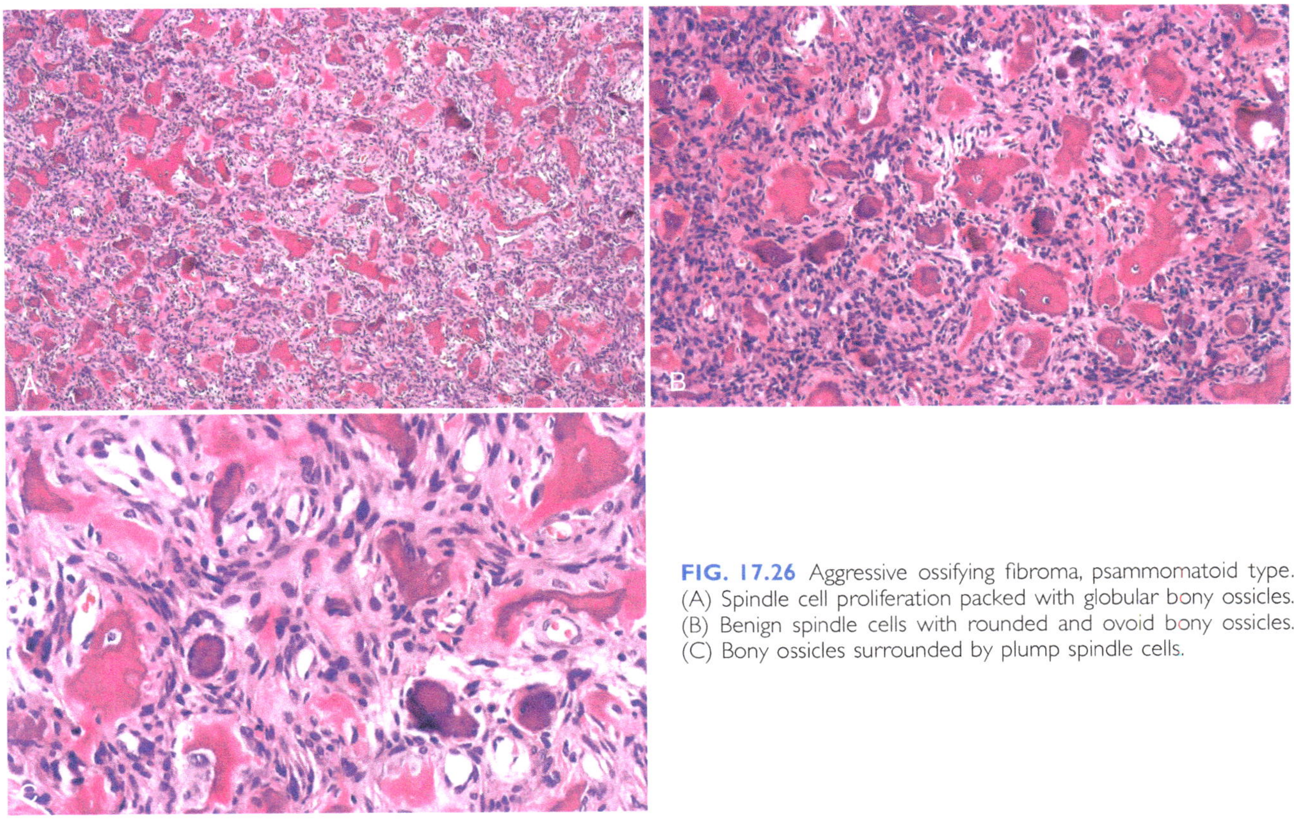

FIG. 17.26 Aggressive ossifying fibroma, psammomatoid type. (A) Spindle cell proliferation packed with globular bony ossicles. (B) Benign spindle cells with rounded and ovoid bony ossicles. (C) Bony ossicles surrounded by plump spindle cells.

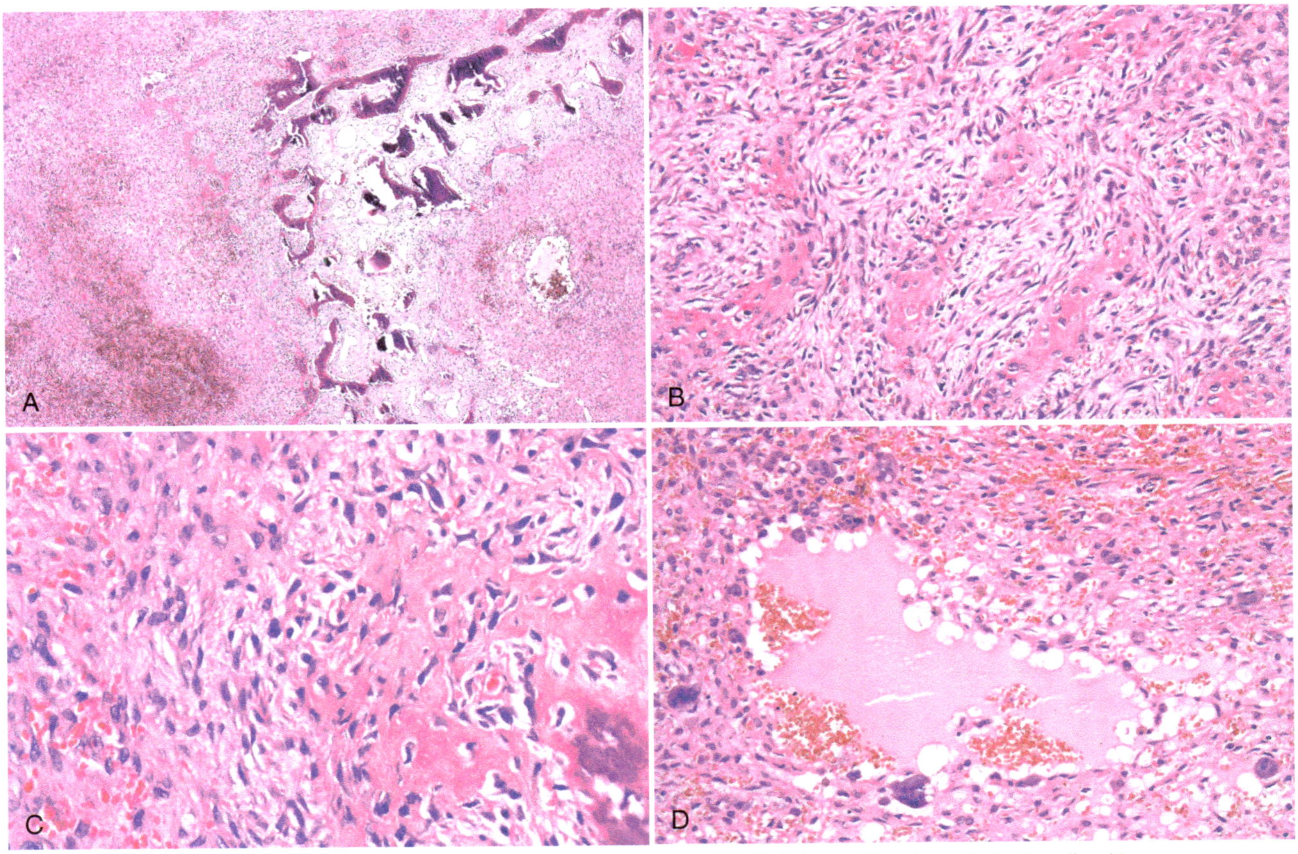

FIG 17.27 Aggressive ossifying fibroma, trabecular type. (A) Cellular proliferation of spindle cells with osteoid *(right)*, woven bone, hemorrhage, and early aneurysmal bone cyst formation. (B) Osteoid is present in poorly delineated spicules, contains plump osteocytes, and is surrounded by plump spindle cells. (C) Plump and slightly atypical osteocytes and osteoblasts, and cellular stroma with spindle and stellate cells. (D) Early aneurysmal bone cystlike areas.

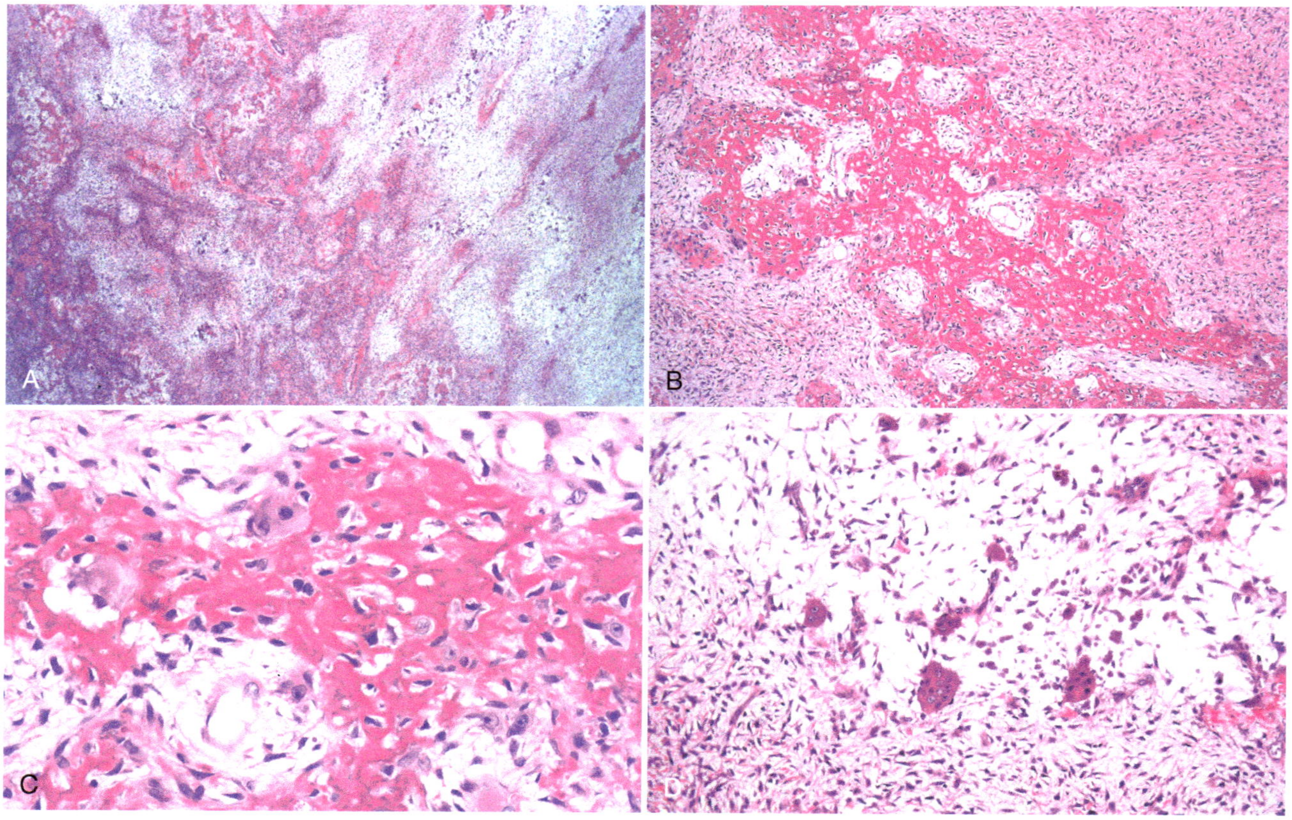

FIG 17.28 Aggressive ossifying fibroma, trabecular type. (A) Spindle cell proliferation with hyper- and hypocellular areas, woven bone formation, and many giant cells in the hypocellular areas. (B) Woven bone with many plump and slightly atypical osteocytes and many osteoclasts. (C) Woven bone with plump, slightly atypical osteocytes, osteoclasts, and stellate and spindle cells within stroma. (D) Clusters of multinucleated giant cells within myxoid stroma.

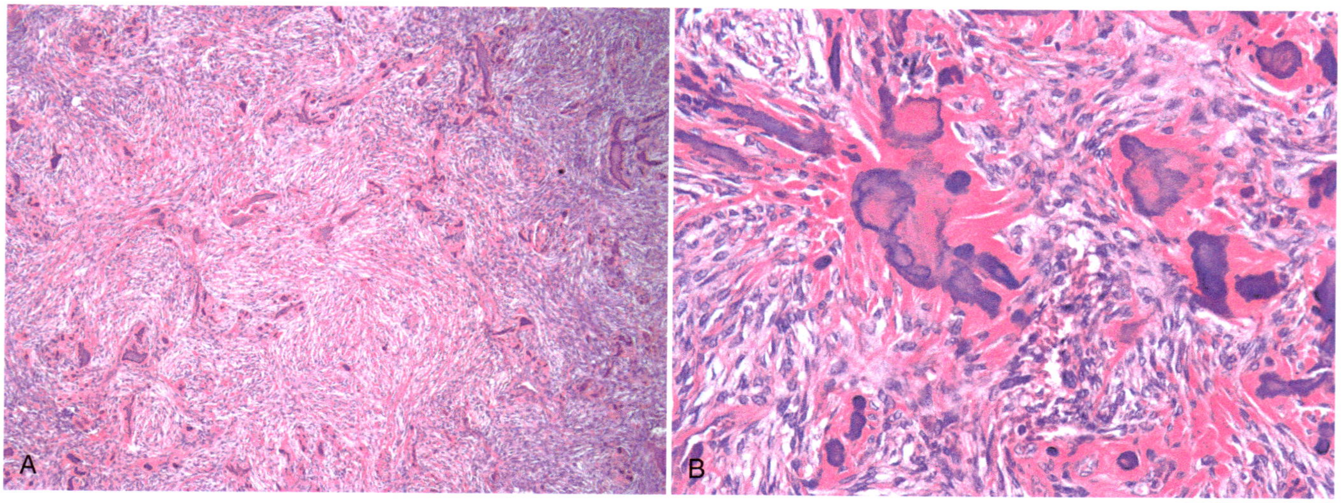

FIG 17.29 Aggressive ossifying fibroma, trabecular type. (A) Slightly storiform and fasciculated pattern of spindle cells and stroma with ossification. (B) Calcified structures are acellular and exhibit the trailing "paintbrush" appearance of osteoid recapitulating Sharpey fibers.

- Desmoplastic fibroma of bone consists of fibrocollagenous tissue with no cementum spherules or osteoid.
- Osteoblastoma shows a proliferation of osteoblasts composed of large cells with eccentric nuclei, often multilayered against the bone, osteoclasts on the same trabeculae, and prominent ectatic vessels; the bone is basophilic, sometimes with many resting and reversal lines.
- Fibroblastic osteosarcoma may be mistaken for aggressive ossifying fibroma, but the former resembles a high grade spindle malignancy and usually produces little woven bone; it is also SATB2+.

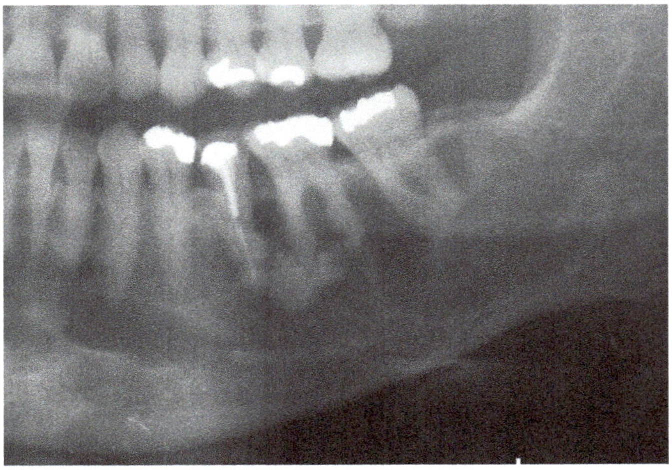

FIG 17.30 Simple bone cyst of the eft mandible that developed within multifocal (florid) cementoosseous dysplasia.

- Low-grade osteosarcoma may resemble fibrous dysplasia, but is positive for SATB2.

Management and Prognosis

- *Fibrous dysplasia:* Surgical recontouring is for aesthetics only although bisphosphonates reduce pain, and calcium and vitamin D supplements maintain bone density. Malignant transformation to osteosarcoma occurs in 1% of monostotic cases and 4% of polyostotic syndromic cases.
- *Cementoosseous dysplasia:* Biopsy confirms the diagnosis although this can often be made without a biopsy, and no further treatment is necessary. However, sclerotic masses of cementum are hypcvascular, extractions may lead to osteomyelitis. Simple bone cysts are associated with long-standing lesions.
- *Cementoossifying fibroma:* Curettage and enucleation may lead to recurrence in up to 14% of cases, but retreatment is curative.
- *Aggressive ossifying fibroma:* Wide excision is the treatment of choice; recurrence is 30% to 50% and may be related to younger age of presentation and the presence of aneurysmal bone cystlike areas (Fig. 17.30).
- *Gigantiform cementoma:* There is no effective treatment at this time.

REFERENCES

Abdelsayed RA, Eversole LR, Singh BS, Scarbrough FE. Gigantiform cementoma: clinicopathologic presentation of 3 cases. *Oral Surg Oral Med Oral Pathol Oral Radiol Endod.* 2001;91:438-444.

Chadwick JW, Alsufyani NA, Lam EW. Clinical and radiographic features of solitary and cemento-osseous dysplasia-associated simple bone cysts. *Dentomaxillofac Radiol.* 2011;40:230-235.

de Mesquita Netto AC, Gomez RS, Diniz MG, et al. Assessing the contribution of HRPT2 to the pathogenesis of jaw fibrous dysplasia, ossifying fibroma, and osteosarcoma. *Oral Surg Oral Med Oral Pathol Oral Radiol.* 2013;115:359-367.

de Noronha Santos Netto J, Machado Cerri J, Miranda AM, Pires FR. Benign fibro-osseous lesions: clinicopathologic features from 143 cases diagnosed in an oral diagnosis setting. *Oral Surg Oral Med Oral Pathol Oral Radiol.* 2013;115:e56-e65.

El-Mofty S. Psammomatoid and trabecular juvenile ossifying fibroma of the craniofacial skeleton: two distinct clinicopathologic entities. *Oral Surg Oral Med Oral Pathol Oral Radiol Endod.* 2002;93:296-304.

El-Mofty SK. Fibro-osseous lesions of the craniofacial skeleton: an update. *Head Neck Pathol.* 2014;8:432-444.

Eversole R, Su L, ElMofty S. Benign fibro-osseous lesions of the craniofacial complex. A review. *Head Neck Pathol.* 2008;2:177-202.

Ferretti C, Coleman H, Dent M, Altini M. Cystic degeneration in fibrous dysplasia of the jaws: a case report. *Oral Surg Oral Med Oral Pathol Oral Radiol Endod.* 1999;88:337-342.

Johnson LC, Yousefi M, Vinh TN, et al. Juvenile active ossifying fibroma. Its nature, dynamics and origin. *Acta Otolaryngol Suppl.* 1991;488:1-40.

Kaplan I, Manor I, Yahalom R, Hirshberg A. Central giant cell granuloma associated with central ossifying fibroma of the jaws: a clinicopathologic study. *Oral Surg Oral Med Oral Pathol Oral Radiol Endod.* 2007;103:e35-e41.

Kumar VV, Ebenezer S, Narayan TV, Wagner W. Clinicopathologic conference: multiquadrant expansile fibro-osseous lesion in a juvenile. *Oral Surg Oral Med Oral Pathol Oral Radiol.* 2012;113:286-292.

MacDonald-Jankowski D. Fibrous dysplasia: a systematic review. *Dentomaxillofac Radiol.* 2009;38:196-215.

Qu N, Yao W, Cui X, Zhang H. Malignant transformation in monostotic fibrous dysplasia: clinical features, imaging features, outcomes in 10 patients, and review. *Medicine (Baltimore).* 2015;94:e369.

Parham DM, Bridge JA, Lukacs JL, et al. Cytogenetic distinction among benign fibro-osseous lesions of bone in children and adolescents: value of karyotypic findings in differential diagnosis. *Pediatr Dev Pathol.* 2004;7:148-158.

Prado Ribeiro AC, Carlos R, Speight PM, et al. Peritrabecular clefting in fibrous dysplasia of the jaws: an important histopathologic feature for differentiating fibrous dysplasia from central ossifying fibroma. *Oral Surg Oral med Oral Pathol Oral Radiol.* 2012;114:503-508.

Riddle ND, Bui MM. Fibrous dysplasia. *Arch Pathol Lab Med.* 2013;137:134-138.

Riminucci M, Liu B, Corsi A, et al. The histopathology of fibrous dysplasia of bone in patients with activating mutations of the Gs alpha gene: site-specific patterns and recurrent histological hallmarks. *J Pathol.* 1999;187:249-258.

Rossbach HC, Letson D, Lacson A, et al. Familial gigantiform cementoma with brittle bone disease, pathologic fractures, and osteosarcoma: a possible explanation of an ancient mystery. *Pediatr Blood Cancer.* 2005;44:390-396.

Slootweg PJ. Juvenile trabecular ossifying fibroma: an update. *Virchows Arch.* 2012;461:699-703.

Su L, Weathers DR, Waldron CA. Distinguishing features of focal cemento-osseous dysplasias and cemento-ossifying fibromas. I. A pathologic spectrum of 316 cases. *Oral Surg Oral Med Oral Pathol Oral Radiol Endod.* 1997;84:301-309.

Su L, Weathers DR, Waldron CA. Distinguishing features of focal cemento-osseous dysplasia and cemento-ossifying fibromas. II. A clinical and radiologic spectrum of 316 cases. *Oral Surg Oral Med Oral Pathol Oral Radiol Endod.* 1997;84:540-549.

Summerlin DJ, Tomich CE. Focal cemento-osseous dysplasia: a clinicopathologic study of 221 cases. *Oral Surg Oral Med Oral Pathol.* 1994;78:611-620.

Tabareau-Delalande F, Collin C, Gomez-Brouchet A, et al. Chromosome 12 long arm rearrangement covering MDM2 and RASAL1 is associated with aggressive craniofacial juvenile ossifying fibroma and extracranial psammomatoid fibro-osseous lesions. *Mod Pathol.* 2015;28:48-56.

Triantafillidou K, Venetis G, Karakinaris G, Iordanidis F. Ossifying fibroma of the jaws: a clinical study of 14 cases and review of the literature. *Oral Surg Oral Med Oral Pathol Oral Radiol.* 2012;114:193-199.

Wang TT, Zhang R, Wang L, et al. Two cases of multiple ossifying fibromas in the jaws. *Diagn Pathol.* 2014;9:75.

Wenig BM, Vinh TN, Smirniotopoulos JG, et al. Aggressive psammomatoid ossifying fibromas of the sinonasal region: a clinicopathologic study of a distinct group of fibro-osseous lesions. *Cancer.* 1995;76:1155-1165.

Woo SB. Central cemento-ossifying fibroma: primary odontogenic or osseous neoplasm? *J Oral Maxillofac Surg.* 2015;73:S87-S93.

PAGET DISEASE OF BONE (OSTEITIS DEFORMANS)

Paget disease of bone is a metabolic bone disease that leads to disorganized deposition of bone that is dense but has poor mechanical strength, and therefore is prone to fractures.

Clinical Findings

- This condition affects approximately 5% of patients of European descent (usually men) older than age 55, with the highest frequency in the United Kingdom and the lowest in Asia, with a positive familial history in 15% of cases. Bone pain is often present and the deposition of bone around skull foramina may lead to neurologic symptoms such as headache and hearing or visual loss. Poor fit of dentures or hats and spacing between teeth may occur from expansion of skull and jaw bones.
- Radiographs in early stages show osteoporotic changes; in the mixed stage there is thickening of bones with mixed radiolucency and radiopacity. Bone sclerosis becomes more marked as the disease progresses ("cotton wool appearance") (Fig. 17.31).
- High levels of bone-specific alkaline phosphatase and urine hydroxyproline are noted.

Etiopathogenesis and Histopathologic Findings

Both genetic and environmental influences have been identified, but the basic defect is one of dysregulation of osteoclastogenesis. Approximately 15% of cases are inherited in an autosomal dominant fashion; sequestosome-1, a gene on 3q35 that encodes p62 (a protein involved in NFκB signaling) is present in 40% to 50% of inherited and 5% to 10% of sporadic cases. The role of paramyxovirus (especially the measles virus) as a trigger is controversial. The increased number and activity of osteoclasts leads to initial resorption of bone and osteolytic appearance (osteoclastic stage), followed by compensatory overproduction of lamellar bone in a haphazard fashion with prominent vascularity (mixed osteoclastic-osteoblastic stage), and finally a "burnt out" stage with fibrosis of connective tissue and dense sclerosis.

- The haphazard deposition of bone results in a mosaic pattern with many resting and reversal lines; numerous giant, irregular-shaped, hypernucleated osteoclasts and many osteoblasts are noted on the surface of bone trabeculae; there is marked hypervascularity in the mixed stage (Fig. 17.32).
- Giant cell tumors occur infrequently in areas of bone affected by the disease.
- Microtubular inclusions are seen on ultrastructural studies.

Differential Diagnosis

- Osteoblastoma may look similar, with many osteoclasts (although these are not usually hypernucleated), osteoblasts, and hypervascular stroma, but radiographs show a diffuse process in Paget disease.

Management and Prognosis

- Treatment is with antiresorptive drugs such as bisphosphonates (first line of treatment), or calcitonin; anti-inflammatory agents for management of pain; and surgery for correction of deformities.
- Less than 1% of cases develop osteosarcoma, usually of the osteoblastic type.

REFERENCES

Campidelli C, Righi A, Maremonti P, et al. Giant cell tumor of the mandible in a patient with Paget's disease. *Otolaryngol Head Neck Surg.* 2007;136:S62-S64.

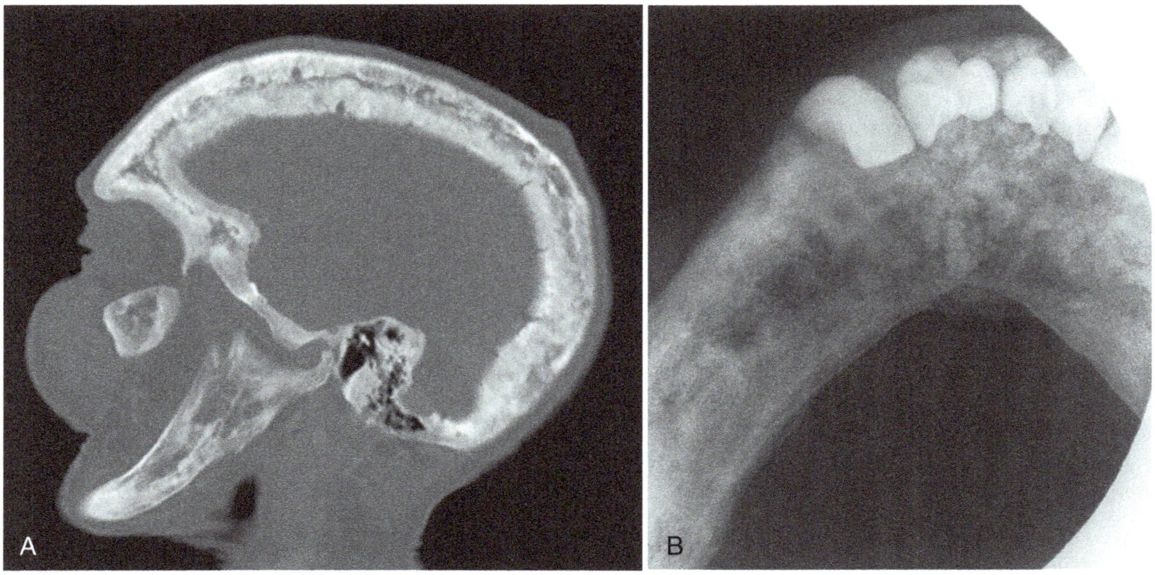

FIG 17.31 Paget disease of bone (osteitis deformans). (A) Sagittal CT shows thickened cranial bones, maxilla and mandible, and an increase in bone density. (B) Occlusal radiograph shows mottled radiolucency/opacity of the mandible. *(From White SC, Pharoah MJ. Oral Radiology: Principles and Interpretation. 6th ed. St Louis, Mosby, 2009.)*

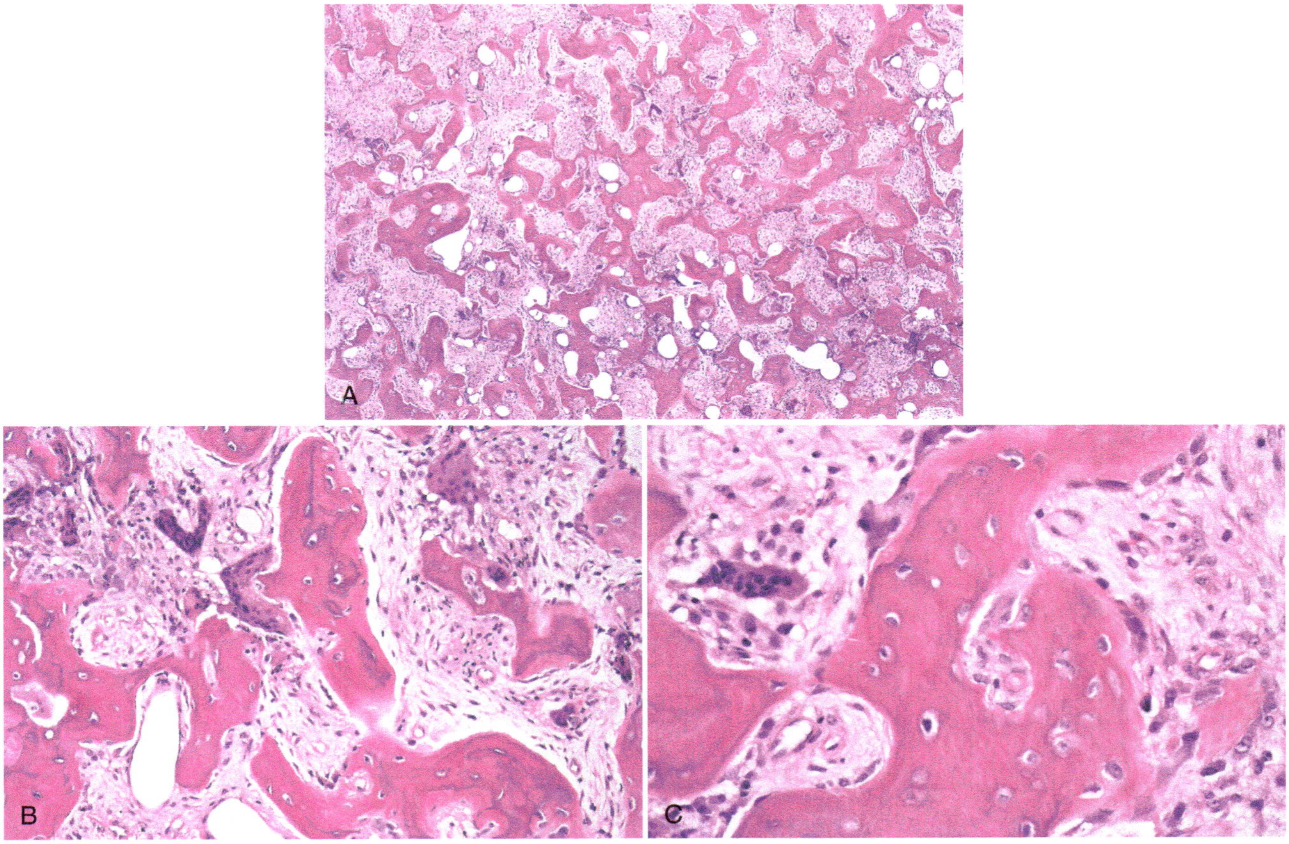

FIG 17.32 Paget disease of bone (osteitis deformans). (A) Interlacing trabeculae of woven bone with many osteoclasts and prominent dilated vessels. (B) Giant hypernucleated osteoclasts with dilated vessels in the stroma. (C) Many osteoblasts are present laying down osteoid. *(A, Courtesy Dr. Charles E. Tomich, Indiana University of School of Dentistry, Indianapolis, Ind.)*

Hansen MF, Seton M, Merchant A. Osteosarcoma in Paget's disease of bone. *J Bone Miner Res.* 2006;21:P58-P63.

Ralston SH. Clinical practice. Paget's disease of bone. *N Engl J Med.* 2013;368:644-650.

Roodman GD. Insights into the pathogenesis of Paget's disease. *Ann N Y Acad Sci.* 2010;1192:176-180.

Seitz S, Priemel M, Zustin J, et al. Paget's disease of bone: histologic analysis of 754 patients. *J Bone Miner Res.* 2009;24:62-69.

CENTRAL GIANT CELL GRANULOMA (CENTRAL GIANT CELL LESION, CENTRAL GIANT CELL REPARATIVE GRANULOMA)

Although giant cell granulomas have been speculated to represent the gnathic variant of the giant cell tumor of long bones, recent molecular studies have shown that they are separate and distinct conditions.

Clinical Findings

- Most cases occur in the first to third decade of life, presenting as a unilocular or multilocular radiolucency of the mandible (75% of cases), usually in the anterior or body (Fig. 17.33A).
- The aggressive type is greater than 5 cm and recurs (primary criteria), or shows at least three of the following secondary criteria: rapid growth, root resorption, tooth displacement, and thinning or perforation of the cortical plate (Fig. 17.33B).

Etiopathogenesis and Histopathologic Features

Cells are derived from mesenchymal stromal cells that differentiate along the monocyte-macrophage-osteoclast lineage. No consistent genetic abnormalities have been noted for jawbone lesions, although one study showed clonality in some lesions using polymorphic human androgen receptor assay (HUMARA). More recently, studies have shown that jaw lesions are distinct from the long bone giant cell tumors in that jaw lesions lack mutations in *H3F3A* that are commonly seen in long bone tumors.

- There is a proliferation of monocytic cells and clusters of multinucleated osteoclast-type giant cells with abundant fresh hemorrhage either in a diffuse or nodular pattern; siderophages and reactive osteoid and woven bone formation are often seen, and monocytic cells often show mitotic activity (Figs. 17.34 and 17.35).
- Central giant cell granuloma is often noted in association with other conditions such as central cementoossifying fibroma and central odontogenic fibroma (see Fig. 17.24).
- Increased vascularity as evidenced by increased expressions of CD34, vascular endothelial growth factor

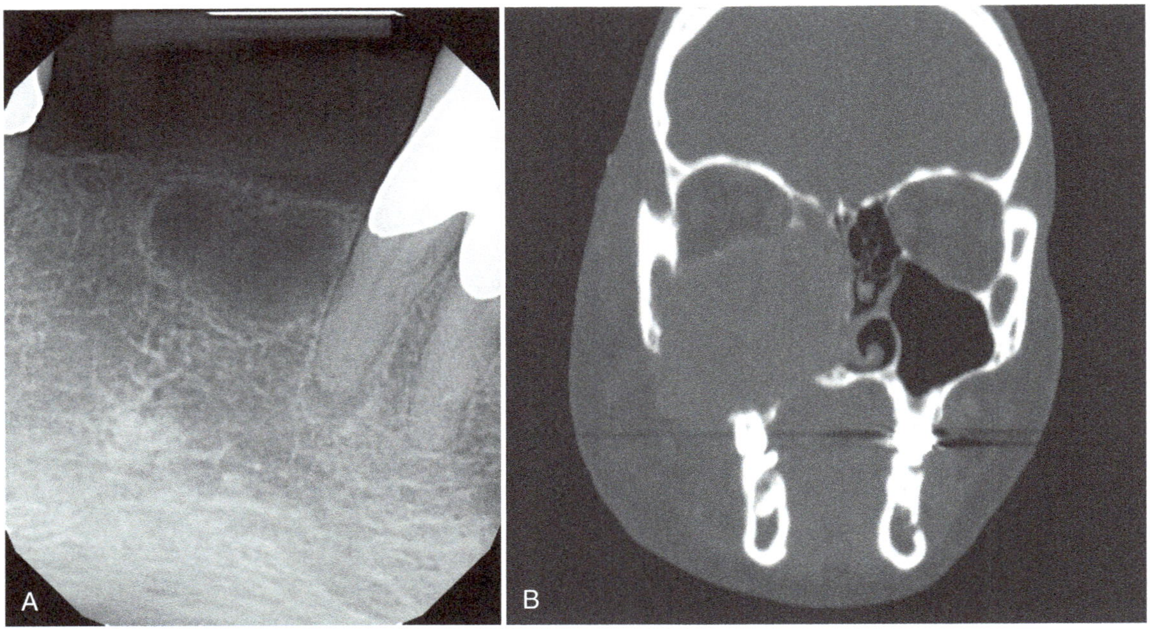

FIG 17.33 (A) Conventional central giant cell granuloma presenting as a solitary discrete radiolucency in the mandible. (B) Aggressive central giant cell granuloma. Recurrent tumor of the right maxilla involving maxillary and ethmoid sinuses, and nasal cavity. *(B, Courtesy Dr. Leonard B. Kaban and Dr. Maria Troulis, Harvard School of Dental Medicine and Massachusetts General Hospital, Boston.)*

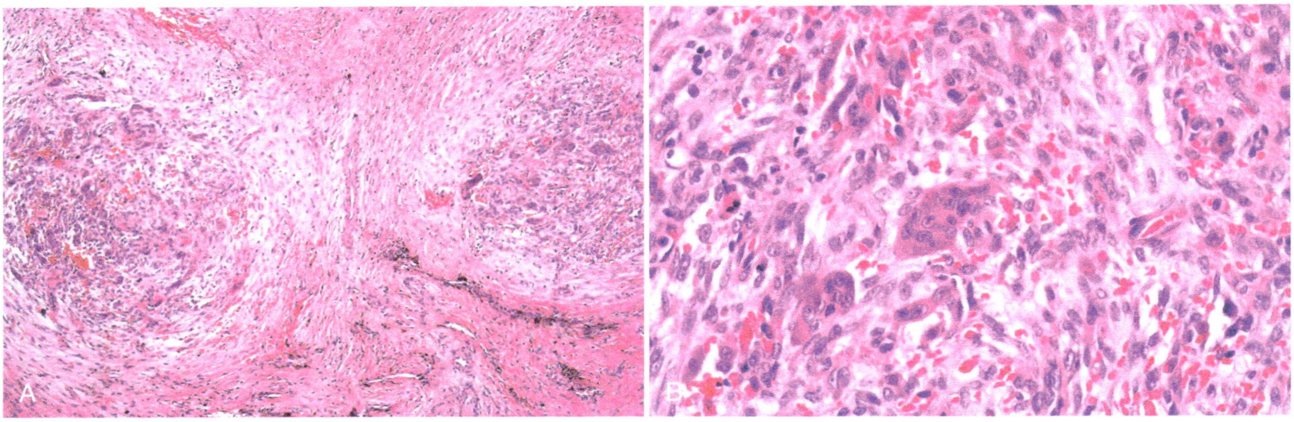

FIG 17.34 Central giant cell granuloma. (A) Nodular aggregates of giant cells and spindled monocytic cells with hemorrhage, fibrosis, and hemosiderin deposits. (B) Monocytic cells with benign nuclei and osteoclast-like giant cells with hemorrhage.

(VEGF), and basic fibroblast growth factor (bFGF) may predict aggressive behavior, but the size of giant cells and the number of nuclei do not.
- Giant cells and stromal cells are positive for glucocorticoid receptors and only 50% are positive for calcitonin receptors; some are positive for parathyroid hormone-related peptide (PTHrP) and PTHrP receptor-1.

Differential Diagnosis

- Brown tumor of hyperparathyroidism is indistinguishable from central giant cell granuloma; high parathormone levels and serum calcium differentiate the two conditions.
- Multiple giant cell lesions are often seen in Noonan syndrome spectrum (formerly referred to as Noonan-like multiple giant cell lesion syndrome) where patients exhibit hypertelorism, down-slanting palpebral fissures, low-set ears, neck webbing, short stature, pectus excavatum, cardiac defects, and cryptorchidism; Noonan syndrome is associated with mutations in *PTPN11* in 50% of cases in addition to mutations in *SOS1* and *RAF1* and other genes in the RAS-MAPK pathway; those with giant cell lesions also exhibit mutations in *PTPN11* and *SOS1* confirming it is a variant of Noonan syndrome.
- Aneurysmal bone cyst consists of large blood-filled spaces lined by multinucleated giant cells. Many cases exhibit mutation in *USP6*.
- Cherubism is distinguished by its typical bilateral presentation in a young child. It is positive for mutation in *SH3BP2*.

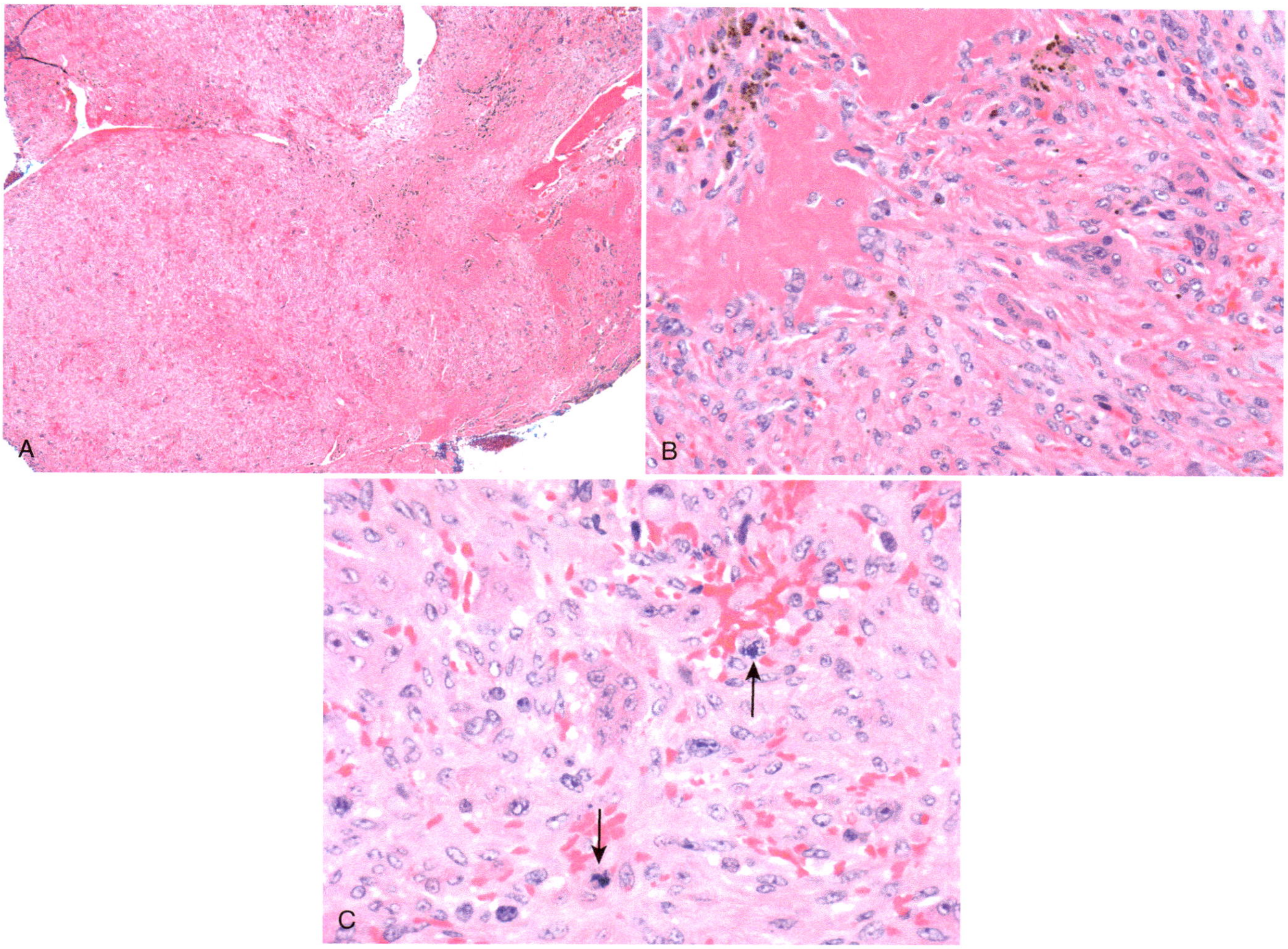

FIG 17.35 Central giant cell granuloma. (A) Monocytic cells, multinucleated giant cells, hemorrhage, and abundant reactive bone. (B) Monocytic cells, giant cells, and reactive bone with osteoblastic rimming, fresh hemorrhage, and siderophages. (C) Mitotic figures are noted within the stromal mononuclear cells *(arrows)*.

- Abundant woven bone deposition may suggest a fibro-osseous lesion, but giant cells are usually only focally present in those lesions.

Management and Prognosis

- Recurrence is noted in 10% to 50% of cases depending on mode of therapy and whether lesions are aggressive or nonaggressive.
- Curettage, enucleation, excision, resection, intralesional steroid injections, and calcitonin nasal spray may be employed with success.
- More recent treatments include enucleation and/or tumor debulking with targeted therapies such as interferon-α, bisphosphonates, denosumab, and imatinib (see Fig. 7.36).

REFERENCES

Amaral FR, Gomes CC, Oliveira CS, et al. Clonality analysis of giant cell lesions of the jaws. *Braz Dent J.* 2010;21:361-364.

Behjati S, Tarpey PS, Presneau N, et al. Distinct H3F3A and H3F3B driver mutations define chondroblastoma and giant cell tumor of bone. *Nat Genet.* 2013;45:1479-1482.

Beneteau C, Cave H, Moncla A, et al. SOS1 and PTPN11 mutations in five cases of Noonan syndrome with multiple giant cell lesions. *Eur J Hum Genet.* 2009;17:1216-1221.

de Lange J, van Rijn RR, van den Burg H, et al. Regression of central giant cell granuloma by a combination of interferon and imatinib: a case report. *Br J Oral Maxillofac Surg.* 2009;47:59-61.

Dewsnup NC, Susarla SM, Abulikemu M, et al. Immunohistochemical evaluation of giant cell tumors of the jaws using CD34 density analysis. *J Oral Maxillofac Surg.* 2008;66:928-933.

Gleason BC, Kleinman PK, Debelenko LV, et al. Novel karyotypes in giant cell-rich lesions of bone. *Am J Surg Pathol.* 2007;31:926-932.

Gomes CC, Diniz MG, Amaral FR, et al. The highly prevalent H3F3A mutation in giant cell tumours of bone is not shared by sporadic central giant cell lesion of the jaws. *Oral Surg Oral Med Oral Pathol Oral Radiol.* 2014;118:583-585.

Houpis CH, Tosios KI, Papavasileiou D, et al. Parathyroid hormone-related peptide (PTHrP), parathyroid hormone/parathyroid hormone-related peptide receptor 1 (PTHR1), and MSX1 protein are expressed in central and peripheral giant cell granulomas of the jaws. *Oral Surg Oral Med Oral Pathol Oral Radiol Endod.* 2010;109:415-424.

Kaban LB, Troulis MJ, Wilkinson MS, et al. Adjuvant antiangiogenic therapy for giant cell tumors of the jaws. *J Oral Maxillofac Surg.* 2007;65:2018-2024.

Karbach J, Coerdt W, Wagner W, Bartsch O. Case report: Noonan syndrome with multiple giant cell lesions and review of the literature. *Am J Med Genet A.* 2012;158A:2283-2289.

Liu B, Yu SF, Li TJ. Multinucleated giant cells in various forms of giant cell containing lesions of the jaws express features of osteoclasts. *J Oral Pathol Med.* 2003;32:367-375.
Peacock ZS, Jordan RC, Schmidt BL. Giant cell lesions of the jaws: does the level of vascularity and angiogenesis correlate with behavior? *J Oral Maxillofac Surg.* 2012;70:1860-1866.
Resnick CM, Margolis J, Susarla SM, et al. Maxillofacial and axial/appendicular giant cell lesions: unique tumors or variants of the same disease? A comparison of phenotypic, clinical, and radiographic characteristics. *J Oral Maxillofac Surg.* 2010;68:130-137.
Roberts AE, Allanson JE, Tartaglia M, Gelb BD. Noonan syndrome. *Lancet.* 2013;381:333-342.
Vered M, Buchner A, Dayan D. Immunohistochemical expression of glucocorticoid and calcitonin receptors as a tool for selecting therapeutic approach in central giant cell granuloma of the jawbones. *Int J Oral Maxillofac Surg.* 2006;35:756-760.
Whitaker SB, Waldron CA. Central giant cell lesions of the jaws. A clinical, radiologic, and histopathologic study. *Oral Surg Oral Med Oral Pathol.* 1993;75:199-208.

CHERUBISM

Clinical Findings

- This is usually diagnosed in the first and second decades of life with patients presenting with swelling of the face or fullness of the mandibular sulcus. There are bilateral multiloculated radiolucencies with the mandible (usually body and ramus) always involved; involvement of the maxilla causes eyes to turn upward, resulting in a cherubic appearance. There is tooth displacement, delayed tooth eruption, and loosening of teeth (Figs. 17.36 and 17.37).
- Grading is as follows: grade 1, mandible involved only, including the coronoid process; grade 2, grade 1 + involvement of maxillary tuberosities, and/or anterior mandible; grade 3, extensive and diffuse involvement of maxilla and mandible.
- Dental abnormalities include missing teeth, taurodontism, and hypercementosis.
- After steady growth in the first and second decades of life, the lesions may become quiescent for a few years and then regress over the ensuing years beginning in adolescence.

Etiopathogenesis and Histopathologic Features

Cherubism is an autosomal dominant condition caused in many, but not all, cases by a mutation in *SH3BP2* on chromosome 4p16 that encodes an adaptor protein 3BP2; TNFα-mediated osteoclastogenesis mediates bone loss.

- There is a proliferation of spindled, fibroblast-like monocytic cells in a delicately fibrous stroma with clusters of osteoclast-type multinucleated giant cells; perivascular hyalinization is seen in up to 50% of cases and there may be hemorrhage (Fig. 17.38).

Differential Diagnosis

- Central giant cell granuloma is a solitary lesion, usually in the anterior mandible and does not show the *SH3BP2* mutation.
- Patients with Noonan syndrome spectrum (previously known as Noonan-like syndrome with multiple giant cell lesions) exhibit multiple giant cell lesions that may be bilateral but have a different clinical phenotype and exhibit mutations in *PTPN11* or *SOS1* (see earlier).

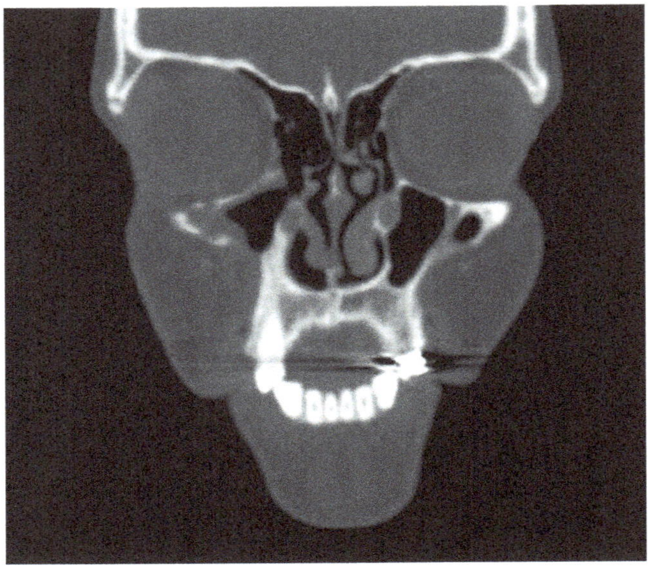

FIG 17.36 Aggressive central giant cell granuloma (same patient as in Fig. 17.33B): coronal CT exhibits resolution of right maxillary lesion 3 years after enucleation and 2 years after completion of treatment with systemic interferon therapy. *(Courtesy Dr. Leonard B. Kaban and Dr. Maria Troulis, Harvard School of Dental Medicine and Massachusetts General Hospital, Boston, MA.)*

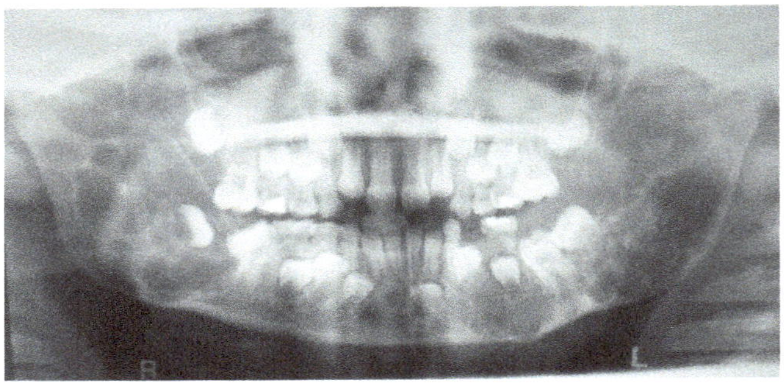

FIG 17.37 Cherubism manifesting with bilateral multiloculated radiolucencies of the mandibular rami and body. *(Courtesy Dr. Bonnie Padwa, Children's Hospital Boston, Boston, Mass.)*

- Aneurysmal bone cyst has blood-filled spaces rimmed by giant cells and exhibits mutation in *USP6.*

Management and Prognosis

- Patients should be on long-term follow-up because many cases will resolve spontaneously. Recontouring of the bone, resection, or curettage should be performed only after teenage when the lesions become quiescent; rare cases have responded to calcitonin but not to antibodies against TNFα.

REFERENCES

Carvalho Silva E, Carvalho Silva GC, Vieira TC. Cherubism: clinicoradiographic features, treatment, and long-term follow-up of 8 cases. *J Oral Maxillofac Surg.* 2007;65:517-522.
Levaot N, Voytyuk O, Dimitriou I, et al. Loss of Tankyrase-mediated destruction of 3BP2 is the underlying pathogenic mechanism of cherubism. *Cell.* 2011;147:1324-1339.
Meng XM, Yu SF, Yu GY. Clinicopathologic study of 24 cases of cherubism. *Int J Oral Maxillofac Surg.* 2005;34:350-356.

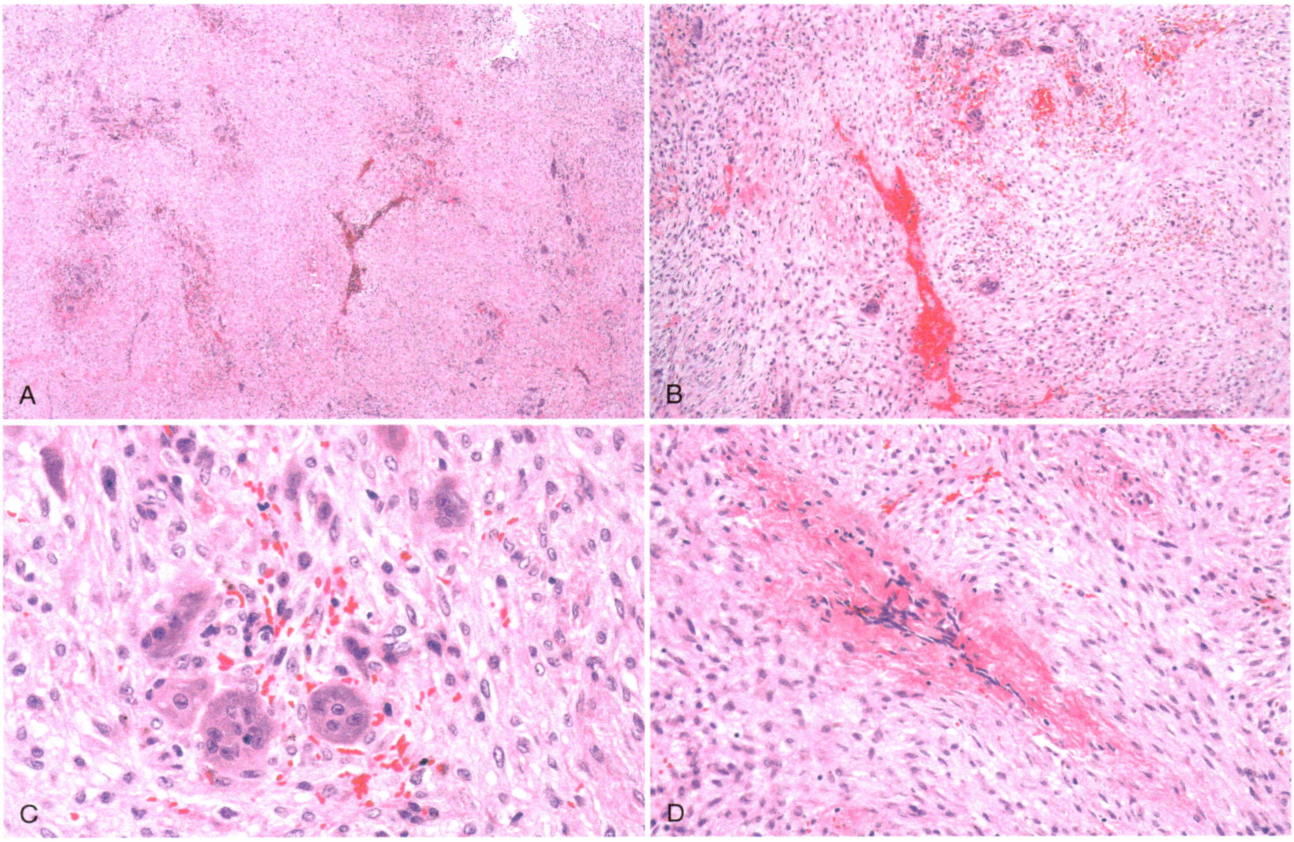

FIG 17.38 Cherubism. (A) Diffuse proliferation of spindled fibroblast-like cells with clusters of multinucleated giant cells in a delicately collagenous stroma. (B) Clusters of giant cells within a delicately collagenous background of spindle cells and fresh hemorrhage. (C) Osteoclast-like multinucleated giant cells and spindled fibroblast-like cells. (D) Perivascular deposits of eosinophilic fibrinoid material.

Mukai T, Ishida S, Ishikawa R, et al. SH3BP2 cherubism mutation potentiates TNF-alpha-induced osteoclastogenesis via NFATc1 and TNF-alpha-mediated inflammatory bone loss. *J Bone Miner Res.* 2014;29:2618-2635.

Papadaki ME, Lietman SA, Levine MA, et al. Cherubism: best clinical practice. *Orphanet J Rare Dis.* 2012;7:S6.

Prescott T, Redfors M, Rustad CF, et al. Characterization of a Norwegian cherubism cohort; molecular genetic findings, oral manifestations and quality of life. *Eur J Med Genet.* 2013;56:131-137.

Roberts AE, Allanson JE, Tartaglia M, Gelb BD. Noonan syndrome. *Lancet.* 2013;381:333-342.

Ueki Y, Tiziani V, Santanna C, et al. Mutations in the gene encoding c-Abl-binding protein SH3BP2 cause cherubism. *Nat Genet.* 2001;28:125-126.

DESMOPLASTIC FIBROMA

This lesion is the intraosseous counterpart of desmoid-type fibromatosis (aggressive fibromatosis or extraabdominal desmoid).

Clinical Findings

- This tumor occurs mostly in those younger than 30 years (85% of cases). There is jaw swelling, displacement and mobility of teeth, and sometimes pain; 85% of lesions occur in the mandible presenting as a well- and sometimes poorly demarcated radiolucency with scalloped borders (in 70% of cases); cortical perforation and extension into soft tissues is seen in 30% of cases.
- Some cases have been associated with tuberous sclerosis.

Etiopathogenesis and Histopathologic Features

This lesion likely arises from mesenchymal stem cells within bone with differentiation toward fibroblasts and myofibroblasts. Although it resembles desmoid-type fibromatosis, nuclear β-catenin is not expressed consistently, unlike desmoid tumors where it is present in 80% to 90% of sporadic cases and 60% to 70% of cases associated with familial adenomatous polyposis syndrome. It is unclear whether the reason for this is because it develops via a different tumorigenic pathway from the usual APC-β-catenin pathway, or because decalcification procedures have rendered immunohistochemical studies unreliable. Trisomy 8 and 20 have been identified in rare cases.

- There is abundant richly collagenous stroma with sweeping fascicles of collagen and in some cases stromal hyalinization; there is usually a mild-to-modest number of spindled fibroblasts and myofibroblasts with minimal to no cytologic atypia, and mitoses may be present (Fig. 17.39).
- Spindle cells are positive for smooth muscle actin in more than 50% of cases, for muscle-specific actin and occasionally for desmin, and are negative for S-100 protein; β-catenin is positive in the cytoplasm in up to

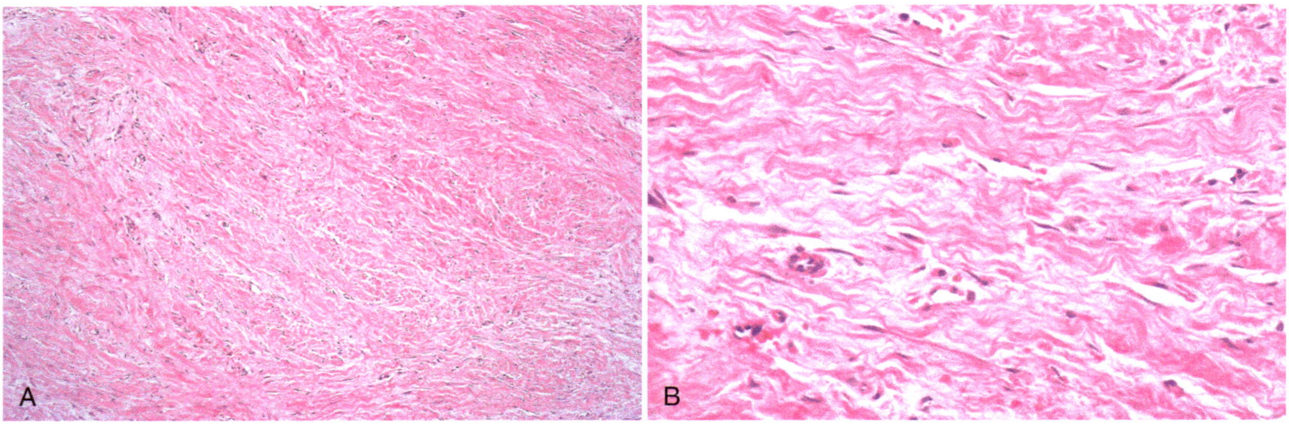

FIG 17.39 Desmoplastic fibroma. (A) Paucicellular tumor with weeping fascicles of dense collagen and scattered spindle cells. (B) Spindle cells have benign morphology.

50% of cases, but nuclear staining is uncommon; Ki-67 index is less than 1%.

Differential Diagnosis

- Central odontogenic fibroma almost always contains odontogenic epithelium, which can be highlighted by keratin studies.
- Central ossifying fibroma may show sweeping fascicles of collagen but cementoosseous material is always identified.
- Other benign spindle cell tumors such as nerve sheath tumors or muscle tumors can be ruled out by appropriate immunohistochemical studies.

Management and Prognosis

- Excision with clear margins is the treatment of choice and there is a 20% recurrence rate; curettage results in 30% recurrence.

REFERENCES

Bridge JA, Swarts SJ, Buresh C, et al. Trisomies 8 and 20 characterize a subgroup of benign fibrous lesions arising in both soft tissue and bone. *Am J Pathol.* 1999;154:729-733.

Carlson JW, Fletcher CD. Immunohistochemistry for beta-catenin in the differential diagnosis of spindle cell lesions: analysis of a series and review of the literature. *Histopathology.* 2007;51:509-514.

Flucke U, Tops BB, van Diest PJ, Slootweg PJ. Desmoid-type fibromatosis of the head and neck region in the paediatric population: a clinicopathological and genetic study of seven cases. *Histopathology.* 2014;64:769-776.

Hauben EI, Jundt G, Cleton-Jansen AM, et al. Desmoplastic fibroma of bone: an immunohistochemical study including beta-catenin expression and mutational analysis for beta-catenin. *Hum Pathol.* 2005;36:1025-1030.

Le Guellec S, Soubeyran I, Rochaix P, et al. CTNNB1 mutation analysis is a useful tool for the diagnosis of desmoid tumors: a study of 260 desmoid tumors and 191 potential morphologic mimics. *Mod Pathol.* 2012;25:1551-1558.

Said-Al-Naief N, Fernandes R, Louis P, et al. Desmoplastic fibroma of the jaw: a case report and review of literature. *Oral Surg Oral Med Oral Pathol Oral Radiol Endod.* 2006;101:82-94.

Salas S, Chibon F, Noguchi T, et al. Molecular characterization by array comparative genomic hybridization and DNA sequencing of 194 desmoid tumors. *Genes Chromosomes Cancer.* 2010;49:560-568.

Tandon S, Garg RK. Intraoral desmoplastic fibroma: a manifestation of tuberous sclerosis. *Fetal Pediatr Pathol.* 2012;31:195-201.

Woods TR, Cohen DM, Islam MN, et al. Desmoplastic fibroma of the mandible: a series of three cases and review of literature. *Head Neck Pathol.* 2015;9:196-204.

OSTEOID OSTEOMA AND OSTEOBLASTOMA

Osteoid osteoma and osteoblastoma represent approximately 10% and 1%, respectively, of primary bone tumors and they exhibit similar histopathology, but osteoid osteoma is usually less than 2 cm and associated with nocturnal pain. The most common location for the osteoid osteoma is the long bones, whereas osteoblastoma is most common in the vertebral column.

Clinical Findings

- Osteoid osteoma: This is most common in the third decade and the majority of patients experience pain that is usually nocturnal and relieved by aspirin or other nonsteroidal antiinflammatory medication. The lesion is usually less than 2 cm and composed of a central radiolucent nidus surrounded by a rim of osteosclerosis.
- Osteoblastoma: This is most common in the third decade with a 4:1 male predilection; 80% occur in the mandible, usually posterior, and patients may also report pain and swelling. It presents as a discrete, generally well-demarcated radiopacity or mixed radiopaque-radiolucent lesion, sometimes with a central radiolucent nidus less than 2 cm in greatest diameter; some are periosteal and not central; an aggressive form grows rapidly to a large size and has poorly demarcated borders radiographically, but may not have a higher recurrence rate.

Etiopathogenesis and Histopathologic Features

This tumor is believed to arise from mesenchymal stem cells that differentiate toward osteoblasts.

- The histopathology of both lesions is similar; there is a proliferation of plump spindle cells and osteoblasts within very vascular stroma, with the deposition of trabeculae of osteoid and woven bone that are surfaced by multiple layers of plump osteoblasts admixed with osteoclasts on the same trabeculae; the bone is basophilic and pagetoid with many resting and reversal lines ("blue bone"), and varies from slender to lacy to thick trabeculae, to large masses of bone; epithelioid

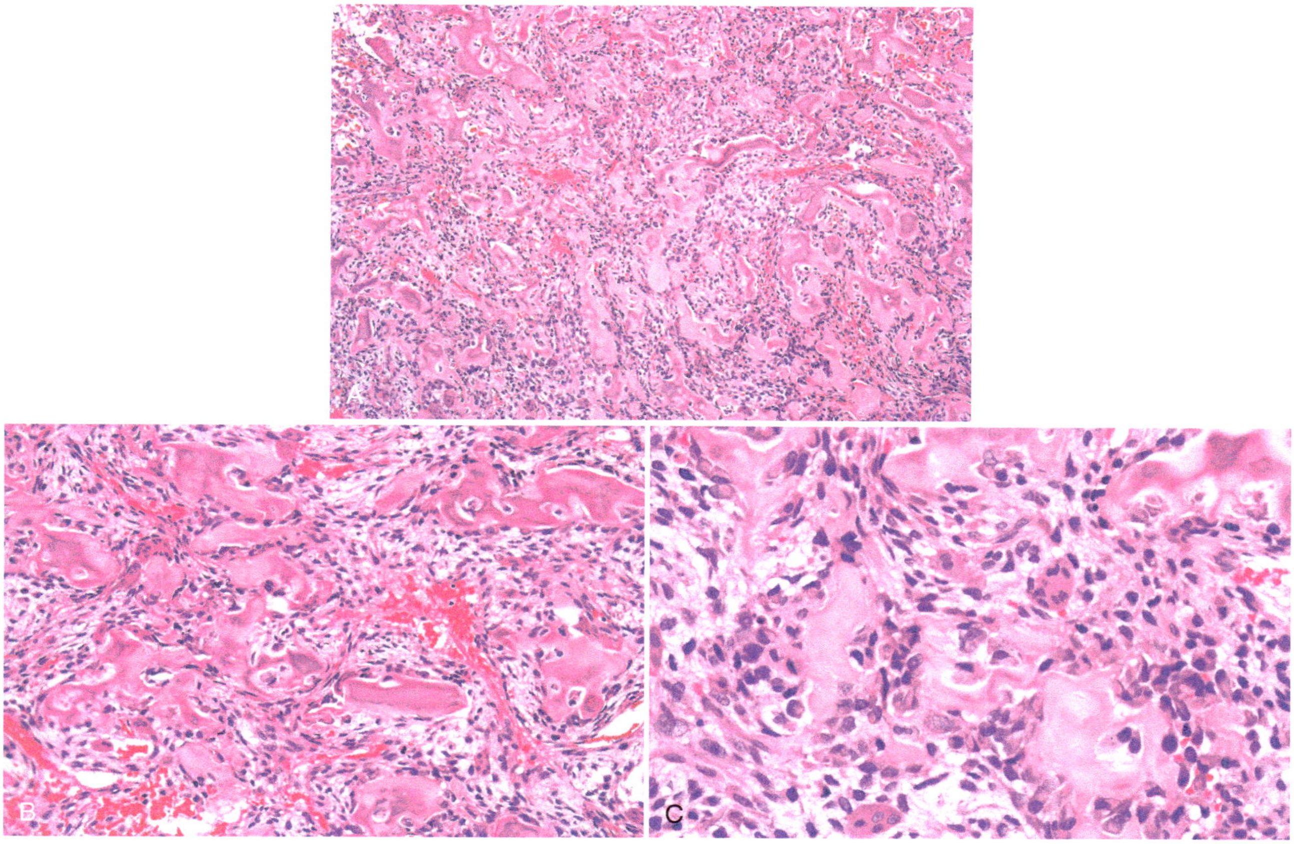

FIG 17.40 Osteoblastoma. (A) Trabeculae of woven bone with a hematoxyphilic hue in a cellular stroma. (B) Proliferation of plump osteoblasts and osteoclasts within a vascular stroma. (C) Multiple layers of osteoblasts with osteoclasts on the same trabeculae.

osteoblasts are present in up to 15% to 25% of cases (Fig. 17.40); cases of osteoid osteoma also show many nerve fibers within the nidus.

- Multinodular epithelioid osteoblastoma consists of nodules and sheets of epithelioid osteoblasts that have abundant eosinophilic cytoplasm and eccentric nuclei with dispersed chromatin, sometimes unassociated with matrix formation; this histopathology is also noted in lesions of "aggressive osteoblastoma."
- Osteoblastoma may be associated with an aneurysmal bone cyst.

Differential Diagnosis

- Osteoblastic osteosarcoma exhibits significant cytologic atypia and it is unclear how this is related to the controversial entity "malignant osteoblastoma."

Management and Prognosis

- Curettage or excision is curative.
- Recurrence is associated less with histopathologic features and more with accessibility of the lesion to complete removal.

REFERENCES

An SY, Shin HI, Choi KS, et al. Unusual osteoid osteoma of the mandible: report of case and review of the literature. *Oral Surg Oral Med Oral Pathol Oral Radiol.* 2013;116:e134-e140.

Della Rocca C, Huvos AG. Osteoblastoma: varied histological presentations with a benign clinical course. An analysis of 55 cases. *Am J Surg Pathol.* 1996;20:841-850.

Harrington C, Accurso BT, Kalmar JR, et al. Aggressive osteoblastoma of the maxilla: a case report and review of the literature. *Head Neck Pathol.* 2011;5:165-170.

Jones AC, Prihoda TJ, Kacher JE, et al. Osteoblastoma of the maxilla and mandible: a report of 24 cases, review of the literature, and discussion of its relationship to osteoid osteoma of the jaws. *Oral Surg Oral Med Oral Pathol Oral Radiol Endod.* 2006;102:639-650.

Lucas DR, Unni KK, McLeod RA, et al. Osteoblastoma: clinicopathologic study of 306 cases. *Hum Pathol.* 1994;25:117-134.

Rahsepar B, Nikgoo A, Fatemitabar SA. Osteoid osteoma of subcondylar region: case report and review of the literature. *J Oral Maxillofac Surg.* 2009;67:888-893.

Yalcinkaya U, Doganavsargil B, Sezak M, et al. Clinical and morphological characteristics of osteoid osteoma and osteoblastoma: a retrospective single-center analysis of 204 patients. *Ann Diagn Pathol.* 2014;18:319-325.

Zon Filippi R, Swee RG, Krishnan Unni K. Epithelioid multinodular osteoblastoma: a clinicopathologic analysis of 26 cases. *Am J Surg Pathol.* 2007;31:1265-1268.

OSTEOSARCOMA (OSTEOGENIC SARCOMA)

Osteosarcoma is the most common primary nonhematopoietic malignancy of bone and the second most common intraosseous malignancy after multiple myeloma in adults.

Gnathic osteosarcomas constitute approximately 6% of all osteosarcomas and are distinct in that they tend to metastasize less frequently, are amenable to surgical excision only without chemotherapy, and exhibit a much higher rate of long term disease-free survival. Anatomically, osteosarcomas may be intramedullary, surface (or juxtacortical), and extraskeletal. Histologically, the vast majority are high-grade and intramedullary. In general, intramedullary gnathic osteosarcomas occur 10 to 20 years later than long bone osteosarcoma.

Clinical Findings

- This occurs most frequently in the fourth decade with a slight male predilection, and is associated with pain, swelling, tooth mobility, and paresthesia; there is a slight mandibular predilection of 2:1. Older patients may have preexisting Paget disease or a history of radiation to the head and neck.
- Radiographs show a mixed radiolucent-radiopaque lesion with poorly demarcated borders (Fig. 17.41A); a sunburst-like or "hair-on-end" osteophytic reaction is seen on radiographs if the periosteum is involved, and some cases destroy the cortex. The presence of bone outside of the medullary space is highly suspicious for osteosarcoma. Intraoral periapical radiographs show widening of the periodontal ligament space.
- Up to 15% of cases may report a prior history of radiation to the head and neck.
- Parosteal osteosarcomas are enlarging masses attached to the surface of the jaw bones, radiographically appearing as a circumscribed radiopacity sometimes with areas of radiolucency (see Fig. 7.41B).

Etiopathogenesis and Histopathologic Features

Osteosarcomas are genetically heterogeneous with complex chromosomal abnormalities such as chromosomal instability with duplications and deletions, and also with mutations of *TP53* (in up to 80% of cases), *RB1*, *MDM2*, *CDK4*, and *RUNX2*. Alternative lengthening of a telomere (ALT) is identified in approximately 85% of cases. Genetic polymorphisms in CTLA-4 and TGF-β1 may also play a role.

Secondary osteosarcoma may develop in preexisting Paget disease of bone or with a history of radiation. Patients who develop osteosarcoma with a history of hereditary retinoblastoma or Li-Fraumeni syndrome, with mutations in *RB1* and *TP53* respectively, have a poorer prognosis.

Intramedullary lesions in the jaws are usually high grade (80% of cases), and the most common is the conventional type composed of chondroblastic, osteoblastic, or fibroblastic components in varying proportions; telangiectatic, small cell, giant cell–rich, epithelioid and dedifferentiated types are rare. Pediatric cases are often primarily osteoblastic. Low-grade osteosarcomas include surface parosteal osteosarcoma and intramedullary low-grade osteosarcoma (fibrous dysplasia–type), which are often difficult to recognize as malignant tumors. Other surface osteosarcomas include intermediate-grade periosteal osteosarcomas, and high grade de novo or dedifferentiated osteosarcomas.

- In osteoblastic osteosarcoma, atypical osteoblasts lay down irregular, lacy, filigreed, basophilic trabeculae of

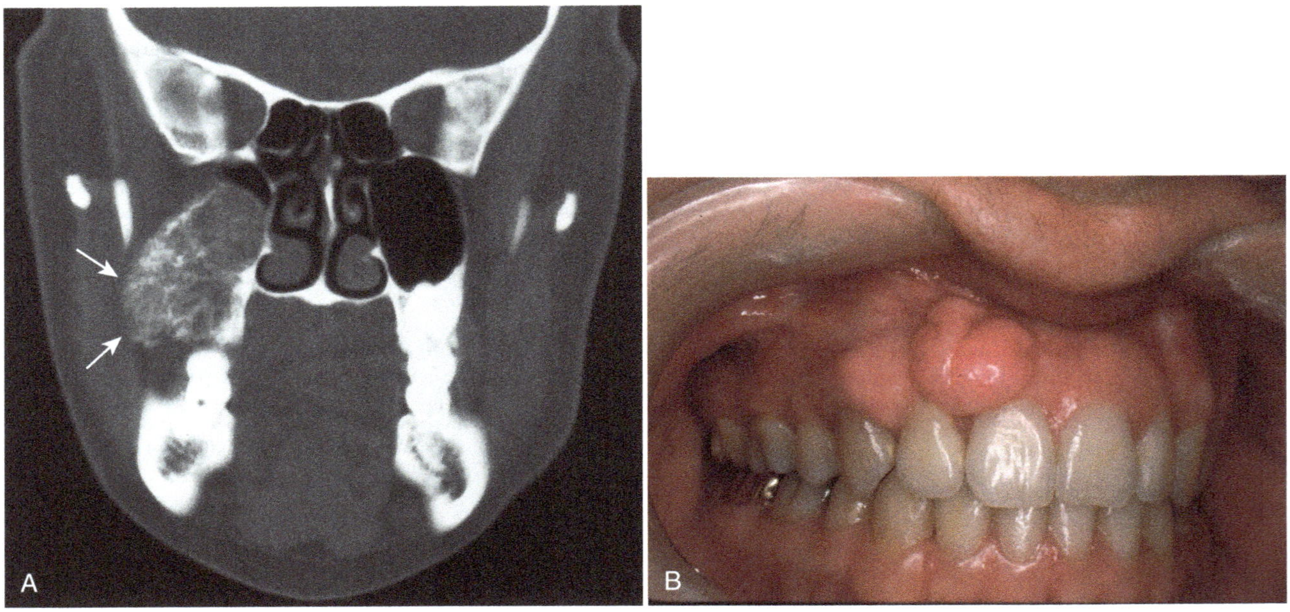

FIG 17.41 (A) Intramedullary osteosarcoma. Coronal CT shows bone-producing tumor of the right maxilla with delicate bone spicules. (B) Parosteal (low-grade) osteosarcoma. Exophytic, nodular tumor on the surface of the bone. *(A, From White SC, Pharoah MJ: Malignant diseases of the jaws. In: Oral Radiology, Principles and Interpretation. 6th ed. St Louis, Mosby, 2008. B, Courtesy Department of Diagnostic Sciences, Baylor College of Dentistry, Houston, Tex.)*

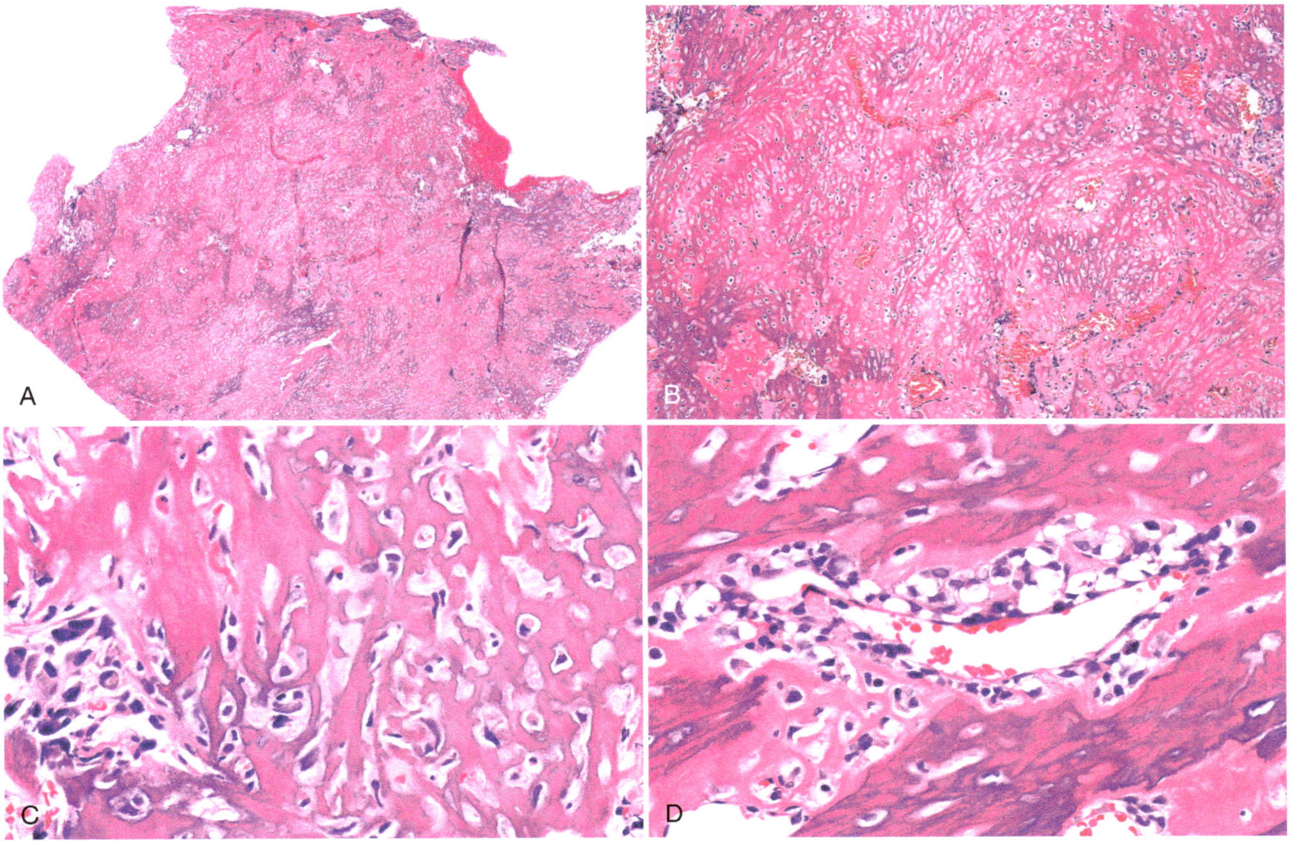

FIG 17.42 Osteoblastic osteosarcoma. (A) Atypical osteoid and woven bone. (B) Interconnected lacy trabeculae of osteoid and woven bone with large lacunae. (C) Woven bone contains many plump, atypical osteoblasts and osteocytes with pleomorphic nuclei. (D) Many atypical osteoblasts and osteocytes within osteoid and woven bone.

malignant osteoid and woven bone. Hyperchromatic, prominent high grade tumors are more cellular, and nuclei are larger and more pleomorphic with irregular contours, mitoses or even necrosis (Fig. 17.42). Atypical cartilage formation is seen in the chondroblastic type, and the fibroblastic type contains atypical spindle cells usually with little osteoid production (Fig. 17.43A–B).

- SATB2, a nuclear matrix protein that regulates osteoblastic differentiation, is a highly sensitive marker for osteoblastic differentiation (close to 100% of cases) (Fig. 17.43C); it is useful for cases where there is little osteoid present, but does not distinguish between benign and malignant bone-forming tumors; MDM2 and CDK4 are also expressed in osteosarcoma in 80% of cases.
- Parosteal (low-grade surface or juxtacortical) osteosarcoma is a low-grade osteosarcoma that is easily mistaken for a benign fibroosseous lesion; thick interconnected trabeculae of bone are surrounded by cellular fibrous tissue containing spindle cells with minimal atypia; very focal osteoblastic rimming is present, and infiltration of the cortex is uncommon; 25% to 50% show cartilage formation with ossification (Figs. 17.44 and 17.45). Dedifferentiation occurs in 15% to 20% of cases and this is associated with a poorer prognosis; MDM2 and CKD4 positivity has been noted in more than 80% of such low-grade lesions, and when seen in high grade surface lesions is usually a sign of dedifferentiation.
- Intramedullary low-grade osteosarcoma lesions are similar to parosteal osteosarcoma with a fibrous dysplasia–like pattern.
- Periosteal osteosarcoma is a chondroblastic osteosarcoma of intermediate grade.
- High-grade surface osteosarcoma is similar to conventional osteosarcoma, exhibits invasion of the medullary spaces in more than 50% of cases, and consists of osteoblastic, chondroblastic, and fibroblastic types predominantly; chondroblastic types are difficult to differentiate from periosteal osteosarcoma.

Differential Diagnosis

- Osteoblasts in osteoblastoma are less atypical; bone trabeculae are more regular in contour and more uniform overall; prominent vasculature and osteoclasts are noted; histopathologic differentiation between the two may be difficult, but osteoblastoma presents as a circumscribed lucent-opaque lesion.
- Aggressive ossifying fibroma, trabecular type, may show atypical osteoblasts but is more uniform in appearance with more mature-appearing osteoid, woven bone and often clusters of multinucleated osteoclast-type giant cells.

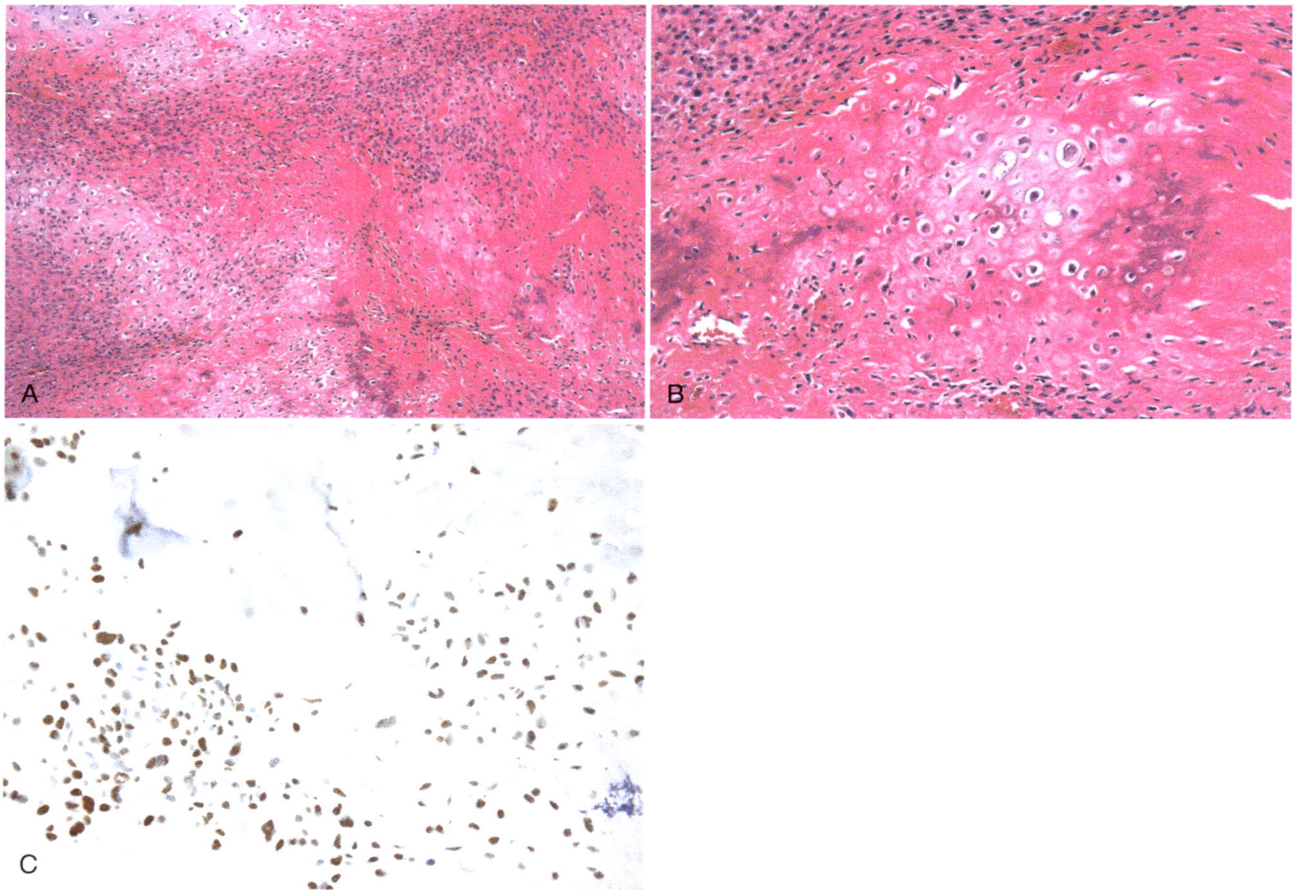

FIG 17.43 Chondroblastic osteosarcoma. (A) Cellular tumor with formation of malignant osteoid and cartilage. (B) Plump atypical osteoblasts noted in *upper left,* with deposition of malignant osteoid and atypical cartilage. (C) SATB2 study is positive within nuclei of osteoblasts.

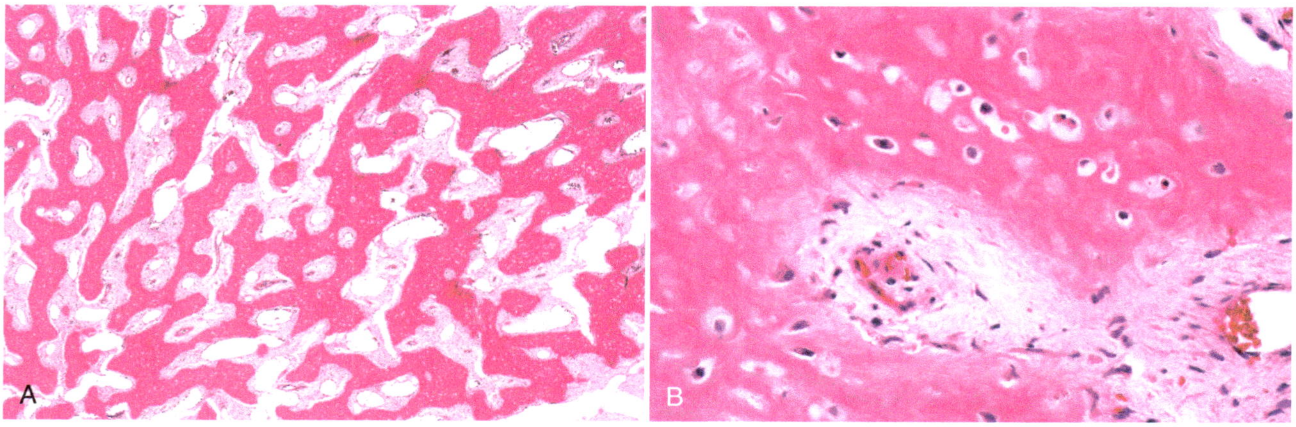

FIG 17.44 Low-grade parosteal osteosarcoma. (A) Interconnected trabeculae of woven bone with delicate hypocellular fibrovascular stroma. (B) Woven bone contains plump osteocytes with minimum cytologic atypia within lacunae and bland-appearing spindle cells in stroma.

- Fibrous dysplasia does not show significant atypia and it may be difficult to distinguish from low-grade fibrous dysplasia–like osteosarcoma; however, the latter is SATB2+.
- Chondrosarcoma does not usually produce malignant osteoid, although lesions may show ossification; chondrosarcomas exhibit mutation of *IDH1* and *IDH2* whereas osteosarcomas exhibit mutation in *SATB2.*

Management and Prognosis

- Gnathic lesions: Wide excision is the treatment of choice and 5-year survival is 60% to 70%; recurrence

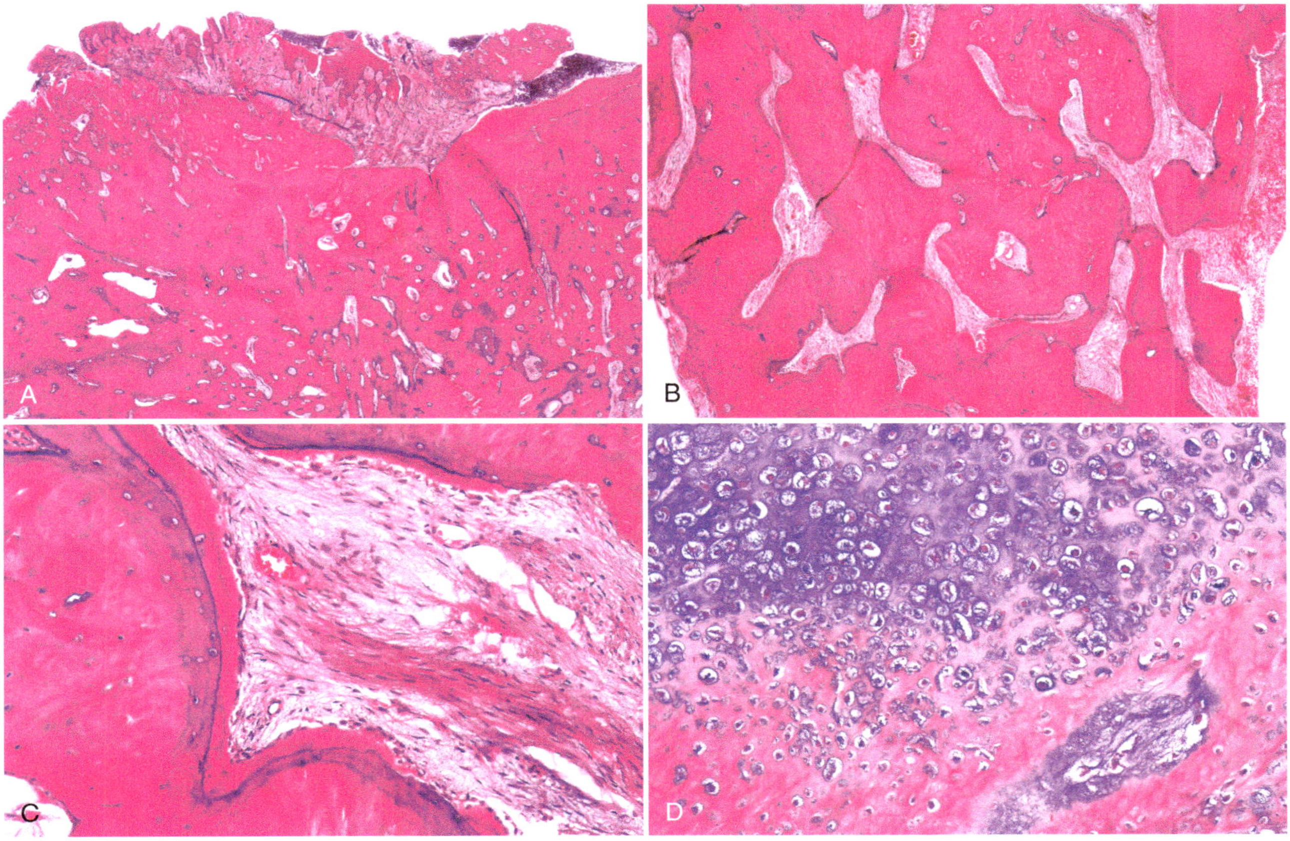

FIG 17.45 Low-grade parosteal osteosarcoma. (A) Sclerotic mass of atypical bone lying beneath surface epithelium, completely replacing the normal cortex. (B) Interconnected broad seams of bone with intervening relatively hypocellular fibrovascular tissue. (C) Bone is rimmed by a single layer of bland-appearing osteoblasts with bland spindle cells in the stroma. (D) Focal area of cartilaginous differentiation.

rate is 20% to 40%, and metastases (usually to the lungs) occur in 10% to 20% of cases. Radiation, neoadjuvant chemotherapy, with/without radiation are other modalities of treatment.

- Prognosis in gnathic lesions is influenced primarily by whether margins are positive, size of tumors, and not by histologic grade or subtype.
- Extragnathic lesions: surgery and adjuvant chemotherapy (usually with methotrexate, doxorubicin [Adriamycin], and cisplatin) is the treatment of choice; overall survival without metastases is 60% to 80%, and 20% to 30% with metastases. Treatment with immune modulators such as mifamurtide is being investigated.
- Prognosis in extragnathic lesions is worsened with high histologic grade, involvement of margins, recurrence, advanced age, in secondary osteosarcomas (such as in patients with Paget disease), and with osteoblastic or chondroblastic subtypes as opposed to fibroblastic and telangiectatic subtypes, which have a better prognosis. Long-term survival is 80% to 90% versus 15% for those who respond (>90% necrosis in tumor) versus those who do not respond to preoperative chemotherapy.
- Parosteal osteosarcoma has a better prognosis with 90% 5-year survival; dedifferentiation is associated with a higher rate of metastasis, especially to the lungs.

REFERENCES

Anderson ME. Update on Survival in Osteosarcoma. *Orthop Clin North Am.* 2016;47:283-292.

Bertoni F, Bacchini P, Staals EL, Davidovitz P. Dedifferentiated parosteal osteosarcoma: the experience of the Rizzoli Institute. *Cancer.* 2005;103:2373-2382.

Demicco EG, Deshpande V, Nielsen GP, et al. Well-differentiated osteosarcoma of the jaw bones: a clinicopathologic study of 15 cases. *Am J Surg Pathol.* 2010;34:1647-1655.

Dujardin F, Binh MB, Bouvier C, et al. MDM2 and CDK4 immunohistochemistry is a valuable tool in the differential diagnosis of low-grade osteosarcomas and other primary fibro-osseous lesions of the bone. *Mod Pathol.* 2011;24:624-637.

Fletcher C, Unni K, Mertens F, eds. *World Health Organization Pathology and Genetics: Tumours of Soft Tissue and Bone.* 3rd ed. Lyon: IARC Press; 2006.

Gadwal SR, Gannon FH, Fanburg-Smith JC, et al. Primary osteosarcoma of the head and neck in pediatric patients: a clinicopathologic study of 22 cases with a review of the literature. *Cancer.* 2001;91:598-605.

Granowski-LeCornu M, Chuang S, Kaban LB, et al. Osteosarcoma of the jaws: factors influencing prognosis. *J Oral Maxillofac Surg.* 2011; 69:2368-2375.

Jasnau S, Meyer U, Potratz J, et al. Craniofacial osteosarcoma: Experience of the cooperative German-Austrian-Swiss osteosarcoma study group. *Oral Oncol.* 2008;44:286-294.

Kansara M, Teng MW, Smyth MJ, Thomas DM. Translational biology of osteosarcoma. *Nat Rev Cancer.* 2014;14:722-735.

Klein MJ, Siegal GP. Osteosarcoma: anatomic and histologic variants. *Am J Clin Pathol.* 2006;125:555-581.

Nissanka EH, Amaratunge EA, Tilakaratne WM. Clinicopathological analysis of osteosarcoma of jaw bones. *Oral Dis.* 2007;13:82-87.

Okada K, Frassica FJ, Sim FH, et al. Parosteal osteosarcoma. A clinicopathological study. *J Bone Joint Surg Am.* 1994;76:366-378.

Okada K, Unni KK, Swee RG, Sim FH. High grade surface osteosarcoma: a clinicopathologic study of 46 cases. *Cancer.* 1999;85:1044-1054.

Paparella ML, Olvi LG, Brandizzi D, et al. Osteosarcoma of the jaw: an analysis of a series of 74 cases. *Histopathology.* 2013;63:551-557.

Wang GD, Zhao YF, Liu Y, et al. Periosteal osteosarcoma of the mandible: case report and review of the literature. *J Oral Maxillofac Surg.* 2011;69:1831-1835.

Wang S, Shi H, Yu Q. Osteosarcoma of the jaws: demographic and CT imaging features. *Dentomaxillofac Radiol.* 2012;41:37-42.

Yoshida A, Ushiku T, Motoi T, et al. MDM2 and CDK4 immunohistochemical coexpression in high-grade osteosarcoma: correlation with a dedifferentiated subtype. *Am J Surg Pathol.* 2012;36:423-431.

SYNOVIAL CHONDROMATOSIS (SYNOVIAL OSTEOCHONDROMATOSIS, SYNOVIAL CHONDROMETAPLASIA)

Clinical Findings

- This is most common in the fifth decade with 2–3:1 female predilection; patients' symptoms are pain and swelling of the temporomandibular joint, crepitus, and in more advanced stages, limited opening of the mouth.
- CT scans and MRIs show the presence of multiple "loose bodies" manifesting as round, ovoid, or irregularly shaped radiopacities of varying sizes within the joint space (>90% in the upper compartment), which is usually enlarged. Panoramic radiographs identify the bodies in only 15% to 30% of cases. There may be accompanying signs of joint disease such as erosions, osteosclerosis, and flattening of the head of the condyle, or even some other pathology such as an osteochondroma. Rare cases exhibit extension into the cranial fossa.

Etiopathogenesis and Histopathologic Features

Synovial chondromatosis is a benign chondroid or osteochondroid proliferation of the synovium of joints, bursa, and tendon sheaths. The prevailing theory is that nodules of cartilage arise within the synovium possibly via a metaplastic process and extrude into the joint space. An alternative theory postulates that synovial cells dislodge from the synovium and proliferate within the joint space with chondroid metaplasia. Fibroblast growth factor-2 may play a role and abnormalities in chromosome 6 have been identified.

Primary synovial chondromatosis arises de novo, whereas secondary synovial chondromatosis arises in association with chronic repetitive trauma, inflammatory joint disease, or other joint disease.

Each of the loose bodies consists of a nodule of mature hyaline cartilage with clustered chondrocytes exhibiting minimal to moderate nuclear atypia and often binucleation and focal ossification. These bodies are sometimes surfaced by synovium or thin fibrous tissue, and mitoses are not encountered; the synovium may exhibit areas of chondroid metaplasia (Fig. 17.46).

- Other pathologies such as osteochondroma may coexist.
- Chondrosarcoma develops in less than 5% of cases, and in such cases BCL2 positivity is lost.

Differential Diagnosis

- Rare cases of malignant transformation have been reported, as has synovial chondrosarcoma; nevertheless, this is one of the rare benign cartilage-producing lesions of the jaws where its clinical presentation is so characteristic that even if there is mild cytologic atypia of chondrocytes, the diagnosis is still synovial chondromatosis.

Management and Prognosis

- All loose bodies must be removed often through open surgery or arthroscopic surgery, and removal of diseased synovium, the meniscus, or even the condyle may be necessary.

REFERENCES

Ardekian L, Faquin W, Troulis MJ, et al. Synovial chondromatosis of the temporomandibular joint: report and analysis of eleven cases. *J Oral Maxillofac Surg.* 2005;63:941-947.

Bertoni F, Unni KK, Beabout JW, Sim FH. Chondrosarcomas of the synovium. *Cancer.* 1991;67:155-162.

Buddingh EP, Krallman P, Neff JR, et al. Chromosome 6 abnormalities are recurrent in synovial chondromatosis. *Cancer Genet Cytogenet.* 2003;140:18-22.

Cai XY, Yang C, Chen MJ, et al. Arthroscopic management for synovial chondromatosis of the temporomandibular joint: a retrospective review of 33 cases. *J Oral Maxillofac Surg.* 2012;70:2106-2113.

Coleman H, Chandraratnam E, Morgan G, et al. Synovial chondrosarcoma arising in synovial chondromatosis of the temporomandibular joint. *Head Neck Pathol.* 2013;7:304-309.

Guarda-Nardini L, Piccotti F, Ferronato G, Manfredini D. Synovial chondromatosis of the temporomandibular joint: a case description with systematic literature review. *Int J Oral Maxillofac Surg.* 2010;39:745-755.

Li Y, Cai H, Fang W, et al. Fibroblast growth factor 2 involved in the pathogenesis of synovial chondromatosis of temporomandibular joint. *J Oral Pathol Med.* 2014;43:388-394.

Meng J, Guo C, Yi B, et al. Clinical and radiologic findings of synovial chondromatosis affecting the temporomandibular joint. *Oral Surg Oral Med Oral Pathol Oral Radiol Endod.* 2010;109:441-448.

Mikami T, Aomura T, Ohira A, et al. Three case reports of synovial chondromatosis of temporomandibular joint: histopathologic analyses of minute cartilaginous loose bodies from joint lavage fluid and comparison with phase II and III cases. *J Oral Maxillofac Surg.* 2012;70:2099-2105.

Shah SB, Ramanojam S, Gadre PK, Gadre KS. Synovial chondromatosis of temporomandibular joint: journey through 25 decades and a case report. *J Oral Maxillofac Surg.* 2011;69:2795-2814.

von Lindern JJ, Theuerkauf I, Niederhagen B, et al. Synovial chondromatosis of the temporomandibular joint: clinical, diagnostic, and histomorphologic findings. *Oral Surg Oral Med Oral Pathol Oral Radiol Endod.* 2002;94:31-38.

Wang Y, Li L, Chen M, Yang C. Osteochondroma with secondary synovial chondromatosis in the temporomandibular joint. *Br J Oral Maxillofac Surg.* 2016;54:454-456.

Xu WH, Ma XC, Guo CB, et al. Synovial chondromatosis of the temporomandibular joint with middle cranial fossa extension. *Int J Oral Maxillofac Surg.* 2007;36:652-655.

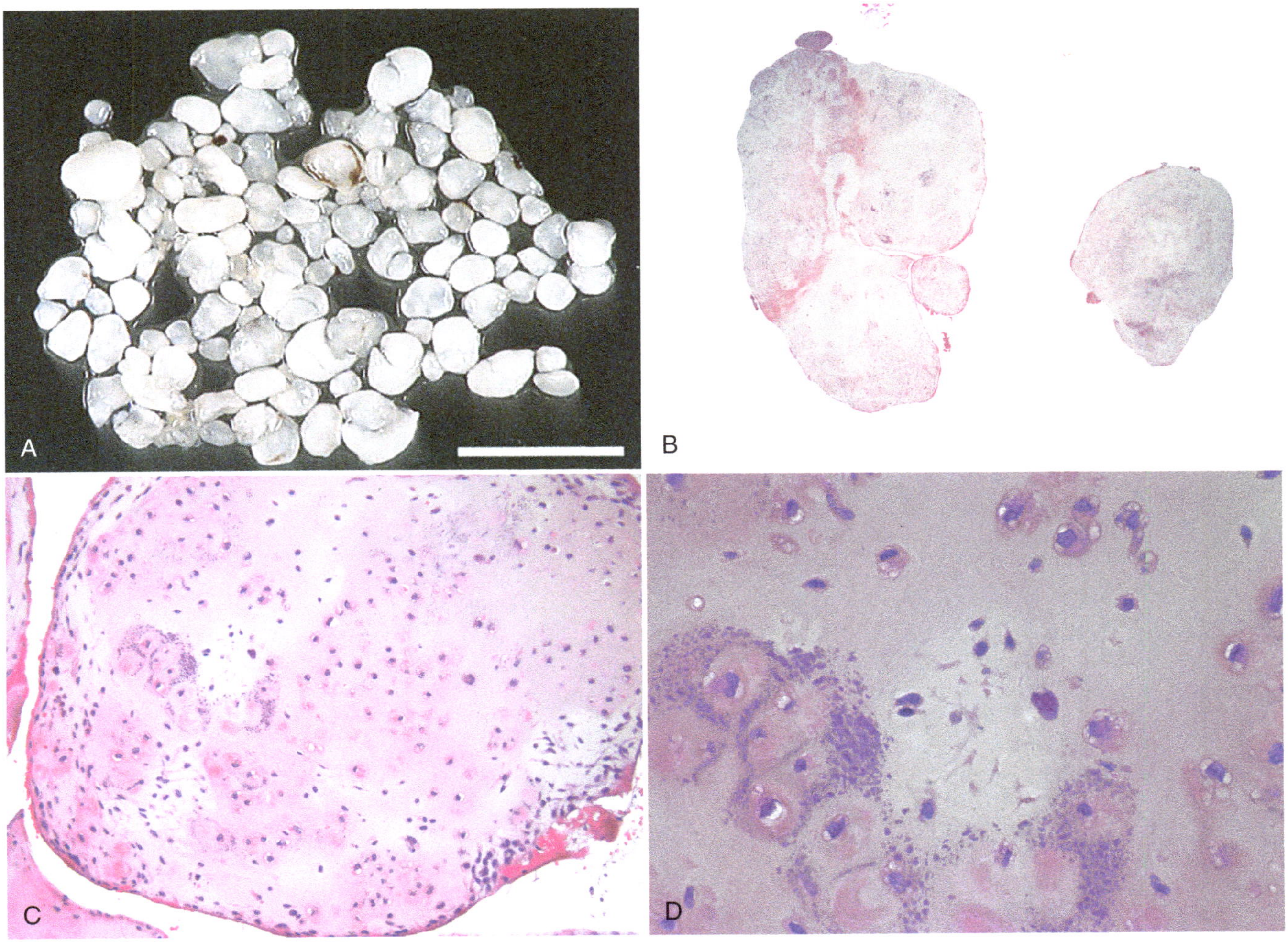

FIG 17.46 Synovial chrondromatosis. (A) Cartilaginous loose bodies. (B) Nodules of cartilage of varying sizes. (C) Mature hyaline cartilage with chondrocytes and dystrophic calcifications. (D) Chondrocytes exhibit mild nuclear atypia and binucleation and there is subtle dystrophic calcification. *(A, From Mikami T, Aomura, Ohira A et al. Three case reports of synovial chondromatosis of temporomandibular joint: histopathologic analyses of minute cartilaginous loose bodies from joint lavage fluid and comparison with phase II and III cases. J Oral Maxillofac Surg. 2012;70:2099–2105. B, Courtesy Dr. Leland Slater, Scripps Oral Pathology Service, San Diego, Calif.)*

CHONDROMYXOID FIBROMA

This most commonly affects the metaphases of long bones.

Clinical Findings

- This is most frequently seen in the second and third decades, and patients experience swelling of the jaw, usually the mandible; it presents as a well-circumscribed radiolucency, occasionally with small radiopacities, sometimes with a sclerotic or scalloped border.

Etiopathogenesis and Histopathologic Features

Rearrangements in chromosome 6 have been identified.

- There is a lobular proliferation of spindle and stellate cells in a myxoid stroma, with the center of the lobules being hypocellular and the periphery being hypercellular. Areas resembling chondroblastoma may be noted in the hypercellular areas composed of epithelioid, polygonal cells with abundant eosinophilic cytoplasm and multinucleated giant cells (Fig. 17.47); entrapped residual osteoid is often present.
- The myxoid stroma is positive for type II collagen and SOX9 is positive within the spindle and stellate cells, confirming they are chondrogenic.

Differential Diagnosis

- Chondrosarcoma exhibits significant cytologic atypia, and well-formed hyaline cartilage is usually noted.
- Chondroblastoma shows a more uniform proliferation of polygonal epithelioid cells with abundant eosinophilic cytoplasm and many giant cells without the extensive myxoid stroma.

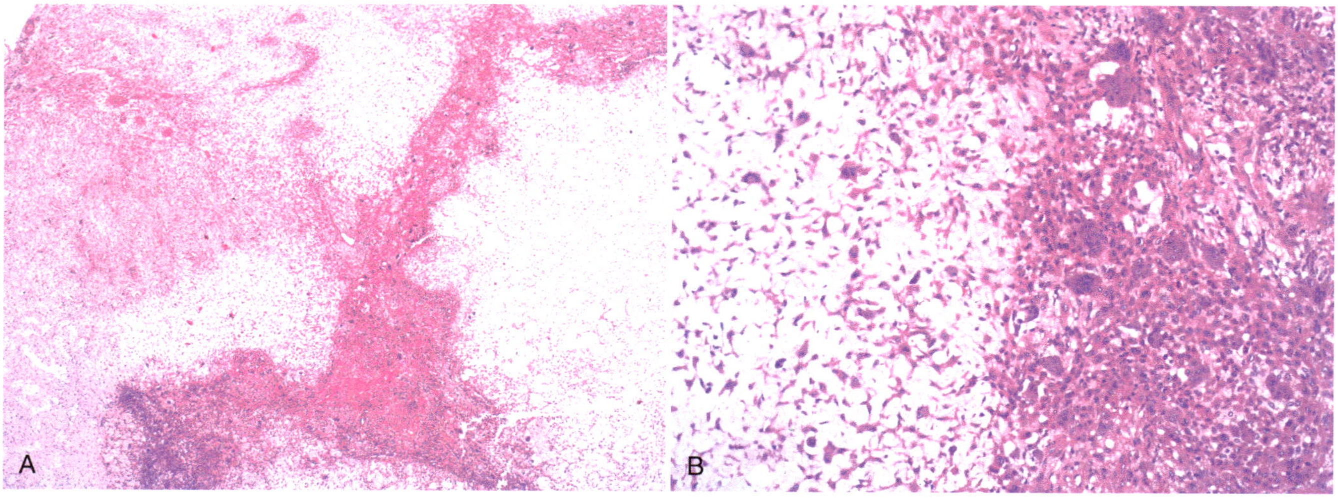

FIG 17.47 Chondromyxoid fibroma. (A) Lobular proliferation of spindle and stellate cells in a myxoid stroma separated by septa that are hypercellular. (B) Proliferation of spindle and stellate cells within myxoid stroma *(left)*, and more cellular chondroblastoma-like areas with large, polygonal cells with abundant eosinophilic cytoplasm, and multinucleated giant cells *(right)*.

Management and Prognosis

- Excision is the treatment of choice.

REFERENCES

Hammad HM, Hammond HL, Kurago ZB, Frank JA. Chondromyxoid fibroma of the jaws. Case report and review of the literature. *Oral Surg Oral Med Oral Pathol Oral Radiol Endod.* 1998;85:293-300.

Khatana S, Singh V, Gupta A. Unilocular anterior mandibular swelling. *Int J Pediatr Otorhinolaryngol.* 2013;77:964-971.

Konishi E, Nakashima Y, Iwasa Y, et al. Immunohistochemical analysis for Sox9 reveals the cartilaginous character of chondroblastoma and chondromyxoid fibroma of the bone. *Hum Pathol.* 2010;41:208-213.

Romeo S, Duim RA, Bridge JA, et al. Heterogeneous and complex rearrangements of chromosome arm 6q in chondromyxoid fibroma: delineation of breakpoints and analysis of candidate target genes. *Am J Pathol.* 2010;177:1365-1376.

Wu CT, Inwards CY, O'Laughlin S, et al. Chondromyxoid fibroma of bone: a clinicopathologic review of 278 cases. *Hum Pathol.* 1998;29:438-446.

CHONDROSARCOMA

Cartilaginous tumors within the jaw bones should be considered chondrosarcomas until proved otherwise because benign intraosseous chondroid tumors such as chondromas are extremely rare. They occur in the anterior maxilla and the condyles as a mass of mature hyaline cartilage. Multiple enchondromas (enchondromatosis) are present in Ollier disease; in Maffucci syndrome, enchondromatosis is associated with cutaneous hemangiomas. In soft tissues cartilaginous rests may be found in the nasopalatine area, within denture-related fibrous hyperplasia (Cutright tumor in epulis fissuratum), and within other neoplasms such as lipomas and pleomorphic adenomas.

Chondrosarcoma is the third most common malignant primary bone neoplasm in adults after myeloma and osteosarcoma and commonly involves the pelvic and long bones. Laryngotracheal and sinonasal tumors are more common than jaw tumors. Primary chondrosarcoma develops de novo, whereas secondary chondrosarcoma develops within a preexisting osteochondroma or enchondroma especially associated with Ollier and Maffucci syndromes.

Clinical Findings

- *Conventional chondrosarcoma:* This is most frequently diagnosed in the fourth decade (slightly younger than extragnathic tumors) with a slight male predilection. There is pain and swelling and the maxilla is affected three to four times more often than the mandible. There is a poorly demarcated destructive radiolucency, with most cases showing coarse calcifications.
- *Mesenchymal chondrosarcoma:* This is most frequently diagnosed in the second decade with the rib and jaw (25% of cases) being the two most common sites; one-third are extraosseous. It also presents with swelling and a poorly demarcated radiolucency usually within the mandible (Fig. 17.48).
- Twenty-five to thirty percent of patients with Ollier disease (enchondromatosis) and Maffucci syndrome (enchondromatosis and vascular lesions) develop chondrosarcoma.

Etiopathogenesis and Histopathologic Features

Mutations of *IDH/1/2* (61% of mutations) and *IDH2* (86% of mutations) are frequent in conventional chondrosarcoma but not in mesenchymal chondrosarcoma, whereas cancer fusion gene *HEY1-NCOA2* has been identified in mesenchymal chondrosarcomas.

The majority of chondrosarcomas are the conventional type, with mesenchymal chondrosarcoma being the second most common. Clear cell, periosteal, and dedifferentiated types are recognized.

- *Conventional chondrosarcoma:* There is a cellular and sometimes lobular proliferation of atypical chondrocytes with deposition of cartilage that permeates medullary spaces; chondrocytic atypia takes the form of binucleation and multinucleation, nuclear

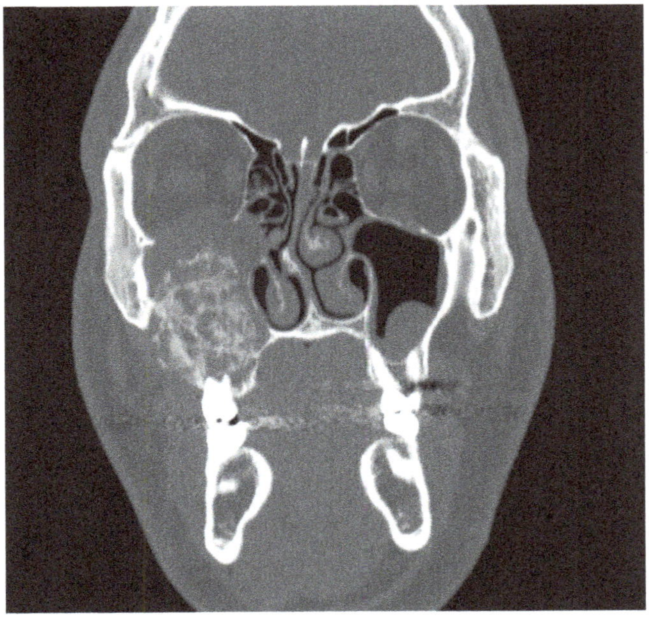

FIG 17.48 Mesenchymal chondrosarcoma. Coronal CT scan shows poorly defined, destructive mass with delicate calcifications of the right maxilla with involvement of the orbita floor. *(From Pellitteri PK, Ferlito A, Fagan JJ, et al: Mesenchymal chondrosarcoma of the head and neck. Oral Oncol. 2007;43:970–975.)*

pleomorphism, hyperchromatism, and more than one chondrocyte within a lacuna; dystrophic ossification is a common finding (Fig. 17.49); some tumors have a myxoid rather than hyaline cartilaginous stroma.

- Grading has prognostic implications: Grade 1 (least atypia): moderate cellularity and slightly atypical cells with occasional binucleation; Grade 2: more atypia and pleomorphism than Grade 1; Grade 3: markedly pleomorphic cells with many mitoses and necrosis.
- Tumor cells are S-100 protein, SOX9, glial fibrillary acidic protein (GFAP), and podoplanin (D2-40) positive, and CD44 is more highly expressed in higher grade tumors with an associated poorer prognosis.

- Clear cell chondrosarcoma is a variant of conventional chondrosarcoma and consists of cells with distinct nuclear membranes, clear cytoplasm, and central nuclei that are atypical; cells with abundant eosinophilic cytoplasm appearing chondroblastoma-like may be present, in addition to osteoclast-type giant cells.
- Dedifferentiated chondrosarcoma consists of a conventional chondrosarcoma with an apposed high grade neoplasm exhibiting pleomorphic or anaplastic spindle and epithelioid cells; it may also arise in an osteochondroma.

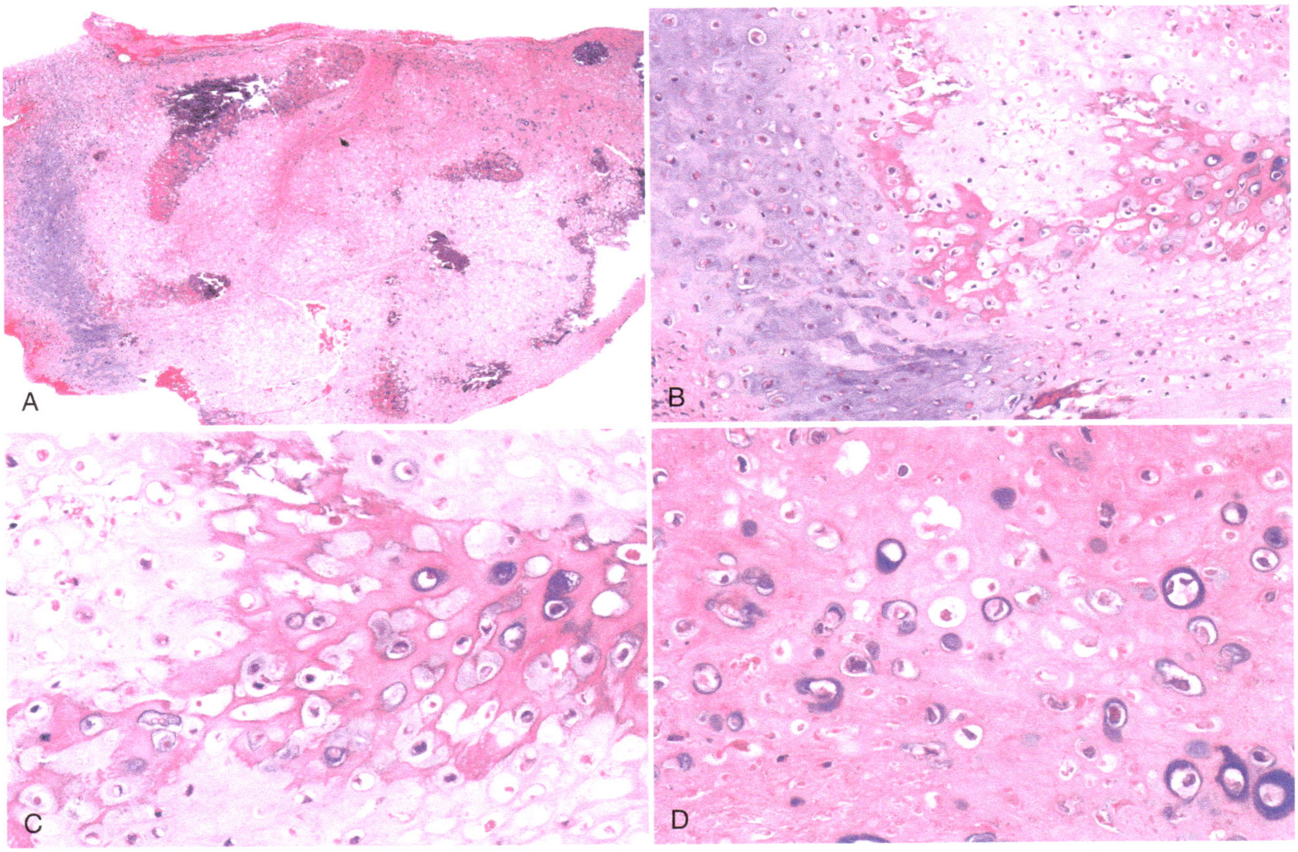

FIG 17.49 Chondrosarcoma, grade 1. (A) Sheets of cartilage with ossification. (B) Hyaline cartilage with ossification. (C) Ossified cartilage exhibiting atypical chondrocytes. (D) Atypical chondrocytes with binucleation and nuclear pleomorphism.

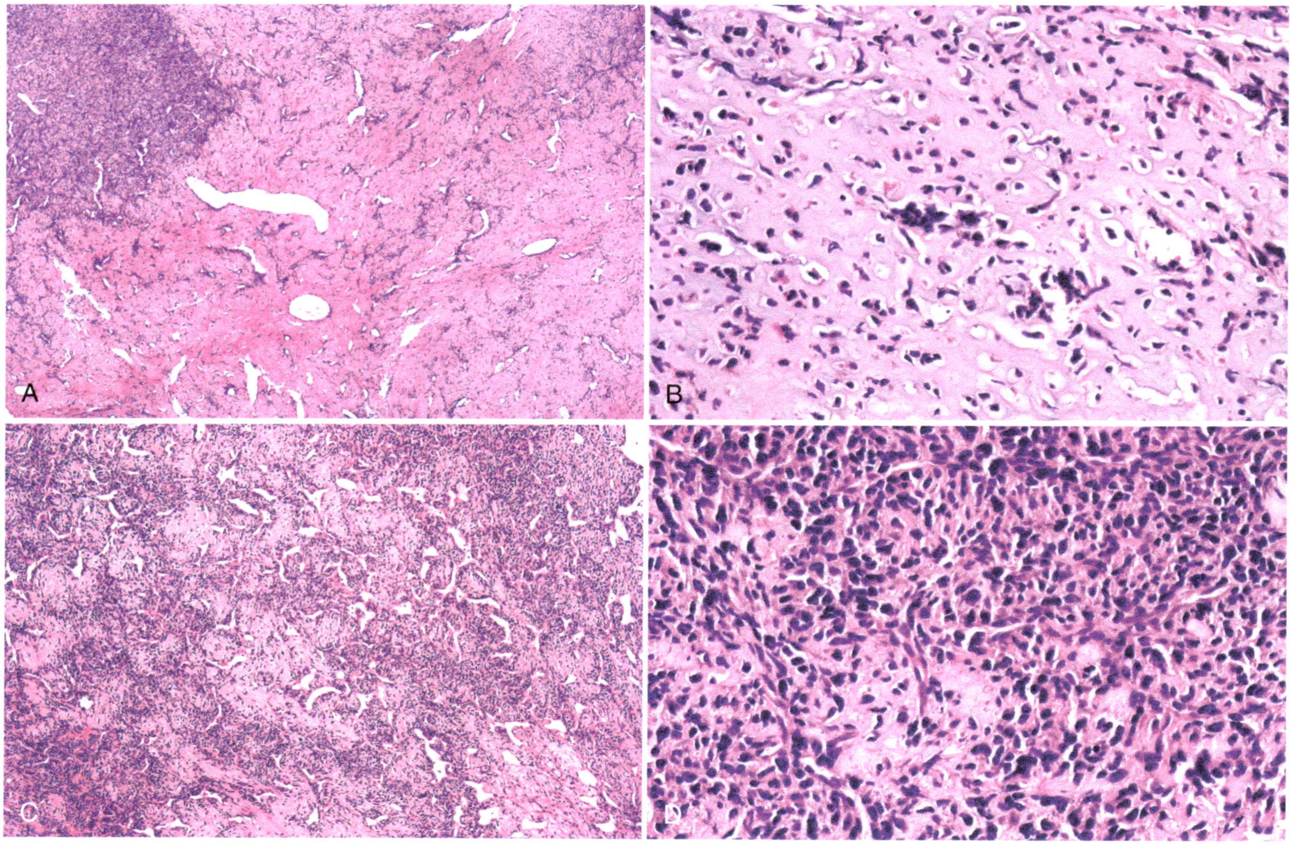

FIG 17.50 Mesenchymal chondrosarcoma. (A) Foci of small hyperchromatic cells juxtaposed with chondroid matrix with spindle cells and dilated vessels (hemangiopericytoma pattern). (B) Atypical chondrocytes with hyperchromatic and pleomorphic nuclei in chondroid matrix. (C) Hyperchromatic small cells clustered around dilated vessels. (D) Atypical small round cells with hyperchromatic nuclei.

- *Periosteal (juxtacortical) chondrosarcoma:* This consists of a conventional chondrosarcoma located on the periosteum.
- *Mesenchymal chondrosarcoma:* There is a biphasic pattern of recognizable chondrosarcoma containing atypical chondrocytes within hyaline cartilage, and a proliferation of small, darkly staining round or spindle cells; these latter cells have indistinct cytoplasmic outlines, scant cytoplasm (that is sometimes clear), and hyperchromatic round to ovoid nuclei. There are often dilated vessels conferring a hemangiopericytoma pattern (Fig. 17.50); foci of ossification are often present.
- The spindle and round cells are CD99+, S-100 protein+ only in the chondroid areas, and SOX9+ in both populations; type II collagen is present in 100% of the matrix.

Differential Diagnosis

- Chondroblastic osteosarcoma is SATB2+.
- The presence of cartilage (may need serial sections to locate this) in mesenchymal chondrosarcoma and of type II collagen rules out other small round cell tumors such as lymphoma, rhabdomyosarcoma, Ewing sarcoma, neuroblastoma, and malignant solitary fibrous tumor.
- Chondroid chordoma is keratin, EMA, S100 protein and vimentin positive, and podoplanin (D2-40) and GFAP negative; physaliferous cells typical for chordoma may be present.

Management and Prognosis

- Wide en bloc resection with or without adjuvant radiotherapy and chemotherapy is the recommended treatment, and the recurrence rate is 30% to 40% with metastases often to the lungs and death from disease.
- Grade 1 and combined grades 2 and 3 tumors have recurrence rates of 89% and 53%, respectively.
- Five-year survival is 85% to 95% for juxtacortical/periosteal lesions, 70% to 75% for conventional and myxoid tumors, 50% for mesenchymal subtypes, and less than 35% for dedifferentiated chondrosarcoma.

REFERENCES

Fletcher C, Unni K, Mertens F, eds. *World Health Organization Pathology and Genetics: Tumours of Soft Tissue and Bone.* 3rd ed. Lyon, France: IARC Press; 2006.

Gadwal SR, Fanburg-Smith JC, Gannon FH, Thompson LD. Primary chondrosarcoma of the head and neck in pediatric patients: a clinicopathologic study of 14 cases with a review of the literature. *Cancer.* 2000;88:2181-2188.

Giuffrida AY, Burgueno JE, Koniaris LG, et al. Chondrosarcoma in the United States (1973 to 2003): an analysis of 2890 cases from the SEER database. *J Bone Joint Surg Am.* 2009;91:1063-1072.

Heyse TJ, Malcherczyk D, Moll R, et al. CD44: survival and metastasis in chondrosarcoma. *Osteoarthritis Cartilage.* 2010;18:849-856.

Kerr DA, Lopez HU, Deshpande V, et al. Molecular distinction of chondrosarcoma from chondroblastic osteosarcoma through IDH1/2 mutations. *Am J Surg Pathol.* 2013;37:787-795.

Kim MJ, Cho KJ, Ayala AG, Ro JY. Chondrosarcoma: with updates on molecular genetics. *Sarcoma.* 2011;2011:405-437.

Knott PD, Gannon FH, Thompson LD. Mesenchymal chondrosarcoma of the sinonasal tract: a clinicopathological study of 13 cases with a review of the literature. *Laryngoscope.* 2003;113:783-790.

Koch BB, Karnell LH, Hoffman HT, et al. National cancer database report on chondrosarcoma of the head and neck. *Head Neck.* 2000;22:408-425.

Meijer D, de Jong D, Pansuriya TC, et al. Genetic characterization of mesenchymal, clear cell, and dedifferentiated chondrosarcoma. *Genes Chromosomes Cancer.* 2012;51:899-909.

Muller S, Soder S, Oliveira AM, et al. Type II collagen as specific marker for mesenchymal chondrosarcomas compared to other small cell sarcomas of the skeleton. *Mod Pathol.* 2005;18:1088-1094.

Pellitteri PK, Ferlito A, Fagan JJ, et al. Mesenchymal chondrosarcoma of the head and neck. *Oral Oncol.* 2007;43:970-975.

Pontes HA, Pontes FS, de Abreu MC, et al. Clinicopathological analysis of head and neck chondrosarcoma: three case reports and literature review. *Int J Oral Maxillofac Surg.* 2012;41:203-210.

Saito K, Unni KK, Wollan PC, Lund BA. Chondrosarcoma of the jaw and facial bones. *Cancer.* 1995;76:1550-1558.

Staals EL, Bacchini P, Bertoni F. Dedifferentiated central chondrosarcoma. *Cancer.* 2006;106:2682-2691.

Wang L, Motoi T, Khanin R, et al. Identification of a novel, recurrent HEY1-NCOA2 fusion in mesenchymal chondrosarcoma based on a genome-wide screen of exon-level expression data. *Genes Chromosomes Cancer.* 2012;51:127-139.

LANGERHANS CELL HISTIOCYTOSIS

This disease has diverse clinical manifestations ranging from a single lesion that may regress to severe multisystem involvement that may be fatal.

Clinical Findings

Approximately 60% to 70% of patients have restricted single-system disease, either unifocal or multifocal, affecting the bone, skin, and lymph nodes. Endocrine abnormalities such as diabetes insipidus or growth disorders are noted if the pituitary-hypothalamus axis is affected. The bones and skin are the two most common sites involved by multisystem disease and a patient with involvement of the liver, spleen, lungs, and bone marrow is designated MS^{RO+} (multisystem, risk-organ positive), which is associated with a worse prognosis. Single-system and multisystem disease are commonly seen in children with 50% to 70% presenting with multisystem disease, whereas single-system disease affects adults more often with involvement of bones (50% of cases), lungs (40% of cases), and skin (7% of cases). Pulmonary Langerhans cell histiocytosis in young adults in the third decade is a particular form of single-system disease that is associated with smoking, may regress with cessation of smoking, or may progress to end-stage pulmonary fibrosis.

- Over 80% of this condition occurs in children in the first and second decades of life and the jaw bones are the third most commonly affected site after the skull bones and the femur (the vertebrae is the second most common site in adults). The mandible is involved in 75% of cases and there is loosening of teeth in a localized area, pain and swelling. Radiographs show either a periapical radiolucency, "floating teeth" because of severe bone loss or a radiolucency unassociated with teeth (Fig. 17.51). Rarely lesions occur in soft tissue only.

Etiopathogenesis and Histopathologic Features

This is a neoplasm of Langerhans cells with a strong inflammatory component. Activating *BRAF, V600E,* and *MAP2K1* mutations have been identified in greater than 50% and 10% to 28% of cases, respectively.

- Sheets of epithelioid histiocyte-like cells are present with abundant, pale eosinophilic cytoplasm, and grooved or reniform ("coffee bean") nuclei; variable numbers of eosinophils are present (Fig. 17.52A–B); T cells, macrophages, and multinucleated giant cells are also often present.
- Cells are positive for S100 protein, CD1a (in a membranous pattern), and CD207 (langerin) (Fig. 17.52C); Birbeck granules (tennis racket–shaped pentilaminar bodies) are a typical ultrastructural finding, and langerin is an antibody directed against a transmembrane protein on the Birbeck granule, which is a subdomain of the endosomal recycling compartment (Fig. 17.52D).

Differential Diagnosis

- Traumatic ulcerative granuloma (eosinophilic granuloma of tongue) contains many CD68+ mononuclear cells and eosinophils, but does not contain Langerhans cells.
- Nonspecific macrophage-dense infiltrates in periapical lesions do not usually contain significant numbers of eosinophils and do not show positivity for markers for Langerhans cells.

Management and Prognosis

- Patients with apparently solitary jaw bone lesions should be evaluated for multifocal or multisystem disease, which is identified in close to 70% of adult patients.
- Curettage is often curative for solitary bone lesions; other treatments include indomethacin (bone lesions are often positive for prostaglandin E2), and intralesional methylprednisolone injections. Radiation and chemotherapy are modalities often employed for cranial bone sites at risk for central nervous system involvement. Recurrence for jaw bone lesions is 7%.
- Patients with multisystem disease are treated with chemotherapy such as methotrexate and vinblastine; in general, patients with MS^{RO+} disease who are refractory to the first six weeks of chemotherapy have a very poor prognosis.
- Because of the presence of activating mutations in *BRAF* and *MAP2K1,* new targeted therapies such as RAF and MEK1 inhibitors may be clinically useful.

REFERENCES

Abla O, Egeler RM, Weitzman S. Langerhans cell histiocytosis: current concepts and treatments. *Cancer Treat Rev.* 2010;36:354-359.

Annibali S, Cristalli MP, Solidani M, et al. Langerhans cell histiocytosis: oral/periodontal involvement in adult patients. *Oral Dis.* 2009;15:596-601.

Cantu MA, Lupo PJ, Bilgi M, et al. Optimal therapy for adults with Langerhans cell histiocytosis bone lesions. *PLoS ONE.* 2012;7:e43257.

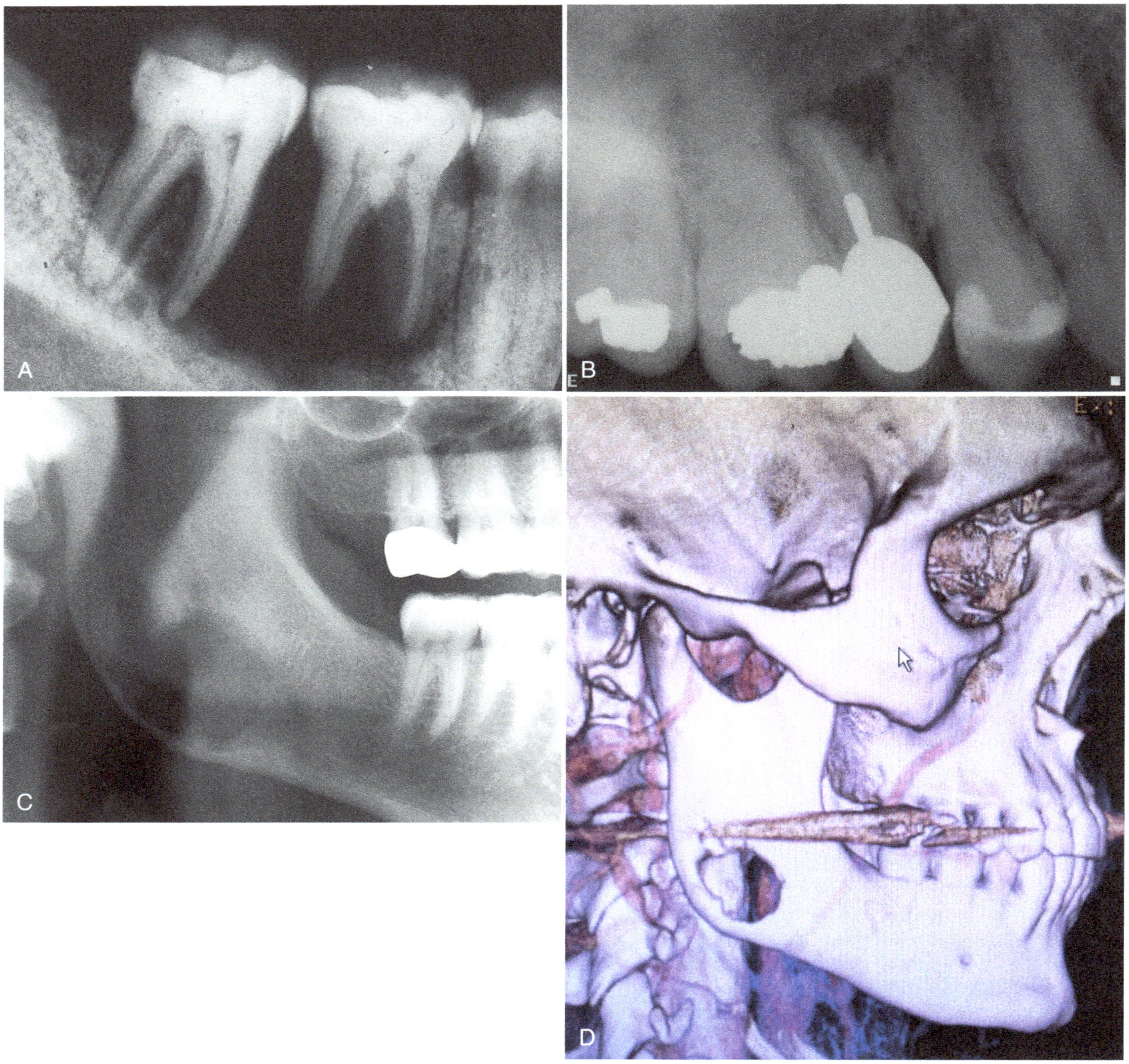

FIG 17.51 Langerhans cell histiocytosis. (A) Focal severe bone loss and radiolucency giving the impression of floating teeth. (B) Nondescript periapical radiolucency associated with endodontically treated right second maxillary premolar. (C) Solitary poorly demarcated radiolucency of the right angle of the mandible. (D) 3-D reconstruction of image C showing through-and-through perforation of the mandible. *(B, Courtesy Dr. Carlene Tsai, private practice, Salem, Mass. C and D, Courtesy Dr. Sam Diamantis, private practice, Lowell, Mass.)*

Cleveland DB, Goldberg KM, Greenspan JS, et al. Langerhans' cell histiocytosis: report of three cases with unusual oral soft tissue involvement. *Oral Surg Oral Med Oral Pathol Oral Radiol Endod.* 1996;82:541-548.

Eckardt A, Schultze A. Maxillofacial manifestations of Langerhans cell histiocytosis: a clinical and therapeutic analysis of 10 patients. *Oral Oncol.* 2003;39:687-694.

Favara BE, Feller AC, Pauli M, et al. Contemporary classification of histiocytic disorders. The WHO Committee on Histiocytic/Reticulum Cell Proliferations. Reclassification Working Group of the Histiocyte Society. *Med Pediatr Oncol.* 1997;29:157-166.

Putters TF, de Visscher JG, van Veen A, Spijkervet FK. Intralesional infiltration of corticosteroids in the treatment of localised langerhans' cell histiocytosis of the mandible Report of known cases and three new cases. *Int J Oral Maxillofac Surg.* 2005;34:571-575.

Rollins BJ. Genomic alterations in Langerhans cell histiocytosis. *Hematol Oncol Clin North Am.* 2015;29:839-851.

Satter EK, High WA. Langerhans cell histiocytosis: a review of the current recommendations of the Histiocyte Society. *Pediatr Dermatol.* 2008;25:291-295.

Windebank K, Nanduri V. Langerhans cell histiocytosis. *Arch Dis Child.* 2009;94:904-908.

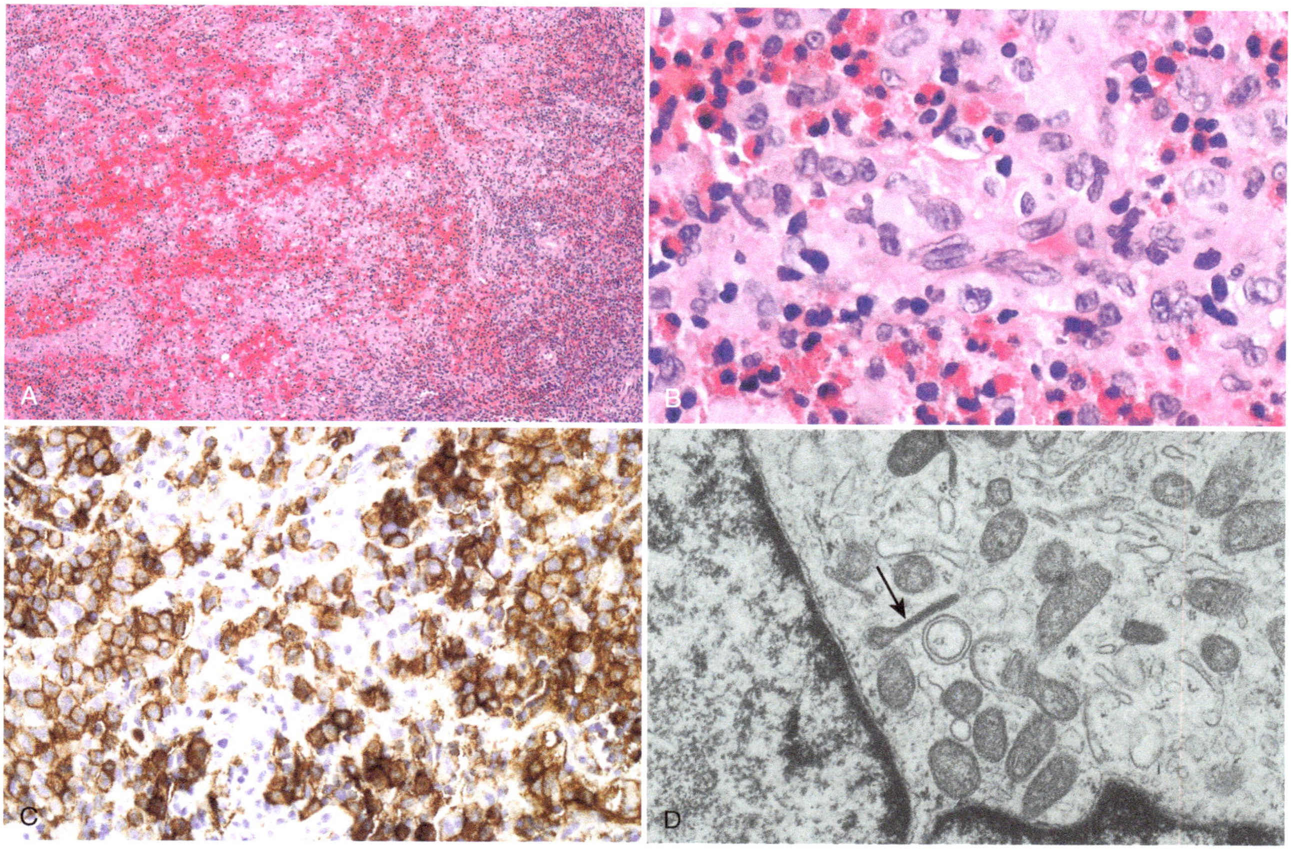

FIG 17.52 Langerhans cell histiocytosis. (A) Sheets of pale epithelioid cells. (B) Langerhans cells have abundant pale cytoplasm and grooved, reniform ("coffee bean") nuclei; many eosinophils are present. (C) Cells show membranous positivity for CD1a. (D) Birbeck granule is a racket-shaped pentilaminar body within the cytoplasm of histiocytes *(arrow)*.

EWING SARCOMA/PRIMITIVE NEUROECTODERMAL TUMOR

This aggressive sarcoma is the second most common bone tumor in children after osteosarcoma.

Clinical Findings

- It is seen most frequently in the second and third decades with a slight male predilection, often with pain and swelling; cortical perforation results in a visible soft tissue tumor (Fig. 17.53). It presents as a poorly delineated radiolucency usually in the mandible; extraskeletal tumors affecting the soft tissues have been reported and 20% of patients exhibit metastases at the time of diagnosis.

Etiopathogenesis and Histopathologic Features

Ewing sarcoma is characterized by a translocation that fuses *EWSR1* on chromosome 22q12 with *FLI1* on chromosome 11q24 forming *EWSR1-FLI1* in 85% to 90% of cases; in 10% of cases the fusion gene is *EWS-ERG*. The putative cell of origin is a multipotential mesenchymal stem cell induced to proliferate by such fusion gene products.

- This is a cellular tumor composed of sheets of fairly monotonous cells with indistinct cell borders, scant cytoplasm, and small round nuclei with dispersed, granular chromatin and inconspicuous nucleoli; a smaller population of cells with hyperchromatic nuclei likely represent cells undergoing apoptosis; necrosis is often present and mitotic figures and Homer-Wright rosettes may be seen (Fig. 17.54A–C).
- Cells often contain abundant glycogen that is periodic acid–Schiff positive and diastase labile, and there is membranous positivity for CD99 and nuclear positivity for FLI1 (Fig. 17.54D); 20% to 30% of tumor cells are positive for keratin.
- An adamantinomatous variant exhibits trabeculae of tumor cells with palisading of the peripheral tumor cells, focal keratin pearl formation, and prominent stroma fibrosis; in addition to being CD99+, the cells are positive for keratin, sometimes synaptophysin, and show diffuse nuclear positivity for p40.

Differential Diagnosis

- Many other small blue round cell tumors enter into the differential diagnosis such as lymphoma, neuroblastoma, and rhabdomyosarcoma; these are ruled

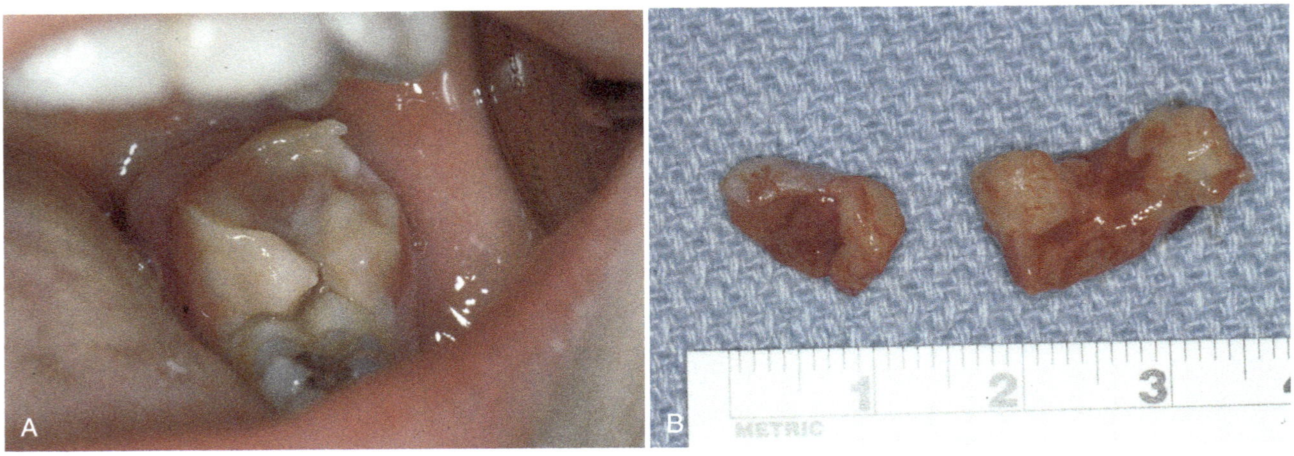

FIG 17.53 Ewing sarcoma. (A) Fleshy ulcerated mass growing out of the mandibular alveolus. (B) Tumor has a fleshy appearance (from patient shown in A).

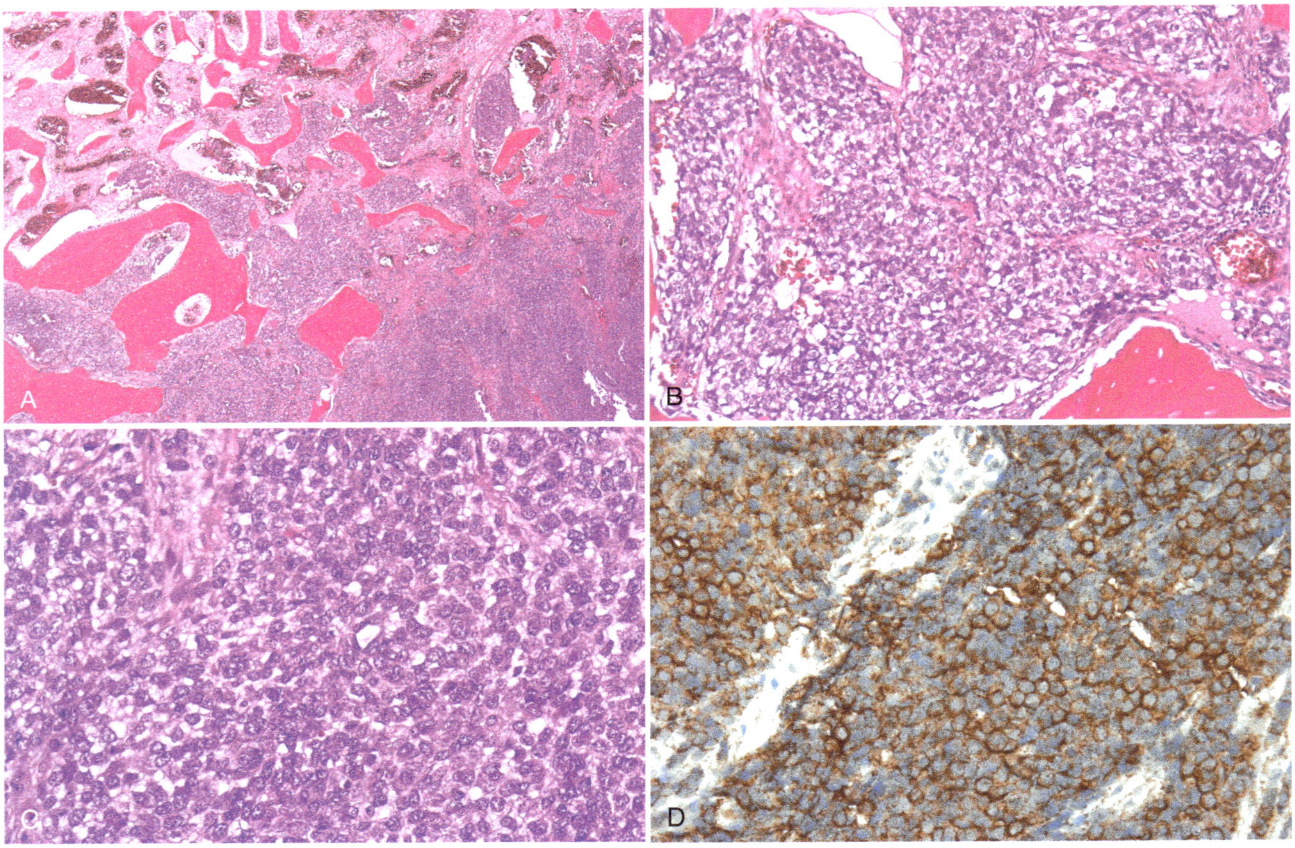

FIG 17.54 Ewing sarcoma. (A) Sheets of small round cells infiltrating bone trabeculae, some of which are fragments of sequestra. (B) Sheets of small round cells with pale to clear cytoplasm. (C) Small cells with pale to clear cytoplasm and round nuclei with dispersed, granular chromatin and inconspicuous nucleoli. (D) Membranous staining of tumor cells with CD99.

out with immunohistochemical, polymerase chain reaction, and fluorescent in situ hybridization studies.

Management and Prognosis

- Local disease is treated with wide resection and/or radiation; neoadjuvant and adjuvant multiagent chemotherapy help to control metastases; 5-year survival is 55% to 65% for localized disease and 20% to 30% for metastatic disease.
- Poor prognostic indicators are large tumor volume, presence of metastases at the time of biopsy, and the presence of greater than 10% of viable tumor cells in the resection specimen postchemotherapy.

REFERENCES

Bishop JA, Alaggio R, Zhang L, et al. Adamantinoma-like Ewing family tumors of the head and neck: a pitfall in the differential diagnosis of basaloid and myoepithelial carcinomas. *Am J Surg Pathol.* 2015;39: 1267-1274.

Gaspar N, Hawkins DS, Dirksen U, et al. Ewing sarcoma: current management and future approaches through collaboration. *J Clin Oncol.* 2015;33:3036-3046.

Gu M, Antonescu CR, Guiter G, et al. Cytokeratin immunoreactivity in Ewing's sarcoma: prevalence in 50 cases confirmed by molecular diagnostic studies. *Am J Surg Pathol.* 2000;24:410-416.

Hafezi S, Seethala RR, Stelow EB, et al. Ewing's family of tumors of the sinonasal tract and maxillary bone. *Head Neck Pathol.* 2011;5:8-16.

Karimi A, Shirinbak I, Beshkar M, et al. Ewing sarcoma of the jaws. *J Craniofac Surg.* 2011;22:1657-1660.

Tsokos M, Alaggio RD, Dehner LP, Dickman PS. Ewing sarcoma/ peripheral primitive neuroectodermal tumor and related tumors. *Pediatr Dev Pathol.* 2012;15:108-126.

18 HEMATOLYMPHOID TUMORS OF THE ORAL CAVITY

Elizabeth A. Morgan and Olga K. Weinberg

CHAPTER CONTENTS

Non-Hodgkin lymphoma (NHL) is the second most common malignancy to arise in the oral cavity after squamous cell carcinoma, yet only accounts for 3.5% of all oral cavity malignancies. Among all lymphomas, oral cavity NHLs are rare, representing approximately 2% of all extranodal lymphomas. Most patients are older although immunosuppressed patients may be of a younger age. Patients often have presenting symptoms clinically of a discrete mass, sometimes ulcerated, with loosening of teeth, and pain, dysesthesia, or paresthesia. The most commonly affected sites are the palatal mucosa, gingiva, tongue, buccal mucosa, and floor of mouth; many cases (almost half in some studies) exhibit underlying bone involvement (Fig. 18.1). Diffuse large B-cell lymphoma is the most common subtype with frequencies ranging from 50% to 68%. Immunosuppressed patients, particularly patients with HIV infection, often develop a distinctive type of this lymphoma known as plasmablastic lymphoma, which was first described in the oral cavity. The majority of other oral cavity NHLs fall into the category of mature B-cell NHLs such as follicular lymphoma and marginal zone lymphoma; T-cell NHLs are infrequent and only extranodal NK/T-cell lymphoma, nasal type will be discussed briefly. In certain geographic locations, Burkitt lymphoma shows a predilection for facial structures, including the jaw.

The term "plasma cell neoplasm" refers to clonal expansions of malignant plasma cells and includes diseases primarily affecting the bone marrow such as multiple myeloma, solitary plasmacytoma in bone, or plasmacytoma arising in extramedullary sites, which may or may not subsequently develop into systemic multiple myeloma. Approximately 14% of patients with multiple myeloma have an oral manifestation. The head and neck region is the most common site of involvement of extramedullary plasmacytomas, including oral cavity lesions.

Finally, acute myeloid leukemia may infrequently manifest as diffuse gingival infiltrates of blasts or discrete tumor masses within the oral cavity. This may be the presenting manifestation of the leukemia, may occur during the course of disease or at relapse, or may represent the first sign of transformation from an underlying myelodysplastic or myeloproliferative neoplasm. This phenomenon is most commonly associated with acute myeloid leukemia exhibiting monocytic or myelomonocyticdifferentiation.

DIFFUSE LARGE B-CELL LYMPHOMA

Diffuse large B-cell lymphoma (DLBCL) comprises 30% to 40% of adult NHL in Western countries and a higher percentage in developing countries. Up to 40% of DLBCLs present in extranodal sites, and it is the most common type of oral cavity NHL. It usually represents a de novo process but can transform from an underlying low-grade lymphoma. Gene expression profiling has identified two distinct molecular subtypes termed germinal center B-cell (GCB) and activated B-cell (ABC) types with different prognoses. Many of the oral DLBCLs tend to be the non-GCB type.

Clinical Findings

- This occurs in the sixth and seventh decades, but may also be seen in younger adults.
- Lesions present as an enlarging painless mass, frequently occur on the palatal mucosa, and may be ulcerated and painful.

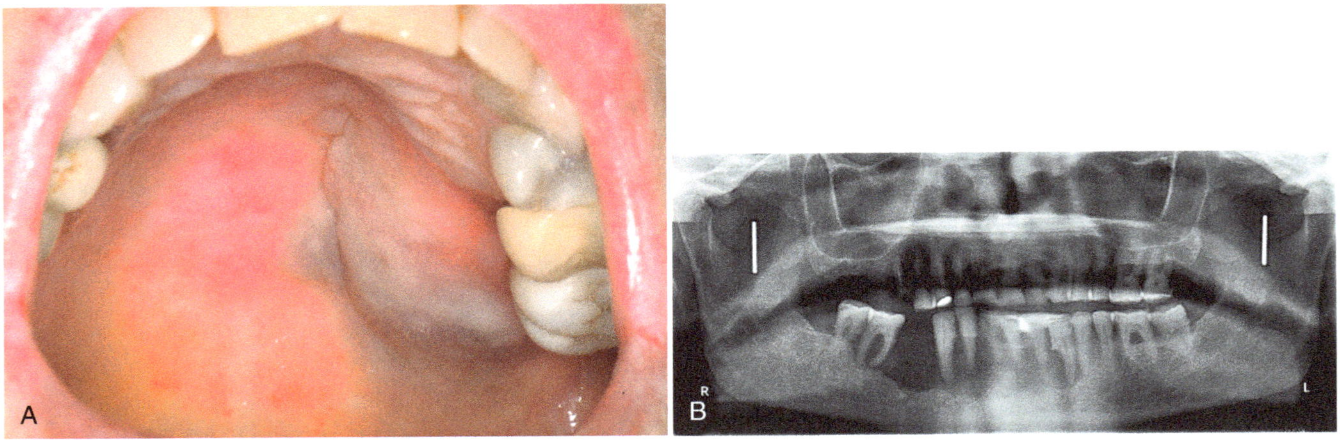

FIG 18.1 (A) Lymphoma of the palatal mucosa presenting as a diffuse swelling. (B) Lymphoma of the right mandible presenting as a poorly demarcated radiolucency extending from the left mandibular canine to the right molars; a nonhealing socket developed after extraction of the loose right first molar.

- B symptoms (fever, weight loss, and night sweats) are uncommon.

Histopathologic Features

- There is a diffuse proliferation of large lymphoid cells effacing underlying tissue architecture; multiple morphologic variants may be seen, including centroblastic (large cells with moderate amounts of cytoplasm, and large, open nuclei with multiple peripheral nucleoli), immunoblastic (large cells with abundant amphophilic cytoplasm, and large nuclei with large central nucleoli), and anaplastic; areas of frank necrosis may be present (Fig. 18.2A–B).
- Lesional cells express B-cell markers CD19, CD20, and PAX5 (Fig. 18.2C); monotypic surface immunoglobulin light chain expression may be detected by flow cytometry.
- The expression of CD10, BCL6, and MUM1 varies depending on subtype (GCB versus ABC) (Fig. 18.2D); several immunohistochemistry-based algorithms have been developed as a tool for assigning subtype.
- In situ hybridization for Epstein-Barr virus (EBV)–encoded RNA (EBER) may be positive in some cases, particularly in older patients; however, EBER reactivity is not common and should prompt evaluation for lesions outlined in the Differential Diagnosis section later.
- The proliferation index is variable and may be moderate to as high as 90% (Fig. 18.2E).

Differential Diagnosis

- *Burkitt lymphoma:* There is a monotonous infiltrate of intermediate-sized B cells in a background of numerous macrophages containing cytoplasmic particles of cellular debris ("tingible-body macrophages"), which imparts a moth-eaten appearance at low-power known as a "starry-sky" pattern; cells express CD10 and lack BCL2; the proliferation index is greater than 95%; endemic cases in particular may show reactivity for EBER; *MYC* translocation is detected (typically t(8;14)(q24;q32)) without concurrent *BCL2* or *BCL6* translocation.
- *Plasmablastic lymphoma:* Cells are uniformly positive for CD138 and EBER and negative for CD20; oral lesions are most commonly seen in the setting of immunosuppression such as HIV/AIDS.
- *EBV-positive mucocutaneous ulcer:* This ulcer contains cells that exhibit Hodgkin-like features in a polymorphous inflammatory background with strong expression of CD30 and EBER, and weak expression of CD20; it typically occurs in older patients, is self-limited, and runs an indolent course (see Chapter 4).
- *Myeloid sarcoma (acute myeloid leukemia):* Given the morphologic overlap between the two entities, immunophenotyping is essential to confirm the B-cell origin of the infiltrate.
- *Extranodal NK/T-cell lymphoma, nasal type:* This lymphoma tends to occur in those living in East Asia and South and Central America; a presenting symptom is an ulcerated, necrotic mass in the nasal and nasopharyngeal mucosa, and oral sites include Waldeyer ring and the palatal mucosa presenting as midline destructive disease; there is an infiltrate of large, irregular lymphoid cells with angiodestruction and abundant necrosis/apoptosis, and there is a high proliferation index; cells are typically positive for CD3 in a cytoplasmic pattern (but negative for surface CD3 by flow cytometry), CD2, CD56, and EBER, and negative for T-cell antigens CD5, CD4, and CD8; cells are also often positive for granzyme B and/or TIA-1.

Management and Prognosis

- High-grade B-cell lymphoma, with *MYC* and *BCL2* and/or *BCL6* rearrangements: Cases falling into this category are also known as "double-" or "triple-hit" lymphomas because they show a *MYC* rearrangement as well as *BCL2* and/or *BCL6* rearrangements. Cases that morphologically resemble DLBCL but show these genetic changes are placed into this category.
- DLBCLs are aggressive but potentially curable with multiagent chemotherapy.
- Multivariable analysis of patients with oral and maxillofacial DLBCL show age, clinical stage, and performance status to be significant prognostic factors.

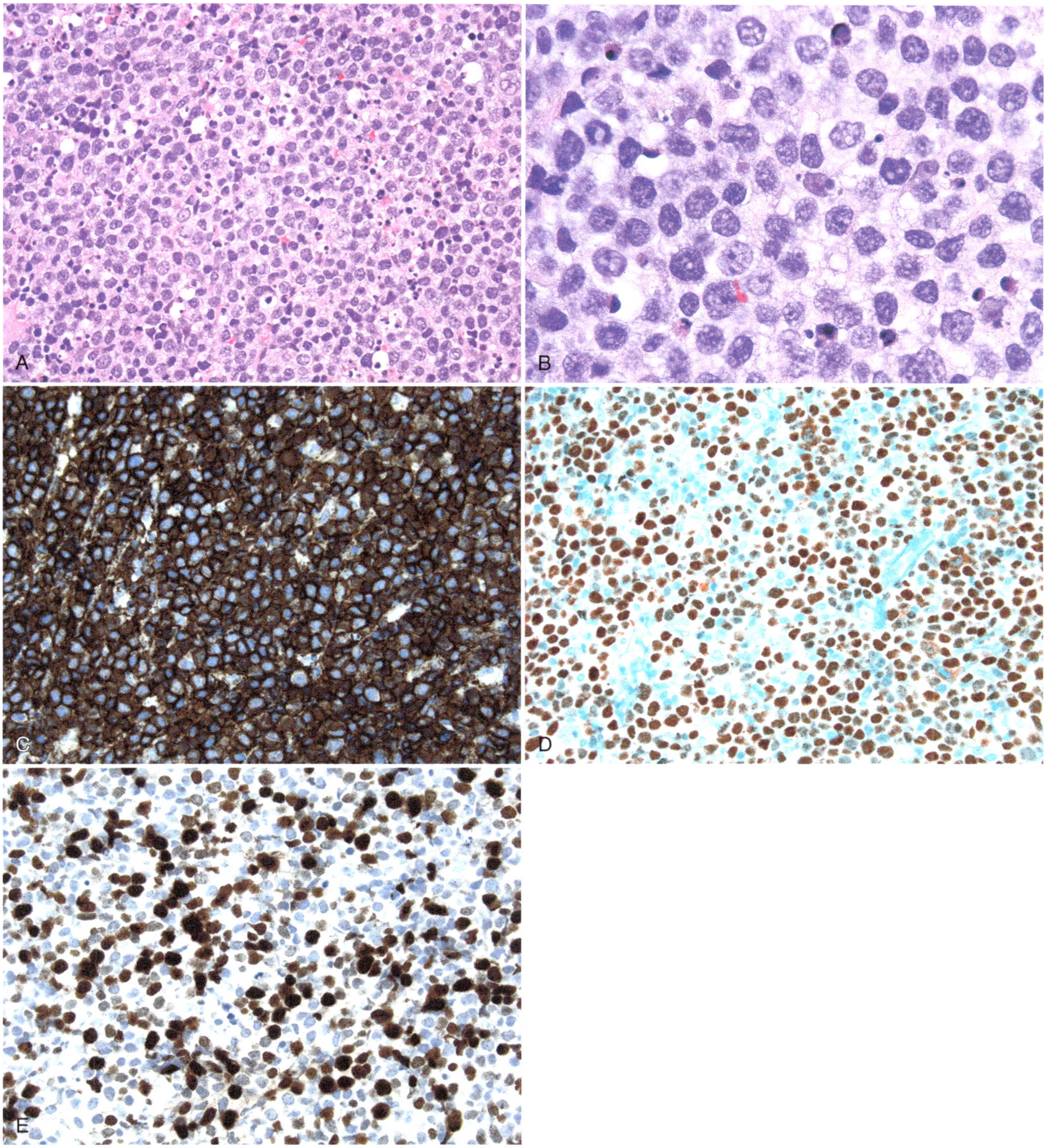

FIG 18.2 Diffuse large B-cell lymphoma (DLBCL). (A) The infiltrate exhibits a diffuse pattern of growth with effacement of underlying tissue architecture. (B) Higher magnification reveals that the tumor cells are large in size with round nuclei and variably distinct nucleoli. (C) The lymphoid cells are shown to be of B-cell origin by diffuse reactivity for CD20. (D) BCL6 may be strongly positive in tumor cell nuclei, as in this case. (E) The Ki67 proliferation index is variable among different cases of DLBCL; in this example approximately 40% of tumor cell nuclei are reactive.

REFERENCES

Alizadeh AA, Eisen MB, Davis RE, et al. Distinct types of diffuse large B-cell lymphoma identified by gene expression profiling. *Nature.* 2000;403:503-511.

Bhattacharyya I, Chehal HK, Cohen DM, Al-Quran SZ. Primary diffuse large B-cell lymphoma of the oral cavity: Germinal center classification. *Head Neck Pathol.* 2010;4:181-191.

Dojcinov SD, Venkataraman G, Pittaluga S, et al. Age-related EBV-associated lymphoproliferative disorders in the western population: A spectrum of reactive lymphoid hyperplasia and lymphoma. *Blood.* 2011;117:4726-4735.

Dojcinov SD, Venkataraman G, Raffeld M, et al. EBV positive mucocutaneous ulcer–a study of 26 cases associated with various sources of immunosuppression. *Am J Surg Pathol.* 2010;34:405-417.

Freeman C, Berg JW, Cutler SJ. Occurrence and prognosis of extranodal lymphomas. *Cancer.* 1972;29:252-260.

Friedberg JW. Double-hit diffuse large B-cell lymphoma. *J Clin Oncol.* 2012;30:3439-3443.

Guevara-Canales JO, Morales-Vadillo R, Cava-Vergiu CE, et al. Survival in patients with oral and maxillofacial diffuse large B-cell lymphoma. *Braz Oral Res.* 2013;27:349-355.

Guevara-Canales JO, Morales-Vadillo R, Sacsaquispe-Contreras SJ, et al. Malignant lymphoma of the oral cavity and the maxillofacial region: overall survival prognostic factors. *Med Oral Patol Oral Cir Bucal.* 2013;18:e619-e626.

Hans CP, Weisenburger DD, Greiner TC, et al. Confirmation of the molecular classification of diffuse large B-cell lymphoma by immunohistochemistry using a tissue microarray. *Blood.* 2004;103:275-282.

Kolokotronis A, Konstantinou N, Christakis I, et al. Localized B-cell non-Hodgkin's lymphoma of oral cavity and maxillofacial region: a clinical study. *Oral Surg Oral Med Oral Pathol Oral Radiol Endod.* 2005;99:303-310.

Owosho AA, Bilodeau EA, Surti U, Craig FE. Large B-cell lymphoma of the base of the tongue and oral cavity: A practical approach to identifying prognostically important subtypes. *Oral Surg Oral Med Oral Pathol Oral Radiol.* 2014;118:338-347.

Sehn LH, Gascoyne RD. Diffuse large B-cell lymphoma: Optimizing outcome in the context of clinical and biologic heterogeneity. *Blood.* 2015;125:22-32.

PLASMABLASTIC LYMPHOMA

Plasmablastic lymphoma (PBL) is an aggressive variant of DLBCL originally described in the HIV-positive population. In initial reports, the majority of the patients presented with oral lesions. Subsequent reports have demonstrated that PBL can also rarely occur in the HIV-negative population, most commonly in the setting of immunosuppression such as posttransplantation. In the HIV-negative setting, PBL frequently arises in an extraoral location.

Clinical Findings

- PBL involving the oral cavity typically presents as a lesion of the gingiva or palatal mucosa, similar to other oral lymphomas; secondary bony involvement is uncommon.
- Approximately 50% of patients present with advanced stage disease, although only a third demonstrate bone marrow involvement.
- The presence of B symptoms is variable.

Histopathologic Features

- There is a diffuse proliferation of large lymphoid cells with variable appearance; some show typical immunoblastic features with prominent central nucleoli, whereas others resemble mature plasma cells or exhibit plasmablastic features (namely vesicular chromatin, prominent nucleoli, and eccentrically placed nuclei) (Figs. 18.3A–C); there is a background of numerous apoptotic bodies and tingible-body macrophages.
- Lesional cells express plasma cell markers including CD138, CD38, and MUM1; CD30 and EMA are frequently positive; cells are mostly negative for, or show weak expression of, CD45 and B-cell markers such as CD20 and PAX5; monotypic cytoplasmic immunoglobulin light chain is detected in 50% to 70% of cases; Ki67 proliferation index is usually very high (>90%); HHV8 and BCL6 are negative.
- EBER is positive in almost all of the HIV-associated oral lesions, and in approximately 50% of the lesions occurring in the HIV-negative setting (Fig. 18.3D).
- CD56 expression is more common in cases associated with HIV than in HIV-negative cases.

Differential Diagnosis

- *Anaplastic (plasmablastic) plasmacytoma:* Correlation with clinical findings is essential; EBER-positivity favors PBL, although rare cases of EBV-positive plasmacytoma in immunocompetent patients have been reported.
- *Burkitt lymphoma:* Shared features include EBER-positivity, high proliferation index, and tingible-body macrophages; unlike PBL, BL cells are intermediate in size without plasmacytoid features and are strongly positive for CD45, CD20, and BCL6.
- *Diffuse large B-cell lymphoma:* Unlike PBL, DLBCL will show strong expression of CD45 and CD20 and typically a lower proliferation index.

Management and Prognosis

- Most are treated with multiagent chemotherapy, but PBL is an aggressive tumor and many patients die within the first year.
- In one study, univariate analysis showed older age (60 years or older), advanced stage/bone marrow involvement, high Ki67 proliferation index (>80%), and HIV-negative status were associated with worse overall survival.

REFERENCES

Boy SC, van Heerden MB, Raubenheimer EJ, van Heerden WF. Plasmablastic lymphomas with light chain restriction - plasmablastic extramedullary plasmacytomas? *J Oral Pathol Med.* 2010;39:435-439.

Castillo JJ, Winer ES, Stachurski D, et al. Clinical and pathological differences between human immunodeficiency virus-positive and human immunodeficiency virus-negative patients with plasmablastic lymphoma. *Leuk Lymphoma.* 2010;51:2047-2053.

Castillo J, Pantanowitz L, Dezube BJ. HIV-associated plasmablastic lymphoma: lessons learned from 112 published cases. *Am J Hematol.* 2008;83:804-809.

Delecluse HJ, Anagnostopoulos I, Dallenbach F, et al. Plasmablastic lymphomas of the oral cavity: A new entity associated with the human immunodeficiency virus infection. *Blood.* 1997;89:1413-1420.

Gaidano G, Cerri M, Capello D, et al. Molecular histogenesis of plasmablastic lymphoma of the oral cavity. *Br J Haematol.* 2002;119:622-628.

Guan B, Zhang X, Hu W, et al. Plasmablastic lymphoma of the oral cavity in an HIV-negative patient. *Ann Diagn Pathol.* 2011;15:436-440.

Hansra D, Montague N, Stefanovic A, et al. Oral and extraoral plasmablastic lymphoma: similarities and differences in clinicopathologic characteristics. *Am J Clin Pathol.* 2010;134:710-719.

Loghavi S, Khoury JD, Medeiros LJ. Epstein-Barr virus-positive plasmacytoma in immunocompetent patients. *Histopathology.* 2015;67:225-234.

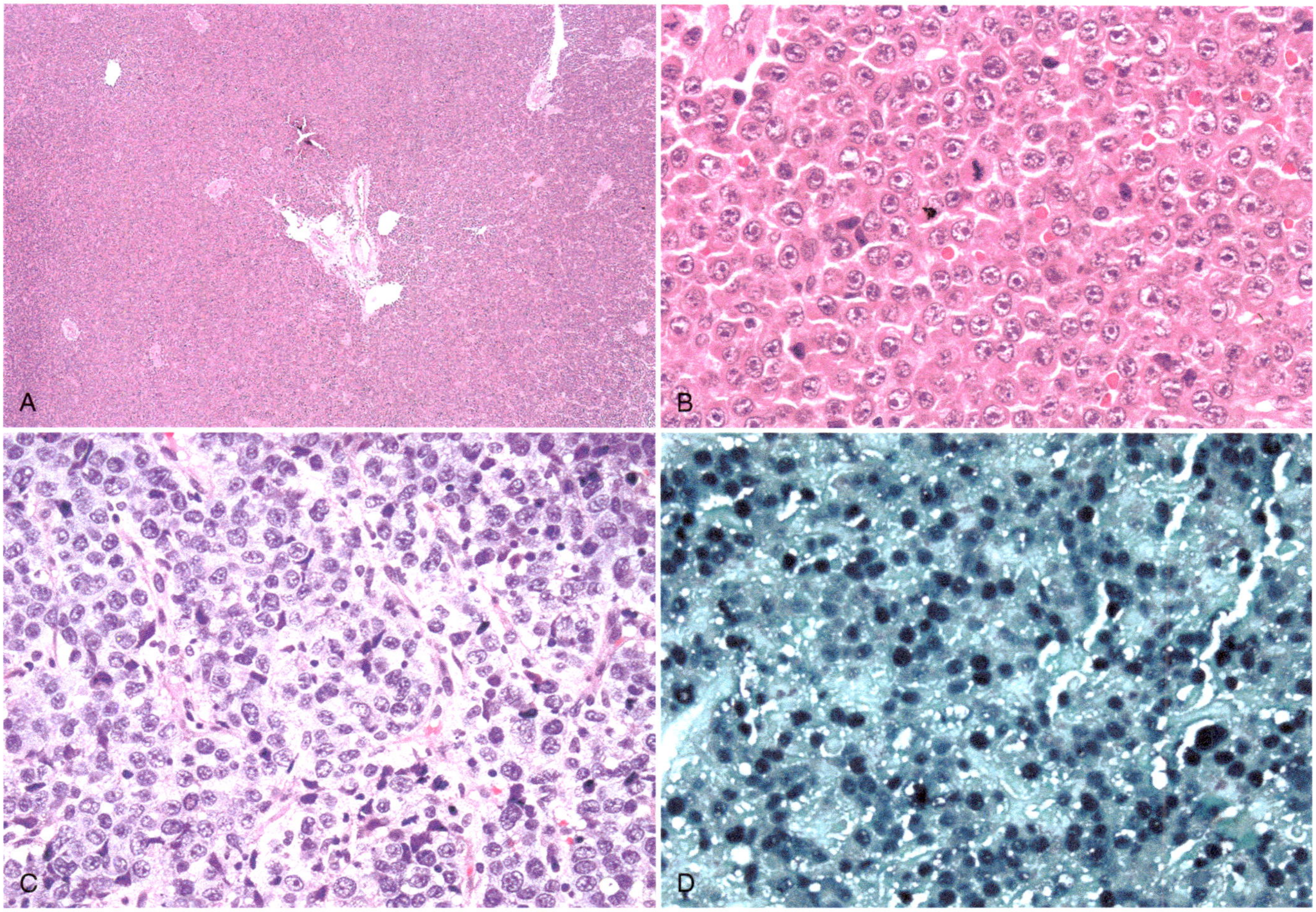

FIG 18.3 Plasmablastic lymphoma (PBL). (A) Low-power view shows diffuse infiltration with near-complete destruction of the underlying tissue. (B) Some cases of PBL show plasmacytic features including eccentrically placed nuclei, variably prominent nucleoli, and abundant cytoplasm. Frequent mitotic figures are seen in this highly proliferative tumor. (C) Other cases of PBL do not show plasmacytic features but instead consist of diffuse sheets of large-sized cells with irregular nuclei, distinct nucleoli, and a high nuclear:cytoplasmic ratio. (D) EBER in situ hybridization is positive in most cases of HIV-associated PBL.

Kane S, Khurana A, Parulkar G, et al. Minimum diagnostic criteria for plasmablastic lymphoma of oral/sinonasal region encountered in a tertiary cancer hospital of a developing country. *J Oral Pathol Med.* 2009;38:138-144.

Rafaniello Raviele P, Pruneri G, Maiorano E. Plasmablastic lymphoma: A review. *Oral Dis.* 2009;15:38-45.

Tsachouridou O, Christoforidou A, Metallidis S, et al. Plasmablastic lymphoma of the oral cavity, a B cell-derived lymphoma associated with HIV infection: a case series. *Eur Arch Otorhinolaryngol.* 2012;269:1713-1719.

Vega F, Chang CC, Medeiros LJ, et al. Plasmablastic lymphomas and plasmablastic plasma cell myelomas have nearly identical immunophenotypic profiles. *Mod Pathol.* 2005;18:806-815.

FOLLICULAR LYMPHOMA

Follicular lymphoma (FL) accounts for 20% of all lymphomas and predominantly occurs in adults with a median age greater than 50 years. Most adults show symptoms of widespread disease but 10% to 20% have a localized stage I or II disease at initial diagnosis. FL primarily involves lymph nodes, although the spleen and bone marrow may also be involved. Fewer than 10% of all FLs show extranodal involvement with common sites including gastrointestinal tract, skin, head and neck, breast, and testis. Oral cavity involvement is rare, and FL is estimated to account for 8.7% to 15% of all oral NHL.

Clinical Findings

- In the oral cavity, the mean age of presentation is in the eighth decade with a 3:1 male predominance; most cases involve the palatal mucosa (75% of cases).
- Most lesions are low-grade at presentation.

Histopathologic Features

- Most cases of FL have a predominantly follicular pattern with back-to-back follicles that replace the nodal architecture (Fig. 18.4A); the abnormal follicles exhibit attenuated mantle zones and are composed of a mixture of centrocytes (lymphoid cells with cleaved nuclei and condensed chromatin) and centroblasts.
- CD21 highlights the follicular dendritic cell (FDC) meshwork underlying neoplastic follicles (Fig. 18.4B); diffuse areas demonstrate an absence of CD21 expression.

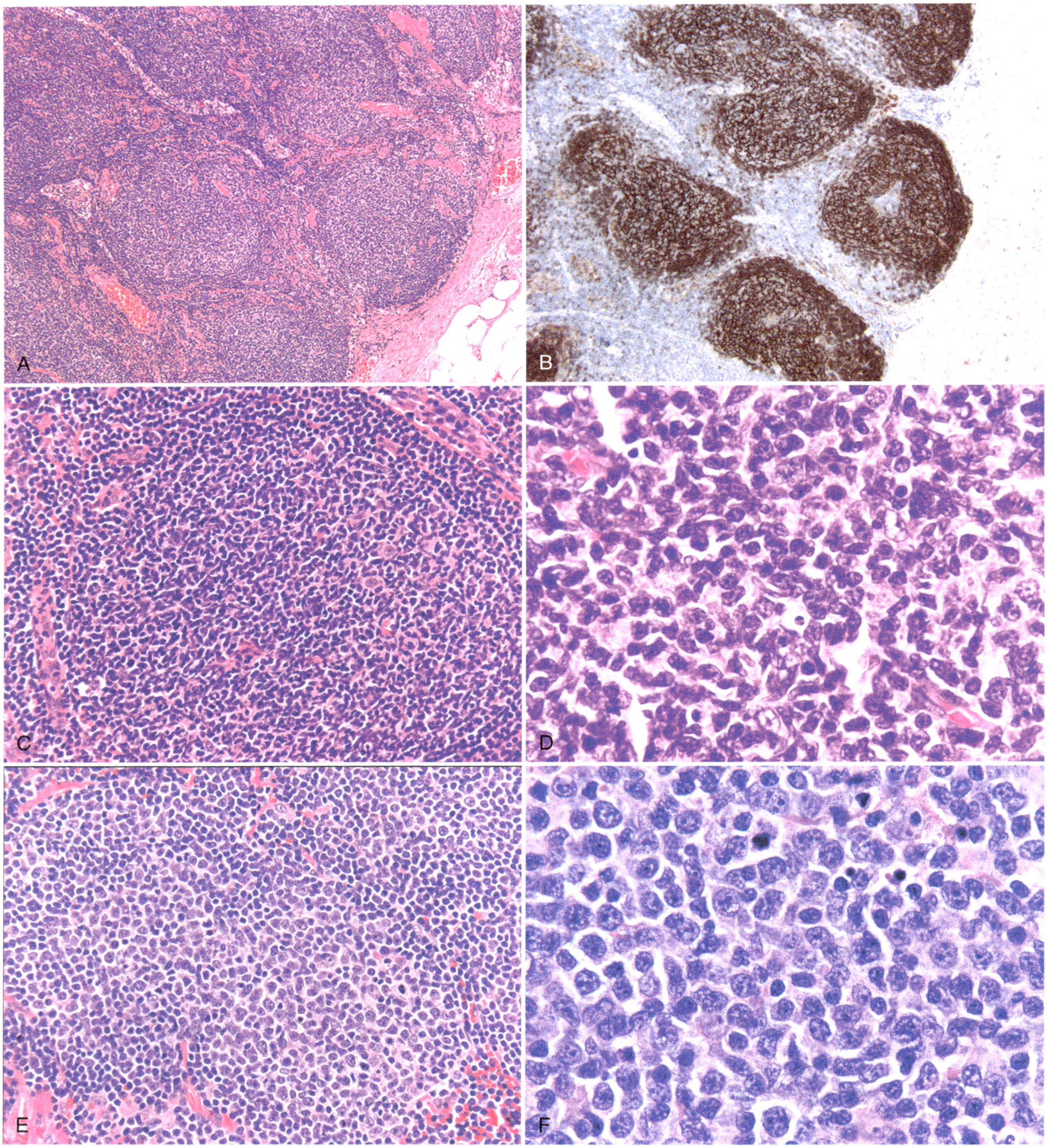

FIG 18.4 Follicular lymphoma (FL). (A) Low-power view shows the well-circumscribed nodules characteristic of FL. (B) CD21 highlights the follicular dendritic cell meshworks underlying the nodules in this case, revealing a follicular growth pattern; an absence of CD21 reactivity in an area with lesional B-cells would signify a diffuse pattern of growth. (C) The nodules of low-grade FL are composed of cleaved centrocytes in contrast to the small round lymphocytes in the surrounding mantle zone. (D) Centrocytes are cleaved (elongated) cells with condensed chromatin. (E) High-grade FL is diagnosed when there are greater than 15 centroblasts per high-powered field, as seen in this case. (F) Centroblasts are larger cells with round to ovoid nuclei, open chromatin, and distinct nucleoli.

- Grading of follicular lymphoma is based on the number of centroblasts present in neoplastic follicles: grade 1 = 0–5 centroblasts/high-powered field (hpf) (Fig. 18.4C–D); grade 2 = 6–15 centroblasts/hpf; grade 3 = greater than 15 centroblasts/hpf (Fig. 18.4E–F); grade 3 is subdivided into grade 3A (admixed centrocytes and centroblasts) and grade 3B (sheets of centroblasts); diffuse areas may be present as defined by an absence of underlying FDC meshworks; if grade 3 cytology is present in an architecturally diffuse area, this should be classified as DLBCL.
- Lesional B cells express the B-cell markers CD19, CD20, and PAX5, and show coexpression of BCL2, BCL6, and CD10.
- Grade 3 FL can be CD10– and lack BCL2 expression.
- Monotypic surface immunoglobulin light chain expression is detected by flow cytometry.
- The majority of FLs show a characteristic *IGH-BCL2* translocation: t(14;18)(q32;q21).

Differential Diagnosis

- *Reactive follicular hyperplasia:* Reactive follicles will show well-defined mantle zones and admixed tingible-body macrophages; germinal center cells will not coexpress BCL2, and molecular analysis will show a polyclonal pattern of immunoglobulin heavy chain gene rearrangements.
- *Marginal zone lymphoma:* May show reactive follicles reminiscent of FL nodules, but the follicles in marginal zone lymphoma demonstrate reactive features as described above and are usually a minor component of the lesion; the majority of the marginal zone lymphoma infiltrate consists of neoplastic B cells in the interfollicular space.

Management and Prognosis

- Prognosis of FL is related to the extent of disease present at diagnosis; histologic grade also correlates with grade 1–2 cases being more indolent (but not curable), whereas grade 3 shows a more aggressive course.
- Localized lesions may be treated with radiation, systemic disease may warrant chemotherapy, and these regimens will differ depending on grade.

REFERENCES

Argyris PP, Dolan M, Piperi E, et al. Oral follicular lymphomas. A short report of 8 cases with assessment of the IGH/BCL2 gene fusion with fluorescence in situ hybridization. *Oral Surg Oral Med Oral Pathol Oral Radiol.* 2013;116:343-347.

Bosga-Bouwer AG, van den Berg A, Haralambieva E, et al. Molecular, cytogenetic, and immunophenotypic characterization of follicular lymphoma grade 3B; a separate entity or part of the spectrum of diffuse large B-cell lymphoma or follicular lymphoma? *Hum Pathol.* 2006;37:528-533.

Freedman A. Follicular lymphoma: 2014 update on diagnosis and management. *Am J Hematol.* 2014;89:429-436.

Kemp S, Gallagher G, Kabani S, et al. Oral non-Hodgkin's lymphoma: review of the literature and World Health Organization classification with reference to 40 cases. *Oral Surg Oral Med Oral Pathol Oral Radiol Endod.* 2008;105:194-201.

Weinberg OK, Ma L, Seo K, et al. Low stage follicular lymphoma: Biologic and clinical characterization according to nodal or extranodal primary origin. *Am J Surg Pathol.* 2009;33:591-598.

EXTRANODAL MARGINAL ZONE LYMPHOMA OF MUCOSA-ASSOCIATED LYMPHOID TISSUE (MALT LYMPHOMA)

MALT lymphomas comprise approximately 8% of all B-cell NHL. Presentation is usually at stage I or II disease. These lymphomas arise from a wide variety of extranodal sites, most commonly the gastrointestinal tract, often in the setting of chronic inflammatory or autoimmune disorders. Other locations where MALT lymphomas frequently occur include the thyroid, salivary glands, ocular adnexa, trachea, larynx, lung, skin, breast, thymus, liver, and dura mater. MALT lymphomas arising in the oral cavity are very rare, with fewer than 20 cases reported in the literature, and in a large series of 108 cases of MALT lymphoma, all 10 reported head and neck cases were located outside of the oral cavity.

Clinical Findings

- Most cases occur with a median age in the seventh decade with a slight female predominance; presents as a painless mass on the palatal mucosa, lip, sublingual gland, and buccal mucosa.
- There is a frequent association with Sjögren syndrome.

Histopathologic Features

- The characteristic marginal zone B cells are small to medium in size with slightly irregular nuclei, moderately dispersed chromatin and inconspicuous nucleoli, and frequently display abundant pale cytoplasm (imparting a monocytoid appearance) (Fig. 18.5A); plasmacytic differentiation is frequently seen (Fig. 18.5B).
- In glandular tissues, lymphocytes often invade epithelium to form lymphoepithelial lesions.
- Lymphoma cells may colonize reactive germinal centers, imparting a nodular appearance at low power.
- Lesional B cells express B cell markers CD19, CD20, and PAX5 (Fig. 18.5C); they may express CD79a and may exhibit aberrant coexpression of CD43; they are negative for CD5 and CD10.
- If plasmacytic differentiation is present, immunohistochemical and/or in situ hybridization often shows monotypic heavy and light chain restriction supporting the clonal (neoplastic) nature of the infiltrate (Fig. 18.5D–E).

Differential Diagnosis

- *Reactive follicular hyperplasia:* Because reactive follicles can be seen in both entities, features favoring a diagnosis of MALT include monocytoid B cells surrounding the follicles, the presence of plasmacytic differentiation showing heavy and light chain restriction, and lymphoepithelial lesions.
- *Follicular lymphoma:* The follicles in FL are often present in a back-to-back architectural arrangement and lack reactive features such as tingible-body macrophages; follicles will show aberrant BCL2 expression.

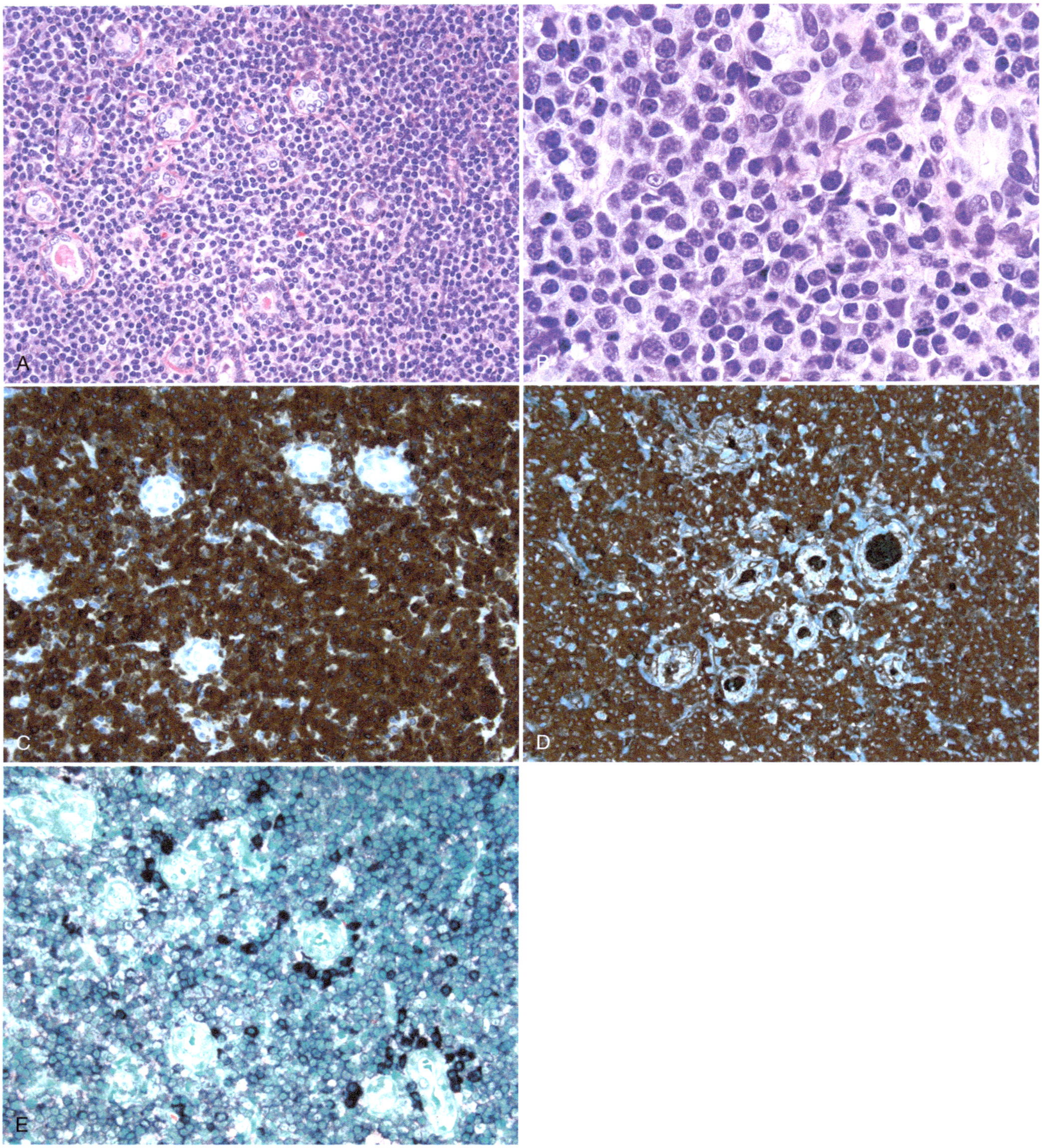

FIG 18.5 Extranodal marginal zone lymphoma of mucosa-associated lymphoid tissue (MALT). (A) The infiltrate consists of predominantly small-sized lymphoid cells surrounding and focally invading glandular structures. (B) The tumor cells in MALT lymphoma often exhibit plasmacytic differentiation. (C) The lymphoid cells are shown to be of B-cell origin by diffuse reactivity for CD20. (D) An immunostain for IgG demonstrates heavy chain restriction within this infiltrate. (E) In situ hybridization for immunoglobulin kappa light chain exhibits dark cytoplasmic reactivity in the plasma cells, and weaker (blush) reactivity in the lymphoid cells, confirming plasmacytic differentiation in this case.

Management and Prognosis

- MALT lymphomas are usually indolent and sensitive to radiation therapy.
- Recurrences can occur in other extranodal sites.

REFERENCES

Benson-Mitchell R, Warwick-Brown N, Chappell ME. Non-Hodgkin's lymphoma presenting as an isolated temporal soft tissue swelling. *J Laryngol Otol.* 1996;110:161-162.

Ferry JA. Extranodal lymphoma. *Arch Pathol Lab Med.* 2008;132: 565-578.

Isaacson PG, Spencer J. Malignant lymphoma of mucosa-associated lymphoid tissue. *Histopathology.* 1987;11:445-462.

McLellan M, Hasserjian R, Emerick K. Marginal zone B-cell lymphoma of the head and neck: A rare case and review. *Laryngoscope.* 2010;120:S165.

Thieblemont C, Bastion Y, Berger F, et al. Mucosa-associated lymphoid tissue gastrointestinal and nongastrointestinal lymphoma behavior: Analysis of 108 patients. *J Clin Oncol.* 1997;15:1624-1630.

Thieblemont C, Berger F, Dumontet C, et al. Mucosa-associated lymphoid tissue lymphoma is a disseminated disease in one third of 158 patients analyzed. *Blood.* 2000;95:802-806.

Yamagata K, Onizawa K, Kojima H, Yoshida H. Treatment of localized oral MALT lymphoma by rituximab: A case report. *Oral Maxillofac Surg.* 2008;12:227-230.

MANTLE CELL LYMPHOMA

Mantle cell lymphoma (MCL) comprises approximately 6% to 10% of all lymphomas. Although the majority of cases of MCL arise in lymph nodes, many patients have extranodal involvement, with spleen, gastrointestinal tract, and Waldeyer ring being the most commonly affected sites. Oral cavity involvement is rare with fewer than 20 cases reported in the literature.

Clinical Findings

- This typically occurs in older patients in the sixth and seventh decades with equal gender distribution, and often occurs as a mass in the palatal region, in addition to the floor of mouth and tongue.

Histopathologic Features

- MCL shows a variety of growth patterns; in the oral cavity, the most frequent patterns are diffuse and nodular (Fig. 18.6A).
- In typical MCL, the cells are small to medium in size with slightly to markedly irregular nuclear contours and inconspicuous nucleoli (Fig. 18.6B). Hyalinized small vessels and epithelioid histiocytes are frequently present in the background.
- Two morphologically defined, aggressive variants are identified: the *blastoid* variant shows cells with a blast-like morphology with open chromatin and distinct nucleoli; the *pleomorphic* variant consists of cells with pleomorphic nuclear features.
- Lesional B cells express B-cell markers CD19, CD20, and PAX5 (Fig. 18.6C); bright monotypic surface immunoglobulin light chain expression is detected by flow cytometry.
- Lesional cells are positive for CD5, cyclin D1, SOX11, BCL2, and CD43, and are usually negative for CD10, BCL6, and CD23 (Fig. 18.6D–E).
- The proliferation index informs prognosis; a Ki67 proliferation rate and mitotic count (number mitotic figures per 10 high-powered fields) should be reported.
- The *CCND1-IGH* translocation t(11;14)(q13;q32) is present in almost all cases and is considered a primary genetic event.

Differential Diagnosis

- *Chronic lymphocytic leukemia/small lymphocytic lymphoma (CLL/SLL):* CLL/SLL is also a CD5+ small-sized B-cell NHL, but will be negative for cyclin D1 expression by immunohistochemistry, and will not show a *CCND1-IGH* translocation.

Management and Prognosis

- Mantle cell lymphoma usually has an aggressive course with a median survival of 3 to 5 years.

REFERENCES

Bosch F, Lopez-Guillermo A, Campo E, et al. Mantle cell lymphoma: presenting features, response to therapy, and prognostic factors. *Cancer.* 1998;82:567-575.

Guggisberg K, Jordan RC. Mantle cell lymphoma of the oral cavity: Case series and comprehensive review of the literature. *Oral Surg Oral Med Oral Pathol Oral Radiol Endod.* 2010;109:98-104.

Scheller K, Becker S, Scheller C. Symmetric palatal swelling as the first clinical manifestation of a mantle cell non-Hodgkin's lymphoma: a case report and review of literature. *J Oral Maxillofac Pathol.* 2011;15:311-315.

Vose JM. Mantle cell lymphoma: 2013 update on diagnosis, risk-stratification, and clinical management. *Am J Hematol.* 2013;88: 1082-1088.

Zhou Y, Wang H, Fang W, et al. Incidence trends of mantle cell lymphoma in the United States between 1992 and 2004. *Cancer.* 2008;113:791-798.

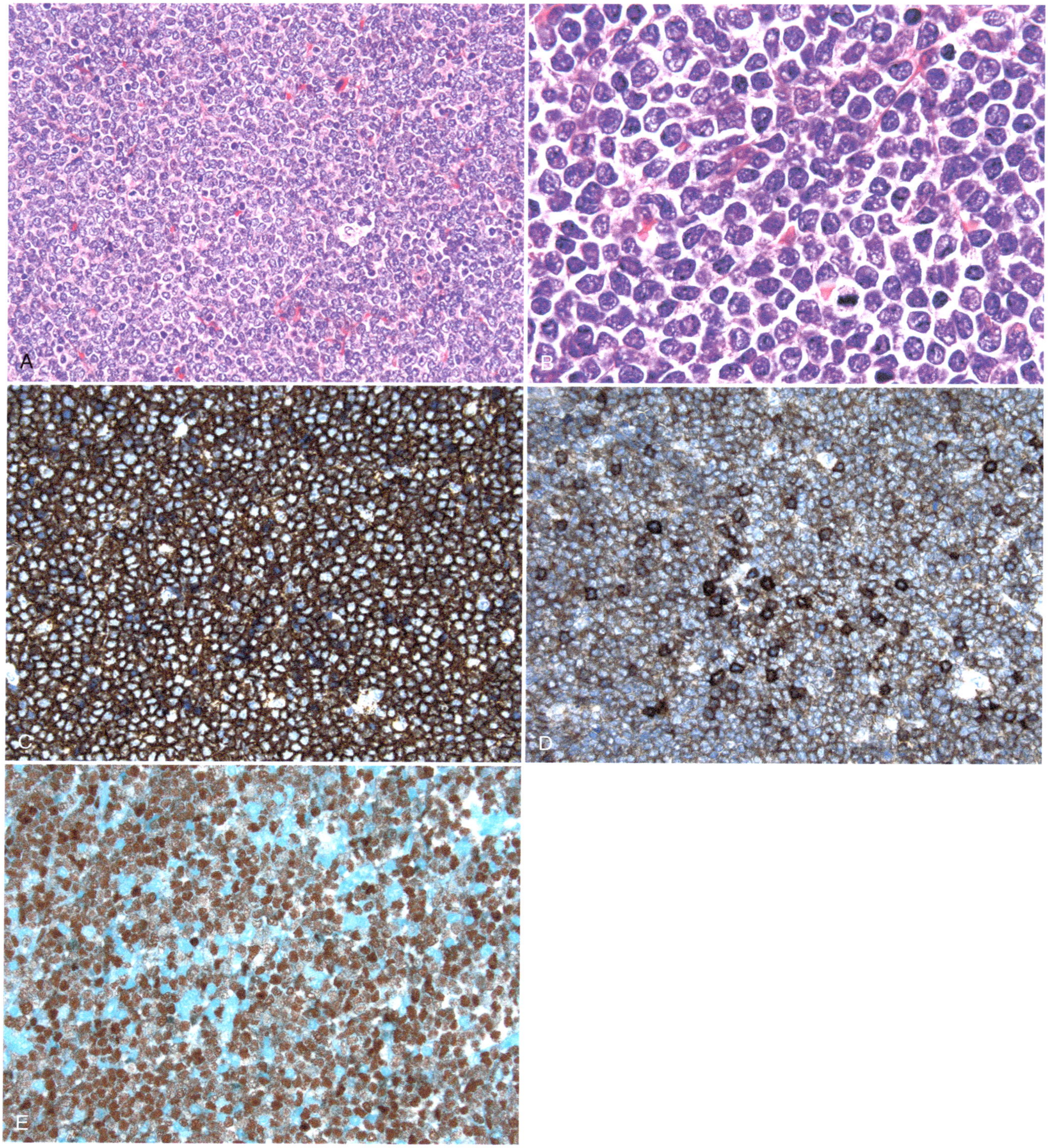

FIG 18.6 Mantle cell lymphoma (MCL). (A) The infiltrate consists of a diffuse population of small-sized lymphoid cells. Scattered mitotic figures are appreciated in this typical case. An epithelioid histiocyte is present near the center of the field. (B) The lymphoid cells exhibit irregular nuclear contours. (C) Diffuse reactivity for CD20 is indicative of a B-cell origin. (D) An immunostain for CD5 shows weak staining in the neoplastic infiltrate and strong reactivity in the admixed reactive T cells. (E) Nuclear positivity for cyclin D1 distinguishes MCL from CLL/SLL.

CHRONIC LYMPHOCYTIC LEUKEMIA/ SMALL LYMPHOCYTIC LYMPHOMA

- B-cell chronic lymphocytic leukemia/small lymphocytic lymphoma (CLL/SLL) is one of the most common lymphoproliferative disorders of adults in the Western world. Although most patients with CLL/SLL will ultimately demonstrate peripheral blood and bone marrow involvement (leukemic involvement or "CLL"), some cases exhibit exclusively nodal disease (lymphomatous involvement or "SLL") at the time of diagnosis. Both of these entities are now considered as a single disease with different patterns of tissue expression. In one study, CLL/SLL comprised 10 of 58 cases (17%) of extranodal NHLs of the oral cavity and maxillofacial region, seven of which were in the oral cavity proper (maxillary mucosa or minor salivary glands).

Clinical Findings

- Most cases occur in older individuals and the most common sites are maxillary mucosa or the minor salivary glands; most present with early stage disease.

Histopathologic Features

- A pseudofollicular architectural pattern is usually seen, characterized by both a diffuse infiltrate of the lesional cells in addition to admixed pale-staining aggregates of cells called "proliferation centers"; proliferation centers are only seen in CLL/SLL (Fig. 18.7A).
- The lesional lymphocytes are small in size, contain round nuclei with a clumped "soccer ball" chromatin pattern, and exhibit scant cytoplasm; the proliferation centers contain slightly larger cells with more open chromatin and slightly more cytoplasm, including

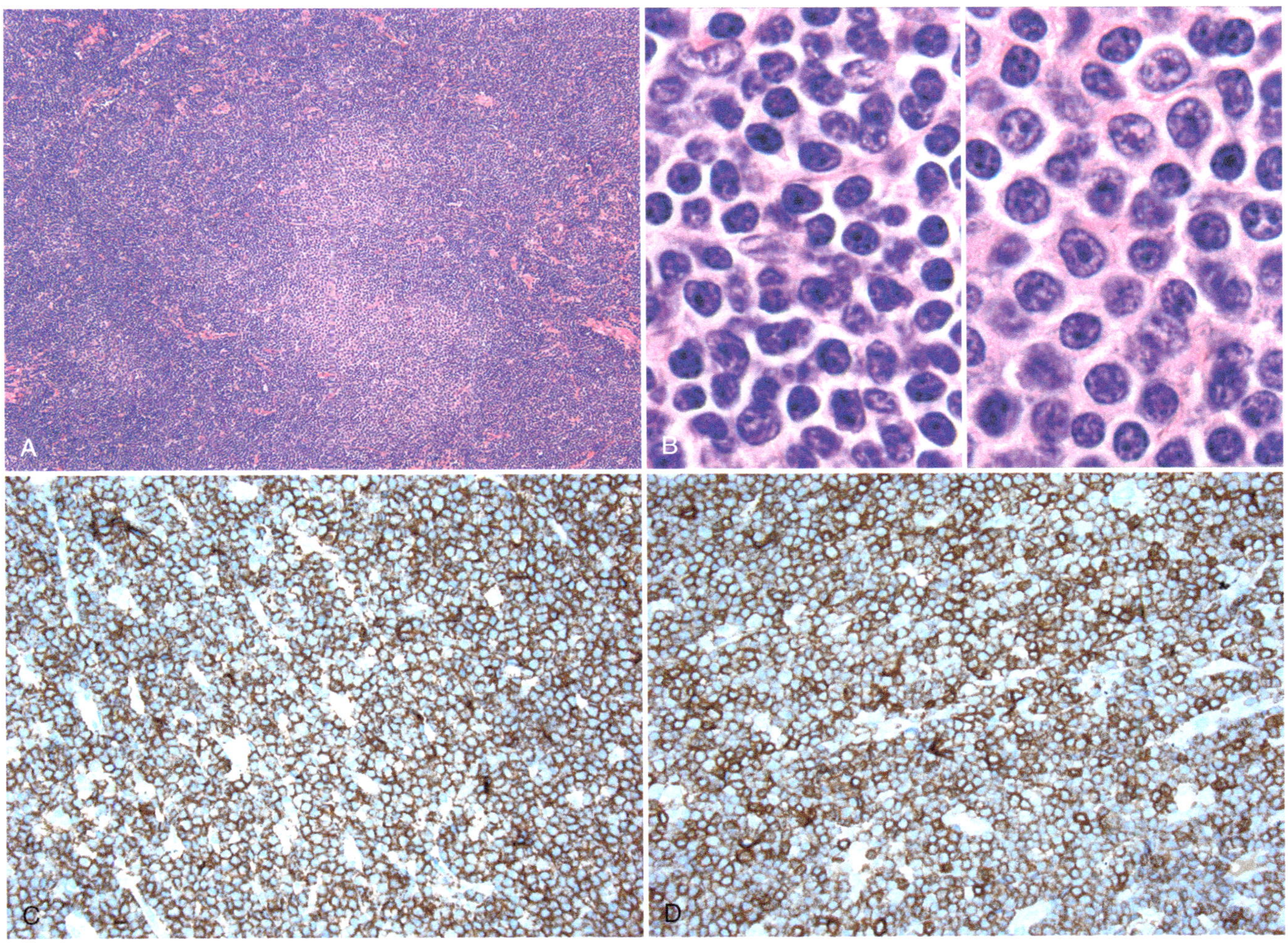

FIG 18.7 Chronic lymphocytic leukemia/small lymphocytic lymphoma (CLL/SLL). (A) The infiltrate consists of a diffuse population of small-sized lymphoid cells. A characteristic feature of CLL/SLL is the presence of irregularly shaped, pale staining aggregates of prolymphocytes and paraimmunoblasts (proliferation centers), seen in the center of the image. (B) The *left panel* shows the morphologic features of CLL/SLL cells, including small size, clumped "soccer ball" chromatin, and small nucleoli. The *right panel* shows the cells of the proliferation centers, which are larger in size with more open chromatin and prominent nucleoli. (C) Diffuse reactivity for CD20 is indicative of a B-cell origin. (D) An immunostain for CD5 shows diffuse dim positivity, characteristic of CLL/SLL.

prolymphocytes and paraimmunoblasts, accounting for the paler appearance at low power (Fig. 18.7B).

- Proliferation centers typically show an increased proliferation index compared to the surrounding, smaller lesional cells.
- The lesional B cells express B-cell markers CD19, CD20 (characteristically dim), and PAX5 (Fig. 18.7C); dim monotypic surface immunoglobulin light chain expression is detected by flow cytometry.
- CLL/SLL cells demonstrate expression aberrant coexpression of the T-cell markers CD5 and CD43 and are typically positive for CD23; cyclin D1 and CD10 are negative (Fig. 18.7D).

Differential Diagnosis

- *Mantle cell lymphoma:* MCL is also a CD5+ small-sized B-cell NHL, but unlike CLL/SLL the tumor cells of MCL will demonstrate expression of cyclin D1 by immunohistochemistry, and a *CCND1-IGH* translocation will be present by karyotype and/or fluorescence in situ hybridization.

Management and Prognosis

- The clinical course of CLL/SLL is extremely variable because of the heterogeneity of the disease, with survival ranging from months to years and largely dependent on the clinical stage; typically, CLL/SLL is considered to be indolent, but incurable without allogeneic stem cell transplantation.
- Transformation to an aggressive lymphoma, most frequently diffuse large B-cell lymphoma (known as Richter syndrome or transformation), occurs in 5% to 10% of cases.

REFERENCES

Alessandrini M, Micarelli A, Mugnaini F, et al. Unusual case of oral chronic lymphocytic leukemia presenting as recurrent epistaxis and asymptomatic intraoral swelling. *Rev Stomatol Chir Maxillofac.* 2012;113:455-457.

Ben-Ezra J, Burke JS, Swartz WG, et al. Small lymphocytic lymphoma: a clinicopathologic analysis of 268 cases. *Blood.* 1989;73:579-587.

Inamdar KV, Bueso-Ramos CE. Pathology of chronic lymphocytic leukemia: An update. *Ann Diagn Pathol.* 2007;11:363-389.

Triantafillidou K, Dimitrakopoulos J, Iordanidis F. Gkagkalis A. Extranodal non-Hodgkin lymphomas of the oral cavity and maxillofacial region: a clinical study of 58 cases and review of the literature. *J Oral Maxillofac Surg.* 2012;70:2776-2785.

BURKITT LYMPHOMA

Burkitt lymphoma (BL) is an aggressive form of B-cell NHL with three variants: endemic, sporadic, and immunodeficiency-associated. Endemic cases occur in equatorial Africa and Papua New Guinea, most commonly in children and adolescents. Typical sites of involvement of endemic BL include facial structures such as the jaw and orbit, and the majority are associated with EBV infection. Sporadic BL affects patients throughout the world, particularly children and young adults, and most frequently occurs at extranodal sites particularly the gastrointestinal tract. Presentation within the oral cavity is rare in sporadic BL; in a large survey of Western cases of lymphoma arising within oral and paraoral regions, BL accounted for fewer than 2% of all cases. BL arising in the setting of immunodeficiency is most frequently associated with HIV infection. Detection of EBV in cases of either sporadic or immunodeficiency-associated BL is less frequent than in the endemic form, ranging from 10% to 30% of cases.

Clinical Findings

- Patients with the endemic form of BL often present with a rapidly enlarging mass causing facial asymmetry; within the oral cavity, there may be loosening of teeth, swelling, or ulceration.

Histopathologic Features

- Due to the high mitotic rate and apoptotic activity, numerous tingible-body macrophages are admixed within the infiltrate imparting a "starry sky" pattern (Fig. 18.8A).
- BL cells are intermediate-sized lymphocytes with round nuclei, coarse chromatin and multiple small basophilic nucleoli (Fig. 18.8B).
- Lesional B cells express pan B-cell markers such as CD19, CD20, and PAX5; monotypic surface immunoglobulin light chain expression is detected by flow cytometry.
- The B cells coexpress BCL6 and CD10, and are negative for BCL2 and TdT.
- The Ki67 proliferation index is nearly 100% (Fig. 18.8C).
- EBV infection can be demonstrated by EBER positivity.
- The characteristic genetic lesion is an *MYC* translocation (typically t(8;14)(q24;q32)) without concurrent *BCL2* or *BCL6* translocation, which results in overexpression of the MYC nuclear protein (Fig. 18.8D).

Differential Diagnosis

- *Diffuse large B-cell lymphoma:* Typically DLBCL shows large-sized cells with prominent nucleoli, does not have a "starry sky" pattern at low power, has a lower mitotic index, and is frequently BCL2+.
- High-grade B-cell lymphoma, with *MYC* and *BCL2* and/or *BCL6* rearrangements: Cases falling into this category are also known as "double-" or "triple-hit" lymphomas because they show a *MYC* rearrangement as well as *BCL2* and/or *BCL6* rearrangements. Cases that morphologically resemble BL but show these genetic changes are placed into this category.

Management and Prognosis

- Intensive combination chemotherapy results in a high cure rate.

REFERENCES

Balasubramaniam R, Goradia A, Turner LN, et al. Burkitt lymphoma of the oral cavity: an atypical presentation. *Oral Surg Oral Med Oral Pathol Oral Radiol Endod.* 2009;107:240-245.

Boffano P, Gallesio C, Benech R, Berrone S. Bilateral oral non-endemic Burkitt lymphoma. *J Craniofac Surg.* 2013;24:1057-1058.

Castellarin P, Pozzato G, Tirelli G, et al. Oral lesions and lymphoproliferative disorders. *J Oncol.* 2010;2010:202305. doi:10.1155/2010/202305.

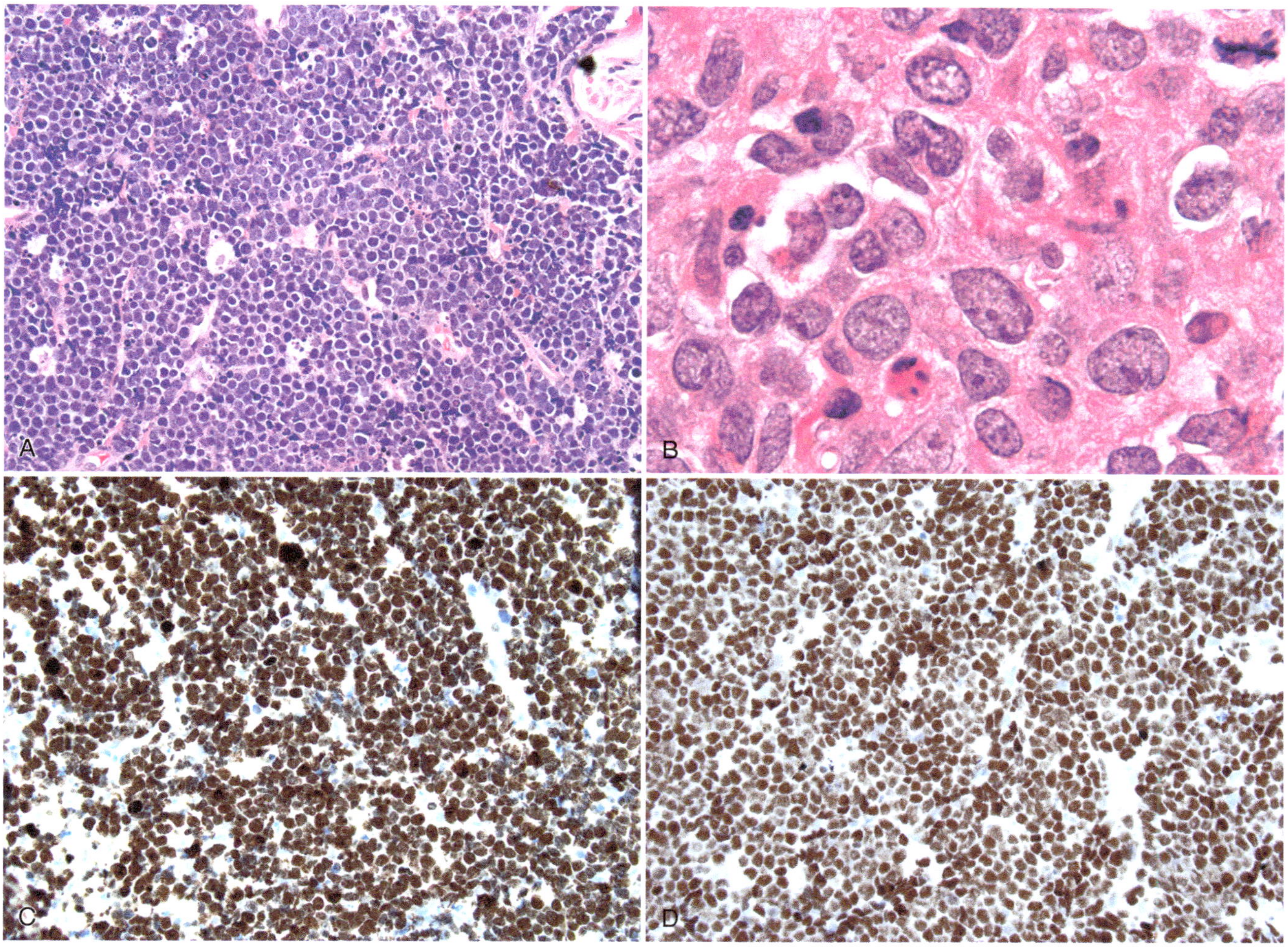

FIG 18.8 Burkitt lymphoma. (A) Low-power evaluation reveals a diffuse infiltrate of intermediate-sized cells with admixed tingible-body macrophages, imparting a "starry-sky" appearance. (B) High-power view reveals multiple small basophilic nucleoli within lesional cell nuclei, and admixed mitotic figures and apoptotic bodies. (C) The Ki67 proliferation index is nearly 100%. (D) There is frequent over-expression of the nuclear MYC protein because of the underlying MYC translocation, permitting detection by immunohistochemistry.

Epstein JB, Epstein JD, Le ND, Gorsky M. Characteristics of oral and paraoral malignant lymphoma: a population-based review of 361 cases. *Oral Surg Oral Med Oral Pathol Oral Radiol Endod.* 2001;92:519-525.

Jaradat JM, Potluri A, Bilodeau EA. B-cell lymphoma, unclassifiable, with features intermediate between diffuse large B-cell lymphoma and Burkitt lymphoma: report of a case in the oral cavity. *Indian J Dent Res.* 2013;24:384-386.

Kikuchi K, Inoue H, Miyazaki Y, et al. Adult sporadic Burkitt lymphoma of the oral cavity: A case report and literature review. *J Oral Maxillofac Surg.* 2012;70:2936-2943.

PLASMA CELL NEOPLASM

Plasma cell neoplasm (PCN) is a general term for the proliferation of malignant monoclonal plasma cells. Clinicopathologic variants include solitary plasmacytoma of bone, extramedullary plasmacytoma, smoldering myeloma, multiple myeloma, and plasma cell leukemia.

Clinical Findings

- PCN is usually seen in the sixth and seventh decades with a female predominance; it may manifest in jaw bones as a solitary lesion (solitary plasmacytoma of bone) or more commonly as one of multiple bony lesions in patients with multiple myeloma; patients with solitary bony involvement at presentation almost always progress to multiple myeloma; bony lesions may cause lip/chin numbness, bone pain, hypercalcemia, and fractures.
- Imaging and physical exam findings include lytic, punched-out lesions in the jaw bones and calvaria (Fig. 18.9A); extension into the soft tissue forming fleshy masses (Fig. 18.9B–C); waxy, yellowish, firm amyloid nodules, especially of the tongue (Fig. 18.9D).
- Patients with multiple myeloma demonstrate an M-component in peripheral blood and urine in 99% of cases; 50% are IgG and 20% to 25% are IgA; monoclonal light chain (Bence Jones protein) is found in serum or urine in 75% of cases.

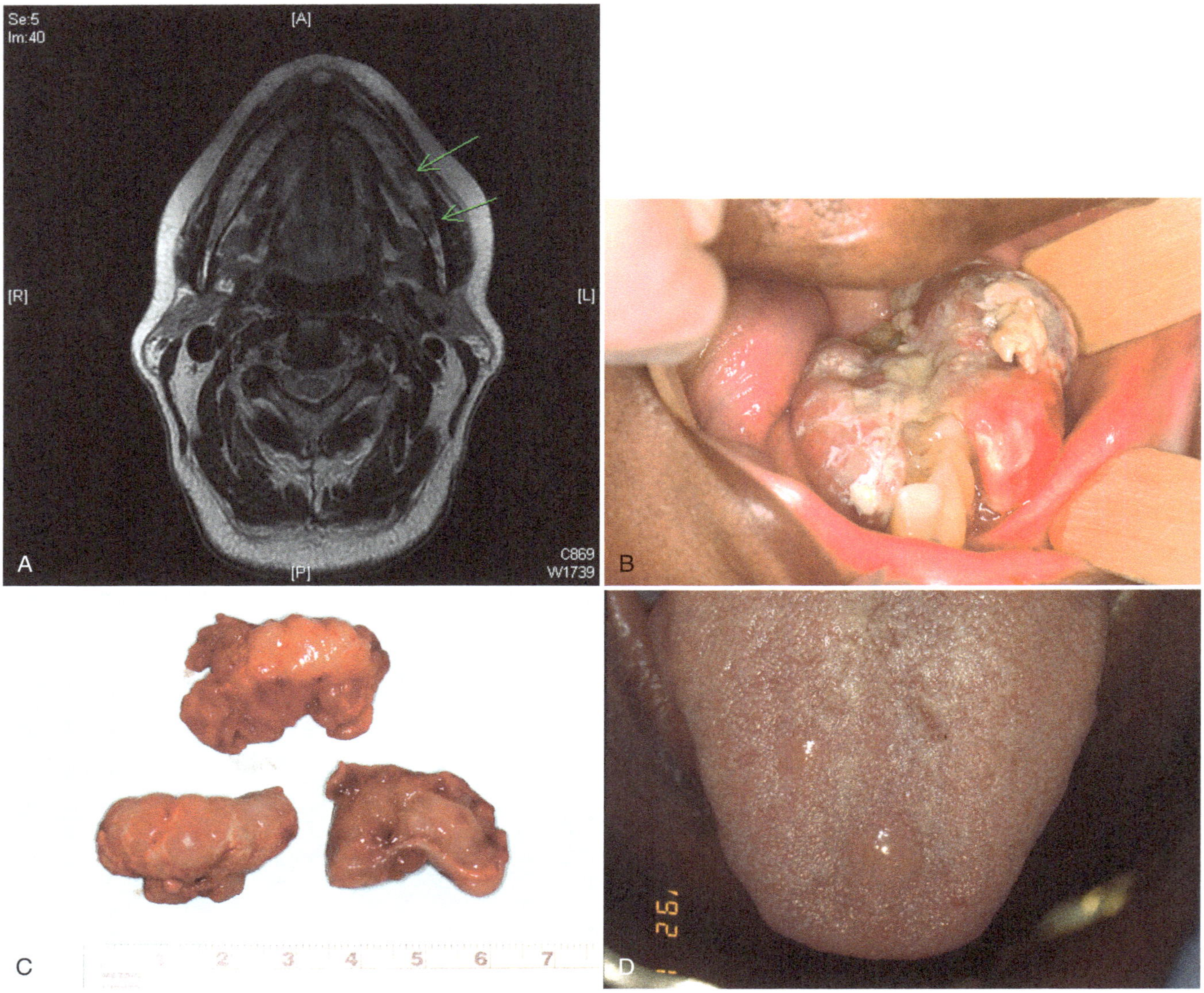

FIG 18.9 Plasma cell neoplasm (clinical findings): (A) There are multiple punched-out lytic lesions of the mandible. (B) This tumor presented as a large, rapidly growing soft tissue mass. (C) Gross specimen from patient shown in B exhibited a fleshy appearance. (D) This patient with multiple myeloma presented with multiple yellow, waxy amyloid nodules of the tongue.

- Solitary extramedullary plasmacytoma (SEP) is a rare tumor that commonly arises in the upper aerodigestive tract, and approximately 5% occur in the oral cavity involving the soft palate, tongue, and gingiva; it consists of a collection of clonal plasma cells occurring at a solitary soft tissue site without evidence of systemic multiple myeloma, but approximately 20% of patients will progress to multiple myeloma.

Histopathologic Features

- These lesions show plasma cells occuring in sheets. Well-differentiated lesions will exhibit plasma cells with abundant amphophilic cytoplasm, eccentric nuclei, clumped chromatin ("clock face" appearance), and a perinuclear hof (prominent Golgi apparatus) (Fig. 18.10A–B); Russell bodies (eosinophilic bodies filled with immunoglobulin) may be noted and significant nuclear atypia can be seen.
- Cells are positive for CD38, CD138, and CD79a with light chain restriction, which can be demonstrated by immunohistochemistry or in situ hybridization (Fig. 18.10C–D); they are usually negative for CD20 and CD45; approximately 70% demonstrate aberrant expression of CD56.
- In general there is no evidence of EBV infection; however, rare cases of EBV-positive plasmacytoma in immunocompetent patients have been reported.

Differential Diagnosis

- *Plasmablastic lymphoma:* Oral lesions typically occur in the setting of HIV infection and involve the soft tissue of the gingiva or palatal mucosa; bone involvement is

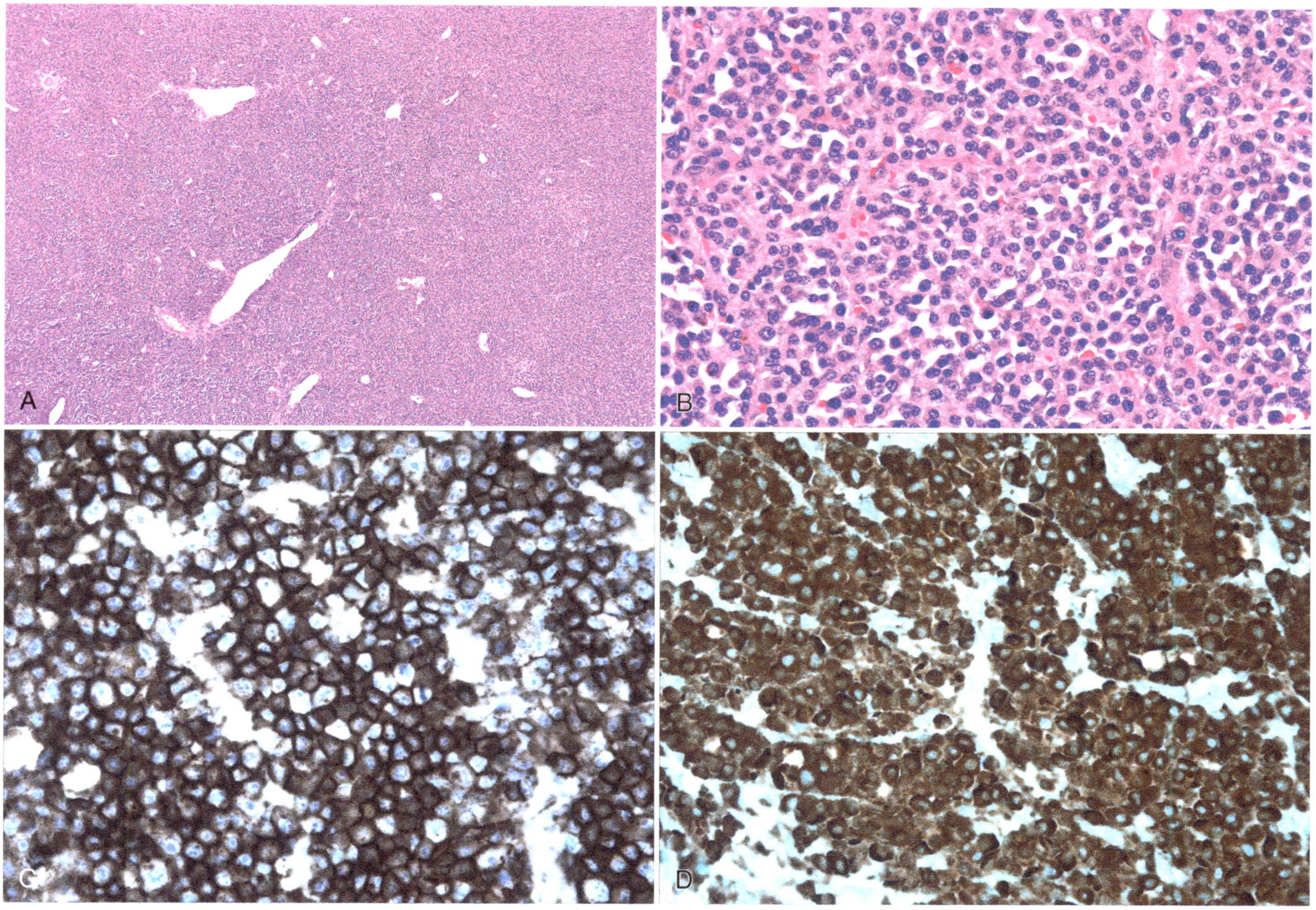

FIG 18.10 Plasma cell neoplasm (histologic findings): (A) There is diffuse infiltration by tumor cells with destruction of underlying architecture. (B) There are sheets of plasma cells with eccentrically placed nuclei. (C) Lesional cells demonstrate strong expression of CD138. (D) In this case, clonality is demonstrated by uniform expression of immunoglobulin lambda light chain.

infrequent; tingible-body macrophages impart a "starry sky" appearance and there may be frank necrosis; cells are plasmablasts or immunoblasts with abundant cytoplasm, large nuclei, prominent central nucleoli, or peripheral nucleoli; immunophenotypic profile is similar to plasma cells (expression of CD138 and CD38; CD20−), but the majority of HIV-associated oral cases are positive for EBER.

- *Poorly differentiated carcinoma:* The lesional cells in PCN with anaplastic features may no longer resemble typical plasma cells and can mimic a poorly differentiated carcinoma, which often also expresses CD138; demonstration of light-chain restriction by immunohistochemistry or in situ hybridization will confirm a diagnosis of PCN.

Management and Prognosis

- Plasmacytoma is usually treated with radiation with or without excision.
- Systemic myeloma treatment includes chemotherapy, bisphosphonates, thalidomide and related drugs, corticosteroids, bortezomib, and/or autologous stem cell transplantation.

REFERENCES

Cardoso RC, Gerngross PJ, Hofstede TM, et al. The multiple oral presentations of multiple myeloma. *Support Care Cancer.* 2014;22:259-267.

Elias HG, Scott J, Metheny L, Quereshy FA. Multiple myeloma presenting as mandibular ill-defined radiolucent lesion with numb chin syndrome: a case report. *J Oral Maxillofac Surg.* 2009;67:1991-1996.

Epstein JB, Voss NJ, Stevenson-Moore P. Maxillofacial manifestations of multiple myeloma. an unusual case and review of the literature. *Oral Surg Oral Med Oral Pathol.* 1984;57:267-271.

Kemp S, Gallagher G, Kabani S, et al. Oral non-Hodgkin's lymphoma: review of the literature and World Health Organization classification with reference to 40 cases. *Oral Surg Oral Med Oral Pathol Oral Radiol Endod.* 2008;105:194-201.

Loghavi S, Khoury JD, Medeiros LJ. Epstein-Barr virus-positive plasmacytoma in immunocompetent patients. *Histopathology.* 2015;67:225-234.

Pisano JJ, Coupland R, Chen SY, Miller AS. Plasmacytoma of the oral cavity and jaws: a clinicopathologic study of 13 cases. *Oral Surg Oral Med Oral Pathol Oral Radiol Endod.* 1997;83:265-271.

Romano A, Marescalco MS, Liardo C, et al. Oral lesion as unusual first manifestation of multiple myeloma: Case reports and review of the literature. *Case Rep Hematol.* 2014;2014:529452. doi:10.1155/2014/529452.

Seoane J, De la Cruz A, Pomareda M, et al. Primary extramedullary plasmacytoma of the palate. *Otolaryngol Head Neck Surg.* 1999;120:530.

Solomides CC, Miller AS, Christman RA, et al. Lymphomas of the oral cavity: histology, immunologic type, and incidence of Epstein-Barr virus infection. *Hum Pathol.* 2002;33:153-157.

Straetmans J, Stokroos R. Extramedullary plasmacytomas in the head and neck region. *Eur Arch Otorhinolaryngol.* 2008;265:1417-1423.

van der Waal RI, Huijgens PC, van der Valk P, van der Waal I. Characteristics of 40 primary extranodal non-Hodgkin lymphomas of the oral cavity in perspective of the new WHO classification and the International Prognostic Index. *Int J Oral Maxillofac Surg.* 2005;34:391-395.

Vega F, Chang CC, Medeiros LJ, et al. Plasmablastic lymphomas and plasmablastic plasma cell myelomas have nearly identical immunophenotypic profiles. *Mod Pathol.* 2005;18:806-815.

ACUTE MYELOID LEUKEMIA

Acute myeloid leukemia (AML) is a clonal neoplastic proliferation composed of myeloid blasts. AML most frequently involves the bone marrow cavity, but can also occur at extramedullary sites. Although extramedullary AML is most often found in lymph nodes or skin, head and neck manifestations also occur and within this anatomic region the oral cavity is most frequently involved.

Clinical Findings

- AML within the oral cavity typically presents as a diffuse gingival infiltrate causing boggy gingival swelling (see Chapter 5, Fig. 5.23C); less commonly, discrete tumor nodules (also known as myeloid sarcoma) may form.
- Gingival infiltrations are frequently associated with AML with myelomonocytic or monocytic/monoblastic differentiation.
- Intraoral myeloid sarcoma tumors arise most commonly in the maxillary and mandibular gingivae.
- AML within the oral cavity may be seen at presentation, during the course of disease or at relapse, or may represent transformation of an underlying myelodysplastic or myeloproliferative neoplasm.

Etiopathogenesis and Histopathologic Features

- There are diffuse sheets of immature myeloid cells with round to ovoid nuclei, finely dispersed chromatin, distinct nucleoli, and scant to moderate amounts of cytoplasm, which may contain granules (Fig. 18.11A–B).
- Expression of markers of monocytic differentiation (CD43, CD68, and lysozyme) is highly sensitive but not specific; classic markers of immaturity such as CD34 and CD117 are often negative, particularly in cases with monocytic differentiation; myeloperoxidase positivity is helpful in cases with granulocytic differentiation (Fig. 18.11C–E).

Differential Diagnosis

- *Diffuse large B-cell lymphoma:* Given the morphologic overlap between the two entities, immunophenotyping is essential to confirm the myeloid or monocytic lineage of the leukemic infiltrates/masses.
- *Burkitt lymphoma:* Both tumors may show a "starry sky" background of tingible-body macrophages; immunophenotyping is essential to distinguish the two entities.
- *Histiocytic proliferations in association with inflammatory conditions:* In contrast to a reactive infiltrate, myeloid sarcoma will exhibit immature nuclear features and often shows distortion/destruction of the underlying architecture.

Management and Prognosis

- The prognostic significance of extramedullary infiltrates in AML has been controversial but likely is associated with worse prognosis.

REFERENCES

Amin KS, Ehsan A, McGuff HS, Albright SC. Minimally differentiated acute myelogenous leukemia (AML-M0) granulocytic sarcoma presenting in the oral cavity. *Oral Oncol.* 2002;38:516-519.

Chang H, Brandwein J, Yi QL, et al. Extramedullary infiltrates of AML are associated with CD56 expression, 11q23 abnormalities and inferior clinical outcome. *Leuk Res.* 2004;28:1007-1011.

Hicsonmez G, Cetin M, Tuncer AM, et al. Children with acute myeloblastic leukemia presenting with extramedullary infiltration: The effects of high-dose steroid treatment. *Leuk Res.* 2004;28:25-34.

Papamanthos MK, Kolokotronis AE. Skulakis HE, Acute myeloid leukemia diagnosed by intraoral myeloid sarcoma. a case report. *Head Neck Pathol.* 2010;4:132-135.

Tomas Carmona I, Cameselle Teijeiro J, Diz Dios P, et al. Intraalveolar granulocytic sarcoma developing after tooth extraction. *Oral Oncol.* 2000;36:491-494.

Xie Z, Zhang F, Song E, et al. Intraoral granulocytic sarcoma presenting as multiple maxillary and mandibular masses: a case report and literature review. *Oral Surg Oral Med Oral Pathol Oral Radiol Endod.* 2007;103:e44-e48.

Zhou J, Bell D, Medeiros LJ. Myeloid sarcoma of the head and neck region. *Arch Pathol Lab Med.* 2013;137:1560-1568.

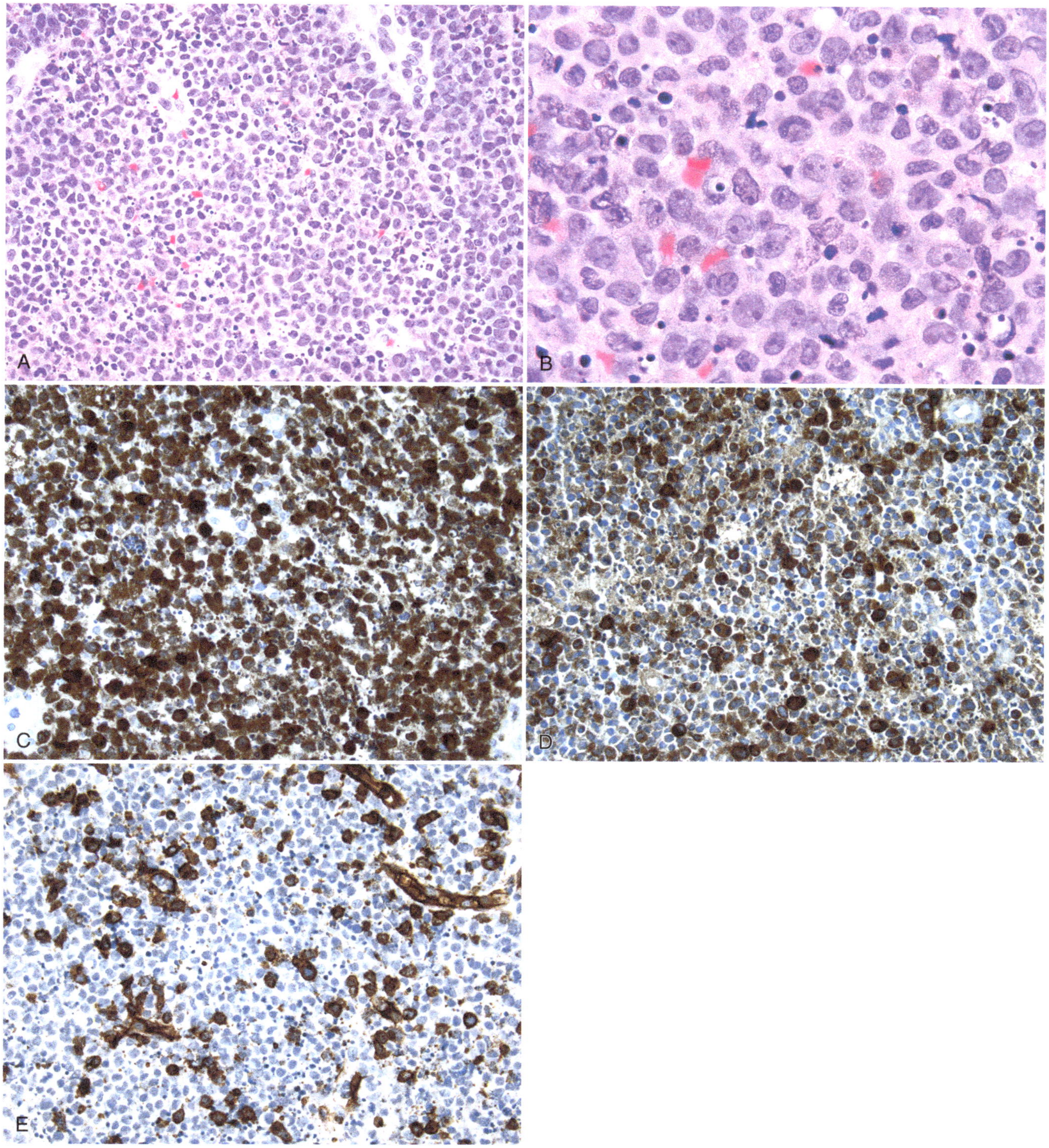

FIG 18.11 Extramedullary involvement by acute myeloid leukemia. (A) The tumor cells form a diffuse, sheet-like infiltrate with destruction of underlying tissue architecture. Numerous apoptotic bodies and mitotic figures attest to the high proliferative rate. (B) The tumor cells are large in size with ovoid to folded nuclei, dispersed chromatin, distinct nucleoli, and pale cytoplasm. In this case, the leukemic cells show myelomonocytic differentiation, including diffuse positivity for lysozyme (C) and subset expression of myeloperoxidase (D) and CD34 (E).

EXTRANODAL NK/T-CELL LYMPHOMA, NASAL TYPE

Extranodal NK/T-cell lymphoma is a lymphoma of natural killer (NK) cells, or less commonly, cytotoxic T cells. It is more common in East Asian and South and Central American countries with a predilection for the nasal cavity and paranasal sinuses (80% of cases); other extranodal sites include the skin and gastrointestinal tract; lymphadenopathy is seen in 10% to 20% of patients. All cases are associated with EBV infection. Heterozygous deletion of 6q21 and/or *PRDM1*, leading to downregulation of *PRDM1*, may be seen. Although T-cell receptor genes are germline in the majority of cases, up to 25% of cases demonstrate a monoclonal T-cell receptor gene rearrangement.

Clinical Findings

- This condition is most frequently seen in the fifth decade with a 2:1 male predilection
- Pain, bleeding, and nasal obstruction are common presenting symptoms and invasion of the hard palate leads to presentation in the oral cavity simulating midline destructive disease; it may also involve Waldeyer ring.
- There may be invasion of facial skin, the orbit, and nasopharynx.

Histopathologic Features

- The lymphoid cells may vary in size from small to large and contain moderate-to-scant cytoplasm with irregular nuclei, and small nucleoli; mitotic figures are readily noted and a background of lymphocytes, plasma cells, histiocytes and neutrophils is usually present (Fig. 18.12A–B).
- Angiocentricity and angioinvasion by tumor cells resulting in necrosis are characteristic features that are present in up to 70% of cases.
- Lesional cells are typically positive for CD2, CD3 in a cytoplasmic pattern (negative for surface CD3 by flow cytometry), and CD56, and negative for CD5 (Fig. 18.12C–D); 70% of cases are negative for both CD4 and CD8; lesional cells are frequently positive for granzyme B and TIA-1; tumors comprised of large cells may be positive for CD30.
- EBER positivity is required for the diagnosis (Fig. 18.12E).

Differential Diagnosis

- Granulomatosis with polyangiitis (formerly called Wegner granulomatosis) is characterized by a mixed cellular infiltrate, vasculitis, necrosis, and sometimes granulomas, but the constituent lymphocytes do not exhibit atypia or EBV positivity; patients are also positive for serum antineutrophil cytoplasmic antibodies.
- Peripheral T-cell lymphoma, not otherwise specified (PTCL,NOS), expresses surface CD3 and typically TCR-βF1 and may show selective loss of pan-T-cell antigens such as CD5 or CD7; CD56 and EBER expression are less common but may be seen, CD56 being associated most frequently with PTCL,NOS of γ-δ type; almost all cases show a clonal T-cell receptor gene rearrangement.
- Fungal/mycobacterial infection may also show angioinvasion and necrosis, but there is no atypical lymphoid infiltrate and organisms are identified by histochemical studies.

Management and Prognosis

- Localized disease is treated by radiation therapy and an aggressive chemotherapy regimen consisting of steroid (dexamethasone), methotrexate, ifosfamide, L-asparaginase, and etoposide.
- Patients with widespread disease have a worse prognosis, with a 5-year overall survival rate of approximately 50%.

REFERENCES

Gualco G, Domeny-Duarte P, Chioato L, et al. Clinicopathologic and molecular features of 122 Brazilian cases of nodal and extranodal NK/T-cell lymphoma, nasal type, with EBV subtyping analysis. *Am J Surg Pathol.* 2011;35:1195-1203.

Huang X, Sun Q, Fu H, et al. Both c-Myc and Ki-67 expression are predictive markers in patients with extranodal NK/T-cell lymphoma, nasal type: a retrospective study in China. *Pathol Res Pract.* 2014;210: 351-356.

Huang YH, Wu QL, Zong YS, et al. Nasopharyngeal extranodal NK/T-cell lymphoma, nasal type: retrospective study of 18 consecutive cases in Guangzhou, China. *Int J Surg Pathol.* 2011;19:51-61.

Li S, Feng X, Li T, et al. Extranodal NK/T-cell lymphoma, nasal type: a report of 73 cases at MD Anderson Cancer Center. *Am J Surg Pathol.* 2013;37:14-23.

Liang L, Zhang Z, Wang Y, et al. The genetic deletion of 6q21 and PRDM1 and clinical implications in extranodal NK/T cell lymphoma, nasal type. *Biomed Res Int.* 2015;2015:435423. doi:10.1155/2015/435423.

Meng W, Zhou Y, Zhang H, et al. Nasal-type NK/T-cell lymphoma with palatal ulcer as the earliest clinical manifestation: a case report with literature review. *Pathol Oncol Res.* 2010;16:133-137.

Ng SB, Lai KW, Murugaya S, et al. Nasal-type extranodal natural killer/T-cell lymphomas: a clinicopathologic and genotypic study of 42 cases in Singapore. *Mod Pathol.* 2004;17:1097-1107.

Susarla SM, Sharaf BA, Faquin W, et al. Extranodal natural killer T-cell lymphoma, nasal type, with minimal osseous involvement: report of a case and literature review. *J Oral Maxillofac Surg.* 2010;68:674-681.

Tse E, Kwong YL. How I treat NK/T-cell lymphomas. *Blood.* 2013; 121:4997-5005.

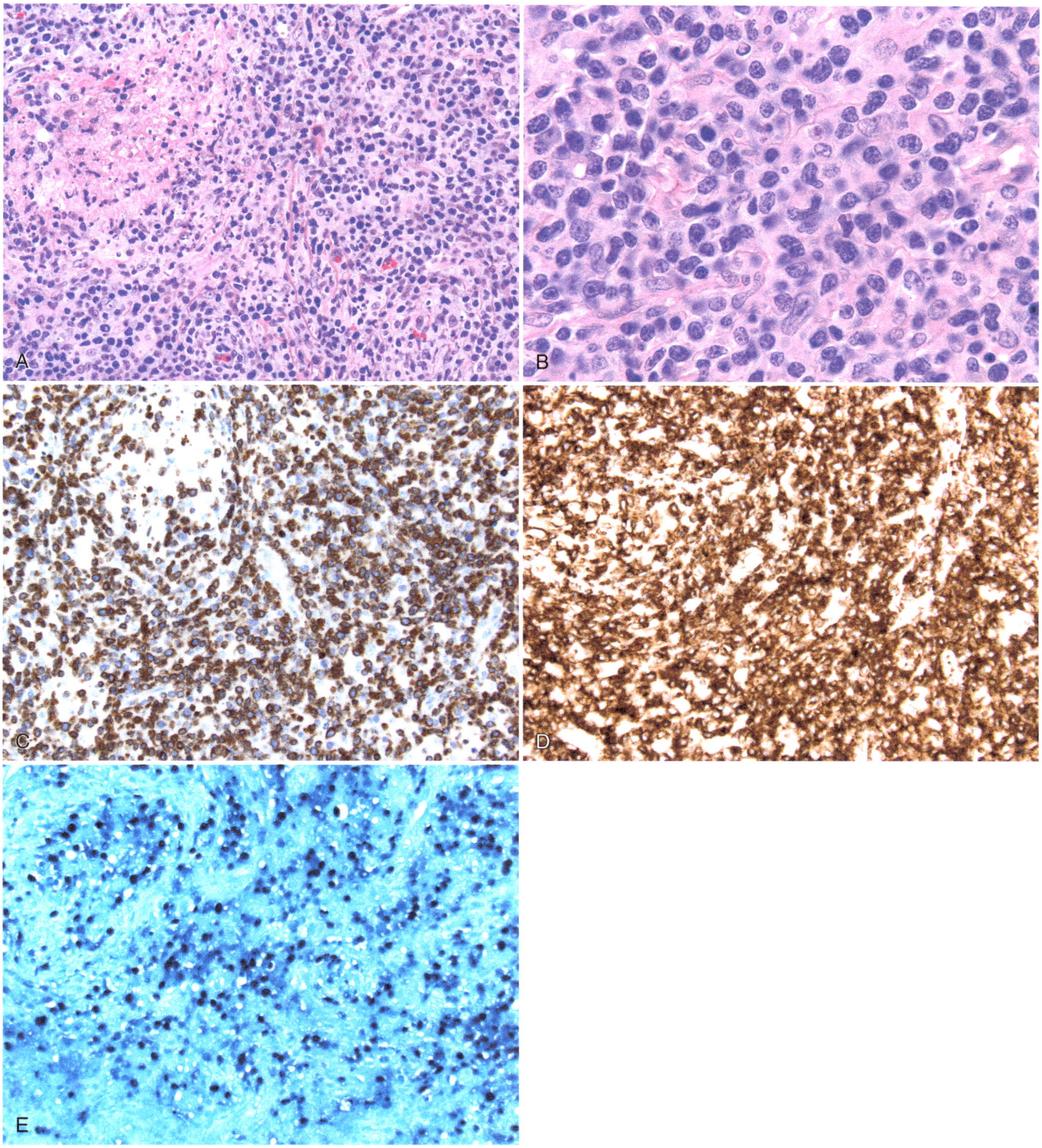

FIG 18.12 Extranodal NK/T-cell lymphoma, nasal type. (A) The infiltrate exhibits a diffuse pattern of growth with marked angiodestruction *(upper left corner)*. (B) The tumor cells are variable in size (ranging from small to intermediate to large) with irregular, elongated nuclei, and indistinct nucleoli. (C) The cells show cytoplasmic CD3 expression by immunohistochemistry, but will be negative for surface CD3 expression by flow cytometry. (D) CD56 is diffusely positive. (E) EBER in situ hybridization is uniformly positive in the lesional cells.

APPENDIX A

PHARMACOLOGIC THERAPY FOR COMMON MUCOSAL CONDITIONS

Medication	How to Prescribe
Topical Immunosuppressive Agents (gels or creams are the most useful; preparations with the same concentration of drug vary in strength, depending on the preparation)	
Class I steroid • Clobetasol propionate 0.05% gel/cream • Betamethasone dipropionate 0.05% gel Class II steroid • Fluocinonide 0.05% gel/cream • Betamethasone dipropionate 0.05% cream • Budesonide 0.025% cream Class III steroid • Triamcinolone 0.1% dental paste[a] (not appropriate for diffuse lesions) Class IV or V steroid • Fluocinolone acetonide 0.025% ointment • Desonide 0.05% ointment Nonsteroidal agents • Tacrolimus 0.1% ointment • Pimecrolimus 1% cream	Dry area, apply to affected site 3–4 times a day; no food or drink for 20 min after OR Saturate a strip of gauze with the gel and apply to affected site for 20–30 min, 2–3 times a day OR Place gel in gingival stent and wear for 20–30 min, 2–3 times a day Note: Use only the class V or lower steroid on the vermilion, if expecting long-term use; the other steroids may cause irreversible atrophy of the vermilion and skin; tacrolimus and pimecrolimus may be used on the vermilion
Swishes • Dexamethasone elixir 0.5 mg/5 mL • Prednisolone syrup (15 mg/5 mL) • Tacrolimus solution (5 mg/mL) • Clobetasol 0.05% solution • Cyclosporine solution (100 mg/mL) • Budesonide (3-mg capsule contents dissolved in 5 mL of water)	Dispense 300 mL or other volume Swish 5 mL (dexamethasone, tacrolimus, cyclosporine, or budesonide), or 15 mL of prednisolone for 3–5 min (timed) and spit out, 3–4 times a day; no food or drink for 20 min after
• Tetracycline 0.25% solution • Minocycline 0.2% or 1% solution	Dispense 300 mL; swish 5–15 mL for 3 min (timed) and spit out, 3–4 times a day; no food or drink for 20 min after
Nasal spray such as fluticasone, betamethasone, and budesonide may be used orally	1–2 puffs onto affected sites 2–3 times daily
Intralesional steroid injection with triamcinolone	5–10 mg of triamcinolone per square centimeter of ulceration
Systemic Immunosuppressive Therapy[b]	
Prednisone	0.75–1.0 mg/kg for 7–10 days with a rapid taper over 2–3 wk, or a slow taper depending on the severity of disease; short-term side effects include restlessness, insomnia, increased appetite, hyperlipidemia, hypertension, and hyperglycemia
Pentoxifylline (especially for aphthous ulcers)	400–800 mg, 3 times daily
Hydroxychloroquine (especially for lichen planus)	100–200 mg twice daily; macular pigment deposits may lead to visual impairment
Dapsone (especially for mucous membrane pemphigoid)	25 mg to begin, increasing to 75–100 mg daily; anemia (or even more serious hemolytic anemia) is significant side effect; patients are susceptible to hemolytic anemia if glucose-6-phosphate dehydrogenase deficient
Mycophenolate mofetil (especially for pemphigus)	500–1500 mg, twice daily; monitor for myelosuppression and alterations in renal and liver function; gastrointestinal upset is a common side effect
Colchicine (especially for aphthous ulcers)	0.6 mg, once or twice daily; myelosuppression and gastrointestinal upset are significant side effects
Azathioprine	1–2 mg/kg daily; myelosuppression and liver toxicity are significant side effects; patient should be screened for adequate thiopurine methyltransferase
Thalidomide (especially for aphthous ulcers)	50–100 mg, 2–3 times a day to begin; begin taper to maintenance dose (which may be weekly) or discontinue completely; drowsiness, paresthesia, and thromboembolic events are significant side effects

Continued

Medication	How to Prescribe
Topical Pain Medications	
Viscous lidocaine 2% swish Benzydamine hydrochloride 0.15% swish Dyclonine hydrochloride 0.5% or 1% swish Dyclonine hydrochloride 0.2 mg or 0.3 mg lozenge (nonprescription) Benzocaine 10% cream (nonprescription)	Swish and spit out 5–15 mL, 3–4 times a day for pain

[a]Methylcellulose adhesive base can be mixed with the other, stronger topical steroids.
[b]Topical therapy should be started concomitantly with systemic therapy.

APPENDIX B

ANTIFUNGAL AND ANTIVIRAL THERAPY

Antifungal Medication	How to Prescribe
Nystatin 100,000 U/mL[a]	Dispense 300 mL; swish and spit out (or swallow) 5 mL 3–4 times a day for 7–10 days
Nystatin pastilles 200,000 U/pastille	Dissolve 1–2 pastilles in mouth 3–4 times a day for 7–10 days
Amphotericin B suspension 100 mg/mL	Dispense 300 mL; swish and spit out 5 mL 3–4 times a day for 7–10 days
Amphotericin 10-mg lozenges	Dissolve 1–2 tablets in mouth 3–4 times a day for 7–10 days
Clotrimazole 10-mg troches[a]	Suck on one troche 3–5 times a day for 7–10 days (troches do not dissolve if there is prominent hyposalivation)
Ketoconazole 200–400 mg daily	Take 1 or 2 tablets twice a day for 7–10 days
Miconazole 50 mg dissolving tablets daily	Dissolve in mouth once a day for 7–10 days
Fluconazole 100–200 mg daily Itraconazole 100–200 mg daily Voriconazole 200 mg twice a day Posaconazole 100 mg daily	Fluconazole: Use as directed for 3–4 days (depending on the severity of the infection); long-term therapy may lead to resistance to fluconazole. Culture and sensitivity should be performed, and itraconazole, voriconazole, and posaconazole are alternatives; may be taken 1–2 times a week for prophylaxis if on long-term immunosuppressive therapy.
Mycostatin/triamcinolone cream	Apply to corners of mouth 3–4 times a day or for angular cheilitis
Clotrimazole/betamethasone cream Iodoquinol/hydrocortisone 1% cream Miconazole 2% gel Miconazole/hydrocortisone	Paint onto denture base 3 times a day and wear denture; add erythromycin gel if there is residual lesion, because *Staphylococcus aureus* may be involved.
Denture soaks: Nystatin 100,000 U/mL Chlorhexidine digluconate 0.12–2% 3% sodium hypochlorite diluted in water (1:10) 2% sodium benzoate	Soak denture in solution overnight. Dentures should never be worn overnight.

[a]Contains cariogenic sugars and may lead to caries if used long term.

Therapy for Herpes Simplex Virus Infection

Anti-Herpes Simplex Virus Medications	How to Prescribe
Acyclovir 200 mg	200–400 mg 5 times a day for 5–7 days
Valacyclovir 500 mg	500–1000 mg twice a day for 5–7 days 2000 mg twice a day for 1 day (herpes labialis)
Famciclovir	250–500 mg 2–3 times a day for 5–7 days 1500 mg for 1 day (herpes labialis)
For long-term suppression:	
Acyclovir	400 mg twice a day
Valacyclovir	500–1000 mg once a day OR 500 mg twice a day
Famciclovir	500 mg twice a day
Topical anti-herpes virus therapy (mostly for herpes labialis): Acyclovir 5% cream (available with 1% hydrocortisone) Penciclovir 1% cream Docosanol 10% cream	Apply at first prodrome 6–8 times a day (every 2 h while awake)

INDEX

NOTE: Page numbers followed by f or t indicate figures or tables, respectively.

T

U

V